Infectious Diseases: In Context

SECOND EDITION

Infectious Diseases: In Context

SECOND EDITION

VOLUME 1

African Sleeping Sickness to Lyme Disease

Thomas Riggs, Editor

GALE
A Cengage Company

Farmington Hills, Mich • San Francisco • New York • Waterville, Maine
Meriden, Conn • Mason, Ohio • Chicago

GALE
A Cengage Company

Infectious Diseases: In Context, Second Edition

Thomas Riggs, Editor

Project Editor: Tracie Moy

Acquisitions Editor: Jessica Bomarito

Editorial Staff: Mike Tyrkus

Rights Acquisition and Management: Ashley M. Maynard and Carissa Poweleit

Imaging: John L. Watkins

Product Design: Kristine A. Julien

Composition: Amy Darga

Manufacturing: Rita Wimberley

Cover photographs: 3D rendering influenza virus, Rost9/Shutterstock.com; Vaccinating a child, CNKO2/Shutterstock.com; Tick crawling on human skin, Henrik Larsson/Shutterstock.com; Vaccine containers, Paula Bronstein/Getty Images; Hand in glove collects water sample, PRESSLAB/Shutterstock.com; Hands of old woman suffering from leprosy, NikomMaelao Production/Shutterstock.com; Fumigation machine to kill mosquitoes carrying Zika, BOONJAEM/Shutterstock.com.

Inside art: 3D rendering Influenza Virus H1N1, Rost9/Shutterstock.com.

LIBRARY OF CONGRESS CATALOGING-IN-PUBLICATION DATA

Names: Riggs, Thomas J., editor.
Title: Infectious diseases : in context / Thomas J. Riggs, editor.
Description: Second edition. | Farmington Hills, Mich : Gale, A Cengage Company, [2018] | Includes bibliographical references and index.
Identifiers: LCCN 2018002810 | ISBN 9781410381286 (set : alk. paper) | ISBN 9781410381293 (vol. 1 : alk. paper) | ISBN 9781410381309 (vol. 2 : alk. paper) | ISBN 9781410381316 (ebook)
Subjects: MESH: Communicable Diseases | Encyclopedias
Classification: LCC RC111 | NLM WC 13 | DDC 616.003—dc23
LC record available at https://lccn.loc.gov/2018002810

Gale
27500 Drake Rd.
Farmington Hills, MI 48331-3535

978-1-4103-8128-6 (set)
978-1-4103-8129-3 (vol. 1)
978-1-4103-8130-9 (vol. 2)

This title is also available as an e-book.
978-1-4103-8131-6

Contact your Gale sales representative for ordering information.

Printed in the United States
1 2 3 4 5 6 7 22 21 20 19 18

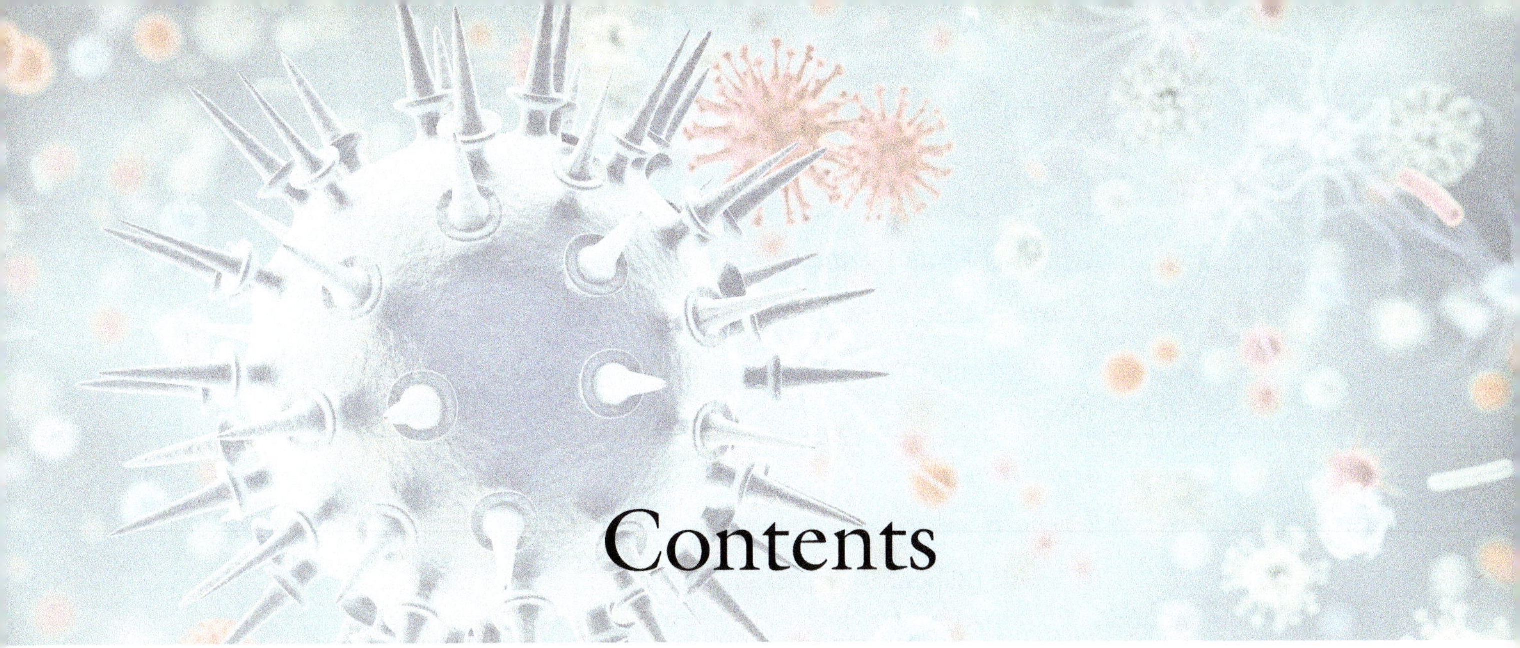

Contents

VOLUME 2

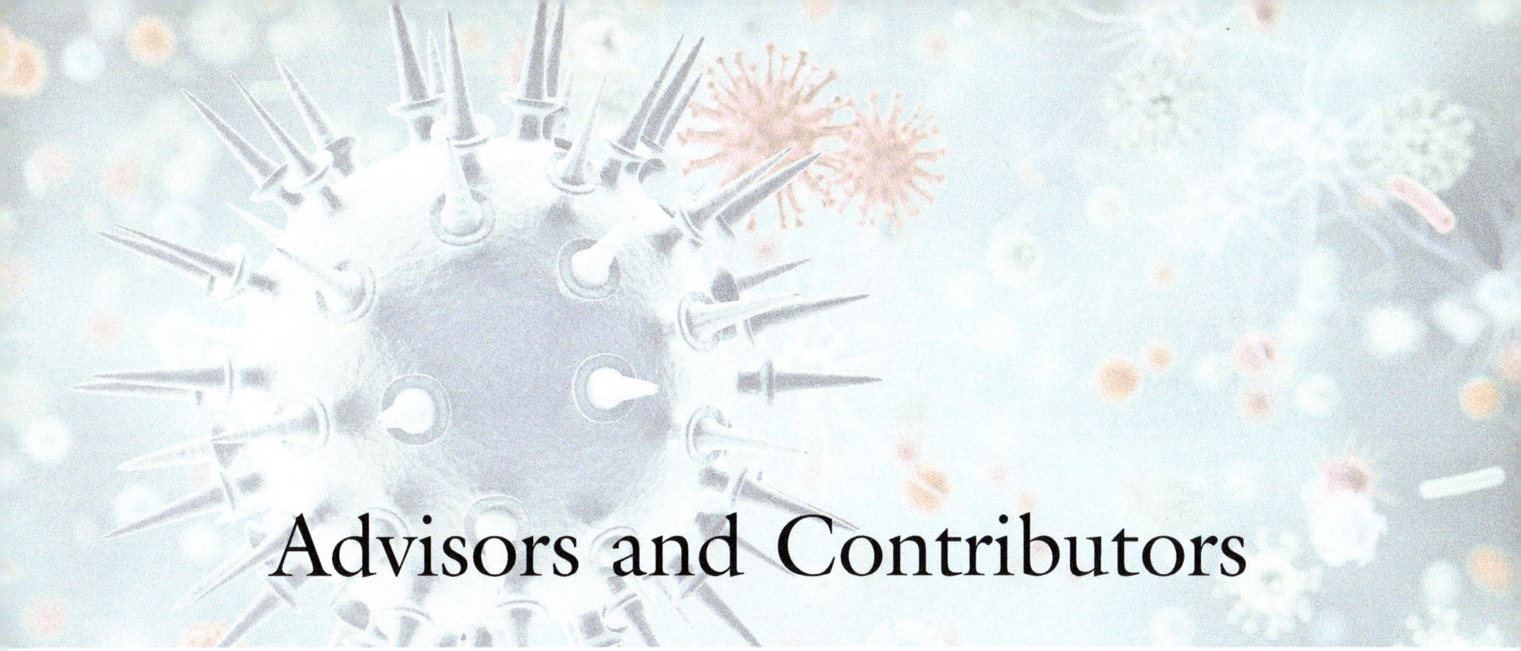

Advisors and Contributors

While compiling this volume, the editors relied on the expertise and contributions of the following scientists, scholars, and researchers, who served as advisors, academic reviewers, or contributors for *Infectious Diseases: In Context.*

Susan Aldridge, Ph.D.
Independent scholar and writer
London, United Kingdom

William Arthur Atkins, M.S.
Independent scholar and writer
Pekin, Illinois

Stephen A. Berger, M.D.
Founder and Medical Advisor
Tel Aviv Medical Center
Tel Aviv, Israel

Agnieszka Caruso, PhD
Canon Biomedical
Rockville, Maryland

Laura J. Cataldo, PhD
Independent Scholar
Myersville, Maryland

L. S. Clements, MD, PhD
Assistant Professor of Pediatrics
University of South Alabama College of Medicine
Mobile, Alabama

Bryan Davies, LLB
Writer and Journalist
Ontario, Canada

Paul Davies, PhD
Director
Science Research Institute
Adjunct Professor
Paris-Sorbonne
Paris, France

Larry Gilman, PhD
Independent Scholar and Journalist
Sharon, Vermont

Tony Hawas, MA
Writer and Journalist
Brisbane, Australia

Brian D. Hoyle, PhD
Microbiologist
Nova Scotia, Canada

Kenneth T. LaPensee, PhD, MPH
Epidemiologist and Medical Policy Specialist
Hampton, New Jersey

Adrienne Wilmoth Lerner, JD
Independent Scholar
Jacksonville, Florida

Ted McDermott, MFA
Writer and Journalist
Butte, Montana

Caryn Neumann, PhD
Senior Lecturer, Interdisciplinary and Communication Studies
Miami University
Oxford, Ohio

James Overholtzer, MA
Independent Scholar
Seattle, Washington

Anna Marie Roos, PhD
Reader and Programme Leader, School of History & Heritage
University of Lincoln
Lincoln, United Kingdom

Kausalya Santhanam, PhD
Founder
SciVista IP & Scientific Communication
India

Claire Skinner, MFA
Writer and Editor
Tucson, Arizona

Constance K. Stein, PhD
Director of Cytogenetics and Associate Professor
SUNY Upstate Medical University
Syracuse, New York

Samuel D. Uretsky, PharmD
Independent Researcher and Writer
New York, New York

Malini Vashishta, PhD
Independent Scholar and Medical Writer
Windsor, California

Jack Woodall, PhD
Former Director, Nucleus for the Investigation of Emerging Infectious Diseases
Institute of Medical Biochemistry,
Center for Health Sciences
Federal University of Rio de Janeiro
Rio de Janeiro, Brazil

Melanie Barton Zoltán, MS
Independent Scholar
Amherst, Massachusetts

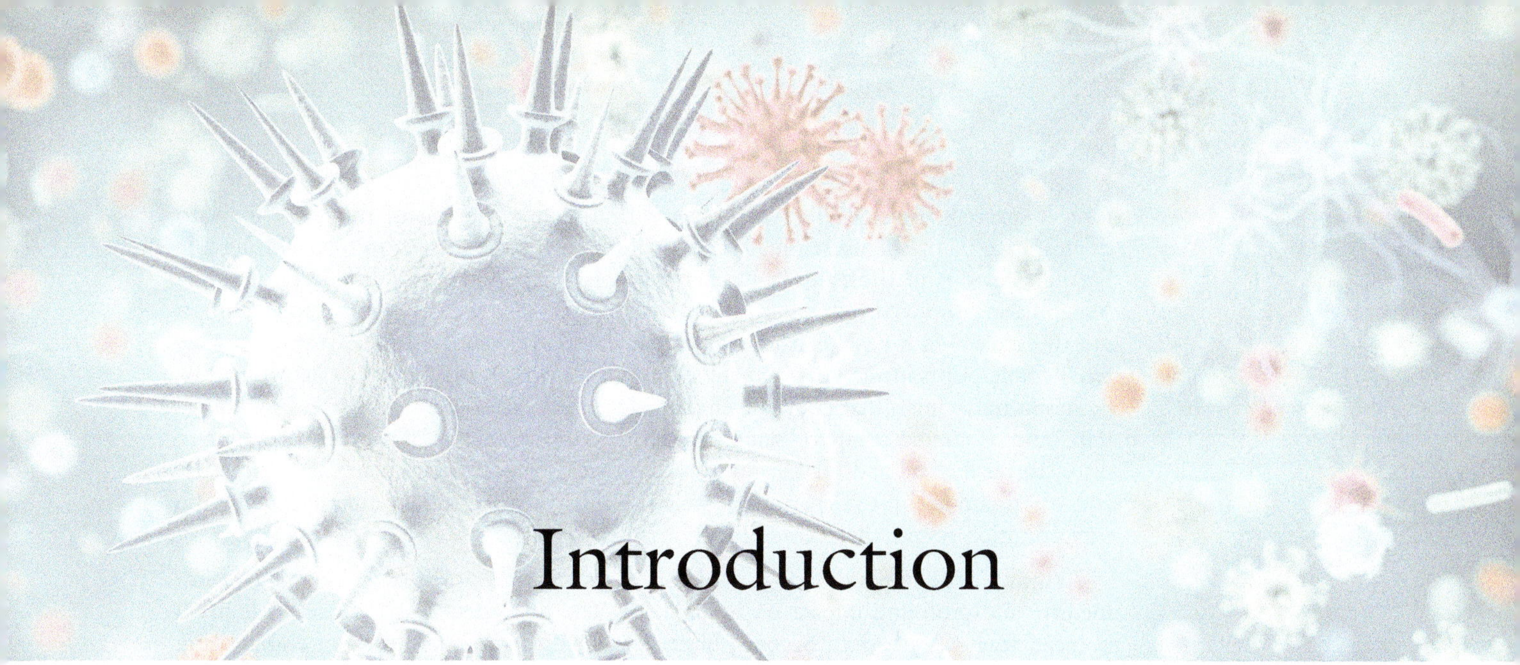

Introduction

Ever since humankind's ancestors first descended from the trees and adopted a bipedal lifestyle in the East African savanna, our species has been victim to two major biothreats: large carnivores and seemingly invisible microbial pathogens. Competing large carnivores were dispatched relatively quickly by *Homo sapiens*, which literally means "wise man," but microorganisms remained invisible and completely unknown to early humans. Yet our species needed to develop a sophisticated innate and adaptive immune system to defend against these microorganisms. Throughout history our forbearers must have fallen prey to a multitude of endemic and epidemic microbial diseases, and infections have taken a terrible toll on human populations.

When the first modern humans appeared in Africa about 170,000 years ago, they lived a predatory existence as scattered bands of hunter-gatherers. However, humans lacked the speed, agility, size, strength, and endowment of traditional weapons featured by most large carnivores such as fangs, thick hides, large claws, and powerful jaws. Our species had to learn to become predators by deploying their relatively few but ultimately decisive assets. Humans possessed three major advantages over their carnivorous competitors: 1) unusually large brains to cooperate and learn through their communication skills; 2) apposable thumbs for tool making; and 3) knowledge of the many uses of fire to survive. Remarkably, the capacity to maintain and control fire was passed down from our closest primate ancestor, *Homo erectus*, which acquired the skill over 1 million years earlier. In addition to providing light, warmth, and some protection against large predators, fire presented an opportunity to limit intestinal parasites by cooking meat before eating it. Helminthic intestinal parasites slowly sap the strength and vitality of their human hosts. Living a life relatively free from parasitism provided humans with a major advantage over other mammals.

Becoming predators had its advantages, but frequent nicks and scratches and intermittent bleeding episodes must have inevitably accompanied this lifestyle. Our thin skins and the lack of decent footwear likely made minor injuries commonplace when chasing prey. Those fortunate enough to possess rapid clotting capacity and an early and intense innate immune response following injury enjoyed an evolutionary advantage over bleeders and poor wound-healers. Regrettably, what were considered survival traits for our ancestors are a liability in modern times. We are now plagued by an excessive risk of clotting tendencies (including deep venous thrombosis, strokes, and myocardial infarction). Likewise, our overly reactive immune responses and propensity to overcompensate from inflammatory stimuli contribute to accelerating incidence of localized and systemic inflammatory states such as sepsis, asthma, multiple sclerosis, and inflammatory bowel disease.

Humans spread out over time from East Africa about 35,000 years ago to populate much of the world's tropical and temperate climates. Yet the entire human population expanded very little for tens of thousands of years. Our collective fate as a species was forever altered about 8,000 years ago with the first successful human efforts to domesticate plants. This seminal event in human history first took place along the Fertile Crescent in the Middle East and was later copied elsewhere, when feasible. Manipulating the environment to maintain favored plant life for human consumption greatly accelerated the yields from a given parcel of land compared to searching for scattered edible plants in the environment. These first agrarian societies were later joined by domesticated animals that could be employed to carry heavy loads, as a source of animal milk, and as animal meat for slaughter. Horses and oxen could also be harnessed to plows to till the soil and further improve crop yields. Jump on a horse's back and later add wheel-and-axel-fitted chariots or wagons, and you have the essential elements of a transportation system that existed for thousands of years.

Putting aside our wandering, predatory ways to settle down as farmers had an immediate and profound impact on humankind. The first effect was food security and a reduced fear of starvation. Second, high crop yields provided women of childbearing age ready access to food, resulting in increased fertility and fecundity rates. Third, a steady source of nutrition freed up at least some members of a farm community to perform more specialized labor. Individuals with a penchant for tool making could become full-time tool makers, good weavers could become permanent weavers, people with a talent for pottery making became full-time pottery makers, and so on. Food could now be provided by someone else in a specialized workforce.

The agrarian lifestyle necessitated human habitation living within fixed dwellings near the fields. Gone were the days of small, nomadic bands of humans scattered over the land hunting for food. People now became close-knit members of towns crowded together in proximity to each other and their animals. This living arrangement created a novel risk for humankind. Some of the deadliest epidemics in history are zoonotic infections, which are infectious diseases found in animals that spread and adapt to replicate in human hosts. Domesticated farm animals serve as unrecognized and unwanted reservoirs for zoonotic infections. These animals have gradually acquired some form of immune defense or tolerance to the manifest disease produced by these microorganisms. When the infections "jump" species and infect their human overseers, massive and potentially lethal epidemics can occur.

This has occurred numerous times in the past and continues in the early 21st century in such diseases as the H7N9 bird flu strain passed from chickens to humans and the Middle Eastern Respiratory Syndrome–associated coronavirus infections spread from camels to humans. Many other examples of zoonotic epidemic diseases are recorded in history. For example, the smallpox virus in humans was likely derived from the camel pox virus and is probably the single greatest killer of humankind throughout history. The black plague in 14th-century Europe was likely derived from city-dwelling, peri-domestic rats. When the bacterial pathogen *Yersinia pestis* first jumped species to humans it caused infection of the lymph glands (bubonic plague) and then via the respiratory tract (pneumonic plague). This disease killed millions over a five-year period in Europe, tearing at the very fabric of Western civilization. Bovine tuberculosis from infected, unpasteurized cow's milk was likely the origin of the first human cases of tuberculosis. Tuberculosis has become a common cause of death ever since. This single chronic lung infection has killed, and continues to kill, over a million patients worldwide each year.

Increasingly our forefathers migrated to crowded population centers, and the human population exploded. This trend continues in the 21st century. We are still on the ascending limb of an exponential expansion of human population. Evidence indicates that it took tens of thousands of years for our species to reach our first billion around 1830 CE. It took about 100 years to reach the second billion in 1930. Yet it took only 12 years to go from 6 billion (1999) to 7 billion people (2011), and it will be an estimated 13 years until we reach 8 billion people. For the first time in history, the majority of people now reside in cities. Many megacities (defined as greater than 10 million inhabitants) are bursting at the seams with overstretched needs for clean water, sufficient goods and services, adequate sewage disposal, and enough living space to handle the expanding population needs.

Living in densely populated spaces facilitates the spread of microbial pathogens by the respiratory tract by sharing a common airspace in poorly ventilated rooms. Food preparation and distribution into large cities under suboptimal sanitary conditions and inadequate sewage disposal puts city dwellers at great risk of foodborne illness and waterborne outbreaks. Even urban mosquito-borne outbreaks are an increasing risk in megacities in developing countries due to poor water drainage systems and standing water sources from old tires and other debris from human activities. As cities get larger and people accumulate under confined spaces, the risk of contagion rises. With ready access to international flights, we are increasingly susceptible to a major epidemic event. A newly reassorted influenza virus strain or a similar respiratory virus will most likely be the cause of the next pandemic. This is one reason why so much effort is going into finding a universal vaccine option to protect people from this potentially deadly virus. Deliberate release of a genetically enhanced hybrid virus as a weapon of bioterrorism is also a possibility. A pan-resistant, highly transmissible bacterial pathogen that has evolved resistance to all major antibiotics is also a possibility.

Remarkably, the existence of pathogenic microorganisms was entirely unknown until 1683, when Dutch microscopist Antoni van Leeuwenhoek (1632–1723) peered down his glass lens magnifier to first identify bacteria. It took almost 200 years to confirm their pathogenic significance by the establishment of the germ theory of disease by Louis Pasteur (1822–1895), Robert Koch (1843–1910), and many others. At least 1,500 known species of microbial pathogens have been identified that can harm humans. To be a pathogen, the microorganism must possess the ability to evade host barrier defenses and immune clearance mechanisms. Further, it must be able to replicate faster that the innate and acquired clearance capacity to remove pathogens from the patient. The struggle continues between the human host and microbial pathogens even in the 21st century.

Consider that, as of 2018, up to one-third of the entire human population was latently infected with tuberculosis. This mycobacterial organism can reawaken and spread within the host if his or her immune defenses fail them. Reactivation of tuberculosis can spread to unsuspecting people living close to the infected patient at any time. The upper airways of up to 60 percent of children in day care centers are colonized with the common respiratory pathogen *Streptococcus pneumoniae. Staphylococcus aureus* is found in the nose of least one-third of humans, and 5 to 10 percent are colonized by *Neisseria meningitidis.* These constant microbial treats are countered by a continuously acting array of innate and acquired host defenses that hold back potential invaders. Patients born with primary immune deficiencies do not have to wait long to be recognized because of the usual onslaught of opportunistic pathogens to which we are all exposed, but they are more susceptible. In addition to endemic infectious disease risks, epidemic diseases continue to plague us on a regular basis. Despite concerted vaccine-induced mitigation strategies, annual influenza epidemics exact a toll on human populations. As of 2018 Brazil was experiencing an entirely newly recognized epidemic of microcephaly and Guillain-Barré syndrome from a previously unknown mosquito-borne flavivirus known as Zika virus. At the same time, the ancient scourge of Yellow Fever, which is caused by a similar, but highly lethal flavivirus, has reappeared and become epidemic in regions of Brazil.

The detailed study of pathogenic microbiology teaches us that, while we are controlling some pathogens, many others are not under our thumb and can still cause us harm. Smallpox and possibly polio have likely been eliminated by concerted control efforts featuring vaccine eradication strategies. We have been less effective eliminating pathogens with antimicrobial chemotherapy. The promise of precision medicine with ready access to molecular biology tools to eradicate pathogens remains an attractive but not as yet unproven method to vanquish our microbial adversaries. We still need new ideas in our continuing efforts to control microorganisms.

This book describes in some detail the nature of essentially all the common microbial pathogens known to infect humans. Content experts who prepared each chapter use a templated format, which provides a succinct yet thorough and up-to-date summary of each pathogen and its clinical infectious disease manifestations. The book provides a detailed and ready access reference text of pathogenic microbiology.

Steven Opal, M.D.
Professor of Medicine, Infectious Disease Division,
Alpert Medical School of Brown University

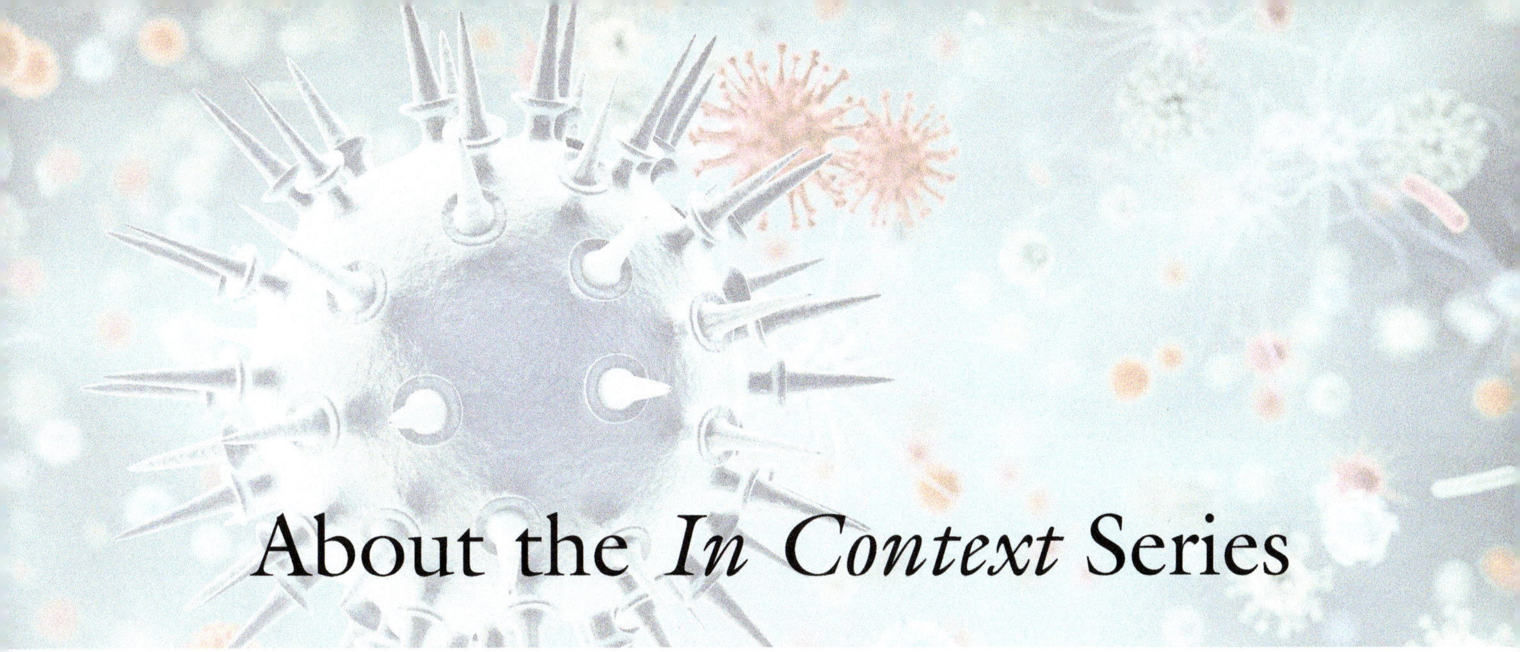

About the *In Context* Series

Written by subject matter experts and aimed primarily at high school students and an interested general readership, the *In Context* series serves as an authoritative reference guide to essential concepts of science, the impacts of recent changes in scientific consensus, and the effects of science on social, political, and legal issues.

In Context books align with, and support, national science standards and high school science curriculums. Cross-curricular in nature, the series addresses the intersections of science and the humanities, and facilitates higher-level thinking that is critical to student achievement. Original essays written by subject matter experts and supplemental primary source documents serve the requirements of high school and international baccalaureate programs. Entries are designed to present foundational concepts, provide insights on leading social issues, and spur critical thinking about connections between science and society.

In Context books also give special coverage to the impact of science on daily life, commerce, travel, and the future of industrialized and impoverished nations. Entries include Words to Know sidebars designed to facilitate understanding and increase reading retention without overwhelming readers with scientific terminology.

Entries include standardized subheads tailored to the subject matter of each book. To facilitate further research, each entry includes a listing of resources (books, periodicals, and websites) and references to related entries.

In addition to maps, charts, tables and graphs, each *In Context* title has approximately 250 topic-related images that visually enrich the content. Each *In Context* title includes a chronology of major events related to the topic, a topic-specific glossary, a bibliography, and an index especially prepared to coordinate with the volume topic.

Disclaimer: This information is not a tool for self-diagnosis or a substitute for professional care.

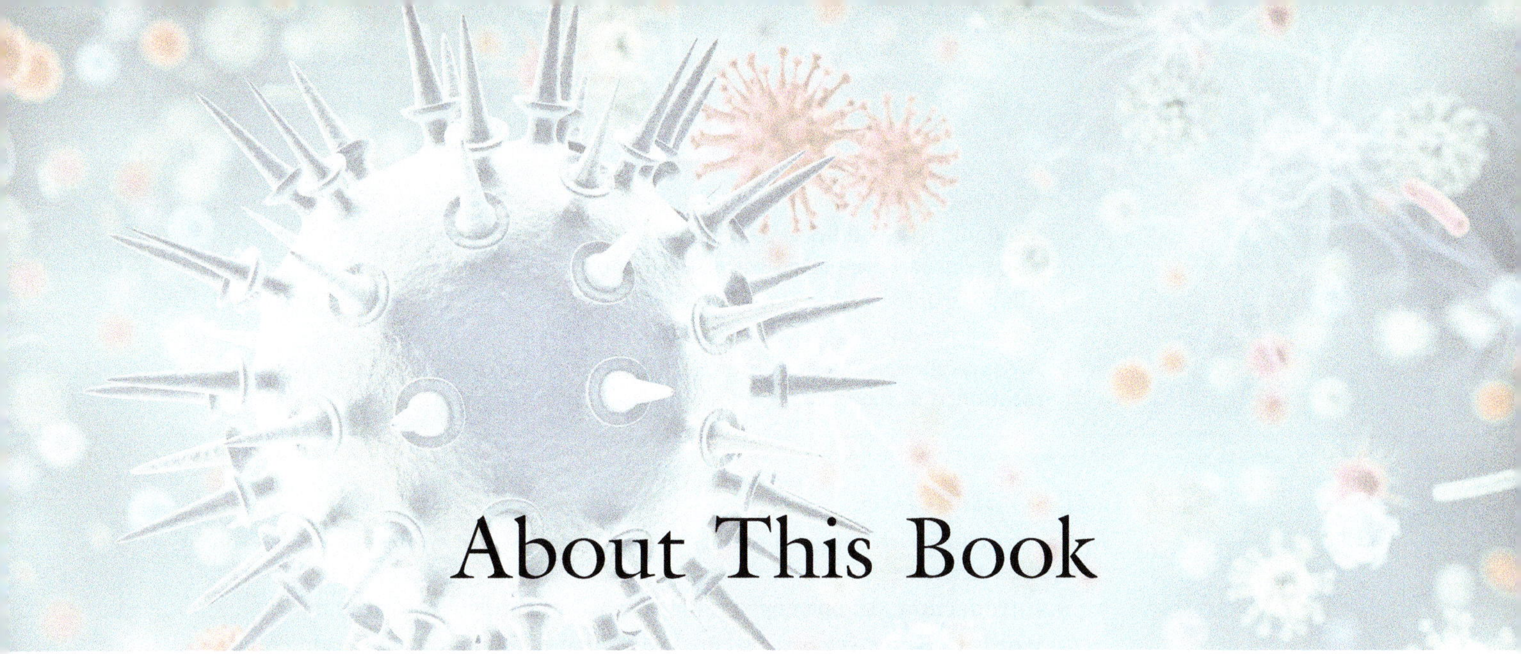

About This Book

The goal of *Infectious Diseases: In Context* is to help high school and early college-age students understand the essential facts and deeper cultural connections of topics and issues related to the scientific study of infectious disease.

The relationship of science to complex ethical and social considerations is evident, for example, when considering the general rise of infectious diseases that sometimes occurs as an unintended side effect of the otherwise beneficial use of medications. Approximately one-quarter of the world's population is infected with tuberculosis (TB). Although for most people the infection is inactive, the organism causing some new cases of TB is evolving toward a greater resistance to the antibiotics that were once effective in treating TB. These statistics take on a social dimension given that TB disproportionately affects social groups such as the elderly, minorities, and people infected with human immunodeficiency virus (HIV). In 2017 TB was a leading cause of death for individuals infected with HIV.

To encourage the reader to explore the relationship between science and culture, as space allows, we have included primary sources that enhance the content of *In Context* entries. Drawn from popular media, accessible scholarly journals, and historical sources, these documents include firsthand accounts from patients and medical professionals, in-depth case studies, foundational works of scientific thought, and government documents that shed light on the topics under study. In keeping with the philosophy that much of the benefit from using primary sources derives from the reader's own process of inquiry, the contextual material introducing each primary source provides an unobtrusive introduction and springboard to critical thought.

General Structure

Infectious Diseases: In Context, Second Edition is a collection of more than 260 entries that provide insight into increasingly important and urgent topics associated with the study of infectious disease.

The articles in the book are meant to be understandable by anyone with a curiosity about topics related to infectious disease, and the second edition of *Infectious Diseases: In Context* has been designed with ready reference in mind:

- Entries are arranged alphabetically rather than by chronology or scientific subfield.
- The **chronology** (timeline) includes many of the most significant events in the history of infectious disease and advances of science. Where appropriate, related scientific advances are included to offer additional context.

- An extensive glossary provides readers with a ready reference for content-related terminology. In addition to defining terms within the text, specific Words to Know sidebars are placed within each entry.
- A bibliography section (citations of books, periodicals, and websites) offers additional resources to those resources cited within each entry.
- A **comprehensive general index** guides the reader to topics and people mentioned in the book.

Entry Structure

In Context entries are designed so that readers may navigate entries with ease. Toward that goal, entries are divided into easy-to-access sections:

- **Introduction**: An opening section designed to clearly identify the topic.
- **Words to Know** sidebar: Essential terms that enhance readability and critical understanding of entry content.
- Established but flexible **rubrics** customize content presentation and identify each section, enabling the reader to navigate entries with ease. Inside *Infectious Diseases: In Context* entries, readers will find two key schemes of organization. Most entries contain internal discussions of **Disease History, Characteristics, and Transmission**, followed by **Scope and Distribution**, then a summary of **Treatment and Prevention**. General social or science topics may have a simpler structure discussing, for example, **History and Scientific Foundations**. Regardless, the goal of *In Context* entries is a consistent, content-appropriate, and easy-to-follow presentation.
- **Impacts and Issues**: Key scientific, political, or social considerations related to the entry topic.
- **Bibliography**: Citations of books, periodicals, and websites used in preparation of the entry or that provide a stepping stone to further study.
- **"See also" references** clearly identify other content-related entries.

Infectious Diseases: In Context Special Style Notes

Please note the following regarding topics and entries included in *Infectious Diseases: In Context*:

- Primary source selection and the composition of sidebars are not attributed to authors of signed entries to which the sidebars may be associated. In all cases the sources for sidebars containing external content (e.g., a CDC policy position or medical recommendation) are clearly indicated.
- The Centers for Disease Control and Prevention (CDC) includes parasitic diseases with infectious diseases, and the editors have adopted this scheme.
- A detailed understanding of biology and chemistry is neither assumed nor required for *Infectious Diseases: In Context*. Accordingly, students and other readers should not be intimidated or deterred by the sometimes complex names of chemical molecules or biological classification. Where necessary, sufficient information regarding chemical structure or species classification is provided. If desired, more information can easily be obtained from any basic chemistry or biology reference.

Bibliography Citation Formats (How to Cite Articles and Sources)

In Context titles adopt the following citation format:

BIBLIOGRAPHY

Books

Magill, Gerard, ed. *Genetics and Ethics: An Interdisciplinary Study.* New York: Fordham University Press, 2003.

Verlinsky, Yury, and Anver Kuliev. *Practical Preimplantation Genetic Diagnosis.* New York: Springer, 2005.

Periodicals

Byrd, Allyson L., and Julia A. Segre. "Adapting Koch's Postulates." *Science* 351, no. 6270 (January 15, 2016): 224–226. This article can also be found online at http://science.sciencemag.org/content/351/6270/224 (accessed January 16, 2018).

Eldin, Carole, et al. "From Q Fever to *Coxiella burnetii* Infection: A Paradigm Change." *Clinical Microbiology Reviews* 30, no. 1 (January 2017): 115–190.

Websites

ADEAR. Alzheimer's Disease Education and Referral Center. National Institute on Aging. http://www.alzheimers.org/generalinfo.htm (accessed January 23, 2018).

"Discussion by the Genetics and Public Policy Center." PGD: Preimplantation Genetic Diagnosis. http://dnapolicy.org/downloads/pdfs/policy_pgd.pdf (accessed January 23, 2006).

Genetics and Public Policy Center. http://dnapolicy.org/index.jhtml.html (accessed January 23, 2018).

There are, however, alternative citation formats that may be useful to readers and examples of how to cite articles in often used alternative formats are shown below.

APA Style

Books

Kübler-Ross, Elizabeth. (1969) *On Death and Dying.* New York: Macmillan. Excerpted in K. Lee Lerner and Brenda Wilmoth Lerner, eds. (2006) *Medicine, Health, and Bioethics: Essential Primary Sources*, Farmington Hills, Mich.: Thomson Gale.

Periodicals

Venter, J. Craig, et al. (2001, February 16). "The Sequence of the Human Genome." *Science*, vol. 291, no. 5507, pp. 1304–51. Excerpted in K. Lee Lerner and Brenda Wilmoth Lerner, eds. (2006) *Medicine, Health, and Bioethics: Essential Primary Sources*, Farmington Hills, Mich.: Thomson Gale.

Websites

Johns Hopkins Hospital and Health System. "Patient Rights and Responsibilities." Retrieved January 14, 2006 from http://www.hopkinsmedicine.org/patients/JHH/patient_rights.html. Excerpted in K. Lee Lerner and Brenda Wilmoth Lerner, eds. (2006) *Medicine, Health, and Bioethics: Essential Primary Sources*, Farmington Hills, Mich.: Thomson Gale.

Chicago Style

Books

Kübler-Ross, Elizabeth. *On Death and Dying.* New York: Macmillan, 1969. Excerpted in K. Lee Lerner and Brenda Wilmoth Lerner, eds. *Medicine, Health, and Bioethics: Essential Primary Sources*, Farmington Hills, MI: Thomson Gale, 2006.

Periodicals

Venter, J. Craig, et al. "The Sequence of the Human Genome." *Science* (2001): 291, 5507, 1304–1351. Excerpted in K. Lee Lerner and Brenda Wilmoth Lerner, eds. *Medicine, Health, and Bioethics: Essential Primary Sources*, Farmington Hills, MI: Thomson Gale, 2006.

Websites

Johns Hopkins Hospital and Health System. "Patient Rights and Responsibilities." http://www.hopkinsmedicine.org/patients/JHH/patient_rights.html (accessed January 14, 2006). Excerpted in K. Lee Lerner and Brenda Wilmoth Lerner, eds. *Medicine, Health, and Bioethics: Essential Primary Sources*, Farmington Hills, MI: Thomson Gale, 2006.

MLA Style

Books

Kübler-Ross, Elizabeth. *On Death and Dying*, New York: Macmillan, 1969. Excerpted in K. Lee Lerner and Brenda Wilmoth Lerner, eds. *Medicine, Health, and Bioethics: Essential Primary Sources*, Farmington Hills, Mich.: Thomson Gale, 2006.

Periodicals

Venter, J. Craig, et al. "The Sequence of the Human Genome." *Science*, 291 (16 February 2001): 5507, 1304–51. Excerpted in K. Lee Lerner and Brenda Wilmoth Lerner, eds. *Terrorism: Essential Primary Sources*, Farmington Hills, Mich.: Thomson Gale, 2006.

Web Sites

"Patient's Rights and Responsibilities." Johns Hopkins Hospital and Health System. 14 January 2006. http://www.hopkinsmedicine.org/patients/JHH/patient_rights.html. Excerpted in K. Lee Lerner and Brenda Wilmoth Lerner, eds. *Terrorism: Essential Primary Sources*, Farmington Hills, Mich.: Thomson Gale, 2006.

Style (Natural and Social Sciences)

Books

Kübler-Ross, Elizabeth. *On Death and Dying*, (New York: Macmillan, 1969). Excerpted in K. Lee Lerner and Brenda Wilmoth Lerner, eds. *Medicine, Health, and Bioethics: Essential Primary Sources*, (Farmington Hills, Mich.: Thomson Gale, 2006).

Periodicals

Venter, J. Craig, et al. "The Sequence of the Human Genome." *Science*, 291 (16 February 2001): 5507, 1304–1351. Excerpted in K. Lee Lerner and Brenda Wilmoth Lerner, eds. *Medicine, Health, and Bioethics: Essential Primary Sources*, (Farmington Hills, Mich.: Thomson Gale, 2006).

Websites

Johns Hopkins Hospital and Health System. "Patient's Rights and Responsibilities." available from http://www.hopkinsmedicine.org/patients/JHH/patient_rights.html; accessed14 January 2006. Excerpted in K. Lee Lerner and Brenda Wilmoth Lerner, eds. *Medicine, Health, and Bioethics: Essential Primary Sources*, (Farmington Hills, Mich.: Thomson Gale, 2006).

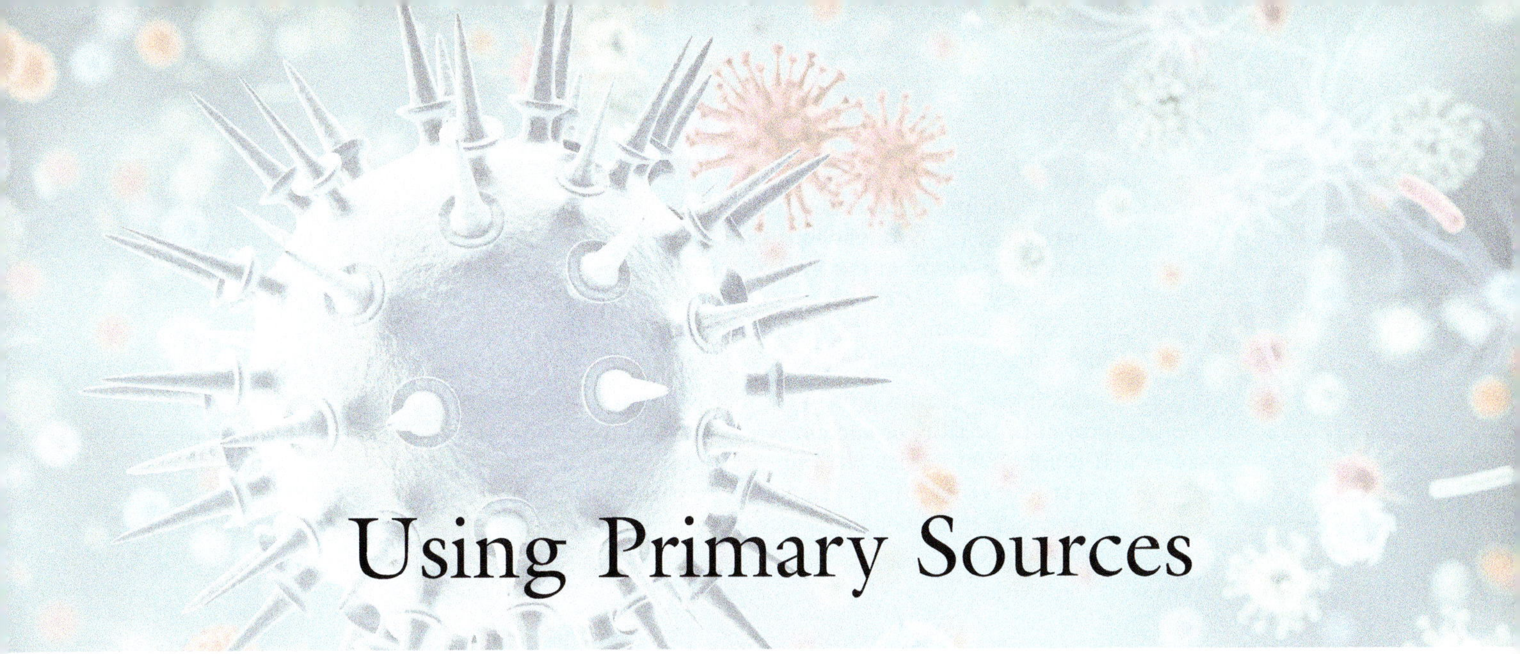

Using Primary Sources

The definition of what constitutes a primary source is often the subject of scholarly debate and interpretation. Although primary sources come from a wide spectrum of resources, they are united by the fact that they individually provide insight into the historical *milieu* (context and environment) during which they were produced.

Primary sources include materials such as newspaper articles, press dispatches, autobiographies, essays, letters, diaries, speeches, song lyrics, posters, works of art—and in the 21st century, Web logs (blogs)—that offer direct, first-hand insight or witness to events of their day.

Categories of primary sources include:

- Documents containing firsthand accounts of historic events by witnesses and participants. This category includes diary or journal entries, letters, email, newspaper articles, interviews, memoirs, and testimony in legal proceedings.
- Documents or works representing the official views of both government leaders and leaders of other organizations. These include primary sources such as policy statements, speeches, interviews, press releases, government reports, research studies, and legislation.
- Works of art, including (but certainly not limited to) photographs, poems, and songs, including advertisements and reviews of those works that help establish an understanding of the cultural environment with regard to attitudes and perceptions of events.
- Secondary sources. In some cases, secondary sources or tertiary sources may be treated as primary sources. For example, if an entry written many years after an event, or to summarize an event, includes quotes, recollections, or retrospectives (accounts of the past) written by participants in the earlier event, the source can be considered a primary source.

Analysis of Primary Sources

The primary material collected in this volume is not intended to provide a comprehensive or balanced overview of a topic or event. Rather, the primary sources are intended to generate interest and lay a foundation for further inquiry and study.

In order to properly analyze a primary source, readers should remain skeptical and develop probing questions about the source. Using historical documents requires that readers analyze them carefully and extract specific information. However, readers must also read "beyond the text" to garner larger clues about the social impact of the primary source.

In addition to providing information about their topics, primary sources may also supply a wealth of insight into their creator's viewpoint. For example, when reading a news article about an outbreak of disease, consider whether the reporter's words also indicate something about his or her origin, bias (an irrational disposition in favor of someone or something), prejudices (an irrational disposition against someone or something), or intended audience.

Students should remember that primary sources often contain information later proven to be false, or contain viewpoints and terms unacceptable to future generations. It is important to view the primary source within the historical and social context existing at its creation. If, for example, a newspaper article is written within hours or days of an event, later developments may reveal some assertions in the original article as false or misleading.

Test New Conclusions and Ideas

Whatever opinion or working hypothesis readers form, it is critical that they then test that hypothesis against other facts and sources related to the incident. For example, it might be wrong to conclude that factual mistakes are deliberate unless evidence can be produced of a pattern and practice of such mistakes with an intent to promote a false idea.

The difference between sound reasoning and preposterous conspiracy theories (or the birth of urban legends) lies in the willingness to test new ideas against other sources, rather than rest on one piece of evidence such as a single primary source that may contain errors. Sound reasoning requires that arguments and assertions guard against argument fallacies that utilize the following:

- false dilemmas (only two choices are given when in fact there are three or more options);
- arguments from ignorance (*argumentum ad ignorantiam*; because something is not known to be true, it is assumed to be false);
- possibilist fallacies (a favorite among conspiracy theorists who attempt to demonstrate that a factual statement is true or false by establishing the possibility of its truth or falsity. An argument where "it could be" is usually followed by an unearned "therefore, it is.");
- slippery slope arguments or fallacies (a series of increasingly dramatic consequences is drawn from an initial fact or idea);
- begging the question (the truth of the conclusion is assumed by the premises);
- straw man arguments (the arguer mischaracterizes an argument or theory and then attacks the merits of their own false representations);
- appeals to pity or force (the argument attempts to persuade people to agree by sympathy or force);
- prejudicial language (values or moral goodness, good and bad, are attached to certain arguments or facts);
- personal attacks (*ad hominem*; an attack on a person's character or circumstances);
- anecdotal or testimonial evidence (stories that are unsupported by impartial observation or data that is not reproducible);
- *post hoc* (after the fact) fallacies (because one thing follows another, it is held to cause the other);
- the fallacy of the appeal to authority (the argument rests upon the credentials of a person, not the evidence).

Despite the fact that some primary sources can contain false information or lead readers to false conclusions based on the information presented, they remain an invaluable resource regarding past events. Primary sources allow readers and researchers to come as close as possible to understanding the perceptions and context of events and thus to more fully appreciate how and why misconceptions occur.

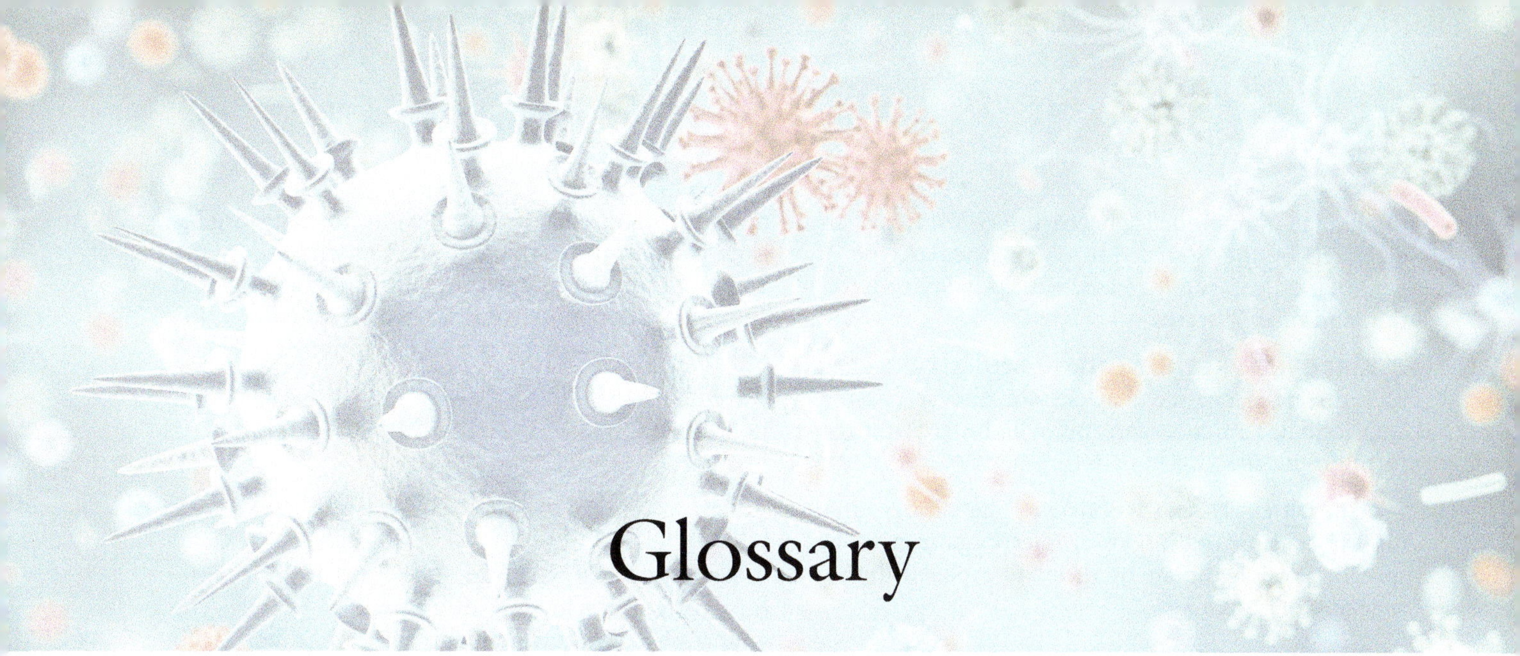

Glossary

A

ABIOGENESIS: Also known as spontaneous generation. The incorrect theory that living things can be generated from nonliving things.

ABIOTIC: The portion of an ecosystem that is not living, such as water or soil.

ABSCESS: A pus-filled sore, usually caused by a bacterial infection. It results from the body's defensive reaction to foreign material. Abscesses are often found in the soft tissue under the skin in areas such as the armpit or the groin. However, they may develop in any organ, and they are commonly found in the breast and gums. If they are located in deep organs such as the lung, liver, or brain, abscesses are far more serious and call for more specific treatment.

ACARACIDES: Chemicals that kill mites and ticks.

ACQUIRED (ADAPTIVE) IMMUNITY: The ability to resist infection that develops according to circumstances and is targeted to a specific pathogen. There are two types of acquired immunity, known as active and passive. Active immunity is either humoral, involving production of antibody molecules against a bacterium or virus, or cell-mediated, where T-cells are mobilized against infected cells. Infection and immunization can both induce acquired immunity. Passive immunity is induced by injection of the serum of a person who is already immune to a particular infection.

ACQUIRED IMMUNODEFICIENCY SYNDROME (AIDS):A disease of the immune system caused by the human immunodeficiency virus (HIV). It is characterized by the destruction of a particular type of white blood cell and increased susceptibility to infection and other diseases.

ACTIVE INFECTION: An infection that is currently producing symptoms or in which the infective agent is multiplying rapidly. In contrast, a latent infection is one in which the infective agent is present but not causing symptoms or damage to the body or reproducing at a significant rate.

ACUTE INFECTION: An infection of rapid onset and of short duration that either resolves or becomes chronic.

ADAPTIVE IMMUNITY: Another term for acquired immunity, referring to the resistance to infection that develops through life and is targeted to a specific pathogen. There are two types of adaptive immunity, known as active and passive. Active immunity is either humoral, involving production of antibody molecules against a bacterium or virus, or cell-mediated, in which T cells are mobilized against infected cells. Infection and immunization can both induce acquired immunity. Passive immunity is induced by injection of the serum of a person who is already immune to a particular infection.

ADHESION: Physical attraction between different types of molecules.

AEROBES: Aerobic microorganisms require the presence of oxygen for growth. Molecular oxygen functions in the respiratory pathway of the microbes to produce the energy necessary for life. Bacteria, yeasts, fungi, and algae are capable of aerobic growth.

AEROSOL: Particles of liquid or solid dispersed as a suspension in gas.

AGGREGATIONS: When blood clots (becomes solid, usually in response to injury), cells called platelets form clumps called aggregations. An instrument called an aggregometer measures the degree of platelet aggregation in blood.

AIDS (ACQUIRED IMMUNODEFICIENCY SYNDROME): A disease of the immune system caused by the human immunodeficiency virus (HIV). It is characterized by the destruction of a particular type of white blood cell and increased susceptibility to infection and other diseases.

AIRBORNE PRECAUTIONS: Procedures designed to reduce the chance that certain disease-causing (pathogenic) microorganisms will be transmitted through the air.

AIRBORNE TRANSMISSION: The ability of a disease-causing (pathogenic) microorganism to be spread through the air by droplets expelled during sneezing or coughing.

ALLELE: Any of two or more alternative forms of a gene that occupy the same location on a chromosome.

ALLERGY: An excessive or hypersensitive response of the immune system to substances (allergens) in the environment. Instead of fighting off a disease-causing foreign substance, the immune system launches a complex series of actions against the particular irritating allergen. The immune response may be accompanied by a number of stressful symptoms, ranging from mild to life threatening. In rare cases an allergic reaction leads to anaphylactic shock—a condition characterized by a sudden drop in blood pressure, difficulty in breathing, skin irritation, collapse, and possible death.

ALPHAVIRUS: A genus of small, spherical RNA viruses. The genus contains some of the most important human and animal pathogens, such as chikungunya virus; Sindbis virus; Semliki Forest virus; Western, Eastern, and Venezuelan equine encephalitis viruses; and the Ross River virus. Alphaviruses are transmitted by arthropods, in particular mosquitoes.

ALVEOLUS: A tiny air sac located within the lungs. The exchange of oxygen and carbon dioxide takes place within these sacs.

AMEBIC DYSENTERY: An inflammation of the intestine caused by the parasite *Entamoeba histolytica*. The severe form of the malady is characterized by the formation of localized lesions (ulcers) in the intestine, especially in the region known as the colon; abscesses in the liver and the brain; vomiting; severe diarrhea with fluid loss leading to dehydration; and abdominal pain. Also referred to as amebiasis or amoebiasis.

AMERICAN TYPE CULTURE COLLECTION (ATCC): A not-for-profit bioscience organization that maintains the world's largest and most diverse collection of microbiological life. Many laboratories and institutions maintain their own stockpile of microorganisms, usually those that are in frequent use in the facility. Some large culture collections are housed and maintained by universities or private enterprises, but none of these rivals the ATCC in terms of size.

AMPLIFICATION: A process by which something is made larger or the quantity of something is increased.

ANADROMOUS: Fish that migrate from ocean (salt) water to fresh water, such as salmon.

ANAEROBIC BACTERIA: Bacteria that grow without oxygen; also called anaerobic bacteria or anaerobes. Anaerobic bacteria can infect deep wounds, deep tissues, and internal organs where there is little oxygen. These infections are characterized by abscess formation, foul-smelling pus, and tissue destruction.

ANTHELMINTIC: Medicines that rid the body of parasitic worms.

ANTHRAX: A disease that is caused by the bacterium *Bacillus anthracis*. The bacterium can enter the body via a wound in the skin (cutaneous anthrax), via contaminated food or liquid (gastrointestinal anthrax), or via inhalation (inhalation anthrax).

ANTIBACTERIAL: A substance that reduces or kills germs (bacteria and other microorganisms but not viruses). Also often a term used to describe a drug used to treat bacterial infections.

ANTIBIOTIC: A drug, such as penicillin, used to fight infections caused by bacteria. Antibiotics act only on bacteria and are not effective against viruses.

ANTIBIOTIC RESISTANCE: The ability of bacteria to resist the actions of antibiotic drugs.

ANTIBIOTIC SENSITIVITY: The susceptibility of a bacterium to an antibiotic. Each type of bacteria can be killed by some types of antibiotics and not be affected by other types. Different types of bacteria exhibit different patterns of antibiotic sensitivity.

ANTIBODIES: Proteins found in the blood that help fight against foreign substances called antigens. Antigens, which are usually proteins or polysaccharides, stimulate the immune system to produce antibodies, or Y-shaped immunoglobulins. The antibodies inactivate the antigen and help remove it from the body. While antigens can be the source of infections from pathogenic bacteria and viruses, organic molecules detrimental to the body from internal or environmental sources also act as antigens. Genetic engineering and the use of various mutational mechanisms allow the construction of a vast array of antibodies (each with a unique genetic sequence).

ANTIBODY-ANTIGEN BINDING: Antibodies are produced by the immune system in response to antigens (material perceived as foreign). The antibody response to a particular antigen is highly specific and often involves a physical association between the two molecules. Biochemical and molecular forces govern this association.

ANTIBODY RESPONSE: The specific immune response that utilizes B cells to kill certain kinds of antigens.

ANTIFUNGAL: Antifungals (also called antifungal drugs) are medicines used to fight fungal infections. They are of two kinds, systemic and topical. Systemic antifungal drugs are medicines taken by mouth or by injection to treat infections caused by a fungus. Topical antifungal drugs are medicines applied to the skin to treat skin infections caused by a fungus.

ANTIGEN: A substance, usually a protein or polysaccharide, that stimulates the immune system to produce antibodies. While antigens can be the source of infections from pathogenic bacteria and viruses, organic molecules detrimental to the body from internal or environmental sources also act as antigens.

ANTIGENIC DRIFT: The gradual accumulation of mutations in genes, such as in gene coding for surface proteins, over a given period.

ANTIGENIC SHIFT: An abrupt and major genetic change, such as in gene coding for surface proteins of a virus.

ANTIMICROBIAL: Slows the growth of bacteria or is able to kill bacteria. Antimicrobial materials include antibiotics (which can be used inside the body) and disinfectants (which can only be used outside the body).

ANTIRETROVIRAL (ARV) DRUGS: Drugs that prevent the reproduction of a type of virus called a retrovirus. The human immunodeficiency virus (HIV), which causes acquired immunodeficiency syndrome (AIDS), is a retrovirus. These ARV drugs are therefore used to treat HIV infections. These medicines cannot prevent or cure HIV infection, but they help to keep the virus in check.

ANTIRETROVIRAL (ARV) THERAPY: A form of drug therapy that prevents the reproduction of a type of virus called a retrovirus. Human immunodeficiency virus (HIV), which causes acquired immunodeficiency syndrome (AIDS), is a retrovirus. ARV drugs are used to treat HIV infections and keep the virus in check, but they cannot prevent or cure the infection.

ANTISENSE DRUG: A drug that binds to messenger RNA (mRNA), thereby blocking gene activity. Some viruses have mRNA as their genetic material, so an antisense drug can inhibit their replication.

ANTISEPTIC: A substance that prevents or stops the growth and multiplication of microorganisms in or on living tissue.

ANTITOXIN: An antidote to a toxin that neutralizes the toxin's poisonous effects.

ANTIVIRAL DRUGS: Compounds that are used to prevent or treat viral infections, via the disruption of an infectious mechanism used by the virus, or to treat the symptoms of an infection.

ARACHNID: An arthropod that belongs to class Arachnida, such as a spider or scorpion. Arachnids have eight legs, which differentiates them from six-legged insects.

ARBOVIRUS: A virus that is typically spread by blood-sucking insects, most commonly mosquitoes. Over 100 types of arboviruses cause disease in humans. Yellow fever and dengue fever are two examples.

ARENAVIRUS: A virus that belongs in a viral family known as Arenaviridae. The name arenavirus derives from the appearance of the spherical virus particles when cut into thin sections and viewed using a transmission electron microscope. The interior of the particles is grainy or sandy in appearance, due to the presence of ribosomes that have been acquired from the host cell. The Latin designation *arena* means "sandy."

ARTHROPOD: A member of the largest single animal phylum, consisting of organisms with segmented bodies, jointed legs or wings, and exoskeletons.

ARTHROPOD-BORNE DISEASE: A disease caused by one of a phylum of organisms characterized by exoskeletons and segmented bodies.

ARTHROPOD-BORNE VIRUS: A virus caused by one of a phylum of organisms characterized by exoskeletons and segmented bodies.

ASEPSIS: Without germs, more specifically without microorganisms.

ASPIRATION: The drawing out of fluid from a part of the body; it can cause pneumonia when stomach contents are transferred to the lungs through vomiting.

ASSAY: A determination of an amount of a particular compound in a sample (e.g., to make chemical tests to determine the relative amount of a particular substance in a sample). A method used to quantify a biological compound.

ASYMPTOMATIC: A state in which an individual does not exhibit or experience symptoms of a disease.

ATAXIA: An unsteadiness in walking or standing that is associated with brain diseases such as kuru or Creutzfeldt-Jakob disease.

ATOPY: An inherited tendency toward hypersensitivity toward immunoglobulin E, a key component of the immune system, which plays an important role in asthma, eczema, and hay fever.

ATROPHY: Decreasing in size or wasting-away of a body part or tissue.

ATTENUATED STRAIN: A bacterium or virus that has been weakened. Often used as the basis of a vaccine against the specific disease caused by the bacterium or virus.

AUTOCLAVE: A device designed to kill microorganisms on solid items and in liquids by exposure to steam at a high pressure.

AUTOIMMUNE DISEASE: A disease in which the body's defense system attacks its own tissues and organs.

AUTOIMMUNITY: A condition in which the immune system attacks the body's cells, causing tissue destruction. Autoimmune diseases are classified as either general, in which the autoimmune reaction takes place simultaneously in a number of tissues, or organ specific, in which the autoimmune reaction targets a single organ. Autoimmunity is accepted as the cause of a wide range of disorders and is suspected to be responsible for many more. Among the most common diseases attributed to autoimmune disorders are rheumatoid arthritis, systemic lupus erythematosus (lupus), multiple sclerosis, myasthenia gravis, pernicious anemia, and scleroderma.

AUTOINFECTION: The reinfection of the body by a disease organism already in the body, such as eggs left by a parasitic worm.

B

B CELL: Also known as B lymphocyte; a kind of cell produced in bone marrow that secretes antibodies.

BABESIOSIS: An infection of the red blood cells caused by *Babesia microti*, a form of parasite (parasitic sporozoan).

BACILLUS ANTHRACIS: The bacterium that causes anthrax.

BACTEREMIA: This condition occurs when bacteria enter the bloodstream through, for example, a wound or an infection or through a surgical procedure or injection. Bacteremia may cause no symptoms and resolve without treatment, or it may produce fever and other symptoms of infection. In some cases, bacteremia leads to septic shock, a potentially life-threatening condition.

BACTERIA: Single-celled microorganisms that live in soil, water, plants, and animals and whose activities range from the development of disease to fermentation. They play a key role in the decay of organic matter and the cycling of nutrients. Bacteria exist in various shapes, including spherical, rod-shaped, and spiral. Some bacteria are agents of disease. Different types of bacteria cause many sexually transmitted infections, including syphilis, gonorrhea, and chlamydia. Bacteria also cause diseases such as typhoid, dysentery, and tetanus. Bacterium is the singular form of bacteria.

BACTERIOCIDAL: The treatment of a bacterium such that the organism is killed. A bactericidal treatment is always lethal and is also referred to as sterilization.

BACTERIOLOGICAL STRAIN: A bacterial subclass of a particular tribe and genus.

BACTERIOPHAGE: A virus that infects bacteria. When a bacteriophage that carries the diphtheria toxin gene infects diphtheria bacteria, the bacteria produce diphtheria toxin.

BACTERIOSTATIC: Refers to a treatment that restricts the ability of the bacterium to grow.

BASIDIOSPORE: A fungal spore of Basidiomycetes. Basidiomycetes are classified under the Fungi kingdom as belonging to the phylum Mycota (i.e., Basidiomycota), class Mycetes (i.e., Basidiomycetes). Fungi are frequently parasites that decompose organic material from their hosts, such as the parasites that grow on rotten wood, although some may cause serious plant diseases such as smuts (Ustomycetes) and rusts (Teliomycetes). Some live in a symbiotic relationship with plant roots (Mycorrhizae). A cell type termed *basidium* is responsible for sexual spore formation in Basidiomycetes, through nuclear fusion followed by meiosis, thus forming haploid basidiospores.

BED NET: A type of netting that provides protection from diseases caused by insects such as flies and mosquitoes. It is often used when sleeping to allow air to flow through its mesh structure while preventing insects from biting.

BIFURCATED NEEDLE: A bifurcated needle is a needle that has two prongs with a wire suspended between them. The wire is designed to hold a certain amount of vaccine. Development of the bifurcated needle was a major advance in vaccination against smallpox.

BIOINDICATOR: A living organism whose status in an ecosystem offers an idea of the health of its environment.

BIOFILM: A population of microorganisms that forms following the adhesion of bacteria, algae, yeast, or fungi to a surface. These surface growths can be found in natural settings, such as on rocks in streams, and in infections, such as those that occur on catheters. Microorganisms can colonize living and inert natural and synthetic surfaces.

BIOINFORMATICS: The development of new database methods to store genomic information (information related to genes and the genetic sequence), computational software programs, and methods to extract, process, and evaluate this information. Also known as computational biology, bioinformatics also refers to the refinement of existing techniques to acquire the genomic data. Finding genes and determining their function, predicting the structure of proteins and sequence of ribonucleic acid (RNA) from the available sequence of deoxyribonucleic acid (DNA), and determining the evolutionary relationship of proteins and DNA sequences are aspects of bioinformatics.

BIOLOGICAL WARFARE: As defined by the United Nations, the use of any living organism, such as a bacterium or virus, or an infective component, such as a toxin, to cause disease or death in humans, animals, or plants. In contrast to bioterrorism, biological warfare is the state-sanctioned use of biological weapons on an opposing military force or civilian population.

BIOLOGICAL WEAPON: A weapon that contains or disperses a biological toxin, disease-causing microorganism, or other biological agent intended to harm or kill plants, animals, or humans.

BIOMAGNIFICATION: The increasing concentration of compounds at a higher trophic level or the tendency of organisms to accumulate certain chemicals to a concentration larger than that occurring in their inorganic, nonliving environment, such as soil or water, or, in the case of animals, larger than in their food.

BIOMODULATOR: Short for biologic response modulator. An agent that modifies some characteristic of the immune system, which may help in the fight against infection.

BIOSAFETY LABORATORY: A laboratory that deals with all aspects of potentially infectious agents or biohazards.

BIOSAFETY LEVEL 4 FACILITY: A specialized biosafety laboratory that deals with dangerous or exotic infectious agents or biohazards that are considered high risks for spreading life-threatening diseases, either because the disease is spread through aerosols or because there is no therapy or vaccine to counter the disease.

BIOSHIELD PROJECT: A joint effort between the US Department of Homeland Security and the Department of Health and Human Services. The program was tasked with improving treatment of diseases caused by biological, chemical, and radiological weapons.

BIOSPHERE: The sum of all life-forms on Earth and the interaction among those life-forms.

BIOTECHNOLOGY: Use of biological organisms, systems, or processes to make or modify products.

BIOWEAPON: A weapon that uses bacteria, viruses, or poisonous substances made by bacteria or viruses.

BLOOD-BORNE PATHOGENS: Disease-causing agents carried or transported in the blood. Blood-borne infections are those in which the infectious agent is transmitted from one person to another via contaminated blood.

BLOODBORNE: Via the blood. For example, bloodborne pathogens are pathogens (disease-causing agents) carried or transported in the blood. Bloodborne infections are those in which the infectious agent is transmitted from one person to another via contaminated blood. Infections of the blood can occur as a result of the spread of an ongoing infection caused by bacteria such as *Yersinia pestis*, *Haemophilus influenzae*, or *Staphylococcus aureus.*

BOTULINUM TOXIN: One of the most poisonous substances known. The toxin, which can be ingested or inhaled, and which disrupts transmission of nerve impulses to muscles, is naturally produced by the bacterium *Clostridium botulinum*. Certain strains of *C. baratii* and *C. butyricum* can also produce the toxin.

BOTULISM: An illness produced by a toxin that is released by the soil bacterium *Clostridium botulinum.*

One type of toxin is also produced by *Clostridium baratii*. The toxins affect nerves and can produce paralysis. The paralysis can affect the functioning of organs and tissues that are vital to life.

BROAD SPECTRUM: A series of objects or ideas with great variety between them. In medicine the term is often applied to drugs that act on a large number of different disease-causing agents.

BROAD-SPECTRUM ANTIBIOTICS: Drugs that kill a wide range of bacteria rather than just those from a specific family. For example, Amoxicillin is a broad-spectrum antibiotic that is used against many common illnesses such as ear infections.

BRONCHIOLITIS: An inflammation (-itis) of the bronchioles, the small air passages in the lungs that enter the alveoli (air sacs).

BUBO: A swollen lymph gland, usually in the groin or armpit, characteristic of infection with bubonic plague.

BUSHMEAT: The meat of terrestrial wild and exotic animals, typically those that live in parts of Africa, Asia, and the Americas; also known as wild meat.

C

CADAVER: The body of a deceased human, especially one designated for scientific dissection or other research.

CAMPYLOBACTERIOSIS: Campylobacteriosis is a bacterial infection of the intestinal tract of humans. The infection, which typically results in diarrhea, is caused by members of the genus *Campylobacter*. In particular, *Campylobacter jejuni* is the most common cause of bacterial diarrhea in the United States, with more occurrences than salmonella (another prominent disease-causing bacteria associated with food poisoning). Worldwide, approximately 5 to 14 percent of all diarrhea may be the result of campylobacteriosis.

CAPSID: The protein shell surrounding a virus particle.

CARBOLIC ACID: An acidic compound that, when diluted with water, is used as an antiseptic and a disinfectant.

CARCINOGEN: Any biological, chemical, or physical substance or agent that can cause cancer. There are more than 100 different types of cancer, which can be distinguished by the type of cell or organ that is affected, the treatment plan employed, and the cause of the cancer. Most of the carcinogens that are commonly discussed come from chemical sources artificially produced by humans. Some of the better-known carcinogens are the pesticide DDT (dichlorodiphenyltrichloroethane), asbestos, and the carcinogens produced when tobacco is smoked.

CASE FATALITY RATE: The rate of patients suffering disease or injury that die as a result of that disease or injury during a specific period of time.

CASE FATALITY RATIO: A ratio indicating the amount of people who die as a result of a particular disease, usually expressed as a percentage or as the number of deaths per 1,000 cases.

CATALYST: Substance that speeds up a chemical process without actually changing the products of reaction.

CD4+ T CELLS: A type of T cell found in the immune system that are characterized by the presence of a CD4 antigen protein on their surface. These are the cells most often destroyed as a result of HIV infection.

CELL CYCLE AND CELL DIVISION: The series of stages that a cell undergoes while progressing to division is known as cell cycle. For an organism to grow and develop, the organism's cells must be able to duplicate themselves. Three basic events must take place to achieve this duplication: the deoxyribonucleic acid (DNA), which makes up the individual chromosomes within the cell's nucleus must be duplicated; the two sets of DNA must be packaged into two separate nuclei; and the cell's cytoplasm must divide itself to create two separate cells, each complete with its own nucleus. The two new cells —products of the single original cell—are known as daughter cells.

CELL MEMBRANE: The cell is bound by an outer membrane that, as described by a membrane model termed the fluid mosaic model, is composed of a phospholipid lipid bilayer with proteins—molecules that also act as receptor sites—interspersed within the phospholipid bilayer. Varieties of channels exist within the membrane. In eukaryotes (cells with a true nucleus) there are a number of internal cellular membranes that can partition regions within the cells' interior. Some of these membranes ultimately become continuous with the nuclear membrane. Bacteria and viruses do not have inner membranes.

CENTERS FOR DISEASE CONTROL AND PREVENTION (CDC): One of the primary public health institutions in the world. The CDC is headquartered in Atlanta,

Georgia, with facilities at nine other sites in the United States. The centers are the focus of US government efforts to develop and implement prevention and control strategies for diseases, including those of microbiological origin.

CESTODE: A class of worms characterized by flat, segmented bodies, commonly known as tapeworms.

CHAGAS DISEASE: A human infection that is caused by a microorganism that establishes a parasitic relationship with a human host as part of its life cycle. The disease is named for the Brazilian physician Carlos Chagas, who in 1909 described the involvement of the flagellated protozoan known as *Trypanosoma cruzi* in a prevalent disease in South America.

CHAIN OF TRANSMISSION: The route by which an infection is spread from its source to a susceptible host. An example of a chain of transmission is the spread of malaria from an infected animal to humans via mosquitoes.

CHANCRE: A sore that occurs in the first stage of syphilis at the place where the infection entered the body.

CHEMILUMINESCENT SIGNAL: The production of light from a chemical reaction. A variety of tests to detect infectious organisms or target components of the organisms relies on the binding of a chemical-containing probe to the target and the subsequent development of light following the addition of a reactive compound.

CHEMOTHERAPY: The treatment of a disease, infection, or condition with chemicals that have a specific effect on its cause, such as a microorganism or cancer cell. The first modern therapeutic chemical was derived from a synthetic dye. Sulfonamide drugs developed in the 1930s, penicillin and other antibiotics of the 1940s, hormones developed in the 1950s, and later drugs that interfere with cancer cell metabolism and reproduction have all been part of the chemotherapeutic arsenal.

CHICKENPOX: Chickenpox (also called varicella disease and sometimes spelled chicken pox) is a common and extremely infectious childhood disease that can also affect adults. It produces an itchy, blistery rash that typically lasts about a week and is sometimes accompanied by a fever.

CHILDBED FEVER: A bacterial infection occurring in women following childbirth, causing fever and, in some cases, blood poisoning and possible death.

CHLORINATION: A chemical process that is used primarily to disinfect drinking water and spills of microorganisms. The active agent in chlorination is the element chlorine, or a derivative of chlorine (e .g., chlorine dioxide). Chlorination is a swift and economical means of destroying many, but not all, microorganisms that are a health threat in fluids such as drinking water.

CHRONIC: Chronic infections persist for prolonged periods of time—months or even years—in the host. This lengthy persistence is due to a number of factors, which can include masking of the disease-causing agent (e.g., bacteria) from the immune system, invasion of host cells, and the establishment of an infection that is resistant to antibacterial agents.

CHRONIC FATIGUE SYNDROME (CFS): A condition that causes extreme tiredness. People with CFS have debilitating fatigue that lasts for six months or longer. They also have many other symptoms. Some of these symptoms are pain in the joints and muscles, headache, and sore throat. CFS appears to result from a combination of factors.

CILIA: Specialized arrangements of microtubules that have two general functions. They propel certain unicellular organisms, such as paramecium, through the water. In multicellular organisms, if cilia extend from stationary cells that are part of a tissue layer, they move fluid over the surface of the tissue.

CIRRHOSIS: A chronic, degenerative, irreversible liver disease in which normal liver cells are damaged and are then replaced by scar tissue. Cirrhosis changes the structure of the liver and the blood vessels that nourish it. The disease reduces the liver's ability to manufacture proteins and process hormones, nutrients, medications, and poisons.

CLINICAL TRIALS: According to the National Institutes of Health, a clinical trial is "a research study to answer specific questions about vaccines or new therapies or new ways of using known treatments." These studies allow researchers to determine whether new drugs or treatments are safe and effective. When conducted carefully, clinical trials can provide fast and safe answers to these questions.

CLOACA: The cavity into which the intestinal, genital, and urinary tracts open in vertebrates such as fish, reptiles, birds, and some primitive mammals.

CLUSTER: A grouping of individuals contracting an infectious disease or foodborne illness very close in time or place.

COCCIDIUM: Any single-celled animal (protozoan) belonging to the subclass Coccidia. Some coccidia species can infest the digestive tract, causing coccidiosis.

COHORT: A group of people (or any species) sharing a common characteristic. Cohorts are identified and grouped in cohort studies to determine the frequency of diseases or the kinds of disease outcomes over time.

COHORTING: The practice of grouping people with similar infections or symptoms together to reduce transmission to others.

COLONIZATION: The process of occupation and increase in number of microorganisms at a specific site.

COLONIZE: To persist and grow at a given location.

COMMUNITY-ACQUIRED INFECTION: An infection that develops outside of a hospital, in the general community. It differs from hospital-acquired infections in that those who are infected are typically in better health than hospitalized people.

CONGENITAL: Existing at the time of birth.

CONJUNCTIVITIS: An inflammation or redness of the lining of the white part of the eye and the underside of the eyelid (conjunctiva) that can be caused by infection, allergic reaction, or physical agents such as infrared or ultraviolet light. Conjunctivitis (also called pink eye) is one of the most common eye infections in children and adults in the United States. Luckily, it is also one of the most treatable infections. Because it is so common in the United States and around the world and is often not reported to health organizations, accurate statistics are not available for conjunctivitis.

CONTACT PRECAUTIONS: Actions developed to minimize the transfer of microorganisms directly by physical contact and indirectly by touching a contaminated surface.

CONTAGIOUS: A disease that is easily spread among a population, usually by casual person-to-person contact.

CONTAMINATION: The unwanted presence of a microorganism or compound in a particular environment. That environment can be in the laboratory setting, for example, in a medium being used for the growth of a species of bacteria during an experiment. Another environment can be the human body, where contamination by bacteria can produce an infection. Contamination by bacteria and viruses can occur on several levels and their presence can adversely influence the results of experiments. Outside the laboratory, bacteria and viruses can contaminate drinking water supplies, foodstuffs, and products, thus causing illness.

COWPOX: A disease that is caused by the cowpox or catpox virus. The virus is a member of the orthopoxvirus family. Other viruses in this family include the smallpox and vaccinia viruses. Cowpox is a rare disease and is mostly noteworthy as the basis of the formulation, over 200 years ago, of an injection by Edward Jenner that proved successful in curing smallpox.

CREPITANT: A crackling sound that accompanies breathing, a common symptom of pneumonia or other diseases of the lungs.

CREUTZFELDT-JAKOB DISEASE (CJD): A transmissible, rapidly progressing, fatal neurodegenerative disorder related to bovine spongiform encephalopathy (BSE), commonly called mad cow disease.

CULL: The selection, often for destruction, of a part of an animal population. Often done just to reduce numbers, a widespread cull was carried out during the epidemic of bovine spongiform encephalopathy (BSE or mad cow disease) in the United Kingdom during the 1980s.

CULTURE: A single species of microorganism that is isolated and grown under controlled conditions. The German bacteriologist Robert Koch first developed culturing techniques in the late 1870s. Following Koch's initial discovery, medical scientists quickly sought to identify other pathogens. In the 21st century bacteria cultures are used as basic tools in microbiology and medicine.

CULTURE AND SENSITIVITY: Laboratory tests that are used to identify the type of microorganism causing an infection and the compounds to which the identified organism is sensitive and resistant. In the case of bacteria, this approach permits the selection of antibiotics that will be most effective in dealing with the infection.

CUTANEOUS: Pertaining to the skin.

CYST: A closed cavity or sac or the dormant stage of life of some parasites when they live inside an enclosed area, covered by a tough outer shell.

CYTOKINE: One of a family of small proteins that mediate an organism's response to injury or infection. Cytokines operate by transmitting signals between cells in an organism. Minute quantities of cytokines are secreted, each by a single cell type, to regulate functions in other cells by binding with specific receptors. Their interactions with the receptors produce secondary signals that inhibit or enhance the action of certain genes within the cell. Unlike endocrine hormones, which can act throughout the body, most cytokines act locally near the cells that produced them.

CYTOTOXIC: Able to kill cells. Cytotoxic drugs kill cancer cells but may also have applications in killing bacteria.

D

DEBRIDEMENT: The medical process of removing dead, damaged, or infected tissue from pressure ulcers, burns, and other wounds to speed healing of the surrounding healthy tissue.

DEFINITIVE HOST: The organism in which a parasite reaches reproductive maturity.

DEGRADATION (CELLULAR): The destruction of host cell components, such as DNA, by infective agents such as bacteria and viruses.

DEHYDRATION: The loss of water and salts essential for normal bodily function. It occurs when the body loses more fluid than it takes in. Water is important to the human body because it makes up about 70 percent of the muscles, around 75 percent of the brain, and approximately 92 percent of the blood. A person who weighs about 150 pounds (68 kilograms) will contain about 80 quarts (just over 75 liters) of water. About 2 cups of water are lost each day just from regular breathing. If the body sweats more and breathes more heavily than normal, the human body loses even more water. Dehydration occurs when that lost water is not replenished.

DEMENTIA: From the Latin word dement, meaning "away mind," a progressive deterioration and eventual loss of mental ability that is severe enough to interfere with normal activities of daily living. Dementia lasts more than six months, has not been present since birth, and is not associated with a loss or alteration of consciousness. It is a group of symptoms caused by gradual death of brain cells. Dementia is usually caused by degeneration in the cerebral cortex, the part of the brain responsible for thoughts, memories, actions, and personality. Death of brain cells in this region leads to the cognitive impairment that characterizes dementia.

DEMOGRAPHICS: The characteristics of human populations or specific parts of human populations, most often reported through statistics.

DEOXYRIBONUCLEIC ACID (DNA): A double-stranded, helical molecule that forms the molecular basis for heredity in most organisms.

DERMATOPHYTE: A parasitic fungus that feeds off keratin, a protein that is abundant in skin, nails, and hair and therefore often causes infection of these body parts.

DIAGNOSIS: Identification of a disease or disorder.

DIARRHEA: To most individuals, diarrhea means an increased frequency or decreased consistency of bowel movements; however, the medical definition is more exact than this explanation. In many developed countries, the average number of bowel movements is three per day. However, researchers have found that diarrhea, which is not a disease, best correlates with an increase in stool weight; a stool weight above 10.5 ounces (300 grams) per day generally indicates diarrhea. This is mainly due to excess water, which normally makes up 60 to 85 percent of fecal matter. In this way, true diarrhea is distinguished from diseases that cause only an increase in the number of bowel movements (hyperdefecation) or incontinence (involuntary loss of bowel contents). Diarrhea is also classified by physicians into acute, which lasts one to two weeks, and chronic, which continues for longer than four weeks. Viral and bacterial infections are the most common causes of acute diarrhea.

DIATOM: Algae are a diverse group of simple, nucleated, plantlike aquatic organisms that are primary producers. Primary producers are able to utilize photosynthesis to create organic molecules from sunlight, water, and carbon dioxide. Ecologically vital, algae account for roughly half of the photosynthetic production of organic material on Earth in both freshwater and marine environments. Algae exist either as single cells or as multicellular organizations. Diatoms are microscopic, single-celled algae that have intricate glass-like outer cell walls partially composed of silicon. Different species of diatom can be identified based on the structure of these walls. Many diatom species are planktonic, suspended in the water column moving at the mercy of water currents. Others remain attached to submerged surfaces. One bucketful of water may contain millions of diatoms. Their abundance makes them important food sources in aquatic ecosystems.

DIMORPHIC: The occurrence of two different shapes or color forms within the species, usually occurring as sexual dimorphism between males and females.

DINOFLAGELLATE: Microorganisms that are regarded as algae. Their wide array of exotic shapes and, sometimes, armored appearance, is distinct from other algae. The closest microorganisms in appearance are the diatoms.

DIPHTHERIA: A potentially fatal, contagious bacterial disease that usually involves the nose, throat, and air passages but may also infect the skin. Its most striking feature is the formation of a grayish membrane covering the tonsils and upper part of the throat.

DISINFECTANT: Disinfection and the use of chemical disinfectants is one key strategy of infection control. Disinfectants reduce the number of living microorganisms, usually to a level that is considered safe for the particular environment. Typically, this entails the destruction of those microbes that are capable of causing disease.

DISSEMINATED: The previous distribution of a disease-causing microorganism over a larger area.

DISSEMINATION: The spreading of a disease in a population or over a large geographic area or the spreading of disease organisms in the body.

DISTAL: From the same root word as distant, the medical word for distant from some agreed-on point of reference. For example, the hand is at the distal end of the arm from the trunk.

DNA: Deoxyribonucleic acid, a double-stranded, helical molecule that is found in almost all living cells and that determines the characteristics of each organism.

DNA FINGERPRINTING: A range of techniques used to show similarities and dissimilarities between the deoxyribonucleic acid (DNA) present in different individuals or organisms.

DNA PROBES: Substances or agents that bind directly to a predefined specific sequence of nucleic acids in deoxyribonucleic acid (DNA).

DORMANT: Inactive but still alive. A resting, nonactive state.

DROPLET: A drop of water or other fluid that is fewer than 5 microns (a millionth of a meter) in diameter.

DROPLET TRANSMISSION: The spread of microorganisms from one space to another (including from person to person) via droplets that are larger than 5 microns in diameter. Droplets are typically expelled into the air by coughing and sneezing.

DRUG RESISTANCE: Develops when an infective agent, such as a bacterium, fungus, or virus, develops a lack of sensitivity to a drug that would normally be able to control or even kill it. This tends to occur with overuse of anti-infective agents, which selects out populations of microbes most able to resist them, while killing off those organisms that are most sensitive. The next time the anti-infective agent is used, it will be less effective, leading to the eventual development of resistance.

DYSENTERY: An infectious disease that has ravaged armies, refugee camps, and prisoner-of-war camps throughout history. The disease is still a major problem in developing countries with primitive sanitary facilities.

DYSPLASIA: Abnormal changes in tissue or cell development.

E

ECOLOGY: The study of the relationships among communities of living things.

ECTOPARASITES: Parasites that cling to the outside of their host rather than their host's intestines. Common points of attachment are the gills, fins, or skin of fish.

ELBOW BUMP: A personal greeting that involves two people touching elbows instead of shaking hands. It is recommended by the World Health Organization for use by researchers handling highly infectious organisms such as Ebola virus.

ELECTROLYTES: Compounds that ionize in a solution. Electrolytes dissolved in the blood play an important role in maintaining the proper functioning of the body.

ELECTRON: A fundamental particle of matter carrying a single unit of negative electrical charge.

EMBRYONATED: When an embryo has been implanted in a female animal.

EMERGING INFECTIOUS DISEASE: A new infectious disease such as severe acute respiratory syndrome (SARS) or West Nile virus, as well as a previously known disease such as malaria, tuberculosis, or bacterial pneumonia that is appearing in a new form that is resistant to drug treatments.

ENCEPHALITIS: A type of acute brain inflammation, most often due to infection by a virus.

ENCEPHALOMYELITIS: Simultaneous inflammation of the brain and spinal cord.

ENCEPHALOPATHY: Any abnormality in the structure or function of the brain.

ENCYSTED LARVAE: Larvae that are not actively growing and dividing and are more resistant to environmental conditions.

ENDEMIC: Present in a particular area or among a particular group of people.

ENDOCYTOSIS: A process by which host cells allow the entry of outside substances, including viruses, through their cell membranes.

ENTERIC: Involving the intestinal tract or relating to the intestines.

ENTEROBACTERIAL: Infections Infections caused by a group of bacteria that dwell in the intestinal tract of humans and other warm-blooded animals. The bacteria are all Gram-negative and rod-shaped. As a group they are termed Enterobacteriaceae. A prominent member of this group is Escherichia coli. Other members are the various species in the genera Salmonella, Shigella, Klebsiella, Enterobacter, Serratia, Proteus, and Yersinia.

ENTEROPATHOGEN: A virus or pathogen that invades the large or small intestine, causing disease.

ENTEROTOXIN: A class of toxin produced by bacteria. Unlike exotoxins, which are released by bacteria, enterotoxins reside with the bacterial cells.

ENTEROVIRUS: A group of viruses that contain ribonucleic acid as their genetic material. They are members of the picornavirus family. The various types of enteroviruses that infect humans are referred to as serotypes, in recognition of their different antigenic patterns. The different immune response is important, as infection with one type of enterovirus does not necessarily confer protection to infection by a different type of enterovirus. There are 64 different enterovirus serotypes. The serotypes include polio viruses, coxsackie A and B viruses, echoviruses, and a large number of what are referred to as non-polio enteroviruses.

ENZOOTIC: Affecting animals, naturally present in an environment, and occurring at regular intervals.

ENZYMES: Molecules that act as critical catalysts in biological systems. Catalysts are substances that increase the rate of chemical reactions without being consumed in the reaction. Without enzymes, many reactions would require higher levels of energy and higher temperatures than exist in biological systems. Enzymes are proteins that possess specific binding sites for other molecules (substrates). A series of weak binding interactions allows enzymes to accelerate reaction rates. Enzyme kinetics is the study of enzymatic reactions and mechanisms. Enzyme inhibitor studies have allowed researchers to develop therapies for the treatment of diseases, including AIDS.

ENZYME-LINKED IMMUNOSORBENT ASSAY (ELISA): A technique used to detect antibodies or infectious agents in a sample. The procedure involves interactions via serial binding to a solid surface, usually a polystyrene multiwell plate. The result is a colored product that correlates to the amount of analyte present in the original sample.

EPIDEMIC: From the Greek epidemic, meaning "prevalent among the people," it is most commonly used to describe an outbreak of an illness or a disease in which the number of individual cases significantly exceeds the usual or expected number of cases in any given population.

EPIDEMIOLOGIST: One who studies the various factors that influence the occurrence, distribution, prevention, and control of disease, injury, and other health-related events in a defined human population. By the application of various analytical techniques, including mathematical analysis of the data, the probable cause of an infectious outbreak can be pinpointed.

EPIDEMIOLOGY: The study of the various factors that influence the occurrence, distribution, prevention, and control of disease, injury, and other health-related events in a defined human population. By the application of various analytical techniques, including mathematical analysis of the data, the probable cause of an infectious outbreak can be pinpointed.

EPIZOOTIC: The abnormally high occurrence of a specific disease in animals in a particular area, similar to a human epidemic.

EPSTEIN-BARR VIRUS (EBV): Part of the family of human herpes viruses. Infectious mononucleosis (IM) is the most common disease manifestation of this virus, which, once established in the host, can never be completely eradicated. Little can be done to treat EBV; most methods can only alleviate resultant symptoms.

EQUID: A mammal of the horse family, such as a horse, donkey, mule, or zebra.

ERADICATE: To get rid of; the permanent reduction to zero of global incidence of a particular infection.

ERADICATION: The process of destroying or eliminating a microorganism or disease.

ERYTHEMA: Skin redness due to excess blood in capillaries (small blood vessels) in the skin.

ESCHAR: Any scab or crust forming on the skin as a result of a burn or disease. Scabs from cuts or scrapes are not eschars.

ETIOLOGY: The study of the cause or origin of a disease or disorder.

EX SITU: A Latin term meaning "from the place" or removed from its original place.

EXECUTIVE: Order Presidential orders that implement or interpret a federal statute, administrative policy, or treaty.

EXOTOXIN: A toxic protein produced during bacterial growth and metabolism and released into the environment.

EYE DROPS: Saline-containing fluid that is added to the eye to cleanse the eye or as the solution used to administer antibiotics or other medication.

F

FASCIA: A type of connective tissue made up of a network of fibers. It is best thought of as being the packing material of the body. Fascia surrounds muscles, bones, and joints and lies between the layers of skin. It functions to hold these structures together, protecting them and defining the shape of the body. When surrounding a muscle, fascia helps prevent a contracting muscle from catching or causing excessive friction on neighboring muscles.

FEBRILE: Pertaining to a fever.

FECAL-ORAL ROUTE: The spread of disease through the transmission of minute particles of fecal material from one organism to the mouth of another. This can occur by drinking contaminated water; eating food exposed to animal or human feces, such as food from plants watered with unclean water; or preparing food without practicing proper hygiene.

FECES: Solid waste excreted from a living body.

FIBROBLAST: A cell type that gives rise to connective tissue.

FILOVIRUS ANY: RNA virus that belongs to the family Filoviridae. Filoviruses infect primates. Marburg virus and Ebola virus are filoviruses.

FLAGELLUM: A hairlike structure in a cell that serves as an organ of locomotion.

FLAVIVIRUS: A single genus of ribonucleic acid (RNA) viruses that belong to the family Flaviviridae. Flaviviruses are found in arthropods but can infect humans and animals. Examples are dengue, yellow fever, West Nile, Japanese encephalitis, and Zika.

FLEA: Any parasitic insect of the order Siphonaptera. Fleas can infest many mammals, including humans, and can act as carriers (vectors) of disease.

FLORA: In microbiology, the collective microorganisms that normally inhabit an organism or system. Human intestines, for example, contain bacteria that aid in digestion and are considered normal flora.

FOCUS: In medicine, a primary center of some disease process (for example, a cluster of abnormal cells). Foci is plural for focus (more than one focus).

FOMITE: An object or a surface to which infectious microorganisms such as bacteria or viruses can adhere and be transmitted. Papers, clothing, dishes, and other objects can all act as fomites. Transmission is often by touch.

FOOD PRESERVATION: Any one of a number of techniques used to prevent food from spoiling, such as canning, pickling, drying or freeze-drying, irradiation, pasteurization, smoking, and the addition of chemical additives. Food preservation has become an increasingly important component of the food industry as fewer people eat foods produced on their own lands and as consumers expect to purchase and consume foods that are out of season.

FULMINANT INFECTION: An infection that appears suddenly and whose symptoms are immediately severe.

G

GAMETOCYTE: A germ cell with the ability to divide for the purpose of producing gametes, either male gametes called spermatocytes or female gametes called oocytes.

GAMMA GLOBULIN: A group of soluble proteins in the blood, most of which are antibodies that can mount a direct attack on pathogens and can be used to treat various infections.

GANGRENE: The destruction of body tissue by a bacteria called Clostridium perfringens or a combination of Streptococci and Staphylococci bacteria. C. perfringens is widespread; it is found in soil and the intestinal tracts of humans and animals. It becomes dangerous only when its spores germinate, producing toxins and destructive enzymes, and germination occurs only in an anaerobic environment (one almost totally devoid of oxygen). While gangrene can develop in any part of the body, it is most common in fingers, toes, hands, feet, arms, and legs, the parts of the body most susceptible to restricted blood flow. Even a slight injury in such an area is at high risk of causing gangrene. Early treatment with antibiotics, such as penicillin, and surgery to remove the dead tissue will often reduce the need for amputation. If left untreated, gangrene results in amputation or death.

GASTROENTERITIS: An inflammation of the stomach and the intestines. Commonly called the stomach flu.

GENE: The fundamental physical and functional unit of heredity. Whether in a microorganism or in a human cell, a gene is an individual element of an organism's genome and determines a trait or characteristic by regulating biochemical structure or metabolic process.

GENE THERAPY: The treatment of inherited diseases by corrective genetic engineering of the dysfunctional genes. It is part of a broader field called genetic medicine, which involves the screening, diagnosis, prevention, and treatment of hereditary conditions in humans. The results of genetic screening can pinpoint a potential problem to which gene therapy can sometimes offer a solution. Genetic defects are significant in the total field of medicine, with up to 15 out of every 100 newborn infants having a hereditary disorder of greater or lesser severity. More than 2,000 genetically distinct inherited defects have been classified as of 2018, including diabetes, cystic fibrosis, hemophilia, sickle cell anemia, phenylketonuria, Down syndrome, and cancer.

GENETIC ENGINEERING: The altering of the genetic material of living cells to make them capable of producing new substances or performing new functions. When the genetic material within the living cells (i.e., genes) is working properly, the human body can develop and function smoothly. However, should a single gene (even a tiny segment of a gene) go awry, the effect can be dramatic deformities, disease, and even death are possible.

GENOME: All of the genetic information for a cell or organism. The complete sequence of genes within a cell or virus.

GENOTYPE: The genetic information that a living thing inherits from its parents that affects its makeup, appearance, and function.

GEOGRAPHIC FOCALITY: The physical location of a disease pattern, epidemic, or outbreak; the characteristics of a location created by interconnections with other places.

GEOGRAPHIC INFORMATION SYSTEM (GIS): A system for archiving, retrieving, and manipulating data that has been stored and indexed according to the geographic coordinates of its elements. The system generally can utilize a variety of data types, such as imagery, maps, tables, etc.

GEOGRAPHIC MEDICINE: Also called geomedicine, the study of how human health is affected by climate and environment.

GERM THEORY OF DISEASE: A fundamental tenet of medicine that states that microorganisms, which are too small to be seen without the aid of a microscope, can invade the body and cause disease.

GLOBAL OUTBREAK ALERT AND RESPONSE NETWORK (GOARN): A collaboration of resources for the rapid identification, confirmation, and response to outbreaks of international importance.

GLOBALIZATION: The integration of national and local systems into a global economy through increased trade, manufacturing, communications, and migration.

GLOMERULONEPHRITIS: Inflammation of the kidneys. Mostly it affects the glomeruli, the small capsules in the kidney where blood flowing through capillaries transfers body wastes to urine.

GLYCOPROTEIN: A protein that contains a short chain of sugar as part of its structure.

GRAM-NEGATIVE BACTERIA: Bacteria whose cell walls are composed of an inner and outer membrane that are separated from one another by a region called the periplasm. The periplasm also contains a thin but rigid layer called the peptidoglycan.

GRANULOCYTE: Any cell containing granules (small, grain-like objects). The term is often used to refer to a type of white blood cell (leukocyte).

GROUP A STREPTOCOCCUS (GAS): A type (specifically a serotype) of the Streptococcus bacteria, based on the antigen contained in the cell wall.

GUILLAIN-BARRÉ SYNDROME: A rare condition in which the body's immune system attacks the nerves. It can cause muscle weakness, nerve tingling, and paralysis and may be triggered by an infection.

H

HARM-REDUCTION STRATEGY: In public health, a public policy scheme for reducing the amount of harm caused by a substance such as alcohol or tobacco. The phrase may refer to any medical strategy directed at reducing the harm caused by a disease, substance, or toxic medication.

HELMINTH: A representative of various phyla of wormlike animals.

HELMINTHIC DISEASE: An infection by parasitic worms such as hookworms or flatworms, known as helminths. A synonym for helminthic is verminous.

HELSINKI DECLARATION: A set of ethical principles governing medical and scientific experimentation on human subjects. It was drafted by the World Medical Association and was originally adopted in 1964.

HEMAGGLUTININ: Often abbreviated as HA, hemagglutinin is a glycoprotein, a protein that contains a short chain of sugar as part of its structure.

HEMOLYSIS: The destruction of blood cells, an abnormal rate of which may lead to lowered levels of these cells. For example, hemolytic anemia is caused by destruction of red blood cells at a rate faster than they can be produced.

HEMORRHAGE: Very severe, massive bleeding that is difficult to control.

HEMORRHAGIC FEVER: A high fever caused by viral infection that features a high volume of bleeding. The bleeding is caused by the formation of tiny blood clots throughout the bloodstream. These blood clots, also called microthrombi, deplete platelets and fibrinogen in the bloodstream. When bleeding begins, the factors needed for the clotting of the blood are scarce. Thus, uncontrolled bleeding (hemorrhage) ensues.

HEPA (HIGH-EFFICIENCY PARTICULATE AIR) FILTER: A filter that is designed to nearly totally remove airborne particles that are 0.3 microns (millionth of a meter) in diameter or larger. Such small particles can penetrate deeply into the lungs if inhaled.

HEPADNAVIRIDAE: A family of hepadnaviruses composed of two genera, Avihepadnavirus and Orthohepadnavirus. Hepadnaviruses have partially double-stranded DNA, and they replicate their genome in the host cells using an enzyme called reverse transcriptase. Because of this, they are also termed retroviruses. The viruses invade liver cells (hepatocytes) of vertebrates. When hepadna retroviruses invade a cell, a complete viral double-stranded (ds) DNA is made before it randomly inserts in one of the host's chromosomes. Once part of the chromosomal DNA, the viral DNA is then transcribed into an intermediate messenger RNA (mRNA) in the hosts' nucleus. The viral mRNA then leaves the nucleus and undergoes reverse transcription, which is mediated by the viral reverse transcriptase.

HEPATITIS AND HEPATITIS VIRUSES: Hepatitis is an inflammation of the liver, a potentially life-threatening disease most frequently caused by viral infections but that may also result from liver damage caused by toxic substances such as alcohol and certain drugs. There are five major types of hepatitis viruses: hepatitis A (HAV), hepatitis B (HBV), hepatitis C (HCV), hepatitis D (HDV), and hepatitis E (HEV).

HERD IMMUNITY: A resistance to disease that occurs in a population when a proportion of them have been immunized against it. The theory is that it is less likely that an infectious disease will spread in a group where some individuals are unlikely to contract it.

HERPESVIRUS: A family of viruses, many of which cause disease in humans. The herpes simplex 1 and herpes simplex 2 viruses cause infection in the mouth or on the genitals. Other common types of herpesvirus include chickenpox, Epstein-Barr virus, and cytomegalovirus. Herpesvirus is notable for its ability to remain latent, or inactive, in nerve cells near the area of infection, and to reactivate long after the initial infection. Herpes simplex 1 and 2, along with chicken pox, cause familiar skin sores. Epstein-Barr virus causes mononucleosis. Cytomegalovirus also causes a flu-like infection but can be dangerous to the elderly, infants, and those with weakened immune systems.

HETEROPHILE ANTIBODY: An antibody found in the blood of someone with infectious mononucleosis, also known as glandular fever.

HIGH-LEVEL DISINFECTION: A process that uses a chemical solution to kill all bacteria, viruses, and other disease-causing agents except for bacterial endospores and prions. High-level disinfection should be distinguished from sterilization, which removes endospores (a bacterial structure that is resistant to radiation, drying, lack of food, and other conditions potentially lethal to the bacteria) and prions (misshapen proteins that can cause disease) as well.

HIGHLY ACTIVE ANTIRETROVIRAL THERAPY (HAART): The name given to the combination of drugs given to people with human immunodeficiency virus (HIV) infection to slow or stop the progression of their condition to AIDS (acquired immunodeficiency syndrome). HIV is a retrovirus, and the various components of HAART block its replication by different mechanisms.

HISTAMINE: A hormone that is chemically similar to the hormones serotonin, epinephrine, and norepinephrine. A hormone is generally defined as a chemical produced by a certain cell or tissue that causes a specific biological change or activity to occur in another cell or tissue located elsewhere in the body. Specifically, histamine plays a role in localized immune responses and in allergic reactions.

HISTOCOMPATIBILITY: The histocompatibility molecules (proteins) on the cell surfaces of one individual of a species are unique. Thus, if the cell is transplanted into another person, the cell will be recognized by the immune system as being foreign. The histocompatibility molecules act as antigens in the recipient and so can also be called histocompatibility antigens or transplantation antigens. This is the basis of the rejection of transplanted material.

HISTOPATHOLOGY: The study of diseased tissues. A synonym for histopathology is pathologic histology.

HIV (HUMAN IMMUNODEFICIENCY VIRUS): The virus that causes acquired immunodeficiency syndrome (AIDS).

HOMOZYGOUS: A condition in which two alleles for a given gene are the same.

HORIZONTAL GENE TRANSFER: A major mechanism by which antibiotic resistance genes get passed between bacteria. It accounts for many hospital-acquired infections.

HORIZONTAL TRANSMISSION: The transmission of a disease-causing microorganism from one person to another, unrelated person by direct or indirect contact.

HOST: An organism that serves as the habitat for a parasite or possibly for a symbiont. A host may provide nutrition to the parasite or symbiont, or it may simply provide a place in which to live.

HOST FOCALITY: The tendency of some animal hosts, such as rodents carrying hantavirus and other viruses, to exist in groups in specific geographical locations and act as a local reservoir of infection.

HUMAN GROWTH HORMONE: A protein that is made and released from the pituitary gland, which increases growth and manufacture of new cells.

HUMAN IMMUNODEFICIENCY VIRUS (HIV): A class of viruses known as the retroviruses. These viruses are known as RNA viruses because they have RNA (ribonucleic acid) as their basic genetic material instead of DNA (deoxyribonucleic acid).

HUMAN T-CELL LEUKEMIA VIRUS (HTLV): Also known as human T-cell lymphotropic viruses, human T-cell leukemia viruses are divided into two known types: HTLV-1 and HTLV-2. HTLV-1 is often carried by people with no obvious symptoms, though it can cause a number of maladies, such as abnormalities of the T cells and B cells, a chronic infection of the myelin covering of nerves that causes degeneration of the nervous system, sores on the skin, and inflammation of the inside of the eye. HTLV-2 infection usually does not produce any symptoms. However, in some people a cancer of the blood known as hairy cell leukemia can develop.

HYBRIDIZATION: The process of combining two or more different molecules or organisms to create a new molecule or organism. Often called a hybrid organism.

HYGIENE: Health practices that minimize the spread of infectious microorganisms between people or between other living things and people. Inanimate objects and surfaces such as contaminated cutlery or a cutting board may be a secondary part of this process.

HYPERENDEMIC: Endemic (commonly present) in all age groups of a population. A related term is holoendemic, meaning a disease that is present more in children than in adults.

HYPERINFECTION: An infection that is caused by a very high number of disease-causing microorganisms. The infection results from an abnormality in the immune system that allows the infecting cells to grow and divide more easily than would normally be the case.

I

IATROGENIC: Any infection, injury, or other disease condition caused by medical treatment.

IMMUNITY HUMORAL REGULATION: One way in which the immune system responds to pathogens is by producing soluble proteins called antibodies. This is known as the humoral response and involves the activation of a special set of cells known as the B lymphocytes, because they originate in the bone marrow. The humoral immune response helps in the control and removal of pathogens such as bacteria, viruses, fungi, and parasites before they enter host cells. The antibodies produced by the B cells are the mediators of this response.

IMMIGRATION: The relocation of people to a different region or country from their native lands. Also, the movement of organisms into an area where they were previously absent.

IMMUNE GLOBULIN: A type of protein found in blood. The immune globulins (also called immunoglobulins) are Y-shaped globulins that act as antibodies, attaching themselves to invasive cells or materials in the body so that they can be identified and attacked by the immune system. There are five immune globulins, designated IgM, IgG, IgA, IgD, and IgE.

IMMUNE RESPONSE: The body's production of antibodies or some types of white blood cells in response to foreign substances.

IMMUNE SYNAPSE: Before they can help other immune cells respond to a foreign protein or pathogenic organism, helper T cells must first become activated. This process occurs when an antigen-presenting cell submits a fragment of a foreign protein, bound to a Class II MHC molecule (virus-derived fragments are bound to Class I MHC molecules), to the helper T cell. Antigen-presenting cells are derived from bone marrow and include both dendritic cells and Langerhans cells, as well as other specialized cells. Because T cell responses depend on direct contact with their target cells, their antigen receptors, unlike antibodies made by B cells, exist bound to the membrane only. In the intercellular gap between the T cell and the antigen-presenting cell, a special pattern of various receptors and complementary ligands forms that is several microns in size.

IMMUNE SYSTEM: The body's natural defense system that guards against foreign invaders and that includes lymphocytes and antibodies.

IMMUNO-BASED TEST: A medical technology that tests for the presence of a disease by looking for a reaction between disease organisms that may be present in a tissue or fluid sample and antibodies contained in the test kit.

IMMUNOCOMPROMISED: Having an immune system with reduced ability to recognize and respond to the presence of foreign material.

IMMUNODEFICIENCY: When part of the body's immune system is missing or defective, thus impairing the body's ability to fight infections. As a result, the person with an immunodeficiency disorder will have frequent infections that are generally more severe and last longer than usual.

IMMUNOGENICITY: The capacity of a host to produce an immune response to protect itself against infectious disease.

IMMUNOLOGY: The study of how the body responds to foreign substances and fights off infection and other disease. Immunologists study the molecules, cells, and organs of the human body that participate in this response.

IMMUNOSUPPRESSION: A reduction of the ability of the immune system to recognize and respond to the presence of foreign material.

IMPETIGO: A very localized bacterial infection of the skin. It tends to afflict primarily children but can occur in people of any age. Impetigo caused by the bacteria Staphylococcus aureus (or staph) affects children of all ages, while impetigo caused by the bacteria called group A streptococci (Streptococcus pyogenes or strep) is most common in children ages two to five years.

IMPORTED CASE OF DISEASE: An instance of disease in which an infected person who is not yet showing symptoms travels from his or her home country to another country and develops symptoms of the disease there.

IN SITU: A Latin term meaning "in place" or in the body or natural system.

INACTIVATED VACCINE: A vaccine that is made from disease-causing microorganisms that have been killed or made incapable of causing the infection. The immune system can still respond to the presence of the microorganisms.

INACTIVATED VIRUS: A virus that is incapable of causing disease but still stimulates the immune system to respond by forming antibodies.

INCIDENCE: The number of new cases of a disease or an injury that occur in a population during a specified period of time.

INCUBATION PERIOD: The time between exposure to a disease-causing virus or bacterium and the appearance of symptoms of the infection. Depending on the microorganism, the incubation time can range from a few hours, such as with food poisoning due to Salmonella, to a decade or more, such as with acquired immunodeficiency syndrome (AIDS).

INFECTION CONTROL: Policies and procedures used to minimize the risk of spreading infections, especially in hospitals and health care facilities.

INFECTION CONTROL PROFESSIONAL (ICP): A nurse, doctor, laboratory worker, microbiologist, public health official, or other specialist in the prevention and control of infectious disease. ICPs develop methods to control infection and instruct others in their use. These methods include proper handwashing; correct wearing of protective masks, eye guards, gloves, and other specialized clothing; vaccination; monitoring for infection; and investigating ways to treat and prevent infection. Courses and certifications are available for those wishing to become ICPs.

INFORMED CONSENT: An ethical and informational process in which a person learns about a procedure or clinical trial, including potential risks or benefits, before deciding to voluntarily participate in a study or undergo a particular procedure.

INNATE IMMUNITY: Resistance against disease that an individual is born with, as distinct from acquired immunity, which develops with exposure to infectious agents.

INOCULUM: A substance such as a virus, bacterial toxin, or viral or bacterial component that is added to the body to stimulate the immune system, which then provides protection from an infection by the particular microorganism.

INPATIENT: A patient who is admitted to a hospital or clinic for treatment, typically requiring the patient to stay overnight.

INSECTICIDE: A chemical substance used to kill insects.

INTERMEDIATE HOST: An organism infected by a parasite while the parasite is in a developmental, not sexually mature form.

INTERMEDIATE-LEVEL DISINFECTION: A form of disinfection that kills bacteria, most viruses, and mycobacteria.

INTERNATIONAL HEALTH REGULATIONS: Regulations introduced by the World Health Organization (WHO) that aim to control, monitor, prevent, protect against, and respond to the spread of disease across national borders while avoiding unnecessary interference with international movement and trade.

INTERTRIGO: A skin rash, often occurring in obese people on parts of the body symmetrically opposite each other. Sometimes called eczema intertrigo, it is caused by irritation of skin trapped under hanging folds of flesh such as pendulous breasts.

INTRAVENOUS: In the vein. For example, the insertion of a hypodermic needle into a vein to instill a fluid, withdraw or transfuse blood, or start an intravenous feeding.

IONIZING RADIATION: Any electromagnetic or particulate radiation capable of direct or indirect ion production in its passage through matter. In general use: Radiation that can cause tissue damage or death.

IRRADIATION: A method of preservation that treats food with low doses of radiation to deactivate enzymes and to kill microorganisms and insects.

ISOLATION: Within the health community, precautions taken in the hospital to prevent the spread of an infectious agent from an infected or colonized patient to susceptible people. Isolation practices are designed to minimize the transmission of infection.

ISOLATION AND QUARANTINE: Public health authorities rely on isolation and quarantine as two important tools among the many they use to fight disease outbreaks. Isolation is the practice of keeping a disease victim away from other people, sometimes by treating them in their homes or by the use of elaborate isolation systems in hospitals. Quarantine separates people who have been exposed to a disease but have not yet developed symptoms from the general population. Both isolation and quarantine can be entered voluntarily by patients when public health authorities request it, or it can be compelled by state governments or by the federal Centers for Disease Control and Prevention.

J

JAUNDICE: A condition in which a person's skin and the whites of the eyes are discolored a shade of yellow due to an increased level of bile pigments in the blood as a result of liver disease. Jaundice is sometimes called icterus, from a Greek word for the condition.

K

KERITITIS: Sometimes called corneal ulcers, an inflammation of the cornea, the transparent membrane that covers the colored part of the eye (iris) and pupil of the eye.

KOCH'S POSTULATES: A series of conditions that must be met for a microorganism to be considered the cause of a disease. German microbiologist Robert Koch (1843–1910) proposed the postulates in 1890.

KOPLIK SPOTS: Red spots with a small blue-white speck in the center found on the tongue and the insides of the cheeks during the early stages of measles. Also called Koplik's sign, they are named after American pediatrician Henry Koplik (1858–1927).

L

LARVAE: Immature forms (wormlike in insects; fishlike in amphibians) of an organism capable of surviving on its own. Larvae do not resemble the parent and must go through metamorphosis, or change, to reach the adult stage.

LATENT: Potential or dormant, as in a condition that is not yet manifest or active.

LATENT INFECTION: An infection already established in the body but not yet causing symptoms or having ceased to cause symptoms after an active period.

LATENT VIRUS: Viruses that can incorporate their genetic material into the genetic material of the infected host cell. Because the viral genetic material can then be replicated along with the host material, the virus becomes effectively "silent" with respect to detection by the host. Latent viruses usually contain the information necessary to reverse the latent state. The viral genetic material can leave the host genome to begin the manufacture of new virus particles.

LEGIONNAIRES' DISEASE: A type of pneumonia caused by Legionella bacteria. The bacterial species responsible for Legionnaires' disease is L. pneumophila. Major symptoms include fever, chills, muscle aches, and a cough that is initially nonproductive. Definitive diagnosis relies on specific laboratory tests for the bacteria, bacterial antigens, or antibodies produced by the body's immune system. As with other types of pneumonia, Legionnaires' disease poses the greatest threat to people who are elderly, ill, or immunocompromised.

LENS: An almost clear, biconvex structure in the eye that, along with the cornea, helps to focus light onto the retina. It can become infected, causing inflammation, for example, when contact lenses are improperly used.

LEPTOSPIRE: Also called a leptospira, any bacterial species of the genus Leptospira. Infection with leptospires causes leptospirosis.

LESION: The tissue disruption or the loss of function caused by a particular disease process.

LIPOPOLYSACCHARIDE (LPS): A molecule that is a constituent of the outer membrane of gram-negative bacteria. LPS is also be referred to as endotoxin. It helps protect the bacterium from host defenses and can contribute to illness in the host.

LIVE VACCINE: A virus or bacteria that has been weakened (attenuated) to cause an immune response in the body without causing disease. Live vaccines are preferred to killed vaccines, which use a dead virus or bacteria, because they cause a stronger and longer-lasting immune response.

LOW-LEVEL DISINFECTION: A form of disinfection that is capable of killing some viruses and some bacteria.

LYMPHADENOPATHY: Any disease of the lymph nodes, or the glandlike bodies that filter the clear intercellular fluid called lymph to remove impurities..

LYMPHATIC SYSTEM: The body's network of organs, ducts, and tissues that filters harmful substances out of the fluid that surrounds body tissues. Lymphatic organs include the bone marrow, thymus, spleen, appendix, tonsils, adenoids, lymph nodes, and Peyer's patches (in the small intestine). The thymus and bone marrow are called primary lymphatic organs, because lymphocytes are produced in them. The other lymphatic organs are called secondary lymphatic organs. The lymphatic system is a complex network of thin vessels, capillaries, valves, ducts, nodes, and organs that runs throughout the body, helping protect and maintain the internal fluids system of the entire body by both producing and filtering lymph and by producing various blood cells. The three main purposes of the lymphatic system are to drain fluid back into the bloodstream from the tissues, to filter lymph, and to fight infections.

LYMPHOCYTE: A type of white blood cell, such as a B or T lymphocyte, that functions as part of the lymphatic and immune systems by stimulating antibody formation to attack specific invading substances.

M

M PROTEIN: An antibody found in unusually large amounts in the blood or urine of patients with multiple myeloma, a form of cancer that arises in the white blood cells that produce antibodies.

MACAQUE: Any short-tailed monkey of the genus Macaca. Macaques, including rhesus monkeys, are often used as subjects in medical research because they are relatively affordable and resemble humans in many ways.

MACULOPAPULAR: A macule is any discolored skin spot that is flush or level with the surrounding skin surface; a papule is a small, solid bump on the skin. A maculopapular skin disturbance is one that combines macules and papules.

MAJOR HISTOCOMPATIBILITY COMPLEX (MHC): The proteins that protrude from the surface of a cell that identify the cell as "self." In humans, the proteins coded by the genes of the major histocompatibility complex (MHC) include human leukocyte antigens (HLA), as well as other proteins. HLA proteins are present on the surface of most of the body's cells and are important in helping the immune system distinguish "self" from "non-self" molecules, cells, and other objects.

MALAISE: A general or nonspecific feeling of unease or discomfort, often the first sign of disease infection.

MALIGNANT: A general term for cells that can dislodge from the original tumor and invade and destroy other tissues and organs.

MATERIEL: A French-derived word for equipment, supplies, or hardware.

MEASLES: An infectious disease caused by a virus of the paramyxovirus group. It infects only humans, and the infection results in life-long immunity to the disease. It is one of several exanthematous (rash-producing) diseases of childhood, the others being rubella (German measles), chickenpox, and scarlet fever. The disease is particularly common in both preschool and young school children.

MENINGITIS: An inflammation of the meninges, the three layers of protective membranes that line the spinal cord and the brain. Meningitis can occur when there is an infection near the brain or spinal cord, such as a respiratory infection in the sinuses, the mastoids, or the cavities around the ear. Disease organisms can also travel to the meninges through the bloodstream. The first signs may be a severe headache and neck stiffness followed by fever, vomiting, a rash, and, then, convulsions leading to loss of consciousness. Meningitis generally involves two types: nonbacterial meningitis, or aseptic meningitis, and bacterial meningitis, or purulent meningitis.

MENINGITIS BELT: The Meningitis Belt is an area of Africa south of the Sahara Desert, stretching from the Atlantic to the Pacific coast, where meningococcal meningitis is common.

MEROZOITE: The motile, infective stage of malaria responsible for disease symptoms.

MESSENGER RIBONUCLEIC ACID (MRNA): A molecule of RNA that carries the genetic information for producing one or more proteins; mRNA is produced by copying one strand of DNA, but in eukaryotes it is able to move from the nucleus to the cytoplasm (where protein synthesis takes place).

MICROBICIDE: A compound that kills microorganisms such as bacteria, fungi, and protozoa.

MICROCEPHALY: A rare neurological condition in which the head of a baby is significantly smaller than that of other children of the same age and sex. This can cause developmental delays, intellectual disability, and movement and coordination difficulties. When detected at birth, it results from abnormal growth in the womb.

MICROFILIAE: Live offspring produced by adult nematodes within the host's body.

MICROORGANISM: With only a single currently known exception (i.e., Epulopiscium fishelsonia, a bacterium that is billions of times larger than the bacteria in the human intestine and is large enough to view without a microscope), microorganisms are minute organisms that require microscopic magnification to view. To be seen, they must be magnified by an optical or electron microscope. The most common types of microorganisms are viruses, bacteria, blue-green bacteria, some algae, some fungi, yeasts, and protozoans.

MIGRATION: In medicine, the movement of a disease symptom from one part of the body to another, apparently without cause.

MIMICKED: In biology, mimicry is the imitation of another organism, often for evolutionary advantage. A disease that resembles another (for whatever reason) is sometimes said to have mimicked the other. Pathomimicry is the faking of symptoms by a patient, also called malingering.

MINIMAL INHIBITORY CONCENTRATION (MIC): The lowest level of an antibiotic that prevents growth of the particular type of bacteria in a liquid food source after a certain amount of time. Growth is detected by clouding of the food source. The MIC is the lowest concentration of the antibiotic at which the no cloudiness occurs.

MITE: A tiny arthropod (insect-like creature) of the order Acarina. Mites may inhabit the surface of the body without causing harm or may cause various skin ailments by burrowing under the skin. The droppings of mites living in house dust are a common source of allergic reactions.

MMR (MEASLES, MUMPS, RUBELLA) VACCINE: A vaccine given to protect someone from measles, mumps, and rubella. The vaccine is made up of viruses that cause the three diseases. The viruses are incapable of causing the diseases but can still stimulate the immune system.

MONO SPOT TEST: A blood test used to check for infection with the Epstein-Barr virus, which causes mononucleosis.

MONOCLONAL ANTIBODIES: Antibodies produced from a single cell line that are used in medical testing and, increasingly, in the treatment of some cancers.

MONONUCLEAR LEUKOCYTE: A type of white blood cell active in the immune system.

MONOVALENT VACCINE: A vaccine that is active against just one strain of a virus, such as the one that is in common use against the poliovirus.

MORBIDITY: From the Latin morbus, "sick," it refers to both the state of being ill and the severity of the illness. A serious disease is said to have high morbidity.

MORPHOLOGY: The study of form and structure of animals and plants. Also, the outward physical form possessed by an organism.

MORTALITY: The condition of being susceptible to death. The term mortality comes from the Latin word mors, which means death. Mortality can also refer to the rate of deaths caused by an illness or injury (e.g., "Rabies has a high mortality rate").

MOSQUITO COILS: Spirals of inflammable paste that, when burned, steadily release insect repellent into the air. They are often used in Asia, where many coils release octachlorodipropyl ether, which can cause lung cancer.

MOSQUITO NETTING: Fine meshes or nets hung around occupied spaces, especially beds, to keep out disease-carrying mosquitoes. Mosquito netting is a cost-effective way of preventing malaria.

MRSA (METHICILLIN-RESISTANT STAPHYLOCOCCUS AUREUS): Bacteria resistant to most penicillin-type antibiotics, including methicillin.

MUCOCUTANEOUS: A region of the body in which mucosa (mucous membrane) transitions to skin. Mucocutaneous zones occur in animals, at the body orifices. In humans mucocutaneous zones are found at the lips, nostrils, conjunctivae, urethra, vagina (in females), foreskin (in males), and anus.

MULTIBACILLARY: The more severe form of leprosy (Hansen's disease). It is defined as the presence of more than five skin lesions on the patient with a positive skin-smear test. The less severe form of leprosy is called paucibacillary leprosy.

MULTIDRUG RESISTANCE: A phenomenon that occurs when an infective agent loses its sensitivity against two or more of the drugs that are used against it.

MULTIDRUG THERAPY: The use of a combination of drugs against infection, each of which attacks the infective agent in a different way. This strategy can help overcome resistance to anti-infective drugs.

MUTABLE VIRUS: A virus whose DNA changes rapidly so that drugs and vaccines against it may not be effective.

MUTATION: A change in an organism's deoxyribonucleic acid (DNA) that occurs over time and may render it less sensitive to the drugs that are used against it.

MYALGIA: Muscular aches and pain.

MYCOBACTERIA: A genus of bacteria that contains the bacteria causing leprosy and tuberculosis. The bacteria have unusual cell walls that are harder to dissolve than the cell walls of other bacteria.

MYCOTIC: Having to do with or caused by a fungus. Any medical condition caused by a fungus is a mycotic condition, also called a mycosis.

MYCOTIC DISEASE: A disease caused by fungal infection.

N

NATIONAL ELECTRONIC TELECOMMUNICATIONS SYSTEM FOR SURVEILLANCE (NETSS): A computerized public health surveillance information system that provides the US Centers for Disease Control and Prevention (CDC) with weekly data regarding cases of nationally notifiable diseases.

NECROPSY: A medical examination of a dead body; also called an autopsy.

NECROTIC TISSUE: Dead tissue in an otherwise living body. Tissue death is called necrosis.

NEEDLESTICK INJURY (NSI): Any accidental breakage or puncture of the skin by an unsterilized medical needle (syringe) is a needlestick injury. Health care providers are at particular risk for needlestick injuries, which may transmit disease, because of the large number of needles they handle.

NEGLECTED TROPICAL DISEASE: Many tropical diseases are considered to be neglected because, despite their prevalence in less-developed areas, new vaccines and treatments are not being developed for them. Malaria was once considered to be a neglected tropical disease, but recently a great deal of research and money have been devoted to its treatment and cure.

NEMATODE: Also known as a roundworm; a type of helminth characterized by a long, cylindrical body.

NEURAMINIDASE (NA): A glycoprotein, which is a protein that contains a short chain of sugar as part of its structure.

NEUROTOXIN: A poison that interferes with nerve function, usually by affecting the flow of ions through the cell membrane.

NEUTROPHIL: A type of white blood cell that phagocytizes foreign microorganisms, releasing a bacteria-killing chemical known as lysozyme. Neutrophils are prominent in the inflammatory response.

NOBEL PEACE PRIZE: An annual prize bequeathed by Swedish inventor Alfred Nobel (1833–1896) and awarded by the Norwegian Nobel Committee to an individual or organization that has "done the most or the best work for fraternity between the nations, for the abolition or reduction of standing armies and for the holding and promotion of peace congresses."

NODULE: A small, roundish lump on the surface of the skin or of an internal organ.

NONGOVERNMENTAL ORGANIZATION (NGO): A voluntary organization that is not part of any government; often organized to address a specific issue or perform a humanitarian function.

NORMAL FLORA: The bacteria that normally inhabit some part of the body, such as the mouth or intestines. Normal flora are essential to health.

NOROVIRUS: A type of virus that contains ribonucleic acid as the genetic material and causes an intestinal infection known as gastroenteritis. A well-known example is Norwalk-like virus.

NOSOCOMIAL INFECTION: An infection that is acquired in a hospital. More precisely, the US Centers for Disease Control and Prevention (CDC) in Atlanta, Georgia, defines a nosocomial infection as a localized infection or an infection that is widely spread throughout the body that results from an adverse reaction to an infectious microorganism or toxin that was not present at the time of admission to the hospital.

NOTIFIABLE DISEASE: A disease that the law requires be reported to health officials when diagnosed. Also called a reportable disease.

NUCLEOTIDE: The basic unit of a nucleic acid. It consists of a simple sugar, a phosphate group, and a nitrogen-containing base.

NUCLEOTIDE SEQUENCE: A particular ordering of the chain structure of nucleic acid that provides the necessary information for a specific amino acid.

NUCLEUS, CELL: Membrane-enclosed structure within a cell that contains the cell's genetic material and controls its growth and reproduction. (Plural: nuclei.)

NUTRITIONAL SUPPLEMENTS: Substances necessary to health, such as calcium or protein, that are taken in concentrated form to compensate for dietary insufficiency, poor absorption, unusually high demand for that nutrient, or other reasons.

NYMPH: In aquatic insects, the larval stage.

O

ONCOGENIC VIRUS: A virus capable of changing the cells it infects so that the cells begin to grow and divide uncontrollably.

OOCYST: A spore phase of certain infectious organisms that can survive for a long time outside the organism and therefore continue to cause infection and resist treatment.

OOPHORITIS: An inflammation of the ovary, which happens in certain sexually transmitted diseases.

OPPORTUNISTIC INFECTION: An infection that occurs in people whose immune systems are diminished or are not functioning normally. Such infections are opportunistic insofar as the infectious agents take advantage of their hosts' compromised immune systems and invade to cause disease.

OPTIC SOLUTION: Any liquid solution of a medication that can be applied directly to the eye.

ORAL REHYDRATION THERAPY: Restoring body water levels by giving the patient fluids through the mouth (orally). Often, a special mixture of water, glucose, and electrolytes called oral rehydration solution is given.

ORCHITIS: Inflammation of one or both testicles. Swelling and pain are typical symptoms. Orchitis may be caused by various sexually transmitted diseases or escape of sperm cells into the tissues of the testicle.

OUTBREAK: The appearance of new cases of a disease in numbers greater than the established incidence rate or the appearance of even one case of an emergent or rare disease in an area.

OUTPATIENT: A person who receives health care services without being admitted to a hospital or clinic for an overnight stay.

OVA: Mature female sex cells produced in the ovaries. (Singular: ovum.)

OVIPOSITION: Ovum is Latin for "egg." To oviposition is to position or lay eggs, especially when done by an insect.

P

PANCREATITIS: An inflammation of the pancreas, an organ that is important in digestion. Pancreatitis can be acute (beginning suddenly, usually with the patient recovering fully) or chronic (progressing slowly with continued, permanent injury to the pancreas).

PANDEMIC: An epidemic that occurs in more than one country or population simultaneously. Pandemic means "all the people."

PAPULAR: A small, solid bump on the skin; papular means pertaining to or resembling a papule.

PAPULE: A small, solid bump on the skin.

PARAMYXOVIRUS: A type of virus that contains ribonucleic acid as the genetic material and has proteins on its surface that clump red blood cells and assist in the release of newly made viruses from the infected cells. Measles virus and mumps virus are two types of paramyxoviruses.

PARASITE: An organism that lives in or on a host organism and that gets its nourishment from that host. The parasite usually gains all the benefits of this relationship, while the host may suffer from various diseases and discomforts or show no signs of the infection. The life cycle of a typical parasite usually includes several developmental stages and morphological changes as the parasite lives and moves through the environment and one or more hosts. Parasites that remain on a host's body surface to feed are called ectoparasites, while those that live inside a host's body are called endoparasites. Parasitism is a highly successful biological adaptation. There are more known parasitic species than nonparasitic ones, and parasites affect just about every form of life, including most all animals, plants, and even bacteria.

PAROTITIS: Inflammation of the parotid gland. There are two parotid glands, one on each side of the jaw, at the back. Their function is to secret saliva into the mouth.

PAROXYSM: In medicine, a fit, convulsion, or seizure. Paroxysm may also be a sudden worsening or recurrence of disease symptoms.

PASTEURIZATION: Pasteurization is a process in which fluids such as wine and milk are heated for a predetermined time at a temperature that is below the boiling point of the liquid. The treatment kills any microorganisms that are in the fluid but does not alter the taste, appearance, or nutritive value of the fluid.

PATHOGEN: A disease-causing agent, such as a bacterium, a virus, a fungus, or another microorganism.

PATHOGENIC: Causing or capable of causing disease.

PAUCIBACILLARY: An infectious condition, such as a certain form of leprosy, characterized by few, rather than many, bacilli, which are a rod-shaped type of bacterium.

PCR (POLYMERASE CHAIN REACTION): A widely used technique in molecular biology involving the amplification of specific sequences of genomic DNA.

PERMETHRIN: A synthetic chemical used as insecticide. It is commonly used for insect control and can be found on food, crops, livestock, pets, and clothing. It affects the nervous system of the insects, resulting in death if consumed or touched by them. Humans and pets are more resistant to the effects but should still avoid consuming food covered with it, touching it, or breathing it.

PERSISTENCE: The length of time a disease remains in a patient. Disease persistence can vary from a few days to life-long.

PESTICIDE: A substance used to reduce the abundance of pests or any living thing that causes injury or disease to crops.

PHAGOCYTOSIS: The process by which certain cells engulf and digest microorganisms and consume debris and foreign bodies in the blood.

PHENOTYPE: The visible characteristics or physical shape produced by a living thing's genotype.

PLAGUE: A contagious disease that spreads rapidly through a population and results in a high rate of death.

PLASMID: A circular piece of DNA that exists outside of the bacterial chromosome and copies itself independently. Scientists often use bacterial plasmids in genetic engineering to carry genes into other organisms.

PLEURAL CAVITY: The lungs are surrounded by two membranous coverings, the pleura. One of the pleura is attached to the lung, the other to the ribcage. The space between the two pleura, the pleural cavity, is normally filled with a clear lubricating fluid called pleural fluid.

PNEUMONIA: Inflammation of the lung accompanied by filling of some air sacs with fluid (consolidation). Pneumonia can be caused by a number of infectious agents, including bacteria, viruses, and fungi.

POSTEXPOSURE PROPHYLAXIS: Treatment with drugs immediately after exposure to an infectious microorganism. The aim of this approach is to prevent an infection from becoming established.

POSTHERPETIC NEURALGIA: Neuralgia is pain arising in a nerve that is not the result of any injury. Postherpetic neuralgia is neuralgia experienced after infection with a herpesvirus, namely Herpes simplex or Herpes zoster.

POTABLE: Water that is clean enough to drink safely.

PREVALENCE: The actual number of cases of disease or injury that exists in a population.

PRIMARY HOST: An organism that provides food and shelter for a parasite while allowing it to become sexually mature. A secondary host is one occupied by a parasite during the larval or asexual stages of its life cycle.

PRIONS: Proteins that are infectious. Indeed, the name prion is derived from "proteinaceous infectious particles." The discovery of prions and confirmation of their infectious nature overturned a central dogma that infections were caused only by intact organisms, particularly microorganisms such as bacteria, fungi, parasites, or viruses. Because prions lack genetic material, the prevailing attitude was that a protein could not cause disease.

PRODROMAL SYMPTOMS: The earliest symptoms of a disease.

PRODROME: A symptom indicating the disease's onset; it may also be called a prodroma. For example, painful swallowing is often a prodrome of infection with a cold virus.

PROPHYLAXIS: Pre-exposure treatment (e.g., immunizations) to prevent the onset or recurrence of a disease.

PROSTRATION: A condition marked by nausea, disorientation, dizziness, and weakness caused by dehydration and prolonged exposure to high temperatures; also called heat exhaustion or hyperthermia.

PROTOZOA: Single-celled, animal-like microscopic organisms that live by taking in food rather than making it by photosynthesis and must live in the presence of water. (Singular: protozoan.) Protozoa are a diverse group of single-celled organisms, with more than 50,000 different types represented. The vast majority are microscopic, many measuring less than 5 one-thousandth of an inch (0.005 millimeters), but some, such as the freshwater Spirostomun, may reach 0.17 inches (3 millimeters) in length, large enough to enable it to be seen with the naked eye.

PRURITIS: The medical term for itchiness.

PRURULENT: Containing, discharging, or producing pus.

PUERPERAL: An interval of time around childbirth, from the onset of labor through the immediate recovery period after delivery.

PUERPERAL FEVER: A bacterial infection present in the blood (septicemia) that follows childbirth. The Latin word puer, meaning "boy" or "child," is the root of this term. Puerperal fever was much more common before the advent of modern aseptic practices, but infections still occur. Louis Pasteur showed that puerperal fever is most often caused by Streptococcus bacteria, which is now treated with antibiotics.

PULMONARY: Having to do with the lungs or respiratory system. The pulmonary circulatory system delivers deoxygenated blood from the right ventricle of the heart to the lungs and returns oxygenated blood from the lungs to the left atrium of the heart. At its most minute level, the alveolar capillary bed, the pulmonary circulatory system is the principle point of gas exchange between blood and air that moves in and out of the lungs during respiration.

PURULENT: Any part of the body that contains or releases pus. Pus is a fluid produced by inflamed, infected tissues and is made up of white blood cells, fragments of dead cells, and a liquid containing various proteins.

PUSTULE: A reservoir of pus visible just beneath the skin. It is usually sore to the touch and surrounded by inflamed tissue.

PYELONEPHRITIS: Inflammation caused by bacterial infection of the kidney and associated blood vessels.

PYROGENIC: A substance that causes fever. The word pyrogenic comes from the Greek word pyr, meaning fire.

Q

QUANTITATED: An act of determining the quantity of something, such as the number or concentration of bacteria in an infectious disease.

QUARANTINE: The practice of separating from the general population people who have been exposed to an infectious agent but have not yet developed symptoms. In the United States, this can be done voluntarily or involuntarily by the authority of states and the federal Centers for Disease Control and Prevention.

R

RALES: French term for a rattling sound in the throat or chest.

RASH: A change in appearance or texture of the skin. A rash is the popular term for a group of spots or red, inflamed skin that is usually a symptom of an underlying condition or disorder. Often temporary, a rash is only rarely a sign of a serious problem.

REASSORTMENT: A condition resulting when two or more different types of viruses exchange genetic material to form a new, genetically different virus.

RECEPTOR: Protein molecules on a cell's surface that act as a "signal receiver" and allow communication between cells.

RECOMBINANT DNA: DNA that is cut using specific enzymes so that a gene or DNA sequence can be inserted.

RECOMBINATION: A process during which genetic material is shuffled during reproduction to form new combinations. This mixing is important from an evolutionary standpoint because it allows the expression of different traits between generations. The process involves a physical exchange of nucleotides between duplicate strands of deoxyribonucleic acid (DNA).

RED TIDE: Red tides are a marine phenomenon in which water is stained a red, brown, or yellowish color because of the temporary abundance of a particular species of pigmented dinoflagellate (these events are known as blooms). Also called phytoplankton, or planktonic algae, these single-celled organisms of the class Dinophyceae move using a taillike structure called a flagellum. They also photosynthesize, and it is their photosynthetic pigments that can tint the water during blooms. Dinoflagellates are common and widespread. Under appropriate environmental conditions, various species can grow very rapidly, causing red tides. Red tides occur in all marine regions with a temperate or warmer climate.

REEMERGING DISEASE: Many diseases once thought to be controlled are reappearing to infect humans again. These are known as reemerging diseases because they have not been common for a long period of time and are starting to appear again among large population groups.

REEMERGING INFECTIOUS DISEASE: Illnesses such as malaria, diphtheria, tuberculosis, and polio that were once nearly absent from the world but are starting to cause greater numbers of infections once again. These illnesses are reappearing for many reasons. Malaria and other mosquito-borne illnesses increase when mosquito-control measures decrease. Other diseases are spreading because people have stopped being vaccinated, as happened with diphtheria after the collapse of the Soviet Union. A few diseases are reemerging because drugs to treat them have become less available or drug-resistant strains have developed.

REHYDRATION: Dehydration is excessive loss of water from the body; rehydration is the restoration of water after dehydration.

REITER'S SYNDROME: Named after German doctor Hans Reiter (1881–1969), a form of arthritis (joint inflammation) that appears in response to bacterial infection in some other part of the body. Also called Reiter syndrome, Reiter disease, or reactive arthritis.

RELAPSE: A return of symptoms after the patient has apparently recovered from a disease.

REPLICATE: To duplicate something or make a copy of it. All reproduction of living things depends on the replication of DNA molecules or, in a few cases, RNA molecules. Replication may be used to refer to the reproduction of entire viruses and other microorganisms.

REPLICATION: A process of reproducing, duplicating, copying, or repeating something, such as the duplication of DNA or the recreation of characteristics of an infectious disease in a laboratory setting.

REPORTABLE DISEASE: By law, occurrences of some diseases must be reported to government authorities when observed by health care professionals. Such diseases are called reportable diseases or notifiable diseases. Cholera and yellow fever are examples of reportable diseases.

RESERVOIR: The animal or organism in which a virus or parasite normally resides.

RESISTANCE: Immunity developed within a species (especially bacteria) via evolution to an antibiotic or other drug. For example, bacteria may acquire of genetic mutations that render them invulnerable to the action of antibiotics.

RESISTANT BACTERIA: Microbes that have lost their sensitivity to one or more antibiotic drugs through mutation.

RESISTANT ORGANISM: An organism that has developed the ability to counter something trying to harm it. Within infectious diseases, the organism, such as a bacterium, has developed a resistance to drugs, such as antibiotics.

RESPIRATOR: Any device that assists a patient in breathing or takes over breathing entirely for them.

RESTRICTION ENZYME: A special type of protein that can recognize certain DNA sequences and cut DNA to isolate specific genes. These DNA fragments may be joined together to create new stretches of DNA.

RETROVIRUS: Viruses in which the genetic material consists of ribonucleic acid (RNA) instead of the usual deoxyribonucleic acid (DNA). Retroviruses produce an enzyme known as reverse transcriptase that can transform RNA into DNA, which can then be permanently integrated into the DNA of the infected host cells.

REVERSE TRANSCRIPTASE: An enzyme that makes it possible for a retrovirus to produce deoxyribonucleic acid (DNA) from ribonucleic acid (RNA).

RHINITIS: An inflammation of the mucous lining of the nose. A nonspecific term that covers infections, allergies, and other disorders whose common feature is the location of their symptoms. These symptoms include infected or irritated mucous membranes, producing a discharge, congestion, and swelling of the tissues of the nasal passages. The most widespread form of infectious rhinitis is the common cold.

RIBONUCLEIC ACID (RNA): Any of a group of nucleic acids that carry out several important tasks in the synthesis of proteins. Unlike DNA (deoxyribonucleic acid), it has only a single strand. Nucleic acids are complex molecules that contain a cell's genetic information and the instructions for carrying out cellular processes. In eukaryotic cells, the two nucleic acids, ribonucleic acid (RNA) and deoxyribonucleic acid (DNA), work together to direct protein synthesis. Although it is DNA that contains the instructions for directing the synthesis of specific structural and enzymatic proteins, several types of RNA actually carry out the processes required to produce these proteins. These include messenger RNA (mRNA), ribosomal RNA (rRNA), and transfer RNA (tRNA). Further processing of the various RNAs is carried out by another type of RNA called small nuclear RNA (snRNA). The structure of RNA is similar to that of DNA, however, instead of the base thymine, RNA contains the base uracil in its place.

RING VACCINATION: The vaccination of all susceptible people in an area surrounding a case of an infectious disease. Because vaccination makes people immune to the disease, the hope is that the disease will not spread from the known case to other people. Ring vaccination was used in eliminating the smallpox virus.

RNA VIRUS: A virus whose genetic material consists of either single- or double-stranded ribonucleic acid (RNA) rather than deoxyribonucleic acid (DNA).

ROUNDWORM: Also known as nematodes, a type of helminth characterized by long, cylindrical bodies. Roundworm infections are diseases of the digestive tract and other organ systems that are caused by roundworms. Roundworm infections are widespread throughout the world, and humans acquire most types of roundworm infection from contaminated food or by touching the mouth with unwashed hands that have come into contact with the parasite larva. The severity of infection varies considerably from person to person. Children are more likely to have heavy infestations and are also more likely to suffer from malabsorption and malnutrition than adults.

ROUS SARCOMA VIRUS: Named after American doctor Francis Peyton Rous (1879–1970), a virus that can cause cancer in some birds, including chickens. It was the first known virus capable of causing cancer.

RUMINANTS: Cud-chewing animals with a four-chambered stomachs and even-toed hooves.

S

SANITATION: The use of hygienic recycling and disposal measures that prevent disease and promote health through sewage disposal, solid waste disposal, waste material recycling, and food processing and preparation.

SCHISTOSOMES: Blood flukes.

SEIZURE: A sudden disruption of the brain's normal electrical activity accompanied by altered consciousness or other neurological and behavioral abnormalities. Epilepsy is a condition characterized by recurrent seizures that may include repetitive muscle jerking called convulsions. Seizures are traditionally divided into two major categories: generalized seizures and focal seizures. Within each major category, however, there are many different types of seizures. Generalized seizures come about due to abnormal neuronal activity on both sides of the brain, whereas focal seizures, also named partial seizures, occur in only one part of the brain.

SELECTION: A process that favors one feature of organisms in a population over another feature found in the population. This occurs through differential reproduction—those with the favored feature produce more offspring than those with the other feature, such that they become a greater percentage of the population in the next generation.

SELECTION PRESSURE: The influence of various factors on the evolution of an organism. An example is the overuse of antibiotics, which provides a selection pressure for the development of antibiotic resistance in bacteria.

SELECTIVE PRESSURE: The tendency of an organism that has a certain characteristic to be eliminated from an environment or to increase in number. An example is the increased prevalence of bacteria resistant to multiple kinds of antibiotics.

SENTINEL: An epidemiological method in which a subset of the population is surveyed for the presence of communicable diseases. Also, an animal used to indicate the presence of disease within an area.

SENTINEL SURVEILLANCE: A method in epidemiology where a subset of the population is surveyed for the presence of communicable diseases. Also, a sentinel is an animal used to indicate the presence of disease within an area.

SEPSIS: A bacterial infection in the bloodstream or body tissues. Sepsis is a very broad term covering the presence of many types of microscopic disease-causing organisms. It is also called bacteremia. Closely related terms include septicemia and septic syndrome.

SEPTIC: Infected with bacteria, particularly in the bloodstream.

SEPTICEMIA: Prolonged fever, chills, anorexia, and anemia in conjunction with tissue lesions.

SEQUENCING: Finding the order of chemical bases in a section of DNA.

SEROCONVERSION: The development in the blood of antibodies to an infectious organism or agent. Typically, seroconversion is associated with infections caused by bacteria, viruses, and protozoans. But seroconversion also occurs after the deliberate inoculation with an antigen in the process of vaccination. In the case of infections, the development of detectable levels of antibodies can occur quickly, in the case of an active infection, or can be prolonged, in the case of a latent infection. Seroconversion typically heralds the development of the symptoms of the particular infection.

SEROLOGIC TEST: A test of the blood or other body fluid, such as spinal fluid, in which serum or the body fluids collected are used to look for antibodies.

SEROTYPE: Also known as a serovar, a class of microorganism based on the types of antigens (molecules that elicit an immune response) presented on the surface of the microorganism. A single species may have thousands of serotypes with medically distinct behaviors.

SEXUALLY TRANSMITTED INFECTION (STI): STIs vary in their susceptibility to treatment, their signs and symptoms, and the consequences if they are left untreated. Some are caused by bacteria. These usually can be treated and cured. Others are caused by viruses and can typically be treated but not cured.

SHED: To cast off or release. In medicine, the release of eggs or live organisms from an individual infected with parasites is often referred to as shedding.

SHOCK: A medical emergency in which the organs and tissues of the body are not receiving an adequate flow of blood. This condition deprives the organs and tissues of oxygen (carried in the blood) and allows the buildup of waste products. Shock can result in serious damage or even death.

SOCIOECONOMIC: Concerning both social and economic factors.

SOUTHERN BLOT ANALYSIS: An electrophoresis technique in which pieces of deoxyribonucleic acid (DNA) that have resulted from enzyme digestion are separated from one another on the basis of size, followed by the transfer of the DNA fragments to a flexible membrane. The membrane can then be exposed to various probes to identify target regions of the genetic material.

SPECIAL PATHOGENS BRANCH: A group within the US Centers for Disease Control and Prevention (CDC) whose goal is to study highly infectious viruses that produce diseases within humans.

SPIROCHETE: A bacterium shaped like a spiral. Spiral-shaped bacteria live in contaminated water, sewage, soil, and decaying organic matter, as well as inside humans and animals.

SPONGIFORM: The clinical name for the appearance of brain tissue affected by prion diseases, such as Creutzfeldt-Jakob disease or bovine spongiform encephalopathy (mad cow disease). The disease process leads to the formation of tiny holes in brain tissue, giving it a spongy appearance.

SPONTANEOUS: Generation Also known as abiogenesis, the incorrect and discarded assumption that living things can be generated from nonliving things.

SPORE: A dormant form assumed by some bacteria, such as anthrax, that enables the bacterium to survive high temperatures, dryness, and lack of nourishment for long periods of time. Under proper conditions, the spore may revert to the actively multiplying form of the bacteria.

SPOROZOAN: The fifth phylum of the kingdom Protista, known as Apicomplexa, comprises several species of obligate intracellular protozoan parasites classified as sporozoa or sporozoans, because they form reproductive cells known as spores. Many sporozoans are parasitic and pathogenic species, such as Plasmodium falciparum, Plasmodium malariae, Plasmodium vivax, Toxoplasma gondii, Pneumocystis carinii, Cryptosporidium parvum and Cryptosporidium muris, The sporozoa reproduction cycle has both asexual and sexual phases. The asexual phase is schizogony (from the Greek, meaning "generation through division"), in which merozoites (daughter cells) are produced through multiple nuclear fissions. The sexual phase is sporogony (i.e., generation of spores) and is followed by gametogony, or the production of sexually reproductive cells termed gamonts.

SPOROZOITE: Developmental stage of a protozoan (e.g., a malaria protozoan), during which it is transferred from vector (with malaria, a mosquito) to a human host.

STAINING: The use of chemicals to identify target components of microorganisms.

STANDARD PRECAUTIONS: The safety measures taken to prevent the transmission of disease-causing bacteria. These measures include proper handwashing; wearing gloves, goggles, and other protective clothing; proper handling of needles; and sterilization of equipment.

STERILIZATION: The complete killing or elimination of living organisms in the sample being treated. Sterilization is absolute. After the treatment, the sample is either devoid of life or the possibility of life (as from the subsequent germination and growth of bacterial spores), or living organisms are still present or could grow if they were present.

STRAIN: A subclass or a specific genetic variation of an organism.

STREP THROAT: An infection caused by group A Streptococcus bacteria. The main target of the infection is the mucous membranes lining the pharynx. Sometimes the tonsils are also infected (tonsillitis). If left untreated, the infection can develop into rheumatic fever or other serious conditions.

STREPTOCOCCUS: A genus of bacteria that includes species such as Streptococci pyogenes, a species of bacteria that causes strep throat.

SUPERINFECTION: A new infection that occurs in a patient who already has some other infection. For example, a bacterial infection appearing in a person who already had viral pneumonia would be a superinfection.

SURVEILLANCE: The systematic analysis, collection, evaluation, interpretation, and dissemination of data. Public health surveillance assists in the identification of health threats and the planning, implementation, and evaluation of responses to those threats.

SYLVATIC: Meaning "pertaining to the woods," the term refers to diseases such as plague that are spread by animals including ground squirrels and other wild rodents.

SYSTEMIC: Any medical condition that affects the whole body (i.e., the whole system) is systemic.

T

T CELL: An immune-system white blood cell that enables antibody production, suppresses antibody production, or kills other cells. When a vertebrate encounters substances capable of causing it harm, a protective system known as the immune system comes into play. This system is a network of many different organs that work together to recognize foreign substances and destroy them. The immune system can respond to the presence of a disease-causing agent (pathogen) in two ways. Immune cells called the B cells can produce soluble proteins (antibodies) that can accurately target and kill the pathogen. This branch of immunity is called humoral immunity. In cell-mediated immunity, immune cells known as the T cells produce special chemicals that can specifically isolate the pathogen and destroy it.

TAPEWORM: Parasitic flatworms of class Cestoidea, phylum Platyhelminthes, that live inside the intestine. Tapeworms have no digestive system but absorb predigested nutrients directly from their surroundings.

T CELL VACCINE: A vaccine that relies on eliciting cellular immunity, rather than humoral antibody-based immunity, against infection. T cell vaccines are being developed against the human immunodeficiency virus (HIV) and hepatitis C.

TICK: Any blood-sucking parasitic insect of suborder Ixodides, superfamily Ixodoidea. Ticks can transmit a number of diseases, including Lyme disease and Rocky Mountain spotted fever.

TOGAVIRUS: is a single-stranded ribonucleic acid (RNA) virus.

TOPICAL: Any medication that is applied directly to a particular part of the body's surface(e.g., a topical ointment).

TOXIC: Something that is poisonous and that can cause illness or death.

TOXIN: A poison produced by a living organism.

TOXOID: A bacterial toxin that has been altered chemically to make it incapable of causing damage but still capable of stimulating an immune response. Toxoids are used to stimulate antibody production, which is protective in the event of exposure to the active toxin.

TRANSFUSION-TRANSMISSIBLE INFECTIONS: Any infection that can be transmitted to a person by a blood transfusion (addition of stored whole blood or blood fractions to a person's own blood). Some diseases that can be transmitted in this way are acquired immunodeficiency syndrome (AIDS), hepatitis B, hepatitis C, syphilis, malaria, and Chagas disease.

TRANSMISSION: Microorganisms that cause disease in humans and other species are known as pathogens. The transmission of pathogens to a human or other host can occur in a number of ways, depending on the microorganism.

TREMATODES: Also called flukes, a type of parasitic flatworm. In humans flukes can infest the liver, lung, and other tissues.

TRICLOSAN: A chemical that kills bacteria.

TRISMUS: The medical term for lockjaw, a condition often associated with tetanus, which is an infection by the Clostridium tetani bacillus. In trismus or lockjaw, the major muscles of the jaw contract involuntarily.

TROPHOZOITE: The amoeboid, vegetative stage of the malaria protozoa.

TYPHUS: A disease caused by various species of Rickettsia, characterized by fever, rash, and delirium. Insects such as lice and chiggers transmit typhus. Two forms of typhus, epidemic typhus and scrub typhus, are fatal if untreated.

U

ULCER: An open sore on the inside or outside of the body that is accompanied by disintegration or necrosis of the surrounding tissue.

ULCERATIVE STI: Any kind of sexually transmitted infection (STI) that results in genital ulcers. This includes herpes, syphilis, chancroid, and gonorrhea. Herpes is the most common.

UNIVERSAL PRECAUTION: An infection-control strategy in which all human blood and other material is assumed to be potentially infectious, specifically with organisms such as human immunodeficiency virus (HIV) and hepatitis B virus. The precautions are aimed at preventing contact with blood or the other materials.

V

VACCINATION: The inoculation, or use of vaccines, to prevent specific diseases within humans and animals by producing immunity to such diseases. It is the introduction of weakened or dead viruses or microorganisms into the body to create immunity by the production of specific antibodies.

VACCINE: A substance that is introduced to stimulate antibody production and thus provide immunity to a particular disease.

VACCINIA VIRUS: A usually harmless virus that is closely related to the virus that causes smallpox, a dangerous disease. Infection with the vaccinia virus confers immunity against smallpox, so vaccinia virus has been used as a vaccine against smallpox.

VARICELLA ZOSTER IMMUNE GLOBULIN (VZIG): A preparation that can give people temporary protection against chickenpox after exposure to the Varicella virus. It is used for children and adults who are at risk of complications of the disease or who are susceptible to infection because they have weakened immunity.

VARICELLA ZOSTER VIRUS (VZV): A member of the alpha herpes virus group and is the cause of both chickenpox (also known as varicella) and shingles (herpes zoster).

VARIOLA VIRUS: The virus that causes smallpox. It is one of the members of the poxvirus group (family Poxviridae). The virus particle is brick shaped and contains a double strand of deoxyribonucleic acid (DNA). The variola virus is among the most dangerous of all the potential biological weapons.

VARIOLATION: The premodern practice of deliberately infecting a person with smallpox to make them immune to a more serious form of the disease. It was dangerous but did confer immunity on survivors.

VECTOR: Any agent that carries and transmits parasites and diseases. Also, an organism or a chemical used to transport a gene into a new host cell.

VECTOR-BORNE DISEASE: One in which the pathogenic microorganism is transmitted from an infected individual to another individual by an arthropod or other agent, sometimes with other animals serving as intermediary hosts. The transmission depends on the attributes and requirements of at least three different living organisms: the pathologic agent, either a virus, protozoa, bacteria, or helminth (worm); the vector, commonly arthropods such as ticks or mosquitoes; and the human host.

VENEREAL DISEASE: Diseases that are transmitted by sexual contact. They are named after Venus, the Roman goddess of female sexuality.

VESICLE: A membrane-bound sphere that contains a variety of substances in cells.

VIRAL SHEDDING: The movement of the herpes virus from the nerves to the surface of the skin. During shedding the virus can be passed on through skin-to-skin contact.

VIRION: A mature virus particle consisting of a core of ribonucleic acid (RNA) or deoxyribonucleic acid (DNA) surrounded by a protein coat. This is the form in which a virus exists outside of its host cell.

VIRULENCE: The ability of a disease organism to cause disease. A more virulent organism is more infective and liable to produce more serious disease.

VIRUS: Essentially nonliving repositories of nucleic acid that require the presence of a living prokaryotic or eukaryotic cell for the replication of the nucleic acid. There are a number of different viruses that challenge the human immune system and that may produce disease in humans. A virus is a small, infectious agent that consists of a core of genetic material—either deoxyribonucleic acid (DNA) or ribonucleic acid (RNA)—surrounded by a shell of protein. Very simple microorganisms, viruses are much smaller than bacteria that enter and multiply within cells. Viruses often exchange or transfer their genetic material (DNA or RNA) to cells and can cause diseases such as chickenpox, hepatitis, measles, and mumps.

VISCERAL: Pertaining to the viscera. The viscera are the large organs contained in the main cavities of the body, especially the thorax and abdomen—for example, the lungs, stomach, intestines, kidneys, or liver.

W

WATERBORNE DISEASE: Diseases that are caused by exposure to contaminated water. The exposure can occur by drinking the water or having the water come in contact with the body. Examples of waterborne diseases are cholera and typhoid fever.

WAVELENGTH: A distance of one cycle of a wave; for instance, the distance between the peaks on adjoining waves that have the same phase.

WEAPONIZATION: The use of any bacterium, virus, or other disease-causing organism as a weapon of war. Among other terms, it is also called germ warfare, biological weaponry, and biological warfare.

WEIL'S DISEASE: Named after German doctor Adolf Weil (1848–1916), a severe form of leptospirosis or seven-day fever, which is a disease caused by infection with the corkscrew-shaped bacillus Leptospira interrogans.

WILD VIRUS: A genetic description referring to the original form of a virus, first observed in nature. It may remain the most common form in existence, but mutated forms develop over time and sometimes become the new wild virus.

Z

ZOONOSES: Diseases of microbiological origin that can be transmitted from animals to people. The causes of the diseases can be bacteria, viruses, parasites, or fungi.

ZOONOTIC: A disease that can be transmitted between animals and humans. Examples of zoonotic diseases are anthrax, plague, and Q fever.

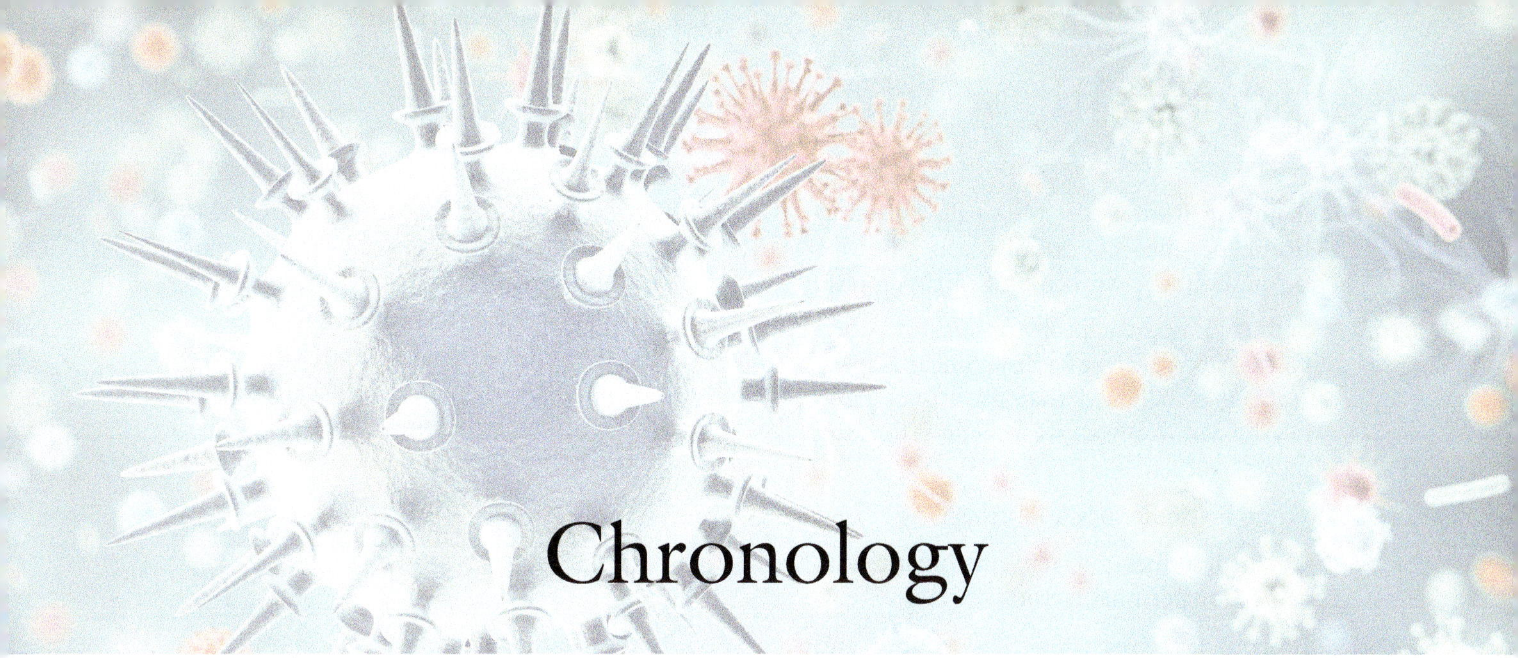

Chronology

BC

c. 2500 The characteristic symptoms of malaria are first described in Chinese medical writings.

c. 1000 Hindu physicians exhibit broad clinical knowledge of tuberculosis. In India, the Laws of Manu consider it to be an unclean, incurable disease and an impediment to marriage.

c. 430 Plague of Athens caused by unknown infectious agent. One-third of the population (increased by those fleeing the Spartan army) die.

c. 400 Hippocrates (460–370 BCE), Greek physician, and his disciples establish their medical practice based on reason and experiment. They attribute disease to natural causes and use diet and medication to restore the body's balance of humors.

c. 400 Hippocratic texts recommend irrigation with fresh water as a treatment for septic wounds.

c. 300 A medical school is set up in Alexandria, where the first accurate anatomical observations using dissection are made. The principal exponents of the school are Greek physician Herophilus (c. 335 BCE–c. 280 BCE) and Greek physician Erasistratus (c. 304 BCE–c. 250 BCE).

c. 300 Herophilus, Greek anatomist, establishes himself as the first systemic anatomist and the first to perform human dissections.

91 Greek scientific medicine takes hold in Rome when the physician Asclepiades (c. 130 BCE–40 BCE) of Bithynia settles in the West.

AD

c. 30 Aulus Cornelius Celsus, Roman encyclopedist, writes his influential book *De Re Medicina*. The work contains descriptions of many conditions and operations and is probably drawn mostly from the collection of writings of the school of Hippocrates. It is rediscovered during the 15th century and becomes highly influential.

c. 75 Dioscorides (c. 40–c. 90), Greek physician, writes the first systematic pharmacopoeia. His *De Materia Medica* in five volumes provides accurate botanical and pharmacological information. It is preserved by the Arabs and, when translated into Latin and printed in 1478, becomes a standard botanical reference.

150 Claudius Galen (129–c. 210), Greek physician, says that pus formation is required for wound healing. This proves to be incorrect and hinders the treatment of wounds for centuries.

c. 160 Bubonic plague (termed "barbarian boils") sweeps China.

c. 160 Galen, in his *De Usu Partium*, describes the pineal gland as a secretory organ that is important to thinking. He names it the pineal because it resembles a pine cone.

c. 166 Plague in Rome (possibly smallpox or bubonic plague) eventually kills millions throughout the weakening Roman empire.

167 Stabiae, a popular health resort for tuberculosis sufferers, is established near Naples, Italy. It is believed that the fumes from nearby Mt. Vesuvius are beneficial for lung ulcers.

170 Galen first describes gonorrhea.

c. 200 Galen describes internal inflammations as caused by personal factors.

c. 370 Basil of Caesarea (330–379) founds and organizes a large hospital at Caesarea (near Palestine).

c. 400 Fabiola, a Christian noblewoman, founds the first nosocomium, or hospital, in Western Europe. After establishing the first hospital in Rome, she establishes a hospice for pilgrims in Porto, Italy.

430 Earliest recorded plague in Europe is an epidemic that breaks out in Athens, Greece.

c. 500 During this century the "plague of Justinian" kills about 1 million people.

529 Benedict of Nursia founds the monastery at Monte Cassino in central Italy. It becomes, if not an actual medical school, at least an important center of scholarship in which medicine played a great part. It also acquires great fame throughout the West, and its medical teachings are spread by the Benedictines to their monasteries scattered all over Europe.

610 In China Ch'ao Yuan-fang (550–630) writes a treatise on the causes and symptoms of diseases. Medical knowledge spreads from China to Japan via the Korean peninsula.

644 Rotharus, King of Lombardy (c. 606–652; also called Rothari), issues his edict ordering the segregation of all lepers.

c. 700 Benedictus Crispus, archbishop of Milan from 681 to about 730, writes his *Commentarium Medicinale*, an elementary practical manual in verse. It describes the use of medicinal plants for curing illnesses.

c. 850 Christian physician Sabur ibn Sahl of Jundishapur compiles a 22-volume work on antidotes that dominates Islamic pharmacopeia for the next 400 years.

c. 850 Islamic philosopher Al-Kindi (813–873) writes his *De Medicinarum Compositarum Gradibus*, which attempts to base dosages of medicine on mathematical measurements.

c. 875 Bertharius (c. 810–883), the abbot of Montcasino from 857 to 884, writes two treatises, *De Innumeris Remediorum Utilitatibus* and *De Innumeris Morbis*, that give insight into the kind of medicine practiced in the monasteries.

896 Abu Bakr al-Razi (c. 845–c. 930; also known as Rhazes), Persian physician and alchemist, distinguishes between the specific characteristics of measles and smallpox. He is also believed to be the first to classify all substances into the great classification of animal, vegetable, and mineral.

c. 900 First medical books written in Anglo-Saxon appear, including *Lacnunga* and *Leech Book of Bald*.

c. 955 Jewish "prince of medicine," Isaac Israeli (c.855–955), dies. He writes classic works on fever and uroscopy, as well as *Guide of the Physicians*.

c. 980 Abu al-Qasim Al-Zahrawi (936–1013), known as Abucasis, creates a system and method of human dissection along with the first formal specific surgical techniques.

c. 1000 Ibn Sina (c. 980–1037), or Avicenna, publishes *Al-Quanun*, or Canon of Medicine, where he held that medicines could be discovered and tried by experiment or by reasoning.

1137 St. Bartholomew's hospital is founded in London.

1140 Bologna, Italy, begins to develop as a major European medical center. In the next century, the Italian physician Taddeo Alderotti (c. 1233–1303) opens a school of medicine there.

1200 Physicians in Italy begin to write case histories that describe symptoms and observable pathology of diseases.

c. 1267 Roger Bacon (1214–1292), English philosopher and scientist, asserts that natural phenomena should be studied empirically.

1302 First formally recorded postmortem or judicial autopsy is performed in Bologna, Italy, by Italian physician Bartolomeo da Varignana. A postmortem is ordered by the court in a case of suspected poisoning.

1333 Public botanical garden is established in Venice, Italy, to grow herbs that have medical uses.

1345 First apothecary shop or drug store opens in London.

1348 The beginning of a three-year epidemic caused by *Yersinia pestis* kills almost one-third of the population of urban Europe. In the aftermath of the epidemic, measures are introduced by the Italian government to improve public sanitation, marking the origin of public health.

1374 As the plague spreads, the Republic of Ragusa places the first quarantines on crews of ships thought to be infected.

1388 Richard II (1367–1400), king of England, establishes the first sanitary laws in England.

1489 Typhus is first brought to Europe by soldiers who had been fighting in Cyprus.

1491 First anatomical book to contain printed illustrations is German physician Johannes de Ketham's *Fasciculus Medicinae.*

1492 Venereal diseases, smallpox, and influenza are brought by the Columbus expedition (and subsequent European explorers) to the New World. Millions of native peoples eventually die from these diseases because of a lack of prior exposure to stimulate immunity. In some regions whole villages succumb, and across broader regions up to 95 percent of the native population dies.

1525 Gonzalo Hernandez de Oviedo y Valdes (1478–1557) of Spain publishes the first systematic description of the medicinal plants of Central America.

1525 Paracelsus (1493–1541), Swiss physician and alchemist, begins the use of mineral substances as medicines.

1527 Paracelsus publicly burns the writings of Galen in Basel, Switzerland. He rejects the traditional medical methods as irrational, and he founds iatrochemistry, asserting that the body is linked in some way to the laws of chemistry.

1528 Italian physician Girolamo Fracastoro (c. 1478–1553), also known as Fracastorius, describes an epidemic of typhus among French troops invading Naples.

1530 Fracastorius writes his poem called "Syphilis" (*Syphilis sive Morbus Gallici*), which gives the definitive name to the sexually transmitted infection that is spreading throughout Europe.

1536 Paracelsus publishes his surgical treatise, *Chirurgia Magna.*

1543 Andreas Vesalius (1514–1564), Dutch anatomist, publishes his *De Corporis Humani Corporis Fabrica*, the first accurate book on human anatomy. Its illustrations are of the highest level of both realism and art, and the result revolutionizes biology.

1546 Fracastorius writes his *De Contagione et Contagiosis Morbis*, which contains new ideas on the transmission of contagious diseases and is considered the scientific beginning of that study.

1567 A book on miner's tuberculosis by Paracelsus is posthumously published.

1602 Felix Platter (1536–1614), Swiss anatomist, publishes his *Praxis Medica*, which is the first modern attempt at the classification of diseases.

1621 Johannes Baptista van Helmont (1577–1635), Dutch physician and alchemist, writes his *Ortus Medicinae* in which he becomes one of the founders of modern pathology. He studies the anatomical changes that occur in disease.

1624 Adriaan van den Spigelius (1578–1625), Dutch anatomist, publishes the first account of malaria.

1640 Juan del Vigo introduces cinchona into Spain. Native to the Andes, the bark of this tree is processed to obtain quinine, used in the treatment of malaria.

1642 First treatise on the use of cinchona bark (quinine powder) for treating malaria is written by Spanish physician Pedro Barba (1608–1671).

1648 René Descartes (1596–1650), French philosopher and mathematician, writes *De Homine*, the first European textbook on physiology. He considers the body to be a material machine and offers his mechanist theory of life.

1648 Willem Piso (1611–1678), Dutch physician and botanist (also called Le Pois), points out the effectiveness of ipecac against dysentery in his book *De Medicina Brasiliensi*. He is among the first to become acquainted with tropical diseases, and he distinguishes between yaws and syphilis.

1660 The Royal Society of London is founded in England with Henry Oldenburg (c. 1618–1677) as secretary and Robert Hooke (1635–1702) as curator of experiments. Two years later, in 1662, King Charles II (1630–1685) grants it a royal charter, and it becomes known as the "Royal Society of London for the Promotion of Natural Knowledge."

1665 Bubonic plague epidemic in London kills 75,000 people. It is during this scourge that English scientist and mathematician Isaac Newton (1642–1727) leaves school in London and stays at his mother's farm in the country. There he formulates his laws of motion.

1665 First drawing of the cell is made by Robert Hooke (1635–1703), English physicist. While observing a sliver of cork under a microscope, Hooke notices it is composed of a pattern of tiny rectangular holes he calls "cells" because each looks like a small, empty room. Although he does not observe living cells, the name is retained.

1665 Hooke publishes his landmark book on microscopy, *Micrographia*. Containing some of the most beautiful drawings of microscopic observations ever made, his book led to many discoveries in related fields.

1666 Robert Boyle (1627–1691), English physicist and chemist, publishes *The Origine of Formes and Qualities* in which he begins to explain all chemical reactions and physical properties through the existence of small, indivisible particles or atoms.

1668 Francesco Redi (1626–1697), Italian physician, conducts experiments to disprove spontaneous generation. He shows that maggots are not born spontaneously but come from eggs laid by flies. He publishes his *Esperienze Intorno all Generazione degli Insetti.*

1671 Michael Ettmüller (1644–1683), German physician, attributes the contagiousness of tuberculosis to sputum.

1672 French physician Le Gras introduces ipecac into Europe. The root of the Brazilian plant ipecacuanha is used to cure dysentery.

1674 Antoni van Leeuwenhoek (1632–1723), Dutch biologist and microscopist, observes "animacules" in lake water viewed through a ground glass lens. This observation of what will eventually be known as bacteria represents the start of the formal study of microbiology.

1675 John Josselyn, English botanist, publishes an account of the plants and animals he encounters while living in America and indicates that tuberculosis existed among Native Americans before the arrival of Europeans.

1677 Antoni van Leeuwenhoek (1632–1723), Dutch biologist and microscopist, discovers spermatozoa and describes them in a letter he publishes in *Philosophical Transactions* in 1679. That year Johan Ham also sees them microscopically, but the semen he observes comes from a patient suffering from gonorrhea, and Ham concludes that spermatozoa are a consequence of the disease.

1700 Bernardino Ramazzini (1633–1714), Italian physician, publishes the first systematic treatment on occupational diseases. His book, *De Morbis Artificum*, opens an entirely new department of modern medicine—diseases of trade or occupation and industrial hygiene.

1721 The word *antiseptic* first appears in print.

1730 British physician George Martine (1702–1743) performs the first tracheostomy on a patient with diphtheria.

1735 Botulism first described.

1748 British physician John Fothergill (1712–1780) describes diphtheria in "Account of the Putrid Sore Throat."

1762 Marcus Anton von Plenciz Sr. (1705–1786), Austrian physician, expresses the idea that all infectious diseases are caused by living organisms and that there is a specific organism for each disease.

1767 William Heberden (1710–1801), English physician, demonstrates that chickenpox is not a mild form of smallpox but a different disease.

1780 George Adams (1750–1795), English engineer, devises the first microtome. This mechanical instrument cuts thin slices for examination under a microscope, thus replacing the imprecise procedure of cutting by handheld razor.

1789 Polio is first described by English physician Michael Underwood (1736–1820) in England.

1796 Edward Jenner (1749–1823) uses cowpox virus to develop a smallpox vaccine. By modern standards, this was human experimentation, as Jenner injected healthy eight-year-old James Phillips with cowpox and then after a period of months with smallpox.

1798 Government legislation is passed to establish hospitals in the United States devoted to the care of ill mariners. This initiative leads to the establishment of a Hygienic Laboratory that eventually grows to become the National Institutes of Health (NIH).

1800 Marie-François-Xavier Bichat (1771–1802) publishes his first major work, *Treatise on Tissues*, which establishes histology as a new scientific discipline. Bichat distinguishes 21 kinds of tissue and relates particular diseases to particular tissues.

1801 A hospital is established in London to treat the victims of typhus.

1802 English chemist John Dalton (1766–1844) introduces modern atomic theory into the science of chemistry.

1814 The Royal Hospital for Diseases of the Chest is founded in London in an attempt to keep consumptive patients (people with tuberculosis) segregated.

1816 The stethoscope, which is an important tool for diagnosing pneumonia, is introduced by René Laënnec (1781–1826).

1817 Start of first cholera pandemic, which spreads from Bengal to China in the east and to Egypt in the west.

1818 William Charles Wells (1757–1817), Scottish American physician, suggests the theory of natural selection in an essay dealing with human color variations. He notes that dark-skinned people seem more resistant to tropical diseases than lighter-skinned people. Wells also calls attention to selection carried out by animal breeders. Jerome Lawrence, James Cowles Prichard (1786–1848), and others make similar suggestions but do not develop their ideas into a coherent and convincing theory of evolution.

1818 Xavier Bichat (1771–1802), French physician, publishes his first major work, *Trait, des membranes en general*, in which he propounds the notion of tissues. This work also founds histology, distinguishing 21 kinds of tissue and relating disease to them.

1820 First United States *Pharmacopoeia* is published.

1824 Start of second cholera pandemic, which penetrates as far as Russia and also reaches England, North America, the Caribbean, and Latin America.

1826 Pierre Bretonneau (1778–1862), French physician, describes and names diphtheria in his specification of diseases.

1829 Salicin, the precursor of aspirin, is purified from the bark of the willow tree.

1831 Charles Darwin (1809–1882), English naturalist, begins his historic voyage on the HMS *Beagle* (1831–1836). His observations during the voyage lead to his theory of evolution by means of natural selection.

1835 Jacob Bigelow (1787–1879), American physician, publishes his book *On Self-Limited Diseases*, in which he states the commonsense idea that some diseases will simply run their course and subside without the benefit of any treatment from a physician.

1836 Theodor Schwann (1810–1882), German physiologist, carries out experiments that refute the theory of the spontaneous generation. He also demonstrates that alcoholic fermentation depends on the action of living yeast cells. The same conclusion is reached independently by French physicist Charles Cagniard de la Tour (1777–1859).

1837 Pierre-François-Olive Rayer (1793–1867), French physician, is the first to describe the disease glanders as found in humans and to prove that it is not a form of tuberculosis.

1838 Angelo Dubini (1813–1902), Italian physician, discovers *Ankylostoma duodenale*, the cause of hookworm disease, in the intestinal tract.

1838 Matthias Jakob Schleiden (1804–1881) notes that the nucleus first described by Scottish botanist Robert Brown (1773–1858) is a characteristic of all plant cells. Schleiden describes plants as a community of cells and cell products. He helps establish cell theory and stimulates Theodor Schwann's recognition that animals are also composed of cells and cell products.

1839 Third cholera pandemic begins with entry of British troops in Afghanistan and travels to Persia, Central Asia, Europe, and the Americas.

1841 Friedrich Gustav Jacob Henle (1809–1885), German pathologist and anatomist, publishes his *Allegemeine Anatomie*, which becomes the first systematic textbook of histology (the study of minute tissue structure and includes the first statement of the germ theory of communicable disease).

1842 Edwin Chadwick (1800–1890), a pioneer in sanitary reform, reports that deaths from typhus in 1838 and 1839 in England exceeded those from smallpox.

1842 Oliver Wendell Holmes (1809–1894), American physician, recommends that surgeons wash their hands using calcium chloride to prevent spread of infection from corpses to patients.

1843 First outbreak of polio in the United States occurs.

1843 Gabriel Andral (1797–1876), French physician, is the first to urge that blood be examined in cases of disease.

1846 American Medical Association establishes a code of ethics for physicians that declares their obligation to treat victims of epidemic diseases even at a risk to their own lives.

1847 A series of yellow fever epidemics sweeps the American Southern states. The epidemics recur for more than 30 years.

1847 The first sexually transmitted infection clinic is opened at the London Docks Hospital.

1849 John Snow (1813–1858), English physician, first states the theory that cholera is a waterborne disease. During a cholera epidemic in London in 1854, Snow breaks the handle of the Broad Street Pump, thereby shutting down the main source of disease transmission during the outbreak.

1849 Snow publishes the groundbreaking paper "On the Transmission of Cholera."

1855 Third, or modern, pandemic of plague probably begins in Yunan province, China.

1857 Louis Pasteur demonstrates that lactic acid fermentation is caused by a living organism. Between 1857 and 1880, he performs a series of experiments that refute the doctrine of spontaneous generation. He also introduces vaccines for fowl cholera, anthrax, and rabies, based on attenuated strains of viruses and bacteria.

1858 Rudolf Ludwig Carl Virchow (1821–1902), German physician, publishes his landmark paper "Cellular Pathology" and establishes the field of cellular pathology.

Virchow asserts that all cells arise from preexisting cells (*Omnis cellula e cellula*). He argues that the cell is the ultimate locus of all disease.

1859 Darwin publishes his landmark book *On the Origin of Species by Means of Natural Selection.*

1861 Carl Gegenbaur (1826–1903), German anatomist, confirms Theodor Schwann's suggestion that all vertebrate eggs are single cells.

1862 First demonstration of pasteurization.

1864 Fourth cholera pandemic starts and revisits locations of previous pandemics.

1865 An epidemic of rinderpest kills 500,000 cattle in Great Britain. Government inquiries into the outbreak pave the way for the development of contemporary theories of epidemiology and the germ theory of disease.

1865 French physiologist Claude Bernard (1813–1878) publishes *Introduction to the Study of Human Experimentation*, which advocates, "Never perform an experiment which might be harmful to the patient even if advantageous to science."

1866 Austrian botanist and monk Johann Gregor Mendel (1822–1884) discovers the laws of heredity and writes the first of a series of papers on heredity (1866–1869). The papers formulate the laws of hybridization. Mendel's work is disregarded until 1900, when Dutch botanist Hugo de Vries (1848–1935) rediscovers it. Unbeknownst to both Darwin and Mendel, Mendelian laws provide the scientific framework for the concepts of gradual evolution and continuous variation.

1867 British surgeon Joseph Lister (1827–1912) publishes a study that implicates microorganisms with infection. Based on this, his use of early disinfectants during surgery markedly reduces postoperative infections and death.

1867 Robert Koch (1843–1910), German bacteriologist, establishes the role of bacteria in anthrax, providing the final piece of evidence in support of the germ theory of disease. Koch goes on to formulate postulates that, when fulfilled, confirm bacteria or viruses as the cause of an infection.

1868 Carl August Wunderlich (1815–1877), German physician, publishes his major work on the relation of animal heat or fever to disease. He is the first to recognize that fever is not itself a disease but rather a symptom.

1869 Johann Friedrich Miescher (1844–1895), Swiss physician, discovers nuclein, a new chemical isolated from the nuclei of pus cells. Two years later he isolates nuclein from salmon sperm. This material comes to be known as nucleic acid.

1871 German biologist Ferdinand Julius Cohn (1828–1898) coins the term *bacterium.*

1871 First US city to use a filter on its public water supply is Poughkeepsie, New York. The evidence mounts that much disease is spread by contaminated drinking water.

1873 Franz Anton Schneider describes cell division in detail. His drawings include both the nucleus and chromosomal strands.

1875 Cohn publishes a classification of bacteria in which the genus name *Bacillus* is used for the first time.

1875 Koch's postulates used for the first time to demonstrate that anthrax is caused by *Bacillus anthracis*, validating the germ theory of disease.

1877 Louis Pasteur first distinguishes between aerobic and anaerobic bacteria.

1877 Paul Ehrlich (1854–1915), German bacteriologist, recognizes the existence of the mast cells of the immune system.

1877 Koch describes new techniques for fixing, staining, and photographing bacteria.

1877 Wilhelm Friedrich Kühne (1837–1900), German physiologist, proposes the term *enzyme* (meaning "in yeast"). Kühne establishes the critical distinction between enzymes, or "ferments," and the microorganisms that produce them.

1878 Lister publishes a paper describing the role of a bacterium he names *Bacterium lactis* in the souring of milk.

1878 Koch publishes his landmark findings on the etiology or cause of infectious disease.

Koch's postulates state that the causative microorganism must be located in a diseased animal and that, after it is cultured or grown, it must then be capable of causing disease in a healthy animal. Finally, the newly infected animal must yield the same bacteria as those found in the original animal.

1878 Thomas Burrill (1839–1916), American botanist, demonstrates that a plant disease (pear blight) is caused by a bacterium (*Micrococcus amylophorous*).

1879 Albert Neisser (1855–1916), German physician, identifies the bacterium *Neiserria gonorrhoeoe* as the cause of gonorrhea.

1880 C. L. Alphonse Laveran (1845–1922), French physician, isolates malarial parasites in erythrocytes of infected people and demonstrates that the organism can replicate in the cells.

1880 The first issue of the journal *Science* is published by the American Association for the Advancement of Science.

1881 Fifth cholera pandemic begins and is widespread in China and Japan in the Far East, as well as Germany and Russia in Europe, although the disease does not spread in North America.

1881 *Streptococcus pneumoniae*, a major cause of bacterial pneumonia, is discovered independently by Pasteur and US Army physician George Sternberg (1838–1915).

1882 Angelina Fanny Hesse (1850–1934) and Walther Hesse (1846–1911) in Koch's laboratory develop agar as a solid grow medium for microorganisms. Agar replaces gelatin as the solid growth medium of choice in microbiology.

1882 Friedrich August Johannes Loffler (1852–1915), German bacteriologist, and F. Schulze discover the bacterium causing glanders, a contagious and destructive disease of animals, especially horses, that can be transmitted to humans.

1883 German-Swiss pathologist Edwin Klebs (1834–1913) and German bacteriologist Friedrich Loeffler (1852–1915) independently discover *Corynebacterium diphtheriae*, the bacterium that causes diphtheria.

1883 Koch discovers *V. cholerae* as the causative agent of cholera in Egypt.

1883 Surgical gowns and headgear begin to be used by surgeons.

1884 Élie Metchnikoff (1845–1916), Russian microbiologist, discovers the antibacterial activity of white blood cells, which he calls phagocytes, and formulates the theory of phagocytosis. He also develops the cellular theory of vaccination.

1884 Danish bacteriologist Hans Christian Gram (1853–1938) develops the Gram stain, a method of categorizing bacteria into one of two groups (Gram positive and Gram negative) based on the chemical reaction of the bacteria cell walls to a staining procedure.

1884 Pasteur and coworkers publish a paper titled *A New Communication on Rabies.* Pasteur proves that the causal agent of rabies can be attenuated and that the weakened virus can be used as a vaccine to prevent the disease. This work serves as the basis of future work on virus attenuation, vaccine development, and the concept that variation is an inherent characteristic of viruses.

1885 Francis Galton (1822–1911) devises a new statistical tool, the correlation table.

1885 Pasteur inoculates a boy, Joseph Meister, against rabies. Meister had been bitten by a dog infected with rabies, and the treatment saved his life. This is the first time Pasteur uses an attenuated (weakened) germ on a human being.

1885 Russian hematologist Antonin Filatov makes the first formal description of mononucleosis.

1885 Theodor Escherich (1857–1911), German-Austrian pediatrician, identifies a bacterium inhabiting the human intestinal tract that he names *Bacterium coli* and shows that the bacterium causes infant diarrhea and gastroenteritis. The bacterium is subsequently named *Escherichia coli.*

1886 Italian physician Camillo Golgi (c. 1843–1926) describes two forms of malaria, with fever occurring every two and every three days, respectively.

1887 Julius Richard Petri (1852–1921), German microbiologist, develops a culture dish that has a lid to exclude airborne contaminants. The innovation is subsequently termed the Petri dish.

1888 Galton publishes *Natural Inheritance*, considered a landmark in the establishment of biometry and statistical studies of variation. Galton also proposes the Law of Ancestral Inheritance, a statistical description of the relative contributions to heredity made by previous generations.

1888 Martinus Wilhelm Beijerinck (1851–1931), Dutch botanist, uses a growth medium enriched with certain nutrients to isolate the bacteria *Rhizobium*, demonstrating that nutritionally tailored growth media are useful in bacterial isolation.

1888 The diphtheria toxin is discovered by French physician Émile Roux (1853–1933) and French bacteriologist Alexandre Yersin (1863–1943).

1888 The Institute Pasteur is formed in France.

1890 Emil von Behring (1854–1917), German bacteriologist, uses his new discovery of antitoxins to develop an antitoxin for diphtheria—a disease that usually brought death to the children it attacked.

1891 First child is treated with the diphtheria antitoxin.

1891 Ehrlich discovers that methyl blue dye immobilizes malaria bacterium and begins searching for other, more potent microbial dyes.

1891 Ehrlich proposes that antibodies are responsible for immunity.

1891 Prussian State dictates that even jailed prisoners must give consent prior to treatment (for tuberculosis).

1891 Koch proposes the concept of delayed type hypersensitivity.

1892 Dmitry Ivanovsky (1864–1920), Russian microbiologist, demonstrates that filterable material causes tobacco mosaic disease. The infectious agent is subsequently showed to be the tobacco mosaic virus. Ivanovsky's discovery heralds the field of virology.

1892 First vaccine for diphtheria becomes available.

1892 Neisser, the discoverer of gonorrhea bacteria, injects human subjects with syphilis, prompting debate and leading to regulations on human experimentation.

1892 German physician Richard Pfeiffer (1858–1945) discovers *Haemophilius influenzae*, a cause of both pneumonia and influenza.

1894 Yersin isolates *Yersinia (Pasteurella) pestis*, the bacterium responsible for bubonic plague.

1894 German physicist Wilhelm Conrad Röntgen, 1845–1923) discovers X-rays.

1895 German chemist Heinrich Dreser (1860–1924), working for the Bayer Company in Germany, produces a drug he thought to be as effective an analgesic as morphine, but without its harmful side effects. Bayer begins mass production of diacetylmorphine and in 1898 markets the new drug under the brand name "heroin" as a cough sedative.

1896 Edmund Beecher Wilson (1856–1939), American zoologist, publishes the first edition of his highly influential treatise *The Cell in Development and Heredity.* Wilson calls attention to the relationship between chromosomes and sex determination.

1896 William Joseph Dibdin (1850–1925), English engineer, and his colleague improve the sewage disposal systems in England with the introduction of a bacterial system of water purification. These improvements greatly reduce the number of waterborne diseases such as cholera and typhoid fever.

1897 American physician William Welch describes and names *Plasmodium falciparum*, a protozoan parasite and cause of malaria.

1898 First state-run sanatorium for tuberculosis in the United States opens in Massachusetts.

1898 Loeffler and German bacteriologist Paul Frosch (1860–1928) publish their *Report on Foot-and-Mouth Disease*. They prove that this animal disease is caused by a filterable virus and suggest that similar agents might cause other diseases.

1898 Beijerinck discovers and names the causative agent of the tobacco mosaic disease. He describes it as a new type of microscopically visible organism that eventually comes to be known as a virus.

1898 The First International Congress of Genetics is held in London.

1898 The transmission of plague by flea-infested rodents is shown by French bacteriologist Paul-Louis Simond (1858–1947).

1899 A meeting to organize the Society of American Bacteriologists is held at Yale University. The society will later become the American Society for Microbiology.

1899 George Henry Falkiner Nuttall (1862–1937), American biologist, first summarizes the role of insects, arachnids, and myriapods as transmitters of bacterial and parasitic diseases.

1899 Start of the sixth cholera pandemic, which affects the Far East, apart from sporadic outbreaks in parts of Europe.

1900 Austrian biologist Karl Landsteiner (1868–1943) discovers the blood-agglutination phenomenon and the four major blood types in humans.

1900 Pandemic plague becomes widely disseminated throughout the world, reaching Europe, North and South America, India, the Middle East, Africa, and Australia.

1900 Ehrlich proposes the theory concerning the formation of antibodies by the immune system.

1900 Walter Reed (1851–1902), American surgeon, discovers that the yellow fever virus is transmitted to humans by a mosquito. This is the first demonstration of a viral cause of a human disease.

1901 Joseph Everett Dutton (1874–1905), English physician, and his colleague J. L. Todd discover the parasite *Trypanosoma gambiense* that is responsible for African sleeping sickness.

1902 Ronald Ross (1857–1932), a British officer with the Indian Medical Service, receives the Nobel Prize for identifying mosquitoes as the transmitter of malaria.

1904 Ehrlich discovers a microbial dye called trypan red that helps destroy the trypanosomes that cause such diseases as sleeping sickness. This is the first such active agent against trypanosomes (parasitic protozoa).

1905 Fritz Richard Schaudinn (1871–1906), German zoologist, discovers *Treponema pallidum*, the organism or parasite causing syphilis. His discovery of this almost invisible parasite is due to his consummate technique and staining methods.

1905 Jules Bordet (1870–1961), Belgian bacteriologist, and his colleague, Octave Gengou (1875–1957), discover the bacillus of whooping cough (*B. pertussis*). Bordet goes on to discover a method of immunization against this dreaded childhood disease.

1906 Charles Nicolle (1866–1936) of the Pasteur Institute in Paris shows a link between typhus and lice.

1906 The Pure Food and Drugs Act is passed in the United States, beginning the organization that would become the Food and Drug Administration (FDA).

1906 Viennese physician Clemens von Pirquet (1874–1929) coins the term *allergy* to describe the immune reaction to certain compounds.

1907 Laveran identifies malaria parasites (protozoa) in blood.

1907 Charles Franklin Craig (1872–1950), American physician, and Percy Moreau Ashburn (1872–1940), American surgeon, work in the Philippines and are the first to prove that dengue fever (also called breakbone fever) is caused by a virus.

1907 Clemens Peter Pirquet von Cesenatico (1874–1929), Austrian physician, first introduces the cutaneous, or skin, reaction test for the diagnosis of tuberculosis.

1907 English biologist William Bateson (1861–1926) urges his colleagues to adopt the term *genetics* to indicate the importance of the new science of heredity.

1909 Sigurd Orla-Jensen (1870–1949) proposes that the physiological reactions of bacteria are primarily important in their classification.

1909 American zoologist and geneticist Thomas Hunt Morgan (1866–1945) selects the fruit fly *Drosophila* as a model system for the study of genetics. Morgan and his coworkers confirm the chromosome theory of heredity and realize the significance of the fact that certain genes tend to be transmitted together. Morgan postulates the mechanism of "crossing over." His associate, Alfred Henry Sturtevant (1891–1970) demonstrates the relationship between crossing over and the rearrangement of genes in 1913.

1909 Walter Reed General Hospital opens in Washington, D.C.

1909 Danish botanist Wilhelm Johannsen (1857–1927) argues the necessity of distinguishing between the appearance of an organism and its genetic constitution. He invents the terms *gene* (carrier of heredity), *genotype* (an organism's genetic constitution), and *phenotype* (the appearance of the actual organism).

1910 Howard Taylor Ricketts (1871–1910), discoverer of the *Rickettsia* genus of bacteria, dies of the *Rickettsia*-caused disease typhus while investigating an outbreak in Mexico City.

1910 Ehrlich announces his discovery of an effective treatment for syphilis. He names this new drug Salvarsan (now arsphenamine). His discovery marks the first chemotherapeutic agent for a bacterial disease.

1911 The first known retrovirus, Rous sarcoma virus, is discovered by Peyton Rous (1879–1970), who also showed that the virus could induce cancer.

1912 The United States Public Health Service is established.

1913 Béla Schick (18771967) designs a skin test that determines immunity to diphtheria.

1914 Frederick William Twort (1877–1950), English bacteriologist, and Felix H. D'Herelle (1873–1949), Canadian-Russian physician, independently discover bacteriophage, viruses that destroy bacteria.

1915 A typhus epidemic in Serbia causes 150,000 deaths.

1915 Stanislaus von Prowazek (1875–1915), Czech parasitologist, dies of typhus when investigating an outbreak in a Russian prisoner of war camp, having identified *R. prowazekii*, the causative agent.

1915 US Public Health Office allows induction of pellagra in Mississippi prisoners.

1916 D'Herelle carries out further studies of the agent that destroys bacterial colonies and gives it the name bacteriophage (bacteria-eating agent). D'Herelle and others unsuccessfully attempt to use bacteriophages as bactericidal therapeutic agents.

1917 D'Arcy Wentworth Thompson (1860–1948) publishes *On Growth and Form*, which suggests that the evolution of one species into another occurs as a series of transformations involving the entire organism rather than a succession of minor changes in parts of the body.

1918 Global influenza pandemic kills more people than numbers of soldiers who died fighting during World War I (1914–1918). By the end of 1918, more than 25 million people die from virulent strain of Spanish influenza.

1918 American geneticist Thomas Hunt Morgan (1866–1945) and coworkers publish *The Physical Basis of Heredity*, a survey of the remarkable development of the new science of genetics.

1919 James Brown uses blood agar to study the destruction of blood cells by the bacterium *Streptococcus*. He observes three reactions that he designates alpha, beta, and gamma.

1919 The Health Organization of the League of Nations was established for the prevention and control of disease around the world.

1920 Data on diphtheria is gathered for the first time in the United States, showing approximately 13,000 deaths per year.

1920 Sprunt and Evans coined the term *infectious mononucleosis*, as they described the abnormal mononuclear leukocytes observed in patients with the condition.

1921 Otto Loewi (1873–1961), German American physiologist, discovers that acetylcholine functions as a neurotransmitter. It is the first such brain chemical to be so identified.

1922 British parasitologist John Stephens (1865–1946) describes *P. ovale*.

1924 Albert Jan Kluyver (1888–1956), Dutch microbiologist and biochemist, publishes *Unity and Diversity in the Metabolism of Microorganisms*. He demonstrates that different microorganisms have common metabolic pathways of oxidation, fermentation, and synthesis of certain compounds. Kluyver also states that life on Earth depends on microbial activity.

1924 The last urban epidemic of plague in the United States begins in Los Angeles.

1926 American chemist James B. Sumner (1887–1955) publishes a report on the isolation of the enzyme urease and his proof that the enzyme is a protein. This idea is controversial until 1930 when American biochemist John Howard Northrop (1891– 1987) confirms Sumner's ideas by crystallizing pepsin. Sumner, Northrop, and Wendell Meredith Stanley (1904–1971) ultimately share the Nobel Prize in Chemistry in 1946.

1927 Thomas Rivers (1888–1962), American bacteriologist and virologist, publishes a paper that differentiates bacteria from viruses, establishing virology as a field of study that is distinct from bacteriology.

1928 British bacteriologist Frederick Griffith (1877–1941) discovers that certain strains of pneumococci could undergo some kind of transmutation of type. After injecting mice with living R type pneumococci and heat-killed S type, Griffith is able to isolate living virulent bacteria from the infected mice. Griffith suggests that some unknown "principle" had transformed the harmless R strain of the pneumococcus to the virulent S strain.

1928 Philip (1894–1972) and Cecil Drinker (1887–1958) of Harvard School of Public Health introduce the "iron lung" for treatment of paralytic polio.

1928 Scottish biochemist Alexander Fleming (1881–1955) discovers penicillin. In his published report (1929), Fleming observes that the mold *Penicillium notatum* inhibits the growth of some bacteria. This is the first antibacterial, and it opens a new era of "wonder drugs."

1929 Fleming publishes his account of the bacteriolytic power of penicillin.

1929 Scientist Francis O. Holmes introduces the technique of "local lesion" as a means of measuring the concentration of tobacco mosaic virus. The method becomes extremely important in virus purification.

1929 Willard Myron Allen (1904–1993), American physician, and George Washington Corner (1889–1981), American anatomist, discover progesterone. They demonstrate that it is necessary for the maintenance of pregnancy.

1930 Max Theiler (1899–1972), South African–born American virologist, demonstrates the advantages of using mice as experimental animals for research on animal viruses. Theiler uses mice in his studies of the yellow fever virus.

1930 British geneticist Ronald A. Fisher (1890–1962) publishes *Genetical Theory of Natural Selection*, a formal analysis of the mathematics of selection.

1930 United States Food, Drug, and Insecticide Administration is renamed the Food and Drug Administration (FDA).

1932 At Tuskegee, Alabama, African American sharecroppers become unknowing and unwilling subjects of experimentation on the untreated natural course of syphilis. Even after penicillin came into use in the 1940s, the men remained untreated.

1932 William J. Elford (1900–1952) and Christopher H. Andrewes (1896–1988) develop methods of estimating the sizes of viruses by using a series of membranes as filters. Later studies prove that the viral sizes obtained by this method were comparable to those obtained by electron microscopy.

1933 "Regulation on New Therapy and Experimentation" decreed in Germany.

1934 Discovery of chloroquine is announced by scientist Hans Andersag (1902–1955) at Bayer in Germany.

1934 J. B. S. Haldane (1892–1964), British geneticist, presents the first calculations of the spontaneous mutation frequency of a human gene.

1934 John Marrack (1886–1976) begins a series of studies that leads to the formation of the hypothesis governing the association between an antigen and the corresponding antibody.

1935 Wendall Meredith Stanley (1904–1971), American biochemist, discovers that viruses are partly protein-based. By purifying and crystallizing viruses, he enables scientists to identify the precise molecular structure and propagation modes of several viruses.

1936 George P. Berry (1898–1986) and Helen M. Dedrick report that the Shope virus could be "transformed" into myxomatosis/Sanarelli virus. This virological curiosity was variously referred to as "transformation," "recombination," and "multiplicity of reactivation." Subsequent research suggests that it is the first example of genetic interaction between animal viruses, but some scientists warn that the phenomenon might indicate the danger of reactivation of virus particles in vaccines and in cancer research.

1937 American researcher H. R. Cox (1907–1986) cultures *Rickettsiae* in the yolks of fertilized hens' eggs, opening the door to research into a vaccine.

1938 American biochemist Emory L. Ellis (1906–2003) and German American biophysicist Max Delbrück (1906–1981) perform studies on phage replication that mark the beginning of modern phage work. They introduce the "one-step growth" experiment, which demonstrates that, after bacteriophages attack bacteria, replication of the virus occurs within the bacterial host during a "latent period," after which viral progeny are released in a "burst."

1939 Ernest Chain (1906–1979), German-born British biochemist, and Howard Florey (1898–1968), Australian pathologist and pharmacologist, refine the purification of penicillin, allowing the mass production of the antibiotic.

1939 Swiss chemist Paul Müller (1899–1965) discovers the insecticidal properties of DDT.

1939 American virologist Richard E. Shope (1901–1966) reports that the swine influenza virus survived between epidemics in an intermediate host. This discovery is an important step in revealing the role of intermediate hosts in perpetuating specific diseases.

1941 American scientists George W. Beadle (1903–1989) and Edward L. Tatum (1909–1975) publish their classic study on the biochemical genetics titled *Genetic Control of Biochemical Reactions in Neurospora*. Beadle and Tatum irradiate red bread mold *Neurospora* and prove that genes produce their effects by regulating particular enzymes. This work leads to the one-gene-one-enzyme theory.

1941 Norman M. Gregg (1892–1966) of Australia discovers that rubella (German measles) during pregnancy can cause congenital abnormalities. Children of mothers who had rubella during their pregnancy are found to suffer from blindness, deafness, and heart disease.

1941 The term *antibiotic* is coined by Russian American microbiologist Selman Waksman (1888–1973).

1942 Jules Freund (1890–1960) and Katherine McDermott identify adjuvants (e.g., paraffin oil) that act to boost antibody production.

1942 Italian microbiologist Salvador E. Luria (1912–1991) and Delbrück demonstrate statistically that inheritance of genetic characteristics in bacteria follows the principles of genetic inheritance proposed by Darwin. For their work, the two, along with American bacteriologist Alfred Day Hershey (1908–1997), are awarded the 1969 Nobel Prize in Medicine or Physiology.

1942 Neil Hamilton Fairley (1891–1966), Australian physician, wins a Fellowship to the Royal Society for work on anemia caused by the rupture of red blood cells in malaria.

1943 At University of Cincinnati Hospital, experiments are performed using mentally disabled patients.

1943 Penicillin starts to become available as a therapy for Allied troops.

1944 Oswald T. Avery (1877–1955), Colin M. MacLeod (1909–1972), and Maclyn McCarty (1911–2005) publish a landmark paper on the pneumococcus transforming principle. The paper is titled "Studies on the Chemical Nature of the Substance Inducing Transformation of Pneumococcal Types." Avery suggests that the transforming principle seems to be deoxyribonucleic acid (DNA), but contemporary ideas about the structure of nucleic acids suggest that DNA does not possess the biological specificity of the hypothetical genetic material.

1944 Waksman introduces streptomycin.

1944 To combat battle fatigue during World War II (1939–1945), nearly 200 million amphetamine tablets are issued to American soldiers stationed in Great Britain during the war.

1944 The United States Public Health Service Act is passed.

1944 University of Chicago Medical School professor Alf Alving conducts malaria experiments on more than 400 Illinois prisoners.

1945 Joshua Lederberg (1925–2008) and Tatum demonstrate genetic recombination in bacteria.

1946 Physicists Felix Bloch (1905–1983) and Edward Mills Purcell (1912–1997) develop nuclear magnetic resonance (NMR) as a viable tool for observation and analysis.

1946 American geneticist Hermann J. Muller (1890–1967) is awarded the Nobel Prize in Medicine or Physiology for his contributions to radiation genetics.

1946 Delbrück and W. T. Bailey Jr. publish a paper titled "Induced Mutations in Bacterial Viruses." Despite some confusion about the nature of the phenomenon in question, this paper establishes the fact that genetic recombinations occur during mixed infections with bacterial viruses. Hershey and American scientist R. Rotman make the discovery of genetic recombination in bacteriophage simultaneously and independently. Hershey and his colleagues prove that this phenomenon can be used for genetic analyses. They construct a genetic map of phage particles and show that phage genes can be arranged in a linear fashion.

1946 Nazi physicians and scientists are tried by international court at Nuremberg, Germany.

1947 Four years after the mass production and use of penicillin, microbial resistance is detected.

1947 Nuremberg Code is issued regarding voluntary consent of human subjects.

1948 American scientist Barbara McClintock (1902–1992) publishes her research on transposable regulatory elements ("jumping genes") in maize. Her work was not appreciated until similar phenomena were discovered in bacteria and fruit flies in the 1960s and 1970s. McClintock was awarded the Nobel Prize in Physiology or Medicine in 1983.

1948 Chloramphenicol and tetracycline are shown to be effective treatments for typhus.

1948 James V. Neel (1915–2000), American geneticist, reports evidence that the sickle-cell disease is inherited as a simple Mendelian autosomal recessive trait.

1948 The World Health Organization (WHO) is formed. WHO subsequently becomes the principle international organization managing public health–related issues on a global scale. Headquartered in Geneva, Switzerland, by 2002 WHO becomes an organization of more than 190 member countries. It contributes to international public health in areas including disease prevention and control, promotion of good health, addressing disease outbreaks, initiatives to eliminate diseases (e.g., vaccination programs), and development of treatment and prevention standards.

1949 John F. Enders (1897–1985), Thomas H. Weller (1915–2008), and Frederick C.

Robbins (1916–2003) publish "Cultivation of Polio Viruses in Cultures of Human Embryonic Tissues." The report by is a landmark in establishing techniques for the cultivation of poliovirus in cultures on non-neural tissue and for further virus research. The technique leads to the polio vaccine and other advances in virology.

1949 Macfarlane Burnet (1899–1985), Australian virologist, and his colleagues begin studies that lead to the immunological tolerance hypothesis and the clonal selection theory. Burnet receives the 1960 Nobel Prize in Physiology or Medicine for this research.

1950 Dr. Joseph Stokes of the University of Pennsylvania infects 200 women prisoners with viral hepatitis.

1950 American microbial ecologist Robert Hungate (1906–2004) develops the roll-tube culture technique, which is the first technique that allows anaerobic bacteria to be grown in culture.

1951 Esther M. Lederberg (1922–2006), American microbiologist, discovers a lysogenic strain of *Escherichia coli* K12 and isolates a new bacteriophage called lambda.

1951 Rosalind Franklin (1920–1958), English chemist, obtains sharp X-ray diffraction photographs of deoxyribonucleic acid (DNA).

1951 The eradication of malaria from the United States is announced.

1951 University of Pennsylvania under contract with US Army conducts psychopharmacological experiments on hundreds of Pennsylvania prisoners.

1952 Hershey and American biologist Martha Chase (1927–2003) publish their landmark paper "Independent Functions of Viral Protein and Nucleic Acid in Growth of Bacteriophage." The famous "blender experiment" suggests that DNA is the genetic material.

1952 James T. Park and Jack L. Strominger (1925–) demonstrate that penicillin blocks the synthesis of the peptidoglycan of bacteria. This represents the first demonstration of the action of a natural antibiotic.

1952 Karl Maramorosch (1915–2016), Austrian-born American virologist, demonstrates that some viruses can multiply in both plants and insects. This work leads to new questions about the origins of viruses.

1952 Joshua and Esther Lederberg develop the replica plating method that allows for the rapid screening of large numbers of genetic markers. They use the technique to demonstrate that resistance to antibacterial agents such as antibiotics and viruses is not induced by the presence of the antibacterial agent.

1952 Polio peaks in the United States, with 57,268 cases recorded.

1952 Italian American virologist Renato Dulbecco (1914–2012) develops a practical method for studying animal viruses in cell cultures. His so-called plaque method is comparable to that used in studies of bacterial viruses, and the method proves to be important in genetic studies of viruses. These methods are described in his paper "Production of Plaques in Monolayer Tissue Cultures by Single Particles of an Animal Virus."

1952 Franklin completes a series of X-ray crystallography studies of two forms of DNA. Her colleague, Maurice Wilkins (1916–2004), gives information about her work to James Watson (1928–).

1952 Waksmanis awarded the Nobel Prize in Physiology or Medicine for his discovery of streptomycin, the first antibiotic effective against tuberculosis.

1952 William G. Gochenour demonstrates that pretibial fever (also called Fort Bragg Fever) is not caused by a virus but rather is an infection caused by a microorganism called *Leptospira*.

1952 William Hayes isolates a strain of *E. coli* that produces recombinants thousands of times more frequently than previously observed. The new strain of K12 is named Hfr (high-frequency recombination) by Hayes.

1953 Watson and British molecular biologist Francis Crick (1916–2004) publish two landmark papers in the journal *Nature*: "Molecular Structure of Nucleic Acids: A Structure for Deoxyribonucleic Acid," and "Genetical Implications of the Structure of Deoxyribonucleic Acid." Watson and Crick propose a double helical model for DNA and call attention to the genetic implications of their model. Their model is based, in part, on the X-ray crystallographic work of Franklin and the biochemical work of Erwin Chargaff (1905–2002). Their model explains how the genetic material is transmitted.

1953 Jonas Salk (1914–1995), American virologist, begins testing a polio vaccine composed of a mixture of killed viruses.

1954 Enders, Weller, and Robbins receive the Nobel Prize in Physiology or Medicine for their work on poliovirus

1954 Enders and Thomas Peebles (1921–2010), American pediatrician, develop the first vaccine for measles. A truly practical and successful vaccine requires more time.

1954 Salk produces the first successful anti-poliomyelitis vaccine, which prevents paralytic polio. It is soon (1955) followed by the development of the first oral vaccine by Polish American virologist Albert Bruce Sabin (1906–1993).

1954 Weller isolated the varicella zoster virus from chickenpox lesions.

1955 Fred L. Schaffer and Carlton E. Schwerdt report on their successful crystallization of the polio virus. Their achievement is the first successful crystallization of an animal virus.

1955 Salk's inactivated polio vaccine is approved for use.

1955 National Institutes of Health organizes a Division of Biologics Control within the FDA following death from faulty polio vaccine.

1956 Alfred Gierer and Gerhard Schramm demonstrate that naked RNA from tobacco mosaic virus is infectious. Subsequently, infectious RNA preparations are obtained for certain animal viruses.

1956 Niels Kaj Jerne (1911–1994), Danish-English immunologist, proposes the clonal selection theory of antibody selection to explain how white blood cells are able to produce a large range of antibodies.

1956 Researchers start hepatitis experiments on mentally disabled children at the Willowbrook State School.

1957 Alick Isaacs (1921–1967), Scottish virologist, demonstrates that antibodies act only against bacteria. This means that antibodies are not one of the body's natural forms of defense against viruses. This knowledge eventually leads to the discovery of interferon this same year by Isaacs and his colleague Jean Lindenmann (1924–2015) of Switzerland. They find that the generation of a small amount of protein is the body's first line of defense against a virus.

1957 Isaacs and Lindenmann publish their pioneering report on the drug interferon, a protein produced by interaction between a virus and an infected cell that can interfere with the multiplication of viruses.

1957 French biologist François Jacob (1920–2013) and French microbial geneticist Élie Wollman (1917–2008) demonstrate that the single linkage group of *Escherichia coli* is circular and suggest that the different linkage groups found in different Hfr strains result from the insertion at different points of a factor in the circular linkage group that determines the rupture of the circle.

1957 The World Health Organization advances the oral polio vaccine developed by Sabin as a safer alternative to the Salk vaccine.

1958 Beadle, Tatum, and Joshua Lederberg are awarded the Nobel Prize in Physiology or Medicine. Beadle and Tatum were honored for the work in *Neurospora* that led to the one-gene-one-enzyme theory. Lederberg was honored for discoveries concerning genetic recombination and the organization of the genetic material of bacteria.

1958 American geneticist and molecular biologists Matthew Meselson (1930–) and

Franklin Stahl (1929–) publish their landmark paper "The Replication of DNA in *Escherichia coli,*" which demonstrated that the replication of DNA follow the semiconservative model.

1959 Sabin announces successful results from testing live attenuated polio vaccine. His vaccine eventually is preferred over the Salk vaccine, because it can be administered orally and offers protection with a single dose.

1959 English biochemist Rodney Porter (1917–1985) begins studies that lead to the discovery of the structure of antibodies. Porter receives the 1972 Nobel Prize in Physiology or Medicine for this research.

1959 American biologist Robert L. Sinsheimer reports that bacteriophage ÛX174, which infects *Escherichia coli*, contains a single-stranded DNA molecule rather than the expected double-stranded DNA. This provides the first example of a single-stranded DNA genome.

1959 Sydney Brenner (1927–) and Robert W. Horne publish a paper titled "A Negative Staining Method for High Resolution Electron Microscopy of Viruses." The two researchers develop a method for studying the architecture of viruses at the molecular level using the electron microscope.

1961 Crick, Brenner, and others propose that a molecule called transfer RNA uses a three-base code in the manufacture of proteins.

1961 French pathologist Jacques Miller (1931–) discovers the role of the thymus in cellular immunity.

1961 Jewish American biochemist and geneticist Marshall Warren Nirenberg (1927–2010) synthesizes a polypeptide using an artificial messenger RNA (a synthetic RNA containing only the base uracil) in a cell-free protein-synthesizing system. The resulting polypeptide only contains the amino acid phenylalanine, indicating that UUU was the codon for phenylalanine. This important step in deciphering the genetic code is described in the landmark paper by Nirenberg and German biochemist J. Heinrich Matthaei (1929–), "The Dependence of Cell-Free Synthesis in *E. coli* upon Naturally Occurring or Synthetic Polyribonucleotides." This work establishes the messenger concept and a system that could be used to work out the relationship between the sequence of nucleotides in the genetic material and amino acids in the gene product.

1961 Noel Warner establishes the physiological distinction between the cellular and humoral immune responses.

1962 Watson, Crick, and Wilkins are awarded the Nobel Prize in Physiology or Medicine for their work in elucidating the structure of DNA.

1962 United States Congress passes Kefauver-Harris Drug Amendments that shift the burden of proof of clinical safety to drug manufacturers. For the first time drug manufacturers had to prove their products were safe and effective before they could be sold.

1963 Sabin's live polio vaccine is approved for use.

1964 British pathologist Michael Epstein (1921–) and Irish virologist Yvonne Barr (1921–2016) discover the Epstein-Barr virus that is the cause of mononucleosis.

1964 Retrovir is developed as a cancer treatment. While not useful for cancer, the drug subsequently becomes the first drug approved for the treatment of acquired immunodeficiency syndrome (AIDS).

1964 World Medical Association adopts Helsinki Declaration.

1965 Anthrax vaccine adsorbed (AVA) is approved for use in the United States.

1965 Jacob, André Lwoff (1902–1994), and Jacques Monod (1910–1976) are awarded the Nobel Prize in Physiology or Medicine for their discoveries concerning genetic control of enzymes and virus synthesis.

1966 Bruce Ames (1928–), American biochemist, develops a test to screen for compounds that cause mutations, including those that are cancer causing. The so-called Ames test utilizes the bacterium *Salmonella typhimurium.*

1966 Daniel Carleton Gajdusek (1923–2008), American pediatrician, transfers for the first time a viral disease of the central nervous system from humans to another species. The viral disease kuru is found in New Guinea and is spread by the ritual eating of the deceased's brains.

1966 FDA and National Academy of Sciences begin investigation of effectiveness of drugs previously approved because they were thought safe.

1966 Nirenberg and Har Gobind Khorana (1922–2011) lead teams that decipher the genetic code. All of the 64 possible triplet combinations of the four bases (the codons) and their associated amino acids are determined and described.

1966 Merck, Sharp, and Dohme Laboratories began research into a varicella-zoster vaccine.

1966 *New England Journal of Medicine* article exposes unethical Tuskegee syphilis study.

1966 NIH Office for Protection of Research Subjects ("OPRR") is created.

1966 Paul D. Parman and Harry M. Myer Jr. develop a live-virus rubella vaccine.

1967 A hemorrhagic fever outbreak in Marburg, Germany, occurs. The virus responsible is subsequently named the marburg virus, and the disease is called marburg hemorrhagic fever.

1967 British physician Maurice Henry Pappworth (1910–1994) publishes "Human Guinea Pigs," advising that "no doctor has the right to choose martyrs for science or for the general good."

1968 FDA administratively moves to Public Health Service.

1968 American molecular biologist Mark Ptashne (1940–) and biochemist Walter Gilbert (1932–) independently identify the bacteriophage genes that are the repressors of the lac operon.

1968 Robert W. Holley (1922–1993), Khorana, and Nirenberg are awarded the Nobel Prize in Physiology or Medicine for their interpretation of the genetic code and its function in protein synthesis.

1968 Werner Arber (1929–), Swiss microbiologist, discovers that bacteria defend themselves against viruses by producing DNA-cutting enzymes. These enzymes quickly become important tools for molecular biologists.

1969 By Executive Order, the United States renounces first use of biological weapons and restricts future weapons research programs to issues concerning defensive responses (e.g., immunization, detection, etc.).

1969 Jonathan R. Beckwith (1935–), American molecular biologist, and colleagues isolate a single gene.

1969 Delbrück, Hershey, and Luria are awarded the Nobel Prize in Physiology or Medicine for their discoveries concerning the replication mechanism and the genetic structure of viruses.

1969 US Surgeon General William Stewart (1921–2008) announces, "The time has come to close the book on infectious diseases."

1970 First outbreak of drug-resistant tuberculosis recorded in the United States.

1970 American geneticist Howard Martin Temin (1934–1994) and American biologist David Baltimore (1938–) independently discover reverse transcriptase in viruses. Reverse transcriptase is an enzyme that catalyzes the transcription of RNA into DNA.

1972 Biological and Toxin Weapons Convention (BWC) is signed. BWC prohibits the offensive weaponization of biological agents (e.g., anthrax spores). It also prohibits the transformation of biological agents with established legitimate and sanctioned purposes into agents of a nature and quality that could be used to effectively induce illness or death.

1972 Introduction of amoxicillin, a drug related to penicillin, which is a treatment of choice for bacterial pneumonia.

1972 Michiaka Takahashi (1928–2013), Japanese virologist, isolates the varicella virus from a three-year-old patient and named it

Oka, after the patient's name. The isolated virus is later used by Merck to develop a vaccine.

1972 Paul Berg (1926–) and researcher Herbert Boyer (1936–) produce the first recombinant DNA molecules.

1972 Recombinant technology emerges as one of the most powerful techniques of molecular biology. Scientists can splice together pieces of DNA to form recombinant genes. As the potential uses, therapeutic and industrial, became increasingly clear, scientists and venture capitalists establish biotechnology companies.

1973 Concerns about the possible hazards posed by recombinant DNA technologies, especially work with tumor viruses, leads to the establishment of a meeting at Asilomar, California. The proceedings of this meeting are subsequently published by the Cold Spring Harbor Laboratory as a book titled *Biohazards in Biological Research.*

1973 Boyer and Stanley Cohen (1922–) create recombinant genes by cutting DNA molecules with restriction enzymes. These experiments mark the beginning of genetic engineering.

1974 National Research Act establishes "The Common Rule" for protection of human subjects.

1974 Peter C. Doherty (1940–) and Rolf Zinkernagel (1944–) discover the basis of immune determination of self and nonself.

1975 César Milstein (1927–2002), Argentinian biochemist, and Georges J. F. Köhler (1946–1995), German immunologist, create monoclonal antibodies.

1975 Baltimore, Dulbecco, and Temin share the Nobel Prize in Physiology or Medicine for their discoveries concerning the interaction between tumor viruses and the genetic material of the cell and the discovery of reverse transcriptase.

1975 HHS promulgates Title 45 of Federal Regulations titled "Protection of Human Subjects," requiring appointment and utilization of Institutional Review Board (IRB).

1976 First outbreak of Ebola virus observed in Zaire, resulting in more than 300 cases with a 90 percent death rate.

1976 Swine flu outbreaks identified in soldiers stationed in New Jersey. Virus identified as H1N1 virus causes concern due to its similarities to H1N1 responsible for Spanish Flu pandemic. President Gerald Ford (1913–2006) calls for emergency vaccination program. More than 20 deaths result from Guillain-Barre syndrome related to the vaccine.

1977 Carl R. Woese (1928–2012) and George E. Fox (1945–) publish an account of the discovery of a third major branch of living beings, the Archaea. Woese suggests that an rRNA database could be used to generate phylogenetic trees.

1977 Earliest known AIDS victims in the United States are two homosexual men in New York who are diagnosed as suffering from Kaposi's sarcoma.

1977 Frederick Sanger (1918–2013), British biochemist, develops the chain termination (dideoxy) method for sequencing DNA and uses the method to sequence the genome of a microorganism.

1977 The first known human fatality from H5N1 avian flu occurs in Hong Kong.

1977 The last reported smallpox case is recorded. Ultimately, WHO declares the disease eradicated.

1979 National Commission issues Belmont Report.

1979 The last case of wild poliovirus infection is recorded in the United States.

1980 Congress passes the Bayh-Dole Act. The act is amended by the Technology Transfer Act in 1986.

1980 In *Diamond v. Chakrabarty*, the US Supreme Court rules that a genetically modified bacterium can be patented.

1980 Researchers successfully introduce a human gene, which codes for the protein interferon, into a bacterium.

1980 The FDA promulgates 21 CFR 50.44, prohibiting the use of prisoners as subjects in clinical trials.

1981 AIDS is officially recognized by the US Centers for Disease Control and Prevention (CDC), and the first clinical description of this disease is made. It soon becomes recognized that AIDS is an infectious disease caused by a virus that spreads virtually exclusively by infected blood or body fluids.

1981 First disease-causing human retrovirus, human T-cell leukemia virus, is discovered.

1981 The first cases of AIDS are reported among previously healthy young men in Los Angeles and New York presenting with *Pneumocystis carinii* pneumonia and Kaposi's sarcoma.

1982 FDA approves the first genetically engineered drug, a form of human insulin produced by bacteria.

1983 *Escherichia coli* O157:H7 is identified as a human pathogen.

1983 Luc Montagnier (1932–), French virologist, and Robert Gallo (1937–), American biomedical researcher, discover the human immunodeficiency virus (HIV) that causes AIDS.

1984 Jerne, Kohler, and Milstein are awarded the Nobel Prize in Physiology or Medicine for theories concerning the specificity in development and control of the immune system and the discovery of the principle for production of monoclonal antibodies.

1984 WHO begins a program to control trypanosomiasis.

1985 British geneticist Alec Jeffreys (1950–) develops "genetic fingerprinting," a method of using DNA polymorphisms (unique sequences of DNA) to identify individuals. The method, which has been used in paternity, immigration, and murder cases, is generally referred to as "DNA fingerprinting."

1985 First vaccine for *H. influenzae* type B is licensed for use.

1985 Japanese molecular biologist Susumu Tonegawa (1939–) discovers the genes that code for immunoglobulins. He receives the 1986 Nobel Prize in Physiology or Medicine for this discovery.

1985 American biochemist Kary Mullis (1944–), while working at Cetus Corporation, develops the polymerase chain reaction (PCR), a new method of amplifying DNA. This technique quickly becomes one of the most powerful tools of molecular biology. Cetus patents PCR and sells the patent to Hoffman-LaRoche Inc. in 1991.

1986 Congress passes the National Childhood Vaccine Injury Act, requiring patient information on vaccines and reporting of adverse events after vaccination.

1986 First genetically engineered vaccine approved for human use is the hepatitis B vaccine. The FDA gives its approval.

1986 First license to market a living organism that was produced by genetic engineering is granted by the US Department of Agriculture. It allows Biologics Corporation to sell a virus that is used as a vaccine against a herpes disease in pigs.

1986 International Committee on the Taxonomy of Viruses officially names the AIDS virus as HIV.

1987 An illness outbreak in Prince Edward Island, Canada, which sickens over 100 people and kills 3, leads to the first isolation and identification of domoic acid.

1987 Maynard Olson (1943–) creates and names yeast artificial chromosomes (YACs), which provides a technique to clone long segments of DNA.

1987 US Congress charters a Department of Energy (DOE) advisory committee, the Health and Environmental Research Advisory Committee (HERAC), which recommends a 15-year, multidisciplinary, scientific, and technological undertaking to map and sequence the human genome. DOE designates multidisciplinary human genome centers. National Institute of General Medical Sciences at the National Institutes of Health (NIH NIGMS) begins funding genome projects.

1988 First report of vancomycin-resistant enterococci, a type of *Streptococcus* that is resistant to almost all antibiotics.

1988 The Human Genome Organization (HUGO) is established by scientists to coordinate international efforts to sequence the human genome. The Human Genome Project officially adopts the goal of determining the entire sequence of DNA comprising the human chromosomes.

1988 WHO and its partners announce the Global Polio Eradication Initiative.

1989 Ebola-Reston virus is the source of an outbreak at an animal facility in Virginia. The outbreak becomes the basis for the best-selling book *The Hot Zone.*

1989 Sidney Altman (1939–) and Thomas R. Cech (1947–) are awarded the Nobel Prize in Chemistry for their discovery of ribozymes (RNA molecules with catalytic activity). Cech proves that RNA can function as a biocatalyst as well as an information carrier.

1990 Only 24 cases of diphtheria reported in the United States during preceding 10-year period.

1991 Cholera returns to the Western Hemisphere when an outbreak in Peru spreads to other Latin American countries.

1991 WHO announces CIOMS Guidelines (the International Ethical Guidelines for Biomedical Research Involving Human Subjects).

1992 American biochemist J. Craig Venter (1946–) establishes the Institute for Genomic Research (TIGR) in Rockville, Maryland. TIGR later sequences the genome of *Haemophilus influenzae* and many other bacterial genomes.

1993 An international research team, led by Daniel Cohen of the Center for the Study of Human Polymorphisms in Paris, produces a rough map of all 23 pairs of human chromosomes.

1993 Beginning in April, a five-week contamination of the drinking water supply of Milwaukee, Wisconsin, by *Cryptosporidium parvum* sickens 400,000 people and kills an estimated 104 people.

1993 Hanta virus emerges in the United States in a 1993 outbreak on a Native American reservation in the Four Corners area (corners of Utah, Colorado, New Mexico, and Arizona). The resulting Hanta pulmonary syndrome (HPS) has a 43 percent mortality rate.

1993 Outbreaks in Moscow and St. Petersburg mark the return of epidemic diphtheria to the Western world.

1994 AZT (zidovudine) is approved by the FDA for use in reducing maternal-fetal HIV transmission.

1994 DOE announces the establishment of the Microbial Genome Project as a spin-off of the Human Genome Project.

1994 Ebola-Ivory Coast virus is discovered.

1994 Geneticists determine that DNA repair enzymes perform several vital functions, including preserving genetic information and protecting the cell from cancer.

1994 WHO declares the Americas free of polio.

1994 WHO reports the start of epidemics of plague in Malawi, Mozambique, and India after a 15-year absence.

1995 Edward B. Lewis (1918–2004), Christiane Nüsslein-Volhard (1942–), and Eric F. Wieschaus (1947–), developmental biologists, share the Nobel Prize in Physiology or Medicine to cover discrimination based on genetic information related to illness, disease, or other conditions.

1995 Peter Funch and Reinhardt Kristensen (1948–) create a new phylum, Cycliophora, for a novel invertebrate called *Symbion pandora*, which is found living in the mouths of Norwegian lobsters.

1995 Public awareness of the potential use of chemical or biological weapons by a terrorist group increases following an attack by Aum Shinrikyo, a Japanese cult, which releases sarin gas in a Tokyo subway, killing a dozen people and sending thousands to the hospital.

1995 FDA approves the varicella-zoster vaccine developed by Merck for vaccinations of people 12 months and older.

1995 The Programme Against African Trypanosomiasis (PAAT) is created.

1995 The sequence of *Mycoplasma genitalium* is completed. *M. genitalium*, regarded as the smallest known bacterium, is considered a model of the minimum number of genes needed for independent existence.

1996 H5N1 avian flu virus is identified in Guangdong, China.

1996 International participants in the genome project meet in Bermuda and agree to formalize the conditions of data access. The agreement, known as the "Bermuda Principles," calls for the release of sequence data into public databases within 24 hours.

1996 Scientists report further evidence that individuals with two mutant copies of the CC-CLR-5 gene are generally resistant to HIV infection.

1996 William R. Bishai and coworkers report that SigF, a gene in the tuberculosis bacterium, enables the bacterium to enter a dormant stage.

1997 The DNA sequence of *Escherichia coli* is completed.

1997 William Jacobs Jr. (1955–) and Barry Bloom create a biological entity that combines the characteristics of a bacterial virus and a plasmid (a DNA structure that functions and replicates independently of the chromosomes). This entity is capable of triggering mutations in *Mycobacterium tuberculosis.*

1997 Outbreaks of highly pathogenic H5N1 influenza are reported in poultry at farms and live animal markets in Hong Kong.

1998 A live, orally administered rotavirus vaccine is approved for use in the United States. Use was discontinued in 1999 due to complications in some vaccinated children.

1998 Venter forms a company (later named Celera) and predicts that the company would decode the entire human genome within three years. Celera plans to use a "whole genome shotgun" method, which would assemble the genome without using maps. Venter says that his company would not follow the Bermuda Principles concerning data release.

1998 DOE (Office of Science) funds bacterial artificial chromosome and sequencing projects.

1998 Scientists find that an adult human's brain can, with certain stimuli, replace cells. This discovery heralds potential breakthroughs in neurology.

1998 World Health Organization reports a resurgence in tuberculosis (TB) cases worldwide. TB is killing more people than at any other point in history. Recommends Directly Observed Therapy (DOT) treatment, which is 95 percent effective in curing patients, even in developing nations.

1999 Pharmaceutical research in Japan leads to the discovery of donepezil (Aricept), the first drug intended to help ward off memory loss in Alzheimer's disease and other age-related dementias.

1999 Scientists announce the complete sequencing of the DNA making up human chromosome 22. The first complete human chromosome sequence is published in December 1999.

1999 NIH and the Office for Protection from Research Risks (OPRR) require researchers conducting or overseeing human subjects to ethics training.

1999 The public genome project responds to Venter's challenge with plans to produce a draft genome sequence by 2000. Most of the sequencing is done in five centers, known as the "G5": the Whitehead Institute for Biomedical Research in Cambridge, Massachusetts; the Sanger Centre near Cambridge, England; Baylor College of Medicine in Houston; Washington University in St. Louis; and the DOE's Joint Genome Institute (JGI) in Walnut Creek, California.

2000 On June 26, 2000, leaders of the public genome project and Celera announce the completion of a working draft of the entire human genome sequence. Ari Patrinos of the DOE helps mediate disputes between the two groups so that a fairly amicable joint announcement could be presented at the White House in Washington, D.C.

2000 Office for Protection from Research Risks (OPRR) becomes part of the Department of Health and Human Services, Office of Human Research Protection (OHRP).

2000 The federal government approves irradiation of raw meat, the only technology known to kill *E. coli* O157 bacteria while preserving the integrity of the meat.

2000 The first volume of Annual Review of *Genomics and Human Genetics* is published. Genomics is defined as the new science dealing with the identification and characterization of genes and their arrangement in chromosomes and human genetics as the science devoted to understanding the origin and expression of human individual uniqueness.

2000 The municipal water supply of Walkerton, Ontario, Canada, is contaminated in the summertime by a strain of the bacterium *Escherichia coli* O157:H7, sickening 2,000 people and killing 7.

2000 WHO declares the Western Pacific region, including China, free of polio.

2001 In February the complete draft sequence of the human genome is published. The public sequence data is published in the British journal *Nature*, and the Celera sequence is published in the American journal *Science*. Increased knowledge of the human genome allows greater specificity in pharmacological research and drug interaction studies.

2001 Microbiologists reveal that bacteria possess an internal protein structure similar to that of human cells.

2001 Researchers at Eli Lilly in Minneapolis sequence the genome of *Streptococcus pneumoniae*.

2001 Letters containing a powdered form of *Bacillus anthracis*, the bacteria that causes anthrax, are mailed to government representatives, members of the news media, and others in the United States. More than 20 cases and 5 deaths eventually result. As of August 2007, the case remains open and unsolved.

2001 The Chemical and Biological Incident Response Force (CBIRF) sends a 100-member initial response team into the Dirksen Senate Office Building in Washington alongside Environmental Protection Agency (EPA) specialists to detect and remove anthrax. A similar mission was undertaken at the Longworth House Office Building in October, when samples were collected from more than 200 office spaces.

2001 The Pan African Trypanosomiasis and Tsetse Eradication campaign (PATTEC) begins operation.

2002 Following September 11, 2001, terrorist attacks on the United States, the Public Health Security and Bioterrorism Preparedness and Response Act of 2002 is passed to improve the ability to prevent and respond to public health emergencies.

2002 In June 2002 traces of biological and chemical weapon agents are found in Uzbekistan on a military base used by US troops fighting in Afghanistan. Early analysis dates and attributes the source of the contamination to former Soviet Union biological and chemical weapons programs that used the base.

2002 In the aftermath of the September 11, 2001, terrorist attacks on the United States, the US government dramatically increases funding to stockpile drugs and other agents that could be used to counter a bioterrorist attack.

2002 Scientists determine that stockpiled smallpox vaccine doses can be effective if diluted to one-tenth their original concentration, greatly enhancing the number of doses available to respond to an emergency.

2002 Severe acute respiratory syndrome (SARS) virus is found in patients in China, Hong Kong, and other Asian countries. The newly discovered coronavirus is not identified until early 2003. The spread of the virus reaches epidemic proportions in Asia and expands to the rest of the world.

2002 The Best Pharmaceuticals for Children Act passed to improve safety and efficacy of patented and off-patent medicines for children.

2002 The Defense Advanced Research Projects Agency (DARPA) initiates the Biosensor Technologies program in 2002 to develop fast, sensitive, automatic technologies for the detection and identification of biological warfare agents.

2002 The Pathogen Genomic Sequencing program is initiated by the Defense Advanced Research Project Agency (DARPA) to focus on characterizing the genetic components of pathogens to develop novel diagnostics, treatments, and therapies for the diseases they cause.

2002 The planned destruction of stocks of the smallpox-causing Variola virus at the two remaining depositories in the United States and Russia is delayed over fears that large-scale production of the vaccine might be needed in the event of a bioterrorist action.

2002 WHO declares the 51 countries of its European region free of polio.

2003 Almost 500,000 civic and health care workers at strategic hospitals, governmental facilities, and research centers across the United States are slated to receive smallpox immunizations as part of a strategic plan for ready response to a biological attack using the smallpox virus.

2003 An international research team funded by NINR found that filters made from old cotton saris cut the number of cholera cases in rural Bangladesh villages almost in half. Other inexpensive cloth should work just as well in other parts of the world where cholera is endemic. This simple preventive measure has the potential to make a significant impact on a global health problem.

2003 By early May WHO officials have confirmed reports of more than 3,000 cases of SARS from 18 different countries with 111 deaths attributed to the disease. United States health officials reported 193 cases with no deaths. Significantly, all but 20 of the US cases are linked to travel to infected areas, and the other 20 cases are accounted for by secondary transmission from infected patients to family members and health care workers. Health authorities assert that the emergent virus responsible for SARS will remain endemic (part of the natural array of viruses) in many regions of China well after the current outbreak is resolved.

2003 Canadian scientists at the British Columbia Cancer Agency in Vancouver announce the sequence of the genome of the coronavirus most likely to be the cause of SARS. Within days scientists at the CDC in Atlanta, Georgia, offer a genomic map that confirms more than 99 percent of the Canadian findings.

2003 Differences in outbreaks in Hong Kong between 1997 and 2003 cause investigators to conclude that the H5N1 virus has mutated.

2003 Following approximately five deaths by heart attack correlated to individuals receiving the new smallpox vaccine, US health officials at the CDC announce a suspension of administration of the vaccine to patients with a history of heart disease until the matter can be fully investigated.

2003 Preliminary trials for a malaria vaccine are scheduled to begin in malaria-endemic African areas, where approximately 3,000 children die from the disease every day.

2003 SARS cases in Hanoi reach 22, as a simultaneous outbreak of the same disease occurs in Hong Kong. WHO issues a global alert about a new infectious disease of unknown origin in both Vietnam and Hong Kong.

2003 SARS is added to the list of quarantinable diseases in the United States.

2003 Studies indicate that women with a history of some sexually transmitted infections, including the human papillomavirus, are at increased risk for developing cervical cancer.

2003 Studies show no correlation between immunization schedules and sudden infant death syndrome (SIDS) occurrences.

2003 The first case of an unusually severe pneumonia occurs in Hanoi, Vietnam, and is identified two days later as severe acute respiratory syndrome (SARS) by Italian physician and epidemiologist Carlo Urbani (1956–2003), who formally identifies

SARS as a unique disease and names it. Urbani dies of SARS later that year.

2003 The first case of bovine spongiform encephalopathy (BSE, mad cow disease) in the United States is found in a cow in Washington state. Investigations later reveal that the cow was imported from a Canadian herd, which included North America's first "homegrown" case of BSE six months earlier.

2003 WHO takes the unusual step of issuing a travel warning that describes SARS as a worldwide health threat. WHO officials announce that SARS cases, and potential cases, have been tracked from China to Singapore, Thailand, Vietnam, Indonesia, Philippines, and Canada.

2003 the United States invades Iraq and finds chemical, biological, and nuclear weapons programs, but no actual weapons.

2003 WHO Global Influenza Surveillance Network intensifies work on development of a H5N1 vaccine for humans.

2004 A 35-year-old television producer in the Guangdong province of China is the first person to become ill with SARS since the end of May 2003, the initial outbreak of the newly identified disease. Within two weeks three other people are suspected of having SARS in the region, and teams from WHO return to investigate possible human-to-human, animal-to-human, and environmental sources of transmission of the disease.

2004 Chinese health officials in the Guangdong province of China launch a mass slaughter of civet cats, a cousin of the mongoose considered a delicacy and thought to be a vector of SARS, in an attempt to control the spread of the disease.

2004 Project BioShield Act of 2004 authorizes US government agencies to expedite procedures related to rapid distribution of treatments as countermeasures to chemical, biological, and nuclear attack.

2005 H5N1 virus, responsible for avian flu, moves from Asia to Europe. WHO attempts to coordinate multinational disaster and containment plans. Some nations begin to stockpile antiviral drugs.

2005 WHO reports outbreaks of plague in the Democratic Republic of the Congo.

2005 FDA Drug Safety Board is founded.

2005 US president George W. Bush (1946–) addresses the issue of HIV/AIDS in black women in the United States, acknowledging it as a public health crisis.

2006 European Union bans the importation of avian feathers (non-treated feathers) from countries neighboring or close to Turkey.

2006 Mad cow disease confirmed in an Alabama cow as third reported case in the United States.

2006 More than a dozen people are diagnosed with avian flu in Turkey, but United Nations (UN) health experts assure the public that human-to-human transmission is still rare and only suspected in a few cases in Asia.

2006 Researchers begin human trials for vaginal microbicide gels.

2007 Texas governor Rick Perry (1950–) adds the HPV vaccine to the list of required vaccines for school-age girls.

2007 Four people are hospitalized with botulism poisoning in the United States after more than 90 potentially contaminated meat products, including canned chili, were removed from grocery shelves across the country.

2007 The CDC issues a rare order for isolation when a New Jersey man infected with a resistant strain of tuberculosis flies on multiple trans-Atlantic commercial flights.

2008 The CDC issues a health advisory after a widespread outbreak of measles in the United States.

2008 An outbreak of salmonellosis linked to peppers imported from Mexico causes more than 1,400 to become ill in the United States between April and August.

2008 A case of Marburg Hemorrhagic Fever is diagnosed in the Netherlands. The patient, a Dutch woman, had recently returned from Uganda, where she contracted the virus. WHO calls on Uganda's Ministry of

Health to advise all tourists against entering caves where bats might be present.

2008 WHO reports that there is an outbreak of the H5N1 virus, often called the "bird flu," in Indonesia. Of the 139 confirmed cases of the virus, 113 have people died.

2009 The 2009 flu pandemic is caused by the H1N1 virus, also known as the "swine flu." CDC estimates place the global death toll between 151,700 and 575,000 during the 2008–2009 flu season.2010 Following a destructive earthquake, a cholera outbreak begins in Haiti and the Dominican Republic, affecting more than 800,000 people and killing nearly 10,000 by May 2017.

2010 WHO releases first report on neglected tropical diseases (NTDs) to highlight challenges and draw attention to eradication efforts.

2010 The Affordable Care Act (ACA) is signed into law in the United States. Purposes of the law included making health insurance more affordable and expanding insurance coverage.

2011 WHO Strategic Technical Advisory Group for Neglected Tropical Diseases adopts a roadmap for controlling, eliminating, and eradicating NTDs by 2020.

2011 An outbreak of haemolytic uremic syndrome, a rare condition linked to *Escherichia coli* bacteria, sickens 276 people in Germany.

2011 A measles outbreak in Europe affects 33 countries, with more than 6,500 people contracting the virus. In response, WHO issues new vaccination and travel recommendations for adults and children.

2012 United Nations Foundation launches the Shot@Life program to provide vaccines for children around the globe.

2012 An outbreak of pertussis (whooping cough) sickens 48,277 people in the United States. This is the largest number of cases since 1955.

2012 Contamination at a Massachusetts compounding pharmacy leads to an outbreak of fungal meningitis in the United States. Roughly 800 people become ill, and 76 die.

2012 The first case of Middle East Respiratory Syndrome Coronavirus (MERS-CoV, initially known as "novel virus") is identified in Saudi Arabia. By 2017 more than 2,000 cases have been reported.

2012 Pre-exposure prophylaxis (PrEP) goes on the market. The medication, which is recommended to people with high risk of contracting HIV, lowers the risk of acquiring the disease. 2013 Polio reemerges in Syria as a consequence of civil war. WHO responds with an immunization drive.

2013 First local transmission of chikungunya occurs in the Americas. Mosquitoes in the Caribbean are found to be spreading the virus to humans.

2013 An Ebola outbreak begins in Guinea in December.

2014 The Ebola virus spreads throughout Guinea and to Liberia and Sierra Leone, becoming widespread in both. Cases are reported in other West African nations, and travelers and returning aid workers introduce cases to the United States, Spain, the United Kingdom, and Italy.

2014 WHO releases its first report on antimicrobial resistance.

2014 WHO declares the South-East Asia Region (comprising Bangladesh, Bhutan, Democratic People's Republic of Korea, India, Indonesia, Maldives, Myanmar, Nepal, Sri Lanka, Thailand, and Timor-Leste) free of polio.

2014 The WHO director-general declares the spread of wild poliovirus a Public Health Emergency of International Concern.

2014 FDA announces the approval of a vaccine (Trumenba) for Group B meningococcal disease.

2014 An outbreak of polio in Pakistan results in more than 300 reported cases and new efforts to eradicate the virus in the country. Immunization efforts lead to a reduction in the number of reported cases to five in 2017.

2014 President Barack Obama (1961–) signs Executive Order 13676: Combating Antibiotic-Resistant Bacteria. The order directs federal agencies to address the problem of bacteria that are becoming resistant to the antibiotics commonly used to treat them.

2015 The Pan American Health Organization declare the Americas free of the endemic transmission of rubella.

2015 Chikungunya becomes a notifiable disease in the United States.

2015 A measles outbreak in the United States affects 189 people in 24 states. Most cases occur in individuals who have not received the measles vaccine.

2015 The US government releases the National Action Plan for Combating Multidrug-Resistant Tuberculosis in response to the growing threat of multidrug-resistant ad extensively drug-resistant tuberculosis.

2016 An outbreak of Rift Valley Fever (RVF) in Niger kills 33 people. This is the largest number of RVF fatalities since the 2005–2007 epidemic in Kenya.

2016 WHO declares a public health emergency due to the Zika virus, which is spreading rapidly in the Americas and causing miscarriage, stillbirth, and birth defects, including microcephaly.

2017 A cholera epidemic begins in Yemen in April. By January 2018 WHO estimates that 1 million have contracted the disease and more than 2,000 have died.

2017 An outbreak of norovirus in Yolo County, California, schools causes more than 2,800 people to become ill.

2017 A large outbreak of plague begins in Madagascar in August, causing 2,119 confirmed and suspected cases by early November, when the Madagascar Ministry of Health declares the outbreak contained. During the outbreak WHO advises against any travel or trade restrictions, citing the low risk of international transmission.

2017 An outbreak of Seoul virus in the United States causes 17 people to become ill. Infected rats are found in Colorado, Georgia, Illinois, Iowa, Minnesota, Missouri, Pennsylvania, South Carolina, Tennessee, Utah, and Wisconsin.

2017 A monkeypox outbreak occurs in Nigeria, with 172 suspected and 61 confirmed cases between September and December.

2017 The WHO Strategic Technical Advisory Group for Neglected Tropical Diseases adds chromoblastomycosis and other deep mycoses, scabies and other ectoparasites, and snakebite envenoming to the list of neglected tropical diseases.

2017 WHO declares that the Zika virus is no longer a public health emergency. The disease remains a risk for pregnant women who live in areas where Zika transmission occurs.

2017 The CDC reports that rates of Hepatitis C are rising in the United States as a result of the opioid drug epidemic. Hepatitis C can be transmitted between people who share injection drug paraphernalia.

2017 A listeriosis outbreak linked to contaminated deli meats sickens 1,000 people in South Africa and becomes the largest recorded listeria outbreak.

2018 An outbreak of Lassa fever in Nigeria becomes the largest recorded. WHO reports 317 confirmed cases, 764 suspected cases, and 72 deaths in January and February, more than in all of 2016.

2018 An outbreak of the vaccine-preventable disease yellow fever occurs in Brazil. WHO records 723 confirmed cases and 237 deaths.

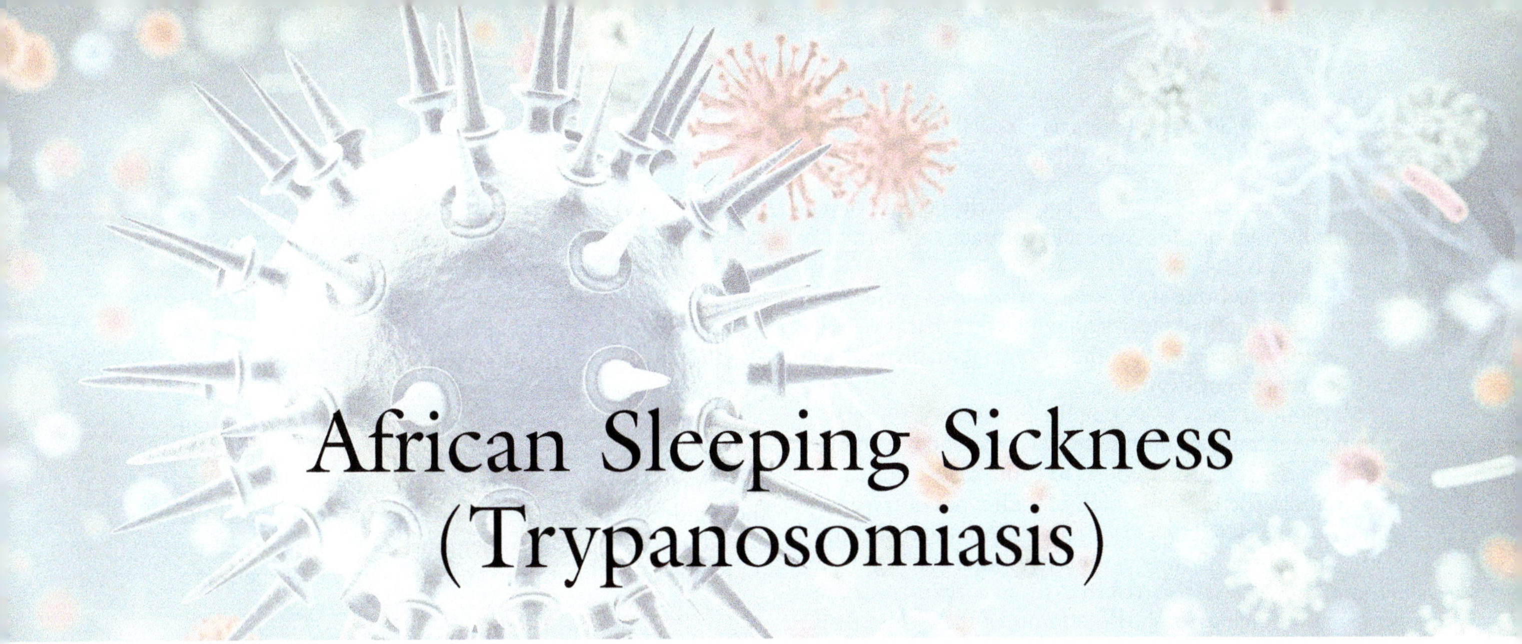

African Sleeping Sickness (Trypanosomiasis)

■ Introduction

Trypanosomiasis (tri-PAN-o-SO-my-a-sis), which is also known as African sleeping sickness because of the semiconscious stupor and excessive sleep that can occur in someone who is infected, is a vector-borne disease passed to humans through the bite of the tsetse fly. The fly bite transfers either *Trypanosoma brucei rhodesiense*, which causes a version of the disease called East African trypanosomiasis, or *T. brucei gambiense*, which causes West African trypanosomiasis. If left untreated, trypanosomiasis is ultimately fatal.

Trypanosomiasis is common in Africa. In the 1960s the disease was almost eradicated, but interruptions in the delivery of public health to affected regions due to government indifference and warfare caused a reemergence of the disease, resulting in tens of thousands of cases every year. The World Health Organization (WHO) estimated that in 2005 there were 50,000 to 70,000 new cases. This is a drop from higher numbers reported during the 1990s. WHO, Médecines Sans Frontières (Doctors Without Borders), and several pharmaceutical companies have jointly been working on national programs in various countries in Africa to bring trypanosomiasis under control. The initiative has resulted in a sharp decline in the number of cases. According to WHO, there were about 10,000 new cases in 2009, fewer than 5,000 in 2014, and approximately 2,100 in 2016.

■ Disease History, Characteristics, and Transmission

Trypanosomiasis has been known for centuries. It was first described in the 14th century in the land-locked region of northwestern Africa that is now known as Mali. The involvement of the trypanosomes and the tsetse fly was discovered by Sir David Bruce (1855–1931) around 1902. A few years later, a massive epidemic that affected millions of Africans and killed 500,000 people called attention to the seriousness of the disease. Shortly afterward the association between trypanosomiasis and the tsetse fly was established.

T. brucei rhodesiense and *T. brucei gambiense* are protozoa. Protozoans are single-celled organisms that are more complex in structure than bacteria and viruses; the organisms are considered to be animals. The protozoa responsible for sleeping sickness are native to Africa. The few cases of trypanosomiasis that occur outside of Africa each year generally result from travelers who acquire the protozoa in Africa, then leave and subsequently develop the disease in another country.

The two protozoans have a complex life cycle. In the animal host, the organisms that are injected by a tsetse fly progressively change their shape to what is described as the stumpy form. This form can infect a tsetse fly when it takes a blood meal from an animal. While inside the gut of the fly, the protozoans change again into a form that can migrate to the salivary glands of the fly. Finally, another change in the organism occurs; the protozoan is now capable of infecting another animal when the tsetse fly seeks a blood meal. This animal-to-human cycle can continue until the chain of transmission (also called the cycle of infection) is interrupted, usually by an organized effort by agencies such as WHO.

T. brucei rhodesiense is naturally carried by antelopes. The antelopes are not harmed by the protozoan and serve as the natural reservoir of the *T. brucei rhodesiense.* Tsetse flies who obtain a blood meal from an antelope can acquire the protozoan, which they can transfer to humans or cows. The resulting infection is lethal in cattle. People who are most likely to become infected are those who come into contact with cattle or antelopes. Thus, those who raise cattle, game wardens, and visitors to East African game reserves and other rural areas are at risk.

T. brucei gambiense does not infect antelope or cattle. It resides in creatures that live in the tropical rain forests found in central and western Africa. The disease caused by this protozoan in humans produces more severe symptoms and more often results in death. Fortunately, because of its isolated distribution, fewer people contract this form of trypanosomiasis.

The infection due to *T. brucei rhodesiense* progresses more swiftly than the longer-lasting infection that is caused by *T. brucei gambiense.* Both infections inevitably lead to death if they are not treated.

Sleeping sickness is a complex disease, with interactions between humans, the tsetse fly vector, and the animal host. This can complicate efforts to control the disease.

Typically, the first indication of both types of trypanosomiasis is the development of redness, pain, and swelling at the site of the fly bite several days after having been bitten. The sore is also referred to as a *chancre.* Some people also develop a rash. Both forms of the disease then progress in two stages. The first stage begins two to three weeks following the bite and the entry of the protozoans into the bloodstream. The symptoms of this stage develop as the trypanosome is carried throughout the body in the bloodstream. The lymphatic system, which is an important part of the immune system, can also become infected. Because at this stage the disease affects the whole body, it is termed the systemic phase. A hallmark of the illness at this point is an extreme fluctuation of body temperature. A person's temperature will cycle from normal to very high and back again, which is a consequence of the immune system's reaction to the protozoan. Additionally, a person may experience a feeling of extreme itchiness and develop a headache. Some people become mentally disoriented. If left untreated, a person can lapse into a coma and die.

West African trypanosomiasis also produces marked swelling of lymph nodes, especially those located behind the ear and at the base of the neck, and swelling of both the spleen and the liver. East African trypanosomiasis can cause the heart to become inflamed and to malfunction.

Some of the symptoms of trypanosomiasis that can occur during the first stage of the illness are a result of the immune reaction to the infection. The immune response remains strong because invading trypanosomes can shift the composition of their outer surface. As the immune system hones in on one surface configuration, that configuration can rapidly change. This trait is known as antigenic variation. The trypanosomes are capable of expressing thousands of different surface profiles during the years that an infection can last. A consequence of the heightened immune response due to the changing surface of the protozoan is the cycling fever, as well as organ damage and weakened blood vessels; the latter aid in the spread of the organism throughout the body.

The second stage of trypanosomiasis involves the nervous system. As the brain becomes affected, a person can experience difficulties in speaking, mental disorientation, and periods of near-unconsciousness or sleep during the daytime (hence the term *sleeping sickness*). During the night insomnia robs a person of sleep. Other symptoms can develop that mimic those of Parkinson's disease; these include difficulty in movement, with difficulty in walking that can require a shuffling motion to avoid falling down, involuntary movement or trembling of arms and legs, and a tightening of muscles. With more time, a person can lapse into a coma and die.

Trypanosomiasis can also be transferred from a pregnant woman to her baby prior to birth or via transfusion with infected blood or a contaminated organ that is transplanted. However, these routes of infection are rare.

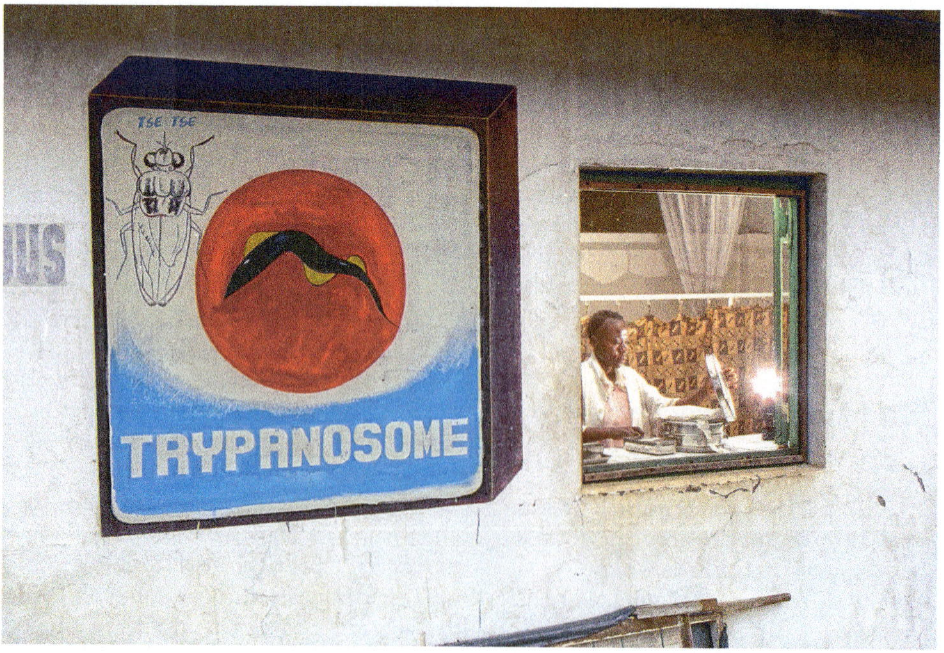

A nurse works in an African sleeping sickness clinic in the Democratic Republic of the Congo. The sign on the building depicts the tsetse fly that transmits the disease. *© Patrick Robert/Sygma/Corbis/Getty Images*

WORDS TO KNOW

CHAIN OF TRANSMISSION Refers to the route by which an infection is spread from its source to susceptible host. An example of a chain of transmission is the spread of malaria from an infected animal to humans via mosquitoes.

EPIDEMIC From the Greek *epidemic*, meaning "prevalent among the people," is most commonly used to describe an outbreak of an illness or disease in which the number of individual cases significantly exceeds the usual or expected number of cases in any given population.

PROTOZOA Single-celled animal-like microscopic organisms that live by taking in food rather than making it by photosynthesis and must live in the presence of water. (Singular: protozoan.) Protozoa are a diverse group of single-celled organisms, with more than 50,000 different types represented. The vast majority are microscopic, many measuring less than 5 one-thousandth of an inch (or 0.005 millimeters), but some, such as the freshwater Spirostomun, may reach 0.17 inches (3 millimeters) in length, large enough to enable it to be seen with the naked eye.

REEMERGING INFECTIOUS DISEASE Illnesses such as malaria, diphtheria, tuberculosis, and polio that were once nearly absent from the world but are starting to cause greater numbers of infections once again. These illnesses are reappearing for many reasons. Malaria and other mosquito-borne illnesses increase when mosquito-control measures decrease. Other diseases are spreading because people have stopped being vaccinated, as happened with diphtheria after the collapse of the Soviet Union. A few diseases are reemerging because drugs to treat them have become less available or drug-resistant strains have developed.

RESERVOIR The animal or organism in which the virus or parasite normally resides.

VECTOR Any agent, living or otherwise, that carries and transmits parasites and diseases. Also, an organism or chemical used to transport a gene into a new host cell.

Scope and Distribution

Trypanosomiasis is prevalent in regions of Africa. East African trypanosomiasis is found in Uganda, Tanzania, Kenya, Malawi, Zaire, Ethiopia, Botswana, and Zimbabwe. West African trypanosomiasis is prevalent in western and central Africa.

According to WHO, in 2002 trypanosomiasis was constantly present in eleven countries and almost as prevalent in an additional twelve countries. In 2007 epidemics were occurring in the Democratic Republic of Congo (DRC), Angola, and Sudan. Between 2007 and 2017, more than 79 percent of reported cases occurred in the DRC. Each year during that period, the DRC had about 1,000 new cases. The Central African Republic ranked next, with between 100 and 200 new cases annually from 2007 to 2017.

Spread of the disease to humans occurs only in Africa, because the tsetse fly is only found on the African continent. On the rare occasions that trypanosomiasis occurs elsewhere in the world, it is usually the result of travel by someone who became infected while in Africa. For example, since 1996 the U.S. Centers for Disease Control and Prevention (CDC) has recorded only thirty-six cases of the disease in the United States, and all involved people who contracted the disease in Africa. A version of trypanosomiasis called Chagas disease, which is caused by *Trypanosoma cruzi*, occurs in South America and sometimes in Central and North America.

Estimating the actual number of cases of trypanosomiasis is difficult. The majority occur in regions of Africa where organized medical care and reporting is scant; therefore, the actual number of cases is likely much higher. For example, in 1998 almost 40,000 cases were reported, but WHO estimated that 300,000 cases were undetected. However, with the eradication efforts that began in 2000, the number of undetected cases has likely dropped. In January 2017 WHO estimated that the number of cases of trypanosomiasis was less than 20,000.

Treatment and Prevention

The diagnosis of trypanosomiasis involves examination of the fluid from either the site of the tsetse fly bite or from a swollen lymph node or blood to detect the presence of infecting protozoa. In addition, fluid can be injected into rats, which can develop an infection. Blood recovered from the rats after several weeks will contain the protozoa.

Medications are available to treat trypanosomiasis. The drug pentamidine is used for the early stage of *T. brucei gambiense* infections, and the drug suramin is used for the early stage of infections caused by *T. brucie rhodesiense.* More advanced stages of both forms of the disease are treated using the drug melarsoprol. Those who do not respond to melarsoprol can be given another drug:

eflornithine. Unfortunately, the drugs can have undesirable side effects. For example, suramin, eflornithine, and pentamidine can cause a fatal reaction in the kidney or liver or inflammation in the brain. These drugs must be used with care and their effects monitored; they are usually only used in a hospital setting. While these drugs can be effective, the CDC does not recommend any particular medication.

Trypanosomiasis cannot clear up on its own. Hospitalization and treatment are necessary. Those who recover from the infection should be monitored for several years afterward to ensure that the infection does not recur.

As of 2017 there was still no vaccine for either form of trypanosomiasis, reflecting the complex life cycle of the protozoan. However, development of drugs that are effective against the disease has been one of the priorities of the Bill & Melinda Gates Foundation. The foundation awarded over $21 million to researchers at the University of North Carolina in 2015 to fund a clinical trial of an orally administered drug called pafuramidine maleate. As of 2017 the trial was ongoing.

Prevention of the disease consists of avoiding contact with the tsetse fly. For example, contact with bushes should be minimized, as the flies often rest there. Bushes and other shrubbery that are near rivers or waterholes are prime spots for tsetse flies and should be avoided. This habitat tends to be rural, so people who spend time traveling or staying in rural areas of regions where trypanosomiasis is prevalent are at risk and should be appropriately cautious.

Clothing can be protective. The clothing should be fairly thick, as the tsetse fly can bite through light fabric. Also, because the fly is attracted to bright colors, clothing should be bland; khaki- or olive-colored clothing is recommended. The clothing should fit tightly at the wrists and ankles to make it harder for flies to enter. Riding in the back of open-air vehicles is unwise; tsetse flies are also attracted to dust. Another wise precaution, which has also proven useful in reducing the incidence of malaria, is the use of protective netting over a bed.

■ Impacts and Issues

The resurgence of trypanosomiasis during the 1970s highlights the vigilance that is necessary to control infectious diseases and prevent their reemergence. The loss of control over trypanosomiasis was due to the interruptions in the monitoring of disease outbreaks, the displacement of people due to regional conflicts, and environmental changes. These problems are ongoing. In particular, the documented warming of the atmosphere will make Africa even more hospitable to the spread of the territory of the tsetse fly, which could increase the geographical distribution of trypanosomiasis.

According to WHO in January 2017, *T. brucei gambiense* was a major health concern in approximately twenty-four countries in Africa, with *T. brucei rhodesiense* present in thirteen African countries. WHO estimated that about 65 million people were at risk of developing the disease in 2017. However, fewer than 4 million people were being monitored and only about 40,000 people were being treated every year. The proportion of people being monitored or treated is smaller than other tropical diseases, even though trypanosomiasis can increase to epidemic proportions and the death rate for those who are not treated is 100 percent.

Epidemics disrupt families as well as national economies, as large numbers of people become unable to work or care for themselves. In 2004 WHO estimated that the number of healthy years of life lost due to premature death and disability caused by trypanosomiasis was 1.5 million. Because many regions of Africa are still agricultural, the rural-based disease affects those who are most important to the economy. Of the 48,000 deaths that occurred in 2004, 31,000 were males, who are often the working family members. Epidemics can decimate the population of a region.

Taking care of those diagnosed with trypanosomiasis is a daunting task for the poor nations, as two-thirds of people diagnosed with the disease already have the advanced stage of the infection, in which the nervous system has been affected. The only treatment that is effective once the central nervous system has been affected—the drug melarsoprol—contains arsenic, and so the treatment itself can sometimes be fatal. Compounding the problem, some strains of the trypanosomes that are resistant to drugs used to treat the disease at an earlier stage have been detected. It seems only a matter of time before these resistant strains become more common, as the resistance gives them a selective advantage over nonresistant trypanosomes.

Treatment can also be hampered by the cost of the drugs. An example is eflornithine. Originally developed as an anticancer compound, the drug has been promising against *T. brucei gambiense*. Beginning in 2000 WHO established partnerships with several manufacturers to provide drugs such as eflornithine, nifurtimox, and melarsoprol for free in countries where the disease is endemic. This partnership was renewed in 2016.

WHO is actively involved in programs intended to monitor and treat trypanosomiasis. For example, since 1975 WHO, the United Nations Children's Fund (UNICEF), the World Bank, and the United Nations Development Program (UNDP) have collaborated on the Special Program for Research and Training in Tropical Diseases. The aim of the program is to develop means of combating infectious diseases, including trypanosomiasis, in a way that is effective and affordable to poorer countries that otherwise are unable to meet the economic and logistical burdens of treatment.

In addition, the WHO Communicable Disease Surveillance and Response unit works with countries experiencing epidemics to set up national programs to control the disease. This can be challenging because governments can treat trypanosomiasis as a low-priority issue until an epidemic strikes. By acting earlier and with a more coordinated national effort, however, epidemics might well be avoided.

PRIMARY SOURCE

September 15, 2015

SOURCE: *"Traveling the Extra Mile to Treat Sleeping Sickness in the DRC." Doctors Without Borders/Médecins Sans Frontières. http://www.doctorswithoutborders.org/article/traveling-extra-mile-treat-sleeping-sickness-drc (accessed November 8, 2017).*

INTRODUCTION: *Traveling by jeep and motorbike, a Doctors Without Borders/Médecins Sans Frontières (MSF) mobile medical team is making its way through a remote and insecure region of Democratic Republic of Congo (DRC) to screen and treat people suffering from sleeping sickness.*

In a small, dark clinic in northeastern DRC, 24-year-old Germaine lies on a cot, too dizzy to walk. She was bitten by a tsetse fly and MSF doctors have diagnosed her with sleeping sickness.

Germaine is one of 42,000 people MSF is aiming to test and treat for the neglected tropical disease over an eight-month period. In May 2015, mobile medical teams, made up of doctors, nurses, and lab technicians, began traveling through dense and unstable regions of Province Orientale, Ango, and Banda Territory, near the border with Central African Republic, visiting villages where disease rates have been historically high.

Reaching Nomads and Refugees

"We are making a big effort to reach people who live beyond the villages," said Rolland Kaya, MSF's head of mission for sleeping sickness. "We are focusing on the most vulnerable and hard-to-reach groups of people, such as refugees and nomads living in the bush. A team of public health sensitizers travels to remote farming and fishing communities to let them know we are in the area. We're encouraging these people to come and get tested because they are most at risk of being bitten and infected by the flies."

Since May, MSF has screened 12,183 people, 91 of whom have so far been diagnosed with sleeping sickness.

With the team working in such remote areas, MSF is also taking the opportunity to provide people with general healthcare, particularly pregnant women, children under five, and adults with malaria symptoms. Since May, the team has treated 6,884 people for malaria.

Too Dizzy to Work

Early symptoms of sleeping sickness include fever, headaches, joint pain, and itching. The drugs used to treat people in the early stages of the disease are relatively easy to administer and non-toxic. The earlier the disease is identified, the better chance there is of a cure.

In the second stage, parasites cross the blood–brain barrier and infect the central nervous system. This is when more obvious signs of the disease appear, including a disturbed sleep cycle, which gives sleeping sickness its name.

Germaine began showing symptoms of sleeping sickness three months ago, after the birth of her third child. Suffering from fatigue and vertigo, she wasn't able to go to the fields to work. "I was so dizzy I would fall to the ground," she recalls. "I had no energy, I couldn't eat, and I could only take sips of water."

Germaine will spend seven days in the clinic to receive injections of the drug pentamadine. "My family couldn't understand what was wrong with me," says Germaine. "They are so relieved that I'm getting treatment and am already starting to feel better."

Sleeping Sickness Caseload Decreasing

Sleeping sickness continues to affect millions of people in 36 countries in sub-Saharan Africa. Most live in remote, rural areas with limited access to health services. Many have been displaced from their homes by war and poverty. These factors all make it difficult to carry out surveillance and to diagnose and treat cases.

However, in the past decade, the number of sleeping sickness cases around the world has dropped, and treatments have improved.

MSF has been actively engaged in treating sleeping sickness for 25 years in DRC, Central African Republic, Republic of Congo, and South Sudan. MSF teams say they have noticed people in DRC becoming more aware of the dangers of the disease, while behavioral changes, linked to insecurity, are also contributing to the fall in cases.

"We believe the decrease in the number of cases we are seeing is linked to people beginning to change their lifestyles due to the insecurity in the area," says MSF health advisor Dr. Turid Piening. "They are abandoning their traditions of hunting and fishing near rivers where tsetse flies gather and are cultivating crops closer to home."

But to eliminate the disease, much more remains to be done, including the development of an easy-to-use rapid test to replace complicated diagnostic procedures, coupled with oral drugs that can be taken at home. Until that happens, MSF is committed to finding, testing, and treating people suffering from this life-threatening disease, however remote the area in which they live.

SEE ALSO *Chagas Disease; Médecins Sans Frontières (Doctors Without Borders); Mosquito-borne Diseases; Reemerging Infectious Diseases*

BIBLIOGRAPHY

Books

Kruel, Donald. *Trypanosomiasis.* New York: Chelsea House, 2007.

Magez, Stefan, and Magdalena Radwanska, eds. *Trypanosomes and Trypanosomiasis.* Vienna: Springer, 2014.

Periodicals

Büscher Philippe, Giuliano Cecchi, Vincent Jamonneau, and Gerardo Priotto. "Human African Trypanosomiasis." *Lancet* (June 30, 2017).

Franco Jose R., Pere P. Simarro, Abdoulaye Diarra, and Jean G. Jannin. "Epidemiology of Human African Trypanosomiasis." *Clin Epidemiol* 6 (2014): 257–275.

Rock Kat S., Steve J. Torr, Crispin Lumbala, and Matt J. Keeling. "Quantitative Evaluation of the Strategy to Eliminate Human African Trypanosomiasis in the Democratic Republic of Congo." *Parasit Vectors* 8, no. 1 (2015): 532.

Websites

"Parasites–African Trypanosomiasis (also known as Sleeping Sickness)." Centers for Disease Control and Prevention. https://www.cdc.gov/parasites/sleepingsickness/index.html (accessed November 6, 2017).

"Trypanosomiasis, Human African (Sleeping Sickness)." World Health Organization. http://www.who.int/mediacentre/factsheets/fs259/en/ (accessed November 6, 2017).

Brian Hoyle

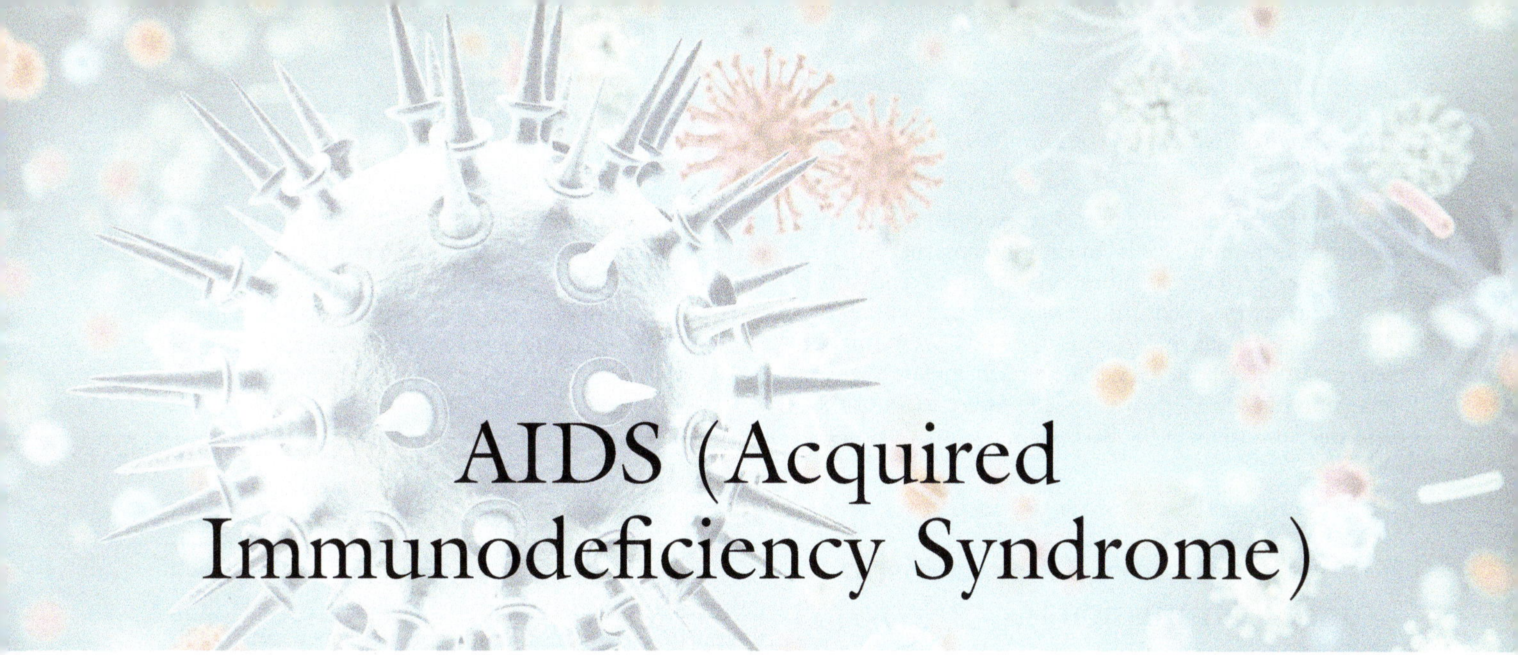

AIDS (Acquired Immunodeficiency Syndrome)

Introduction

First reported in the United States in 1981, acquired immunodeficiency syndrome (AIDS) has since become a major worldwide pandemic. Medical research has demonstrated that AIDS is caused by the human immunodeficiency virus (HIV), a retrovirus, so named because its genes are coded in ribonucleic acid (RNA) instead of the more common deoxyribonucleic acid (DNA). Essentially, the virus causes disease by killing or damaging cells of the human immune system. HIV gradually destroys a person's ability to battle infections and certain types of cancer. This loss of immune system functioning causes victims to be vulnerable to often-deadly opportunistic infections, which are caused by pathogens (disease-causing organisms) that are usually harmless to healthy people.

Because the spread of the AIDS epidemic in the United States and Western Europe has been extensively tracked and analyzed, the most reliable information regarding its transmission, treatment, and prevention comes from research based in these countries. However, the majority of people infected with HIV in the early 21st century live outside of these regions. While modes of transmission of HIV have been determined to be the same across the world, risk patterns among different peoples have varied

Percentage of People Living with HIV (2016)

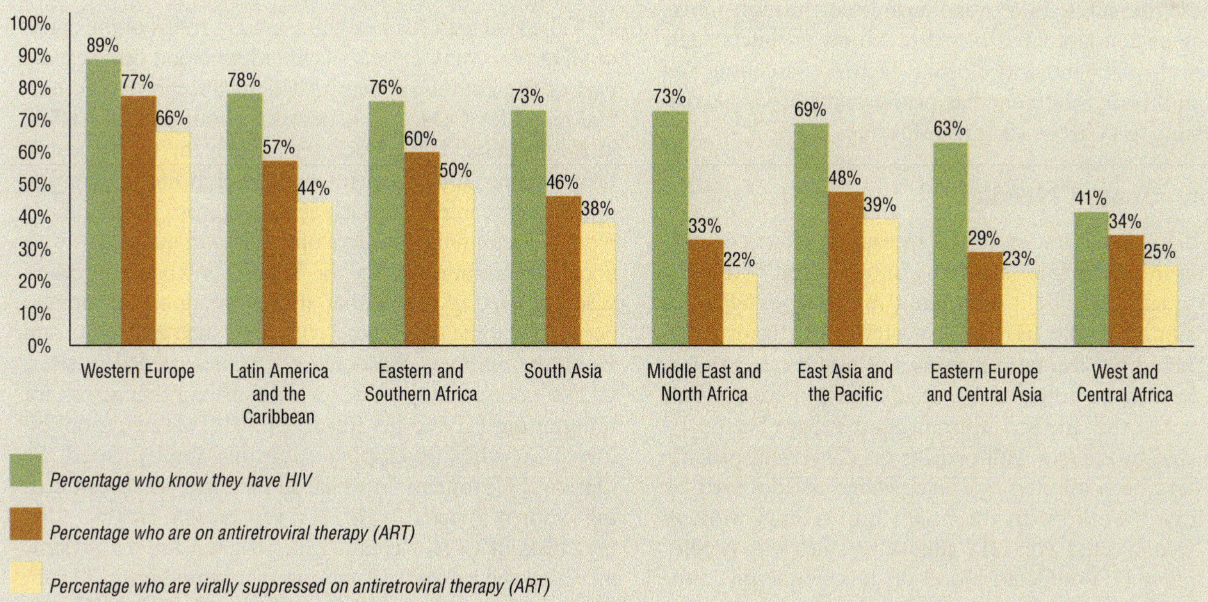

SOURCE: Adapted from UNICEF/UNAIDS. 2017. Available from: https://data.unicef.org/topic/hivaids/global-regional-trends/

according to cultural influences. For example, outside of Western Europe and North America, homosexual activity has been comparatively more circumscribed and suppressed; hence, the major pattern of sexual transmission of HIV occurs among heterosexuals in non-Westernized countries. Although the HIV epidemic acquired its original momentum in the United States, the future focus of the pandemic lies mainly in the developing countries of Africa and Asia.

Disease History, Characteristics, and Transmission

HIV is transmitted by the exchange of body fluids such as blood, semen, and saliva. Therefore, certain behaviors put people at risk for contracting HIV, including sharing drug syringes; engaging in anal, vaginal, or oral sexual contact with an infected person without using a condom; and having sexual contact with someone with unknown HIV status.

The most common way to transmit HIV is by having unprotected sex with an infected partner. The virus can enter the body through the mucous membranes of the vagina, vulva, penis, rectum, or mouth during sexual activity.

Contact with Infected Blood

It is possible to contract HIV through contact with infected blood. This risk has given rise to extensive screening of donated blood for evidence of HIV infection, as well as heat-treatment techniques to destroy HIV in blood products used in medical practice. Prior to these measures, HIV was transmitted through transfusions of contaminated blood or blood products such as serum, platelets, and clotting factors. Screening for HIV and heat treatment has nearly eliminated the risk of getting HIV from such transfusions.

Contaminated Needles

One of the primary means of spreading infection with HIV is the sharing of syringes contaminated with very small quantities of blood among injection drug users from someone who has been infected with the virus.

There have also been rare cases of health care workers who have been infected by accidental punctures with needles or other medical instruments that have been contaminated by contact with patients or, conversely, patients who have been infected by contaminated needles used by health care workers. In the health care setting, workers have been infected with HIV after being stuck with needles containing HIV-infected blood or, less frequently, after infected blood gets into a worker's open cut or a mucous membrane (for example, the eyes or inside of the nose). According to the US Centers for Disease Control (CDC), the transmission of HIV from a health care provider to a patient is very rare when risk-reducing procedures are followed. The CDC reported that six patients were infected by a Florida dentist in the early 1990s. After that initial report, just three additional cases have been reported as of 2018.

Mother-to-Child Transmission

Women can transmit HIV to their babies during pregnancy or birth. About one-quarter to one-third of HIV-positive pregnant women will pass the virus on to their babies. HIV can also be transmitted from infected mothers to babies through breast milk. Available drug treatment for the mother during pregnancy can significantly reduce the probability of such infection. Cesarean section delivery can further reduce mother-to-newborn infection rates to just 1 percent. Drug treatment and cesarean delivery has nearly eradicated mother-to-baby transmission of HIV in the United States. Use of these measures has increased worldwide.

The CDC's Division of Global HIV & TB (DGHT) plays a prominent role in reducing mother-to-child transmission of HIV. The division's program of promoting and enabling antiretroviral therapy (ART) lowers the blood level of circulating HIV in maternal blood—the "viral load"—which is correlated with the transmission risk to the infant during pregnancy, childbirth, and breastfeeding. Increasing the prevalence of ART for mothers globally reduced the number of new infant HIV infections by 60 percent between 2001 and 2016. Still more work is needed to completely stop mother-to-child HIV transmission, such as making sure mothers and babies stay in treatment until breastfeeding is complete and testing babies whose mothers are known to have HIV.

The viral load has been measured in terms of the count of CD4 positive (CD4+) T cells (white blood cells that are part of the immune system that fight infection). The normal range for CD4 cells is between about 500 and 1,500 in the so-called T-cell blood test. When the CD4+ count drops below 200, a patient will develop life-threatening opportunistic infections such as *Pneumocystis* pneumonia, a type of pneumonia that develops mainly in individuals with impaired immune systems, or Kaposi's sarcoma, an otherwise rare type of cancer that affects immunocompromised people. In some developing countries, such as Malawi and Haiti, the numbers of laboratory facilities needed to assess CD4+ counts are too few to test every mother at risk for transmitting HIV to her infant. In 2011 Malawi, soon followed by other developing countries, implemented the Option B+ program, in which all pregnant and breastfeeding women infected with HIV can receive lifelong ART regardless of CD4+ count. This program has dramatically increased the use of ART among at-risk mothers in Malawi and may be instrumental in achieving the World Health Organization's (WHO) goal of eliminating mother-to-child HIV transmission globally.

Saliva and Other Bodily Fluids

Researchers have detected HIV in the saliva of infected people. However, as of 2017 no evidence has been produced that the virus is transmitted by contact with saliva. Laboratory studies indicate that saliva has natural properties that limit the infectivity of HIV, and the concentration of virus in saliva has been found to be very low. Studies of HIV-positive individuals have found no evidence that the virus can be spread through saliva by kissing. Because of the potential for contact with blood during open-mouth kissing, the CDC does not recommend engaging in this activity with a person known to be infected with HIV. However, the risk of acquiring HIV during open-mouth kissing is very low. The CDC has investigated only one case of HIV infection that may be attributed to contact with blood during open-mouth kissing. Nevertheless, the mucous membrane of the mouth can be infected by HIV, and there have been documented instances of HIV transmission through oral sex.

Researchers have found no evidence that HIV is spread through sweat, tears, urine, or feces that is not contaminated with blood.

Biting

In 1997 the CDC published findings from a state health department investigation of an incident that suggested blood-to-blood transmission of HIV by a human bite. There have been other reports in medical literature in which HIV appeared to have been transmitted by a bite. Severe trauma with extensive tissue tearing and damage and presence of blood were reported in each of these instances. Biting is not a common way of transmitting HIV. In fact, there are numerous reports of bites that did not result in HIV infection.

Casual Contact and Environmental Transmission

Extensive studies of families of HIV-infected people have shown conclusively that HIV is not spread through casual contact such as the sharing of food utensils, towels and bedding, swimming pools, telephones, or toilet seats. HIV is not spread by biting insects such as mosquitoes or bedbugs. From the beginning of the AIDS epidemic, some people feared that HIV might be transmitted in other common ways, but no scientific evidence to support these fears has been found. If HIV were being transmitted via other routes (such as through air, water, or insects), the pattern of reported AIDS cases would be much different from what has been observed. For example, if mosquitoes could transmit HIV infection, many more young children and adolescents would have been diagnosed with AIDS. All reported cases suggesting new or potentially unknown routes of transmission are thoroughly investigated by state and local health departments with assistance, guidance, and laboratory support from the CDC. No additional routes of transmission have been recorded as of 2017, despite a national sentinel system (an early warning system using animals or population data to detect the presence of disease) designed to detect just such an occurrence.

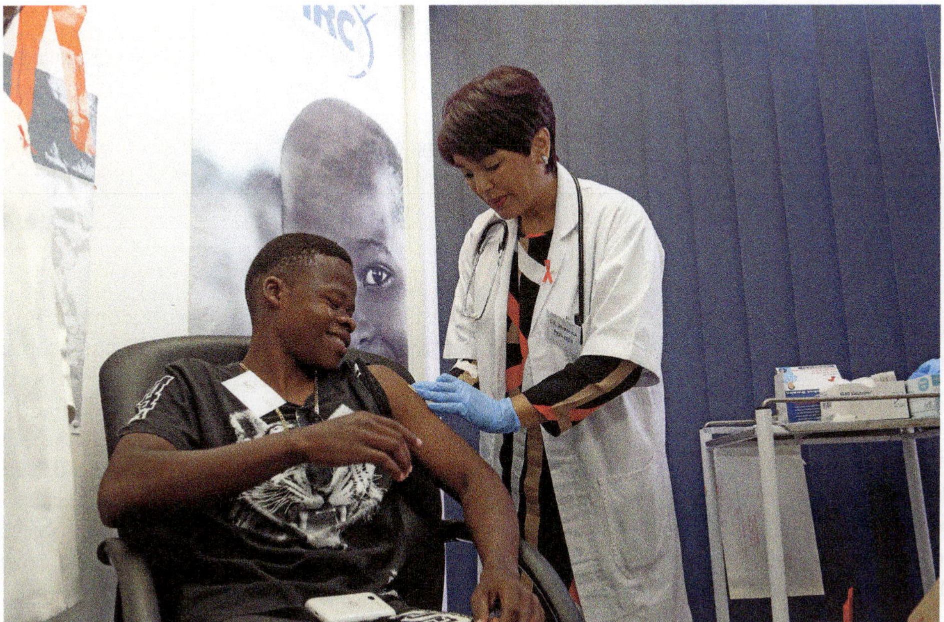

A man receives an injection as part of an experimental AIDS vaccine trial in South Africa in 2016.
© Gallo Images/The Times/Jackie Clausen/Getty Images

WORDS TO KNOW

ANTIBODIES Proteins found in the blood that help fight against foreign substances called antigens. Antigens, which are usually proteins or polysaccharides, stimulate the immune system to produce antibodies, or Y-shaped immunoglobulins. The antibodies inactivate the antigen and help remove it from the body. While antigens can be the source of infections from pathogenic bacteria and viruses, organic molecules detrimental to the body from internal or environmental sources also act as antigens. Genetic engineering and the use of various mutational mechanisms allow the construction of a vast array of antibodies (each with a unique genetic sequence).

ASYMPTOMATIC A state in which an individual does not exhibit or experience symptoms of a disease.

CD4+ T CELLS A type of T cell found in the immune system that are characterized by the presence of a CD4 antigen protein on their surface. These are the cells most often destroyed as a result of HIV infection.

HIGHLY ACTIVE ANTIRETROVIRAL THERAPY (HAART) The name given to the combination of drugs given to people with human immunodeficiency virus (HIV) infection to slow or stop the progression of their condition to AIDS (acquired immunodeficiency syndrome). HIV is a retrovirus, and the various components of HAART block its replication by different mechanisms.

LATENT INFECTION An infection already established in the body but not yet causing symptoms or having ceased to cause symptoms after an active period.

OPPORTUNISTIC INFECTION An infection that occurs in people whose immune systems are diminished or are not functioning normally. Such infections are opportunistic insofar as the infectious agents take advantage of their hosts' compromised immune systems and invade to cause disease.

PANDEMIC An epidemic that occurs in more than one country or population simultaneously. *Pandemic* means "all the people."

REPLICATE To duplicate something or make a copy of it. All reproduction of living things depends on the replication of DNA molecules or, in a few cases, RNA molecules. Replication may be used to refer to the reproduction of entire viruses and other microorganisms.

RETROVIRUS Viruses in which the genetic material consists of ribonucleic acid (RNA) instead of the usual deoxyribonucleic acid (DNA). Retroviruses produce an enzyme known as reverse transcriptase that can transform RNA into DNA, which can then be permanently integrated into the DNA of the infected host cells.

SENTINEL An epidemiological method in which a subset of the population is surveyed for the presence of communicable diseases. Also, an animal used to indicate the presence of disease within an area.

SEXUALLY TRANSMITTED INFECTION (STI) Infections that vary in their susceptibility to treatment, their signs and symptoms, and the consequences if they are left untreated. Some are caused by bacteria. These usually can be treated and cured. Others are caused by viruses and can typically be treated but not cured.

STRAIN A subclass or a specific genetic variation of an organism.

ULCERATIVE STI Any kind of sexually transmitted infection (STI) that results in genital ulcers. This includes herpes, syphilis, chancroid, and gonorrhea. Herpes is the most common.

Households

Although HIV has been transmitted between family members in a household setting, such transmission is very rare. These transmissions are argued to have resulted from contact between skin or mucous membranes and infected blood. To prevent even such rare occurrences, precautions should be taken in all settings, including the home, to prevent exposure to the blood of people who are HIV infected, who are at risk for HIV infection, or whose infection and risk status are unknown. CDC guidelines stipulate that (1) gloves should be worn during contact with blood or other body fluids that could possibly contain visible blood, such as urine, feces, or vomit; (2) cuts, sores, or breaks on both the caregiver's and the patient's exposed skin should be covered with bandages; (3) hands and other parts of the body should be washed immediately after contact with blood or other body fluids, and surfaces soiled with blood should be disinfected appropriately; (4) practices that increase the likelihood of blood contact, such as sharing of razors and toothbrushes, should be avoided; and (5) needles and other sharp instruments should be used only when medically necessary and handled according to recommendations for health care settings.

Businesses and Other Settings

There is no known risk of HIV transmission to coworkers, clients, or consumers from contact in industries such as food-service establishments. Food-service workers known to be infected with HIV need not be restricted from work unless they have other infections or illnesses (such as diarrhea or hepatitis A) for which any food-service worker, regardless of HIV infection status, should be restricted. The CDC recommends that all food-service workers follow recommended standards and practices of good personal hygiene and food sanitation.

In 1985 the CDC issued routine precautions that all personal-service workers (such as hairdressers, barbers, cosmetologists, and massage therapists) should follow, even though there is no evidence of transmission from a personal-service worker to a client or vice versa. Instruments that penetrate the skin (such as tattooing and acupuncture needles, ear piercing devices) should be used once and disposed of or thoroughly cleaned and sterilized. Instruments that are not intended to penetrate the skin but may become contaminated with blood (e.g., razors) should be used for only one client and disposed of or thoroughly cleaned and disinfected after each use. Personal-service workers can use the same cleaning procedures that are recommended for health care institutions.

As of 2017 the CDC reported no instances of HIV transmission through tattooing or body piercing, although hepatitis B virus has been transmitted during some of these practices. One case of HIV transmission from acupuncture has been documented. The medical complications for body piercing appear to be greater than for tattoos. Healing of piercings generally will take weeks, and sometimes even months, and the pierced tissue could conceivably be abraded (torn or cut) or inflamed even after healing. Therefore, a theoretical HIV transmission risk does exist if the unhealed or abraded tissues come into contact with an infected person's blood or other infectious body fluid. Additionally, HIV could be transmitted if instruments contaminated with blood are not sterilized or disinfected between clients.

Sexually Transmitted Infections

Sexually transmitted infections (STIs) such as syphilis, genital herpes, chlamydia, gonorrhea, and bacterial vaginosis appear to increase susceptibility to infection with HIV during sex with infected partners. A study published in the journal *Sexually Transmitted Diseases* in 1992 reported that "having an STD [sexually transmitted disease] more than doubles the risk of an HIV-negative heterosexual person of acquiring HIV during sex with an HIV-positive heterosexual partner." This conclusion applies to ulcerative STIs among HIV-negative partners who have genital herpes, syphilis, or chancroid. In the United States condoms are regulated by the Food and Drug Administration (FDA), and condom manufacturers are required to test each latex condom for defects such as holes prior to packaging. The proper and consistent use of latex or polyurethane condoms when engaging in vaginal, anal, or oral sexual intercourse can greatly reduce the risk of acquiring or transmitting sexually transmitted diseases, including HIV infection.

Only latex or polyurethane condoms provide a highly effective mechanical barrier to HIV. In laboratories, viruses occasionally have been shown to pass through natural membrane ("skin" or lambskin) condoms, which may contain natural pores and are therefore not recommended for disease prevention, although they are documented to be effective for contraception. For condoms to provide maximum protection, they must be used consistently and correctly. Numerous studies among sexually active people have demonstrated that a properly used latex condom provides a high degree of protection against a variety of sexually transmitted diseases, including HIV infection.

Early Signs and Symptoms of HIV Infection

Most people show no early symptoms when initially infected with HIV. In a minority of cases, people may have a flulike illness within a month or two after exposure that could include fever, headache, fatigue, and swollen lymph nodes in the neck and groin. These symptoms usually disappear within a week to a month and are often attributed to some other viral infection. During this early period, people are very contagious, and HIV is present in large quantities in genital fluids.

Long-lasting, debilitating symptoms may not appear for 10 or more years after infection with HIV in adults or within 2 years in children born with HIV infection. This latent period without symptoms varies greatly by individual, ranging from a few months to more than a decade. However, even during the asymptomatic period, the virus is actively multiplying and destroying immune system cells or can be dormant (inactive) within infected cells. The most readily apparent laboratory sign of HIV infection is a gradual decline in the blood concentration of CD4+ cells, which are the immune system's most important infection fighters. HIV slowly disables or destroys these cells without causing symptoms.

As the immune system deteriorates, various complications appear. The first persistent symptoms experienced by many people with HIV include enlarged lymph nodes for more than three months, fatigue, weight loss, frequent fevers and sweats, persistent or frequent yeast infections (oral or vaginal), persistent skin rashes or flaky skin, pelvic inflammatory disease in women that does not respond to treatment, and short-term memory loss. Some people develop frequent and severe herpes infections that cause mouth, genital, or anal sores or a resurgence of the dormant virus that causes chickenpox, known as shingles. Children may fail to thrive and grow.

Acquired Immunodeficiency Syndrome (AIDS)

Usually after a long assault on the immune system, victims reach the most advanced stage of HIV infection, which is known as AIDS. The CDC, the agency responsible for tracking the AIDS epidemic in the United States, has developed official criteria that define AIDS. The CDC's definition of AIDS includes all HIV-infected people who have fewer than 200 CD4+ T cells per cubic millimeter of blood. (Healthy adults usually have CD4+ T-cell counts of 1,000 or more.) In addition, the definition includes 26 clinical conditions, mainly opportunistic infections that affect people with advanced HIV disease. In people with AIDS, these infections are generally severe and can be fatal because the immune system is so ravaged by HIV that the body loses its ability to fight off certain bacteria, viruses, fungi, parasites, and other microbes.

Common symptoms of opportunistic infections in both adults and children with AIDS include persistent coughing and shortness of breath, seizures, lack of coordination, difficult or painful swallowing, confusion or forgetfulness, severe and persistent diarrhea, fever, vision loss, nausea, abdominal cramps, vomiting, weight loss, extreme fatigue, and severe headaches. In addition, children may have severe forms of common childhood bacterial infections such as conjunctivitis (pink eye), otitis media (ear infection), and tonsillitis.

In addition to opportunistic infections, people with AIDS are prone to various cancers that are associated with persistent exposure to certain viruses, such as Kaposi's sarcoma and cervical cancer, or cancers of the immune system known as lymphomas. These cancers are usually more aggressive and difficult to treat in people with AIDS.

As HIV infection progresses and the number of CD4+ T cells declines, people with CD4+ T cells above 200 may experience some of the early symptoms of HIV disease. Conversely, others with their CD4+ T-cell count below 200 may have no symptoms. Victims frequently become so debilitated by the symptoms of AIDS that they are unable to work or do household chores. Other people with AIDS may experience intermittent phases of life-threatening illness followed by periods during which they appear to be reasonably healthy.

A few people known to have been infected with HIV before 1997 have not developed symptoms of AIDS. Scientists are trying to ascertain what factors may account for this lack of progression to AIDS, such as whether their immune systems have particular characteristics, whether they were infected with a less aggressive strain of the virus, or whether their genes may protect them from the effects of HIV. Researchers hope that understanding the body's natural method of controlling infection may produce ideas for protective HIV vaccines that can prevent the disease from progressing in the general population. In 2012 researchers at Joshua Sharp's laboratory at the University of Georgia's Research Center, along with Robert Woods's computational chemistry group at the University of Georgia and Dennis Burton's virology group at Scripps Research, identified people with "natural immunity" to HIV. Such individuals create antibodies that bind with a protein on the viral envelope or surface of HIV known as gp120. This protein enables HIV to find targets everywhere in the body, attach to them, and gain entry into host cells. The antibodies in people with natural immunity attack this and disrupt its functions. Crucially, HIV is not able to mutate to evade the attack.

Diagnosis

Because early HIV infection often causes no symptoms, health care providers can usually diagnose it by testing blood for the presence of antibodies to HIV. HIV antibodies generally do not reach noticeable levels in standard blood tests in the blood for one to three months or more following infection. To determine whether a person has been recently infected, health care providers can screen for the presence of HIV genetic material. This direct screening of HIV is extremely critical to prevent transmission of HIV from recently infected individuals. Such individuals can discuss with health care providers when they should start treatment to help combat HIV and prevent the emergence of opportunistic infections. Early testing also alerts people to avoid high-risk behaviors that could transmit the virus to others. Health care providers often provide counseling to individuals who test HIV positive. People can be tested anonymously at many sites if they are concerned about confidentiality.

The diagnosis of HIV infection is established by using a test to detect HIV nucleic acid or several different types of antibody tests. Individuals who are highly likely to be infected with HIV but have received negative results for a particular test may request additional tests or may be told to repeat antibody testing at a later date, when antibodies are more likely to have developed.

Types of HIV screening tests currently approved by the CDC include HIV-1 nucleic acid laboratory-based tests to detect the actual virus in blood, antigen/antibody (Ag/Ab) laboratory-based tests, and antibody rapid tests. The CDC has posted a chart detailing the strengths and limitations of each of these tests, which vary in terms of run time, cost, and time sensitivity.

Babies born to HIV-infected mothers may or may not be infected with the virus, but all carry their mothers' antibodies to HIV for several months. If these babies lack symptoms, a doctor cannot make a definitive diagnosis of HIV infection using standard antibody tests. Extremely sensitive p24 antigen detection is a dependable method for detecting HIV infection in infants older than six weeks. However, this procedure requires special equipment and consumables that may not be available for purchase. In resource-constrained settings, HIV DNA and RNA polymerase chain reaction (PCR) kits are increasingly affordable and used worldwide.

The CDC recommends that all women undergo HIV testing during prenatal care using an "opt-out" approach, meaning that a pregnant woman will be administered an HIV test during prenatal care unless she refuses to have the test. The CDC also recommends a second test during the third trimester of pregnancy in regions where HIV infection rates are higher.

■ Scope and Distribution

In the United States, as of the end of 2015, nearly 1 million adults and adolescents and more than 2,000 children were living with diagnosed HIV infection; more than 500,000 adults and adolescents were living with AIDS. AIDS has been spreading most rapidly among non-Caucasian populations and is one of the foremost killers of adult African American males between the ages 25 and 44. The CDC reports that the population rate of AIDS is more than eight times higher among African Americans and three times higher among Hispanics than whites in the United States.

As of 2016 WHO estimates that there were almost 37 million adults and children living with HIV globally, with nearly 2 million new infections and 1 million deaths that year.

■ Treatment and Prevention

When AIDS first appeared in the United States, there were no medicines that were effective against HIV, and few treatments existed for the associated opportunistic diseases. Within a relatively short time after the discovery of HIV, researchers began to develop drugs to fight both HIV infection and its associated infections and cancers.

The first group of drugs used to treat HIV infection, nucleoside reverse transcriptase (RT) inhibitors, interrupts an early stage of the virus as it replicates (duplicates). These drugs slow the spread of HIV in the body and delay the start of opportunistic infections. This class of drugs, called nucleoside analogs, includes AZT (azidothymidine), ddC (zalcitabine), ddI (dideoxyinosine), d4T (stavudine), 3TC (lamivudine), abacavir, tenofovir, and emtricitabine. Physicians can also prescribe non-nucleoside reverse transcriptase inhibitors (NNRTIs) to treat HIV infection, such as delavridine, nevirapine, and efravirenz, often in combination with other antiretroviral drugs.

A second class of drugs for treating HIV infection, protease inhibitors (PIs), was later approved. Protease inhibitors interrupt the virus from replicating itself at a later step in its life cycle. They include ritonavir, saquinivir, indinavir, amprenivir, nelfinavir, lopinavir, atazanavir, and fosamprenavir.

A third class of ART drugs are integrase strand transfer inhibitors (INSTIs). These drugs block the action of integrase, a viral enzyme that integrates the HIV genome into the DNA of the host cell. This integration is a crucial step in HIV replication, and blocking it can stop further viral proliferation.

Another class of drugs, HIV fusion inhibitors, includes enfuvirtide, the first approved fusion inhibitor. It works by interfering with HIV-1's (the first-discovered strain of HIV) ability to enter into cells by blocking the merging of the virus with the cell membranes. This inhibition blocks the virus's ability to enter and infect human immune cells. Enfuvirtide was designed for use in combination with other treatments. It reduces the level of HIV infection in the blood and may be active against HIV that has become resistant to certain antiviral treatment schedules.

The CDC has issued new HIV/AIDS treatment guidelines for health care providers regarding how they should initiate ART and the patient journey through various drug treatments over time. The guidelines recommend INSTI-based drug regimens as initial therapy for most patients. NNRTI- and PI-based regimens can be used for certain patients.

The new guidelines take longer-term safety data into account that show that tenofovir alafenamide (TAF) and tenofovir disoproxil fumarate (TDF) have fewer adverse effects on patients. For patients at risk for bone and kidney impairment, TAF is particularly advantageous. TDF does not raise lipid levels as much as other treatments. Patient safety, cost, and access should be considered when choosing between TAF and TDF. Certain other antiretroviral regimens cannot be used for initial therapy in combination with abacavir, TAF, and TDF due to drug-to-drug interactions. Various new combination treatment strategies are being tested in ongoing clinical trials.

The guidelines also emphasize that clinicians should not use monotherapy with any antiretroviral drug because it increases the risk of virologic failure and drug resistance. This is because HIV mutates frequently and is able to evade the drug mechanism of action and eliminate its effectiveness, leaving the virus free to proliferate.

Because HIV can become resistant to any of these drugs, health care providers must use a combination of treatments to effectively suppress the virus. When three or more drugs are used in combination, it is referred to as highly active antiretroviral therapy, or HAART, and can be used by people who are newly infected with HIV, as well as people with AIDS. Researchers have credited HAART as being a major factor in significantly reducing the number of deaths from AIDS in the United States. While HAART is not a cure for AIDS, it has greatly improved the health of many people with AIDS and reduces the amount of virus circulating in the blood to nearly undetectable levels. Researchers, however, have shown that HIV remains present in some places in the body, such as the lymph nodes, brain, testes, and retina of the eye, even in people who have been treated.

Opportunistic Infections

A number of available drugs help treat the opportunistic infections of AIDS. These drugs include foscarnet and ganciclovir to treat CMV (cytomegalovirus) eye infections, fluconazole to treat yeast and other fungal infections, and TMP/SMX (trimethoprim/sulfamethoxazole) or pentamidine to treat a pneumonia known as PCP (*Pneumocystis carinii* pneumonia) that is sometimes associated with AIDS.

Cancers

Health care providers use radiation, chemotherapy, or injections of alpha interferon, a genetically engineered protein that occurs naturally in the human body, to treat Kaposi's sarcoma or other cancers associated with HIV infection.

Prevention

In the absence of a vaccine for HIV, the only means to prevent infection by the virus is to avoid behaviors that put people at risk of infection, such as sharing needles and having unprotected sex. Because many people infected with HIV have no symptoms, there is no way of knowing with certainty whether a sexual partner is infected unless he or she has repeatedly tested negative for the virus and has not engaged in any risky behavior. Abstaining from having sex offers the most protection from AIDS. Using male latex condoms or female polyurethane condoms have been shown in prospective studies to offer partial protection during oral, anal, or vaginal sex. Only water-based lubricants should be used with male latex condoms.

Although some laboratory evidence shows that spermicides can kill HIV, researchers have not found that these products can prevent the transmission of HIV during sex.

Ongoing Research

A significant amount of research in the early 21st century is focused on finding the best ways to prevent and control the spread of HIV. Research is ongoing in all areas of HIV infection, including developing and testing preventive HIV vaccines and new treatments for HIV infection and AIDS-associated opportunistic infections. Researchers also continue to trace how the disease progresses or sometimes fails to progress in different people.

Current research also includes testing chemical barriers, such as topical microbicides (germ-killing compounds) that people can use in the vagina or in the rectum during sex to help prevent HIV transmission. In addition, scientists are examining the effectiveness of other ways of preventing HIV transmission, including controlling other sexually transmitted infections, such as chlamydia, that have a role in making HIV easier to contract.

■ Impacts and Issues

As of 2017 the number of people infected with HIV has been declining due to increasingly effective prevention and prophylactic strategies. Approximately two-thirds of infected people live in Africa, where the epidemic grew exponentially during the 1990s, and one-fifth are in Asia, where the epidemic has been growing most rapidly in the early 21st century. By the end of 2016, nearly 40 million people worldwide were living with HIV infection. Worldwide funding from public and private sources to combat the epidemic initially rose dramatically in an urgent effort to reverse the growth trajectory of the epidemic. Indeed, the global response to the HIV/AIDS epidemic was unparalleled in public health history. As a result of this effort, projections of worldwide HIV infections and deaths were revised downward. However, as of 2017 the amount of funding has declined. Funding to combat HIV in low- and middle-income countries decreased by 7 percent from 2015 to 2016. This reduction in the global HIV response came after a period of flatline funding beginning during the global economic crisis of 2008–2009. It is not clear whether the decrease in HIV infections and deaths can be sustained in the face of resource cuts, particularly on the part of developing countries that bear the greatest burden of HIV.

Data has shown that the primary modes of HIV transmission have not changed significantly over time from those already outlined: unprotected heterosexual intercourse, unprotected anal sex between men, injection-drug use, unsafe medical injections and blood transfusions, and transmission from mother to child during pregnancy, labor and delivery, or breastfeeding. Direct blood contact, such as the sharing of drug-injection equipment, is by far the most efficient means of transmitting the virus.

However, the specific features of the epidemic vary among regions and within countries. The most recent statistics underline global disparities in AIDS deaths. Absent treatment with antiretroviral drugs, it usually takes about 10 years for HIV infection to progress to AIDS. In 2016 approximately 420,000 people died of AIDS-related illnesses in eastern and southern Africa, the region hardest hit by the epidemic, although the death toll fell substantially from 760,000 in 2010. By comparison, in Western Europe and North America, where drug treatment is widely available, comparatively few (an estimated 18,000) people died of AIDS in 2016.

The rate of new infections among children declined by 56 percent among children 0 to 14 years from 2010 to 2016 to about 77,000. Although mother-to-child transmission of HIV at birth is the main route of infection, many of the new infections among children are attributed to child marriage, in which girls are not empowered to assert any desire for safer sex. During 2013–2015 countries such as Ethiopia, Zambia, and Malawi have passed laws against child marriage, in part to help protect children from HIV and prevent child abuse.

Because the rapid growth of the epidemic was more recent in Asia, the number of deaths from AIDS has been comparatively lower than in Africa, given the number of infected people and a similar lack of drug treatment. Still, hundreds of thousands of people have died in Thailand, India, China, and other countries in South and East Asia since 2005. In 2016 there were 270,000 new HIV infections and 170,000 deaths.

Increasingly the mantra of the international community is access for all to effective antiretroviral therapy. Only two approaches to containing the epidemic have been effective: preventing new HIV infections and providing antiretroviral treatment to victims of HIV. As there is no AIDS vaccine, prevention efforts focus on education about sexual and other practices, behavioral change, and outreach to marginalized groups of people, including injection-drug users and sex workers and their clients. Many infected people do not realize that they are infected; others may not seek available care because of the stigma of being HIV positive. Cambodia and Thailand are cited as examples of nations that have prevention programs promoting increased condom use by prostitutes and their clients that have been demonstrably effective.

Significant progress has been made toward WHO goals for reducing AIDS deaths. Numbers of annual AIDS deaths have dropped from 1.9 million globally in 2005 to 1 million in 2016 and are projected to be cut in half again by 2020. Even if ambitious WHO goals for increasing access to antiretroviral treatment are successful, and despite substantial progress toward these goals, only about half of the people globally who need treatment for HIV infection are receiving it. A few countries such as Botswana, Senegal, and Uganda in Africa and Brazil in South America are doing better. Brazil has a universal program for distributing antiretroviral medications. Botswana, with one of the highest adult HIV infection rates in the world (21.9 percent), has a program of routine HIV testing and is also successfully expanding access to drug treatment.

There is some evidence that the global HIV epidemic is starting to slow slightly, both in the rate of new infections and in the AIDS death rate. Behavioral change based on detailed knowledge of the means of viral transmission has been successful in saving millions of lives, and access to modern drug therapy has and can save millions more. Although the ultimate eradication of HIV infection remains a cherished goal of the worldwide medical research community, efforts to change behavior and expand access to currently available treatments will save untold millions of lives until the enigma of HIV infection is finally solved.

SEE ALSO *AIDS: Origin of the Modern Pandemic; Bloodborne Pathogens; Epidemiology; Opportunistic Infection; Public Health and Infectious Disease; Sexually Transmitted Infections*

BIBLIOGRAPHY

Books

Bell, Sigall K., Courtney L. McMickens, and Kevin Selby. *AIDS.* Santa Barbara, CA: Greenwood, 2011.

Johanson, Paula. *HIV and AIDS (Coping in a Changing World).* New York: Rosen, 2007.

World Health Organization. *Preventing HIV/AIDS in Young People.* Geneva: WHO, 2006.

Periodicals

Buehler, Kelsey, Julie Spencer-Rogers, and Kaiping Peng. "HIV/AIDS, Treatment Adherence, and Lifestyle: A Qualitative Study." *Journal of HIV/AIDS & Social Services* 6, no. 4 (October–December 2017): 367–381.

McNeil, Donald G., Jr. "Progress Against AIDS, but Not Enough." *New York Times* (November 8, 2017): D3. This article can also be found online at https://www.nytimes.com/2017/11/20/health/aids-drugs-united-nations.html (accessed December 6, 2017).

Paulson, Michael. "'Brilliant,' 41 and Lost to AIDS: The Theater World Asks Why." *New York Times* (October 15, 2017): AR1. This article can also be found online at https://www.nytimes.com/2017/10/11/theater/michael-friedman-aids-death-theater.html (accessed December 6, 2017).

Websites

"Advantages and Disadvantages of FDA-Approved HIV Assays Used for Screening, by Test Category." Centers for Disease Control and Prevention. https://www.cdc.gov/hiv/pdf/testing/hiv-tests-advantages-disadvantages.pdf (accessed December 5, 2017).

"Epidemiology of HIV Infection through 2016." Centers for Disease Control and Prevention. https://www.cdc.gov/hiv/pdf/library/slidesets/cdc-hiv-surveillance-genepi-2016.pdf (accessed December 5, 2017).

"Factors Increasing the Risk of Acquiring or Transmitting HIV." Centers for Disease Control and Prevention. https://www.cdc.gov/hiv/risk/estimates/riskfactors.html (accessed December 3, 2017).

"Funding for HIV and AIDS." Avert. https://www.avert.org/professionals/hiv-around-world/global-response/funding (accessed December 30, 2017).

"Guidelines for Prevention and Treatment of Opportunistic Infections in HIV-Infected Adults and Adolescents: Recommendations from CDC, the National Institutes of Health, and the HIV Medicine Association of the Infectious Diseases Society of America." Centers for Disease Control and Prevention. https://www.cdc.gov/mmwr/preview/mmwrhtml/rr58e324a1.htm (accessed December 5, 2017.

"HIV and AIDS in Asia and the Pacific Regional Overview." Avert. https://www.avert.org/professionals/hiv-around-world/sub-saharan-africa/overview (accessed January 1, 2018).

"HIV and AIDS in East and Southern Africa Regional Overview." Avert. https://www.avert.org/professionals/hiv-around-world/sub-saharan-africa/overview> (accessed January 1, 2018).

"HIV and AIDS in Western Europe and North America Regional Overview." Avert. https://www.avert.org/professionals/hiv-around-world/western europe and north america/overview (accessed January 1, 2018).

"Impact of an Innovative Approach to Prevent Mother-to-Child Transmission of HIV—Malawi, July 2011–September 2012." Centers for Disease Control and Prevention. https://www.cdc.gov/mmwr/preview/mmwrhtml/mm6208a3.htm (accessed December 2, 2017).

"People with Natural Immunity to HIV May Serve as Basis for New Vaccine." Medical Xpress. https://medicalxpress.com/news/2012–11-people-natural-immunity-hiv-basis.html (accessed December 28, 2017).

"Summary of the Global HIV Epidemic 2016." World Health Organization. http://www.who.int/hiv/data/epi_core_2016.png?ua=1 (accessed December 2, 2017).

"UNICEF Eastern and Southern Africa Overview." UNICEF. https://www.unicef.org/esaro/5482_HIV_AIDS.html (accessed January 1, 2018).

"Update: Investigations of Patients Who Have Been Treated by HIV-Infected Health-Care Workers." Centers for Disease Control and Prevention. https://www.cdc.gov/mmwr/preview/mmwrhtml/mm5753a3.htm (accessed December 2, 2017).

Kenneth T. LaPensee

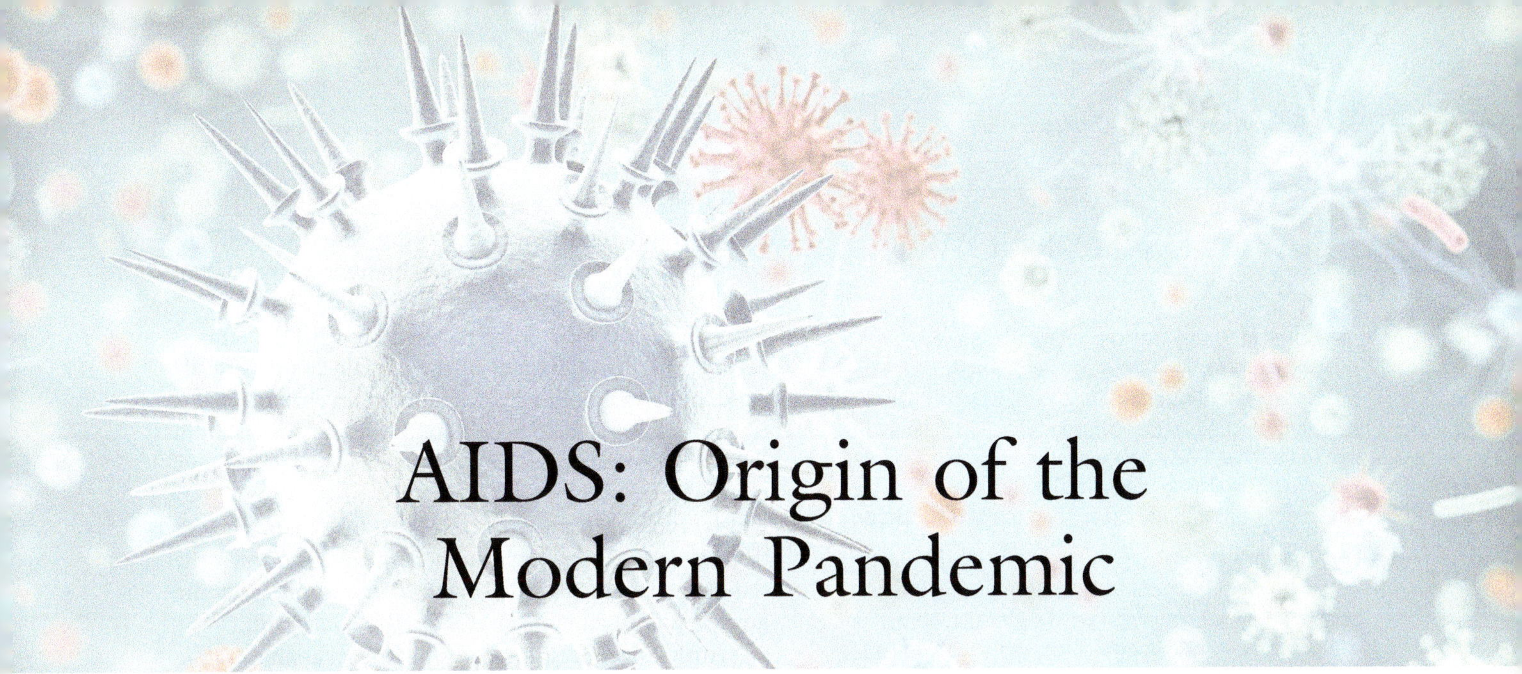

AIDS: Origin of the Modern Pandemic

Introduction

In 2018 the world reached the thirty-seventh year of the modern AIDS pandemic, which has been acknowledged by the United Nations (UN) to be among the deadliest epidemics in human history. A UN organization tasked with uniting efforts to treat and eliminate human immunodeficiency virus (HIV), the Joint United Nations Programme on HIV and AIDS (UNAIDS), estimated in 2017 that 78 million people have been infected with HIV since the beginning of the epidemic in 1981, 35 million of whom have died of illnesses associated with AIDS.

History and Policy Response

Evidence collected by medical archaeologists investigating human remains indicates that HIV jumped from chimpanzees to humans in the Kinshasa, Congo, region (now the Democratic Republic of the Congo) in the 1920s. Chimpanzees carry a related virus, Simian immunodeficiency virus (SIV). Chimps have long been hunted and eaten by people in that area. The virus could have been transmitted to a hunter by a bite. In the 1970s, just previous to the outbreak of AIDS cases in the early 1980s, the HIV virus was unknown. Due to its long latency period, transmission was not associated

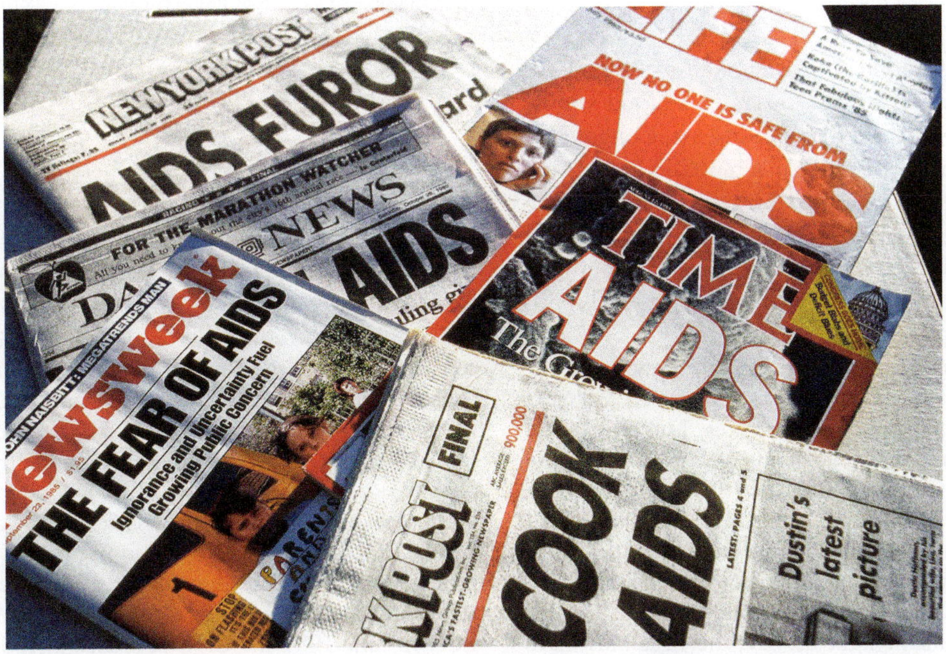

The Centers for Disease Control and Prevention first observed public health trends associated with the emergence of AIDS in 1981. By 1985 the AIDS crisis was at the center of American national discourse.
© Van D. Bucher/Science Source

WORDS TO KNOW

ANTIRETROVIRAL (ARV) DRUGS Drugs that prevent the reproduction of a type of virus called a retrovirus. The human immunodeficiency virus (HIV), which causes acquired immunodeficiency syndrome (AIDS), is a retrovirus. These ARV drugs are therefore used to treat HIV infections. These medicines cannot prevent or cure HIV infection, but they help to keep the virus in check.

IMMUNODEFICIENCY When part of the body's immune system is missing or defective, thus impairing the body's ability to fight infections. As a result, the person with an immunodeficiency disorder will have frequent infections that are generally more severe and last longer than usual.

LATENT INFECTION An infection already established in the body but not yet causing symptoms or having ceased to cause symptoms after an active period.

OPPORTUNISTIC INFECTION An infection that occurs in people whose immune systems are diminished or are not functioning normally. Such infections are opportunistic insofar as the infectious agents take advantage of their hosts' compromised immune systems and invade to cause disease.

PANDEMIC An epidemic that occurs in more than one country or population simultaneously. *Pandemic* means "all the people."

with signs or symptoms serious enough to be noticed. HIV was discovered by researchers in a blood sample collected in 1959 from a man in Kinshasa, Congo. Further genetic analysis of the man's blood indicated that the HIV infection was caused by a single virus in the late 1940s or early 1950s. Thus, it appears that the earliest human infections went unnoticed on a continent where people routinely die from tropical diseases with unusual manifestations.

HIV is a *lentivirus*, a class of viruses that attack the immune system in a way much like that in which SIV attacks the immune systems of other primates. Microbiological research has established that strains of HIV and SIV are closely related. One strain of SIV (SIVcpz) evolved in chimps that can also infect humans. The most widely accepted hypothesis is that SIVcpz was transferred to hunters via the consumption of chimp meat or from chimp blood entering wounds on a hunter's skin. Although the hunter's body would ordinarily fight off SIV, the virus must have adapted to the human host to become HIV-1. The existence of multiple HIV strains is due to multiple instances of SIVcpz transmission from various primate species, specifically the chimpanzee and the sooty mangabey, and adaptation to different human hosts over time. Accordingly, scientists have identified the species of monkeys that harbor the SIV strain that ultimately evolved to HIV-2.

HIV-1 and HIV-2 are the two known HIV strains. HIV-1, the first-identified of these strains, is genetically close to the strain of SIVcpz acquired from chimps. HIV-2 is genetically related to a strain of SIVcpz that is found in the sooty mangabey. However, because chimpanzees prey on monkeys and have been infected by viruses that are carried by them, it has been determined by genetic analysis that SIVcpz did not originate in chimps but rather in the red-capped mangabey (*Cercocebus torquatus*) and the greater spot-nosed monkey (*Cercopithecus nictitans*).

Analyses of medical records in African countries have shown that there had been striking increases in opportunistic infections now known to be AIDS-related during the late 1970s and early 1980s. These included "slim" disease in Zaire (late 1970s) and in Uganda and Tanzania (early 1980s), esophageal candidiasis in Rwanda (from 1983), aggressive Kaposi's sarcoma in Zaire (early 1980s) and in Zambia and Uganda (1982 and 1983), and cryptococcal meningitis in Zaire (late 1970s to early 1980s). Research suggests that, although isolated cases of AIDS may have occurred in Africa earlier, it was probably rare until the late 1970s and early 1980s. Studies further suggest that demographic groups and the routes of disease transmission have been largely similar in Africa and Western nations, implicating sexual activity among young and middle-aged people, blood transfusions, transmission from mother to infant (vertical transmission), and frequent exposure to unsterilized needles as the most likely means of transmitting AIDS.

Available data therefore suggest that the modern AIDS pandemic started in the mid- to late 1970s. By 1980 HIV had spread to North America, South America, Europe, and Australia. During this early stage of the epidemic, transmission of the virus was unhindered by awareness of the disease or any preventive action, and approximately 100,000 to 300,000 persons are estimated to have contracted the infection.

In March 1981, however, a few cases of an aggressive form of Kaposi's sarcoma were documented among young gay men in New York City. This development caused concern because Kaposi's sarcoma was known as a rare, relatively benign cancer that tended to occur in elderly people with immune system impairment. Simultaneously, there was an increase in California and New York in the incidence of *Pneumocystis* pneumonia (PCP), an unusual lung infection. The US Centers for Disease Control and Prevention (CDC) noticed this increase in April while monitoring prescriptions that were dispensed for rare drugs and detected a spike in requests for the drug pentamidine to treat PCP. In June 1981 the CDC published a report outlining the occurrence of five cases of PCP without identifiable cause in Los Angeles. This report marks the beginning of a more general awareness of AIDS. Shortly thereafter the

CDC formed a task force to investigate a syndrome that it called Kaposi's sarcoma (KS) and opportunistic infections (OI), or KSOI.

Speculation among scientists soon centered on whether this apparently new disease was a consequence of the widespread recreational use of amyl nitrate for sexual stimulation among gay men or the possibility of immune system overload in this population due to exposure to repeated sexually transmitted infections such as cytomegalovirus (CMV). CDC officials issued statements indicating that the disease appeared to be limited to gay men and that there was no apparent risk of spreading the disease through contagion.

By 1982, however, AIDS was reported among injection drug users, and disease patterns among a group of gay men in California appeared to support the notion that the disease was sexually transmitted. Later in the year, cases appeared among citizens of Haiti and among persons with hemophilia, a blood disorder that is treated with infusions of blood-clotting factors. After the spreading disease shed its exclusive association with gay men, the CDC characterized the disease as acquired immunodeficiency syndrome (AIDS). This terminology for the ailment was chosen because the immune system impairment that was its hallmark was acquired rather than inherited as in other known immunodeficiencies. AIDS was labeled a syndrome because it was associated with a group of diseases rather than a single disease. By the end of 1982, cases of AIDS began to appear in European countries, and a wasting syndrome dubbed "slim" was reported in Uganda, which was soon linked to AIDS. By the end of the year, more than 600 cases had been reported in the United States.

In 1983 physicians diagnosed the first cases of AIDS among women with no other apparent risk factors, indicating that the disease could be transmitted by heterosexual contact. In view of the evidence that AIDS was an infection that could be transmitted via blood and blood products, the CDC mounted a concerted effort to discover an infectious agent responsible for causing the disease. In May 1983 doctors at the Institute Pasteur in France reported the isolation of a new virus, which they suggested might be the cause of AIDS. Although scant notice was taken of this announcement when it was made, a sample of the virus was sent to the CDC. Several months later the virus was named lymphadenopathy-associated virus (LAV), and a sample of LAV was sent to the National Cancer Institute (NCI). In the meantime, public anxiety over the means of AIDS transmission, viewed by some people as potentially spread through casual contact due to its incidence among children, continued to grow, giving rise to increasingly numerous panic-driven and sometimes cruel interactions involving people either with AIDS or seen as at risk for AIDS. These incidents included evictions of persons with AIDS from housing, families and loved ones abandoning their relatives or partners with AIDS, and use of surgical masks during police work with individuals suspected of having AIDS. The CDC soon issued information that confirmed that there was no evidence for casual transmission and explained the possibility of bloodborne transmission of infection of AIDS from mothers to children.

By 1984 it became clear that the AIDS epidemic had been established in central Africa among populations that were not at risk from homosexuality, drug use, blood transfusion, or hemophilia. In Africa cases often had an aggressive and often fatal form of Kaposi's sarcoma, which had up to this point been endemic to the region but had been easily treatable. The main risk factor in Africa for AIDS appeared to be heterosexual contact. American and European scientists began to focus on the African epidemic, particularly because it appeared more likely to spread throughout the world due to its predominantly heterosexual mode of transmission.

The Institute Pasteur continued to claim that LAV was the cause of AIDS, but a related virus called human T-cell leukemia virus III (HTLV-III) was discovered by a research team in San Francisco. Investigators began to suspect that these viruses were identical. By the end of 1984, the CDC had reported nearly 8,000 AIDS cases and 3,500 deaths from the disease.

In 1985 the US Food and Drug Administration (FDA) confirmed that LAV and HTLV-III were identical and that the virus was indeed the cause of AIDS. The FDA additionally ordered testing of the national blood supply and required that anyone testing positive for the virus would not be allowed to donate blood. Now that the cause

THE FIRST REPORTS OF AIDS

Within an eight-month period from 1980 to 1981, five young men were hospitalized in the Los Angeles area with a rare, severe form of pneumonia caused by the pathogen *Pneumocystis carinii*. In reporting the outbreak to the US Centers for Disease Control and Prevention (CDC), physician Michael S. Gottlieb and his colleagues first documented in medical literature the disease that was to become known as AIDS. The report jarred physicians in New York and San Francisco, who noticed a handful of similar cases occurring at about the same time. In another unusual occurrence, eight young men in the New York area with Kaposi's sarcoma had recently died. Kaposi's sarcoma is a form of skin cancer that was usually seen mainly in elderly persons. Suspecting a new or emerging disease among young men, the CDC formed a task force to investigate the outbreaks. Gottlieb was an assistant professor of medicine at the University of California at Los Angeles (UCLA) in 1981 when he submitted the featured report as its lead author. In 1985 Gottlieb cofounded the American Foundation for AIDS Research (amfAR).

of AIDS could be detected, public bewilderment over AIDS transmission gave way to concern over the dissemination and use of information about HTLV-III/LAV infection. The gay community voiced fears of stigmatization of people found to carry the virus, believing the information would be misused by employers and insurance companies to exclude infected individuals. Incidents of cruelty and prejudice directed toward AIDS victims and perceived risk groups continued to mount, though Haitians were removed from the list of high-risk groups in view of a new understanding of heterosexual and injection-drug transmission risks. The year 1985 ended with more than 20,000 reported US AIDS cases, with more than 15,000 cases reported in other nations.

The International Committee on the Taxonomy of Viruses (ICTV) ruled in May 1986 that the LAV and HTLV-III virus names should be dropped in favor of human immunodeficiency virus (HIV). During that year the director-general of the World Health Organization (WHO), Halfdan T. Mahler (1923–2016), announced that some 10 million people worldwide could already have been infected with HIV by June 1986. The true scope and devastation of the disease had begun to be apparent to the scientific community.

■ Impacts and Issues

In early 2007 officials at UNAIDS estimated that another 50 million people could die from AIDS in India and China alone by the year 2025. In Africa, where research indicates that the epidemic likely began, AIDS will have killed 100 million people by that time if trends continue. Although antiretroviral (ARV) medications have begun to lower expected death rates, AIDS could still kill 40 million additional Africans by 2025. To date, all vaccine development programs have failed, although one small 2017 study of a so-called "therapeutic vaccine" (a vaccine that aims to control an active HIV infection) may have demonstrated limited and preliminary success in a few patients when administered after antiretroviral therapy (ART) had driven down their viral count to undetectable levels.

Prevention programs focused on changing sexual and drug-use behaviors have had increasing success across regions and across cultural and political divides. Introduced in 2011, the UNAIDS Global Plan has had a dramatic impact on providing HIV services to children and women in Uganda. In 2016 nearly all (approximately 115,000 women, or 95 percent) of HIV-positive pregnant women received ART to reduce mother-to-child transmission (MTCT). The UNAIDS effort to prevent MTCT is referred to as the Prevention of Mother-to-Child Transmission (PMTCT) program.

The progress of the PMTCT program in Uganda is clear: between 2009 and 2013, new infections among children were reduced by 50 percent. Much more still needs to be done to expand testing and effective treatment in that country. Just 56 percent of infants exposed to HIV were screened in 2012 and 2013. Of these, only 28 percent received effective treatment in 2013. Uganda had the fourth-highest number of new infections among children of the 22 countries given priority for prevention efforts by UNAIDS.

See Also *AIDS (Acquired Immunodeficiency Syndrome); Antiviral Drugs; Bloodborne Pathogens; Developing Nations and Drug Delivery; Epidemiology; Opportunistic Infection; Public Health and Infectious Disease; Sexually Transmitted Diseases*

BIBLIOGRAPHY

Books

Mayer, Kenneth H., and H. F. Pizer, eds. *The AIDS Pandemic: Impact on Science and Society.* San Diego: Academic Press, 2005.

Periodicals

Cohen, Jon. "AIDS Vaccine May Be 'Functional Cure' for Some." *Science* (February 22, 2017). This article can also be found online at http://www.sciencemag.org/news/2017/02/aids-vaccine-may-be-functional-cure-some (accessed December 23, 2017).

Gottlieb, M. S., et al. "*Pneumocystis* Pneumonia—Los Angeles." *Morbidity and Mortality Weekly Report* 30, no. 21 (June 5, 1981): 1–3.

Hymes, K. B., et al. "Kaposi's Sarcoma in Homosexual Men: A Report of Eight Cases." *Lancet* 2 (September 19, 1981): 598–600.

Sharp, Paul M., and Beatrice H. Hahn. "Origins of HIV and the AIDS Pandemic." *Cold Springs Harbor Perspectives in Medicine* 1 (2011): a006841.

Websites

"Ending AIDS: Progress Towards the 90–90–90 Targets." UNAIDS, July 20, 2017. http://www.unaids.org/en/resources/documents/2017/20170720_Global_AIDS_update_2017 (accessed December 17, 2017).

"Global HIV/AIDS Timeline." Henry J. Kaiser Family Foundation, November 29, 2016. https://www.kff.org/global-health-policy/timeline/global-hivaids-timeline/ (accessed December 23, 2017).

"Milestones in the U.S. HIV Epidemic." Centers for Disease Control and Prevention, 2002. https://stacks.cdc.gov/view/cdc/40914 (accessed December 23, 2017).

"Origin of HIV & AIDS." Avert, December 5, 2017. https://www.avert.org/professionals/history-hiv-aids/origin (accessed December 17, 2017).

Kenneth T. LaPensee

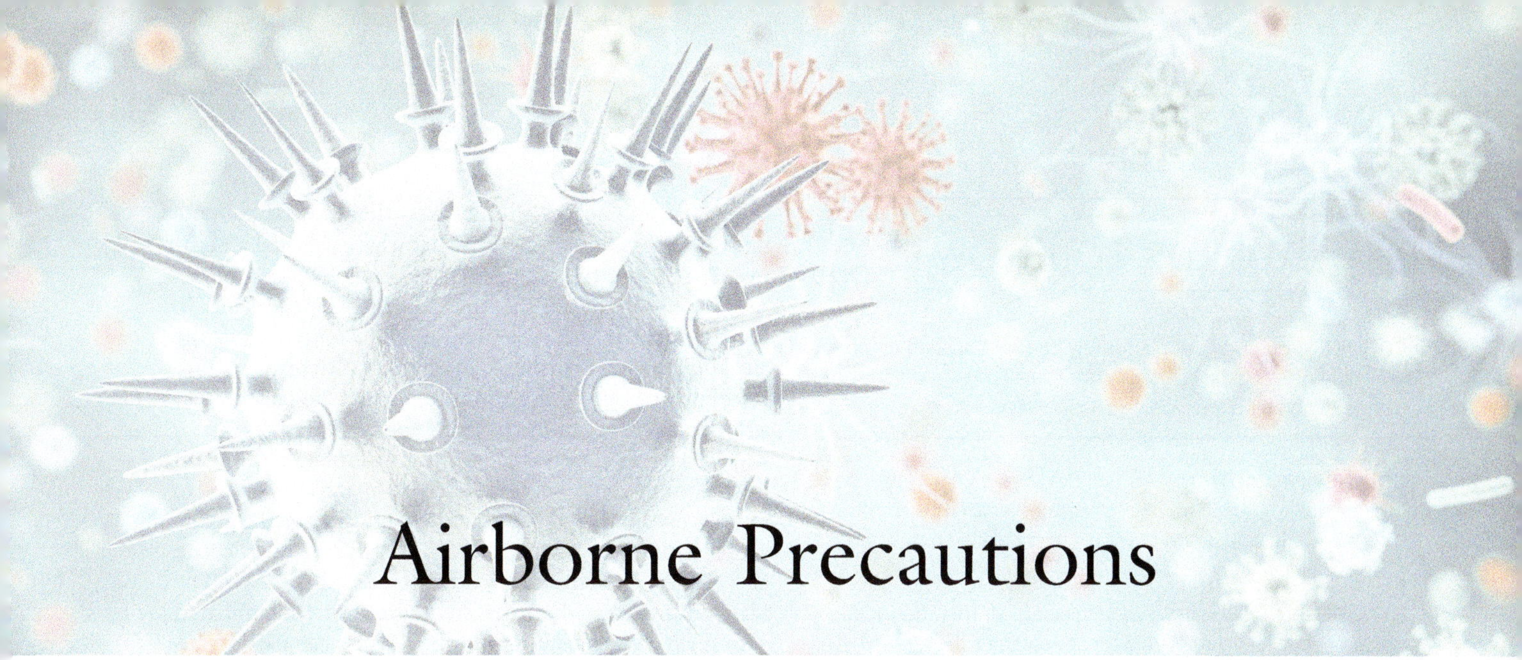

Airborne Precautions

Introduction

Airborne precautions are procedures that are designed to reduce the chance that certain disease-causing (pathogenic) microorganisms will be transmitted through the air.

The precautions relate to airborne, microbe-containing droplets that are less than 5 microns in diameter (a micron is 10^{-6} meters). Such droplets can remain suspended in the air for a long time and so can be transported a considerable distance (such as from room to room) in even a gentle current of air. In addition, particles of this size can be inhaled deeply into the lungs, where the chance of establishing an infection can be increased.

Airborne precautions that involve the treatment of the air and ventilation systems are necessary for patients who have tuberculosis and often for those with herpes zoster (shingles), varicella (chickenpox), and rubeola (measles). The precautions also apply to severe acute respiratory syndrome (SARS). Other diseases do not require these mandated precautions.

History and Scientific Foundations

It has been known since the mid-19th century that some bacteria and viruses can be dispersed into the air and that they can cause infection if they are inhaled or enter a wound. Joseph Lister (1827–1912) realized that operating room procedures that included covering the surgical site with sterile cloth was important in reducing the incidence of infections following surgery. Indeed, the physical isolation of an operating theater from the rest of a hospital and the wearing of a face mask by health care providers is designed in part to limit the airborne spread of microbes.

In the United States regulated airborne precautions were instituted by the Centers for Disease Control and Prevention (CDC). The latest guidelines were issued in 2007. The CDC also formulated separate guidelines that were specific for patients with tuberculosis.

Availability of Hospital Beds

Successful application of airborne precautions depends on the availability of hospital beds. Data from the *World Fact Book* demonstrates the wide disparity in the availability of hospital beds around the world. Data was not available for all countries.

Country	Hospital Beds (per 1,000 people)	Year
Iran (Islamic Republic of)	0.1	2012
Burkina Faso	0.4	2010
Afghanistan	0.5	2012
Egypt	0.5	2011
Bangladesh	0.6	2011
Guatemala	0.6	2011
Cambodia	0.7	2011
India	0.7	2011
Sudan	0.8	2012
Philippines	1.0	2011
Haiti	1.3	2007
Mexico	1.5	2011
Vietnam	2.0	2010
Thailand	2.1	2010
Sweden	2.5	2014
Canada	2.7	2010
United Kingdom	2.9	2011
United States	2.9	2011
Italy	3.4	2011
China	3.8	2011
Switzerland	5.0	2011
Cuba	5.3	2012
Ethiopia	6.3	2011
France	6.4	2011
Hungary	7.2	2011
Austria	7.6	2011
Germany	8.2	2011
Greenland	8.2	2014
Ukraine	9.0	2012
Belarus	11.3	2011
Japan	13.7	2009
Monaco	13.8	2012

SOURCE: US Central Intelligence Agency. *World Fact Book.* Available from: https://www.cia.gov/library/publications/the-world-factbook/fields/2227.html

WORDS TO KNOW

COHORT A group of people (or any species) sharing a common characteristic. Cohorts are identified and grouped in cohort studies to determine the frequency of diseases or the kinds of disease outcomes over time.

CONTACT PRECAUTIONS Actions developed to minimize the person-to-person transfer of microorganisms by direct physical contact and indirectly by inhalation or touching a contaminated surface.

HEPA FILTER A high-efficiency particulate air filter, designed to nearly totally remove airborne particles that are 0.3 microns (millionth of a meter) in diameter or larger. Such small particles can penetrate deeply into the lungs if inhaled.

Applications and Research

The airborne precautions pertain to patient placement in the hospital, transport of the patient from one area of the hospital to another, and the protective breathing gear worn by health care providers when around the patient.

According to the precautions, the affected patients must be housed in a room that has what is termed a negative air pressure relative to the surrounding spaces. Negative air pressure means that the number of air molecules in the room is less than the number of air molecules in the areas adjacent to the room. The result is that air will move into but not out of the room, reducing the chance that airborne microbes in the patient's room will disperse more widely. The air pressure of the room is monitored, the air in the room must be completely changed six to twelve times every hour, and the exhausted air is passed through a special type of air filter called a high-efficiency particulate air (HEPA) filter that traps extremely small particles. The filter ensures that the exhausted air is not contaminated with the pathogenic microbes. The filter is changed at regular intervals and disposed of in a certain way to make sure that the trapped microbes do not pose a further hazard.

The room should be separated from adjacent rooms and hallways by a door, which is left closed when not in use. Ideally, the room should be just for the affected patient. If this is not possible, then more than one patient can be housed in the same room (this is called cohorting). These cohorts should have the same infection that is caused by the same microorganism (there are exceptions for tuberculosis). However, the patients should not have any other infections. If these precautions cannot be met, then another strategy should not be undertaken without the advice of infection control experts.

The precaution concerning respiratory protection is specific. When entering the affected patient's room, health

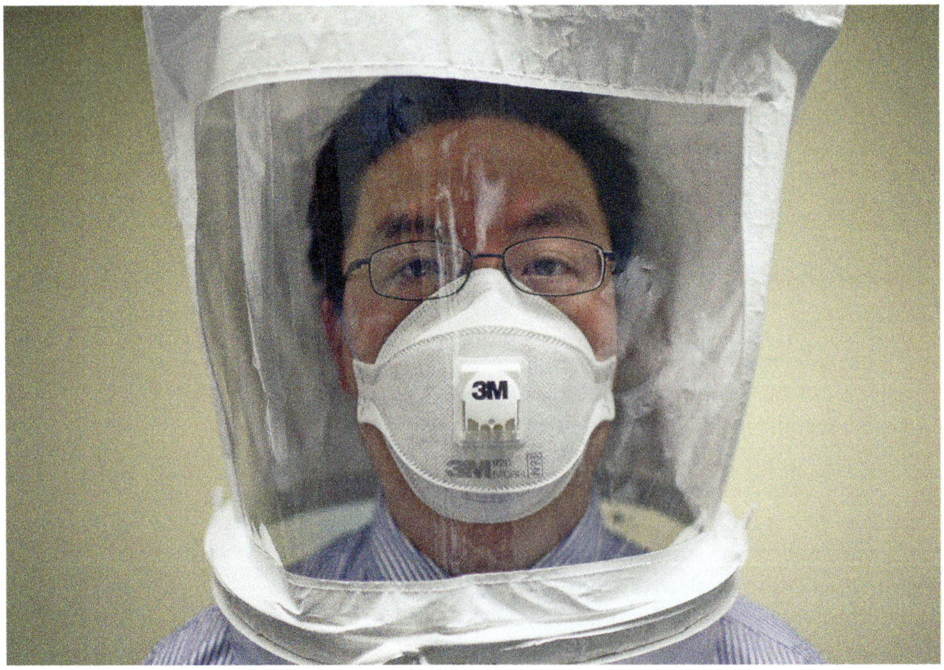

A doctor demonstrates the correct use of an N-95 respirator during a swine flu training in Oakland, California, in 2009. The mask is the best defense against infectious airborne particles. *© Justin Sullivan/Getty Images*

care providers must wear an N-95 respirator, which is a mask certified by the CDC's National Institute for Occupational Safety and Health (NIOSH). The mask is equipped with a filter that can trap over 95 percent of particles that are 0.3 microns or greater in diameter in an aerosol that is free of oil (oil can affect droplet size and is not the sort of aerosol encountered in hospitals).

Anyone who is susceptible to rubeola or chickenpox should not enter the room of a patient with these diseases without an N-95 mask. A person who has a compromised immune system should not have close contact with a person whose illness requires airborne precautions. This applies to other patients as well as visitors and health care personnel.

Airborne precautions also pertain to the movement of patients within the hospital. This movement should only be done when absolutely necessary. During transport a surgical mask is placed over the patient's nose and mouth to minimize the dispersal of droplets.

■ Impacts and Issues

Airborne precautions reduce the spread of certain infections. But this safeguard comes with a price tag. Equipping hospital rooms to be negative pressure rooms, installing and maintaining HEPA filters, and equipping staff with respirators is expensive. Furthermore, the requirements to frequently document compliance with the precautions is an added burden to hospital caretakers.

One example highlighting airborne precautions concerns *Mycobacterium tuberculosis*, which is extremely resistant to antibiotics. According to the World Health Organization (WHO), the extreme drug-resistant tuberculosis (XDR-TB) is virtually untreatable using the present arsenal of drugs. Strains of XDR-TB have been noted in individuals mainly in South Africa but also in Russia, North America, South America, and Asia. According to WHO, people infected with the human immunodeficiency virus (HIV) are particularly susceptible to XDR-TB. As of 2017 prevention and containment through the use of airborne precautions constituted the main line of defense against XDR-TB.

SEE ALSO *Anthrax; Bioterrorism; Contact Precautions; Droplet Precautions; Standard Precautions*

BIBLIOGRAPHY

Books

Delort, Anne-Marie, and Pierre Amato, eds. *Microbiology of Aerosols.* New York: Wiley-Blackwell, 2017.

Kumar, Sandeep, and Jane C. Benjamin. *Pathogenic Bacteria in Bioaerosol of Hospitals: Important of Airborne Pathogen in Hospital.* New York: Lap Lambert Academic, 2013.

Tierno, Philip M. *The Secret Life of Germs: What They Are, Why We Need Them, and How We Can Protect Ourselves against Them.* New York: Atria, 2004.

Periodicals

Graham, Judith. "In Flu Season, Use a Mask. But Which One?" *New York Times* (January 16, 2013). This article can also be found online at https://newoldage.blogs.nytimes.com/2013/01/16/in-flu-seasonuse-a-mask-but-which-one/ (accessed November 6, 2017).

McNeil, Donald G., Jr. "Fearsome Plague Epidemic Strikes Madagascar." *New York Times* (October 7, 2017): A12. This article can also be found online at https://www.nytimes.com/2017/10/06/health/madagascar-plague.html (accessed November 6, 2017).

Websites

"Transmission-Based Precautions." Centers for Disease Control and Prevention. https://www.cdc.gov/infectioncontrol/basics/transmission-based-precautions.html (accessed November 2017).

Brian Hoyle

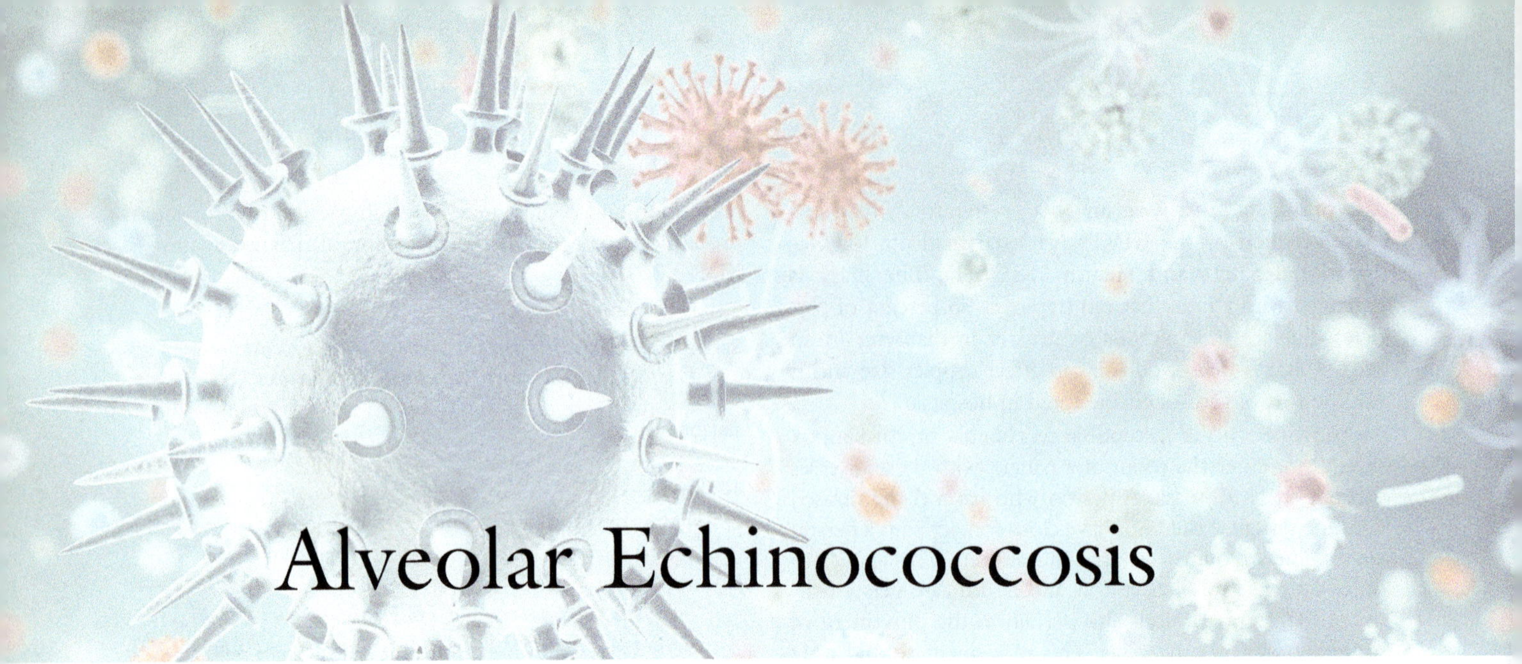

Alveolar Echinococcosis

Introduction

Alveolar echinococcosis (al-VEE-oh-ler ee-keye-ni-kah-KOH-sis) is an infection caused by the tapeworm *Echinococcus multilocularis.* The infection is rare in humans, although is serious when it occurs. If not treated, the infection is nearly always lethal. Tumorlike formations —due to the growth of the larval form of the tapeworm —occur most commonly in the liver but can also be present in the brain, lungs, and elsewhere in the body.

WORDS TO KNOW

LARVAE Immature forms (wormlike in insects; fishlike in amphibians) of an organism capable of surviving on its own. Larvae do not resemble the parent and must go through metamorphosis, or change, to reach the adult stage.

PARASITE An organism that lives in or on a host organism and that gets its nourishment from that host. The parasite usually gains all the benefits of this relationship, while the host may suffer from various diseases and discomforts or show no signs of the infection. The life cycle of a typical parasite usually includes several developmental stages and morphological changes as the parasite lives and moves through the environment and one or more hosts. Parasites that remain on a host's body surface to feed are called ectoparasites, while those that live inside a host's body are called endoparasites. Parasitism is a highly successful biological adaptation. There are more known parasitic species than nonparasitic ones, and parasites affect just about every form of life, including most all animals, plants, and even bacteria.

Disease History, Characteristics, and Transmission

E. multilocularis has a life cycle that consists of an egg phase and a larval phase. The eggs are excreted in the feces of the infected animal. If the feces are eaten by another animal, the eggs can germinate to form the larva, which matures in the intestine. As part of the maturation process, eggs are produced, which are shed in the feces. The cycle can then repeat in another animal.

Humans acquire the infection by ingesting the eggs. This usually occurs in one of two ways. First, food that is contaminated with fox or coyote feces is eaten. This can happen when, for example, a person hiking in the woods eats herbs or berries collected along the route. Second and more commonly, eggs that have stuck to the fur of family pets as they have been shed by the animal (or picked up as the dog or cat has rubbed against vegetation) transfer to the hands of the owner when the animal is petted or groomed and are accidentally ingested when the hands are put into the mouth.

As the larvae of the tapeworm grow, they aggregate (come together) to create tumorlike formations. These typically occur in the liver but can spread elsewhere. The symptoms, which develop slowly over years, include abdominal pain, a feeling of weakness, and loss of weight. The symptoms can be mistaken for the slow growth of a liver tumor or the type of progressive liver damage that can result from the chronic overconsumption of alcohol.

Scope and Distribution

Alveolar echinococcosis is widespread in animal populations in northern latitudes including Europe, China, Russia, Asia, Japan, and North America (primarily in the north-central area of the United States from Montana to Ohio, Alaska, and most of Canada). In these

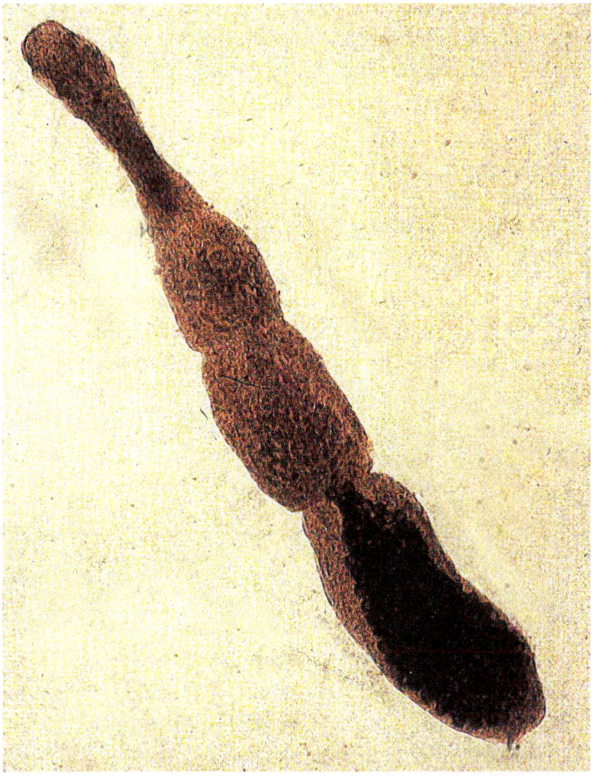

Echinococcus multilocularis photographed at the Ludwig Maximilians University of Munich in 2003. The tapeworm is the parasite that causes alveolar echinococcosis. © *Agency-Animal-Picture/Getty Images*

regions the tapeworm is present in over 50 percent of the fox and coyote populations. Human cases have rarely been reported in North America. In the 20th century only two cases are known to have occurred: one in the state of Minnesota and the other in the western Canadian province of Manitoba. Since 2000 only one more case has been confirmed, in the province of Alberta.

In addition to foxes and coyotes, *E. multilocularis* can be found in the intestinal tract of dogs and cats. The animals can also become infected when they eat rodents, voles, or field mice that are infected with the tapeworm larvae.

Because the infection occurs most often in wild foxes, people who are most at risk are those who spend much of their time outdoors. These include park rangers, trappers, and hunters. Urban and rural veterinarians also run a risk of contact because they handle animals that may carry the tapeworm eggs. There is no evidence of racial or gender association with the infection. The higher tendency of men to be infected could reflect the traditional dominance of men in occupations such as logging and in pursuits like hunting.

The distribution of the infection may be spreading as the territory of wild foxes contracts and they come into closer contact with humans. This is partially due to the expansion of urban areas; the availability of food attracts foxes that had not previously inhabited these areas.

Treatment and Prevention

As of 2017 there is no cure for alveolar echinococcosis. The most common treatment involves surgery to remove the tumorlike larval mass, followed by drug therapy to attempt to prevent the germination of eggs that may still be present in the individual. Drug therapy, typically with the antifungal compound benzimidazole, can be long and expensive.

The best prevention is to lessen the chances of contacting *E. multilocularis.* Avoiding contact with living or dead wild animals unless protective gloves are worn is a sensible precaution. Keeping domestic pets close to home and away from contact with wild animals is another wise move. Washing hands after handling pets is another preventative step but one that is difficult for most people to consistently follow.

The World Health Organization continues to try and develop an effective control strategy to prevent transmission of the tapeworm. As of 2017 its target date was 2020.

Impacts and Issues

The main impact on human health of alveolar echinococcosis is the high death rate of the infection if it is

PERSONAL RESPONSIBILITY AND PREVENTION

The Centers for Disease Control and Prevention recommends that people who live in an area where *E. multilocularis* is often found in rodents and wild canines take the following precautions to avoid infection:

- Don't touch a fox, coyote, or other wild canine, dead or alive, unless you are wearing gloves. Hunters and trappers should wear plastic gloves to avoid exposure.
- Don't keep wild animals, especially wild canines, as pets or encourage them to come close to your home.
- Don't allow your cats and dogs to wander freely or to capture and eat rodents.
- If you think that your pet may have eaten rodents, consult your veterinarian about the possible need for preventive treatments.
- After handling pets, always wash your hands with soap and warm water.
- Fence in gardens to keep out wild animals.
- Do not collect or eat wild fruits or vegetables picked directly from the ground. All wild-picked foods should be washed carefully or cooked before eating.

not treated. The odds of survival for five years if the infection is untreated is only 40 percent versus almost 90 percent if treatment is provided. Even with treatment, persons treated for alveolar echinococcosis often face a diminished quality of life. Furthermore, treatment comes with a high price tag: up to $300,000 per person.

The infection is an example of how political or economic decisions can influence a disease. The clearing of forests to provide more farmland or timber can cause rodent populations to become more concentrated in urban areas, increasing the chances for the spread of *E. multilocularis.*

SEE ALSO *Tapeworm Infections; Vector-Borne Disease; Zoonoses*

BIBLIOGRAPHY

Books

Colbert, Bruce J., and Luis S. Gonzalez III, eds. *Microbiology: Practical Applications and Infection Prevention.* Boston: Cengage Learning, 2016.

Dongyou Liu, ed. *Molecular Detection of Human Parasitic Pathogens.* Boca Raton, FL: Taylor & Francis, 2013.

Periodicals

Brehm, K., and U. Koziol. "*Echinococcus*-Host Interactions at Cellular and Molecular Levels." *Advances in Parasitology* 95 (2017): 147–212.

Budke, Christine M., Adriano Casulli, Peter Kern, and Dominique A. Vuitton. "Cystic and Alveolar Echinococcosis: Successes and Continuing Challenges." *PLOS Neglected Tropical Diseases* 11, no. 4 (2017).

Chauchet, Adrien, et al. "Increased Incidence and Characteristics of Alveolar Echinococcosis in Patients with Immunosuppression-Associated Conditions." *Clinical Infectious Diseases* 59, no. 8 (October 15, 2014): 1095–1104.

Massolo, Alessandro, Stefano Liccioli, Christine Budke, and Claudia Klein. "*Echinococcus multilocularis* in North America: The Great Unknown. *Parasite* 21 (2014): 73–86.

Piarroux, Martine, et al. "Populations at Risk for Alveolar Echinococcosis, France." *Emerging Infectious Diseases* 19, no. 5 (May 2013): 721–728.

Websites

"Alveolar Echinococcosis (AE) FAQs." Centers for Disease Control and Prevention. https://www.cdc.gov/parasites/echinococcosis/gen_info/ae-faqs.html (accessed November 6, 2017).

"Echinococcosis Fact Sheet." World Health Organization, March 2017. http://www.who.int/mediacentre/factsheets/fs377/en/ (accessed November 6, 2017).

Brian Hoyle

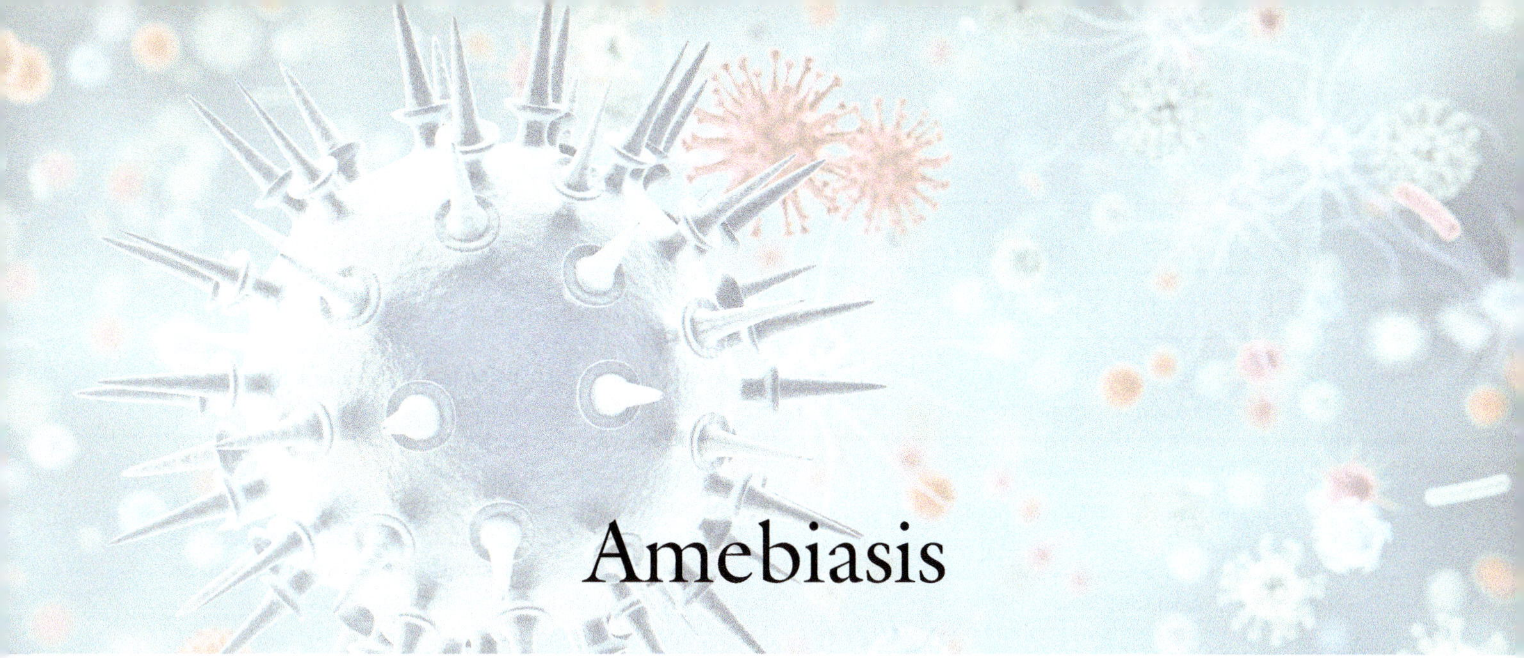

Amebiasis

Introduction

Amebiasis (am-e-BI-a-sis) is an infection that is caused by the one-celled parasite *Entamoeba histolytica*. The infection, which produces an inflammation of the cells lining the intestinal tract, is also referred to as amebic (or amoebic) dysentery.

Amebiasis often results in relatively mild illness, producing diarrhea and abdominal pain. However, the infection can be quite severe, with inflammation being so extensive that the intestinal wall in the colon can become perforated, and damage can occur to both the liver and the brain. In addition, diarrhea can be copious and often accompanied by vomiting, which can lead to dehydration if fluids are not replaced.

Disease History, Characteristics, and Transmission

E. histolytica can occur in two forms. One form is known as a cyst. This form is very tough and can survive harsh conditions of temperature and lack of moisture that would kill the other, growing form of the organism, the trophozoite. This hardiness makes a cyst similar to a bacterial spore. The parasite is excreted in feces as a cyst. It can survive for a long time until it finds itself in a more favorable environment, such as the intestinal tract of another person. There, the cyst can resume growth. The trophozoite is the form that causes amebiasis. Some trophozoites will form cysts and can be excreted, beginning another cycle of infection.

The cysts can also invade the walls of the intestine, where they can germinate into the trophozoite forms. Then, ulcers and diarrhea can be produced. Or, much more seriously, the cysts may enter the bloodstream and can be carried all over the body. Damage to tissues such as the brain and liver can result.

When symptoms develop, they tend to begin about two to four weeks after the parasite has entered the body, although some people develop symptoms in only a few days.

Amebiasis has been known since the early years of the 20th century. Despite this, the diagnosis of amebiasis has not changed, still relying on the visual detection of the cyst in feces from the person suspected of having the infection. This can be a tedious and lengthy process, often requiring days of examination. Complicating diagnosis, the cysts of *E. histolytica* resemble that of other amoeba, *Entamoeba coli* and *Entamoeba dispar*, which are normal and harmless residents of the intestinal tract of warm-blooded animals, including humans. Indeed, *E. histolytica* and *E. dipar* are virtually identical in appearance. This means that many cases of amebiasis are likely diagnosed incorrectly.

Scope and Distribution

Some people who are infected carry *E. histolytica* in their intestinal tract without displaying symptoms. Because the parasite can be excreted along with feces, a person can unknowingly pass the parasite to someone else by handling food with unwashed hands after going to the bathroom, by person-to-person contact (includ-

WORDS TO KNOW

DYSENTERY An infectious disease that has ravaged armies, refugee camps, and prisoner-of-war camps throughout history. The disease is still a major problem in developing countries with primitive sanitary facilities.

TROPHOZOITE The amoeboid, vegetative stage of the malaria protozoa.

AVOIDING INFECTION WITH E. HISTOLYTICA

To avoid infection with *E. histolytica*, the Centers for Disease Control and Prevention (CDC) recommends that a person traveling to a country that has poor sanitary conditions should observe the following with regard to eating and drinking:

- Drink only bottled or boiled (for one minute) water or carbonated (bubbly) drinks in cans or bottles. Do not drink fountain drinks or any drinks with ice cubes. Another way to make water safe is by filtering it through an "absolute 1 micron or less" filter and dissolving iodine tablets in the filtered water. "Absolute 1 micron" filters can be found in camping/outdoor supply stores.
- Do not eat fresh fruit or vegetables that you did not peel yourself.
- Do not eat or drink milk, cheese, or dairy products that may not have been pasteurized.
- Do not eat or drink anything sold by street vendors.

ing sexual intercourse), or by contaminating drinking water with feces. This route of transmission can persist for years after a person has been exposed to the parasite. The persons who subsequently become infected might become ill.

Amebiasis affects about 50 million people worldwide each year, making it one of the two most common causes of intestinal inflammation (the other is caused by *Shigella*). Approximately 100,000 people die of the infection each year. Those most often affected are in poorer health; thus, amebiasis tends to be more common in developing countries, where sanitation is inadequate and where people live in crowded conditions, making the spread of the parasite much easier. However, anyone is susceptible; several hundred cases are reported each year in the United States, for example. In developed countries those who become infected tend to be pregnant women, the young and the elderly, and those whose immune systems have become compromised due to malnourishment or disease, such as acquired immunodeficiency syndrome (AIDS).

■ Treatment and Prevention

Amebiasis is treatable using a combination of drug therapies. Some drugs generically called amebicides kill the organisms that are growing in the intestinal tract, while other drugs can lessen the chance that the infection will spread to tissues such as the liver.

■ Impacts and Issues

Persons who travel to countries where the infection is commonly prevalent, such as parts of Africa, India, Latin America, and Southeast Asia, should take precautions against contracting amebiasis. Precautions include drinking bottled water or boiling drinking water for at

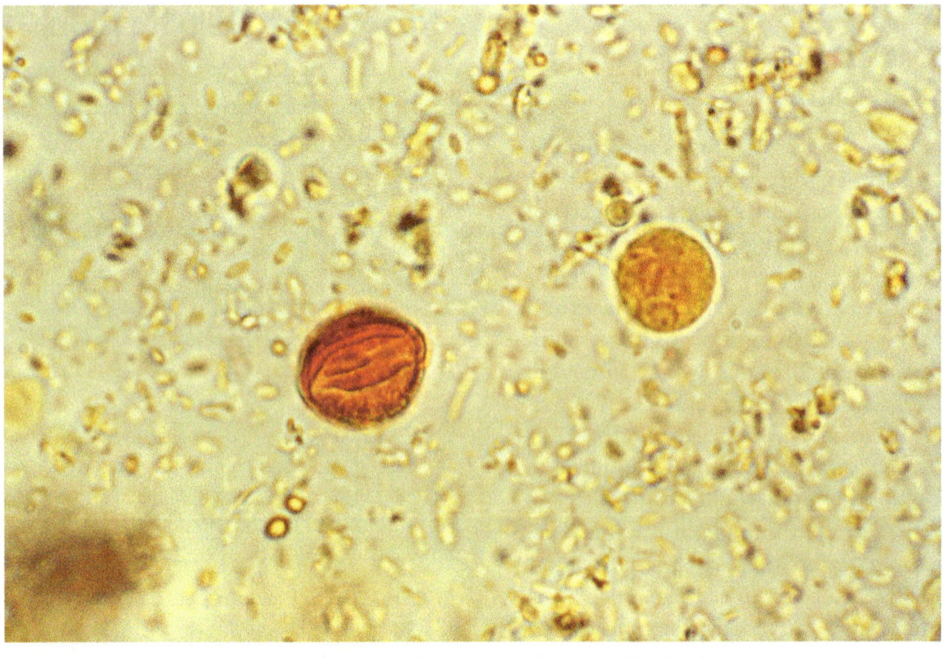

This photomicrograph shows ***Entamoeba histolytica*** cysts. ***Entamoeba histolytica*** is the parasite that causes amebiasis. *© Media for Medical/Getty Images*

least one minute, peeling the skins off fresh fruits and vegetables before eating them, and proper handwashing using soap.

An important issue concerning amebiasis is that the parasite can be excreted in the feces of someone who has no symptoms of the infection. In fact, this is true for the majority of people; estimates are that only one in ten people who are infected actually become sick. While this is a small percent, the fact that millions of people become infected each year still means that a great many people become ill, with many more remaining capable of spreading the infection to others.

Research is ongoing to find more definitive ways of treating amebiasis and in preventing the infection in the first place. As of 2017 there was no vaccine for the infection. A component of *E. histolytica* has been identified as a candidate for a vaccine, but the potential vaccine needs to be confirmed in a clinical trial. A blood test is available that can detect the presence of the parasite. However, because the test detects the presence of antibodies—molecules produced by the immune system that are targeted against the particular invading organism—the test only reveals if someone has ever had an infection, not necessarily an ongoing infection.

The World Health Organization (WHO) recommends that if the presence of amoeba in the feces is confirmed microscopically but the person is not experiencing any symptoms, then it should not be assumed that the person has amebiasis.

On a larger scale, WHO is building an international network, which as of late 2017 totaled over 150 organizations, that together aim to reduce worldwide deaths from diseases such as amebiasis. The group, called the International Network to Promote Household Water Treatment and Safe Storage, plans to implement sustainable and affordable methods of purifying drinking water supplies in communities without access to sanitation or treated water or with water that is improved but from unsafe sources. Although large waterborne outbreaks of amebiasis are uncommon, water treatment and sanitation measures are complementary and are developed together when possible.

In the era of molecular biology, procedures have been developed that can detect the genetic material of *E. histolytica* in feces. However, the test is relatively expensive and requires specialized equipment and training that may not be part of a clinic, especially in an underdeveloped region.

SEE ALSO *Giardiasis; Parasitic Diseases; Sanitation*

BIBLIOGRAPHY

Books

Muriel, Pablo. *Liver Pathophysiology: Therapies and Antioxidants.* Boston: Elsevier, 2017.

Periodicals

Nagata, N., et al. "Predictive Value of Endoscopic Findings in the Diagnosis of Active Intestinal Amebiasis." *Endoscopy* 44, no. 4 (2012): 425–428.

Quach, Jeanie, Joëlle St-Pierre, and Kris Chadee. "The Future for Vaccine Development against *Entamoeba histolytica*." *Human Vaccines & Immunotherapies* 10, no. 6 (2014): 1514–1521.

Singh, Preeti, Bijay Mirdha, Vineet Ahuja, and Sundeep Singh. "Loop-Mediated Isothermal Amplification (LAMP) Assay for Rapid Detection of *Entamoeba histolytica* in Amoebic Liver Abscess. *World Journal of Microbiology and Biotechnology* 29, no. 1 (2013): 27–32.

Websites

"Gastrointestinal Amebiasis." Harvard Health Publishing. https://www.health.harvard.edu/digestive-health/gastrointestinal-amebiasis (accessed November 7, 2017).

"Parasites—Amebiasis—*Entamoea histolytica* Infection." Centers for Disease Control and Prevention. https://www.cdc.gov/parasites/amebiasis/index.html (accessed November 7, 2017).

Brian Hoyle

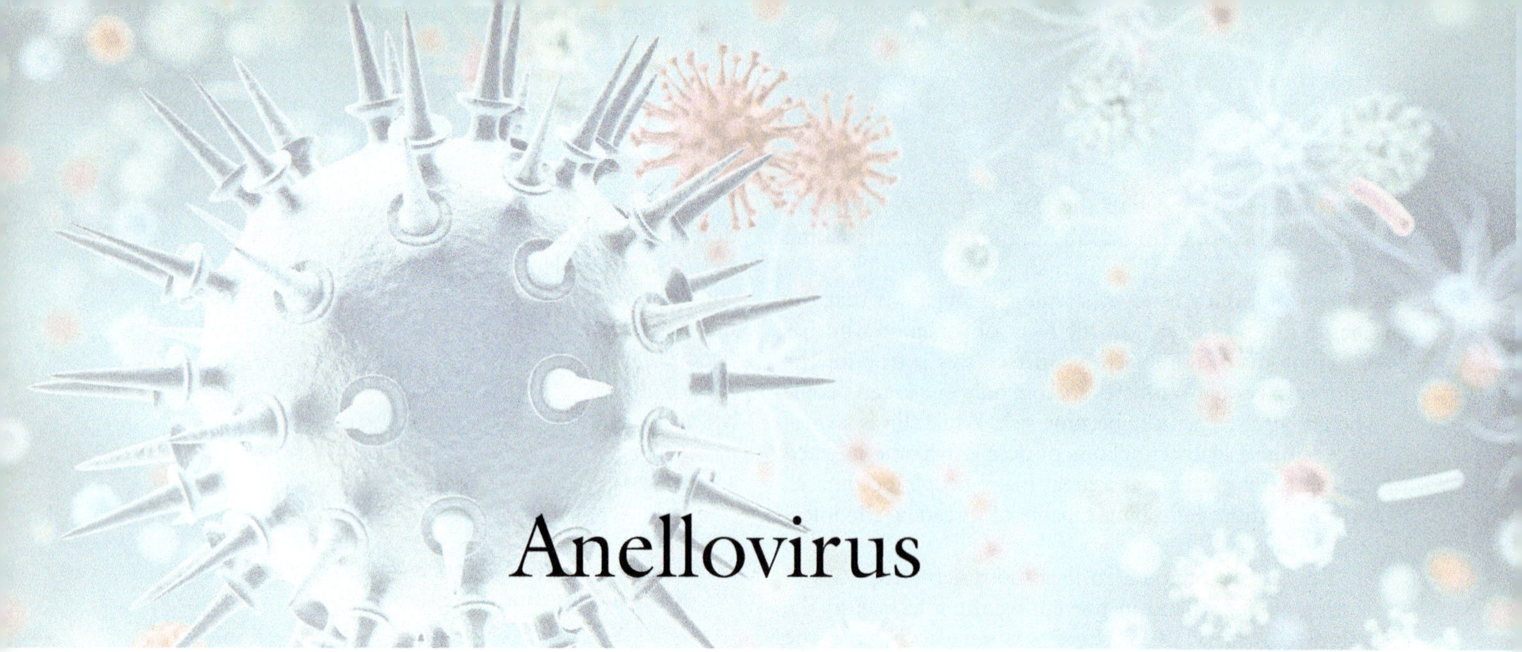

Anellovirus

Introduction

Anelloviruses are a family of viruses described as having a vertebra and a round, non-enveloped capsid (the protein shell of a virus). Within the family Anelloviridae, these relatively small viruses share the characteristic of being single-stranded deoxyribonucleic acid (DNA) viruses.

The three known viruses within Anelloviridae are known to cause chronic viral infections within humans. However, the medical community has yet to associate these particular infections with any specific diseases. The anelloviruses infect a wide number and variety of mammals throughout the world.

This group of viruses was formerly called hepatitis G, but the nomenclature was changed when medical professionals found that anelloviruses do not cause hepatitis. It is known that anelloviruses are highly prevalent in humans and that low-level concentrations are found within humans roughly half the time. The amount of virus contained within any human body increases drastically when the immune system is compromised. The specific concentration of anelloviruses in such patients helps to determine just how compromised the immune system is within those people.

Disease History, Characteristics, and Transmission

The three viruses within anelloviruses are torque teno virus (TTV), torque teno mini virus (TTMV), and torque teno midi virus (TTMDV). Japanese physician T. Nishizawa discovered TTV in 1997 when he described it in a patient with post-transfusion hepatitis. The virus was referred to as the TT virus in reference to the initials of the patient's name. The International Committee on the Taxonomy of Viruses (ICTV) later changed the name to torque teno virus (TTV). Also called transfusion transmitted virus, TTV is found within the genus Alphatorquevirus. Twenty-nine type species are grouped within the genus (torque teno viruses 1–29).

TTV is common in humans, even in healthy people. Approximately 10 percent of people who are blood donors in the United Kingdom and the United States possess TTV. In other countries that percentage can reach as high as 100 percent. The virus is distributed throughout Africa, Asia, Europe, North and South America, and Oceania.

The other two viruses, TTMV and TTMDV, were discovered a few years later (in 2000 and in 2007, respectively). TTMV, previously called TT virus-like mini virus, is found within the genus Betatorquevirus. As with TTV, it is also within the family Anelloviridae. As of April 2015, 12 type species were grouped within the genus (torque teno mini viruses 1–12). TTMV was discovered while studying the earlier-found TTV. Researchers noticed that some (supposed) TTVs were shorter in length than others, which led to the discovery of this second species.

TTMDV, the third member of the group, is a member of the genus Gammatorquevirus. As with the other two, it is also within the family Anelloviridae. It was first isolated in 2005 from patients with acute viral infection syndrome. Since its discovery TTMDV has been found commonly in body fluids such as saliva. Two type species are associated with the genus (torque teno midi viruses 1–2).

Anellovirus infections can be transmitted into humans and other mammals. A 2012 research study published in the journal *PLOS One* found three viruses within anelloviruses (TTV, TTMV, and TTMDV) to have infected humans. The researchers studied children from 2 to 36 months of age while under the care of physicians as pediatric patients.

The *PLOS One* study showed TTV and TTMDV to be associated in children with fever, while TTMV was found to have no association with fever in children.

WORDS TO KNOW

CAPSID The protein shell surrounding a virus particle.

CULTURE A single species of microorganism that is isolated and grown under controlled conditions. The German bacteriologist Robert Koch (1843–1910) first developed culturing techniques in the late 1870s. Following Koch's initial discovery, medical scientists quickly sought to identify other pathogens. In the early 21st century, bacteria cultures are used as basic tools in microbiology and medicine.

DEOXYRIBONUCLEIC ACID (DNA) A double-stranded, helical molecule that forms the molecular basis for heredity in most organisms.

IMMUNE SYSTEM The body's natural defense system that guards against foreign invaders and that includes lymphocytes and antibodies.

PATHOGENIC Something causing or capable of causing disease.

REPLICATION A process of reproducing, duplicating, copying, or repeating something, such as the duplication of DNA or the recreation of characteristics of an infectious disease in a laboratory setting.

RIBONUCLEIC ACID (RNA) Any of a group of nucleic acids that carry out several important tasks in the synthesis of proteins. Unlike DNA, it has only a single strand. Nucleic acids are complex molecules that contain a cell's genetic information and the instructions for carrying out cellular processes. In eukaryotic cells, the two nucleic acids, RNA and DNA, work together to direct protein synthesis. Although it is DNA that contains the instructions for directing the synthesis of specific structural and enzymatic proteins, several types of RNA actually carry out the processes required to produce these proteins. These include messenger RNA (mRNA), ribosomal RNA (rRNA), and transfer RNA (tRNA). Further processing of the various RNAs is carried out by another type of RNA called small nuclear RNA (snRNA). The structure of RNA is very similar to that of DNA, however, instead of the base thymine, RNA contains the base uracil in its place.

■ Scope and Distribution

A 2015 study published in *Archives of Virology* found anelloviruses to be "characterized by an extremely high prevalence, with relatively uniform distribution worldwide and a high level of genomic heterogeneity [similar observable traits though through different genetic mechanisms], as well as an apparent pan-tropism [likelihood to affect many types of tissues] at the host level."

Anellovirus infections have been found commonly within the general population. A 2009 Japanese study concluded that the majority of participants within the study (75 to 100 percent) had been infected with at least one of the three known human anelloviruses. Many had been infected with more than one of the viruses. Young children were especially susceptible to anellovirus infections, with children as young as one month old having shown to be infected. In addition, these viruses were found in almost all parts of the body, from blood plasma and feces to bone marrow, saliva, and breast milk. Many tissues and organs have also been infected, including the kidneys, liver, lungs, lymph nodes, pancreas, spleen, and thyroid gland.

A number of domesticated and wild animals have been found to be infected with anellovirus infections. These include badgers, boars, camels, cats, dogs, a number of rodent species, numerous nonhuman primates, and sea lions. Experiments to learn more about these infections have been most successful when carried out on pigs. Anellovirus infections within pigs have been discovered worldwide.

■ Treatment and Prevention

The viruses within Anelloviridae are known to cause chronic viral infections within humans. However, the medical community has yet to associate these particular infections with any specific diseases within humans. Little information on the prevention and treatment of anelloviruses is available.

A 2014 article in the *Journal of General Virology* asked the following questions about anelloviruses: "Is there any true disease process or identifiable pathology? What are the host cell responses to infection? What are the functions of the encoded viral proteins? How does the virus replicate?" The authors noted the problem that researchers must contend with when answering these questions: "The difficulty in obtaining answers to these and other questions stems, in part, from the lack of suitable *in vitro* [taking place outside a living organism, such as in a test tube] and *in vivo* [taking place inside a living organism] model systems for viral replication."

■ Impacts and Issues

Scientific knowledge concerning anelloviruses remains limited. Specifically, the mechanisms for replication of these viruses are not well known to the medical community, primarily because of an inability to develop an effective system for growing cell cultures.

As of 2018 the viruses within the anellovirus grouping had been scientifically studied for less than two decades. Little is known about how diseases develop as a consequence of these viral infections (what is called pathogenesis).

Although infections from this group of viruses has been medically associated with many diseases (including autoimmune diseases, cancer, hepatitis and related hematological disorders, liver diseases, multiple sclerosis, and respiratory disorders), direct evidence for associating any of these viruses with causing any specific clinical diseases has not yet been determined by the medical community. As of 2018 professionals were still trying to accurately detect, differentiate, and quantify the three viruses (TTV, TTMDV, and TTMV) of anelloviruses.

PRIMARY SOURCE

Increased Prevalence of Anellovirus in Pediatric Patients with Fever

SOURCE: *McElvania TeKippe, Erin, et al. "Increased Prevalence of Anellovirus in Pediatric Patients with Fever."* PLOS ONE *7, no. 11 (2012).*

INTRODUCTION: *Researchers continue to make new discoveries regarding anelloviruses. The following excerpt from the scholarly journal* PLOS ONE *discusses a study linking the anelloviruses torque teno virus (TTV) and torque teno midi virus (TTMDV) to fevers in children.*

Early research on anelloviruses drastically underreported their prevalence in patient specimens. The *Anellovirdae* family of viruses is extremely diverse. They have few conserved regions between species and also within species, making it difficult to design PCR primers that amplify all anelloviruses that might be present in patient specimens. Continued research has revealed a high level of diversity of anellovirus at the nucleotide level, and appreciation of this diversity has led to higher frequency of detection of anelloviruses in patient specimens, including healthy controls. We used conventional end point PCR assays to detect TTV, TTMDV, and TTMV. To ensure that our PCR assays were achieving maximum broad-range detection of individual anellovirus species (TTV, TTMDV, and TTMV) as possible, we used primers that were homologous to sequences within the GC-rich region upstream of the OFR1 transcription start site. This is the most conserved region in the *Anellovirdae* family of viruses but also provides conserved sequences that are unique for each species of viruses. We used multiple forward and reverse primers to maximize the range of detection within each anellovirus species. Synthetic oligonucleotides representing two diverse sequences within each anellovirus species were used as positive controls to ensure that our PCR primers and conditions were suitable for amplification of diverse anellovirus sequences.

In our study we investigated various patient demographic parameters to determine whether they correlated with the presence of anelloviruses in our patient cohort. We were also interested in racial differences in virus distribution. Using univariate analyses, African-American subjects had a significantly higher prevalence of anelloviruses. However, in our population race was highly correlated with febrile status—57% of febrile children were African-American and 43% were Caucasian, while 15% of afebrile controls were African-American and 85% were Caucasian. In multivariate logistic models race was not significant after adjusting for the febrile status. Since race and fever status were so highly collinear, we assessed the effect of race in analyses stratified by maximum temperature. In a subsample of afebrile subjects African-American subjects had significantly higher presence of TTV virus than Caucasian subjects (OR: 4.9, 1.01–23.35, $p = 0.048$). No racial differences were found in febrile patients for TTV or for either febrile or afebrile for TTMDV.

We also investigated the age of patients infected with anellovirus. Based on the concept that anelloviruses cause persistent infection, we hypothesized that older children would be more likely than younger children to be infected due to a longer exposure time to anellovirus-positive family members and other children. We found that children with TTV and TTMDV DNA detected in their plasma or NP specimens were older than uninfected children. This was not the case for TTMV as children in which TTMV DNA was detected were no different in age from those in which TTMV DNA was not detected. After grouping our patient cohort into 6-month age blocks we found that the percentage of anellovirus-positive specimens rose as age increased and peaked at 19–24 months, after which the percent of positive specimens declined. The trend was striking in the TTV and TTMDV-positive plasma and NP specimens and modest in the TTMV-positive plasma and NP specimens. This was a surprising finding because research in the anellovirus field has shown that they are chronic, replicating viruses, with no evidence that they are cleared from the body or enter into a latent life cycle phase. We saw the same trend in plasma and NP specimens tested for all three human anellovirus species suggests that the finding is real and that further analysis is needed to explain this phenomenon. In our study, each patient was sampled only once; however, longitudinal studies in which the onset of anellovirus infection and the viral load could be assessed would allow us to address the question of anellovirus persistence.

Our study showed that DNA from anellovirus species TTV and TTMDV, but not TTMV, were related to fever in young children. Most strikingly we found that the higher the temperature, the larger the percentage of patients that were positive for TTV and TTMDV. Although the relationship is clear, the mechanism by which this happens is unknown. TTV and TTMDV could be causing fevers in children, but we believe it is more likely that fever brought on by other means is creating a permissive environment for anellovirus replication or decreasing the clearance of the viruses. The combination of an inflammatory environment and a weakened immune system could alter the replication and degradation dynamics affecting infection, proliferation, and stability of TTV and TTMDV. To address this question one would need to follow a cohort of patients over time using a quantitative assay to measure viral titers of TTV and TTMDV. This type of experimentation would allow one to study the effect of a patient's first anellovirus infection as well as anellovirus replication dynamics as patients undergo various other febrile illnesses. It would also be interesting to follow anellovirus titers before and after patients have been placed on immunosuppressant drug regimens to study the role of the immune system in anellovirus replication.

In conclusion, our study investigated the interplay between anelloviruses and fever. By high-throughput sequencing we found more anellovirus DNA in the plasma and NP specimens of febrile patients compared to afebrile controls. PCR detection of each anellovirus species showed that TTV and TTMDV, but not TTMV, were more prevalent in febrile patient specimens compared to afebrile controls. Finally, as the temperature of febrile patients increased, so too did the frequency of detection of DNA from TTV and TTMDV. Overall these data argue that the anelloviruses TTV and TTMDV are associated with fever in children.

See Also *Immune Response to Infection; Public Health and Infectious Disease; Viral Disease*

BIBLIOGRAPHY

Books

David, Michael, and Jean-Luc Benoit, eds. *The Infectious Disease Diagnosis: A Case Approach.* Cham, Switzerland: Springer, 2018.

De Villiers, Ethel-Michele, and Harald zur Hausen, eds. *TT Viruses: The Still Elusive Human Pathogens.* Berlin: Springer, 2009.

MacLachlan, N. James, and Edward J. Dubovi. *Fenner's Veterinary Virology.* London: Academic Press, 2016.

Tselis, Alex C., and John Booss, eds. *Neurovirology.* Amsterdam: Elsevier, 2014.

Periodicals

Bernardin, F., et al. "Transfusion Transmission of Highly Prevalent Commensal Human Viruses." *Transfusion* 50, no. 11 (November 2010). This article can also be found online at https://www.ncbi.nlm.nih.gov/pubmed/20497515 (accessed February 1, 2018).

Maggi, F., and M. Bendinelli. "Human Anelloviruses and the Central Nervous System." *Reviews in Medical Virology* 20, no. 6 (November 2010): 392–407. This article can also be found online at https://www.ncbi.nlm.nih.gov/pubmed/20925048 (accessed February 2, 2018).

Ninomiya M., et al. "Development of PCR Assays with Nested Primers Specific for Differential Detection of Three Human Anelloviruses and Early Acquisition of Dual or Triple Infection During Infancy." *Journal of Clinical Microbiology* 46 (2008): 507–514. This article can also be found online at http://jcm.asm.org/content/46/2/507 (accessed February 1, 2018).

Nishiyama, Shoko, et al. "Identification of Novel Anelloviruses with Broad Diversity in UK Rodents." *Journal of General Virology* 95 (July 2014): 1544–1553. This article can also be found online at https://www.ncbi.nlm.nih.gov/pmc/articles/PMC4059270 (accessed February 1, 2018).

Okamoto, H. "History of Discoveries and Pathogenicity of TT Viruses." *Current Topics in Microbiology and Immunology* 331 (2009): 1–20. This article can also be found online at https://www.ncbi.nlm.nih.gov/pubmed/19230554 (accessed February 1, 2018).

Spandole, S., et al. "Human Anelloviruses: An Update of Molecular, Epidemiological and Clinical Aspects." *Archives of Virology* 160, no. 4 (April 2015): 893–908. This article can also be found online at https://www.ncbi.nlm.nih.gov/pubmed/25680568 (accessed February 1, 2018).

TeKippe, Erin McElvania, et al. "Increased Prevalence of Anellovirus in Pediatric Patients with Fever." *PLOS One* (November 30, 2012). This article can also be found online at http://journals.plos.org/plosone/article?id=10.1371/journal.pone.0050937 (accessed February 1, 2018).

Vasilyev, Evgeny V, et al. "Torque Teno Virus (TTV) Distribution in Healthy Russian Population." *Virology Journal* 6 (September 7, 2009). This article can also be found online at https://www.ncbi.nlm.nih.gov/pmc/articles/PMC2745379 (accessed February 1, 2018).

Websites

"Anellovirus." ScienceDirect. https://www.sciencedirect.com/topics/immunology-and-microbiology/anellovirus (accessed February 2, 2018).

Di Bisceglie, Adrian M. "TT Virus and Other Anelloviruses." UpToDate, September 5, 2017. https://www.uptodate.com/contents/tt-virus-and-other-anelloviruses (accessed February 1, 2018).

William Arthur Atkins

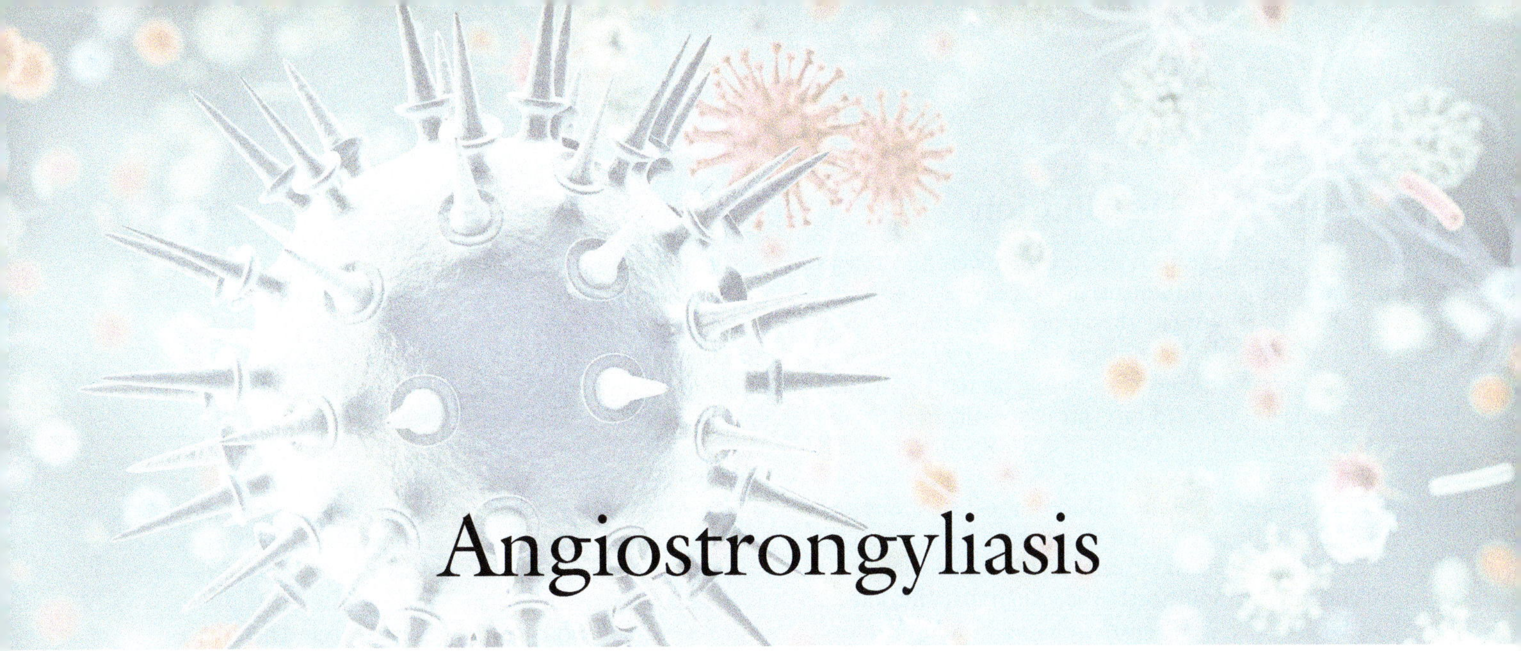

Angiostrongyliasis

■ Introduction

Angiostrongyliasis (ann-gee-o-stronge-uh-luss), also known as rat lungworm, is an infection caused by the internal parasites *Angiostrongylus cantonensis* and *A. costaricensis.* These nematodes (roundworms) are transmitted as eggs or larvae from rats to other animals such as snails, slugs, and some crustaceans. Humans become infected when they ingest the immature parasites, usually after eating undercooked or raw mollusks, crustaceans, and especially snails. An angiostrongyliasis infection often has mild or no symptoms, although some cases result in meningitis. Infection disappears as the worms die in the body.

Most outbreaks of angiostrongyliasis occur in Southeast Asia and the Pacific Islands, although cases have been reported in other countries. The first appearance of the parasites in humans was noted in 1944. Since then there have been numerous reported infections.

■ Disease History, Characteristics, and Transmission

Angiostrongyliasis is caused by the ingestion of one of two parasites, *A. cantonensis* or *A. costaricensis.* Both are parasites of rats and are transmitted to snails and slugs when they eat rat feces. Crustaceans such as prawns can also carry the parasite. Transmission to humans occurs when humans eat undercooked or raw intermittent hosts containing the parasite. Most humans become infected after eating in restaurants that do not cook the animals properly or when they accidentally ingest a snail or slug attached to a salad item that has not been washed properly.

Infection by *A. cantonensis,* which travels to the brain or lungs and eventually dies there, usually results in mild or no symptoms, although eosinophilic meningitis can develop. Meningitis is usually accompanied by headaches, stiff neck, fever, nausea, and vomiting. Infection by *A. costaricensis,* which travels to the digestive tract and dies there, can result in abdominal pain as the dying parasites cause inflammation in the abdomen.

WORDS TO KNOW

HELMINTHIC DISEASE An infection by parasitic worms such as hookworms or flatworms, known as helminths. A synonym for helminthic is verminous.

PARASITE An organism that lives in or on a host organism and gets its nourishment from that host. The parasite usually gains all the benefits of this relationship, whereas the host may suffer from various diseases and discomforts or show no signs of the infection. The life cycle of a typical parasite usually includes several developmental stages and morphological changes as the parasite lives and moves through the environment and one or more hosts. Parasites that remain on a host's body surface to feed are called ectoparasites, whereas those that live inside a host's body are called endoparasites. Parasitism is a highly successful biological adaptation. There are more known parasitic species than nonparasitic ones, and parasites affect just about every form of life, including most animals, plants, and even bacteria.

PCR (POLYMERASE CHAIN REACTION) A widely used technique in molecular biology involving the amplification of specific sequences of genomic DNA.

RESERVOIR The animal or organism in which a virus or parasite normally resides.

Scope and Distribution

Angiostrongylus parasites were first discovered in rats in China in 1933 and in humans in Taiwan in 1944. Infection of rats first spread throughout the Indo-Pacific basin and through Madagascar, Cuba, Egypt, Puerto Rico, and New Orleans. Following the end of World War II in 1945, infected rats spread to Micronesia, Australia, and Polynesia. During the 1950s infected rats were reported in the Philippines, Saipan, New Caledonia, Rarotonga, and Tahiti. During the 1960s infected rats had spread to Thailand, Cambodia, Java, Sarawak, Guam, and Hawaii. As of early 2018 angiostrongyliasis was endemic in Southeast Asia, Australia, the Pacific Islands, and the Caribbean and was becoming more common in parts of Africa.

Despite efforts to educate communities about the dangers of eating raw or undercooked snails, outbreaks of angiostrongyliasis have occurred periodically since 2000. That year students from Chicago traveling through Jamaica became infected with eosinophilic meningitis, which is the presence of more than 10 eosinophils (a type of white blood cell) in every 1 cubic millimeter of cerebrospinal fluid or when eosinophils make up more than 10 percent of all leukocytes in the cerebrospinal fluid. The cause of infection was traced to a salad eaten by all the students that most likely contained secretions from infected slugs or snails.

In August 2006 a number of cases of angiostrongyliasis infection were reported in Beijing, China. Over the course of two months, an outbreak occurred during which the number of infected people rose to 132. The cause of this outbreak was linked to a restaurant chain that served Amazonian snails, known hosts of the parasites. These snails were most likely undercooked. Another outbreak occurred in Dali, China, between October 2007 and March 2008. Thirty-three cases were diagnosed after consumption of raw or undercooked snails.

In 2017 six cases of angiostrongyliasis were confirmed in Hawaii, where roughly 80 percent of land snails carry the parasites that cause the disease. Cases of angiostrongyliasis have increased in the state since approximately 2000, with one to nine confirmed cases each year. There have been two confirmed deaths from the infection since 2007. As of 2018 the state was working to educate the public about the dangers of eating raw or undercooked snails and to educate medical practitioners to identify the disease.

Treatment and Prevention

Diagnosing angiostrongyliasis can be challenging. No single blood test is available to identify *A. cantonensis* or *A. costaricensis.* Doctors make the diagnosis based on factors such as symptoms, travel history, and possible ingestion of raw or undercooked foods such as snails.

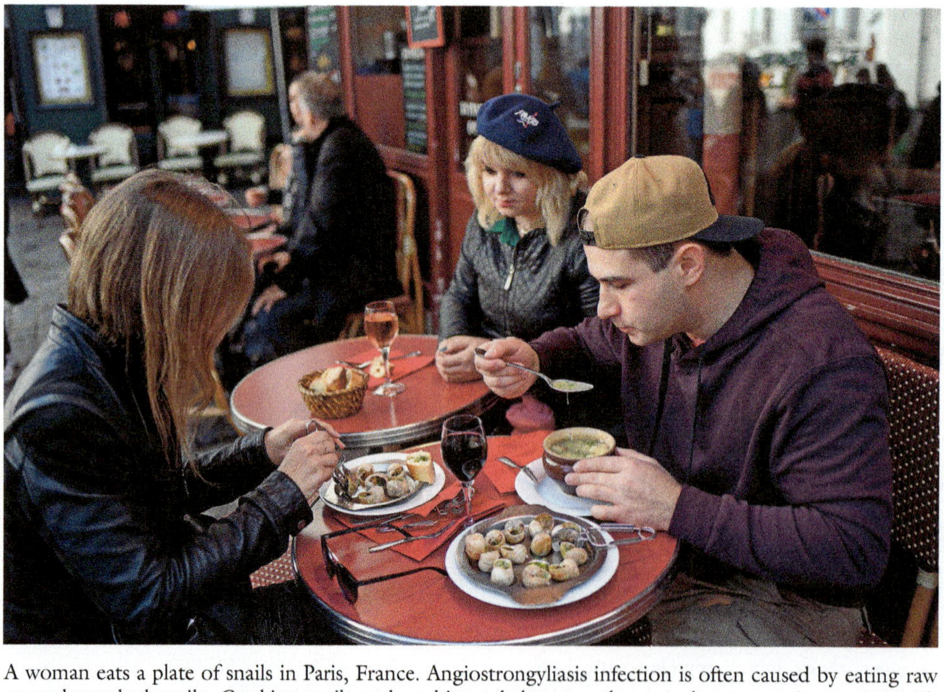

A woman eats a plate of snails in Paris, France. Angiostrongyliasis infection is often caused by eating raw or undercooked snails. Cooking snails and washing salad greens that may have come in contact with snails helps reduce the probability of angiostrongyliasis infection. *© STEPHANE DE SAKUTIN/AFP/Getty Images*

Life Cycle of *Angiostrongylus cantonensis*

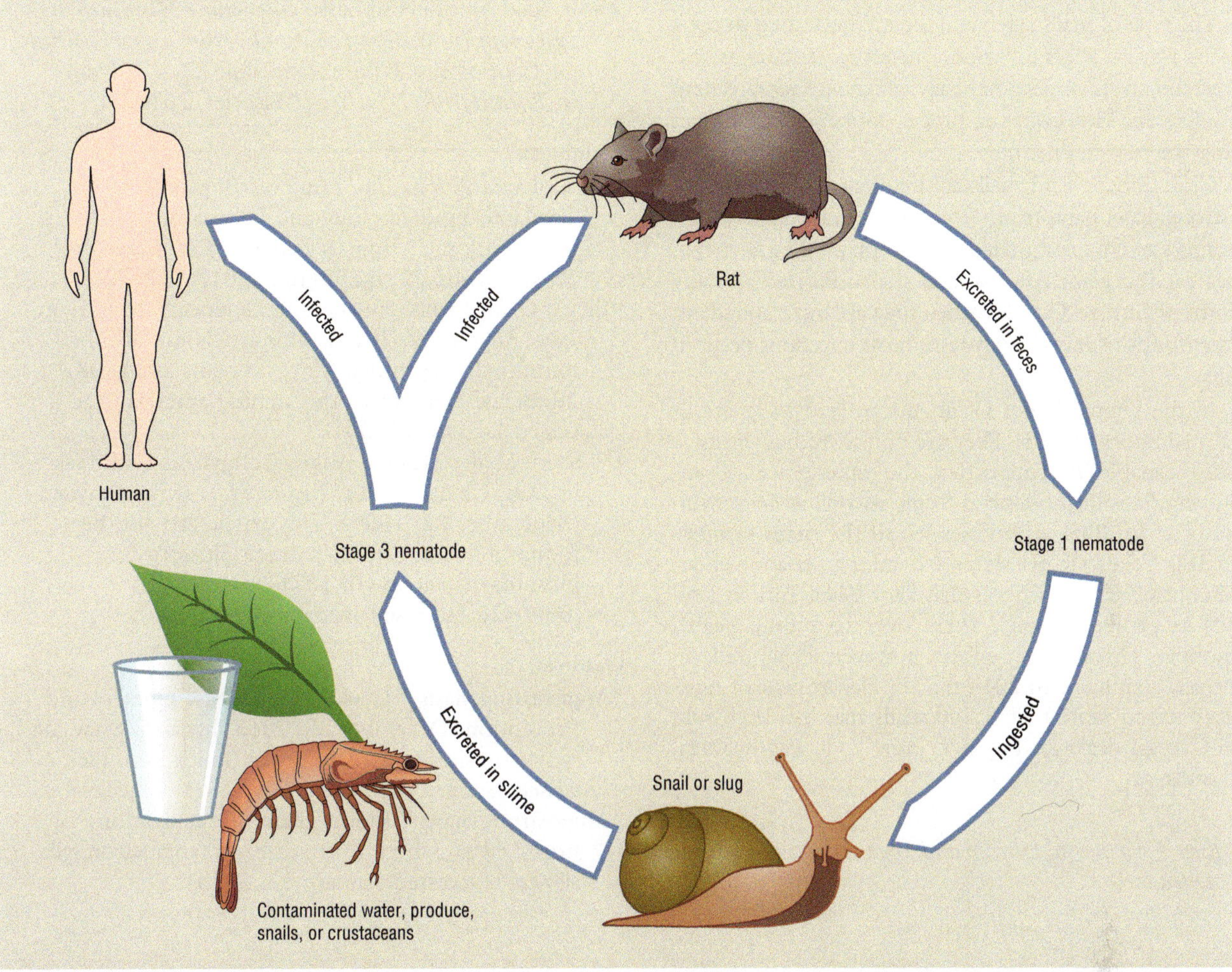

High levels of eosinophils often provide an important diagnostic clue, particularly if they are identified in a patient's cerebrospinal fluid. A polymerase chain reaction (PCR) test can detect the DNA of *A. cantonensis* in a patient's spinal fluid. Such testing, however, is not widely available.

Angiostrongyliasis parasites die within weeks to months. Sometimes the body reacts to the dying parasites, which causes mild symptoms such as abdominal pain. Infected humans usually recover fully without treatment, although treatment may be administered to treat symptoms. Eosinophilic meningitis can also develop and is characterized by neck pain, headaches, and nausea. Although there is no specific treatment for angiostrongyliasis, analgesics or corticosteroids may be administered. Antiparasite medications are not always recommended because they may exacerbate patient symptoms by killing the parasites more rapidly.

Angiostrongyliasis can be prevented by cooking snails, crustaceans, and slugs thoroughly so that the parasite is killed. In addition, careful washing of salad items will prevent infected snails and slugs from being present in salads and potentially being ingested. Although some cases have been attributed to the ingestion of mucus and secretions, some scientists insist that it is still unknown whether transmission can occur following ingestion of mucus from infected snails and slugs. Ingestion of mucus may occur when people who collect snails touch their mouths or nasal passages. Infection can also be prevented by wearing gloves while collecting snails.

■ Impacts and Issues

The main mode of transmission of the parasites that cause angiostrongyliasis is through poor preparation of food. Therefore, infection is more likely to occur in countries with soft regulations on food preparation. People traveling through countries in which rats are infected by the parasites need to be aware of the risks associated with eating food in these countries. Reducing the rodent population in endemic countries also reduces the available population for the initial reservoir of the parasite and thus minimizes the opportunity for infection.

The type of snails eaten and the methods used to cook these snails also affect infection. Therefore, restaurants that sell certain snails could potentially contribute to spreading the infection. However, the proper cooking of snails can render the parasites harmless.

Giant African land snails are frequent hosts of the angiostrongyliasis parasite. In Taiwan angiostrongyliasis occurs most often among children who play with and sometimes eat the giant African land snails during the rainy months of June to October when they are most abundant. In the islands of French Polynesia, most infections occur in adults.

In the United States Giant African land snails are illegal to import as pets. They are considered an invasive species capable of supporting the emergence of angiostrongyliasis in the United States, as well as an agricultural pest. In 2004 authorities seized the snails in more than 100 US exotic pet shops and among private owners. Additionally, several schools that kept Giant African land snails as projects turned them over to public health authorities. Despite such efforts, however, illegal trade in the snails continues. In 2014 the US Department of Agriculture seized more than 1,200 snails that had been sold by a Georgia dealer to buyers in New York, Pennsylvania, and Indiana.

SEE ALSO *Food-Borne Disease and Food Safety; Parasitic Diseases*

BIBLIOGRAPHY

Books

Zhou, Xiao-Nong, et al., eds. *Important Helminth Infections in Southeast Asia: Diversity and Potential for Control and Elimination.* Vol. 72 of *Advances in Parasitology.* New York: Elsevier, 2010.

Periodicals

Eamsobhana, Praphathip. "Angiostrongyliasis in Thailand: Epidemiology and Laboratory Investigations." *Hawaii Journal of Medicine and Public Health* 72, no. 6 (June 2013): 28–32.

"Illegal Giant Snails Threatening America." *New York Post* (August 29, 2014). This article can also be found online at https://nypost.com/2014/08/29/illegal-giant-snails-threatening-america/ (accessed January 12, 2018).

Lv, Shan, et al. "Human Angiostrongyliasis Outbreak in Dali, China." *PLOS Neglected Tropical Diseases* (September 22, 2009). This article can also be found online at http://journals.plos.org/plosntds/article?id=10.1371/journal.pntd.0000520 (accessed January 12, 2018).

Websites

"Angiostrongyliasis." Centers for Disease Control and Prevention, December 28, 2015. https://www.cdc.gov/parasites/angiostrongylus/index.html (accessed January 12, 2018).

"Angiostrongyliasis." World Health Organization. http://www.who.int/ith/diseases/angiostrongyliasis/en/ (accessed January 12, 2018).

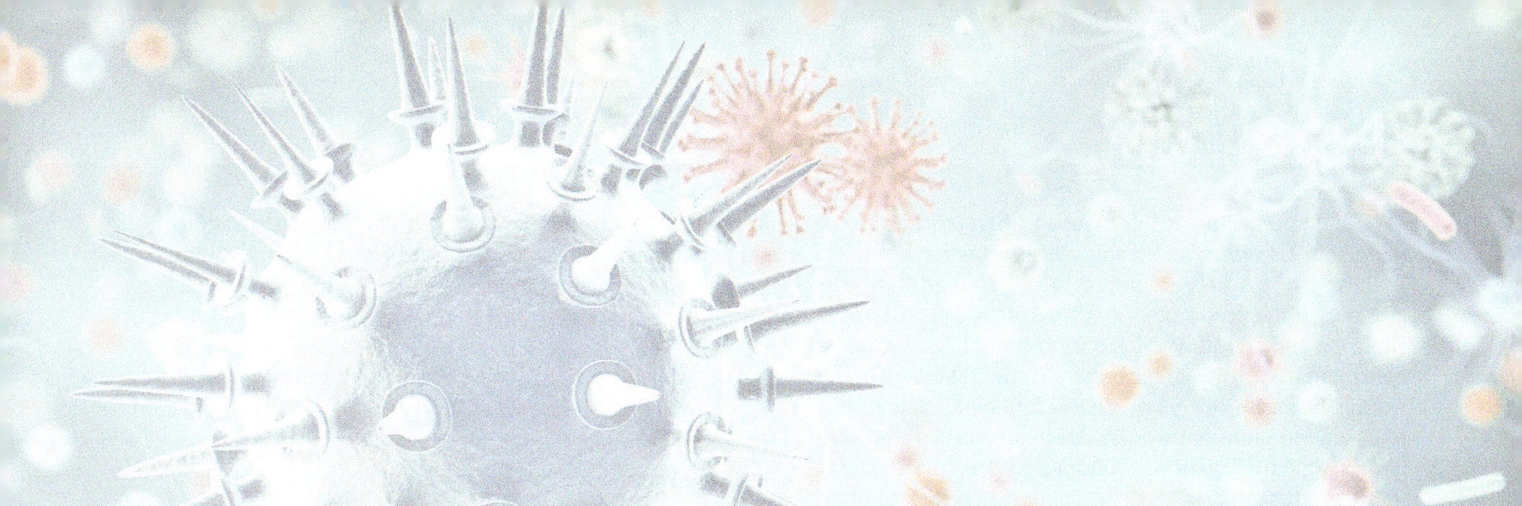

Animal Importation

Introduction

Animal importation is defined as bringing animals into a country. In the United States animal importation is regulated by the US Centers for Disease Control and Prevention (CDC). The prevention of zoonotic diseases (those capable of transmission from animal to human populations) is the primary focus of animal importation regimes. Every nation, as well as supranational bodies such as the European Union, has established protocols concerning the admission of foreign animals into domestic jurisdictions.

In the United States, various governmental departments and agencies assume concurrent jurisdiction for the development, publication, and enforcement of animal importation standards. The primary American bodies that direct these initiatives are the CDC, specifically the National Center for Emerging and Zoonotic Infectious Diseases (NCEZID), and the US Department of Agriculture (USDA).

History and Scientific Foundations

The organized transport of livestock and other domesticated animals has played an important role in human food production since prehistoric times. The empires of Mesopotamia, Greece, and Rome employed successively more sophisticated methods to move desired animals more efficiently between various geographic regions.

The first Industrial Revolution (c. 1780–1830) precipitated a European population surge that generated a corresponding demand for increased food production. After 1820 Britain was the world leader in the importation of cattle, securing both dairy and beef breeds from various parts of Europe to bolster its domestic stock. This burgeoning industry was essentially unregulated. Any sickness or disease noted in an imported cattle herd or among domestic livestock that had contact with imported animals was regarded as a local phenomenon. Contaminated beef was usually disguised by vendors and sold in the normal course of business.

In this laissez-faire industrial environment, the first great cattle epidemics swept both Britain and Europe after 1839. Foot and mouth disease (*Aphthovirus*), bovine pleuropneumonia, and sheep pox were the most common of the epizootic outbreaks that posed significant challenges to veterinary medicine. British veterinarian John Gamgee (1831–1894) was the first expert to propose the comprehensive government regulation of animals entering Britain to prevent "contagionism," his rudimentary appreciation of the viral properties of these newly identified animal plagues.

Bovine Spongiform Encephalopathy (BSE) Cases in North America (2003–February 2015)

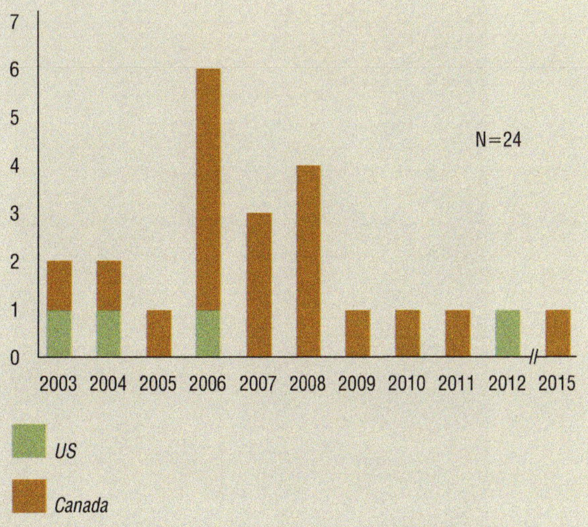

SOURCE: US Department of Agriculture (USDA)

Rinderpest, a highly infectious and fatal bovine virus of the genus *Morbillivirus*, became the impetus for European government regulation of imported cattle. In 1865 rinderpest caused the deaths of more than 400,000 cattle in Britain alone and an estimated 1 million more livestock across continental Europe. That year Britain established the world's first state veterinary service. Rinderpest is transmitted between animals through direct physical contact and has remained a potent agricultural industry threat across modern Africa, where war and political unrest have often prevented effective regulation of cattle imports.

■ Applications and Research

Many types of imported livestock are intended for both breeding and direct food production. Cattle are the most prominent example of a dual-purpose animal. As all cattle breeds are susceptible to myriad highly contagious diseases, both zoonotic and bovine-specific, national import regulation is designed to anticipate such risks through mandatory inspections and reporting provisions.

The most prominent threat to the international animal importation regulatory framework was the discovery of bovine spongiform encephalopathy (BSE) in Britain in 1986. Also known as mad cow disease, BSE is a progressive and fatal neurological condition that destroys the function of an animal's central nervous system. BSE is highly contagious, although the incubation period of the disease is over five years. The precise cause of BSE remains unknown, although there is a scientifically validated relationship between the disease and the presence of infectious proteins known as prions. The disease is most likely transmitted through either direct animal-to-animal contact or through the ingestion of feed prepared from the bone marrow of infected animals.

Creutzfeldt-Jakob disease (CJD) is a condition similar to BSE that occurs in humans. A variant of CJD is capable of being transmitted to humans through the consumption of BSE-contaminated beef. In this form it is called variant Creutzfeldt-Jakob disease (vCJD). It was first classified in the United Kingdom in 1996. According to the CDC and the Texas Department of State Health Services, only four confirmed cases of vCJD had been reported in the United States as of October 2014.

The danger of BSE to both livestock and humans is so sufficiently grave that, when a single cow afflicted with BSE was identified in Washington state in 2003, the Canada–US border was closed to all cattle imports between each nation for 15 months. As BSE has no known treatment or cure except to slaughter and incinerate the affected animal, national border authorities inevitably err on the side of caution when BSE is suspected.

Scientific research involving animal experiments engages additional animal importation issues. The scientific community places a premium on the ability to use monkeys and other nonhuman primates for research purposes, given the physiological similarities between these animals and humans. Primates also represent a significant risk to the human population as disease carriers.

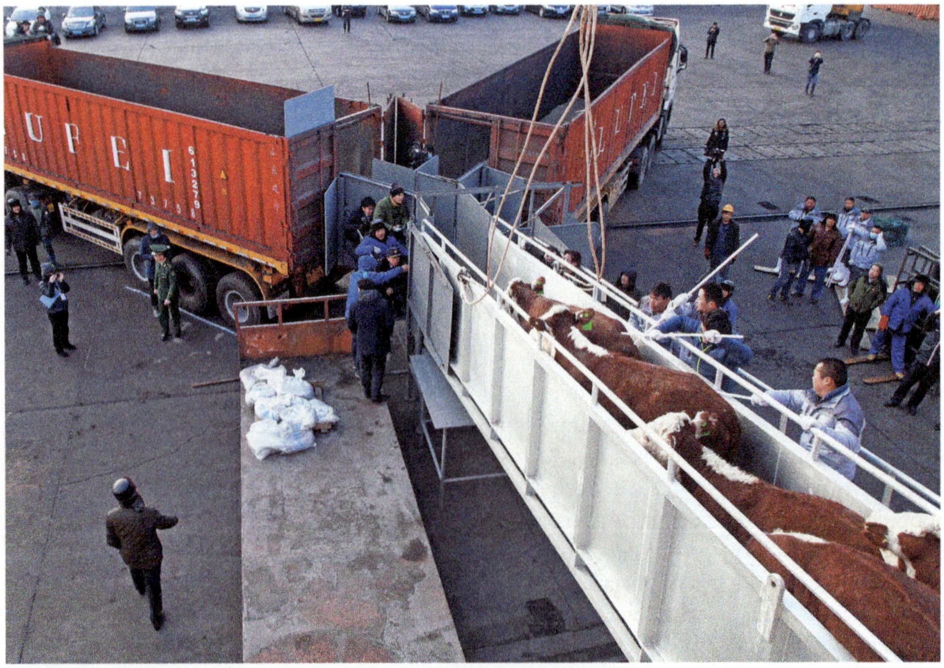

Cattle imported from Australia are seen at the port of Shidao in Weihai, east China's Shandong Province, on February 20, 2017. © Xinhua News Agency/Getty Images

The Ebola and Marburg viruses are the most prominent component of the Filoviridae family. African and Southeast Asian primates are known carriers of the various forms of these viruses. The strain that causes Ebola hemorrhagic fever (EHF) is a remarkably virulent virus that is transmitted by direct contact with a contaminated person or through the exchange of bodily fluids. EHF often triggers a fatal attack on the contaminated person's internal organs.

The four most prolific outbreaks of Ebola occurred in the African nations of Zaire, Sudan, Gabon, and Cote d'Ivoire between 1976 and 1997, killing hundreds of people. In each instance the EHF mortality rates exceeded 60 percent. A typical victim dies within 21 days of contracting this disease.

It was for these reasons that the identification of a new Ebola strain at a primate research facility in Reston, Virginia, in 1989 attracted significant international attention. The discovery touched off a fresh consideration of American research animal importation controls. The Reston animals were monkeys imported from the Philippines. Twenty-one of the animals were determined to have contracted this Ebola strain (later referenced as Ebola Reston, or Ebola-R). Four human handlers became ill from exposure to Ebola-R, but each subsequently recovered.

Because the epidemiology and pathology of Ebola variants remains poorly understood, strict importation rules, including express CDC permission for nonhuman primates, remain in force in the United States. The primary risk concerning a recurrence of Ebola-R in the United States or elsewhere is that this strain may mutate at a future time into a variant that is deadly to the human population. The 1990 Ebola case in the United States was the last confirmed case of Ebola in the country as of 2017. According to the CDC, the most recent case of Ebola in the world as of 2017 was in the remote Likati health zone of the Democratic Republic of the Congo from May to July 2017. Eight humans contracted the virus, four of whom subsequently died from the infection.

WORDS TO KNOW

EPIZOOTIC The abnormally high occurrence of a specific disease in animals in an area, similar to a human epidemic.

PRIONS Proteins that are infectious. Indeed, the name *prion* is derived from "proteinaceous infectious particles." The discovery of prions and confirmation of their infectious nature overturned a central dogma that infections were caused only by intact organisms, particularly microorganisms such as bacteria, fungi, parasites, or viruses. Because prions lack genetic material, the prevailing attitude was that a protein could not cause disease.

QUARANTINE The practice of separating from the general population people who have been exposed to an infectious agent but have not yet developed symptoms. In the United States, this can be done voluntarily or involuntarily by the authority of states and the federal Centers for Disease Control and Prevention.

STRAIN A subclass or specific genetic variation of an organism.

ZOONOSES Diseases of microbiological origin that can be transmitted from animals to people. The causes of diseases can be bacteria, viruses, parasites, or fungi.

■ Impacts and Issues

The transport of pets across national borders is the third significant aspect of animal import regulation. Dogs and cats form the majority of such animals. The number of pet dogs worldwide is difficult to estimate. According to WorldAtlas.com, the two largest domestic dog populations are located in the United States (75.8 million dogs) and Brazil (35.7 million dogs). The sheer number of household pets and the ability of a large number of animal-borne zoonotic diseases to move quickly through a given population to infect both pets and humans has led to rigorous pet importation controls being enacted in most countries.

Exotic or unconventional pets, including large members of the cat family and various reptiles, are governed by species-specific regulations throughout the world. As an example, a turtle with a shell measuring less than 4 inches (10 centimeters) in length may not be imported into the United States without the advance permission of the CDC due to a heightened risk to humans of salmonellosis, a bacterial disease caused by contact with the bacterium *Salmonella*, which may be contracted through the handling of small turtles.

Dogs and cats are subject to similar entry and quarantine regulations in most Western nations. In the United States, a pet cat or dog entering the country must be both quarantined and proven free of any contagious disease. The standard requirement is a certificate from a licensed veterinarian confirming that the animal is free of rabies or any other infectious disease. The USDA possesses the discretion to quarantine any pet entering the United States, but, as a general rule, once rabies certification is available, the animal will not be quarantined. These regulations apply equally to animals imported as pets or for breeding purposes.

The most common zoonotic diseases addressed by import controls are rabies (*Lyssavirus*, transmitted through the bite of an infected animal), ringworm (*Tinea*, a fungal skin disease), and roundworm (*Trichinella spiralis*, a parasitic worm that attacks a mammal's gastrointestinal tract).

See Also *Bovine Spongiform Encephalopathy (Mad Cow Disease); CDC (Centers for Disease Control and Prevention); Ebola; Emerging Infectious Diseases; Globalization and Infectious Disease; Rabies; Ringworm; Roundworm; Zoonoses*

BIBLIOGRAPHY

Books

Blazina, Christopher, Güler Boyraz, and David Shen-Miller, eds. *The Psychology of the Human-Animal Bond: A Resource for Clinicians and Researchers.* New York: Springer, 2013.

Julius, Henri. *Attachment to Pets: An Integrative View of Human-Animal Relationships with Implications for Therapeutic Practice.* Cambridge, MA: Hogrefe, 2013.

Periodicals

Albariño, Cesar G., et al. "Insights into Reston Virus Spillovers and Adaption from Virus Whole Genome Sequences." *PLOS One* 12, no. 5 (May 25, 2017): e0178224. This article can also be found online at http://journals.plos.org/plosone/article?id=10.1371/journal.pone.0178224 (accessed January 26, 2018).

Websites

"Bringing an Animal into the United States." Centers for Disease Control and Prevention, September 1, 2016. https://www.cdc.gov/importation/bringing-an-animal-into-the-united-states/index.html (accessed January 26, 2018).

"Countries with the Most Dogs Worldwide." WorldAtlas.com, April 25, 2017. https://www.worldatlas.com/articles/countries-with-the-most-dogs-worldwide.html (accessed January 26, 2018).

"Import Live Animals." United States Department of Agriculture, January 29, 2018. https://www.aphis.usda.gov/aphis/ourfocus/animalhealth/animal-and-animal-product-import-information/import-live-animals (accessed January 26, 2018).

"Outbreaks Chronology: Ebola Virus Disease." Centers for Disease Control and Prevention, July 28, 2017. https://www.cdc.gov/vhf/ebola/outbreaks/history/chronology.html (accessed January 26, 2018).

"Variant Creutzfeldt-Jakob Disease (vCJD)." Centers for Disease Control and Prevention, February 10, 2015. https://www.cdc.gov/prions/vcjd/index.html (accessed January 26, 2018).

Bryan Davies
William Arthur Atkins

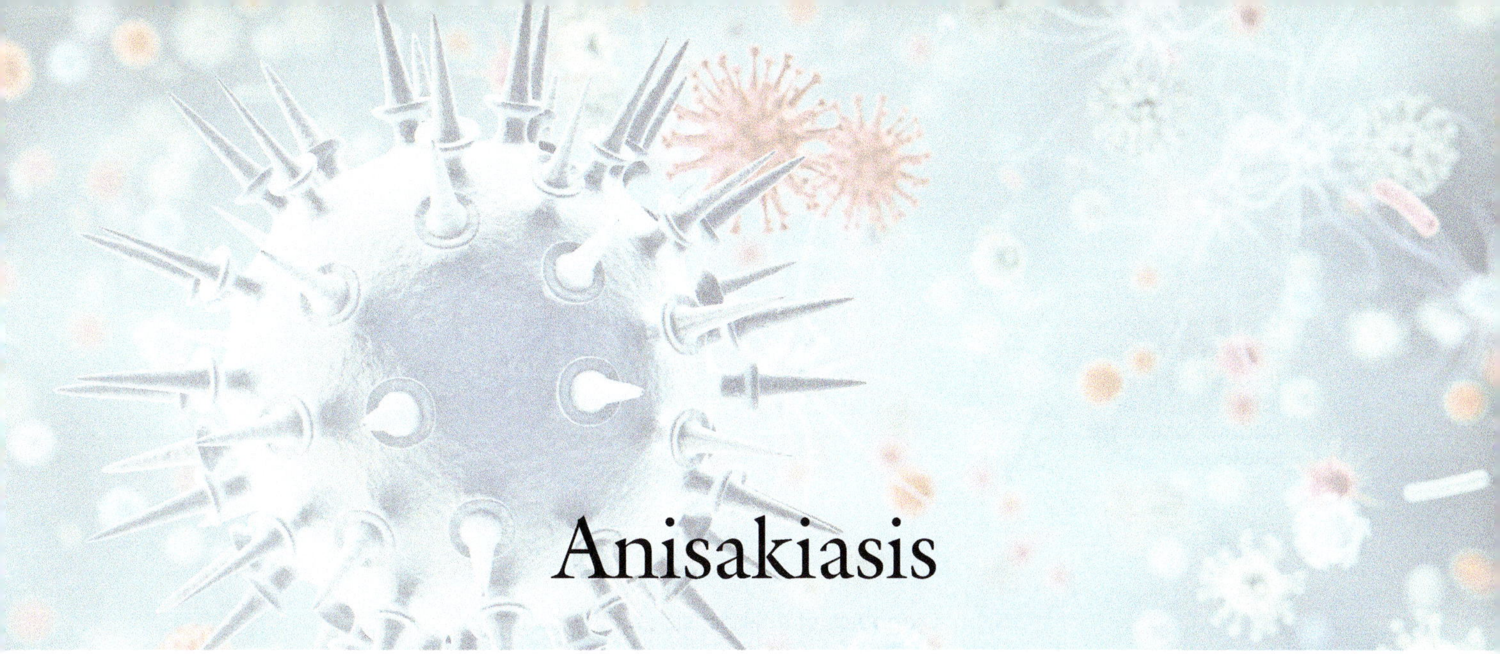

Anisakiasis

Introduction

Anisakiasis is an infection in humans caused by ingesting the larvae of nematodes (parasitic roundworms with long, cylindrical bodies) in raw or undercooked saltwater fish. When the larvae infect humans, the anisakiasis infection causes discomfort to the stomach and intestinal areas. According to the Center for Food Safety and Applied Nutrition (CFSAN), a division of the US Food and Drug Administration (FDA), *Anisakis simplex* (herring worm) and *Pseudoterranova decipiens* (cod or seal worm) are linked to human infections in North America.

Before ingestion into the human body, anisakiads travel through a complex life cycle involving the ingestion by various marine and anadromous fish (those that breed by returning from the sea to the water bodies where they were born) and crustaceans.

Usually marine life infected with *Anisakidae* larvae are only found in seawater because larvae need to grow within waters of higher salinity. It is also uncommon in areas where cetaceans (large ocean mammals such as whales) are not found, such as waters in the southern North Sea (a marginal sea of the Atlantic Ocean on the European continental shelf).

Disease History, Characteristics, and Transmission

Human anisakiasis was first reported in Japan during the middle part of the twentieth century. *Anisakis simplex* and *Pseudoterranova decipiens* is found frequently inside saltwater fish. *P. decipiens* is typically found in temperate and arctic environments.

The characteristics of anisakids include a long, cylindrical (vermiform, or wormlike) body shape. It does not contain segments. The posterior part narrows to a cavity (pseudocoel), with the anus somewhat off-centered. The mouth is encircled by projections, which are used for sensing and feeding.

Transmission of the adult *Anisakis simplex* and *P. decipiens* begins in the stomach of marine mammals, specifically in the mucosa (mucous membranes). The eggs of female anisakids are expelled as feces of infected mammals. The eggs develop into embryos in seawater, where first-stage larvae are formed. The larvae then molt and become second-stage larvae. Upon hatching, free-swimming larvae are ingested by crustaceans, turning into mature, third-stage larvae.

Infected crustaceans are eaten by fish and squid, which become intermediate hosts. Inside fish, anisakids are coil-shaped. When uncoiled, their average length is 0.8 inches (2.0 centimeters). When these fish and squid die, the larvae move into muscle tissues. Anisakids transfer between fish when larger fish eat smaller ones. During these times larvae are infective to humans and marine mammals. Sometimes larvae are ingested by humans when infected seafood is

Anisakis Poisoning Cases in Japan (2007–2016)

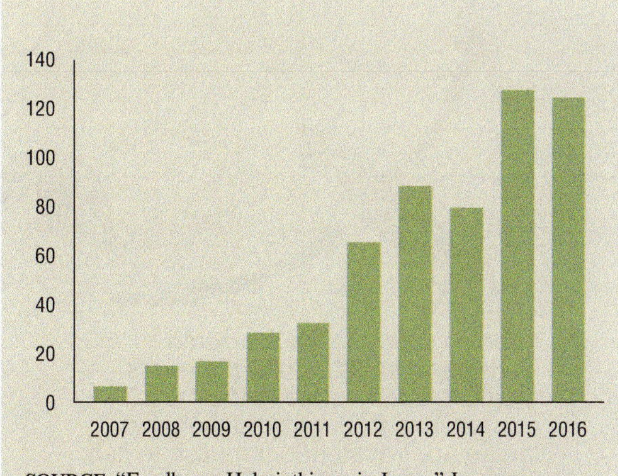

SOURCE: "Foodborne Helminthiases in Japan." Japanese National Institute of Infectious Diseases. 2017. Available from: https://www.niid.go.jp/niid/en/?option=com_content&view=article&id=7225:446te&catid=865:iasr&lang=en

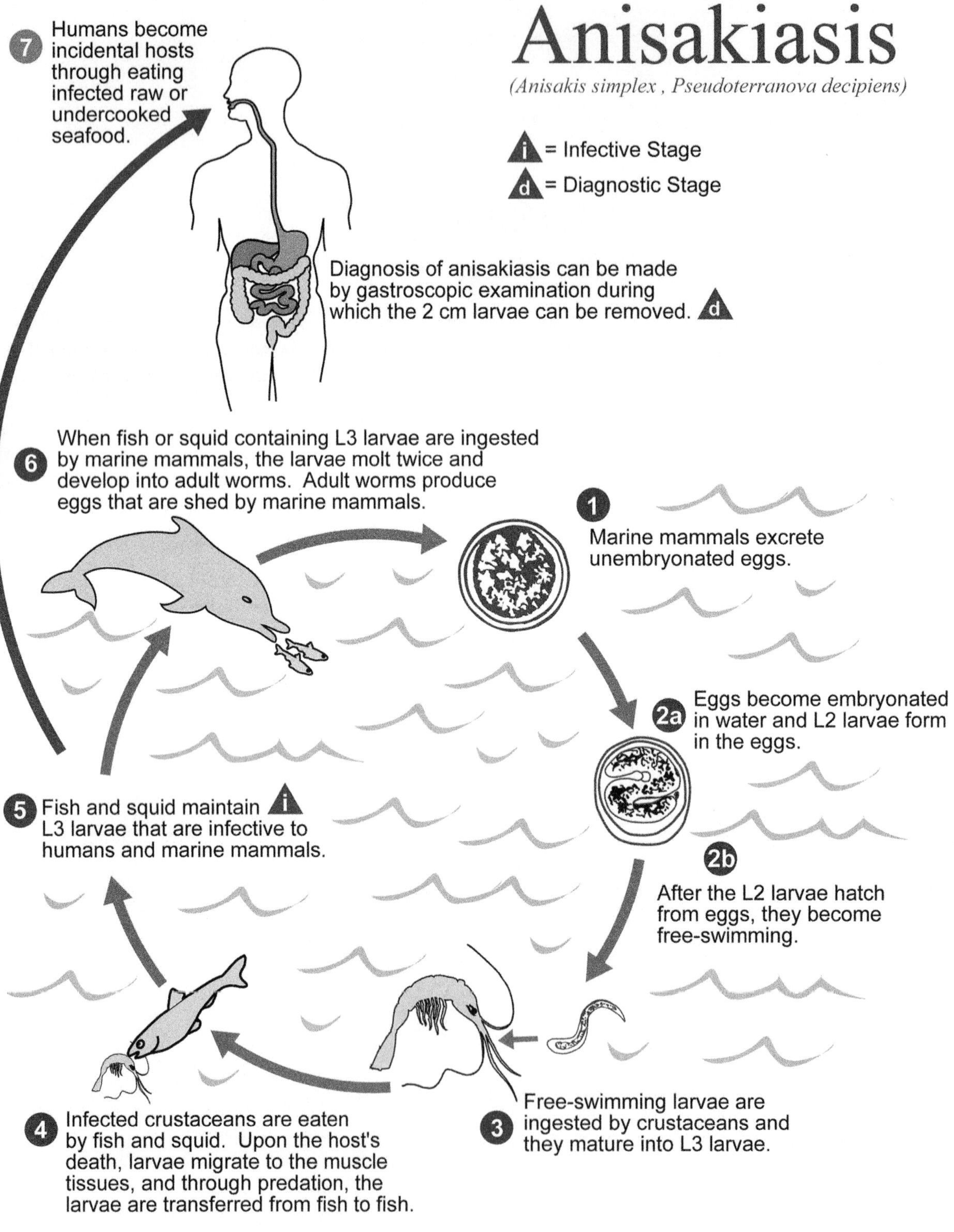
Anisakiasis
(Anisakis simplex , Pseudoterranova decipiens)
i = Infective Stage
d = Diagnostic Stage
7 Humans become incidental hosts through eating infected raw or undercooked seafood.
Diagnosis of anisakiasis can be made by gastroscopic examination during which the 2 cm larvae can be removed. d
6 When fish or squid containing L3 larvae are ingested by marine mammals, the larvae molt twice and develop into adult worms. Adult worms produce eggs that are shed by marine mammals.
1 Marine mammals excrete unembryonated eggs.
2a Eggs become embryonated in water and L2 larvae form in the eggs.
5 Fish and squid maintain i L3 larvae that are infective to humans and marine mammals.
2b After the L2 larvae hatch from eggs, they become free-swimming.
4 Infected crustaceans are eaten by fish and squid. Upon the host's death, larvae migrate to the muscle tissues, and through predation, the larvae are transferred from fish to fish.
3 Free-swimming larvae are ingested by crustaceans and they mature into L3 larvae.

This diagram illustrates the complex life cycle of *Anisakis simplex* and *Pseudoterranova decipiens.* These parasitic roundworms develop in saltwater mammals, crustaceans, and fish or squid before infecting humans. © Smith Collection/Gado/Getty Images eaten raw, is undercooked, or is improperly prepared. After humans ingest third-stage larvae, the larvae attach themselves to, or burrow into, stomach or intestine tissues.

When third-stage larvae are digested by marine mammals, the larvae molt two times and develop into adult worms. These parasites are longer than two centimeters when uncoiled, with a thicker and sturdier body than when inside fish. The adult worms produce eggs that are expelled by marine mammals.

Scope and Distribution

Anisakiasis is found worldwide but is more common in areas where raw fish has traditionally been part of people's diets, including in coastal regions of Spain, the Netherlands, and Japan. In 2017 Japan's Health, Labor and Welfare Ministry stated that the number of reported anisakiasis infections had surged in the early 21st century, with just 4 reported cases in 2004, 79 in 2013, and 126 in 2016 (although the ministry noted the rise in cases could be attributed in part to increased public awareness of the infection). As of 2017 Japan was believed to have the highest rates of anisakiasis infection in the world. However, the growing worldwide popularity of sushi, a traditionally Japanese dish, has led to an increased incidence of anisakiasis in countries where it has historically been rare, including the United States, Europe, and South America. Fish and marine mammals most affected include cod, crabs, cuttlefish, halibut, herring, mackerel, porpoises, rockfish, salmon, seals, sea lions, squid, tuna, and whales.

Treatment and Prevention

Diagnosis cannot be accomplished from stool specimens. Instead, it is made by X-ray images and medical examinations of the patient's stomach and intestines using a flexible endoscope. In addition, microscopic examination of tissue can be made in which larvae are removed through biopsy or during surgery. *Anisakis simplex* and *Pseudoterranova decipiens* cannot survive in human hosts. They eventually die while inside the inflamed tissue.

In some cases invasive treatments may be attempted. Endoscopy may be used for the removal of larvae, especially in emergency cases involving obstruction or rupture of the bowel. Also, nasogastric suction (suction through a tube inserted through the nose and into the stomach) may be used, followed by drugs that target parasitic worms. If such action fails, worms can be removed surgically. Surgical procedures sometimes may be avoided by drug treatments, including albendazole (marketed under Albenza®, Eskazole®, and Zentel® brands), which the FDA first approved for use in 1996.

WORDS TO KNOW

ANADROMOUS Fish that migrate from ocean (salt) water to fresh water, such as salmon.

INTERMEDIATE HOST An organism infected by a parasite while the parasite is in a developmental, not sexually mature form.

NEMATODE Also known as a roundworm; a type of helminth characterized by a long, cylindrical body.

PARASITE An organism that lives in or on a host organism and that gets its nourishment from that host. The parasite usually gains all the benefits of this relationship, while the host may suffer from various diseases and discomforts or show no signs of the infection. The life cycle of a typical parasite usually includes several developmental stages and morphological changes as the parasite lives and moves through the environment and one or more hosts. Parasites that remain on a host's body surface to feed are *ectoparasites*, while those that live inside a host's body are *endoparasites*. Parasitism is a highly successful biological adaptation. There are more known parasitic species than nonparasitic ones, and parasites affect just about every form of life, including most animals, plants, and even bacteria.

Anisakiasis infection can be prevented by heating seafood to a temperature higher than 145°F (63°C) or by freezing it to at least −4°F (−20°C) for at least seven days. Such actions kill the larvae. If fish or shellfish is to be consumed raw or semi-raw, the FDA recommends that the food be blast frozen to −31°F (−35°C) or below for 15 hours or that it be blast frozen to −31°F (−35°C) or below and stored at −4°F (−20°C) or below for 24 hours.

Impacts and Issues

When anisakid worms infect humans, they can produce severe sickness affecting the stomach and intestines within several hours of ingestion. Sometimes the larvae are vomited or coughed up. Symptoms include vomiting, diarrhea, nausea, and severe abdominal pain that may resemble appendicitis, so cases are often misdiagnosed. With the increasing popularity of raw seafood dishes, government and medical organizations have made efforts to educate physicians to consider the possibility of anisakiasis in patients with these symptoms.

If larvae pass into the bowel, major symptoms may occur within one to two weeks because of tissue inflammation. They can also produce a minor chronic disease that causes stomach or intestinal irritation, which may last between weeks and years. These symptoms resemble stomach ulcers and tumors or irritable bowel syndrome.

Fish and shellfish are important foods to maintain a healthy lifestyle. They are high in protein and other essential nutrients. However, the growing international popularity of eating such raw seafood dishes as sushi, sashimi, ceviche, and pickled herring has produced an increase in the number of cases of anisakiasis, a trend that health authorities expect to continue.

SEE ALSO *Cancer and Infectious Disease; Food-Borne Disease and Food Safety; Helminth Disease; Host and Vector; Parasitic Diseases; Tropical Infectious Diseases*

BIBLIOGRAPHY

Books

Adley, Catherine C., ed. *Food-Borne Pathogens: Methods and Protocols.* Totowa, NJ: Humana, 2006.

Guerrant, Richard L., David H. Walker, and Peter F. Weller. *Tropical Infectious Diseases: Principles, Pathogens, and Practice.* Philadelphia: Elsevier Churchill Livingstone, 2006.

Periodicals

Bucci, Cristina, et al. "Anisakis, Just Think about It in an Emergency!" *International Journal of Infectious Diseases* 17, no. 11 (2013): e1071–e1072.

Osumi, Magdalena. "Anisakis Infections from Raw Fish on Rise, Health Ministry Warns." *Japan Times* (May 12, 2016). This article can also be found online at https://www.japantimes.co.jp/news/2017/05/12/national/science-health/anisakis-infections-raw-fish-rise-health-ministry-warns/#.WjQ64baZNN0 (accessed January 18, 2018).

Porter, Tom. "Sushi Fans Warned of Raw Fish Infection Risk." *Newsweek* (May 12, 2017). This article can also be found online at http://www.newsweek.com/sushi-rise-parasitic-infection-608240 (accessed January 18, 2018).

Websites

"Anisakiasis." Centers for Disease Control and Prevention. 2016. https://www.cdc.gov/parasites/anisakiasis/ (accessed December 15, 2017).

"Anisakiasis." Merck Manuals. 2017. https://www.merckmanuals.com/professional/infectious-diseases/nematodes-roundworms/anisakiasis (accessed December 15, 2017).

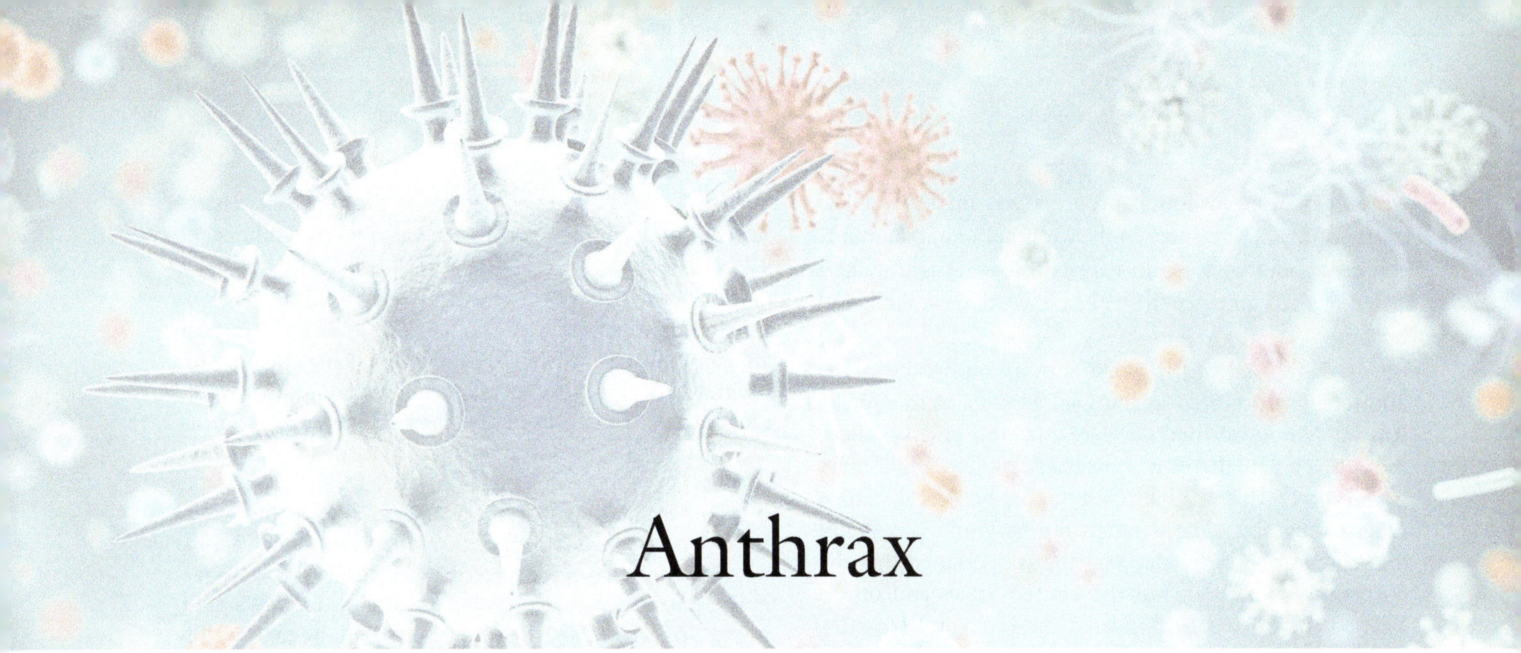

Anthrax

Introduction

Anthrax is an infection typically caused by the bacterium *Bacillus anthracis*, though a second a strain known as *Bacillus cereus*, or rainforest anthrax, was identified in the early 21st century. The name *anthrax*, the Greek word for "coal," refers to the black spots that can appear on the body in the cutaneous form of the disease. Anthrax is usually transmitted through hardy spores that can survive in soil for decades. It exists naturally in many parts of the world as an infection of plant-eating animals such as cattle and sheep. Because its spores are small enough to become airborne, humans can contract it as a lung infection. In this form it is fatal in at least 95 percent of cases that do not receive immediate antibiotic treatment.

Because of the high mortality rate of the inhaled form of the disease, anthrax was developed as a biological weapon by several countries, including Japan, the Soviet Union, the United Kingdom, and the United States, although by the 21st century no nation was known to have retained stocks of weaponized anthrax. A 1972 treaty known as the Convention on the Prohibition of the Development, Production, and Stockpiling of Bacteriological (Biological) and Toxin Weapons and on Their Destruction prohibited the use of anthrax and other diseases in warfare. However, news reports in 2017 suggested that North Korea, a signatory of the 1972 convention, had begun testing methods for loading anthrax on intercontinental ballistic missiles.

Observers have also expressed concern that terrorists might use anthrax as a weapon. Such concerns were heightened when, a week after the September 11, 2001, terror attacks in New York City, letters laced with anthrax were discovered at various congressional and media offices in the United States. Concerns about the intentional spread of anthrax and the infection's high mortality rate led to the development of various treatments as well as a vaccine.

Disease History, Characteristics, and Transmission

History

Anthrax is a naturally occurring disease afflicting livestock and occasionally, through contact with livestock, humans. Scientists believe that anthrax emerged in ancient Egypt and Mesopotamia around 700 BCE. The description of a sooty "morain" in the book of Exodus is reminiscent of anthrax, and the disease is probably the "burning wind of plague" in Homer's *Iliad.* The mass death of horses and cattle (the primary targets of anthrax infection, along with sheep) during the Eurasian campaign of the Huns in 80 CE was also likely due to anthrax.

Records show that in Europe in the 1600s, a cattle disease that was almost certainly anthrax, called the Black Bane, killed about 60,000 cattle. Until the development of antibiotics and an effective veterinary vaccine for anthrax in the mid-20th century, anthrax was one of the most common causes of death for cattle, goats, horses, pigs, and sheep.

In 1876 the German physician Robert Koch (1843–1910) showed that a bacterium was responsible for the disease, making anthrax one of the first diseases to be identified as having a bacterial cause. Koch, who was awarded a Nobel Prize in Medicine in 1905, also discovered the bacterial causes of tuberculosis and cholera. Over the course of the 20th century, the development of vaccines and treatments for anthrax in both animals and humans helped drive down infections drastically, especially in industrialized countries with modern methods for animal processing and vaccination.

But as scientists and doctors reduced naturally occurring anthrax infections, various governments, including those of the United States, the United Kingdom, and the Soviet Union, sought to harness anthrax for use as a weapon of war. Although progress was made over the course of the 20th century in the weaponization of anthrax, concerns about what might happen if it were used militarily led to the signing of the 1972 convention on biological weapons.

In 1979 one of the worst anthrax outbreaks of the 20th century occurred in the Ural Mountains in western Russia. Ninety-six people were infected and 66 died, though the actual toll was probably higher. The Soviet government, which had also instituted a biological warfare program that focused on anthrax during World War II and that continued for decades after the war, claimed that the outbreak was natural. But the United States and others claimed the Soviets had violated the biological weapons convention. In the early 1990s, after the breakup of the Soviet Union, Russian and American scientists were able to study the 1979 outbreak in detail. They concluded that it was caused by an accidental release of anthrax spores from a military facility on the outskirts of the city Sverdlovsk (now called Yekaterinburg).

The potential for even a small quantity of anthrax to disrupt a society and drain its resources was shown in 2001 when attacks using anthrax spores were carried out through the US mail. The attacks began on September 18, a week after the attacks on the World Trade Center and Pentagon. Letters containing anthrax spores in powder form were mailed from a public mailbox in Princeton, New Jersey, and received by several TV networks, the *New York Post*, and the offices of US senators Tom Daschle (1947–) and Patrick Leahy (1940–). Neither of the senators was infected, but five other people were killed by the anthrax and 17 became ill.

Early news reports characterized the 2001 anthrax powder as weapons grade, but in 2006 the US Federal Bureau of Investigation (FBI) confirmed that the powder did not have any of the special technical features that would identify it as coming from a military facility, such as a coating on the spores to prevent them from sticking together. After seven years of investigation, the FBI announced that it believed the person responsible for the outbreak was Bruce Ivins (1946–2008), a former government scientist who committed suicide after being identified as a suspect in the case. Later media reports cast doubt on Ivins's guilt, but as of 2017 no other suspect had been credibly identified.

In 2010 medical workers in the United Kingdom and Germany identified a small outbreak of what they believed to be anthrax, despite the symptoms being different than those of typical anthrax infections. Rather than the black spots that appear in the cutaneous form of anthrax, these patients experienced infection of deeper skin layers. All those infected with this unusual form of anthrax were heroin users, which led doctors and epidemiologists to conclude that the anthrax spores had somehow tainted the heroin being used. They deemed the new form of the disease "injection anthrax."

In the early 21st century, scientists working in Africa also identified the previously unknown anthrax strain *B. cereus* in chimpanzee and other mammal populations in the

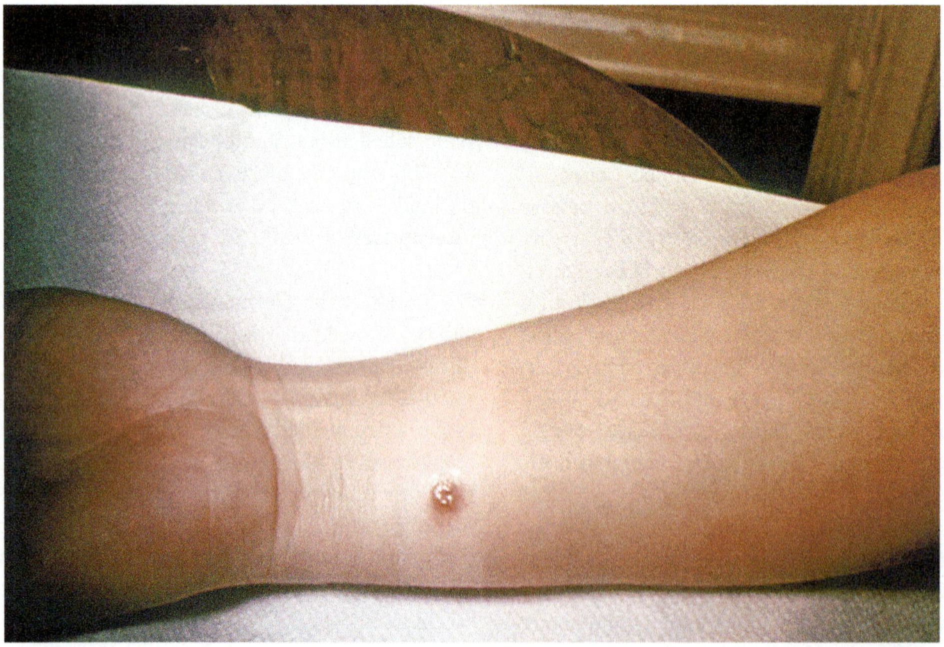

Cetaceous anthrax enters the human host through broken skin, forming a lesion as pictured here. Cetaceous is a more common and much less severe infection than pulmonary anthrax, which enters the human host through the lungs and is fatal in at least 95 percent of cases that do not receive immediate antibiotic treatment. © *CDC/Science Source*

Taï rain forest of the Ivory Coast. In a 2017 article published in *Nature*, Constanze Hoffmann and coauthors argued that this strain of rain forest anthrax could have "severe consequences for local wildlife communities" and "will accelerate the decline and possibly result in the extirpation of local chimpanzee (*Pan troglodytes verus*) populations."

Characteristics

Anthrax bacteria in their vegetative form are shaped like rods about 1 millionth of a meter (1 μm) in diameter and 6 μm long. The vegetative form multiplies inside a host animal. When conditions are not right for anthrax to grow and multiply, such as when temperature, the level of acid, humidity, and nutrient levels are outside the favorable range, some of the vegetative anthrax bacteria sporulate, or take on a spore form. A spore is an extremely small, one-celled reproductive unit that is usually able to survive extreme environmental conditions. Unlike a seed, a spore does not store a significant amount of nutrients. Anthrax spores can survive in soil or as a dry powder for many years, even decades, and are the most common source of anthrax infection.

Once in the body, anthrax spores germinate and multiply. Toxins released by the bacteria cause the immune system to malfunction. In the final phase of infection, the bacteria build rapidly in the blood, doubling in number every 45 minutes to two hours. At death there may be more than 100 million anthrax bacteria per milliliter of blood. (A milliliter is about the size of a small drop.) Toxins from the bacteria break down the blood vessels, causing death by internal bleeding.

After death the bacteria continue to multiply in the carcass. Large numbers of spores are shed to the surrounding soil. The anthrax life cycle is continued when other creatures either eat the flesh of the dead animal or ingest enough of the spores.

There are four basic types of anthrax infection: pulmonary, cutaneous, gastrointestinal (also called enteric), and injection anthrax. Pulmonary or lung infection with anthrax is caused by inhalation of spores. Cutaneous, or skin, infection is caused by entry of spores or bacteria into cuts or sores. Gastrointestinal infection is caused by eating anthrax-contaminated meat. Injection anthrax is caused by the use of needles to inject an anthrax-tainted substance into the body.

Transmission

Anthrax is usually contracted either by taking spores or bacteria into the body through a lesion, such as a cut or open sore; through the bite of a fly; by eating the flesh of an anthrax-infected animal; or by inhaling spores. Direct transmission of anthrax between humans is extremely rare and, according to the US Centers for Disease Control and Prevention (CDC), only occurs when there is physical contact with discharge from skin lesions that is contaminated.

Humans are moderately resistant to anthrax. The infectious dose for inhalation anthrax, measured by spore count, is probably between 2,500 and 760,000 spores, the same range recorded for nonhuman primates. The US Department of Defense estimated that for humans 8,000 to 10,000 spores is the anthrax LD50, or "lethal dose 50," the amount of an agent that will be fatal in about 50 percent of cases. Scientists have shown that, in contaminated industrial settings, people can inhale more than 1,000 anthrax spores per day without contracting the disease. When anthrax is developed as a weapon, it is meant to be delivered in extremely large quantities. For example, 220 pounds (100 kilograms) of spores, often cited as a working figure in discussions of large-scale military use, contain about 10 trillion LD50 doses, which is about 1,300 times the population of the world. However, most of the spores distributed by a weapon would not end up being inhaled.

WORDS TO KNOW

CUTANEOUS Pertaining to the skin.

ENTERIC Involving the intestinal tract or relating to the intestines.

HYPERENDEMIC Endemic (commonly present) in all age groups of a population. A related term is *holoendemic*, meaning a disease that is present more often in children than in adults.

SPORE A dormant form assumed by some bacteria, such as anthrax, that enables the bacterium to survive high temperatures, dryness, and lack of nourishment for long periods. Under proper conditions, the spore may revert to the actively multiplying form of the bacteria.

■ Scope and Distribution

As a naturally occurring disease, anthrax mostly afflicts cattle. In humans it is relatively rare but tends to infect those who work with cattle or other animals, such as veterinarians and livestock producers. Persons in agricultural settings in poor nations account for the vast majority of human anthrax cases worldwide. According to the CDC, anthrax is most commonly found in the Caribbean, Central and South America, sub-Saharan Africa,

WEAPONIZING ANTHRAX

The use of anthrax in modern warfare began in 1915 during World War I (1914–1918), when a German American agent working for the imperial German government set up a secret laboratory in Washington, D.C., to produce anthrax bacteria. These were then used to infect cattle and draft animals being shipped to the Allied armies in Europe. Several hundred Allied military personnel were infected by the anthrax-ridden cattle.

During World War II (1939–1945), anthrax was developed as a major weapon by several countries. A biological warfare unit, Unit 731, was formed in the Japanese Imperial Army, which carried out experiments on thousands of Chinese prisoners of war in the 1930s. In one facility about 4,000 prisoners were killed by biological agents, mostly anthrax. By 1945 Japan had prepared about 880 pounds (400 kilograms) of powdered anthrax spores for use in fragmentation bombs intended to spread the spores in the air. Japan surrendered before using the bombs, but historians estimate that Japan may have killed over a half a million Chinese civilians using other forms of biological warfare. All members of Unit 731 were granted amnesty by the United States after the war in exchange for full disclosure of their wartime activities.

Japan was not the only country to place anthrax in bombs during World War II. In the United States a major offensive biological warfare program was established at Fort Detrick, Maryland, in 1942. Anthrax and a number of other agents were developed as weapons there, and a plant for producing biological weapons was constructed near Terre Haute, Indiana. Thousands of anthrax bombs were produced, but none were used during the war.

The British government, which was cooperating with the United States and Canada in developing anthrax as a weapon, contaminated the Scottish island of Gruinard with anthrax spores in 1942. Due to the long-lived nature of the spores, the island was off-limits for 48 years until it was decontaminated. The difficulty of decontaminating Gruinard shows how a large-scale attack with anthrax spores might render large areas of land uninhabitable. Decontamination of the small island involved soaking it in 308 tons of formaldehyde diluted in seawater and removing tons of topsoil in sealed containers.

In response to a 1969 decision by US president Richard Nixon (1913–1994), the US army destroyed all its antipersonnel biological warfare stocks, including anthrax, in 1971 and 1972, the year the biological weapons convention was first opened for signatures. The treaty took effect three years later, in 1975.

Central Asia, southwestern Asia, southern Europe, and Eastern Europe. The human anthrax rate normally depends on the livestock anthrax rate in a given area. There is about one human cutaneous anthrax case for every 10 anthrax-infected livestock carcasses processed and one enteric case for every 100 to 200 cutaneous cases. Inhalation anthrax is relatively rare; this route of exposure is usually intentional, as in the instances of the deliberately contaminated letters described earlier.

Treatment and Prevention

Prevention of anthrax is based on breaking the cycle of infection, which primarily means controlling its appearance in livestock. Cattle were first successfully inoculated against anthrax in 1880 by French biologist Louis Pasteur (1822–1895). His vaccine, which was completed in 1881, represented a breakthrough in the prevention of anthrax infections in animals. A half century later, Italian veterinarian Max Sterne (1905–1997) improved on Pasteur's vaccine, creating an anthrax live spore vaccine in 1937 that was soon adopted as a routine preventative treatment for animals. As animal infections declined, so did human anthrax infections, especially in industrialized countries such as the United States, where the disease was almost eradicated over the course of the 20th century. Despite being available for almost a century, anthrax vaccination for livestock is not universal and is less common in developing countries because of its expense.

Anthrax vaccination is only recommended for use by certain high-risk populations. The two primary forms of the vaccine for humans are the live attenuated vaccine, which involves the use of spores of *Bacillus anthracis*, and a cell-free filtrate, which contains isolated components of the anthrax bacteria instead of the spores. A live attenuated vaccine was first licensed for use in the Soviet Union in the 1950s. Research suggests that only about 1 percent of such vaccinations lead to serious adverse reactions. There are two kinds of cell-free filtrate anthrax vaccines: anthrax vaccine precipitated (AVP), a form of which has been licensed in the United Kingdom since 1979, and anthrax vaccine adsorbed (AVA), which became available in the United States in 1972 under the name BioThrax®.

The CDC recommends that adults 18 to 65 years of age who are prone to exposure to large amounts to *Bacillus anthracis* or who have already been exposed to anthrax receive the BioThrax® vaccine. In addition, the vaccine is mandatory for some categories of US military personnel and civilian defense contractors, including those assigned to serve on the Korean peninsula. While acknowledging the possibility of allergic reaction to the vaccine, the CDC states that risk for serious harm is very small.

Anthrax infection can be treated with large doses of antibiotics, swallowed (oral) or injected directly into the bloodstream (intravenous). Treatment must begin soon after infection, especially for inhalation anthrax, generally within a day and before symptoms appear. In addition, various antitoxins may be used to treat patients who have been infected with anthrax toxins.

Impacts and Issues

In countries where anthrax is naturally present, it exacts a steady human and economic toll. People contracting the disease may die or live with a decreased quality of life. Animals that contract the disease must be destroyed, and their carcasses are economically worthless.

While efforts to combat naturally occurring cases of anthrax persist in many parts of the world, much of the concern surrounding the infection has to do with its potential for use as a weapon. During the 20th century such concerns pertained to anthrax's potential but unrealized use as a battlefield weapon. While these concerns persist, especially with respect to North Korea, the 21st century has seen growing concern about how anthrax could be used by non-state terrorist organizations against civilian populations. Such concerns grew in the United States and elsewhere in the West after the 2001 anthrax letter mailings.

The US National Academy of Sciences estimated in 2003 that 2.2 pounds (1 kilogram) of anthrax spores sprayed aerially over a large city could kill more than 100,000 people. Anthrax spores could also render hundreds of square miles uninhabitable for many decades by lodging in the soil, causing immense economic damage. An often-overlooked aspect of the use of anthrax as a terrorist weapon is the economic hardship that the dispersal of a small amount of the spores would exact. A report from the CDC titled "The Economic Impact of a Bioterrorist Attack" estimated the costs of dealing with an anthrax incident at a minimum of $26 billion per 100,000 people. In 2001 a flurry of hoax anthrax incidents following the real attacks cost the US government millions of dollars.

The threat of the use of anthrax as a weapon has caused the US government to undertake extraordinary preventive efforts in addition to its military vaccination program. In 2004, as part of a $5.6 billion program called Project BioShield, which was intended to protect the public from biological threats, the federal government ordered 75 million doses ($877 million worth) of a new anthrax vaccine from a private company, VaxGen Inc., to be stockpiled in case of an anthrax attack on the United States. The new vaccine was to have required no more than three separate injections. The US Department of Health and Human Services (HHS) also stockpiled more than a billion antibiotic tablets, enough to treat 20 million people for two months. The new anthrax vaccine was to be delivered in 2006, but the program was delayed and ultimately cancelled after VaxGen was not able to start human clinical trials of its new vaccine on time.

Despite this failure the CDC continued to acquire BioThrax® vaccines in an effort to create a national stockpile. The need for such a stockpile became increasingly urgent in late 2017, as tensions between the United States and North Korea increased and as reports emerged that North Korea was weaponizing anthrax.

SEE ALSO *Biological Weapons Convention; Bioterrorism; Koch's Postulates; War and Infectious Disease; Zoonoses*

BIBLIOGRAPHY

Books

Sarasin, Philipp. *Anthrax: Bioterror as Fact and Fantasy.* Translated by Giselle Weiss. Cambridge, MA: Harvard University Press, 2006.

Swiderski, Richard M. *Anthrax: A History.* Jefferson, NC: McFarland, 2004.

World Organisation for Animal Health, World Health Organization, and Food and Agriculture Organization of the United Nations. *Anthrax in Humans and Animals.* 4th ed. Geneva, Switzerland: World Health Organization, 2008. This report can also be found online at http://apps.who.int/iris/bitstream/10665/97503/1/9789241547536_eng.pdf (accessed January 11, 2018).

Periodicals

Broad, William J. "Anthrax Not Weapons-Grade, Official Says." *New York Times* (September 26, 2006). This article can also be found online at http://www.nytimes.com/2006/09/26/us/26anthrax.html (accessed January 12, 2018).

Enserink, Martin, and Jocelyn Kaiser. "Accidental Anthrax Shipment Spurs Debate over Safety." *Nature* 304 (June 2004): 1726–1727.

Hilts, Philip J. "79 Anthrax Traced to Soviet Military." *New York Times* (November 18, 1994).

Hoffmann, Constanze, et al. "Persistent Anthrax as a Major Driver of Wildlife Mortality in a Tropical Rainforest." *Nature* 548 (2017): 82–86.

Kaufmann, Arnold F., Martin I. Meltzer, and George P. Schmid. "The Economic Impact of a Bioterrorist Attack: Are Prevention and Postattack Intervention Programs Justifiable?" *Emerging Infectious Diseases* 3, no. 2 (June 1997): 83–94. This article can also be found online at https://wwwnc.cdc.gov/eid/article/3/2/97-0201_article (accessed January 12, 2018).

Lipton, Eric. "Bid to Stockpile Bioterror Drugs Stymied by Setbacks." *New York Times* (September 18, 2006). This article can also be found online at http://www.nytimes.com/2006/09/18/washington/18anthrax.html (accessed January 12, 2018).

Rosovitz, M. J., and Stephen H. Leppla. "Virus Deals Anthrax a Killer Blow." *Nature* 418 (August 2002): 825–826. This article can also be found online at https://www.nature.com/articles/418825a (accessed January 12, 2018).

Yong, Ed. "A Strange Type of Anthrax Is Killing Chimpanzees." *Atlantic* (August 2, 2017). This article can also be found online at https://www.theatlantic.com/science/archive/2017/08/a-strange-type-of-anthrax-is-killing-chimpanzees/535521/ (accessed January 11, 2018).

Websites

"Anthrax." Centers for Disease Control and Prevention, January 31, 2017. https://www.cdc.gov/anthrax/index.html (accessed January 11, 2018).

"Britain's 'Anthrax Island.'" British Broadcasting Corporation, July 25, 2001. http://news.bbc.co.uk/2/low/uk_news/scotland/1457035.stm (accessed January 11, 2018).

Engelberg, Stephen. "New Evidence Adds Doubt to FBI's Case against Anthrax Suspect." ProPublica, October 10, 2011. https://www.propublica.org/article/new-evidence-disputes-case-against-bruce-e-ivins (accessed January 11, 2018).

"Guidelines for the Surveillance and Control of Anthrax in Humans and Animals." World Health Organization. http://www.who.int/csr/resources/publications/anthrax/WHO_EMC_ZDI_98_6/en (accessed January 11, 2018).

Sharp, Andy. "North Korea Begins Tests to Load Anthrax onto ICBMs, Report Says." Bloomberg, December 19, 2017. https://www.bloomberg.com/news/articles/2017–12-20/north-korea-begins-tests-to-load-anthrax-onto-icbms-asahi-says (accessed January 11, 2018).

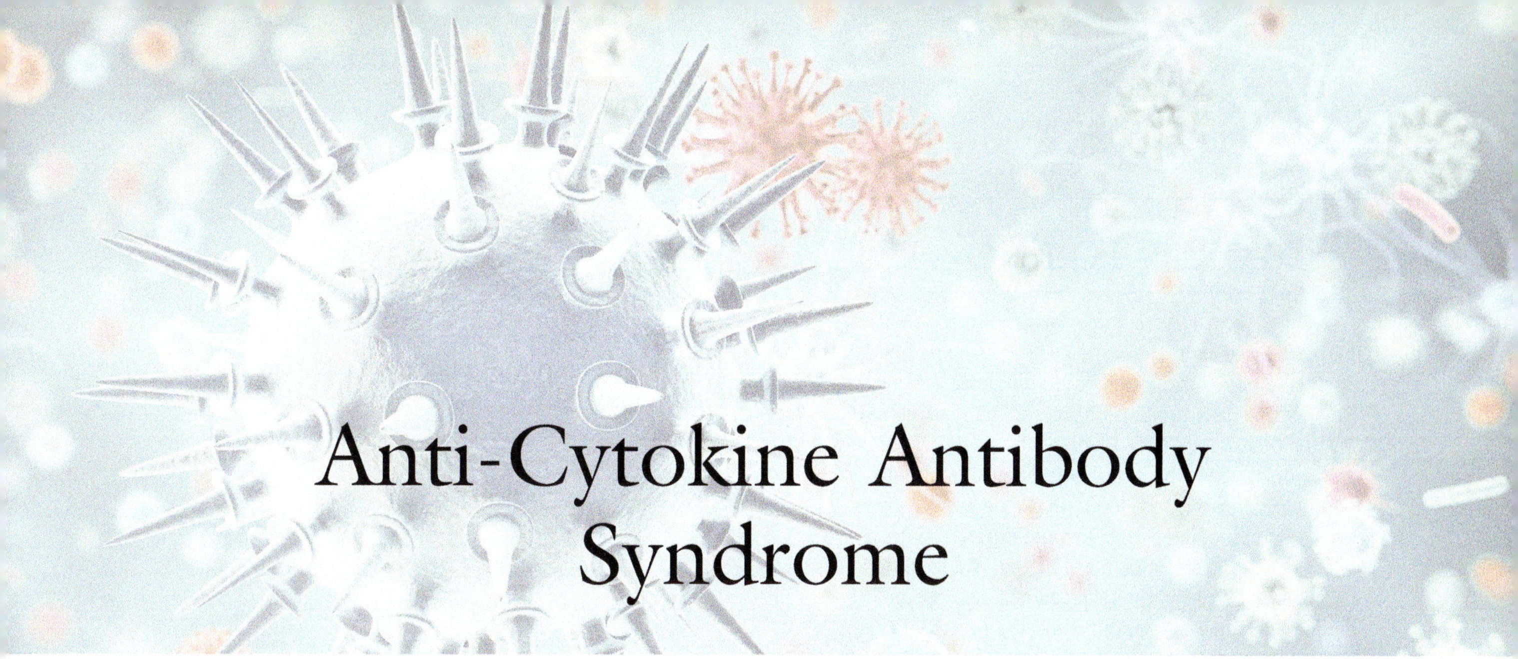

Anti-Cytokine Antibody Syndrome

Introduction

Anti-cytokine antibody syndromes occur when the body develops antibodies to secreted proteins known as cytokines. Cytokines function as signaling protein molecules between cells of the immune system and between immune and nonimmune cells. The term comes from the Greek *cyto* (cell) and *kino* (motion). Although the immune system usually tolerates self molecules (molecules recognized by the immune system as belonging to the organism), autoantibodies to cytokines may develop in many individuals.

Anti-cytokine antibodies are not always associated with disease. They have been detected in healthy individuals as well as in patients with various infections. At low levels they may function to regulate the immune system. However, at higher levels they may compromise the body's ability to fight off infection and leave patients susceptible to disease.

Disease Characteristics and Clinical Findings

The symptoms of anti-cytokine antibody syndromes are diverse and depend on the particular cytokine that is affected. High levels of anti-cytokine antibodies may make a person susceptible to opportunistic infections such as candidiasis, tuberculosis, and cryptosporidiosis. These infections do not occur in healthy individuals but only in those with weakened immune systems. For instance, pulmonary alveolar proteinosis (PAP) is seen in patients with high levels of anti-granulocyte-macrophage colony-stimulating factor (GM-CSF) antibodies, and disseminated nontuberculous mycobacterial disease (NTM) is seen in patients with high levels of anti-interferon autoantibodies. Certain other diseases have been shown to have high titers (concentrations) of anti-cytokine autoantibodies. These include autoimmune polyendocrinopathy, candidiasis, ectodermal dystrophy (APECED) syndrome and thymoma. However, the direct causal link to anti-cytokine autoantibodies has not been established.

Interferon gamma is a key cytokine for defense against pathogens that live inside the cell, such as mycobacteria. In otherwise healthy individuals, antibodies to interferon gamma have been associated with intracellular infections, where the infectious agent lives inside the cell. Extrapulmonary disseminated NTM infections, infections with *Salmonella typhi*, cytomegalovirus, cerebral toxoplasmosis, and reactivation of *Varicella zoster* (an organism that causes shingles) have been identified in patients with elevated levels of these antibodies. According to an article by Sarah K. Browne and coauthors published in the *New England Journal of Medicine*, a 2012 study of 80 patients with high levels of neutralizing antibody to interferon gamma showed a strong association with widespread nontuberous mycobacterial infections. Some of the patients had additional opportunistic infections caused by bacteria and fungi.

Interleukin 6 (IL-6), produced by many cells, is involved in inflammation and is produced in response to tissue damage and infection. In a 2014 study published in the *Annual Review of Immunology*, three patients with high levels of IL-6 neutralizing antibodies were identified. These patients had severe bacterial infections, including *Staphylococcus aureus*, *Streptococcus intermedius*, and *Escherichia coli*. Several healthy individuals were also seen to have high levels of IL-6 neutralizing antibody, suggesting that additional factors may have been involved in the development of infectious diseases in these patients.

Patients with neutralizing antibodies to GM-CSF may develop chronic PAP, a severe condition of lung insufficiency. These patients may also suffer from recurrent common pulmonary infections, as well as opportunistic infections, including a type of cryptococcal meningitis commonly seen in immunocompromised patients. Other diseases seen in these patients include disseminated Nocardia infections in the central nervous system and invasive aspergillosis.

WORDS TO KNOW

ANTIBODIES Proteins found in the blood that help fight against foreign substances called antigens. Antigens, which are usually proteins or polysaccharides, stimulate the immune system to produce antibodies, or Y-shaped immunoglobulins. The antibodies inactivate the antigen and help remove it from the body. While antigens can be the source of infections from pathogenic bacteria and viruses, organic molecules detrimental to the body from internal or environmental sources also act as antigens. Genetic engineering and the use of various mutational mechanisms allow the construction of a vast array of antibodies (each with a unique genetic sequence).

CYTOKINE One of a family of small proteins that mediate an organism's response to injury or infection. Cytokines operate by transmitting signals between cells in an organism. Minute quantities of cytokines are secreted, each by a single cell type, to regulate functions in other cells by binding with specific receptors. Their interactions with the receptors produce secondary signals that inhibit or enhance the action of certain genes within the cell. Unlike endocrine hormones, which can act throughout the body, most cytokines act locally near the cells that produced them.

OPPORTUNISTIC INFECTION An infection that occurs in people whose immune systems are diminished or are not functioning normally. Such infections are opportunistic insofar as the infectious agents take advantage of their hosts' compromised immune systems and invade to cause disease.

PATHOGEN A disease-causing agent, such as a bacterium, a virus, a fungus, or another microorganism.

Treatment

In general, patients with anti-cytokine autoantibodies are first treated with agents that can control the infections. The use of corticosteroids to suppress the immune system can be counterproductive because it may worsen the disease. In the case of PAP caused by anti-GM-CSF antibody, the patient's lung may be lavaged (washed), and recombinant GM-CSF may be given intranasally. Other treatments that have been useful include the immunosuppressive drug cyclophosphamide and plasmapheresis (treatment of blood outside the body). Some success has been obtained by using rituximab, an antibody that blocks antibody-producing B cells.

Impacts and Issues

Anti-cytokine autoantibodies can make otherwise healthy patients susceptible to opportunistic infections, including mycobacterial diseases, various viruses, and candidiasis. In inflammatory diseases, anti-cytokine autoantibodies may play a protective or exacerbating role. Further understanding of the exact role of these antibodies in autoimmune diseases will help develop better treatments for these patients.

See Also *Escherichia coli O157:H7; Opportunistic Infection; Staphylococcus aureus Infection*

BIBLIOGRAPHY

Books

Klenerman, Paul. *The Immune System: A Very Short Introduction.* Oxford, UK: Oxford University Press, 2018.

Shuiping Jiang, ed. *TH17 Cells in Health and Disease.* London: Springer, 2011.

Periodicals

Browne, Sarah K., et al. "Adult-Onset Immunodeficiency in Thailand and Taiwan." *New England Journal of Medicine* 367, no. 8 (2012): 725–734.

Browne, Sarah K. "Anticytokine Autoantibody-Associated Immunodeficiency." *Annual Review of Immunology* 32, no. 1 (2014): 635–657.

Browne, Sarah K., and Steven M. Holland. "Immunodeficiency Secondary to Anti-Cytokine Autoantibodies." *Current Opinion in Allergy and Clinical Immunology* 10, no. 6 (2010): 534–541.

Hanitsch, Leif Gunnar, et al. "Late-Onset Disseminated Mycobacterium avium intracellare Complex Infection (MAC), Cerebral Toxoplasmosis and Salmonella Sepsis in a German Caucasian Patient with Unusual Anti-Interferon-Gamma IgG1 Autoantibodies." *Journal of Clinical Immunology* 35, no. 4 (2015): 361–365.

Kisand, Kai, et al. "Chronic Mucocutaneous Candidiasis in APECED or Thymoma Patients Correlates with Autoimmunity to Th17-Associated Cytokines." *Journal of Experimental Medicine* 207, no. 2 (2010): 299–308.

O'Connell, Elise, et al. "The First US Domestic Report of Disseminated *Mycobacterium avium* Complex and Anti-Interferon Gamma Autoantibodies." *Journal of Clinical Immunology* 34, no. 8 (2014): 928–932.

Rosen, Lindsey B., et al. "Nocardia-Induced Granulocyte Macrophage Colony-Stimulating Factor Is Neutralized by Autoantibodies in Disseminated/Extrapulmonary Nocardiosis." *Clinical Infectious Disease* 60, no. 7 (2015): 1017–1025.

Saijo, Tomomi, et al. "Anti-Granulocyte-Macrophage Colony-Stimulating Factor Autoantibodies Are a Risk Factor for Central Nervous System Infection by *Cryptococcus gattii* in Otherwise Immunocompetent Patients." *Mbio* 5, no. 2 (2014): e00912–e00914.

Walter, Jolan E., et al. "Broad-Spectrum Antibodies against Self-Antigens and Cytokines in RAG Deficiency." *Journal of Clinical Investigation* 125, no. 11 (2015): 4135–4148.

Websites

"Autoimmune Diseases." National Institute of Allergy and Infectious Diseases. https://www.niaid.nih.gov/diseases-conditions/autoimmune-diseases (accessed March 13, 2018).

"Immune System." PubMedHealth. https://www.ncbi.nlm.nih.gov/pubmedhealth/PMHT0025680/ (accessed March 13, 2018).

Malini Vashishtha

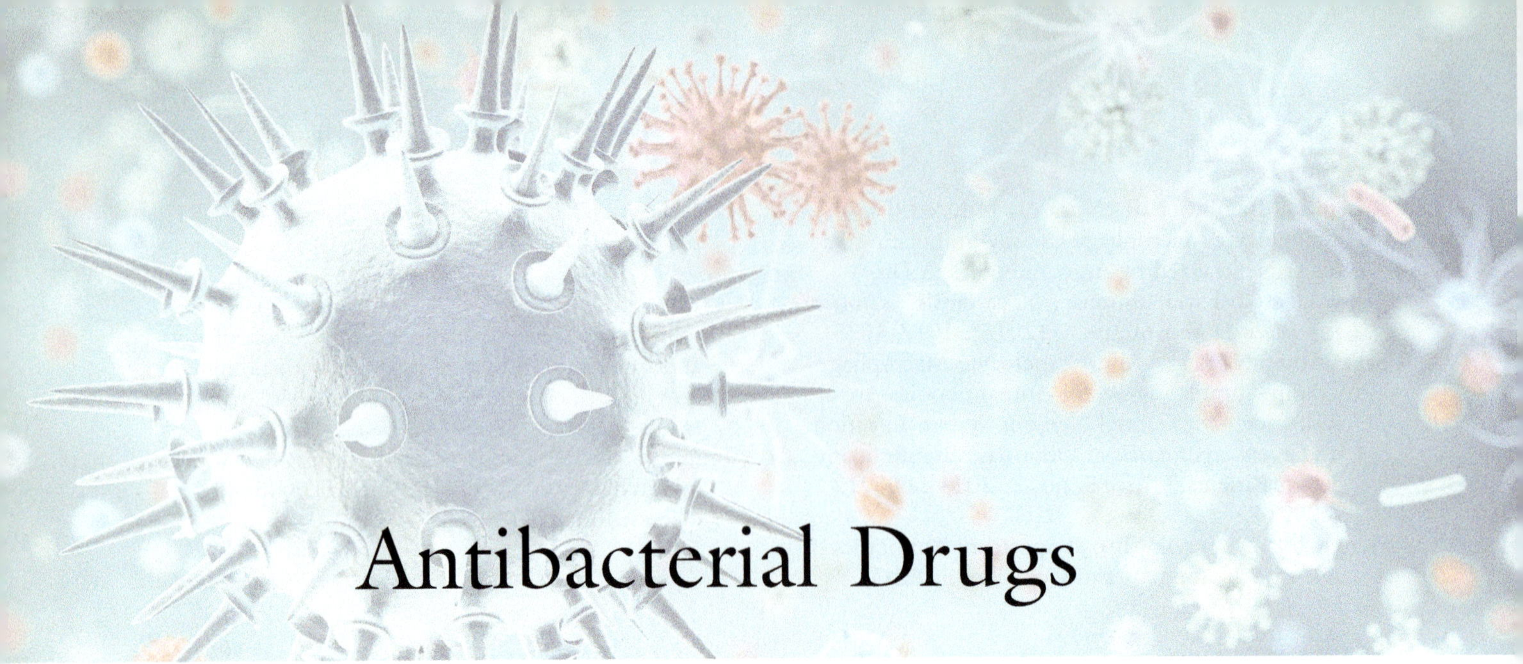

Antibacterial Drugs

Introduction

Antibacterial drugs stop bacterial infections in two ways: they prevent bacteria from dividing and increasing in number or they kill the bacteria. The former drugs, which prevent bacteria from increasing in number but do not kill the bacteria, are termed bacteriostatic drugs. The latter, which kill the infectious bacteria, are known as bactericidal drugs. Both types of drugs can stop an infection.

The terms antibacterial drugs and antibiotics are often used interchangeably. Though the most common antibacterial drugs are the many types of antibiotics, other compounds can also be considered antibacterial. One example is alcohol, which kills bacteria by dissolving the cell membrane. Another example is carbolic acid, which was famously used by Joseph Lister (1827–1912) in the mid-19th century as a spray to prevent bacterial contamination of wounds during operations. Antibacterial agents such as alcohol and carbolic acid are more accurately considered disinfectants (chemicals that kill or inactivate bacteria on surfaces and instruments) rather than antibiotics, which are generally taken internally and can create resistant strains of bacteria.

History and Scientific Foundations

The use of antibacterial drugs is ancient. Thousands of years ago, when the scientific basis of infection and its

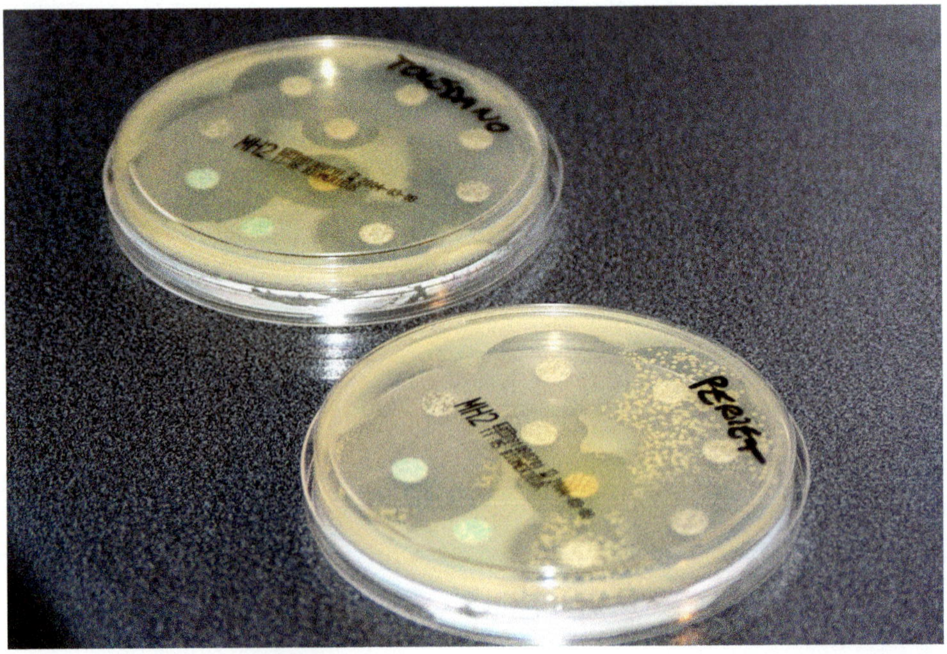

This photograph shows antibiotic testing in a lab. Bacteria in petri dishes are exposed to multiple antibiotics to test their susceptibility. *© BSIP/UIG/Getty Images*

treatment were still unknown, infections were sometimes successfully treated with molds and plants. Centuries later the production of antibiotics by some species of molds and plants was discovered. Indeed, one argument against the large-scale deforestation of regions, such as the Amazon basin, is that there are likely still many antibiotic-producing molds and plants yet to be discovered.

The antibiotic era began in the first decade of the 20th century, when Paul Ehrlich (1854–1915) discovered a compound that proved to be an effective treatment for syphilis. In 1928 Sir Alexander Fleming (1881–1955) discovered the antibiotic penicillin. With recognition of the compound's prowess in killing a wide variety of bacteria, interest in antibiotics soared. In 1941 Selman Waksman (1888–1973) coined the term *antibiotic.* In the ensuing decades, much work focused on the discovery of new antibiotics from natural sources, the laboratory alteration of existing compounds to increase their potency (and, later, to combat the problem of antibiotic resistance), and the synthesis of entirely new antibiotics.

Antibiotics kill bacteria in a variety of ways. Some alter the structure of the bacteria so that the bacteria become structurally weakened and unable to withstand physical stresses, such as pressure, with the result that the bacteria explode. Other antibiotics halt the production of various proteins in a number of ways: inhibiting the decoding of the genes specifying the proteins (transcriptional inhibition); blocking the production of the proteins following the production of the genetic message, messenger ribonucleic acid (mRNA, in a process termed *translational inhibition*); blocking the movement of the manufactured protein to its final location in the bacterium; or blocking the import of compounds that are crucial to the continued survival of the bacterium.

Some antibiotics—described as *broad-spectrum*—are effective against many different bacteria. Other antibiotics—described as *narrow-spectrum*—are very specific in their action and, as a result, affect fewer bacteria.

Penicillin is the classic example of a class of antibiotics known as beta-lactam antibiotics. The term *beta-lactam* refers to the ring structure that is the backbone of these

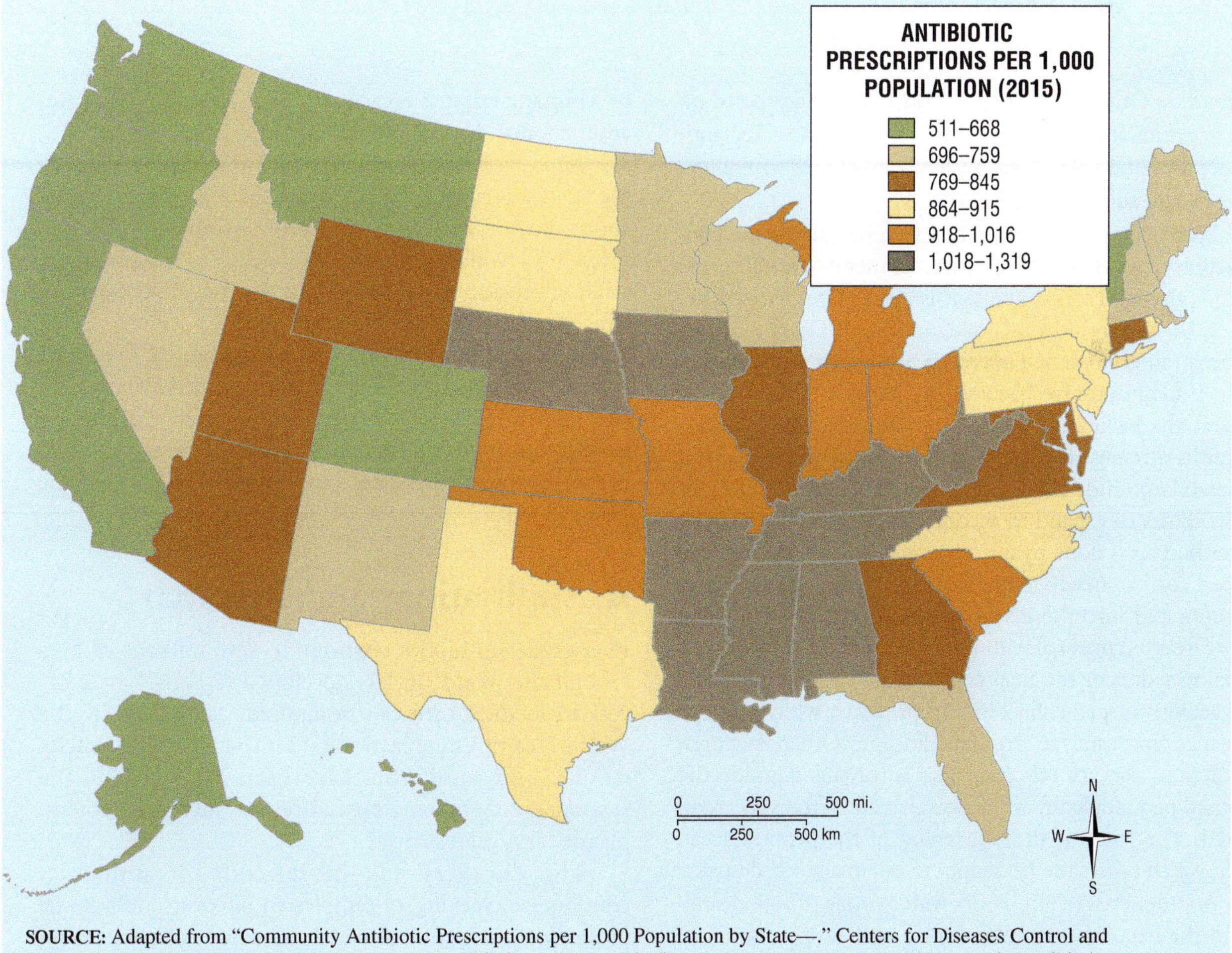

SOURCE: Adapted from "Community Antibiotic Prescriptions per 1,000 Population by State—." Centers for Diseases Control and Prevention. Available from: https://www.cdc.gov/antibiotic-use/community/images/programsmeasurement/Community-antibiotic-map-2015.jpg

WORDS TO KNOW

ANTIBIOTIC A drug, such as penicillin, used to fight infections caused by bacteria. Antibiotics act only on bacteria and are not effective against viruses.

ANTIBIOTIC RESISTANCE The ability of bacteria to resist the actions of antibiotic drugs.

BACTERIOCIDAL A term that refers to the treatment of a bacterium such that the organism is killed. A bacteriocidal treatment is always lethal and is also referred to as sterilization.

BACTERIOSTATIC A term that refers to a treatment that restricts the ability of the bacterium to grow.

BROAD–SPECTRUM ANTIBIOTICS Drugs that kill a wide range of bacteria rather than just those from a specific family. For example, Amoxicillin is a broad-spectrum antibiotic that is used against many common illnesses such as ear infections.

DISINFECTANT Disinfection and the use of chemical disinfectants is one key strategy of infection control. Disinfectants reduce the number of living microorganisms, usually to a level that is considered to be safe for the particular environment. Typically, this entails the destruction of those microbes that are capable of causing disease.

NOSOCOMIAL INFECTION An infection that is acquired in a hospital. More precisely, the Centers for Disease Control and Prevention in Atlanta, Georgia, defines a nosocomial infection as a localized infection or an infection that is widely spread throughout the body that results from an adverse reaction to an infectious microorganism or toxin that was not present at the time of admission to the hospital.

antibiotics. Other classes of antibiotics, which are based on the structure and/or the mechanism of action of the antibiotic, are tetracyclines, rifamycins, quinolones, aminoglycosides, and sulphonamides.

Beta-lactam antibiotics kill bacteria by altering the construction of a portion of the bacterial membrane called the peptidoglycan. This component is a thin layer located between the inner and outer membranes of Gram-negative bacteria (an example is *Escherichia coli*) and a much thicker layer in Gram-positive bacteria (an example is *Bacillus anthracis*, the bacterium that causes anthrax). The peptidoglycan is a tennis-racket-like mesh of sugar molecules and other compounds that is very strong when intact. This network has to expand to accommodate the growth of the bacteria. This is done by introducing breaks in the peptidoglycan so that newly made material can be inserted and incorporated into the existing network, cross-linking the newly inserted material with the older material. Beta-lactam antibiotics disrupt the final cross-linking step by inhibiting the activity of penicillin-binding proteins, which are the enzymes that catalyze the cross-linkage. Other enzymes, autolysins, also are released. The autolysins degrade the exposed peptidoglycan at the sites that are defectively cross-linked. The result is the weakening of the peptidoglycan layer, which causes the bacterium to essentially self-destruct.

Another class of antibiotics with a mode of action similar to the beta-lactam antibiotics are cephalosporins. There have been a number of versions, or generations, of cephalosporins that have improved the ability of these antibiotics to withstand enzyme breakdown. The latest cephalosporins are the fourth generation of these antibiotics.

Aminoglycoside antibiotics bind to certain regions of the cellular structure called ribosomes. Ribosomes are responsible for decoding the information contained in mRNA to produce proteins. By binding to the ribosome, aminoglycoside antibiotics disrupt protein production, which is often lethal for the bacterium.

As a final example, quinolone antibiotics impair an enzyme that unwinds the double helix of deoxyribonucleic acid (DNA). This unwinding must occur so that the genetic information can be used to make proteins and other bacterial components. These antibiotics kill bacteria at the genetic level.

■ Applications and Research

Every year antibiotics continue to save millions of lives around the world. In less developed regions, where access to medical care can be limited, campaigns by the World Health Organization (WHO) and other agencies to distribute antibiotics have been invaluable in the response to epidemics of diseases such as cholera, plague, and yellow fever.

The discovery and manufacture of antibiotics continues. Screening of samples to uncover antibacterial properties has been automated; thousands of samples can be processed each day. Furthermore, the increased knowledge of the molecular details of the active sites of antibiotics and the ability to target specific regions have been exploited in the design of new antibiotics.

Impacts and Issues

In the decades after pencillin's discovery and use, many different antibiotics were discovered or synthesized and introduced for use. The control of bacterial infections became so routine that it appeared that infectious diseases would become a problem of the past. However, this optimism has proven to be premature. Instead, some bacteria have developed resistance to a number of antibiotics. For example, bacterial resistance was first observed only about three years after the commercial introduction and widespread use of penicillin in the late 1940s. Penicillin-resistant staphylococcus bacteria were reported in 1944, and, by the 1950s, a penicillin–resistant strain of *Staphylococcus aureus* became a worldwide problem in hospitals. By the 1960s most staphylococci were resistant to penicillin, and two decades later it was rare to encounter methicillin-resistant *S. aureus* (MRSA). In 2017 MRSA was a daily concern of a hospital's infection control challenge.

Another emerging health care problem is carbapenem-resistant Enterobacteriaceae, or CRE. Carapenems are another class of antibiotics. Bacteria such as *E. coli* that become resistant to carbapenems are difficult to kill. CRE is a big problem in China and other regions of Asia. Without efforts to control these infections, it seems a matter of time before other regions of the globe also are affected.

The effectiveness of an antibiotic to which bacteria have developed resistance can sometimes be restored by slightly modifying a chemical group of antibiotic. For example, the antibiotics ampicillin and amoxicillin are variants of penicillin. However, this strategy usually produces only a short-term benefit because resistance to the altered antibiotic also develops.

One factor contributing to the growth of antibiotic resistance is the overuse or misuse of antibiotics. All the bacteria responsible for an infection may not be killed if an insufficient concentration of an antibiotic is used or if antibiotic therapy is stopped before the prescription has been used completely. The surviving bacteria may possess resistance to the antibiotic, which can sometimes be passed on to other bacteria. For example, tuberculosis has reemerged as a significant health problem, especially for people whose immune systems are compromised, because the tuberculosis bacteria have developed resistance to the antibiotics used to treat them.

Acinetobacter baumannii is another bacterium that has developed resistance to many antibiotics. This bacterium is normally found in soil and water and so is commonly encountered. While *A. baumannii* infections were once confined to hospitals, where they accounted for about 80 percent of all nosocomial (hospital-acquired) infections, the bacterium now has become a growing problem for the military. Multidrug resistant *A. baumanii* has infected more than 3,300 U.S. soldiers wounded in conflicts in Afghanistan and Iraq up to 2009, the last year the Department of Defense publicly reported the number of infections. In military hospitals that handled the evacuated soldiers, the physicians had few treatment options for these infections.

New antibacterial drugs are expected to produce blockbuster sales for their manufacturers, as emerging resistant organisms push the development of new and efficient antibiotics into the forefront. As of 2017 approval is pending for antibiotics that are active against the bacteria that cause intra-abdominal infections, complicated urinary tract infections, and community-acquired bacterial pneumonia, among others. These successes are tempered by the reality that other drugs fail in clinical trials that are more far along in the drug development pathway, after millions of dollars have been spent. In 2014 the development cost of a new drug was estimated to exceed $2.5 billion. This can hamper the drug development pipeline.

See Also *Antibiotic Resistance; Antimicrobial Soaps; MRSA*

BIBLIOGRAPHY

Books

McKenna, Maryn. *Big Chicken: The Incredible Story of How Antibiotics Created Modern Agriculture and Changed the Way the World Eats.* Washington, DC: National Geographic, 2017.

Walsh, Christopher, and Timothy Wencewicz. *Antibiotics: Challenges, Mechanisms, Opportunities.* Washington, DC: ASM, 2016.

Periodicals

Sharma, Monica, Shashank Singh, and Sidharth Sharma. "New Generation Antibiotics/Antibacterials: Deadly Arsenal for Disposal of Antibiotic Resistant Bacteria." *Journal of Microbial & Biochemical Technology* 7, no. 6 (January 2015): 374–379. This article can also be found online at https://www.researchgate.net/publication/288859488_New_Generation_AntibioticsAntibacterials_Deadly_Arsenal_for_Disposal_of_Antibiotic_Resistant_Bacteria (accessed November 8, 2017).

Ventola, C. L. "The Antibiotic Resistance Crisis. Part 1: Causes and Threats." *Pharmacy & Therapeutics* 40, no. 4 (2015): 277–283.

Websites

"Antibiotic/Antimicrobial Resistance." Centers for Disease Control and Prevention. https://www.cdc.gov/drugresistance/index.html (accessed November 8, 2017).

"Antimicrobial Resistance Fact Sheet." World Health Organization, November 2017. http://www.who.int/mediacentre/factsheets/fs194/en/ (accessed November 8, 2017).

"Cost to Develop New Pharmaceutical Drug Now Exceeds $2.5B." *Scientific American*, 2014. https://www.scientificamerican.com/article/cost–to–develop–new–pharmaceutical–drug–now–exceeds–2–5b/ (accessed November 8, 2017).

Brian Hoyle

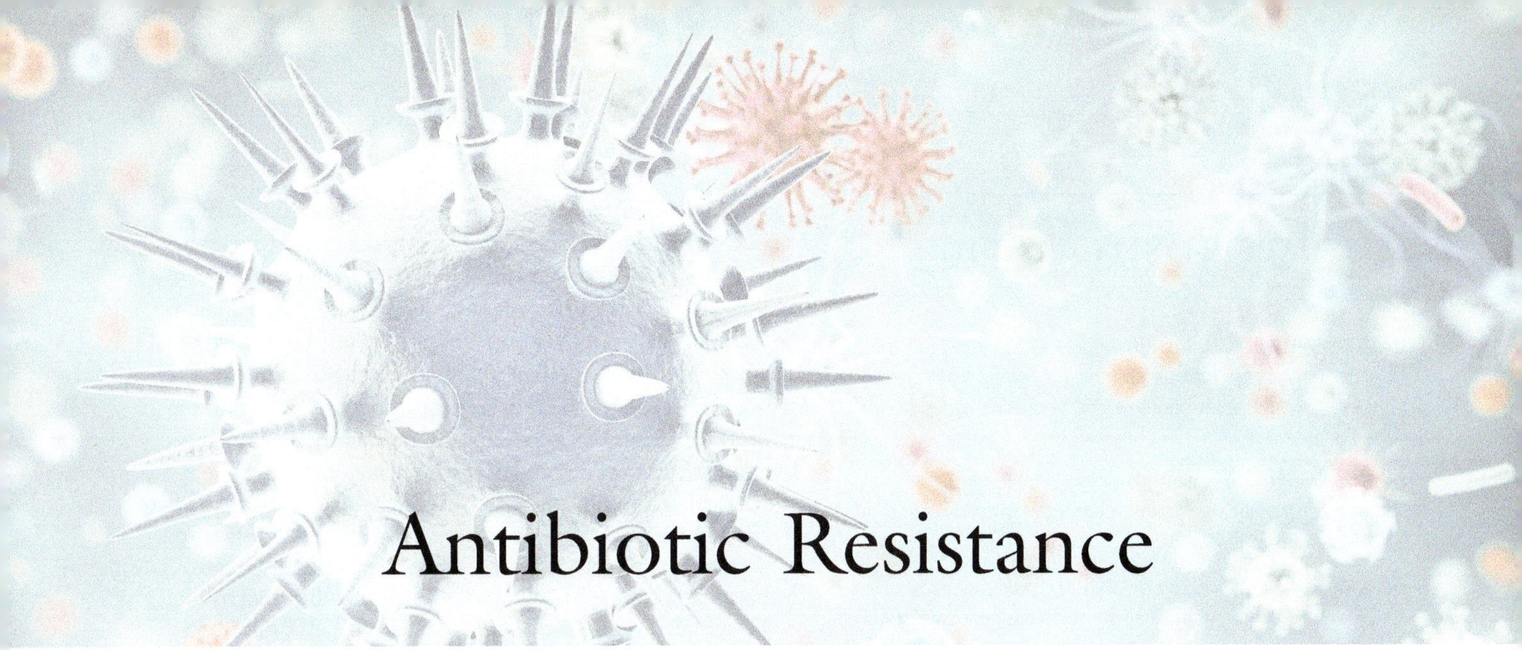

Antibiotic Resistance

Introduction

Antibiotic resistance refers to the change of bacteria from a state in which they are able to be killed by a drug to a state in which they can survive. This phenomenon is proving to be the case for all antibiotics.

The classic example of antibiotic resistance is penicillin. Penicillin was the first antibiotic to be mass-produced for use in treating bacterial infections. Following its introduction during World War II (1939–1945), infections that had until then been difficult to treat became easy to cure. The next few decades were a time of great optimism. Scientists and others believed that most, if not all, bacterial infections would be controlled by penicillin and other antibiotics. In 1969 US Surgeon General William Stewart (1921–2008) proclaimed, "It is time to close the book on infectious diseases. The war against pestilence is over."

This optimism proved to be premature. In fact, there had already been a hint of what was to come. Only three years after the introduction of penicillin, clinical infections caused by a penicillin-resistant form of the Gram-positive bacterium *Staphylococcus aureus* began to be reported. In

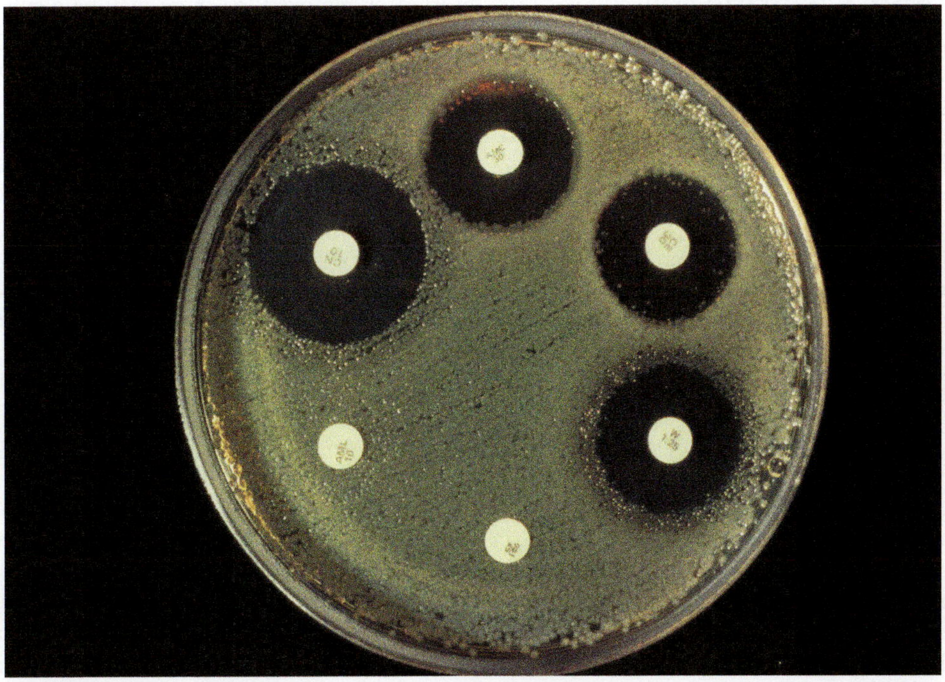

This petri dish contains six different antibacterial pellets surrounded by a culture of *E. coli* bacteria. The absence of bacterial growth around four of the pellets shows that the culture is sensitive to the antibiotic. The presence of bacterial growth around the remaining two pellets shows that the culture is resistant to those antibiotics. *© John Durham/Science Source*

WORDS TO KNOW

BACTERIOPHAGE A virus that infects bacteria. When a bacteriophage that carries the diphtheria toxin gene infects diphtheria bacteria, the bacteria produce diphtheria toxin.

MRSA Methicillin-resistant *Staphylococcus aureus* are bacteria resistant to most penicillin-type antibiotics, including methicillin.

PLASMID A circular piece of DNA that exists outside of the bacterial chromosome and copies itself independently. Scientists often use bacterial plasmids in genetic engineering to carry genes into other organisms.

subsequent decades antibiotic resistance has become a major concern in hospitals and in daily life. The problem does not have a single cause; bacteria have devised a number of ways to overcome antibiotics.

The result, according to 2015 statistics from the US Centers for Disease Control and Prevention (CDC), is the death of 23,000 Americans each year from infections caused by antibiotic-resistant bacteria.

History and Scientific Foundations

By 1947 the antibiotic methicillin had been in widespread use for only two years. Nonetheless, resistance to this penicillin-related antibiotic by *S. aureus* was already known. The bacterium, since dubbed methicillin-resistant *S. aureus*, or MRSA, has become a major problem because it possesses resistance to a variety of other antibiotics commonly used to treat infections.

By 2007 about 50 percent of all hospital infections caused by *S. aureus* in the United States resulted from MRSA, and the bacterium had spread from hospitals into the general community. This bleak picture was followed by some good news. According to the CDC, the number of life-threatening infections caused by MRSA had decreased 54 percent between 2005 and 2011. This decline is likely the result of policies put in place by hospitals to limit the development and spread of MRSA infections. However, MRSA remains a major problem in hospitals specifically and communities in general.

As of 2017 there was only one antibiotic, vancomycin, that was effective against such multiresistant bacteria. However, in 1997 a strain of *S. aureus* that also was resistant to vancomycin was reported in Japan. This resistant bacterium is also present in Europe and North America. While not yet as prevalent as MRSA, the number of cases of infection due to vancomycin-resistant *S. aureus* continues to rise. As of 2014 13 cases of such infections have been confirmed in the United States. The last case, which occurred in March 2012 in Delaware, was especially troubling because it involved someone who had not been hospitalized.

Antibiotic resistance is present in other disease-causing bacteria as well. An important example are bacteria including *Klebsiella* species and *Escherichia coli*, which are members of a family of Gram-negative bacteria termed *Enterobacteriaceae.* These bacteria have become resistant to the antibiotic carbapenem. Carbapenem-resistant Enterobacteriaceae, or CRE, are also resistant to other antibiotics. Healthy individuals are usually resistant to CRE, but hospitalized patients are at risk, which has led to the spread of CRE in many hospitals.

Data from the CDC in 2017 indicated the presence of a type of CRE called *Klebsiella pneumoniae* in at least one hospital in every US state. This is ominous because CRE infections can be fatal in up to half of all patients who become infected, according to the CDC.

Acquisition of resistance has been a consequence of the use of antibiotics in hospitals. The selective pressure on a bacterium in a hospital is to develop antibiotic resistance, as the continued survival of the bacterium depends on its ability to thwart the antibiotic.

Bacteria can also become resistant to an antibiotic purely by chance. Changes in the bacterial deoxyribonucleic acid (DNA) can occur randomly. Portions of DNA may be inserted or removed, or there may be a substitution of some of the building blocks (nucleotides) of the DNA. If the change occurs in a portion of DNA that codes for a bacterial component, the result can be resistance to an antibiotic. For example, a change in the composition of the bacterial membrane may prevent an antibiotic from passing as easily to the inside of the cell, or the enhanced activity of a bacterial enzyme may degrade a particular antibiotic. This spontaneous antibiotic resistance is thought to be responsible for the appearance of drug resistance in the bacterium that causes tuberculosis, which has led to the resurgence of this lung infection.

A second way that antibiotic resistance can be acquired is by the transfer of some of the DNA from the chromosomes of one bacterium to another. This typically occurs when the two bacteria are connected to each other by a hollow tube (a sex pilus). DNA can pass down the tube from the donor bacterium to the recipient bacterium. The process can be interrupted by breaking the tube, and so the transfer of genetic material can often be incomplete.

The third means by which antibiotic resistance develops is the most worrisome. This also involves the transfer of DNA from one bacterium to another, but, instead of the transfer of DNA from the chromosomes of the donor bacterium to the recipient bacterium, the DNA found in a circular piece of DNA—known as a plasmid—is transferred from donor to recipient. Transfer of the plasmid to a new bacterium can easily occur, and the inserted plasmid may not need to be part of the recipient's genome to produce whatever factor is responsible for antibiotic resistance.

Plasmid-mediated transfer can occur at a much higher frequency than the other types of DNA transfer, and, as a result, antibiotic resistance can spread quickly. Furthermore, the DNA transfer can be promoted by selection pressure. For example, the presence of antibiotics can encourage the transfer DNA coding for antibiotic resistance among populations of bacteria.

A plasmid may contain a number of genes that each code for resistance to a certain antibiotic, as well as the genetic information that enables all this information to be deciphered and the necessary resistance factors made. The plasmid only needs to get inside the recipient bacterium for that cell to become resistant to the antibiotics.

There are different mechanisms of antibiotic resistance. Change of the target site of an antibiotic can make the antibiotic less effective or completely ineffective. For example, some Gram-negative bacteria can become resistant to a class of antibiotics called beta-lactam antibiotics by a modification to proteins called penicillin-binding proteins. The modification keeps the beta-lactam antibiotics from disrupting the construction of peptidoglycan, a component that is vital to maintaining the structure of the bacterial membrane. Other mechanisms of antibiotic resistance include the increased ability of the bacterium to pump an antibiotic back out of the cell and the production of enzymes by the bacteria that can destroy the incoming antibiotic.

Laboratory tests can determine whether the bacteria isolated from an infection are resistant to antibiotics; which antibiotics the microbe is resistant to; and, most importantly for treatment, which antibiotics can kill the microbe. Typically, this testing involves adding the bacteria to the surface of a solid nutrient. The bacteria are spread over the surface so that they will grow as a continuous layer. At about the same time, discs of a paper-like material that have been soaked in various concentrations of antibiotics are positioned on the nutrient surface. When the bacteria eventually grow, there will be circular clear zones devoid of bacteria wherever the antibiotic has been effective in killing them. Measurement of the diameter of these zones of growth inhibition can be used to determine how sensitive a particular type of bacteria is to the particular antibiotic. An automated version of this test also exists, but the basic design of the test is similar.

■ Applications and Research

Antibiotic resistance is a race between the development and introduction of an antibiotic and the development of bacterial resistance to the drug. Antibiotic development largely focuses on modifying an existing compound. For some antibiotics, effectiveness can be regenerated relatively easily by modifying the three-dimensional structure of the molecule. Even a slight alteration involving the replacement of one chemical group in the molecule by another can restore the potency of the drug. Unfortunately, this effectiveness tends to be short term. Within several years bacteria can adapt to the modified drug and once again become resistant.

Researchers continue to try and find new mechanisms of antibiotic resistance. By understanding how bacteria become resistant to antibiotics, they hope to discover or design drugs that will kill the bacteria without stimulating the development of resistance. One promising approach is the use of bacteriophages—viruses that specifically infect and make new copies inside of a certain type of bacteria. Different bacteriophages each infect a particular bacterium. Because bacteriophages have been around for millions of years without the development of resistance by the target bacteria, researchers have been experimenting with the use of bacteriophages to deliver a toxic payload of antibacterial compounds. As of 2017 the research seems promising but is still in the experimental stage.

■ Impacts and Issues

Antibiotic discovery or synthesis is a long and costly process. This has hampered antibiotic research because a pharmaceutical company needs to have a reasonable expectation of recouping the dollars spent on drug development before the drug becomes clinically less useful. In 2014 the estimated cost of drug development (which includes drugs other than antibiotics) was $2.9 billion. A 2015 article in the *New York Times* reports that only about 40 new antibiotics were in development compared to 771 new drugs and vaccines for cancer that were at the clinical trial stage.

Antibiotic resistance is a problem that humans have created through the misuse and overuse of antibiotics. For example, it was once common practice to prescribe antibiotics for almost all illnesses, even those caused by viruses. Because viruses are not affected by antibiotics, this approach only served to exert a selection pressure favoring the development of resistance on the bacteria already present. In addition, antibiotics continue to be widely used in the poultry and cattle industries to enhance the weight gain of the birds or livestock. This practice involves giving antibiotics to healthy animals rather than using them to treat infections. It encourages the development of resistant bacteria, and this resistance can be passed to other bacterial populations.

Since 2000 the prevalence of community-associated MRSA (CA-MRSA) has been increasing. CA-MRSA infections are found in healthy people interacting normally in their community, not among those who have been hospitalized within the past year or had recent medical procedures, such as dialysis or surgery. This type of antibiotic resistance is especially challenging for health authorities, as it indicates that antibiotic resistance is capable of developing and spreading in the absence of antibiotic use. Outbreaks of community-associated MRSA have continued to occur globally.

PRIMARY SOURCE

What If Cipro Stopped Working?

SOURCE: *Silbergeld, Ellen K., and Polly Walker. "What If Cipro Stopped Working?"* New York Times *(November 3, 2001). Available online at http://www.nytimes.com/2001/11/03/opinion/what-if-cipro-stopped-working.html.*

INTRODUCTION: *In the following op-ed column published by the* New York Times *during the intense media coverage surrounding the 2001 anthrax attacks on the US Postal Service, the US Senate, and various media outlets, authors Ellen K. Silbergeld and Polly Walker describe the dangers of the careless use of powerful antibiotics. At the time of publication, Silbergeld was professor of epidemiology at the University of Maryland School of Medicine. Walker was associate director of the John Hopkins Center for a Livable Future.*

Cipro, despite its current fame for preventing and treating anthrax, is in danger of becoming a casualty of what might be called the post-antibiotic age. Bayer, the maker of Cipro, also sells a chemically similar drug called Baytril, which is used in large-scale poultry production worldwide. The widespread use of Baytril in chickens has already been shown to decrease Cipro's effectiveness in humans for some types of infections.

Bayer recommends that Baytril be used only to treat infected poultry and says it poses no threat to public health. But the use of antibiotics in agriculture is part of a serious public health problem in the United States. According to the Union of Concerned Scientists, as much as 70 percent of all antibiotics produced in the United States are fed to healthy livestock for "growth promotion," in other words, to increase their weight for market. Not only does this reduce their effectiveness in animals; it poses a real danger to humans.

The discovery and use of antibiotics to treat human disease and save lives is one of the greatest feats of modern medicine. Many of us are alive today because of antibiotics. Just 60 years ago, the discovery of antibiotics revolutionized medicine, tipping the balance in our favor against the sea of pathogens that surrounds us. Now, with the very real threat of biological terrorism, preserving the power of antibiotics is a matter of the highest urgency.

Bacteria have always adapted to our new drugs faster and more efficiently than we can adapt to their genetic changes. Through prudent use, we can preserve the effectiveness of our drugs for use in treating human disease while we search nature and chemistry for new defenses. Yet we are now squandering this precious resource by using powerful antibiotics carelessly for livestock and poultry —mostly for nontherapeutic reasons.

Agribusiness argues that nontherapeutic use of antibiotics is essential to the continued supply of cheap food. But many countries have demonstrated that food can be safely and efficiently produced without robbing the medicine chest. In the European Union, the nontherapeutic use of antibiotics in agriculture has been banned.

The use of antibiotics in food animal production increases the risks of contracting drug-resistant infections from eating animal products. Despite a national network for testing food, every year the Centers for Disease Control and Prevention reports incidents of food poisoning by drug-resistant bacteria. In addition, using antibiotics in agriculture can result in environmental pollution by both drugs and drug-resistant bacteria.

Last month, the New England Journal of Medicine reported that drug-resistant bacteria were present in meat purchased at supermarkets in the Washington, D.C., area. An accompanying editorial recommended that the use of nontherapeutic antibiotics in farm animals be prohibited.

We need better information and more government oversight in this arena. Opinions differ on the amount of antibiotics currently used in animal production. Creating a national tracking system to measure how much of each antibiotic is used and for what purposes—as proposed by the Food and Drug Administration—is a necessary first step. Mandatory reporting of antibiotic use was discussed in January at meetings sponsored by the F.D.A., but no actual legislation or regulations have been proposed.

For Bayer, the maker of Baytril, the need for action is clear. The use of Baytril falls into a gray area between growth promotion and treatment; it is common practice in the poultry industry to add Baytril to drinking water during the last weeks of a flock's life, even if no disease has been diagnosed. Last year, the F.D.A. asked Bayer and Abbott Laboratories, the two producers of the chicken drug, to withdraw their Cipro-like antibiotics from agricultural use voluntarily. Abbott agreed. Bayer did not.

Bayer has committed itself to supporting our national efforts to protect the public health by supplying Cipro at a reduced cost to the federal government. Voluntarily withdrawing Baytril from the market would show that the company is serious about its commitment to the public health.

SEE ALSO *Antibacterial Drugs; MRSA*

BIBLIOGRAPHY

Books

Mirete, Salvador, and Marcos López Pérez, eds. *Antibiotic Resistance Genes in Natural Environments and Long-Term Effects.* New York: Nova Biomedical, 2017.

Salyers, Abigail A., and Dixie D. Whitt. *Revenge of the Microbes: How Bacterial Resistance Is Undermining the Antibiotic Miracle.* Washington, DC: ASM, 2005.

Walsh, Christopher, and Timothy Wencewicz. *Antibiotics: Challenges, Mechanisms, Opportunities.* Washington, DC: ASM, 2016.

Wiles, Siouxsie. *Antibiotic Resistance: The End of Modern Medicine?* Wellington, New Zealand: BWB, 2017.

Periodicals

Emanuel, Ezekiel J. "How to Develop New Antibiotics." *New York Times* (February 24, 2015). This article can also be found online at https://www.nytimes.com/2015/02/24/opinion/how-to-develop-new-antibiotics.html (accessed November 14, 2017).

Limbago, Brandi M., et al. "Report of the 13th Vancomycine-Resistant *Staphylococcus aureus* Isolate from the United States." *Journal of Clinical Microbiology* 52, no. 3 (March 2014): 998–1002.

Lin, Derek M., Britt Koskella, and Henry C. Lin. "Phage Therapy: An Alternative to Antibiotics in the Age of Multi-drug Resistance." *World Journal of Gastrointestinal and Pharmacology and Therapeutics* 8, no. 3 (August 2017): 162–173.

Websites

"Antibiotic Resistance." World Health Organization. http://www.who.int/mediacentre/factsheets/antibiotic-resistance/en (accessed November 15, 2017).

"General Background: About Antibiotic Resistance." Alliance for the Prudent Use of Antibiotics. http://emerald.tufts.edu/med/apua/about_issue/about_antibioticres.shtml (accessed November 15, 2017).

Brian Hoyle

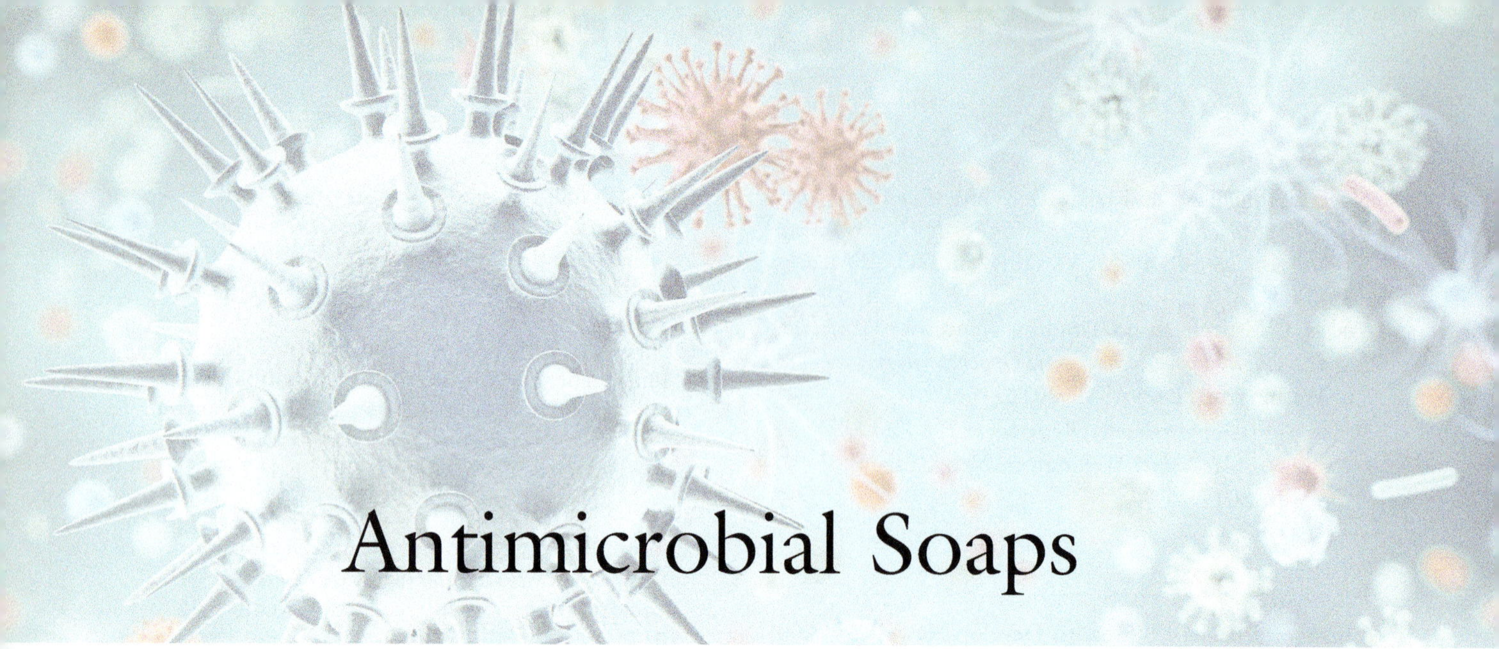

Antimicrobial Soaps

Introduction

Antimicrobial soaps refer to solutions that are designed to lessen the number of living (viable) microorganisms on the surface of the skin. As they are usually rubbed on the skin during handwashing, the most common form of the antimicrobial product is soap. The main target of antimicrobial soaps are the bacteria that commonly live on, or colonize, the surface of the skin. These include bacteria in the genera of *Staphylococcus* and *Streptococcus*. Normally, these bacteria do not cause harm to the host. However, if they gain access to sites inside the body due to a cut or another injury, they can cause serious and even life-threatening diseases. An example is the contamination of implanted heart valves by *Staphylococcus aureus*, which can cause an infection called *endocarditis*. By handwashing with an antimicrobial soap for an adequate length of time (at least one minute) to lessen the number of living *S. aureus* on the skin prior to heart valve surgery, a surgeon can diminish the risk of infecting the patient.

Antimicrobial soaps play an important role in medical settings, and over time they have also become popular for home use. Research has shown, however, that there is no evidence that the antimicrobial compounds most commonly used in soaps are more effective than proper handwashing using just water and soaps that do not include antimicrobial compounds. Moreover, because of fears regarding the development of antibiotic-resistant germs and unanswered questions about the long-term safety of popular antimicrobial compounds such as triclosan (used primarily in liquid soaps) and triclocarban (used primarily in bar soaps), these substances were banned by the US Food and Drug Administration (FDA) in 2016. As of 2017 similar bans were also in place in Europe.

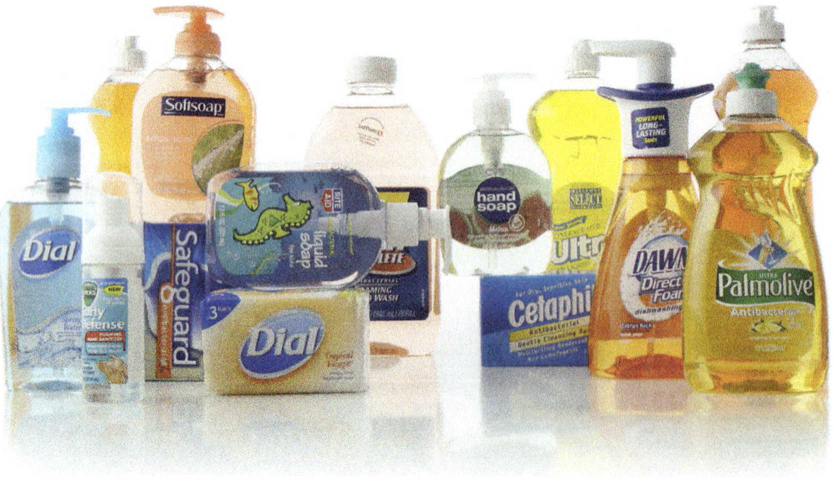

Antibacterial soaps have become common in American homes. In 2016 the US Food and Drug Administration banned the sale of household soaps containing triclosan effective September 2017. © *Julia Ewan/ The Washington Post/Getty Images*

History and Scientific Foundations

The use of antibacterial soap began in the mid-19th century. At that time Viennese physician Ignaz Semmelweiss (1818–1865) noted the markedly higher death rate among hospitalized patients who received care from medical students versus patients cared for by midwives. Semmelweiss determined that it was a common practice for the students to come from dissection and teaching labs to the hospital ward without washing their hands. By instituting a handwashing policy, the high death rate was almost completely eliminated.

With time came the knowledge that bacteria and other disease-causing microorganisms such as fungi could be transferred from person to person on the skin of the caregiver. The use of antimicrobial compounds in soaps gained credence in the several decades following World War II (1939–1945) with the expanded use of antibiotics to treat bacterial diseases. The initial overwhelming success of antibiotics made the incorporation of antimicrobials into other products a health priority.

For many years the principle ingredient most commonly used in antimicrobial soaps was triclosan. The compound contains a phenol ring structure to which chlorine groups are attached. The phenol ring is difficult to break apart, which means that bacteria and fungi are less capable of degrading the triclosan molecule to a form that is inactive. In addition, chlorine has a potent antibacterial and antifungal effect. Triclocarban is another antimicrobial compound once commonly used in soaps. Like triclosan, triclocarban has ring structures and chlorine groups, and its antimicrobial activity is similar to that of triclosan. At the height of its popularity, triclosan was the active ingredient in an estimated 75 percent of antibacterial liquid soaps marketed for home use.

In the early 21st century, researchers began to question the long-term safety and effectiveness of triclosan, triclocarban, and other similar compounds. In 2013, in response to this research, the FDA issued a ruling requiring manufacturers of antimicrobial soaps to provide evidence that their products were more effective than plain soap and water at reducing the chances of infection. Following this action many manufacturers began to phase out the use of triclosan and triclocarban. Absent the submission of the requested evidence from manufacturers, the FDA banned these compounds for use in antibacterial soaps in the United States in 2016.

The European Union also banned the use of triclosan in disinfectants and algaecides products, as well as some types of preservatives. Other countries, including Canada, Australia, and Japan, have not as of 2017.

Applications and Research

Antibacterial soaps are a standard feature of hospitals and other health care facilities, where the need to control the spread of infections is essential. For example, the use of antibacterial soap or other types of skin wash is important in controlling the spread of a type of bacteria designated methicillin-resistant *Staphylococcus aureus* (MRSA) from ward to ward in hospitals. This is because MRSA is resistant to many antibiotics and so can be difficult to treat once present in a hospital. A patient whose immune system is not functioning efficiently can become extremely ill or can die if infected with MRSA.

WORDS TO KNOW

COLONIZATION The process of occupation and increase in number of microorganisms at a specific site.

RESISTANT ORGANISM An organism that has developed the ability to counter something trying to harm it. Within infectious diseases, the organism, such as a bacterium, has developed a resistance to drugs, such as antibiotics.

TRICLOSAN A chemical that kills bacteria.

Impacts and Issues

While antimicrobial soaps initially were effective in controlling the spread of infectious diseases, their overuse or misuse may have promoted the development of bacteria that were resistant to triclosan. Studies with *Escherichia coli* indicated that the genetic alterations that rendered the bacteria resistant to triclosan might have also conferred resistance to other antibacterial compounds, including some antibiotics. In other words, the use of antimicrobial soaps may have driven the bacteria to become more resistant and, therefore, a greater threat to health.

An important reason was the expansion in the use of triclosan-containing soaps in the home. Consumers became more conscious of the possible health threat of microorganisms, and the marketplace responded by formulating products designed for everyday use. Unfortunately, if a microorganism was exposed to a concentration of triclosan that was not enough to kill it or not exposed to the compound long enough due to inadequate washing (the soap needed to be present on the skin for 30 to 45 seconds), the microbe may have survived and become more resistant to the antimicrobial agent. If this resistance was acquired because of a genetic alteration, the trait could be passed to future generations of microorganisms.

Triclosan is capable of blocking the manufacture of fatty acids, molecules vital to the construction of membranes. The altered membrane can make some bacteria resistant to antibiotics that formerly killed them. Studies in the late 20th and early 21st centuries have provided solid evidence that bacteria that become resistant to triclosan were often resistant to other drugs.

The expanded and less controlled use of antimicrobial soaps also became a concern in light of a study published in 2006 that demonstrated how low doses of triclosan in the environment from domestic wastes caused hormonal alterations in the North American bullfrog. This indicated that there may have been detrimental changes associated with the discharge of low levels of antimicrobial soaps into the environment. According to a study by Rolf U. Halden published in *Environmental Science and Technology*, an estimated 375,000 to 2.1 million pounds (170,000 to 970,000 kilograms) of triclosan was discharged from wastewater treatment plants in the United States in 2014.

In September 2016 the FDA announced a ban on the sale of household soaps that contain 19 different antimicrobial ingredients, including triclosan and triclocarban. The decision took effect on September 17, 2017. The ban did not apply to all products, however. Triclosan has been eliminated from soap products sold in the United States, but one brand of toothpaste containing triclosan (Colgate Total) has been determined by the FDA to be safe and is exempt from the ban. Hand sanitizers that are used without water are not subject to the ban. The FDA deferred making a decision on three other antimicrobial compounds —benzalkonium chloride, benzethonium chloride, and chloroxylenol (PCMX)—until more data could be collected. It advocates the use of proper handwashing techniques, using plain soap and water, for home use. Antimicrobial soaps remain approved for use in hospitals, nursing homes, and other medical settings.

PRIMARY SOURCE

FDA Issues Final Rule on Safety and Effectiveness of Antibacterial Soaps

SOURCE: *"FDA Issues Final Rule on Safety and Effectiveness of Antibacterial Soaps." US Food and Drug Administration, September 2, 2016. https://www.fda.gov/newsevents/newsroom/pressannouncements/ucm517478.htm (accessed November 27, 2017).*

INTRODUCTION: *In the following press release, the US Food and Drug Administration (FDA) explains the ban on triclosan and triclocarban in hand and body washes intended for consumer use.*

The U.S. Food and Drug Administration today issued a final rule establishing that over-the-counter (OTC) consumer antiseptic wash products containing certain active ingredients can no longer be marketed. Companies will no longer be able to market antibacterial washes with these ingredients because manufacturers did not demonstrate that the ingredients are both safe for long-term daily use and more effective than plain soap and water in preventing illness and the spread of certain infections. Some manufacturers have already started removing these ingredients from their products.

This final rule applies to consumer antiseptic wash products containing one or more of 19 specific active ingredients, including the most commonly used ingredients — triclosan and triclocarban. These products are intended for use with water, and are rinsed off after use. This rule does not affect consumer hand "sanitizers" or wipes, or antibacterial products used in health care settings.

"Consumers may think antibacterial washes are more effective at preventing the spread of germs, but we have no scientific evidence that they are any better than plain soap and water," said Janet Woodcock, M.D., director of the FDA's Center for Drug Evaluation and Research (CDER). "In fact, some data suggests that antibacterial ingredients may do more harm than good over the long-term."

The agency issued a proposed rule in 2013 after some data suggested that long-term exposure to certain active ingredients used in antibacterial products — for example, triclosan (liquid soaps) and triclocarban (bar soaps) — could pose health risks, such as bacterial resistance or hormonal effects. Under the proposed rule, manufacturers were required to provide the agency with additional data on the safety and effectiveness of certain ingredients used in over-the-counter consumer antibacterial washes if they wanted to continue marketing antibacterial products containing those ingredients. This included data from clinical studies demonstrating that these products were superior to non-antibacterial washes in preventing human illness or reducing infection.

Antibacterial hand and body wash manufacturers did not provide the necessary data to establish safety and effectiveness for the 19 active ingredients addressed in this final rulemaking. For these ingredients, either no additional data were submitted or the data and information that were submitted were not sufficient for the agency to find that these ingredients are Generally Recognized as Safe and Effective (GRAS/GRAE). In response to comments submitted by industry, the FDA has deferred rulemaking for one year on three additional ingredients used in consumer wash products — benzalkonium chloride, benzethonium chloride, and chloroxylenol (PCMX) — to allow for the development and submission of new safety and effectiveness data for these ingredients. Consumer antibacterial washes containing these specific ingredients may be marketed during this time while data are being collected.

Washing with plain soap and running water remains one of the most important steps consumers can take to avoid getting sick and to prevent spreading germs to others.

If soap and water are not available and a consumer uses hand sanitizer instead, the U.S. Centers for Disease Control and Prevention (CDC) recommends that it be an alcohol-based hand sanitizer that contains at least 60 percent alcohol.

Since the FDA's proposed rulemaking in 2013, manufacturers already started phasing out the use of certain active ingredients in antibacterial washes, including triclosan and triclocarban. Manufacturers will have one year to comply with the rulemaking by removing products from the market or reformulating (removing antibacterial active ingredients) these products.

The FDA, an agency within the U.S. Department of Health and Human Services, protects the public health by helping to ensure the safety, effectiveness, and security of human and veterinary drugs, vaccines and other biological products for human use, and medical devices. The agency also is responsible for helping to ensure the safety and security of our nation's food supply, cosmetics, dietary supplements, and products that give off electronic radiation, and for regulating tobacco products.

SEE ALSO *Disinfection; Germ Theory of Disease; Handwashing; Resistant Organisms*

BIBLIOGRAPHY

Books

Bankston, John. *Joseph Lister and the Story of Antiseptics.* Hockessin, DE: Mitchell Lane, 2005.

McDonnell, Gerald E. *Antisepsis, Disinfection, and Sterilization.* 2nd ed. Washington, DC: ASM, 2017.

Periodicals

Carey, Daniel E., and Patrick J. McNamara. "The Impact of Triclosan on the Spread of Antibiotic Resistance in the Environment." *Frontiers in Microbiology* (January 15, 2015). This article can also be found online at https://www.frontiersin.org/articles/10.3389/fmicb.2014.00780/full (accessed November 16, 2017).

Halden, Rol U. "On the Need and Speed of Regulating Triclosan and Tricarban in the United States." *Environmental Science and Technology* 48, no. 7 (April 2014): 3603–3611. This article can also be found online at https://www.ncbi.nlm.nih.gov/pmc/articles/PMC3974611/ (accessed November 27, 2017).

Webber Mark A., et al. "Quinolone-Resistant Gyrase Mutants Demonstrate Decreased Susceptibility to Triclosan." *Journal of Antimicrobial Chemotherapy* 72, no. 10 (October 2017): 2755–2763.

Websites

"5 Things to Know About Triclosan." Food and Drug Administration (FDA). https://www.fda.gov/ForConsumers/ConsumerUpdates/ucm205999.htm (accessed November 17, 2017).

Hartmann, Erica. "Banned Antimicrobial Chemicals Found in Many Household Products." CNN. January 25, 2017. http://www.cnn.com/2017/01/25/health/triclosan-household-items-partner/index.html (accessed November 17, 2017).

Tetro, Jason. "This Natural Chemical May Replace Triclosan and Improve Oral Health. Huffington Post, May 25, 2015. http://www.huffingtonpost.ca/jason-tetro/triclosan-oral-health_b_7421152.html (accessed November 27, 2017).

Brian Hoyle

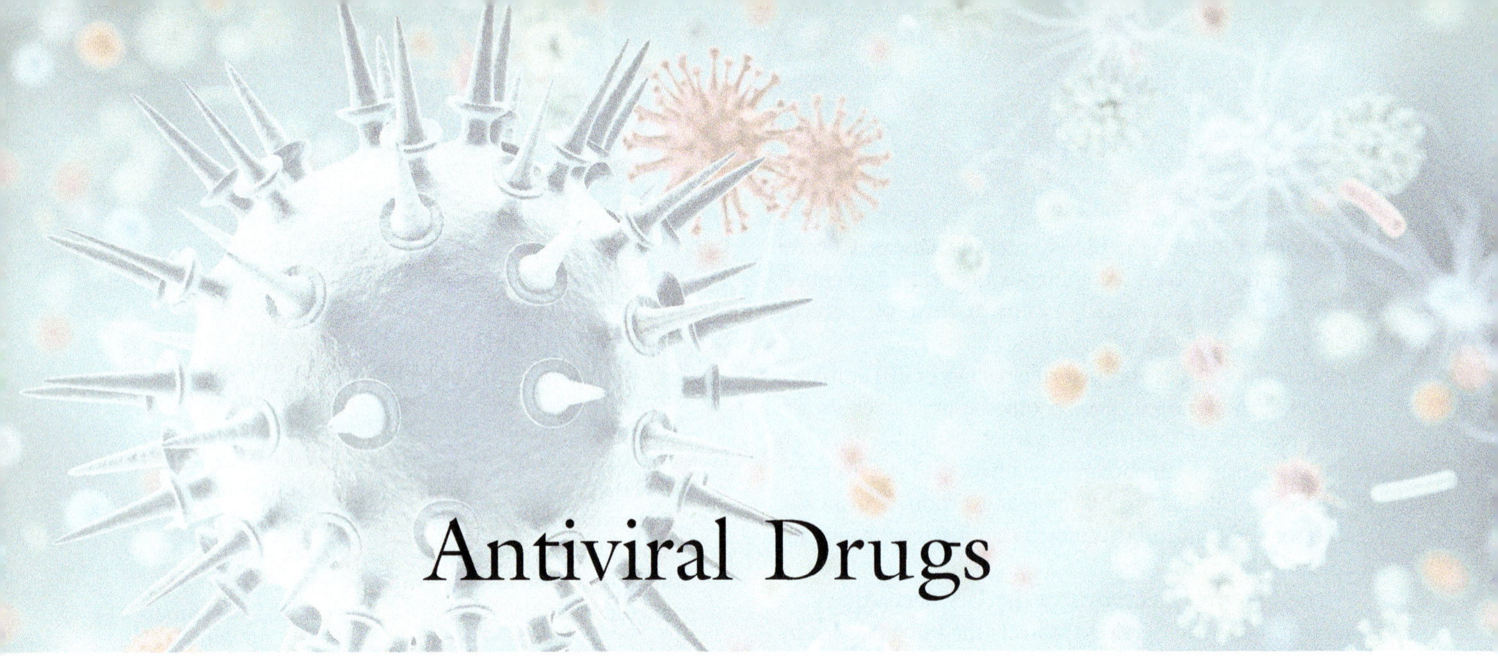

Antiviral Drugs

Introduction

Antiviral drugs are used to prevent or treat viral infections. They are antimicrobial compounds, as are antibiotics. However, antiviral compounds do not have the same mode of action as antibiotics. This is because most antibiotics rely on the ability of the bacteria to grow and divide. Bacteria grow and divide independently. In contrast, viruses must infect a host cell before they can exploit the host cell's genetic machinery to manufacture the components of new virus particles. Antibiotics are useless against viruses, both because viruses are localized inside of another cell or tissue and viruses are not alive in the absence of the host cell.

Antibiotics and antiviral drugs are similar in that specific drugs are designed for specific targets. For example, antiretroviral drugs specifically inhibit infections caused by retroviruses, such as the human immunodeficiency virus (HIV). Other antiviral drugs specifically target other viruses, including herpes viruses and the various hepatitis viruses.

Hepatitis C virus (HCV) provides a good example. The development of direct-acting antivirals (DAAs) has been a boon to the treatment of HCV. DAAs target specific steps in the HCV cycle from infection of a host cell to the manufacture of new virus particles. There are four classes of DAA, and each class focuses on an enzyme that is vital in the HCV cycle. By blocking the function of the enzymes, virus manufacture is halted.

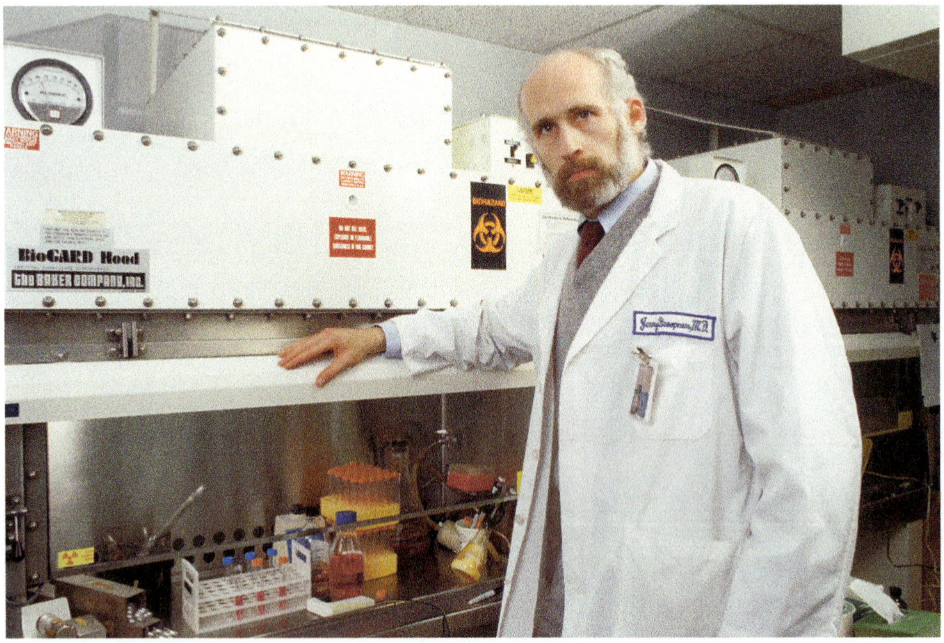

Jerome Groopman is photographed in his lab. Dr. Groopman is a pioneer in the development of AIDS therapies, including the antiviral drug AZT. *© Ira Wyman/Sygma/Getty Images*

WORDS TO KNOW

ANTIBODIES Also called Y-shaped immunoglobulins, proteins found in the blood that help to fight against foreign substances called antigens. Antigens, which are usually proteins or polysaccharides, stimulate the immune system to produce antibodies. The antibodies inactivate the antigen and help to remove it from the body. While antigens can be the source of infections from pathogenic bacteria and viruses, organic molecules detrimental to the body from internal or environmental sources also act as antigens. Genetic engineering and the use of various mutational mechanisms allow the construction of a vast array of antibodies (each with a unique genetic sequence).

ENZYME Molecules that act as critical catalysts in biological systems. Catalysts are substances that increase the rate of chemical reactions without being consumed in the reaction. Without enzymes, many reactions would require higher levels of energy and higher temperatures than exist in biological systems. Enzymes are proteins that possess specific binding sites for other molecules (substrates). A series of weak binding interactions allow enzymes to accelerate reaction rates. Enzyme kinetics is the study of enzymatic reactions and mechanisms. Enzyme inhibitor studies have allowed researchers to develop therapies for the treatment of diseases, including AIDS.

MESSENGER RIBONUCLEIC ACID (MRNA) A molecule of RNA that carries the genetic information for producing one or more proteins; mRNA is produced by copying one strand of DNA, but in eukaryotes it is able to move from the nucleus to the cytoplasm (where protein synthesis takes place).

REPLICATION A process of reproducing, duplicating, copying, or repeating something, such as the duplication of DNA or the recreation of characteristics of an infectious disease in a laboratory setting.

RESISTANCE Immunity developed within a species (especially bacteria) via evolution to an antibiotic or other drug. For example, in bacteria, the acquisition of genetic mutations that render the bacteria invulnerable to the action of antibiotics.

STRAIN A subclass or a specific genetic variation of an organism.

Other antiviral drugs that are used for HCV include interferons (naturally occurring proteins that are produced in response to infection), ribavirin, inhibitors of various enzymes, and molecules that mimic the shape of components of deoxyribonucleic acid (DNA). The latter incorporate into the viral DNA and stop its transcription.

History and Scientific Foundations

The history of antiviral compounds dates back only to the 1960s. Prior to that time, a viral illness had to run its course. In the 1960s antiviral drugs were developed to deal with herpes infections (which include cold sores, genital infection, chickenpox, mononucleosis, and Kaposi's sarcoma). At that time the development of the drugs was more of a trial-and-error process than a directed process. It typically involved growing cultures of a particular type of cell and then infecting the cells with a particular virus. Successful infection is often apparent by a change in the appearance of the host cell. By adding compounds during the infection, researchers could monitor whether the visible signs of infection occurred or not. The absence of changes in the host cells was an indication that the particular compound was a potential antiviral agent.

This process was tedious and time-consuming. Beginning in the 1970s, advances in molecular biology made antiviral drug design more focused. The genetic sequences of disease-causing viruses began to be determined. In addition, researchers discovered that many viruses initiated infection by recognizing and binding to sites on the surface of host cells. As the three-dimensional shapes of these host sites and the molecular details of the binding of the virus were clarified, it became possible to design compounds to block the binding.

The binding of a virus particle to a host cell can be blocked in two ways. In one approach, the target site on the host surface is occupied by an added molecule. Because the site is occupied, the virus is unable to bind to it. In the second approach, the viral recognition site is blocked by the addition of a molecule. The blocking molecule may be an antibody—a protein that is produced by the immune system—that has been manufactured in the laboratory. Then virus particles cannot gain access to the host cell; they are stranded outside the host cells and can be destroyed when they are recognized by the hosts' immune system, which causes antiviral immune molecules to be made and deployed.

This strategy of blocking viral infection early in the infectious process is the basis of some viral vaccines. It can be successful if the host or viral target sites do not change. However, in viral infections such as influenza, the viral site can change from year to year. A vaccine designed for the viral strain that dominates one year may be ineffective the next year, which is why new influenza vaccines need to be produced and administered prior to each flu season.

Some antiviral drugs operate slightly differently, by blocking the uptake of virus into the host cell. Other antiviral drugs prevent the infecting virus from using the host cell's genetic replication (duplication) mechanisms. The numbers of infecting viruses are not reduced, but, because the infection process is blocked, new viruses are not made. Once again, the host's immune system can more easily deal with the stranded viruses.

Two antiviral drugs, idoxuridine and trifluridine, halt viral infection at the genetic level. These drugs act by replacing one of the units (a compound called thymidine) that forms the genetic material. The drugs are able to do this because their structure is similar to the structure of thymidine. The incorporation of either drug produces DNA that does not function. Other drugs mimic other compounds, and their incorporation produces the same result. However, the drugs can also be incorporated into the DNA of the host cells, which disrupts their function. This action can cause side effects, but, if the infection is stopped, it can be worthwhile in the longer term.

Other antiviral drugs, such as acyclovir, target an enzyme produced by the virus, usually early in the infection, that is vital for the replication of the genetic material. The drug binds to the enzyme, which prevents the enzyme from binding to its normal target. As a result, DNA formation stops. Acyclovir is used to treat infections due to herpes simplex viruses and Epstein-Barr virus.

Zidovudine (AZT) acts against HIV by blocking the activity of the reverse transcriptase enzyme. This enzyme makes it possible for the infecting virus to convert its ribonucleic acid (RNA) to DNA, and this DNA is subsequently used by the host cell's replication machinery to produce new viral constituents. The compound can become incorporated into the host cell DNA, which also blocks the replication of viral genetic material. AZT is beneficial in reducing the transmission of HIV from a pregnant woman to her developing fetus and to her newborn during labor or breastfeeding.

Still other antiviral drugs focus on translation—the process whereby the messenger ribonucleic acid (mRNA), which is formed from instructions encoded in DNA, is used to manufacture compounds, such as protein. Some antiviral drugs block mRNA formation and disrupt the translation process. Antiviral therapy also involves molecular tools. The best example is oligonucleotides, which are sequences of the building blocks of genetic material that are deliberately made to be complementary to a target sequence of viral genetic material. The term *complementary* means that the two sequences are able to chemically associate with one another. When the oligonucleotide binds to a stretch of viral genetic material, it prevents that stretch from being used in viral replication. One oligonucleotide-based drug is available for the treatment of eye infections in patients with AIDS.

■ Applications and Research

The different mechanisms of action of different antiviral drugs have been useful in treating a variety of viral infections. For example, acyclovir, which was the first successful antiviral drug developed, is used to treat infections caused by herpes viruses, which include lesions on the genitals, in the mouth, and even in the brain, as well as treating chickenpox and shingles. The antiviral drug ganciclovir has been useful in the treatment of cytomegalovirus-mediated eye infections.

A well-known type of antiviral drug acts against retroviruses, in particular human HIV, the virus that causes AIDS. Most of the antiretroviral drugs that have been developed have focused on combating HIV. The antiviral drug combination known as highly active antiretroviral therapy (HAART) is targeted at blocking the use of the HIV RNA to manufacture DNA (which is then used to make the viral components); blocking the integration of viral genetic material into the host genome; and blocking adhesion of the virus to host cells. This multipronged approach, which was introduced in 1996, can delay the progression of AIDS and, as of 2017, was an important part of treatment for HIV-infected people. It has changed what was once a fatal infection to an infection that, while not cured, can be managed.

Research is progressing on antiviral drugs to block enzymes that cut DNA or RNA or proteins. These enzymes are important in the viral manufacturing process, so their disruption can stop viral replication. Researchers are also exploring ways to block the release of an assembled virus from the host cell. If release can be blocked, new host cells cannot be infected and the infection stops.

Another avenue of research is examining drugs that are used for other purposes to see if they might be effective antiviral drugs. One example is spironolactone, which is used to treat heart failure. A study published in 2016 demonstrated the effectiveness of spironolactone against Epstein-Barr virus.

■ Impacts and Issues

Antiviral drugs are invaluable in the treatment of viral diseases. Millions of people infected with HIV or suffering from the symptoms of AIDS use them. The US National Institutes of Health recommends HAART even if symptoms are absent. HAART is expensive, however. In 2017 the cost of care for an individual receiving HAART therapy in the United States was estimated at $10,000 to $12,000 per year. In the regions that are most affected by AIDS, such as sub-Saharan

Africa, HAART is far less available. Economics and political resistance have affected those most in need of help. Organizations such as the International Center for Research on Women have worked to introduce HAART more widely in Africa and to encourage its use. A 2016 study from South Africa, which has only recently allowed the use of the therapy, reported encouraging results in delaying the development of Kaposi's sarcoma, particularly in women.

Researchers have argued that widespread availability and use of antiretroviral drugs could make AIDS in Africa a treatable (although still chronic) disease, similar to the situation in Europe, Australia, and North America. According to 2017 data from UNAIDS, 19.4 million people in eastern and southern Africa were living with HIV in 2016. Encouragingly, that year 61 percent of HIV-infected adults and 51 percent of HIV-infected children in eastern and southern Africa were receiving antiretroviral treatment. This good news is tempered by the reality that, as of 2017, the prevalence of HIV in adults is 1.2 percent worldwide but 9.0 percent in sub-Saharan Africa. Adolescent girls and women aged 15 to 24 have rates of HIV infection up to eight times higher than males of the same age.

Side effects of antiviral drugs continue to be an issue. For example, Tamiflu®, which is used to combat viral influenza and is approved in the United States for individuals one year and older, has recognized side effects. Most are uncommon and are usually minor, such as nausea, vomiting, and diarrhea. Rare but severe side effects include abnormal functioning of the heart and liver, stomach or intestinal bleeding, seizures, and hallucinations.

See Also *Developing Nations and Drug Delivery; Pandemic Preparedness*

BIBLIOGRAPHY

Books

Sherman, Irwin W. *Drugs That Changed the World: How Therapeutic Agents Shaped Our Lives.* Boca Raton, FL: CRC, 2017.

Watson, Ronald. *Health of HIV Infected People: Food, Nutrition and Lifestyle with Antiretroviral Drugs.* Boston: Elsevier, 2015.

Periodicals

Kharsany, Ayesha B.M., and Quarraisha A. Karim. "HIV Infection and AIDS in Sub-Saharan Africa: Current Status, Challenges and Opportunities." *Open AIDS Journal* 10 (2016): 34–48.

Naidoo, Levashni, et al. "HAART in Hand: The Change in Kaposi's Sarcoma Presentation in KwaZulu-Natal, South Africa." *South African Medical Journal* 106, no. 6 (2016): 611–616.

Sullivan, Con, et al. "Using Zebrafish Models of Human Influenza A Virus Infections to Screen Antiviral Drugs and Characterize Host Immune Cell Responses." *Journal of Visualized Experiments* 119 (2017): e55235.

Verma, Dinesh, Jacob Thompson, and Sankar Swaminathan. "Spironolactone Blocks Epstein-Barr Virus Production by Inhibiting EBV SM Protein Function." *Proceedings of the National Academy of Sciences* 113 (2016): 3609–3614. This article can also be found online at http://www.pnas.org/content/113/13/3609.full.pdf (accessed November 16, 2017).

Websites

"HIV and AIDS in East and Southern Africa Regional Overview." Avert. https://www.avert.org/professionals/hiv-around-world/sub-saharan-africa/overview (accessed November 14, 2017).

Pockros, Paul J. "Direct-Acting Antivirals for the Treatment of Hepatitis C Virus Infection." UpToDate. https://www.uptodate.com/contents/direct-acting-antivirals-for-the-treatment-of-hepatitis-c-virus-infection (accessed November 16, 2017).

Brian Hoyle

Arthropod-Borne Disease

Introduction

Arthropods are members of the invertebrate phylum Arthropoda, which includes insects, arachnids, myriapods, and crustaceans. Arthropod-borne diseases are infections that are transmitted by arthropods, primarily mosquitos and ticks, but also fleas, lice, and flies. These arthropods transmit various pathogens (disease-causing microorganisms), including bacteria, viruses, helminths (parasitic worms), and protozoa, that result in diseases in humans, including malaria, yellow fever, Chagas disease, leishmaniasis, lymphatic filariasis, dengue, California encephalitis, chikungunya, Eastern equine encephalitis, Powassan encephalitis, St. Louis encephalitis, West Nile, Lyme disease, onchocerciasis, and Zika. These and other arthropod-borne diseases can result in a wide range of effects, from mild flu-like symptoms to death. Some survivors of arthropod-borne diseases can suffer chronic, crippling aftereffects.

While arthropod-borne diseases are a major concern worldwide, developing countries are the most affected. These diseases tend to occur primarily in tropical countries—the endemic zones of the pathogens and the arthropods that harbor them. However, these diseases can also spread when people travel between infected and noninfected areas or when infected arthropods are inadvertently transported. Natural disasters, wars, poverty, and overpopulation can facilitate outbreaks of disease, as they may create conditions

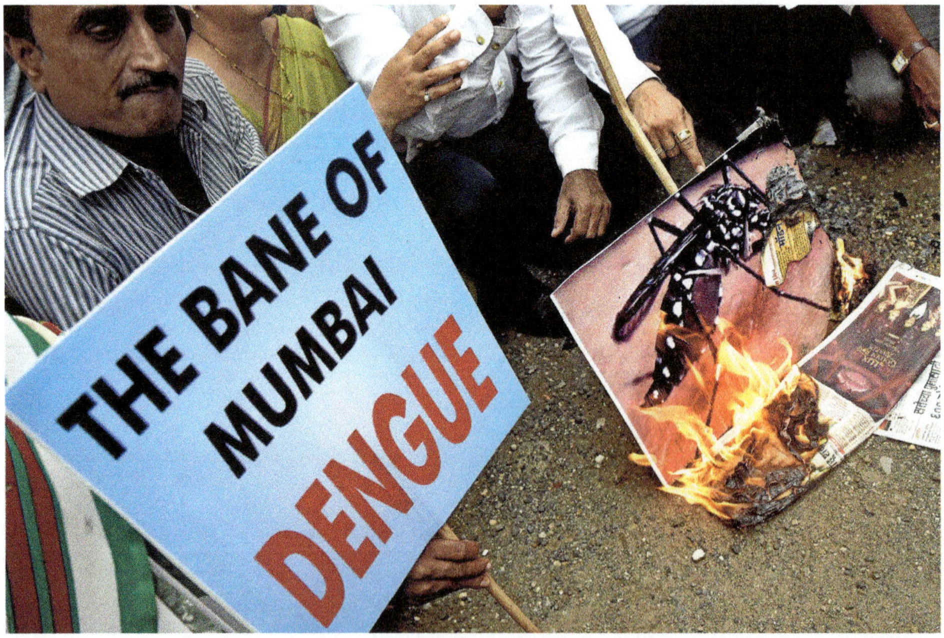

Arthropod-borne diseases occur worldwide, but they are most widespread in tropical and developing countries. In Mumbai, India, around 700 confirmed cases of dengue fever were reported in 2017. Outbreaks of dengue following summer rains are common in the sprawling city of more than 18 million.
© Arijit Sen/Hindustan Times/Getty Images

that are ideal for transmission or may cause a breakdown in the health care and public health systems.

Disease History, Characteristics, and Transmission

Humans contract arthropod-borne diseases when a pathogen, such as a bacterium or virus, is transmitted from its reservoir (natural host) to a human via an infected arthropod vector (disease carrier). Transmission from arthropod to human occurs either mechanically or biologically. In mechanical transmission the arthropod deposits the pathogens onto a surface from which a host either absorbs or ingests them. For example, a housefly may deposit bacteria onto food that is then eaten by a human. In biological transmission the arthropod injects the pathogens directly into the body of the host, as when a mosquito bites a human and transmits malaria or dengue.

The effects of arthropod-borne disease range from mild to severe. Arthropod-borne diseases, such as encephalitis and malaria, are characterized by headaches, fevers, weakness, and anemia. Some diseases can be fatal if they are not treated in a timely manner, and others, while not fatal, may have chronic effects that decrease quality of life.

Arthropod-borne diseases have shaped the course of history. From 1343 to 1351, several forms of plague caused by the bacterium *Yersinia pestis* were likely carried to humans by fleas on black rats. The event, which became known as the black plague or Black Death, killed over two-thirds of the population of urban areas in Asia, one-third of the population of the Middle East, and between one-third and two-thirds of the population of Europe. Epidemic plague largely disappeared in Europe just before the turn of the 19th century, well before the development of antibiotics, but isolated outbreaks of plague still occur. For example, in 2017 a plague outbreak in Madagascar killed 200 people. Scientists debate the reasons for the disappearance of plague, but many point to increased sanitation and the possibility that *Yersinia pestis*-carrying fleas diminished as brown rat populations replaced black rats in Europe.

Until the mid-20th century, arthropod-borne diseases were an endemic health problem. American cities battled outbreaks of mosquito-borne yellow fever. Yellow fever, along with malaria, a disease caused by a *Plasmodium* protozoan also transmitted by mosquitoes, stopped French construction of a canal through Panama during the 1880s when it claimed the lives of more than 20,000 workers. The same diseases claimed an additional 5,000 lives when the United States completed the Panama Canal project two decades later. In the latter half of the 20th century, efforts were focused on prevention and control programs for the arthropod vectors. The programs focused on elimination of arthropod sites as well as restricting the use of chemical insecticides. These programs were largely a success, to the extent that yellow fever, dengue, and most arthropod-borne diseases were no longer major health problems in most parts of the world.

WORDS TO KNOW

ARTHROPOD A member of the largest single animal phylum, consisting of organisms with segmented bodies, jointed legs or wings, and exoskeletons.

ENCEPHALITIS A type of acute brain inflammation, most often due to infection by a virus.

INACTIVATED VACCINE A vaccine that is made from disease-causing microorganisms that have been killed or made incapable of causing the infection. The immune system can still respond to the presence of the microorganisms.

LIVE VACCINE A vaccine that uses a virus or bacterium that has been weakened (attenuated) to cause an immune response in the body without causing disease. Live vaccines are preferred to killed vaccines, which use a dead virus or bacterium, because they cause a stronger and longer-lasting immune response.

PATHOGEN A disease-causing agent, such as a bacterium, a virus, a fungus, or another microorganism.

RESERVOIR The animal or organism in which a virus or parasite normally resides.

VECTOR Any agent that carries and transmits parasites and diseases. Also, an organism or a chemical used to transport a gene into a new host cell.

A global resurgence of arthropod-borne diseases has been attributed to shortcomings in public health infrastructure and rampant use of insecticides and drugs. Thus, arthropod-borne diseases remain a cause for concern with regard to global health, especially in developing countries. According to the World Health Organization (WHO), malaria remains the most widespread arthropod-borne disease in the world, affecting about 500 million people each year, with about 40 percent of the world's population being at risk. Dengue fever, a viral disease transmitted by mosquitoes, increased in prevalence during the late 20th and early 21st centuries. In 2005 it was endemic to more than 100 countries, with about 50 million cases of dengue fever occurring each year. Dengue hemorrhagic fever is a severe form of dengue that affected over 10,000 people in North and South America in 2015.

A more recent addition to the list of mosquito-transmitted diseases is Zika virus. Although the virus itself was first isolated in 1947, the first epidemic was reported 40 years later, in 2007, in Yap, an island in Micronesia. In 2013 an outbreak in French Polynesia affected about

IN CONTEXT: SOCIAL, ETHICAL, AND LEGAL ISSUES

Although remarkable efforts for developing a vaccine against Zika virus are ongoing, medical prevention of the disease was not in sight as of 2018. Amid ongoing indications that microcephaly in newborns is associated with Zika infection, women were advised to avoid pregnancy in Latin American countries that have a high prevalence of Zika virus. This has raised social, ethical, and legal concerns because, in most of the affected countries, there is neither access to affordable and acceptable contraceptive methods or laws that repeal the criminalization of abortion.

32,000 people. In 2015 infants born with microcephaly (a condition that results in an abnormally small head associated with incomplete brain development) and other congenital defects were directly linked to a Zika outbreak in Brazil. WHO has declared Zika a public health emergency.

Some arthropod-borne diseases, including lymphatic filariasis, leishmaniasis, Chagas disease, and onchocerciasis, are mostly prevalent in the tropical areas of Africa, Southeast Asia, and Central and South America.

■ Scope and Distribution

Arthropod-borne diseases occur worldwide, although they are more common in tropical regions such as the Caribbean, Central and South America, Asia, the South Pacific, and Africa. Although many regions in North America, Europe, and Australia are less affected by these diseases, cases of West Nile virus infection and Lyme disease have been consistently recorded in the United States. Some arthropod-borne diseases are endemic to a particular country or locality, while others, such as malaria, are widely spread throughout the world.

Arthropod-borne diseases can be dispersed when infected individuals travel from a locality where they contracted the disease to an area where the disease is absent or less common. In this context, studies show that modern modes of transportation may also hugely facilitate the movement of pathogens and arthropod vectors to new regions and localities. A variety of causes, from accidental transportation in food products to deliberate introduction of a species as a pest control agent, may be responsible for the transfer of an infected arthropod to an uninfected area.

■ Treatment and Prevention

The recommended treatment of an arthropod-borne disease depends on the specific disease and the severity of the infection. Treatment often involves a course of antibiotics, and, in some cases, a vaccine may be available for the specific disease. However, prevention measures are similar for all arthropod-borne diseases.

The most effective prevention method is to avoid being bitten by the arthropod vector in the first place. This can be achieved by wearing clothing that covers bare skin, using insect repellants, avoiding outdoor activities at times when the arthropods are most active, and sleeping under mosquito nets. Common breeding sites for mosquitoes include standing water, drains, and bird baths. Thus, it is important to avoid any activity that causes the formation of small water bodies during mosquito-active seasons. Strengthening arthropod vector control programs is a key initiative of WHO, which has undertaken the Global Vector Control Response 2017–2030 strategy. In addition to providing constant guidance and technical support to regions with heavy burdens of vectors, WHO recognizes the need for access to water and sanitation as important factors in controlling the disease-causing arthropods.

■ Impacts and Issues

Arthropod-borne diseases account for about 17 percent of all infectious diseases globally and cause 700,000 deaths annually. An estimated 3.9 billion people across 128 countries are at risk of contracting dengue, with 96 million affected annually. Malaria is yet another major cause for concern, and an estimated 400,000 deaths occur each year globally, with children under age five being most susceptible. In addition, according to WHO, diseases such as Chagas, yellow fever, and leishmaniasis further affect a large number of people globally.

Arthropod-borne diseases spread rapidly when humans inhabit areas with high densities. This can occur during wars, where soldiers live in close quarters. It can also occur after natural disasters when homes are destroyed and people are forced to live close together in temporary shelters. A rise in the density of the human population leads to an increase in contact between humans and arthropod vectors, causing the rate of infection to rise.

Developing countries are most affected by arthropod-borne diseases, with the burden focused in tropical and subtropical areas. This is primarily the result of poor living conditions, including lack of sanitation and the presence of stagnant water, which may be key areas to address in tropical countries. In addition, lack of access to high-quality health care in many regions limits prevention and treatment of disease, causing an increase in transmission, as well as more serious outcomes when infection does occur.

In the United States, some of the arthropod-borne diseases of major concern are Lyme disease, rickettsia, West Nile fever, malaria, dengue, and Zika virus. The resurgence of and increased vulnerability to arthropod-borne diseases in the United States is attributed to changing land use, climate change, urbanization, and transmission through infected travelers. For example, during an outbreak of dengue in southern Florida in 2009, transmission occurred via infected travelers from Caribbean islands.

Globally one of the most common methods employed to combat arthropod-borne diseases is the use of insecticides to control the insect vectors. However, the sustainability of this method is questionable due to the emergence of insecticide-resistant arthropods. An increase in urban slums, a lack of clean water, and inadequate waste management further provide breeding grounds for the arthropods. The widespread use of insecticides also can have unintended, negative environmental impacts. For example, the widely used insecticide DDT (dichlorodiphenyltrichloroethane) greatly reduced the number of malaria outbreaks in the 1950s and 1960s, but it also caused extensive reduction in bird populations and other negative effects on the natural environment. As of 2018 WHO recommended the use of DDT but encouraged its use to be limited to targeted areas infested with disease-bearing mosquitoes so as to minimize negative environmental effects.

The development of vaccines is a growing area of interest. WHO's Initiative for Vaccine Research was established to guide the development of vaccines for various diseases, and this program supports research on various arthropod-borne diseases, including dengue fever, Japanese encephalitis, malaria, and West Nile virus. In 2013 the Bill & Melinda Gates Foundation adopted Accelerate to Zero, a strategy to address and accelerate progress toward eradication of malaria in Africa and South Asia.

Ongoing research is also addressing various challenges associated with the development of Zika vaccines. The range of vaccines that were in preclinical or clinical stages for Zika virus as of 2018 included inactivated, live, deoxyribonucleic acid (DNA), protein, messenger ribonucleic acid (mRNA), and peptide vaccines.

SEE ALSO *Animal Importation; Bacterial Disease; Chagas Disease; Chikungunya; Cholera; Contact Precautions; Demographics and Infectious Disease; Dengue and Dengue Hemorrhagic Fever; Eastern Equine Encephalitis; Emerging Infectious Diseases; Host and Vector; Japanese Encephalitis; Leishmaniasis; Lyme Disease; Malaria; Microorganisms; Mosquito-Borne Diseases; Rickettsial Disease; River Blindness (Onchocerciasis); Sanitation; St. Louis Encephalitis; Travel and Infectious Disease; Tropical Infectious Diseases; Vaccines and Vaccine Development; War and Infectious Disease; West Nile; Yellow Fever*

BIBLIOGRAPHY

Books

Gubler, Duane J. "The Global Threat of Emergent/Reemergent Vector-Borne Diseases." In *Vector-Borne Diseases: Understanding the Environmental, Human Health, and Ecological Connections: Workshop Summary.* Washington, DC: National Academies Press, 2008.

Mandell, G. L., J. E. Bennett, and R. Dolin. *Principles and Practice of Infectious Diseases.* Vol. 2. Philadelphia: Elsevier, 2005.

Petersen, Lyle R., et al. "Emerging Vector-Borne Diseases in the United States: What Is Next and Are We Prepared?" In *Global Health Impacts of Vector-Borne Diseases: Workshop Summary.* Washington, DC: National Academies Press, 2016.

Periodicals

Fried, Susana T. "Telling Women to Avoid Pregnancy Is Not a Solution for HIV and the Zika Virus." *Guardian* (May 28, 2016). This article can also be found online at https://www.theguardian.com/global-development/2016/may/28/women-avoid-pregnancy-not-solution-hiv-zika-virus-internation-day-action-womens-health-conservative-religious-ideologies (accessed January 24, 2018).

Hill, C. A., et al. "Arthropod-Borne Diseases: Vector Control in the Genomics Era." *Nature Reviews Microbiology* 3 (March 2005): 262–268.

Lagunas-Rangel, Francisco. A., et al. "Current Trends in Zika Vaccine Development." *Journal of Virus Eradication* 3 (2017): 124–127.

Websites

"Dengue." Centers for Disease Control and Prevention. https://www.cdc.gov/dengue/epidemiology/index.html (accessed January 14, 2018).

Fried, Susana T., and Debra J. Lebowitz. "What the Solution Isn't: The Parallel of the Zika and HIV Viruses for Women. Lancet Global Health Blog, February 16, 2016. http://globalhealth.thelancet.com/2016/02/16/what-solution-isnt-parallel-zika-and-hiv-viruses-women (accessed January 24, 2018).

"Malaria—Strategy Overview." Bill & Melinda Gates Foundation. https://www.gatesfoundation.org/What-We-Do/Global-Health/Malaria (accessed January 14, 2018).

"Vector-Borne Diseases." World Health Organization. http://www.who.int/mediacentre/factsheets/fs387/en/ (accessed January 14, 2018).

"West Nile Virus." Centers for Disease Control and Prevention. https://www.cdc.gov/westnile/index.html (accessed January 15, 2018).

"Zika Virus." Centers for Disease Control and Prevention. https://www.cdc.gov/zika/index.html (accessed January 14, 2018).

Tony Hawas
Kausalya Santhanam

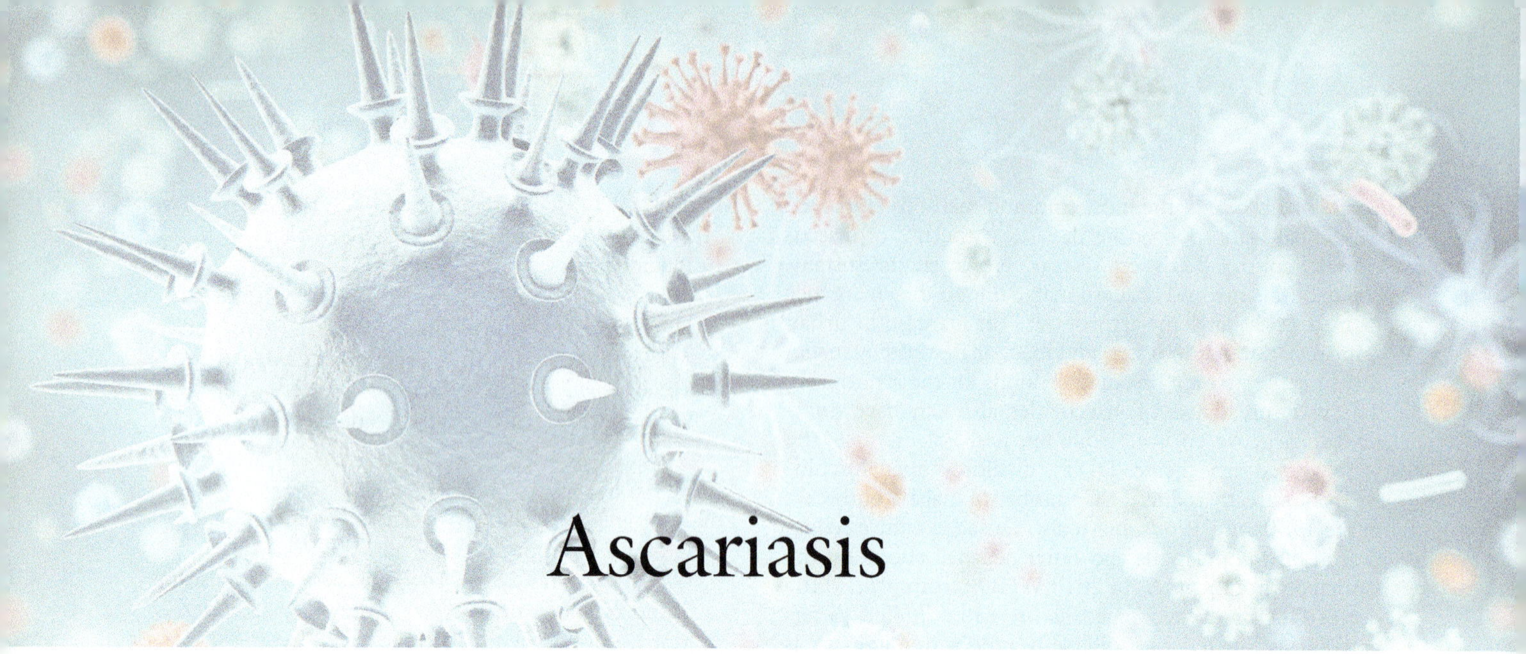

Ascariasis

Introduction

Ascariasis (as-kuh-RYE-uh-sis) is an infection caused by the parasitic nematode, or roundworm, *Ascaris lumbricoides.* It infects humans and other mammals when embryonated eggs are ingested with contaminated food or water. *A. lumbricoides* is considered the largest roundworm that infects the intestines of humans.

Commonly called the giant intestinal roundworm, the parasite can grow up to a length of 6 to 12 inches (15 to 30 centimeters) and a diameter of 0.12 to 0.32 inches (0.3 to 0.8 centimeters) in males and 8 to 14 inches (20 to 36 centimeters) by 0.2 inches (0.5 centimeters) in females. The embryonated eggs are the infectious part of the disease.

Globally, ascariasis is one of the most common worm infections. As of 2017 an estimated 1 billion people were infected with *A. lumbricoides* worldwide, according to the National Center for Biotechnology Information. The World Health Organization (WHO) reports that some 60,000 die of ascariasis each year. Infections are most common among children living in developing tropical and subtropical countries. WHO estimates that up to 10 percent

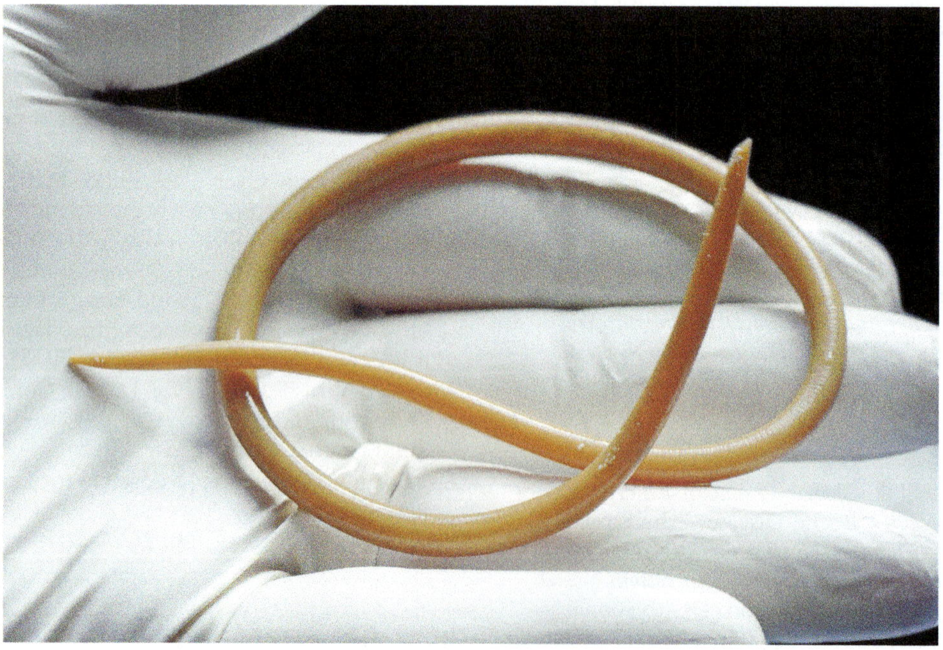

Parasitic roundworm (*Ascaris lumbricoides*), which is considered the largest roundworm that infects the intestines of humans, causes ascariasis, or roundworm infection. *© Clouds Hill Imaging Ltd./Science Source*

WORDS TO KNOW

EMBRYONATED When an embryo has been implanted in a female animal.

FECAL-ORAL ROUTE The spread of disease through the transmission of minute particles of fecal material from one organism to the mouth of another. This can occur by drinking contaminated water; eating food exposed to animal or human feces, such as food from plants watered with unclean water; or preparing food without practicing proper hygiene.

HELMINTH A representative of various phyla of wormlike animals.

PARASITE An organism that lives in or on a host organism and that gets its nourishment from that host. The parasite usually gains all the benefits of this relationship. The host may suffer from various diseases and discomforts or show no signs of the infection. The life cycle of a typical parasite includes several developmental stages and morphological changes as the parasite lives and moves through the environment and one or more hosts. Parasites that remain on a host's body surface to feed are called ectoparasites, whereas those that live inside a host's body are called endoparasites. Parasitism is a highly successful biological adaptation. There are more known parasitic species than nonparasitic ones, and parasites affect just about every form of life, including most all animals, plants, and even bacteria.

of the developing world's population is infected with intestinal worms, many of which are *A. lumbricoides.*

Disease History, Characteristics, and Transmission

Infection occurs via the fecal-oral route, most often when food is contaminated by fecal material containing fertilized eggs. The larvae hatch and burrow into the moist lining (mucosa) of the intestines. They then travel to the lungs, where they mature, usually for 10 to 14 days. They eventually travel through the respiratory tract and up into the throat, where they are swallowed and sent to the small intestines. They mature as worms while attached to the walls of the small intestines.

A mature female can produce about 200,000 eggs per day. Roundworms live approximately one to two years. The time from egg ingestion to egg egression with feces is between two and three months. Upon egress from a host, the eggs become infectious within 18 days to several weeks, with the range dependent on soil conditions such as temperature.

Typically, there are few symptoms, and a person may even be symptom-free when the worms are immature and small. Noticeable symptoms usually occur between 4 and 16 days of ingestion. Common symptoms include diarrhea, fever, inflammation, wheezing, and nonproductive cough. Other serious problems develop whenever the worms live within the lungs (pulmonary symptoms) or throughout the body (neurological disorders). The final symptoms are gastrointestinal distress, nausea, vomiting, fever, nutritional insufficiencies, peritonitis (inflammation of the abdominal wall), enlargement of the liver or spleen, and observation of live worms in stools. In rare cases worms may obstruct the intestines, cause pneumonitis (inflammation of the lungs), or cause eosinophilia (increase in white blood cells).

Humans become infected by direct contact of the worms to skin and through the ingestion of soil and vegetation that contain fecal matter contaminated with eggs. Transmission can also occur when wastewater is recycled onto crop fields as fertilizer, a practice that is common in developing countries.

Scope and Distribution

Roundworm infection is found throughout the world but especially in tropical regions and among the poorest areas with the worst of hygiene conditions. It is pronounced in Africa, especially Nigeria, and in Southeast Asia, especially Indonesia. Although infections were historically prevalent along the rural areas of the American Gulf Coast, incidence has declined, making infections uncommon in the United States. About 2 percent of Americans are estimated to be infected with roundworms. High-risk groups include visitors and travelers to developing countries.

Treatment and Prevention

The diagnosis is easily made when the infected person observes worms in his or her stool or vomit. If that does not happen, stool samples may be taken to medically determine the presence of eggs. Blood counts can also diagnose eosinophilia, and respiratory samples can find pneumonitis and other pulmonary diseases.

TOXOCARIASIS

Nematodes, or roundworms as they are more commonly known, cause not only ascariasis but a wide variety of conditions. Among the most common and overlooked of these is toxocariasis, which humans contract from dogs and cats. In fact, the US Centers for Disease Control and Prevention (CDC) considers toxocariasis so severe, widespread, and poorly treated that the infection is on its list of neglected parasitic infections, along with Chagas disease, cysticercosis, toxoplasmosis, and trichomoniasis.

Two different but closely related nematodes carry the larvae that causes toxocariasis: *Toxocara canis*, which dogs carry, and *T. cati*, which cats carry. Research suggests that nearly all puppies carry *T. canis* and that a quarter of all cats carry *T. cati*. Because of the high rates of these nematodes in domestic animals, nearly 15 percent of the US population and up to 40 percent of the population in other countries is infected with one of the two *Toxocara* strains. The roundworms typically enter a person's bloodstream after he or she ingests dirt containing *Toxocara* larvae.

Toxocariasis is treatable with albendazole, mebendazole, and other drugs. The risk of prevention can be reduced with good pet hygiene. Nevertheless, the CDC and other health organizations have faced difficulty in combatting toxocariasis.

Treatment involves medicines that commonly combat parasitic worms such as albendazole (Albenza®), mebendazole (Ovex®, Vermox®), piperazine (Entacyl®), pyrantel pamoate (Antiminth®, Pin-Rid®, Pin-X®), and thiabendazole (Mintezol®). Corticosteroid medicine is sometimes given to counter inflammation.

Roundworm infection is prevented by using careful and comprehensive hygiene techniques such as protecting food from soil and dirt, thoroughly washing vegetables and fruits, washing hands especially after using the toilet, and other similar sanitary measures.

■ Impacts and Issues

Ascariasis dominates in areas with poor sanitation. According to the Office of Laboratory Security at the Public Health Agency of Canada, roundworm infection is concentrated in moist tropical areas of the world. Within these regions its incidence can be over 50 percent. The group with the highest infection rate in these areas is children aged three to eight years. Ascariasis adds to iron-deficiency anemia, malnutrition, and impairment of growth and intelligence among the people it affects.

Complications that occur as a direct result of roundworm infection are common. The most frequent complication is intestinal tract obstruction. According to WHO and other sources, an estimated 60,000 deaths occur annually in the world, primarily in children. Male children are thought to be more likely to get the disease because of the amount of time they play in dirt.

The disease has generally been neglected in the past because it occurs primarily in poor, rural areas of the world. The affliction has been around for thousands of years. However, aggressive treatment has been attempted in some regions.

See Also *Food-Borne Disease and Food Safety; Globalization and Infectious Disease; Handwashing; Helminth Disease; Travel and Infectious Disease*

BIBLIOGRAPHY

Books

Holland, Celia V., and Malcolm W. Kennedy. *The Geohelminths: Ascaris, Trichuris, and Hookworm.* Boston: Kluwer Academic, 2002.

McDowell, Mary Ann, and Sima Rafati. *Neglected Tropical Diseases—Middle East and North Africa.* Vienna: Springer, 2014.

Singh, Prati Pal, and Vinod P. Sharma. *Water and Health.* New Delhi: Springer, 2014.

Periodicals

Banderker, Ebrahim, et al. "Imaging and Management of Childhood Ascariasis." *Journal of Pediatric Infectious Diseases* 12, no. 1 (2017): 20–29.

Mubarak, Mohammad Yousuf, et al. "Hygienic Behaviors and Risks for Ascariasis among College Students in Kabul, Afghanistan." *American Journal of Tropical Medicine and Hygiene* 97, no. 2 (August 2017): 563–566.

Websites

"Ascariasis." Centers for Disease Control and Prevention, May 24, 2016. https://www.cdc.gov/parasites/ascariasis/ (accessed January 10, 2018).

"Ascariasis." Mayo Clinic. https://www.mayoclinic.org/diseases-conditions/ascariasis/symptoms-causes/syc-20369593 (accessed January 10, 2018).

de Lima Corvino, Daniela F., and Steve S. Bhimji. "Ascariasis." National Center for Biotechnology Information, May 25, 2017. https://www.ncbi.nlm.nih.gov/books/NBK430796/ (accessed January 10, 2018).

"Water Related Diseases." World Health Organization. http://www.who.int/water_sanitation_health/diseases-risks/diseases/ascariasis/en/ (accessed January 10, 2018).

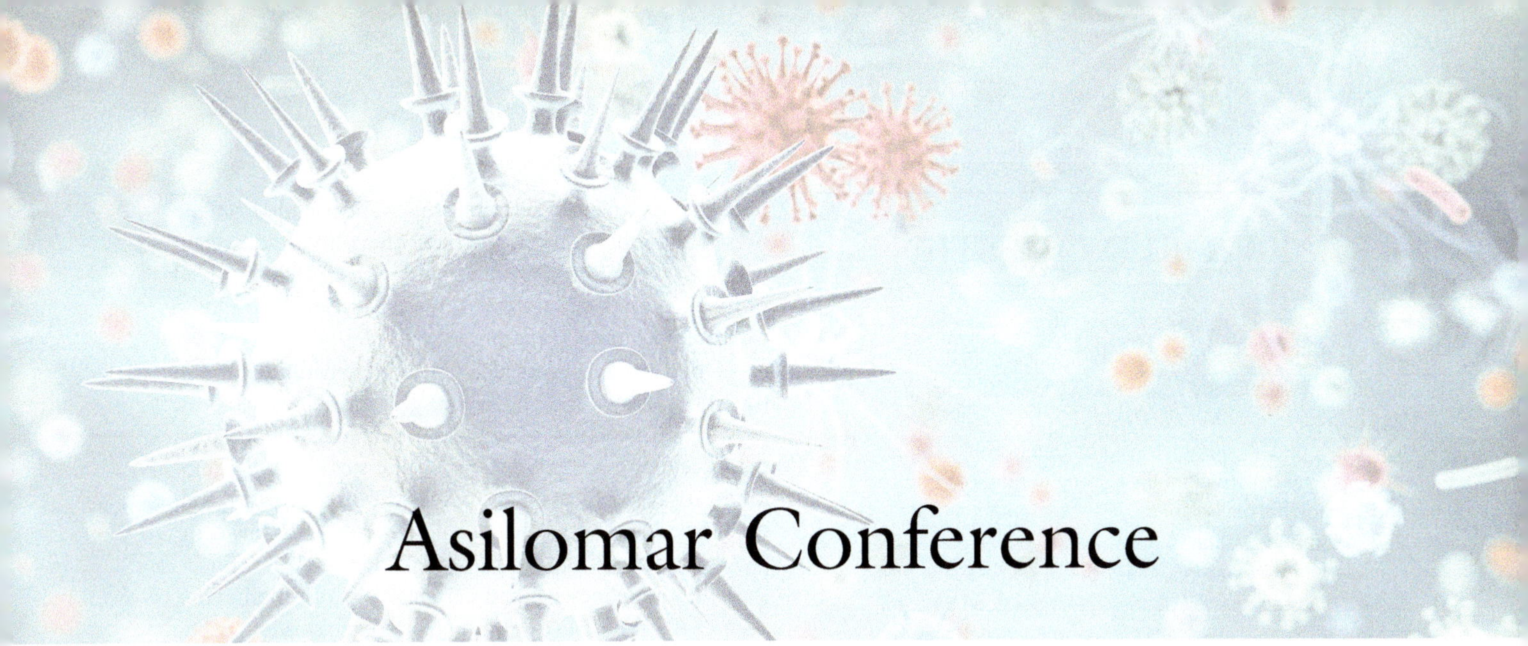

Asilomar Conference

Introduction

The Asilomar Conference of 1975 was held to consider the possible biohazards of then newly developed recombinant DNA technology. This technology involves selectively removing the genetic material (deoxyribonucleic acid, or DNA) from one organism and inserting it into the DNA of a different organism. As a result, the proteins encoded by the inserted genes are expressed in the host organism.

Following the development of recombinant DNA technology in the mid-1970s, researchers successfully transferred DNA into target microorganisms, such as the bacterium *Escherichia coli*, thus enabling the target organism to produce the protein(s) encoded by the inserted DNA. Almost immediately researchers recognized the potential for the deliberate or accidental misuse of this technology to create an organism whose ability to cause disease was enhanced or even created anew.

These early molecular biology researchers took the extraordinary step of declaring a moratorium on recombinant DNA research until they could meet, discuss their concerns, and formulate guidelines to restore confidence in future research. The meeting took place in February 1975 in Asilomar, which is located on the northern coast of California near San Francisco.

History and Scientific Foundations

Recombinant DNA technology has its roots in the 1970 discovery by American microbiologist Hamilton Smith (1931–) of restriction enzymes. (Since that time dozens of different restriction enzymes have been discovered.) Restriction enzymes function by recognizing a unique sequence of nucleotides within a strand of DNA and cutting the DNA at that site. The cut exposes a portion of one of the two nucleotide strands that intertwine to form the DNA double helix. This portion can bind to the corresponding nucleotide on another exposed DNA strand, thereby allowing segments of DNA from different sources to meld.

Following the discovery of restriction enzymes, recombinant DNA technology progressed with astonishing swiftness. In 1972 Paul Berg (1926–), then a faculty member at Stanford University, reported the manufacture of recombinant DNA consisting of an oncogene from a human cancer-causing monkey virus ligated, or joined, into the genetic material of the bacterial virus lambda. The following year Stanley Cohen (1935–) and Herbert Boyer (1936–) were successful in transferring foreign DNA into *E. coli*.

The rapid developments of recombinant DNA technology, combined with Berg's demonstration that a potentially harmful gene could be transferred into a new organism, caused great concern. The specter of the malicious design of a deadly microorganism that was capable of person-to-person transmission, and the realization that the

WORDS TO KNOW

DNA Deoxyribonucleic acid, a double-stranded, helical molecule that is found in almost all living cells and that determines the characteristics of each organism.

RECOMBINANT DNA DNA that is cut using specific enzymes so that a gene or DNA sequence may be inserted.

RESTRICTION ENZYME A special type of protein that can recognize certain DNA sequences and cut DNA to isolate specific genes. These DNA fragments may be joined together to create new stretches of DNA.

REAL-WORLD QUESTIONS

Potential applications of recombinant DNA technology include food crops engineered to produce edible vaccines. This strategy would make vaccines more readily available to children worldwide. Bananas have been the object of considerable research because of their use across many cultures and their ability to adapt to tropical and subtropical environments. Researchers have developed and evaluated transgenic bananas containing inactivated viruses that normally cause cholera, hepatitis B, and diarrhea, as well as transgenic potatoes carrying recombinant vaccines for cholera and intestinal disorders. However, the potential use of these crops remains controversial, and the approach is not yet fully accepted.

technology had outpaced knowledge of its potential pitfalls, prompted the moratorium and the Asilomar Conference.

Impacts and Issues

In February 1975 the leaders of the international molecular biology community met at the Asilomar Conference Center in California. At the time the international molecular biology community consisted of slightly more than 100 researchers, compared to the hundreds of thousands of molecular biology researchers in 2017. The purpose of the gathering was to establish minimum standards for those engaged in recombinant DNA research. Anyone seeking to conduct recombinant DNA research would be required to follow the guidelines.

To rate the risks of recombinant DNA research as minimal, low, moderate, or high, conference delegates considered the type of research being conducted and the equipment and laboratory facilities required to perform the research. As the riskiness of the research increased, such as when using a known pathogen, the stringency of the precautions increased. For example, a low-risk research lab would not require any special ventilation, whereas high-risk research would require a facility designed to contain the organism in the event of a spill or other accident.

The conference's task was difficult because some of the guidelines applied to experiments that had not yet been performed. Still, some realistic guidelines emerged. For example, the scientists decided that the bacteria used in recombinant DNA research should be incapable of surviving outside the controlled environment of the lab. This could be achieved, for example, by genetically crippling the bacteria so that the cells could not make some vital nutrient. As a result, bacterial survival depended on the presence of the nutrient in the artificial food source on which they were grown. In this way, the chance of spread of the recombinant bacteria to the outside world would be extremely remote.

Other risk-related guidelines included banning food in the laboratory; wearing protective gear including a lab coat, gloves, and face mask; scrupulous cleaning of work areas before and after experiments to ensure surfaces and equipment are free of bacteria; and, at the highest risk level, designing a laboratory that is self-contained and thus completely separated from the outside world.

The guidelines banned certain types of experiments, such as the use of highly pathogenic organisms or genetic material known to encode harmful products such as toxins. Then, as now, it was recognized that scientists or organizations bent on designing harmful organisms would circumvent the guidelines. However, the vast majority of the scientific community supported and followed the guidelines developed at the Asilomar Conference.

In June 2017 the US National Institutes of Health (NIH) held a workshop that revisited the relevance of the Asilomar guidelines now that recombinant DNA technology had become mainstream. The NIH judged the guidelines to be still relevant in evaluating the biosafety of new technologies of synthetic biology and genome editing.

Nevertheless, debates over recombinant technologies continue. One example is recombinant influenza virus. Refinements in molecular biology have made it possible to build influenza viruses that can express viral proteins that contain mutations as well as proteins from organisms other than viruses. There is a benefit to this approach, known as *gain of function*, as it might be harnessed to make vaccines. Critics argue that the same approach could be used to deliver toxic molecules via a virus that has been adapted to easily pass from person to person.

In mid-2017 researchers reported using a recently developed gene technology termed *CRISPR-Cas9* to remove a mutated gene from a developing embryo. The success opened the door to the possibility that potentially lethal genetic mutations could one day be safely removed prior to birth. Whether the technology could be used to produce designer babies (genetically modified embryos) is part of the discussion surrounding the advance.

BIBLIOGRAPHY

Books

Doudna, Jennifer A., and Samuel H. Sternberg. *A Crack in Creation: Gene Editing and the Unthinkable Power to Control Evolution*. Boston: Houghton Mifflin Harcourt, 2017.

National Academies of Science, Engineering, Medicine. *Human Genome Editing: Science, Ethics, and Governance*. Washington, DC: National Academies Press, 2017.

Periodicals

Dominguez, Antonia A., Wendell A. Lim, and Lei S. Qi. "Beyond Editing: Repurposing CRISPR-Cas9 for Precision Genome Regulation and Interrogation." *Nature Reviews Molecular Cell Biology* 17, no. 1 (January 2016): 5–15.

Websites

"Back to the Future: Asilomar and the Upcoming *NIH Guidelines* Workshop." National Institutes of Health. https://osp.od.nih.gov/2017/07/05/back-to-the-future-asilomar-and-the-upcoming-nih-guidelines-workshop/ (accessed November 14, 2017).

"What Are Genome Editing and CRISPR-Cas9?" National Institutes of Health. https://ghr.nlm.nih.gov/primer/genomicresearch/genomeediting (accessed November 14, 2017).

Brian Hoyle

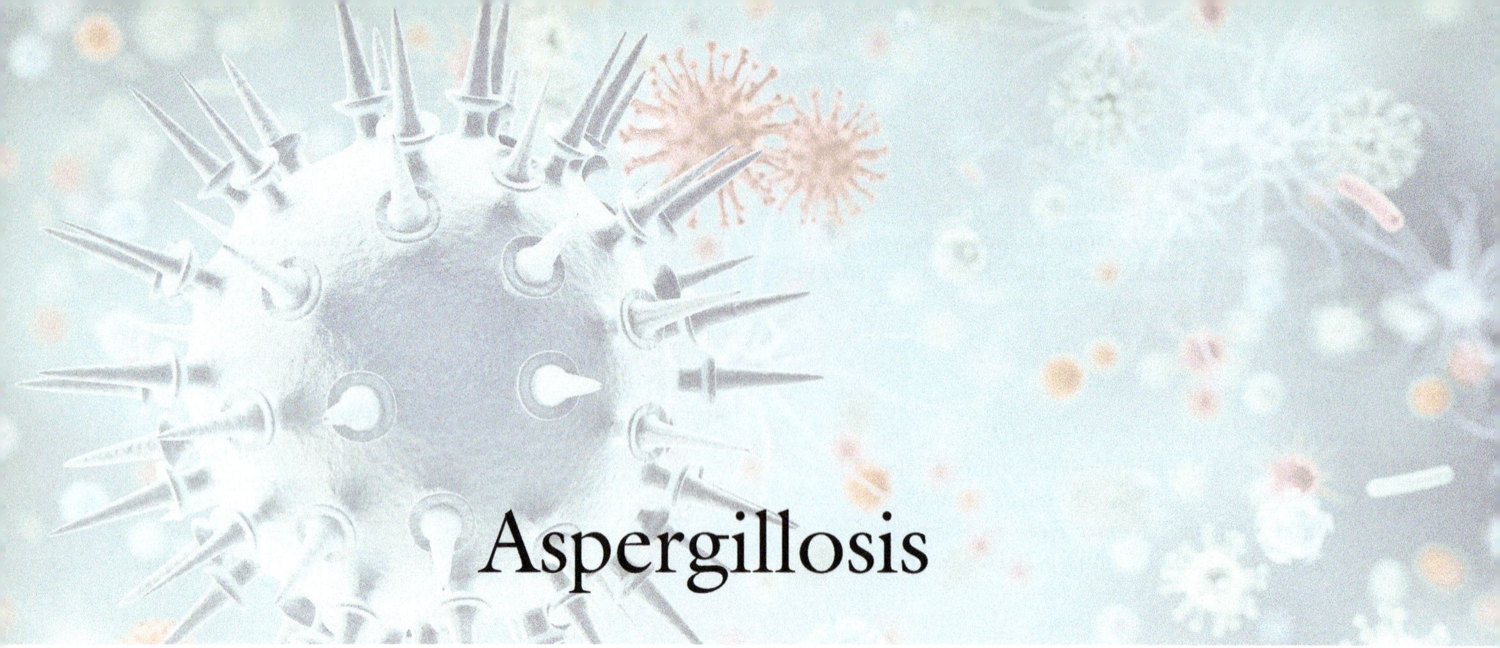

Aspergillosis

Introduction

Aspergillosis is a lung infection or allergic reaction caused by a type of fungus called *Aspergillus.* The fungus, which is found naturally on decaying organic material such as leaves, hay, and compost, can infect the lungs. Pulmonary aspergillosis may remain confined to the lungs or may spread to other parts of the body. A widespread infection can be especially serious and occurs most commonly in people whose immune systems are less capable of fighting off infections.

Disease History, Characteristics, and Transmission

Aspergillosis is most typically caused by *Aspergillus fumigatus* or *A. flavus.* Less commonly, the infection is caused by *A. terreus, A. nidulans,* or *A. niger.*

Inhalation of the spores of *Aspergillus* can lead to the growth of the fungus in the lungs. This growth can cause an allergic reaction called pulmonary aspergillosis. The infection, which can develop along with asthma, can dimin-

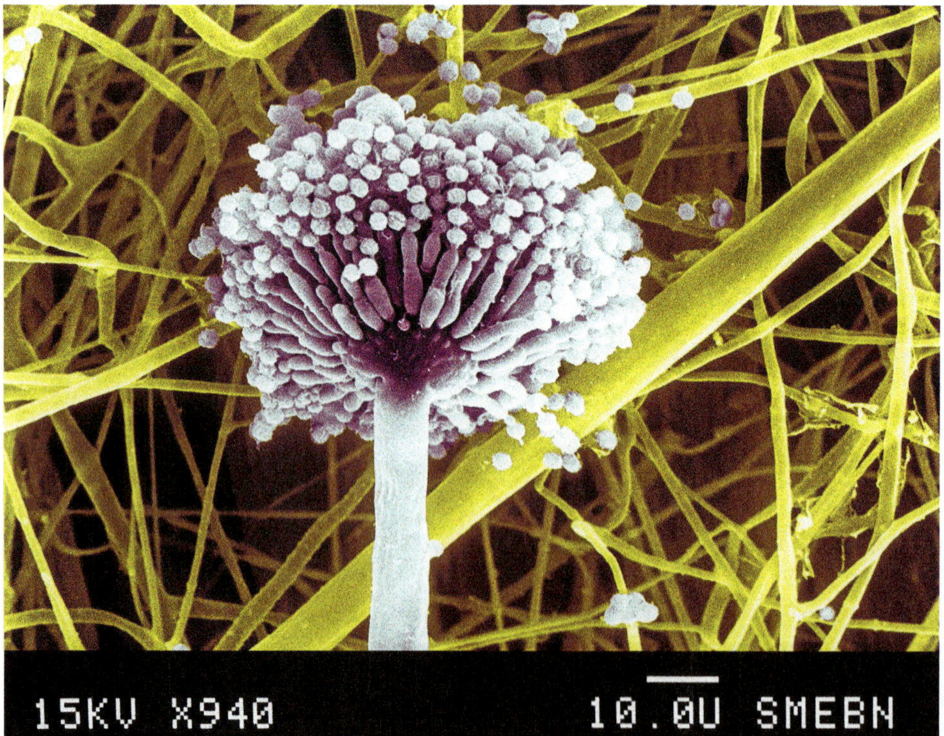

The fungus *Aspergillus niger* is shown under magnification. *A. niger* can cause aspergillosis. © BSIP/UIG/Getty Images ish the ability of the lungs to function. Growth of the fungus also can produce a compact structure called a fungus ball. The ball tends to develop in an area of the lung that has previously been damaged by tuberculosis or some other infection that results in a localized buildup of fluid or infected material.

Pulmonary aspergillosis also can be more invasive, meaning the infection can move from the lungs to other parts of the body. This spread is promoted when the infection is less efficiently cleared due to a compromised immune system, as can occur during treatment for cancer or certain other ailments, following organ transplantation to minimize rejection of the transplant, or in people with acquired immunodeficiency syndrome (AIDS).

The symptoms of aspergillosis include fever, a general feeling of tiredness, cough that may be combined with expelled blood or mucous, wheeziness when breathing, loss of weight, and periodic difficulty in breathing. Additional symptoms may be present in the more invasive type of aspergillosis. These include chills, headaches, chest pain, an increased amount of expelled mucous, a decreased amount of urine, bloody urine, bone pain, inflammation of nerve lining in the brain or spinal cord (meningitis), sinus infection, diminished vision, and heart trouble.

WORDS TO KNOW

IMMUNOCOMPROMISED Having an immune system with reduced ability to recognize and respond to the presence of foreign material.

OPPORTUNISTIC INFECTION An infection that occurs in people whose immune systems are diminished or are not functioning normally. Such infections are opportunistic insofar as the infectious agents take advantage of their hosts' compromised immune systems and invade to cause disease.

PULMONARY Having to do with the lungs or respiratory system. The pulmonary circulatory system delivers deoxygenated blood from the right ventricle of the heart to the lungs and returns oxygenated blood from the lungs to the left atrium of the heart. At its most minute level, the alveolar capillary bed, the pulmonary circulatory system is the principle point of gas exchange between blood and air that moves in and out of the lungs during respiration.

Scope and Distribution

Aspergillosis is global in scope because the fungus that causes the disease is a common environmental organism. The prevalence of aspergillosis is unclear, although it tends to be more prevalent in areas where the population includes more immunosuppressed people. For example, in the early 1990s, the city of San Francisco, which then had a higher proportion of people with AIDS than some other metropolitan areas, had an estimated annual rate of aspergillosis of one to two people per 100,000, according to data from the US Centers for Disease Control and Prevention (CDC). Since then the rate has likely dropped with improved treatments of immunocompromised people, including those with AIDS, although exact figures are unknown because aspergillosis is not a reportable infection in the United States.

Treatment and Prevention

Aspergillosis is diagnosed by the detection of a lung infection. The infection can be imaged using X-rays or a technique called computed tomography (CT). The fungus also can be obtained from a sample of expelled mucous or sputum and grown on various food sources. The food sources can be selected to help distinguish whether the fungus is from the genus *Aspergillus*. In addition, a patient's sputum can be stained and examined using a light microscope to detect fungal cells. The staining method produces a less precise result. It reveals the presence of fungi but is not refined enough to distinguish one genus of fungus from another. However, just knowing the infection is caused by a fungus can be enough to initiate treatment.

Aspergillosis can also be diagnosed by detecting the presence of protein components of the fungus. The proteins function as antigens and stimulate the production of specific antibodies by the immune system. *Aspergillus* antigens can be detected by a skin-based reaction or in a test tube or the well of a plastic assay dish by the formation of a cloudy precipitate that comprises a complex (product) formed between a specific antigen and antibody.

Treatment for aspergillosis varies depending on the nature of the infection. When the infection involves a fungal ball, treatment can be withheld if the infection is not associated with bleeding into the lung. For invasive aspergillosis, treatment is typically with the antifungal drug voriconazole. Drug treatment is usually administered directly into the bloodstream (intravenously) at regular intervals to maintain a constant and effective level of drug in the body. Surgery may be needed to remove the fungal mass. *Aspergillus*-infected heart valves are usually removed, and extended treatment with an antifungal drug follows the surgery.

SELECTIVE SURVEILLANCE

As of 2017 there was no dedicated national surveillance program in the United States to track aspergillosis. However, some US hospitals monitor patients who receive transplants of stem cells and organs because these patients are at higher risk of infection.

People whose illness is due to an allergic reaction to *Aspergillus* do not benefit from the use of an antifungal drug. For them treatment is usually with the antifungal drug itraconazole or with corticosteroids. The latter dampen the response of the immune system and reduce the allergic reaction.

■ Impacts and Issues

The invasive form of aspergillosis can be life-threatening. The seriousness of the infection is especially pronounced in people with a malfunctioning or deliberately suppressed immune system. As of 2017 the death rate from the invasive form of aspergillosis was 59 percent in people who had received a solid organ transplant and who become infected while on immunosuppressive therapy and 25 percent among those who had received a stem cell transplant.

As of 2017 there was no rapid test for the infection. The allergic form of the infection is detected by tests of a person's allergic reaction to exposure to components of the fungus.

Aspergillosis can also affect species other than humans. For example, waterfowl populations can be decimated by aspergillosis outbreaks if the birds feed on decaying grain. Aspergillosis is a common and lethal infection in birds, such as parakeets and parrots.

SEE ALSO *Mycotic Disease; Nosocomial (Healthcare-Associated) Infections; Opportunistic Infection*

BIBLIOGRAPHY

Books

Carvalho, Agostinho. *Immunogenetics of Fungal Diseases.* New York: Springer Berlin Heidelberg, 2017.

Estenson, Joseph. *Aspergillosis: A Reference Guide.* Washington, DC: Capitol Hill Press, 2016.

Periodicals

"Treatment of Aspergillosis: Clinical Practice Guidelines of the Infectious Disease Society of America." *Clinical Infectious Diseases* 46, no. 3 (2008): 327–360.

Websites

"Aspergillosis." Centers for Disease Control and Prevention. https://www.cdc.gov/fungal/diseases/aspergillosis/index.html (accessed November 14, 2017).

Brian Hoyle

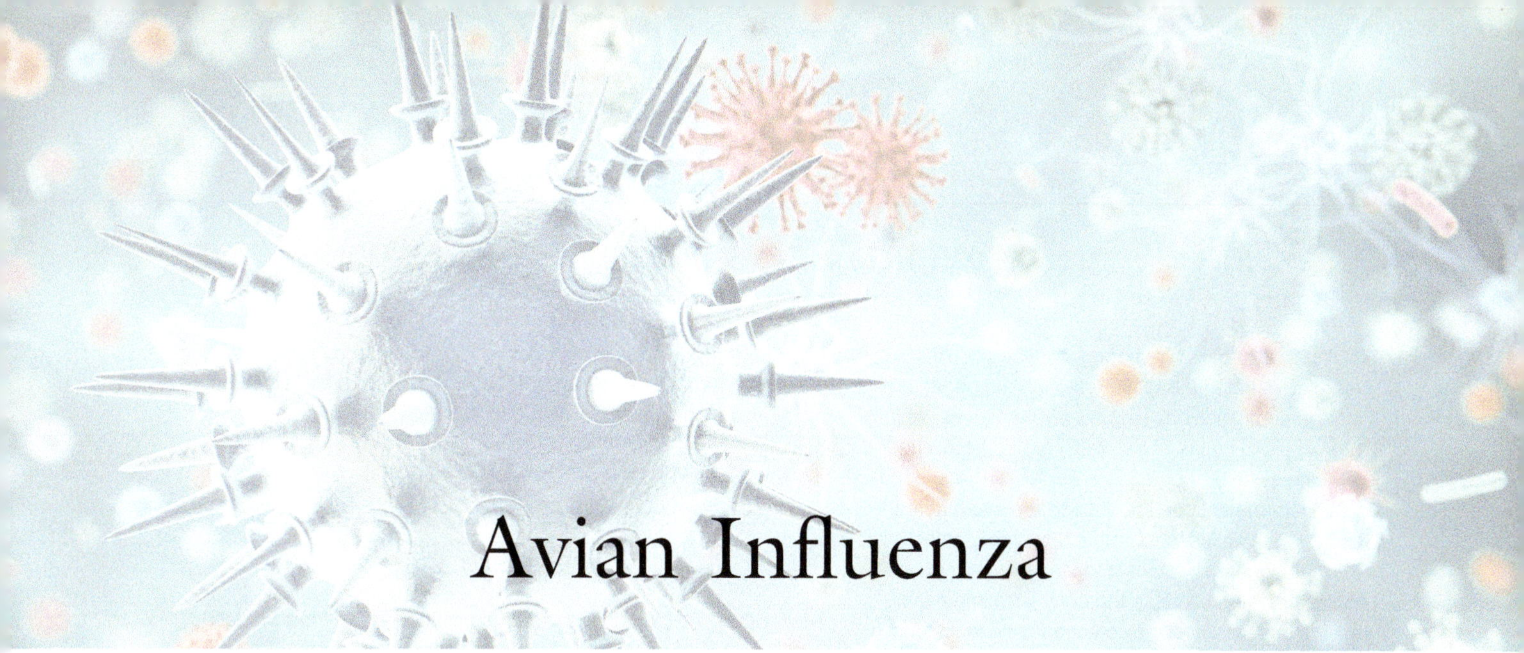

Avian Influenza

Introduction

Avian influenza, also known as avian flu or bird flu, is a type of influenza that is transferred to humans from birds. The virus resides naturally in birds, so birds are the natural host. Avian influenza is an example of a zoonotic infection, an infection that is transferred from a nonhuman species to humans.

If the bird-to-human transfer was the only means of transfer, then avian influenza would not be an important health issue. However, because the virus can spread from person to person, outbreaks of avian influenza can occur.

Avian influenza was first detected in 2003. Whether it existed before then is unknown. Up until about 2007 human cases were rare, with only 916 laboratory-confirmed cases reported to the World Health Organization (WHO). However, scientists think that around 2007 the virus acquired the ability to more easily transfer from birds to humans and establish an infection in humans. This made larger, more widespread outbreaks more likely—a major concern because of the high death rate in people who contract avian influenza. The H5N1 form of the virus (the letters refer to different proteins present on the surface of the

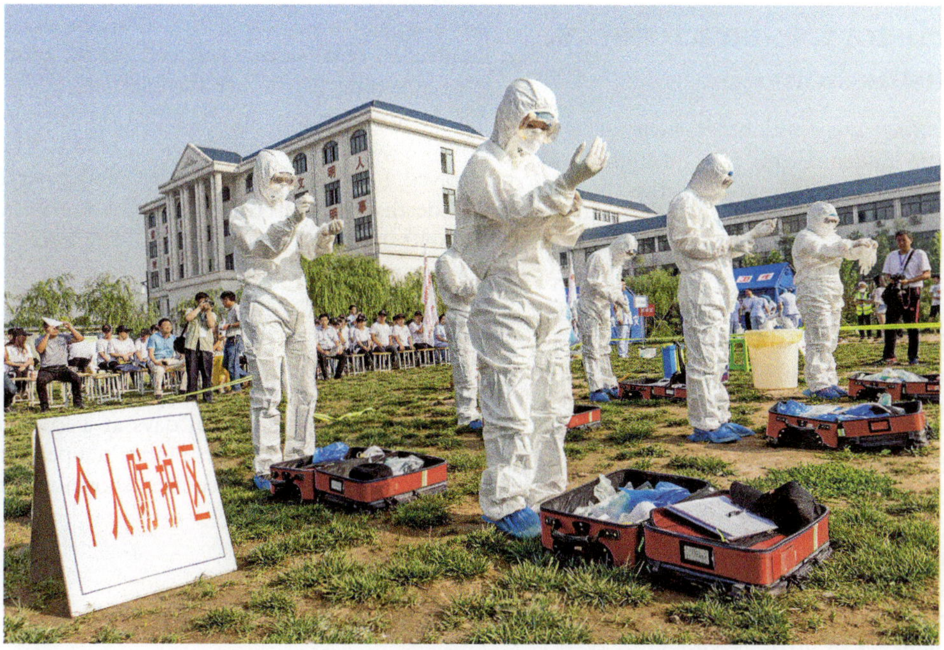

Chinese health professionals conduct a drill designed to prepare for an outbreak of avian influenza. The first outbreak of avian influenza occurred in 1997 in Hong Kong. *© Feature China/Barcroft Images/Barcroft Media/Getty Images*

WORDS TO KNOW

ANTIBODIES also called Y-shaped immunoglobulins, proteins found in the blood that help to fight against foreign substances called antigens. Antigens, which are usually proteins or polysaccharides, stimulate the immune system to produce antibodies. The antibodies inactivate the antigen and help to remove it from the body. While antigens can be the source of infections from pathogenic bacteria and viruses, organic molecules detrimental to the body from internal or environmental sources also act as antigens. Genetic engineering and the use of various mutational mechanisms allow the construction of a vast array of antibodies (each with a unique genetic sequence).

ANTIGEN Usually proteins or polysaccharides, they stimulate the immune system to produce antibodies. The antibodies inactivate the antigen and help to remove it from the body. While antigens can be the source of infections from pathogenic bacteria and viruses, organic molecules detrimental to the body from internal or environmental sources also act as antigens. Genetic engineering and the use of various mutational mechanisms allow the construction of a vast array of antibodies (each with a unique genetic sequence).

CLOACA The cavity into which the intestinal, genital, and urinary tracts open in vertebrates such as fish, reptiles, birds, and some primitive mammals.

HOST An organism that serves as the habitat for a parasite or possibly for a symbiont. A host may provide nutrition to the parasite or symbiont, or it may simply provide a place in which to live.

PANDEMIC An epidemic that occurs in more than one country or population simultaneously. *Pandemic* means "all the people."

STRAIN A subclass or a specific genetic variation of an organism.

virus particle) has a death rate of about 60 percent, according to WHO and the US Centers of Disease Control and Prevention (CDC).

■ Disease History, Characteristics, and Transmission

The term *avian influenza* is a misnomer, as virtually all strains (types) of the influenza virus pass through ducks or other birds before emerging into the human population. Influenza strains differ from one another according to the nature of two surface proteins: hemagglutinin (H) and neuraminidase (N). As of 2017 there were 36 subtypes of the virus, featuring different H and N proteins and different combinations of these proteins.

While most human infection is caused by types H1, H2, and H3, types H5 and H7 cause infections that are more serious. The first outbreak occurred in 1997, when infections caused by H5N1 sickened 18 people and killed 6 in Hong Kong. Subsequently, a handful of cases occurred in Hong Kong, Vietnam, Thailand, Indonesia, and Cambodia from 2003 through 2005. Beginning in 2006 a geographic spread was evident, with cases confirmed in Turkey, Iraq, Egypt, Djibouti, and Azerbaijan. Cases continued to occur in these regions up to 2014, according to WHO. Other regions have also been affected, including Malaysia, where an outbreak in March 2017 was the first reported occurrence in that country in 10 years.

The outbreak first reported in Malaysia in early 2017 was first detected in the northeastern part of the country. The cases all involved chickens. Of the 16 chickens known to be infected, 15 died. The deliberate killing of all chickens in the affected villages controlled the outbreak before any spread to humans occurred. Other measures taken included disinfection of all suspect surfaces and the quarantining of any birds suspected to have the infection.

Another outbreak in 2017 that occurred in China involved another variant of the virus, H7N9. This outbreak involved 1,622 human cases as of November 2017, with 619 deaths. The outbreak is thought to have arisen from chickens imported from Malaysia. The infection had not been detected in the chickens prior to importation.

H5N1 mutates rapidly and has a propensity to acquire genes from other animal species. Birds may excrete the virus from the mouth and cloaca (the excretory vent of a bird) for up to 10 days. H5N1 virus was found to survive in bird feces for at least 35 days at a low temperature (39.2°F [4°C]). At a much higher temperature (98.6°F [37°C]), H5N1 viruses have been shown to survive in fecal samples for six days.

■ Scope and Distribution

Extensive outbreaks involving poultry have occurred in regions of Asia, Africa, Europe, and the Middle East, with millions of birds affected. As of 2017 the number of human cases remained low. The transfer of the virus from birds to humans still seems to be difficult. This is fortunate, given the high fatality rate of the human infection. Nonetheless, the history with other emerging viral infections such as Ebola suggests that the transfer between birds and humans, and the subsequent person-to-person transfer, will become easier. This is because viruses tend to adapt over time to exploit a new host. Numerous outbreaks limited to wild and domestic birds have been reported in Afghanistan, Albania, Austria, Azerbaijan, Bosnia and Herzegovina, Burkina Faso, Croatia, Cyprus, the Czech Republic, Denmark, France, Georgia, Germany, Ghana, Greece, Hungary, India, Iran, Israel, Italy, the Ivory Coast, Jordan, Kazakhstan, Kuwait, Malaysia, Mongolia, Myanmar, the Netherlands, Niger, Nigeria, Pakistan, Poland, the Philippines, Romania, the Russian Federation, Saudi Arabia, Scotland, Serbia, Slovakia, Slovenia, Spain, Sudan, Sweden, Switzerland, Ukraine, and the United Kingdom. In other words, the principal mode of transfer among countries is in the intestines of migrating wild birds.

Avian influenza is characterized by fever greater than 100.4°F (38°C), shortness of breath, and cough. The incubation period is two to four days. Some people have reported a sore throat, conjunctivitis, muscle pain, a rash, and a runny nose. Watery diarrhea or loose stools is noted in approximately 50 percent of cases, a symptom that is uncommon in the more familiar forms of influenza. All patients reported to date have presented with significant lymphopenia (diminished concentration of lymphocytes, white blood cells, in the blood) and marked chest X-ray abnormalities consisting of diffuse, multifocal, or patchy infiltrates (areas of inflammatory cells, foreign organisms, and cellular debris, often indicating pneumonia). Physical examination reveals the patient to be short of breath, with signs of lung inflammation. Myocardial (heart muscle) and hepatic (liver) dysfunction are also reported. Approximately 60 percent of patients have died an average of 10 days after the onset of symptoms.

■ Treatment and Prevention

Diagnosis depends on demonstration of the virus or serum antibody toward the virus in specialized laboratories. Because of intense media reporting (and misinformation), a given patient may be reported repeatedly or a case of unrelated respiratory infection may be mistakenly reported as avian influenza. Thus, only reports issued by qualified centralized laboratories should be considered valid. As of 2017 the antiviral agents recommended by the CDC for treatment of avian influenza were Oseltamivir, Peramivir, and Zanamivir. All three act by inhibiting the binding of the virus to human cells. In April 2007 the Food and Drug Administration (FDA) approved a vaccine for H5N1. While not commonly used (it is being reserved for outbreak), the vaccine could prove valuable when the virus acquires the ability to spread easily from person to person.

■ Impacts and Issues

The main issues with avian influenza are its high death rate in humans and the possibility that the virus will transfer easily from person to person. The fear of those who deal with avian influenza is that the virus will one day convert to a contagious form while retaining its high virulence, a combination that could lead to millions of new cases.

Another disturbing feature of the most recent outbreaks is the age of infected individuals. The common epidemic forms of influenza to date have had greatest impact among the elderly, with most deaths occurring in people over age 65 with underlying heart or lung disease. However, 90 percent of patients with the H5N1 avian influenza virus have been below age 40, with many deaths reported in children. This may be because children have a less well-developed immune system than adults and because young adults tend to be more active and therefore more easily exposed to sources of the virus.

PRIMARY SOURCE

Avian Influenza—Necessary precautions to prevent human infection of H5N1, need for virus sharing

SOURCE: *"Avian Influenza—Necessary Precautions to Prevent Human Infection of H5N1, Need for Virus Sharing." World Health Organization, July 16, 2004. http://www.who.int/csr/don/2004_07_16/en/ (accessed December 6, 2017).*

INTRODUCTION: *The World Health Organization (WHO) publishes* Disease Outbreak News *reports to provide timely outbreak information and foster communication among various national and international public health organizations. As an example, the following report outlines WHO recommendations for combating the threat of pandemic Highly Pathogenic Avian Influenza H5N1.*

WHO continues to be concerned by the simultaneous outbreaks of Highly Pathogenic Avian Influenza H5N1 in several Asian countries.

While these outbreaks thus far remain restricted to poultry populations, they nevertheless increase the chances of virus transmission and human infection of the disease, as well as the possible emergence of a new influenza virus strain capable of sparking a global pandemic.

In this context, WHO reemphasizes the necessity of protecting individuals involved in the culling of H5N1-infected poultry. Workers who might be exposed to H5N1-infected poultry should have proper personal protective equipment (i.e., protective clothing, masks and goggles) since there is a high risk of exposure during the slaughtering process.

In addition to the use of personal protective equipment, WHO is recommending:

- To avoid the co-infection of avian and human influenza, which could allow for the emergence of a pandemic influenza virus, all persons involved in mass culling operations, transportation and burial/incineration of carcasses should be vaccinated with the current WHO-recommended influenza vaccine.
- All persons exposed to infected poultry or to farms under suspicion should be under close monitoring by local health authorities. National authorities should also increase their surveillance of any reported clusters of influenza or influenza-like illness.
- Antiviral treatment should be available on an ongoing basis for treatment of a suspected human infection with a Highly Pathogenic Avian Influenza virus. If antivirals are available in sufficient quantities, prophylactic use should be considered.

Please see the full list of WHO's interim recommendations for the protection of persons involved in the mass slaughter of animals potentially infected with Highly Pathogenic Avian Influenza viruses.

WHO is also urging countries to work on standardized procedures for immediate sharing of all avian influenza virus strains responsible for outbreaks with WHO's international network of laboratories.

WHO is depending on the continued collaboration of the national health and agricultural services to establish routine procedures for immediate sharing of avian influenza virus samples. Without such virus samples, WHO will not be in a position to provide proper vaccine prototype strains and related guidance for vaccine producers.

SEE ALSO *Developing Nations and Drug Delivery; Emerging Infectious Diseases; H5N1; Influenza; Influenza, Tracking Seasonal Influences and Virus Mutation; Influenza Pandemic of 1918; Notifiable Diseases; Pandemic Preparedness; Vaccines and Vaccine Development*

BIBLIOGRAPHY

Books

Bristow, Nancy. *American Pandemic: The Lost Worlds of the 1918 Influenza Pandemic.* Oxford, UK: Oxford University Press, 2017.

Compans, Richard W., and Michael B.A. Oldstone, eds. *Influenza Pathogenesis and Control—Volume 1.* New York: Springer, 2016.

Periodicals

Peeters, Ben, et al. "Genetic versus Antigenic Differences among Highly Pathogenic H5N1 Avian Influenza A Viruses: Consequences for Vaccine Strain Selection." *Virology* 503 (2017): 83–93.

Websites

"Avian and Other Zoonotic Influenza." World Health Organization. http://www.who.int/influenza/human_animal_interface/en (accessed December 6, 2017).

"Information on Avian Influenza." Centers for Disease Control and Prevention. http://www.cdc.gov/flu/avianflu/index.htm (accessed December 6, 2017).

Stephen A. Berger
Brian Hoyle

B Virus (Cercopithecine Herpesvirus 1) Infection

Introduction

B virus, also called Cercopithecine herpesvirus 1, is an infectious virus found in macaques (short-tailed monkeys), such as rhesus macaques, pig-tailed macaques, stump-tailed macaques, and cynomolgus monkeys. The virus, which is a member of the herpes group of viruses, possesses origins and causes diseases similar to those of the herpes simplex virus in humans. When humans are infected with B virus from macaques, they can become ill with severe, sometimes permanent central nervous system (CNS) involvement or death from encephalomyelitis (inflammation of the brain).

The mortality rate for undiagnosed or untreated B virus disease is approximately 80 percent, according to Jeffrey I. Cohen and coauthors of a 2002 article on the virus. However, quick implementation of antiviral therapy for B virus, which was first recommended by the US Centers for Disease Control and Prevention's (CDC) 2002 B Virus Working Group, can help reduce neurological damage and prevent death from infection.

B virus is also called herpes B virus, herpesvirus simiae, and monkey B virus. The last known fatality from B virus in the United States occurred in 1997 at the Yerkes National Primate Research Center, located at Emory Univer-

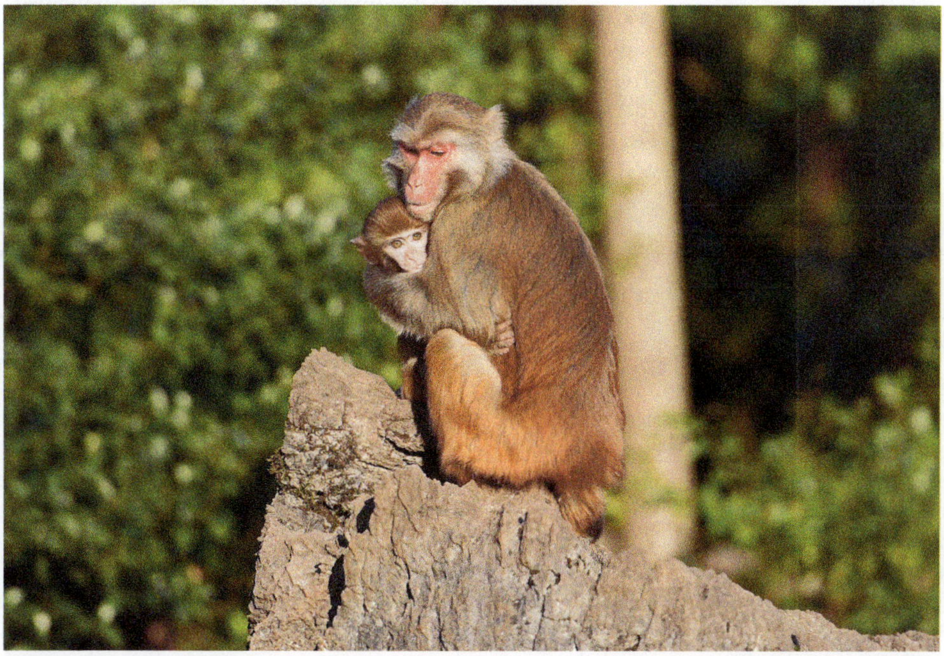

Pictured here is a wild macaque. Macaques infected with B virus sometimes develop herpes-like lesions of the face, mouth, lips, or genitals, but other times they show no symptoms at all. The disease is much more severe in humans, potentially causing death from encephalomyelitis in cases that do not receive antiviral therapy. *© TPG/Getty Images*

WORDS TO KNOW

ENCEPHALOMYELITIS Simultaneous inflammation of the brain and spinal cord.

HERPESVIRUS A family of viruses, many of which cause disease in humans. The herpes simplex 1 and herpes simplex 2 viruses cause infection in the mouth or on the genitals. Other common types of herpesvirus include chickenpox, Epstein-Barr virus, and cytomegalovirus. Herpesvirus is notable for its ability to remain latent, or inactive, in nerve cells near the area of infection, and to reactivate long after the initial infection. Herpes simplex 1 and 2, along with chickenpox, cause skin sores. Epstein-Barr virus causes mononucleosis. Cytomegalovirus also causes a flulike infection but can be dangerous to the elderly, infants, and those with weakened immune systems.

MACAQUE Any short-tailed monkey of the genus *Macaca*. Macaques, including rhesus monkeys, are often used as subjects in medical research because they are relatively affordable and resemble humans in many ways.

sity in Atlanta, Georgia. Biological material from a monkey infected the eye of a worker, and the infection eventually killed the worker.

Because of this incident, the CDC formed a working group to devise recommendations for the evaluation, prevention, and treatment of B virus in humans. The group's report, "Recommendations for Prevention of and Therapy for Exposure to B Virus (*Cercopithecine Herpesvirus* 1)," was published in 2002 in the journal *Clinical Infectious Diseases.*

■ Disease History, Characteristics, and Transmission

The first medically documented case of human B virus infection occurred in 1932 when a rhesus macaque bit a researcher's hand. The worker died two weeks later of encephalomyelitis.

Macaques are primates in the family Cercopithecidae (commonly called Old World monkeys), subfamily Cercopithecinae, and genus *Macaca*. The scientific name of the rhesus macaque is *Macaca mulatta*. The southern pig-tailed macaque is called *M. nemestrina*. The northern pig-tailed macaque is called *M. leonine*. The stump-tailed macaque, or bear macaque, is called *M. arctoides*. The cynomolgus monkey, or crab-eating macaque, is called *M. fascicularis.*

Macaque monkeys infected with B virus usually become infected when oral or genital secretions from other monkeys contact their mucous membranes or skin. Infected monkeys usually have few or no symptoms. When symptoms are present, they usually consist of lesions on the face, genitals, lips, or mouth. Normally, the lesions heal themselves, but they may reappear repeatedly, especially during extended periods of stress or anxiety. This condition is called gingivostomatitis, which is a type of stomatitis, or inflammation of the mucous lining within the mouth, specifically on the tongue, lips, or gums. When the inflammation involves the gums (gingiva), it is called gingivostomatitis.

B virus infection in humans is rare. When it occurs the virus usually comes from cells or tissues (such as in cultures) of monkeys and less frequently from secretions such as saliva, bites, or scratches. The incubation period is generally between two days and five weeks, although most symptoms appear in five days to three weeks. Symptoms are usually limited to the infected areas. They may include itching, numbness, skin lesions, and pain. However, some patients develop serious symptoms in the peripheral or central nervous system. Symptoms may initially include dizziness, headache, nausea, and vomiting and may progress to seizures, respiratory failure, and coma.

Other patients have flu-like symptoms such as chills, fever, and muscle pain. Additional symptoms include itching, weakness, general pain, tingling, or numbness at the infection site. Often humans come down with acute encephalomyelitis (inflammation of the brain and spinal cord), which causes death. Groups of people most at risk from B virus include laboratory workers, veterinarians, and other similar groups who have close contact with macaques or their cell cultures.

■ Scope and Distribution

B virus is found worldwide but is most likely to be found in areas inhabited by Asiatic monkeys of the genus *Macaca* or at locations where they are kept in captivity.

■ Treatment and Prevention

To prevent the transmission of the disease, protective equipment is recommended when working with macaque monkeys, especially virus-positive animals. Protective equipment includes eyewear (such as goggles or glasses with side shields), disposable head coverings, face shields (such as a welder's mask), gloves, disposable shoe covers, and disposable surgical scrubs or fluid-resistant cloth uniforms. Bites, scratches, and exposed mucous membranes, including the eyes, must be cleansed immediately. Culture samples from the macaque and the person who may have been exposed should be sent for B virus diagnostic testing.

THE PROBLEM OF UNWITTING EXPOSURE TO B VIRUS

The native habitat of macaque monkeys spans a vast area of Asia that extends from Afghanistan to China. There, these small, red-faced primates often live in close proximity to humans. However, only 50 cases of transmission have been reported. Of these, only 26 are considered well documented, according to Jeffrey I. Cohen and the coauthors of the 2002 article "Recommendations for Prevention of and Therapy for Exposure to B Virus (*Cercopithecine Herpesvirus* 1)." All 26 of these cases occurred in laboratory settings, where captive monkeys bit, scratched, or threw bodily fluids at caretakers and researchers.

Transmission of B virus typically occurs when infected macaques over 2.5 years of age are ill, are breeding, have suppressed immune systems, or are stressed. According to Cohen and his coauthors, "1 in 50 to 1 in 250 contacts with macaques have the potential to result in exposure to material contaminated with B virus." While the most important time to prevent infection from B virus is right after it occurs, when thorough washing can greatly reduce the chance of transmission, Cohen and his coauthors noted that people sometimes do not know they have been exposed to the virus and do not respond rapidly to prevent transmission. Although numerous procedures exist for stopping the spread of B virus, these procedures are complicated by the fact that infected humans sometimes do not know they have been exposed to the virus until long afterward.

The minutes after exposure are critical. The skin or mucosa affected by bites, scratches, or monkey fluids should be cleansed for a minimum of 15 minutes. If the eyes are contaminated, they should be irrigated with sterile saline solution or water for 15 minutes. Exposed skin should be washed with a chemical antiseptic (such as chlorhexidine or povidone iodine) or detergent soap. After cleansing, wounds should be lightly massaged to increase the effectiveness of the cleaning agent. As soon as possible, antiviral medicine should be started to prevent severe disease or death from B virus.

Impacts and Issues

According to the CDC, workers who handle monkeys directly or handle cultures, bones, or other objects that originate from monkeys are potentially at risk for contracting B virus. Because this work is potentially hazardous, the CDC has written a set of guidelines for the care and maintenance of macaques titled "Guidelines for Prevention of Herpesvirus Simiae (B Virus) Infection in Monkey Handlers."

Although thousands of humans have handled macaques since B virus was first reported, only about 50 cases of human infection had been documented as of 2016, according to the CDC. However, because B virus is potentially deadly, CDC health officials stated that precautions should be instituted to minimize health risks to monkey handlers.

An effective vaccine for B virus, even after years of research, is still unavailable. Because the potential for human death from B virus infection is high and handling and exposure to macaques are rising with increased use of these animals in laboratory settings, a better understanding of the infection is necessary. The mechanism by which the B virus lives within the macaque host is still unclear, and further research is needed to combat this virus.

SEE ALSO *Antiviral Drugs; Personal Protective Equipment; Viral Disease; Zoonoses*

BIBLIOGRAPHY

Books

Bourassa, Erick A. *Infectious Diseases: Pharmacology & Therapeutics.* Seattle: CreateSpace, 2017.

Wayne, Marta L., and Benjamin L. Bolker. *Infectious Disease: A Very Short Introduction.* New York: Oxford University Press, 2015.

Periodicals

Cohen, Jeffrey I., et al. "Recommendations for Prevention of and Therapy for Exposure to B Virus (*Cercopithecine Herpesvirus* 1)." *Clinical Infectious Diseases* 35, no. 10 (2002): 1191–1203. This article can also be found online at https://academic.oup.com/cid/article/35/10/1191/296729 (accessed December 15, 2017).

"Guidelines for Prevention of Herpesvirus Simiae (B Virus) Infection in Monkey Handlers." *Morbidity and Mortality Weekly Report* 36, no. 41 (October 23, 1987): 680+. This article can also be found online at http://www.cdc.gov/mmwr/preview/mmwrhtml/00015936.htm (accessed December 15, 2017).

Huff, Jennifer L., and Peter A. Barry. "B-Virus (*Cercopithecine Herpesvirus* 1) Infection in Humans and Macaques: Potential for Zoonotic Disease." *Emerging Infectious Diseases* 9 (February 2003): 246–250. This article can also be found online at https://wwwnc.cdc.gov/eid/article/9/2/02-0272_article (accessed December 15, 2017).

Kim, W. Ray. "Epidemiology of Hepatitis B in the United States." *Hepatology* 49, no. 5 Suppl. (2009): S28–S34. This article can also be found online at https://www.ncbi.nlm.nih.gov/pmc/articles/PMC3290915/ (accessed December 15, 2017).

Pöhlmann, Stefan, et al. "Herpes B Virus Replication and Viral Lesions in the Liver of a Cynomolgus Macaque Which Died from Severe Disease with Rapid Onset." *Journal of Medical Primatology* 46, no. 5 (October 2017): 256–259.

Websites

"B Virus (Herpes B, Monkey B Virus, Herpesvirus Simiae, and Herpesvirus B)." Centers for Disease Control and Prevention, July 18, 2014. https://www.cdc.gov/herpesbvirus/index.html (accessed December 15, 2017).

"National B Virus Resource Center." Georgia State University. http://www2.gsu.edu/~wwwvir/ (accessed December 15, 2017).

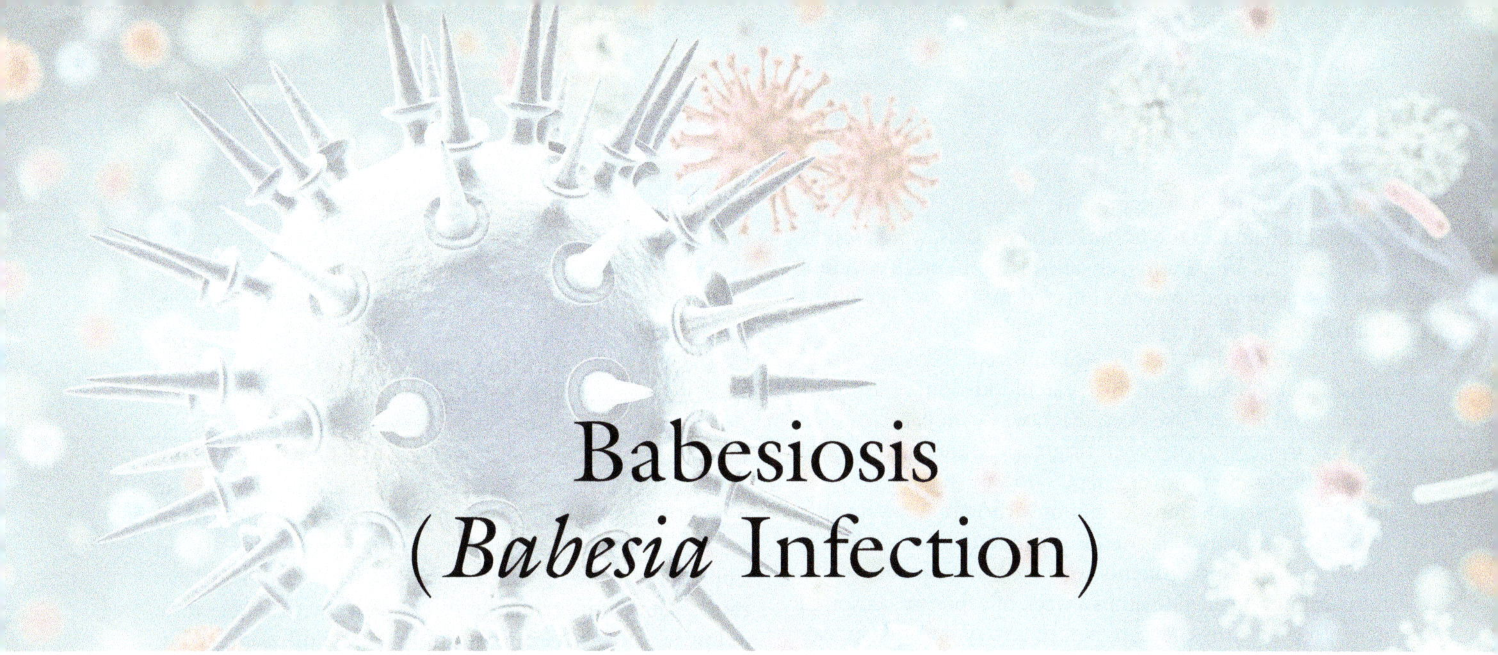

Babesiosis (*Babesia* Infection)

■ Introduction

Babesiosis (bab-EE-see-OH-sis), also known as *Babesia* infection, occurs when humans are bitten by ticks infected with parasites of the genus *Babesia*. Not all *Babesia* infections produce symptoms. When symptoms arise from infection, they usually include fever, chills, muscle aches, and fatigue. In severe cases liver and kidney damage can occur.

Babesiosis was first reported in humans in 1957 and first appeared in the United States in 1969. Because symptoms are either mild or do not arise in individuals with strong immune systems, some people are unaware they are infected. The majority of reported cases occur in people with weakened immune systems.

Babesiosis can be treated using a combination of antibiotics and antiparasitic medications and can be prevented by avoiding tick bites. This is done by covering up bare skin and wearing insect repellent. Advancements in diagnostic technology that identify organisms based on the detection of target regions of their genetic material, including use of the polymerase chain reaction (PCR) technique, have allowed researchers to identify new species of *Babesia* and medical professionals to more definitively diagnose cases of babesiosis.

■ Disease History, Characteristics, and Transmission

Babesiosis was first recognized in humans in 1957 after a Croatian cattle farmer contracted the disease. Prior to that case, babesiosis was thought to affect only animals. Biologist Victor Babes (1854–1926) first discovered the *Babesia* parasite in infected cattle. In 1893 Theobald Smith (1859–1934) and Frederick L. Kilbourne (1858–1936) determined that the parasite was transmitted by ticks, resulting in the disease babesiosis.

Babesiosis was first recorded in the United States in 1969 after an outbreak in Nantucket, Massachusetts. This led to the disease known as Nantucket fever. Since then there have been further outbreaks throughout the United States, mainly in the Northeast. Babesiosis outbreaks have also occurred in parts of Europe.

Babesiosis is caused by several species of parasites belonging to the genus *Babesia*. Although there are a number of species that cause the disease in animals, the most common species that infect humans are *B. microti* and *B. divergens*. The parasite is commonly transmitted from infected animals to humans by blacklegged or deer ticks (*Ixodes scapularis*), the same species that transmits Lyme disease. Infection occurs most commonly between May and October, with the summer months being most active. The ticks feed off infected animals and ingest the parasite.

US Babesiosis Hospital Stays (2011–2014)

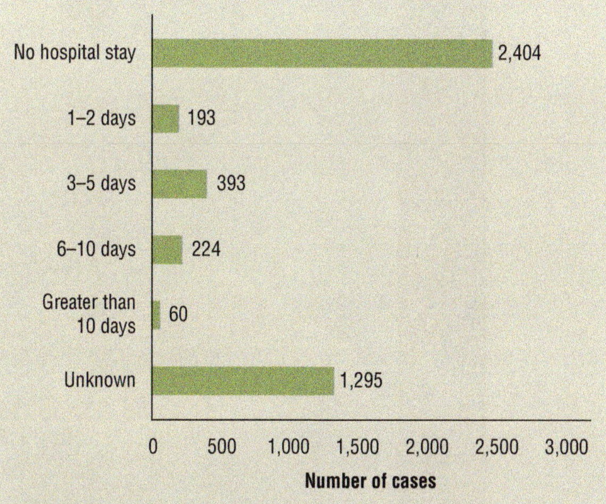

SOURCE: Adapted from "Surveillance for Babesiosis—United States, 2014: Annual Summary." Centers for Disease Control and Prevention. Available from: https://www.cdc.gov/parasites/babesiosis/resources/babesiosis_surveillance_summary_2016.pdf

When a tick bites a human, it transmits the parasite. The parasite then attacks the host's red blood cells, which results in infection. The parasite remains in the bloodstream and can be transmitted from an infected mother to her infant during the course of pregnancy or childbirth.

Babesiosis can also be transmitted through blood transfusions. Because of this risk, blood donors are routinely asked if they have been diagnosed with babesiosis. As of 2017 those who had been diagnosed were blocked from donating blood. However, there is no way to screen donors for the disease, meaning that those who are unaware that they are infected will not be prevented from donating blood. In babesiosis patients who are symptomatic, symptoms commonly begin within a week of exposure, although it may be months or years before any symptoms appear. Common symptoms include fever, chills, sweating, muscle aches, fatigue, an enlarged spleen, and hemolytic anemia.

■ Scope and Distribution

Babesiosis occurs worldwide. It was initially reported predominantly in the United States but is increasingly being reported in Europe, Asia, Africa, and South America. The prevalence of the disease was long underreported in malaria-endemic countries because the clinical presentation is similar to that of malaria and the *Babesia* parasite may be misidentified as *Plasmodium*, the parasite that causes malaria. Advances in identifying the disease and parasite have led to increased reporting in those areas.

In the United States, babesiosis is most common in the northeastern coastal states, including Massachusetts, Connecticut, Rhode Island, and New York. The disease is considered endemic in parts of these states. Babesiosis has also been reported in New Jersey, California, Georgia, Washington, Indiana, and Minnesota. The parasite *B. microti* has been identified as the primary causal agent in the United States, although *B. duncani* has been reported to have caused infections in Washington and California. In Europe the parasite *B. divergens* has been found to have caused infection, primarily in countries with large cattle industries, such as Great Britain, France, and Ireland. *B. divergens* infections have occasionally been identified in Croatia, Sweden, Spain, Portugal, and Switzerland. Although the parasite *B. divergens* has not been identified in the United States, researchers have identified a *B. divergens*–like organism that has caused infections in Missouri, Kentucky, and Washington. PCR also led to the identification of another species of the parasite, *B. venatorum*, which has caused at least three nonfatal cases of babesiosis in Europe.

The majority of babesiosis cases involve people with weak immune systems, such as the elderly, very young children, people with immunodeficiencies, and people whose spleens have been removed. Severe complications such as low blood pressure, liver problems, anemia, and kidney

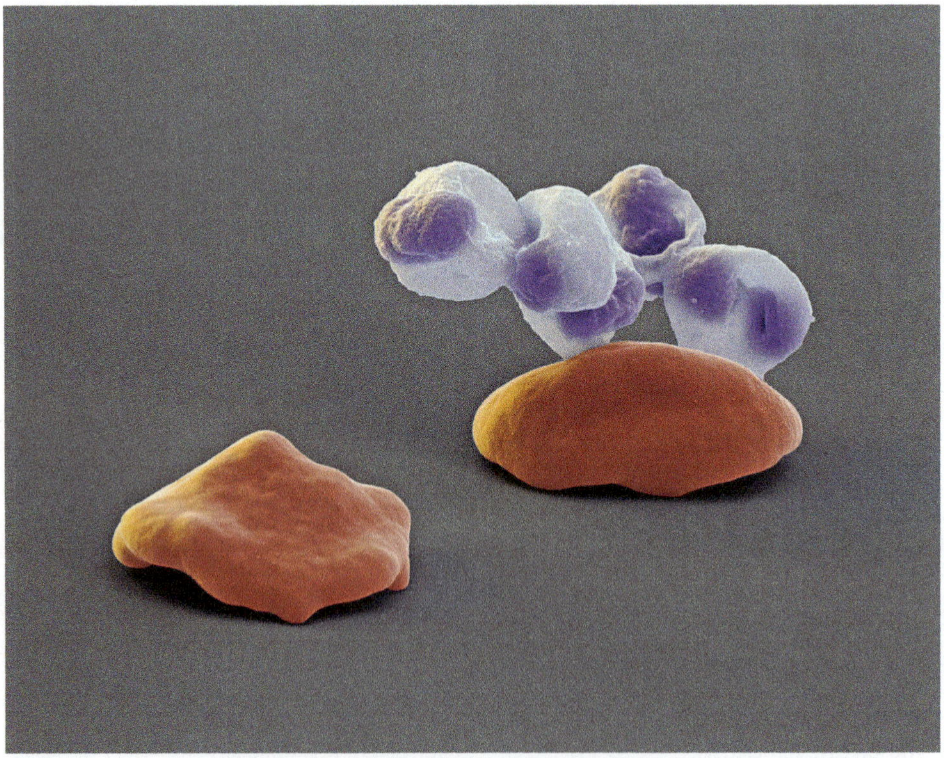

This picture shows five single-celled babesia parasites feeding on a red blood cell. Their feeding will eventually cause the cell to burst and infect other blood cells. *© Eye of Science/Science Source*

failure may occur with this disease. Most people exhibit mild symptoms or show no symptoms at all. Symptoms often go unnoticed so that people are unaware they are infected.

■ Treatment and Prevention

Initially, diagnosis of babesiosis was dependent on identification of *Babesia* parasites in a patient's red blood cells. The PCR technique has since allowed for the identification of *Babesia* DNA in a patient's blood. This technique also identifies the *Babesia* species responsible for the infection. In some cases health providers may send samples to the US Centers for Disease Control and Prevention (CDC) to confirm the diagnosis. Testing for babesiosis is often done in conjunction with testing for other tick-borne diseases, such as Lyme disease and human granulocytic anaplasmosis.

Treatment of babesiosis usually requires removal of the parasites with antiparasitic medications in conjunction with antibiotic therapy. Two treatments are available. The first uses the drugs clindamycin and quinine, but these drugs sometimes are not well tolerated by patients. Another treatment uses the drugs atovaquone and azithromycin. Both treatments have been found to be effective. In some cases, particularly when patients are not symptomatic, no treatment is necessary for the infection to resolve.

No vaccine is available to protect humans from babesiosis. Avoiding contact with ticks is the best way to avoid getting the disease. A variety of measures to avoid tick exposure can be used, including staying away from areas known to be inhabited by ticks, walking in the center of trails, wearing protective clothing (such as socks, long-sleeved shirts, and long pants), and using insect repellents to discourage or kill ticks. Because a tick must remain attached to a human for 36 to 48 hours for the parasite to be transmitted, quick removal of the tick may prevent infection. Therefore, a thorough body check for ticks and the quick removal of any ticks discovered is a wise prevention strategy after any outdoor activity in a tick-infested area. Fine-tipped tweezers are recommended for removing ticks from the body.

WORDS TO KNOW

EMERGING DISEASE A new infectious disease such as severe acute respiratory syndrome (SARS) or West Nile virus, as well as a previously known disease such as malaria, tuberculosis, or bacterial pneumonia that is appearing in a new form that is resistant to drug treatments.

ENDEMIC Present in a particular area or among a particular group of people.

PCR (POLYMERASE CHAIN REACTION) A widely used technique in molecular biology involving the amplification of specific sequences of genomic DNA.

VECTOR Any agent that carries and transmits parasites and diseases. Also, an organism or a chemical used to transport a gene into a new host cell.

■ Impacts and Issues

The most common explanation for the increasing occurrence of babesiosis is an increase in the number of hosts for the parasite. *Babesia* parasites reproduce in mice and other rodents, with the parasites being introduced into the mice while the tick feeds. While deer are not sites for parasite reproduction, they are hosts for adult ticks. As a result, they have an indirect influence on the *Babesia* life cycle because they ensure tick survival. Increased deer populations, particularly in the United States, have resulted in rising populations of ticks. This causes a higher likelihood that the parasite will be transmitted and a higher likelihood of human infection, partially accounting for the increased incidence of babesiosis.

On January 1, 2011, babesiosis became a nationally notifiable disease. This means that health departments in states where the disease is reportable use the National Notifiable Disease Surveillance System to report diagnosed cases to the CDC. By 2014 it was reportable in 31 states. In the United States, there were 1,126 reported cases in 2011, 911 in 2012, 1,761 in 2013, and 1,744 in 2014.

SEE ALSO *Arthropod-Borne Disease; Emerging Infectious Diseases; Host and Vector; Immune Response to Infection; Lyme Disease; Parasitic Diseases*

BIBLIOGRAPHY

Books

Drisdelle, Rosemary. *Parasites: Tales of Humanity's Most Unwelcome Guests.* Berkeley: University of California Press, 2010.

Periodicals

Herwaldt, B. L., et al. "Endemic Babesiosis in Another Eastern State: New Jersey." *Emerging Infectious Diseases* 9 (February 2003): 184–188.

Vannier, Edouard, and Peter J. Krause. "Human Babesiosis." *New England Journal of Medicine* 366 (June 21, 2012): 2397–2407.

Websites

"Babesiosis." Centers for Disease Control and Prevention. https://www.cdc.gov/parasites/babesiosis/ (accessed January 8, 2018).

"Babesiosis." Columbia University Medical Center Lyme and Tick-Borne Diseases Research Center. http://columbia-lyme.org/patients/tbd_babesia.html (accessed January 8, 2018).

"Babesiosis." New York State Department of Health. https://www.health.ny.gov/diseases/communicable/babesiosis/fact_sheet.htm (accessed January 8, 2018).

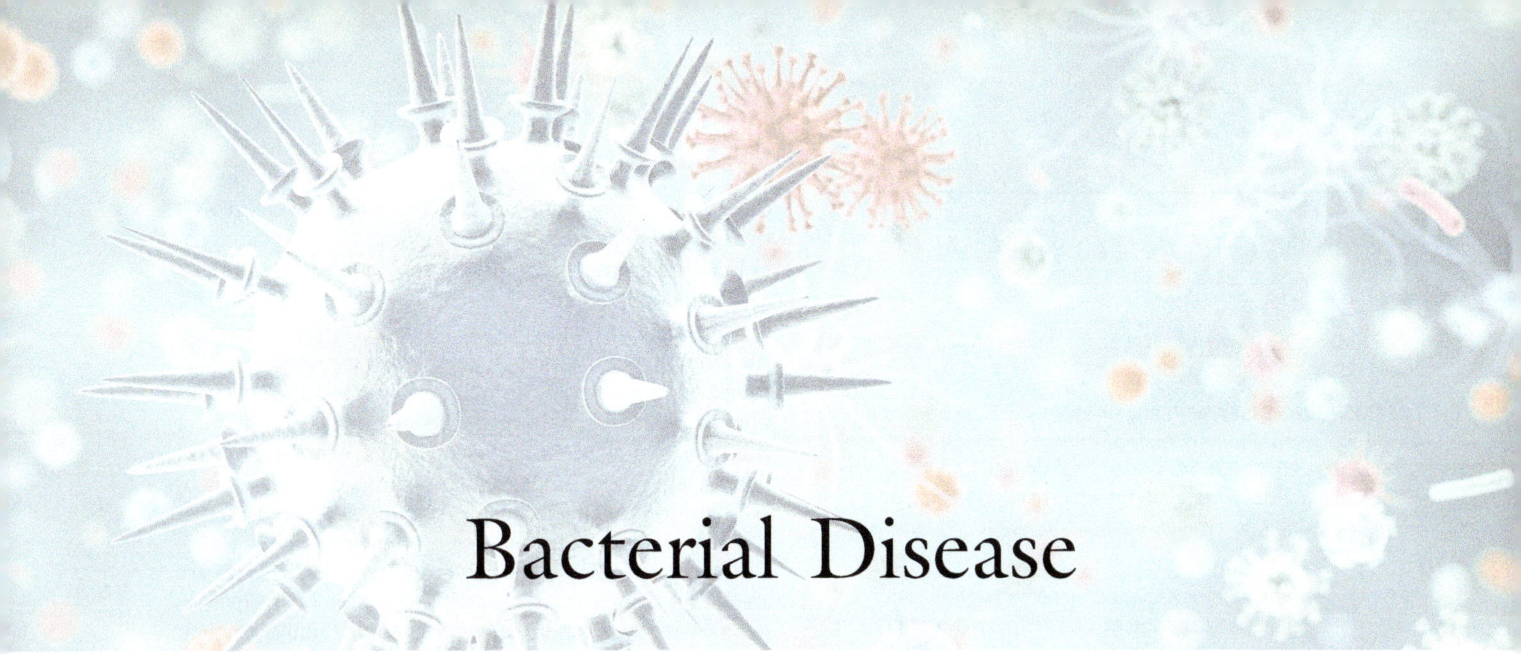

Bacterial Disease

■ Introduction

Bacterial diseases refer to a large variety of diseases caused by bacteria or bacterial components that affect humans, domesticated animals, wildlife, fish, and birds. Most of these diseases are contagious—that is, they can be passed from one member of a species to another member or, in a smaller number of instances, from one species to a different species. Depending on the organism, bacterial disease can be spread in different ways. Examples include contaminated food or water, air currents, infection of an environment that is not normally inhabited by the particular bacterium, and the possession or release of toxins by the bacteria.

■ Disease History, Characteristics, and Transmission

The history and characteristics of bacterial diseases are as varied as the diseases caused. *Bacillus anthracis*, the cause of anthrax, and *Yersinia pestis*, the cause of plague, have been present for millennia. Indeed, references to these diseases can be found in chapters of the Old Testament of the Bible. Other bacterial infections have arisen only recently. One example is the severe diarrheal and potentially kidney-destroying infection caused by the consumption of water or food that is contaminated by *Escherichia coli* strain O157:H7. The effects of

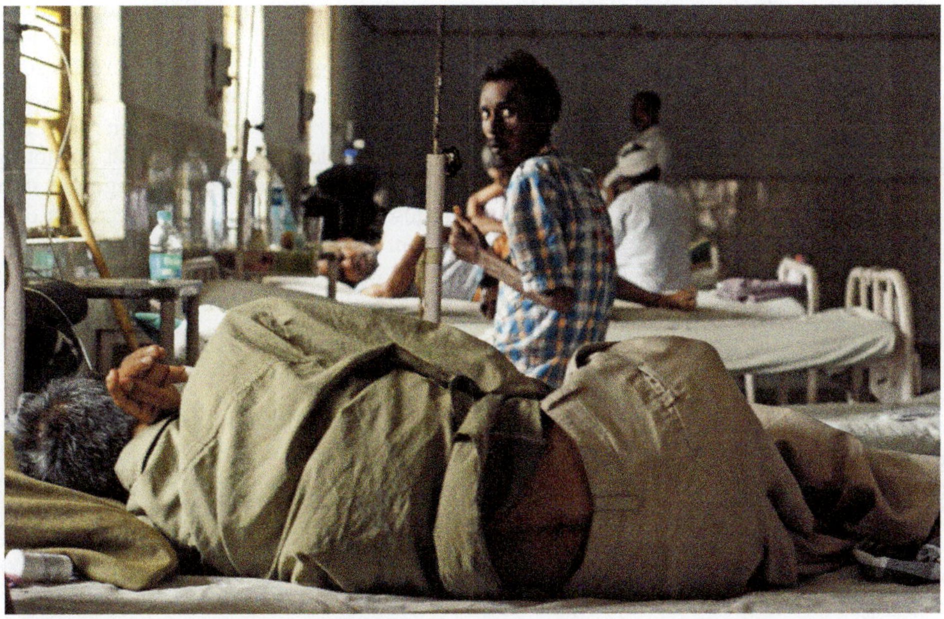

In Ahmedabad, India, in 2007, patients await treatment for tuberculosis, a deadly bacterial disease that has reemerged in the 21st century in multidrug-resistant strains. *© MARINE SIMON/AFP/Getty Images*

WORDS TO KNOW

ANTIBIOTIC RESISTANCE The ability of bacteria to resist the actions of antibiotic drugs.

REEMERGING DISEASE Many diseases once thought to be controlled are reappearing to infect humans again. These are known as reemerging diseases because they have not been common for a long period of time and are starting to appear again among large population groups.

SPORE A dormant form assumed by some bacteria, such as anthrax, that enables the bacterium to survive high temperatures, dryness, and lack of nourishment for long periods of time. Under proper conditions, the spore may revert to the actively multiplying form of the bacteria.

O157:H7 are due to a cell-damaging toxin that can be released by the bacteria. Scientists who have studied this bacterium argue that the strain arose in the 1970s when *E. coli* residing in the intestinal tract (their normal environment) acquired genetic material that coded for the production of a destructive toxin from related bacteria, *Shigella*.

Some bacterial diseases depend on the number of infecting bacteria present and, therefore, are related to the growth of the bacteria. One example is the intestinal upset, diarrhea, and vomiting that results from the growth of *Campylobacter* following the ingestion of contaminated food or water. Poultry is a particularly important source of this infection because the bacterium is a normal inhabitant of the intestinal tract of poultry. Release of intestinal contents during slaughter contaminates over 50 percent of the poultry sold each year in the United States, according to the US Food and Drug Administration. The symptoms of *Campylobacter* can take a few days to develop, as the bacteria need time to reach sufficient numbers in the intestinal tract.

Other bacterial infections, particularly those involving toxins, require the presence of only a few bacteria, and growth of the bacteria is not necessary to produce the disease if the toxin has already been produced when the bacteria are ingested.

Bacterial diseases also vary in their methods of establishing infection. Some bacteria readily cause infections because they are contagious—they can be easily passed from person to person or can be easily spread to humans via a vector (another organism that transmits the bacteria from their normal host to a susceptible recipient). An example of a contagious bacterial disease is plague, which is caused by *Yesinia pestis* and which is passed to people via the bite of an infected flea. Throughout history plague has claimed millions of lives. In contrast, other bacteria cause infections opportunistically—that is, they are not normally infectious but can cause disease under certain circumstances. An example is *Pseudomonas aeruginosa*, a species normally found in soil that is normally of little consequence to humans. However, in burn victims, the organism can infect the damaged skin. In addition, people who have cystic fibrosis and whose lungs contain deposits of a thick mucus can be susceptible to recurring *P. aeruginosa* infections that can progressively compromise lung function.

Another means by which a few types of bacteria are able to cause infection is via their production of an environmentally hardy structure known as a spore. Similar to plant spores, bacterial spores are designed to help a bacterium survive tough environmental challenges, which can include temperatures that are too high or low for growth and lack of moisture. In a more hospitable environment, the spore can germinate, and bacterial growth and division will resume. Bacteria in the genus *Bacillus* can form spores and, when they germinate, cause disease. A well-known example is *B. anthracis*, which causes anthrax. Inhalation of only about 10 spores can be sufficient to cause pulmonary anthrax.

Bacterial diseases can be caused by bacteria that have become resistant to antibiotics used to treat them. Examples include methicillin-resistant *Staphylococcus aureus* (MRSA), carbapenem-resistant *Enterobacteriaceae* (CRE), and vancomycin-resistant *Enterococci* (VRE)

Scope and Distribution

Bacterial disease occurs virtually worldwide, with the exceptions of the North Pole and South Pole and at very high altitudes. Even temperate waters can harbor disease-causing (pathogenic) bacteria, such as *Vibrio cholerae*, the cause of cholera.

Helicobacter pylori is a resident in the stomach of about half of all people in the world. Most do not become sick. However, the bacterium can damage the stomach lining and cause ulcers. Antibiotics are effective at eliminating the infection.

Vaccine-Preventable Bacterial Diseases in the Post-Vaccine Era

Disease	Deaths	Year
Diphtheria	2,500	2011
Haemophilus influenzae type b disease	199,000	2008
Neonatal tetanus	59,000	2008
Pertussis	195,000	2008
Pneumococcal disease	476,000	2008
Tetanus	63,000	2008

SOURCE: World Health Organization.

Treatment and Prevention

Antibiotics are the standard treatment for bacterial infections caused by organisms sensitive to their actions. The type of antibiotic and the concentration required to kill the target bacteria depend on the organism. Frequently, bacteria develop resistance to a variety of antibiotics. Vaccines continue to be a valuable means of preventing bacterial diseases, such as diphtheria, meningococcal disease, and pertussis (whooping cough).

Bacterial diseases can be prevented in a variety of ways. Avoiding the source of the organism (for example, not drinking contaminated water), practicing good hygiene such as regular handwashing with an antibacterial soap, and maintaining a balanced and healthy diet to keep the body's immune system efficient are a few examples of good preventive measures.

Impacts and Issues

Bacterial diseases have been responsible for countless millions of deaths and continue to be a significant problem. In the late 20th century, it was thought that many bacterial infections had been brought under control with the discovery or synthesis of a variety of effective antibiotics. However, this optimism has been short-lived. Antibiotic resistance is looming as one of the great medical challenges of the 21st century. As of 2017 vaccines are available for tuberculosis, diphtheria, whooping cough, tetanus, *Haemophilus influenzae* type B, cholera, typhoid, and bacterial pneumonia.

While progress is being made to lessen the occurrence of some bacterial diseases, the threat posed by the deliberate malicious use of disease-causing bacteria remains. Biological warfare has been practiced for centuries. In the 20th century a number of countries, including the United States, experimented with the use of bacteria as a weapon. In the early 21st century, this threat has moved from governments to organizations and individuals.

The specter of bioterrorism and the often-frenzied reporting of bacterial disease outbreaks has spawned a growing apprehension in many people about diseases that are, in fact, not common. For example, the fear of the bacteria that cause necrotizing fasciitis, termed the "flesh-eating bacteria" by the media, is out of proportion to the handful of cases that occur in North America each year.

A more realistic concern is the emergence or reemergence of bacterial diseases that do pose a health threat. One example is the reemergence of tuberculosis. The emerging strains are also more antibiotic resistant than their predecessors. In developing nations, multidrug-resistant tuberculosis and extremely drug-resistant tuberculosis are considered an emergency by agencies such as the World Health Organization (WHO). WHO and other agencies, including the US Centers for Disease Control and Prevention, have spearheaded surveillance and notification campaigns designed to detect and respond rapidly to such outbreaks.

SEE ALSO *Airborne Precautions; Antibiotic Resistance; Bioterrorism; Climate Change and Infectious Disease; Culture and Sensitivity; Emerging Infectious Diseases; Vaccines and Vaccine Development*

BIBLIOGRAPHY

Books

Henderson, Cary G., ed. Enterococci *and Bacterial Diseases: Risk Factors, Molecular Biology and Antibiotic Resistance.* Hauppauge, NY: Nova Science, 2017.

Kudva, Indira T., et al., eds. *Virulence Mechanisms of Bacterial Pathogens.* Washington, DC: ASM, 2016.

Periodicals

Cabral, Maria P., et al. "Design of Live Attenuated Bacterial Vaccines Based on D-Glutamate Auxotrophy." *Nature Communications* 8 (May 2017).

Websites

"Antibiotic/Antimicrobial Resistance." Centers for Disease Control and Prevention. https://www.cdc.gov/drugresistance/index.html (accessed November 14, 2017).

Brian Hoyle

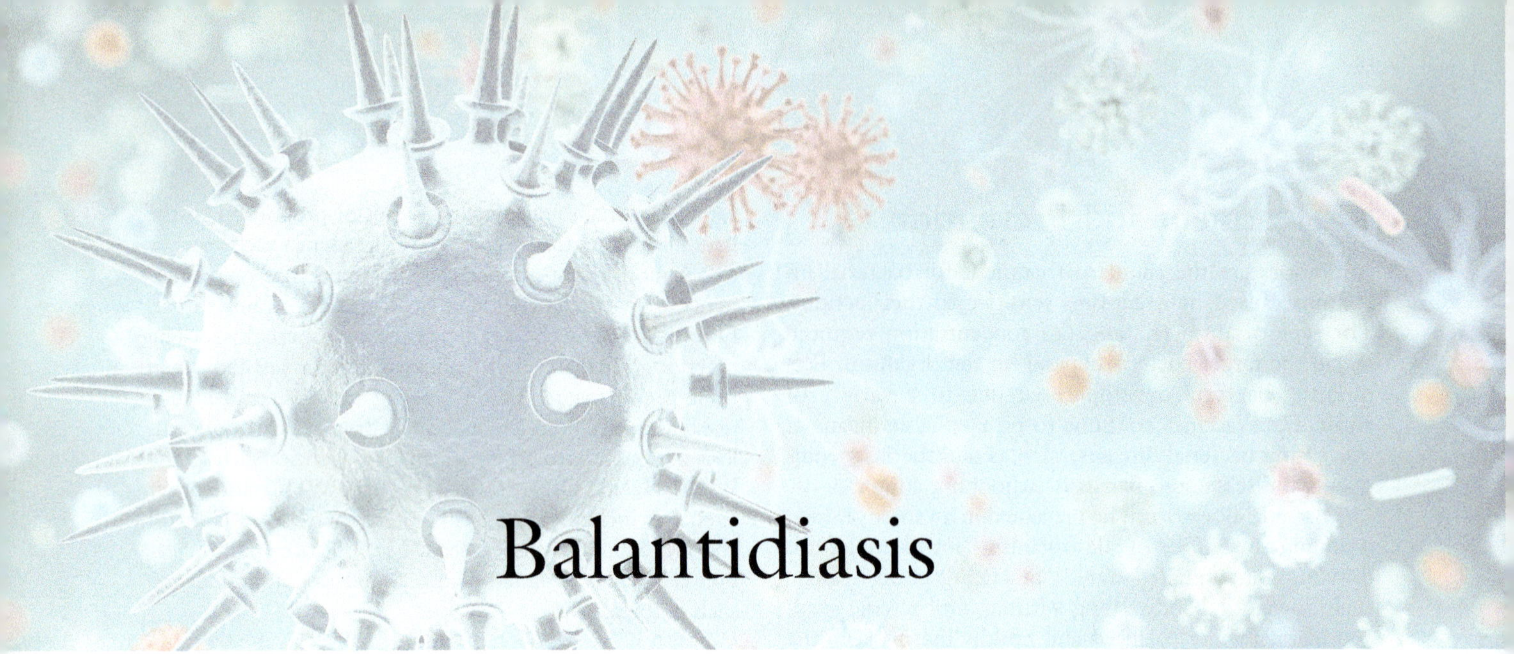

Balantidiasis

■ Introduction

Balantidiasis (ba-lan-ti-DYE-a-sis) is an intestinal infection caused by ingestion of the protozoan parasite *Balantidium coli.* The parasite is transmitted from animal reservoirs to humans by oral contact with fecal matter. This transmission occurs when unwashed food or unclean water is ingested or if hands are not washed after handling animals. While balantidiasis infection is rare, and most cases are asymptomatic, some cases result in diarrhea, dysentery, colitis, abdominal pain, weight loss, and death. Treatment is effective and involves a short course of antibiotics, which eradicates the parasite.

Balantidiasis occurs worldwide but is more common in areas where humans live in close contact with livestock and particularly in areas with poor sanitation or other health problems. Infection is best prevented by treating water, washing food and hands, and reducing contact with livestock. Improving community sanitation standards, as well as educating communities about the importance of sanitation, can also help reduce infection.

■ Disease History, Characteristics, and Transmission

Balantidiasis is an intestinal infection caused by the parasite *Balantidium coli.* Humans are infected when they ingest *B. coli* cysts—immobile, protected forms of the parasite. Once in the body, these cysts break open and a

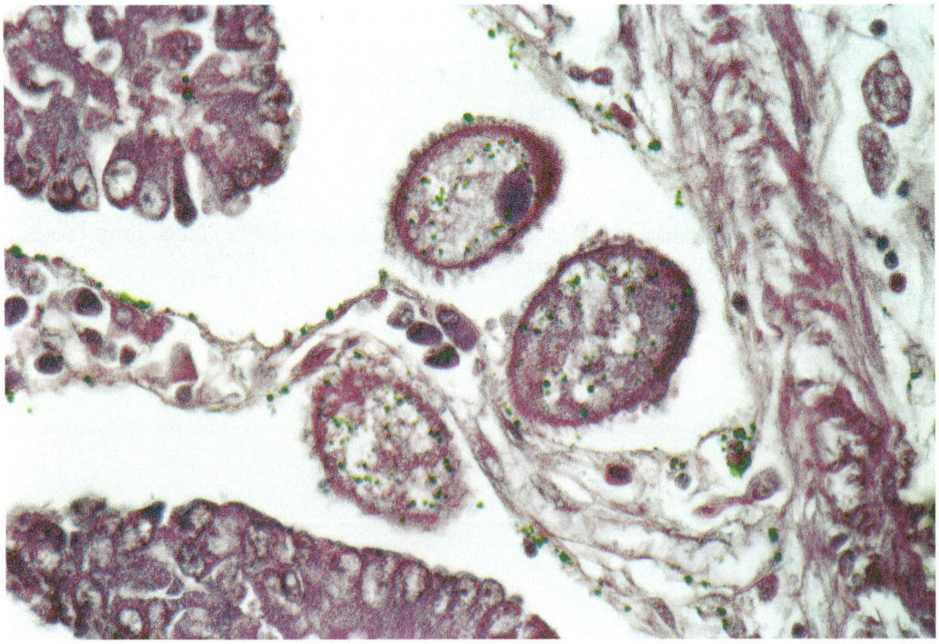

Balantidium coli, shown here, is the protozoan parasite that causes balantidiasis. *© Michael Abbey/Science Source*

mobile stage called a trophozoite is released. The trophozoite feeds on bacteria within the intestine or enters the intestinal lining and secretes a tissue-destroying substance. As a result, sores (ulcers) and abscesses develop in the intestinal lining. New cysts are formed by the trophozoites and are excreted from the body in the feces. The cysts are well protected and can remain outside the body under favorable conditions for many weeks.

B. coli are transmitted to humans from animal reservoirs such as livestock, rodents, and non-human primates. The most common reservoirs are pigs, which are often infected with *B. coli*, but tend to be asymptomatic. Transmission occurs when humans ingest food or water contaminated with the feces of infected animals or when the mouth comes in contact with something contaminated with feces, such as unwashed hands.

Balantidiasis infection is uncommon in humans, and most cases are asymptomatic. However, asymptomatic humans are still capable of spreading the infection. When symptoms do appear, the most common are diarrhea, dysentery, abdominal cramps, and inflammation of the colon. In severe cases, perforation of the intestinal wall may occur, which can be fatal.

WORDS TO KNOW

RESERVOIR The animal or organism in which a virus or parasite normally resides.

TROPHOZOITE The amoeboid, vegetative stage of the malaria protozoa.

Scope and Distribution

Balantidiasis infection occurs worldwide, although it is more common in tropical and subtropical regions, as well as in developing countries. It also is more common in regions where livestock, particularly pigs, are kept in conjunction with poor water systems and poor sanitation. Bolivia, Brazil, the Philippines, southern Iran, and Papua New Guinea have all had outbreaks of balantidiasis. Infection rates are similar for males and females.

Treatment and Prevention

Balantidiasis is usually diagnosed through detection of *B. coli* in a stool sample from the patient. It can also be diagnosed by examining samples collected by scraping intestinal ulcers to detect trophozoites. Treatment of balantidiasis is usually effective and is administered to both symptomatic and asymptomatic patients. Asymptomatic patients are treated to prevent them from spreading infection to others. Symptomatic patients are treated because untreated balantidiasis can become chronic and lead to dehydration, abdominal bleeding, and perforation of the intestinal wall, any of which—left untreated—can be fatal. Treatment usually involves oral administration of one of the following antibiotics: tetracycline, metronidazole, and iodoquinol. Tetracycline is the treatment of choice, but it is not recommended for pregnant women and children under the age of eight.

The most effective methods to prevent infection by *B. coli* involve improving sanitation. This includes boiling contaminated water prior to using it, washing hands after handling pigs or using the toilet, effectively washing and cooking food prior to eating, and preventing water sources from coming into contact with animal and human feces. As the most common mode of infection is from pigs to humans, reducing contact between pigs and humans will reduce infection. This can be achieved by preventing pigs from sharing human water sources, washing hands after handling pigs, and putting up barriers between pig and human living areas.

Impacts and Issues

Balantidiasis infection most commonly occurs in communities in which sanitation is poor. This situation often arises due to a lack of resources to provide adequate sanitation, as well as a lack of education about sanitary living. Infections by the parasite *B. coli* have also been found to cause more severe infection in people who are already debilitated. This may be due to malnourishment, coinciding parasitic infections, or a weakened immune system.

Efforts to improve sanitation and health in communities may lead to a reduction in the prevalence of infection. Installing hygienic measures such as potable water sources, toilets separate from living areas, and separate housing for livestock and humans will greatly reduce the likelihood of transmission of *B. coli* between animals and humans. In addition, educating people on the risks associated with poor hygiene may also help prevent transmission. Addressing other health issues within communities, such as coexisting parasitic infections and malnourishment, will help improve the overall health of the community and will aid in reducing the severity of any infections that do occur.

See Also *Dysentery; Handwashing; Parasitic Diseases; Sanitation*

BIBLIOGRAPHY

Books

Bennett, John E., Raphael Dolin, and Martin J. Blaser, eds. *Principles and Practice of Infectious Diseases.* Vol. 2. Philadelphia: Elsevier, 2015.

Engelkirk, Paul G., and Janet Duben-Engelkirk. *Laboratory Diagnosis of Infectious Diseases: Essentials of Diagnostic Microbiology*. Baltimore: Lippincott Williams & Wilkins, 2008.

Periodicals

Schuster, F.L., and L. Ramirez-Avila. "Current World Status of *Balantidium coli*." *Clinical Microbiology Reviews* 21, no. 4 (October 2008): 626–638. this article can also be found online at http://cmr.asm.org/content/21/4/626.full (accessed November 10, 2017).

Websites

"Balantidiasis." National Organization for Rare Disorders (NORD). https://rarediseases.org/rare-diseases/balantidiasis/ (accessed November 10, 2017).

"Parasites—Balantidiasis (also known as Balantidium coli infection)." Centers for Disease Control and Prevention. https://www.cdc.gov/parasites/balantidium/ (accessed November 10, 2017).

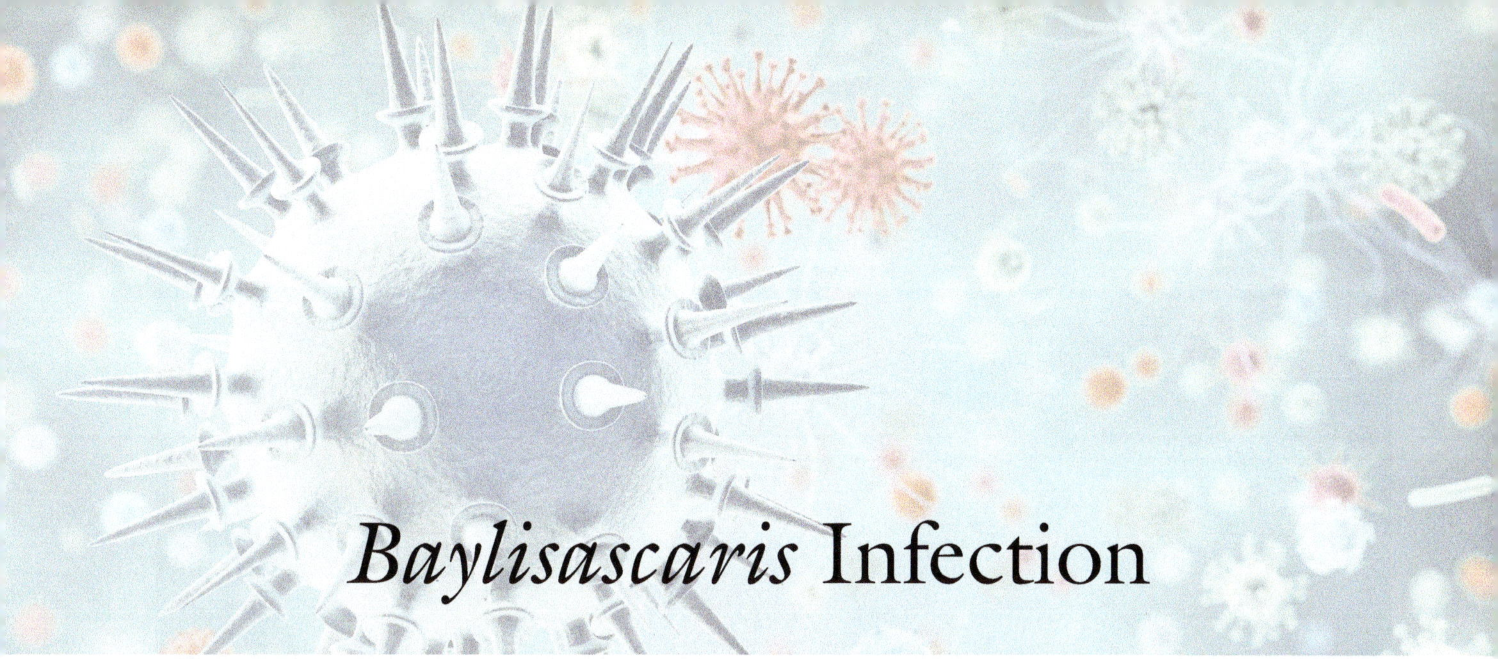

Baylisascaris Infection

■ Introduction

Baylisascaris (bay-liss-AS-kuh-ris) is an intestinal infection caused by the *Baylisascaris procyonis* larvae of roundworms that infect raccoons, their primary host. According to the US Centers for Disease Control and Prevention (CDC), the infection has also been diagnosed as secondarily infecting more than 90 animal species, both domesticated and wild, including birds, mice, rabbits, and humans. Initially, raccoon roundworms grow within the intestine of raccoons. Millions of microscopic eggs produced by the mature worms are passed with the raccoon's feces. The raccoon is not generally affected by being infested with the worms. However, infestation inside humans may cause serious illness or death.

Generally, two to four weeks after being released into the environment through the feces, the eggs are considered infectious to animals and humans. The group of large raccoon roundworms is a very robust species that can survive environments such as harsh cold and hot temperatures. With enough moisture, *Baylisascaris procyonis* can survive for years.

■ Disease History, Characteristics, and Transmission

According to the CDC, the first human fatality in the United States due to *Baylisascaris* occurred in 1984 and involved a ten-month-old infant living in rural Pennsylvania.

Common characteristics of adult *Baylisascaris* worms include a length of 5 to 8 inches (13 to 20 centimeters) and a width of about 0.5 inches (1.3 centimeters). The worm is whitish-tan in color and has a cylindrically shaped body that narrows at both ends.

Human transmission occurs when infective eggs in water are consumed or upon contact with soil or objects contaminated with egg-containing raccoon feces. Upon ingestion, eggs hatch into larvae within the intestines. They travel throughout the body, often affecting the muscles and organs, especially the brain.

Symptoms generally take from two to three weeks to appear, up to a maximum of two months. Common symptoms include skin irritations, nausea, tiredness, lack of muscle control, and inability to focus. More severe symptoms include brain and eye damage, liver enlargement, loss of muscle control, blindness, and coma. Death can occur.

Symptom severity depends on the number of eggs ingested and where the larvae spread. Approximately several thousand eggs are needed to cause infection. A few eggs cause little or no symptoms, while large numbers can cause serious problems.

Raccoons are infected in two ways. In the direct cycle, raccoons, especially young raccoons, ingest the *Baylisascaris* eggs while feeding and grooming. In the indirect cycle,

WORDS TO KNOW

HELMINTH A representative of various phyla of wormlike animals.

HOST An organism that serves as the habitat for a parasite or possibly for a symbiont. A host may provide nutrition to the parasite or symbiont, or it may simply provide a place in which to live.

INTERMEDIATE HOST An organism infected by a parasite while the parasite is in a developmental, not sexually mature form.

ZOONOSES Diseases of microbiological origin that can be transmitted from animals to people. The causes of the disease may be bacteria, viruses, parasites, or fungi.

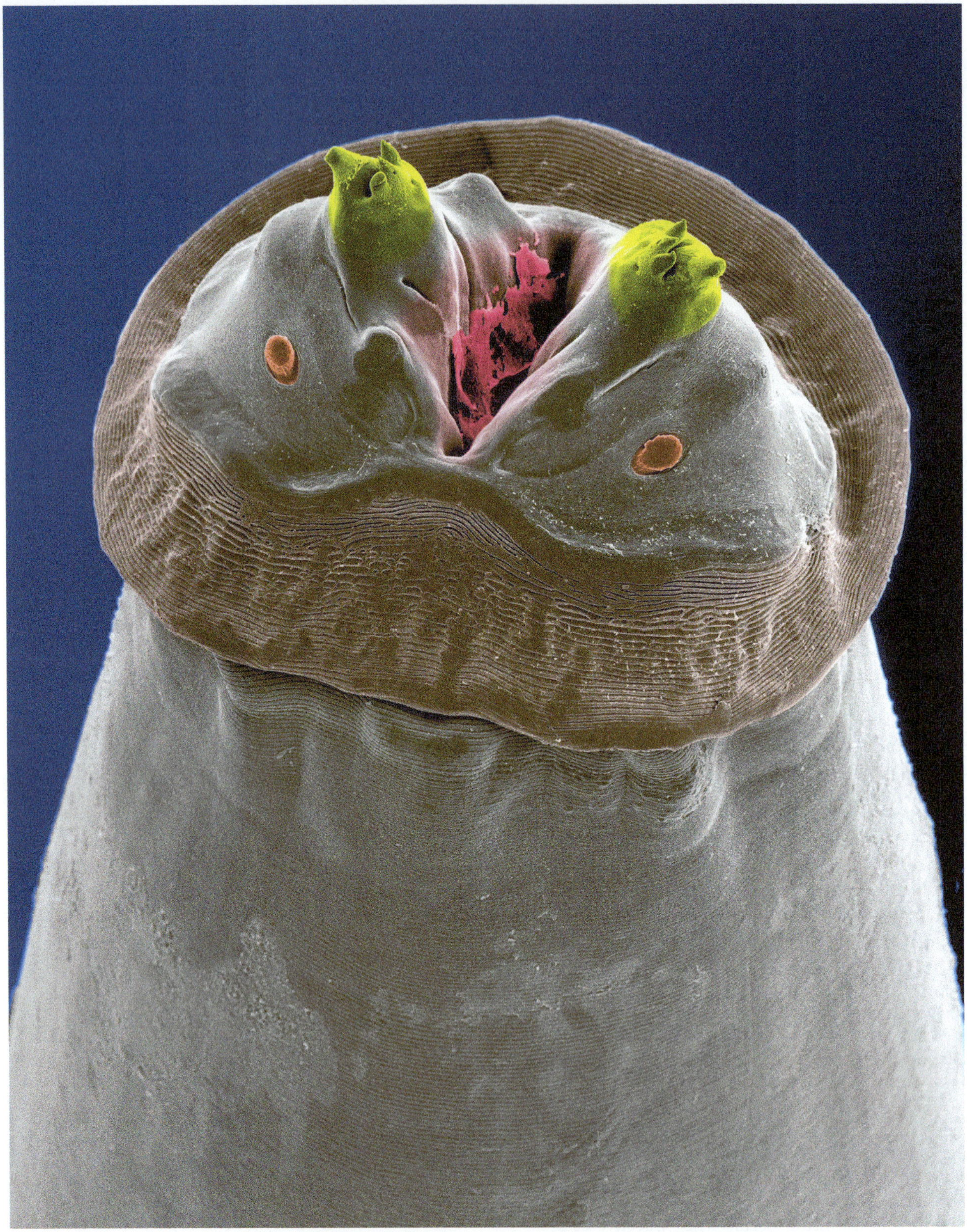

A colored scanning electron micrograph (SEM) of *Baylisascaris procyonis*, a roundworm found in the intestines of raccoons. Pictured here is a parasite's mouth region that attaches to the intestinal wall. *© Dennis Kunkel Microscopy/Science Source*

eggs are eaten by intermediate hosts such as armadillos, birds, chipmunks, dogs, mice, rabbits, and squirrels. Within the host, the eggs hatch, and the larvae travel into the intestines, liver, and lungs and, later, into the head, neck, or chest. Adult raccoons then eat the intermediate host, and the *Baylisascaris* larvae are released and sent to the intestine to mature.

There are usually no outward symptoms visible when raccoons are infected. Symptoms can be observed, however, when intermediate hosts are infected. When in their brains, larvae can cause behavioral changes, destroy the brain, or kill the host. Early symptoms include awkwardness in walking and climbing, sight problems, and a tilting head. Later symptoms include loss of fear of humans; behaviors such as rolling on the ground, laying on one side, and feet paddling; and finally a comatose state and death.

Scope and Distribution

Raccoons are commonly found throughout the United States. Through the end of the 20th century, the occurrence of *Baylisascaris* infection was largely isolated within the Midwest, the Northeast, the Middle Atlantic, and the West Coast. However, beginning in 2002 cases were documented in states such as Florida and Georgia. According to Anita D. Sircar and coauthors of a 2016 study published in *Morbidity and Mortality Weekly Report*, the expansion of *Baylisascaris* to new geographic areas likely indicated an increase in human exposure to infection. However, as of 2017, increased exposure had not led to a significant rise in reports of human infection.

Treatment and Prevention

Baylisascaris can infect humans who come into contact with animal feces and do not properly wash their hands. Careful decontamination procedures after contact can aid in prevention. Dark, tubular droppings with a strong odor may continue to harbor infectious larvae even after months, as larvae can survive severe heat and cold, as well as harsh chemicals.

To disinfect contaminated areas, feces should be immediately buried, burned, or isolated in a landfill. Wearing gloves, a face mask, and protective clothing can prevent further contamination. Known infected surfaces should be cleaned with high temperatures, such as with boiling water, or treated with strong disinfectants. Feeding and interacting with stray raccoons should also be avoided.

It is difficult to diagnose *Baylisascaris* infection. Medical professionals often first eliminate other infections with similar symptoms. There are no known treatments to lessen the illness.

As of 2017 there was no definitive commercial serologic (blood) test to diagnose the infection. Drugs and vaccines were not available to effectively kill larvae. Laser surgery has been successful in killing larvae within the eyes. However, damage already present is likely permanent.

HIDDEN DANGERS OF TREATING WILD ANIMALS AS PETS

The most effective way to prevent *Baylisascaris* infection is to avoid the primary host of *Baylisascaris procyonis* roundworms: raccoons. Raccoons are native to North America and are common throughout much of the United States, in both rural and dense urban areas. Due to their adaptability, it can be difficult to discourage racoons from inhabiting areas near people's homes. The U.S. Centers for Disease Control and Prevention (CDC) recommends a number of measures to discourage raccoons from entering backyards or homes, where they are likely to spread *Baylisascaris*-carrying feces.

The most important precaution is to treat raccoons as what they are: wild animals, not pets. This means never feeding raccoons or keeping them as pets. Homeowners should instead stop raccoons from scavenging for food and finding places to den by keeping garbage cans tightly shut; ensuring basements, crawl spaces, and attics are inaccessible; covering sandboxes; eliminating fishponds and bird feeders; and cleaning up outdoor areas where raccoons might den, such as in dense brush.

Impacts and Issues

Baylisascaris infection is an emerging helminthic zoonosis (an increasingly common worm infection acquired from animals) and therefore a growing public health concern. Due to increased human encroachment into raccoon habitat, raccoons have had increasing contact with humans, which exacerbates the problem.

People most likely to become infected include children and persons who spend more time outdoors than other groups and are therefore more likely to swallow infected substances. Hikers, taxidermists, veterinarians, trappers, wildlife handlers, and other similar groups who spend large amounts of time outdoors near raccoons and their habitats are also at increased risk.

According to the CDC, exposure and infection rates are likely much larger in humans than is medically reported. Rates of infection have been widely found in the United States to be up to 82 percent in adults in the American Midwest, Northeast, and West Coast and 93.5 percent in juveniles, according to a report by Charles E. Gilbert for the Epidemiology and Toxicology Institute. Many veterinarians advise against keeping raccoons as pets due to the high rate of roundworm infection in raccoons. One adult female worm can produce hundreds of thousands of eggs daily, and an infected raccoon can deposit as many as 45 million eggs each day.

Raccoons are among the most common wild animals in the United States. Their proximity to humans makes *Baylisascaris* infection a potentially major infectious disease. However, as of 2017 the prevalence of infection in the US population was not known, and its identity as a growing public health problem was underrecognized.

Due to several factors, including the low infective dose, the wide availability of the host (raccoons), and the lack of a definitive, effective treatment for human infection, *Baylisascaris procyonis* is considered a potential agent of bioterrorism.

See Also *Handwashing; Host and Vector; Public Health and Infectious Disease; Roundworm (Ascariasis) Infection*

BIBLIOGRAPHY

Books

Scheld, W. Michael, et al. *Infections of the Central Nervous System.* 4th ed. Philadelphia: Wolters Kluwer Health, 2014.

Periodicals

Fernandez, Sonia. “Undetected Infection: Raccoon Roundworm—a Hidden Human Parasite?” *Current* (July 24, 2017). This article can also be found online at http://www.news.ucsb.edu/2017/018138/undetected-infection (accessed December 17, 2017).

Gompper, Matthew E., and Amber N. Wright. “Altered Prevalence of Raccoon Roundworm (*Baylisascaris procyonis*) Owing to Manipulated Contact Rates of Hosts.” *Journal of Zoology* 266, no. 2 (June 2005): 215–219.

Kreston, Rebecca. “Baylisascariasis! The Tragic Parasitic Implications of Raccoons in Your Backyard.” *Discover* (March 29, 2012). This article can also be found online at http://blogs.discovermagazine.com/bodyhorrors/2012/03/29/baylisascariasis/#.WjgSkFQ-dN1 (accessed December 17, 2017).

Sircar, Anita D., et al. “Raccoon Roundworm Infection Associated with Central Nervous System Disease and Ocular Disease.” *Morbidity and Mortality Weekly Report* 65, no. 35 (September 9, 2016): 930–933. This article can also be found online at https://www.cdc.gov/mmwr/volumes/65/wr/mm6535a2.htm (accessed December 17, 2017).

Young, Bob. “King County Toddler May Have Rare Disease Linked to Roundworms Found in Raccoon Droppings.” *Seattle Times* (May 8, 2017). This article can also be found online at https://www.seattletimes.com/seattle-news/health/king-county-toddler-may-have-rare-disease-linked-to-roundworms-found-in-raccoon-droppings/ (accessed December 17, 2017).

Websites

“Baylisascaris Infection.” Centers for Disease Control and Prevention. https://www.cdc.gov/parasites/baylisascaris/ (accessed December 17, 2017).

Gilbert, Charles E. “Concern with Communicable (Infectious) Diseases of Raccoons.” Epidemiology and Toxicology Institute. http://www.epidemiologyandtoxicology.org/raccoons.html (accessed December 17, 2017).

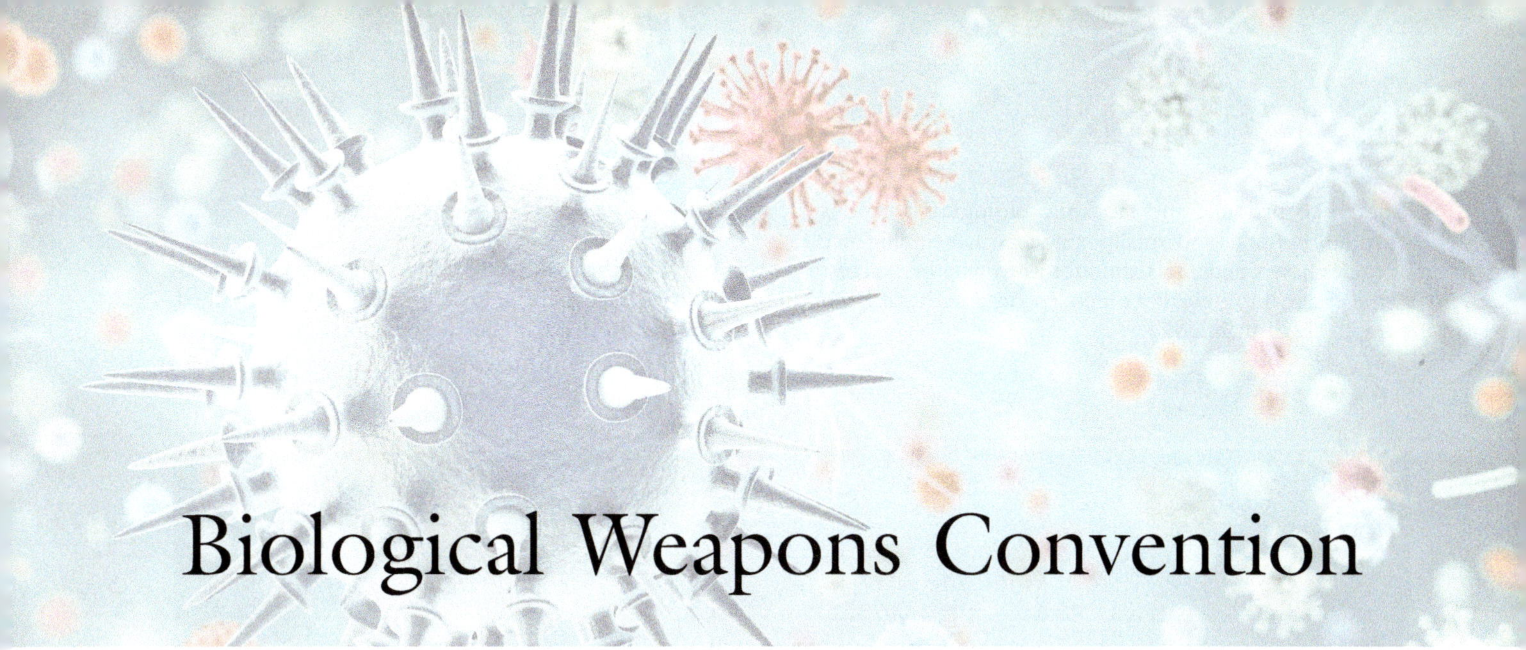

Biological Weapons Convention

Introduction

The Biological Weapons Convention (BWC), more properly but less widely known as the Convention on the Prohibition of the Development, Production and Stockpiling of Bacteriological (Biological) and Toxin Weapons and on Their Destruction, is an international agreement that prohibits the development and stockpiling of biological weapons. The language of the BWC, drafted in 1972, describes biological weapons as "repugnant to the conscience of mankind."

History and Scientific Foundations

The BWC broadly prohibits the development of pathogens and biological toxins that do not serve a protective immunological role, have beneficial industrial use, or prove useful in medical treatment.

The BWC prohibits the offensive weaponization of biological agents such as anthrax spores. It also prohibits the transformation of biological agents with established, legitimate, and sanctioned purposes into agents of a nature and quality that could be used to effectively induce illness or death. In addition to offensive weaponization of microorganisms or toxins, prohibited research procedures include concentrating a strain of bacterium or virus and altering the size of aggregations of potentially harmful biologic agents, such as by refining anthrax spores to sizes small enough to be widely carried in air currents. The BWC also prohibits producing strains capable of withstanding normally adverse environmental conditions, such as disbursement from a weapons blast, and the manipulation of other factors that make biologic agents effective weapons.

In 1969 the United States renounced by executive order the first use of biological weapons and restricted future weapons research programs to issues concerning defensive responses, such as immunization and detection.

Applications and Research

Although the BWC disarmament provisions stipulated that biological weapons stockpiles were to have been destroyed by 1975, most Western intelligence agencies openly questioned whether all stockpiles were in fact destroyed. For example, even though it was a signatory party to the 1972 BWC, the former Soviet Union maintained a well-funded and high-intensity biological weapons program throughout the 1970s and 1980s that

WORDS TO KNOW

BACTERIUM A single-celled microorganism. Plural: *bacteria.*

EXECUTIVE ORDER Presidential orders that implement or interpret a federal statute, administrative policy, or treaty.

PATHOGEN A disease-causing agent, such as a bacterium, a virus, a fungus, or another microorganism.

SPORE A dormant form assumed by some bacteria, such as anthrax, that enable the bacterium to survive high temperatures, dryness, and lack of nourishment for long periods. Under proper conditions, the spore may revert to the actively multiplying form of the bacteria.

STRAIN A subclass or a specific genetic variation of an organism.

TOXIN A poison produced by a living organism.

WEAPONIZATION The use of any bacterium, virus, or other disease-causing organism as a weapon of war. Among other terms, it is also called germ warfare, biological weaponry, and biological warfare.

worked to produce and stockpile biological weapons including anthrax and smallpox agents. US intelligence agencies have openly raised doubt as to whether successor Russian biological weapons programs have been completely dismantled.

Impacts and Issues

According to the United Nations Office at Geneva, as of January 2018 there were 180 countries recognized as parties to the BWC. The latest country to become a

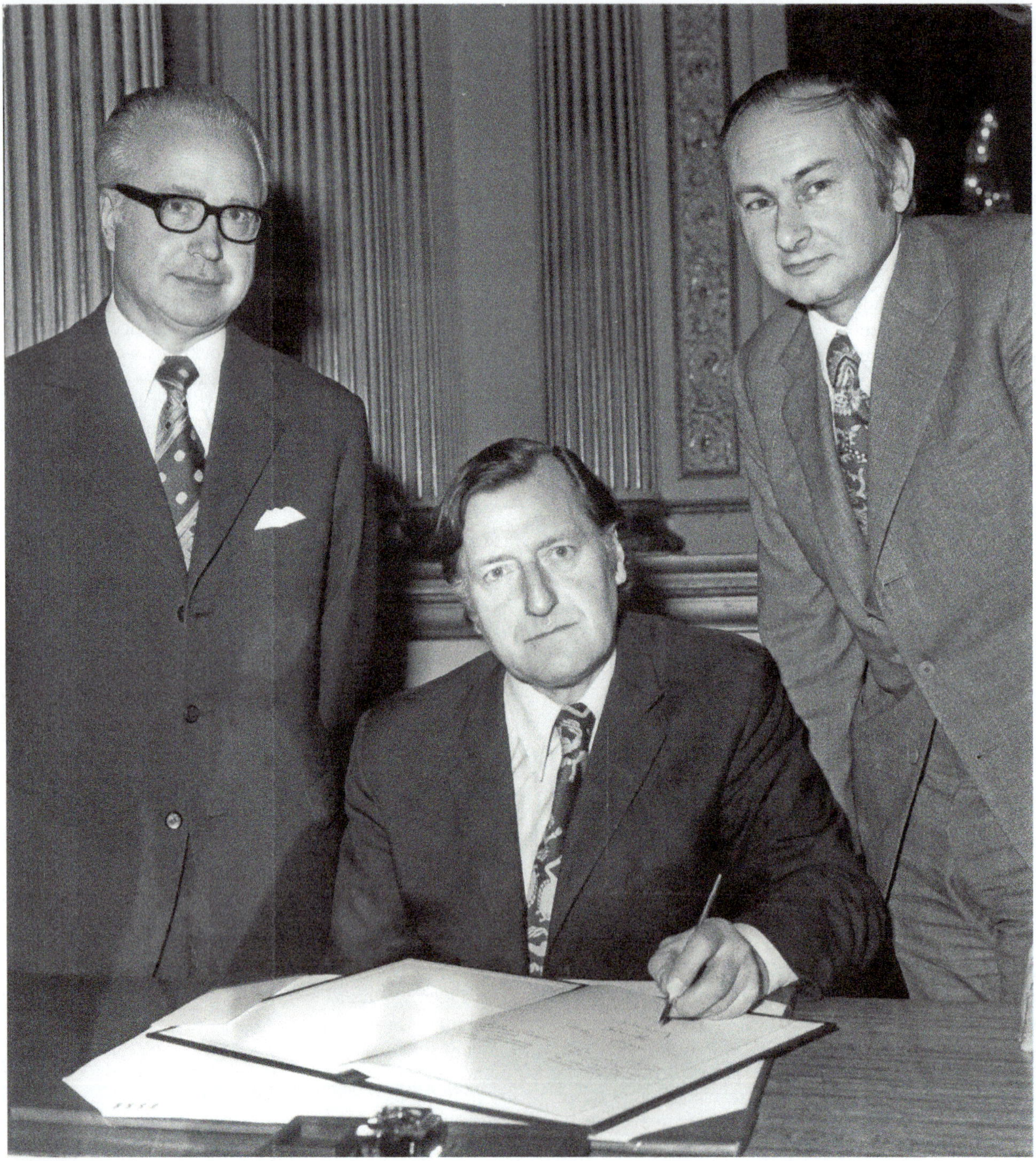

The United States, the United Kingdom, and the Soviet Union ratified the Biological Weapons Convention on March 3, 1975. This photo shows the signing of ratification documents by Nikolai Lunkov, Russian ambassador; David Ennals, British Minister of State; and Ronald Spiers, American ambassador at the Foreign and Commonwealth Office. *© Keystone Pictures USA/ZUMAPRESS/Alamy Stock Photo*

TERRORISM AND BIOLOGICAL WARFARE

The USA PATRIOT Act (commonly called the Patriot Act) is an acronym for the Uniting and Strengthening America by Providing Appropriate Tools Required to Intercept and Obstruct Terrorism Act of 2001. The bill was signed into law by US president George W. Bush (1946–) on October 26, 2001. According to the act, research facilities that handled certain chemical and biological agents were required to institute new employee screening and security procedures.

The Patriot Act was introduced to improve counterterrorism efforts by providing law enforcement with new tools to detect and prevent terrorism. Section 817 of the Patriot Act is titled "Expansion of the Biological Weapons Statute" and expands on chapter 10 of title 18 in the United States Code, providing new laws to prevent terrorist acts involving biological weapons.

The specific changes made by the Patriot Act include making it unlawful to possess biological agents, toxins, or delivery systems unless there is a reasonably justified purpose and making it unlawful for a restricted person to possess biological agents, toxins, and delivery systems that are classified as select agents.

Laboratories that operate within the United States or that are funded by the United States must comply with the new regulations regarding prohibiting access to selected agents by restricted individuals. Each organization is required to develop its own screening or application forms to obtain the required information on people working (or seeking work) in its laboratories to certify the workers' right to access to selected agents.

The US Centers for Disease Control and Prevention (CDC) regulates "the possession, use, and transfer of select agents and toxins that have the potential to pose a severe threat to public health and safety. The CDC Select Agent Program oversees these activities and registers all laboratories and other entities in the United States of America that possess, use, or transfer a select agent or toxin."

On March 18, 2005, the US Department of Health and Human Services (HHS) and US Department of Agriculture (USDA) published final rules for the possession, use, and transfer of select agents and toxins (42 C.F.R. Part 73, 7 C.F.R. Part 331, and 9 C.F.R. Part 121) in the *Federal Register.*

member of the BWC is the State of Palestine. According to the US Arms Control Association, as of September 2017 an additional six countries were listed as signatories, including the Central African Republic, Egypt, Haiti, Somalia, Syria, and Tanzania. Although they had signed the BWC, they had not yet ratified it. Another 11 countries had neither signed nor ratified the convention.

Recent US intelligence estimates compiled from various agencies indicate that certain countries are still actively involved in the development of biological weapons. The US Office of Technology Assessment and the US Department of State identify and report on states potentially developing biological weapons.

Although there have been several international meetings designed to strengthen the implementation and monitoring of BWC provisions, verification procedures remain the responsibility of an ad hoc commission of scientists. Broad international efforts to coordinate and strengthen enforcement of BWC provisions remain elusive.

At the Eighth Review Conference of the Biological Weapons Convention on November 7, 2016, Secretary-General Ban Ki-moon (1944–) stated, "The deliberate release of a biological agent would be a global health and humanitarian catastrophe. Yet there are glaring gaps in our ability to both prevent and respond to this nightmare scenario." He added, "I also encourage States parties to address the vital question of how to promote advances in life sciences that benefit all humanity, while safeguarding against their use for malicious purposes."

SEE ALSO *Anthrax; Bioterrorism; War and Infectious Disease*

BIBLIOGRAPHY

Books

Carus, W. Seth. *A Short History of Biological Warfare: From Pre-history to the 21st Century.* Washington, DC: National Defense University Press, 2017.

Johnson, Kristy Young, and Paul Matthew Nolan. *Biological Weapons: Recognizing, Understanding, and Responding to the Threat.* Hoboken, NJ: Wiley, 2016.

Tu, Anthony. *Chemical and Biological Weapons and Terrorism.* Boca Raton, FL: CRC, 2018.

Vargo, Marc E. *The Weaponizing of Biology: Bioterrorism, Biocrime and Biohacking.* Jefferson, NC: McFarland, 2017.

Periodicals

Pal, Mahendra, et al. "An Overview on Biological Weapons and Bioterrorism." *American Journal of Biomedical Research* 5, no. 2 (2017): 24–34. The article can also be found online at https://www.researchgate.net/profile/Mahendra_Pal2/publication/316189350_An_Overview_on_Biological_Weapons_and_Bioterrorism/links/58f8f149a6fdcc770be54143/An-Overview-on-Biological-Weapons-and-Bioterrorism.pdf (accessed January 29, 2018).

Websites

"Biological Weapons." United Nations Office for Disarmament Affairs. https://www.un.org/disarmament/wmd/bio/ (accessed January 29, 2018).

"Biological Weapons Convention Signatories and States-Parties." Arms Control Association, September 27, 2017. https://www.armscontrol.org/factsheets/bwcsig (accessed January 29, 2018).

Hooker, Edmond, "Biological Warfare." eMedicine-Health, November 20, 2017. https://www.emedicinehealth.com/biological_warfare/article_em.htm (accessed January 29, 2018).

"Latest Information." United Nations Office at Geneva. https://www.unog.ch/bwc/news (accessed January 29, 2018).

"Secretary-General Warns of Glaring Gaps in Ability to Prevent, Respond to Catastrophic Biological Attack, at Review Conference Opening." United Nations, November 7, 2016. https://www.un.org/press/en/2016/sgsm18256.doc.htm (accessed January 29, 2018).

Paul Davies
William Arthur Atkins

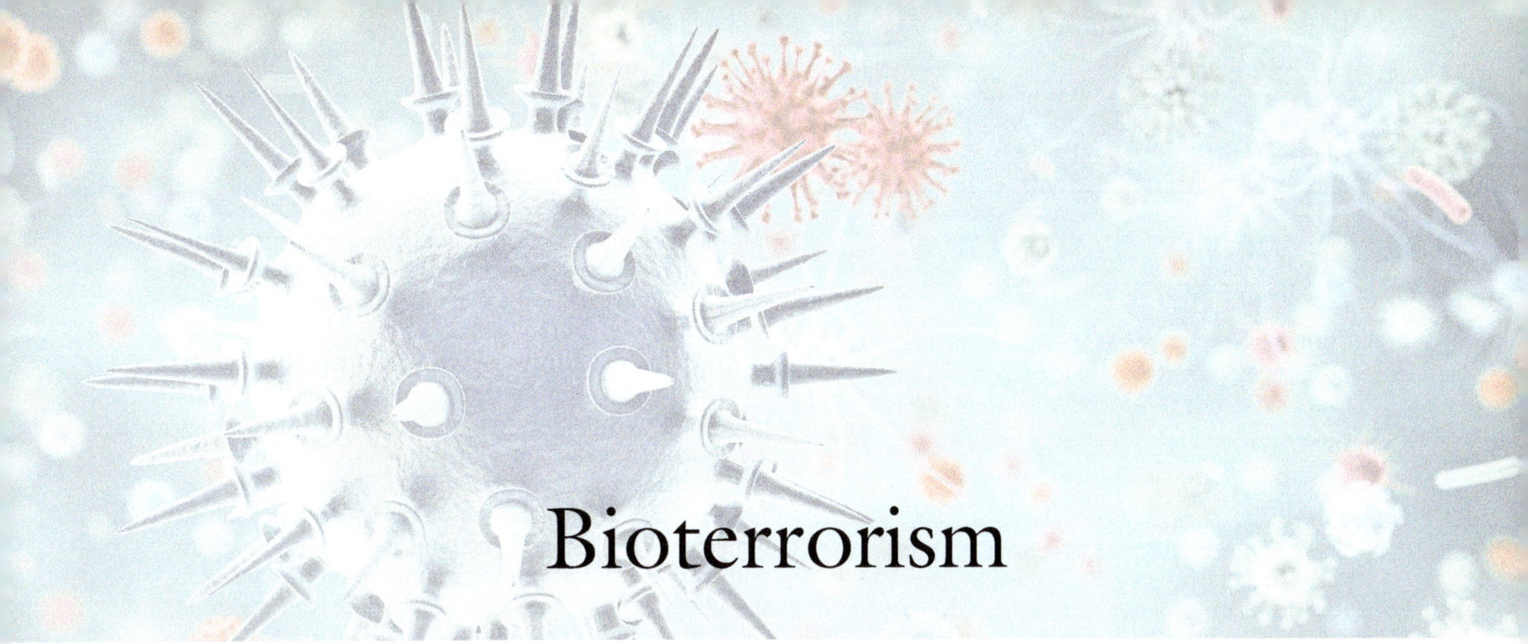

Bioterrorism

Introduction

After years of back-burner, low-priority research, work on defensive measures against bioterrorism began in earnest in the United States soon after the anthrax attacks in 2001. The anthrax attacks, dubbed "Amerithrax" by the US Federal Bureau of Investigation (FBI), began just one week after the deadly September 11 attacks on New York City and Washington, D.C. Envelopes contaminated with a powder containing anthrax were mailed to news media offices and two US senators, killing 5 people and infecting 17 others.

Scientists have continued to develop strategies designed to protect nation-states against a potentially limitless variety of biological weapons. The psychological impact of the anthrax attacks of late 2001 was enormous compared to the number of people actually killed and sickened dur-

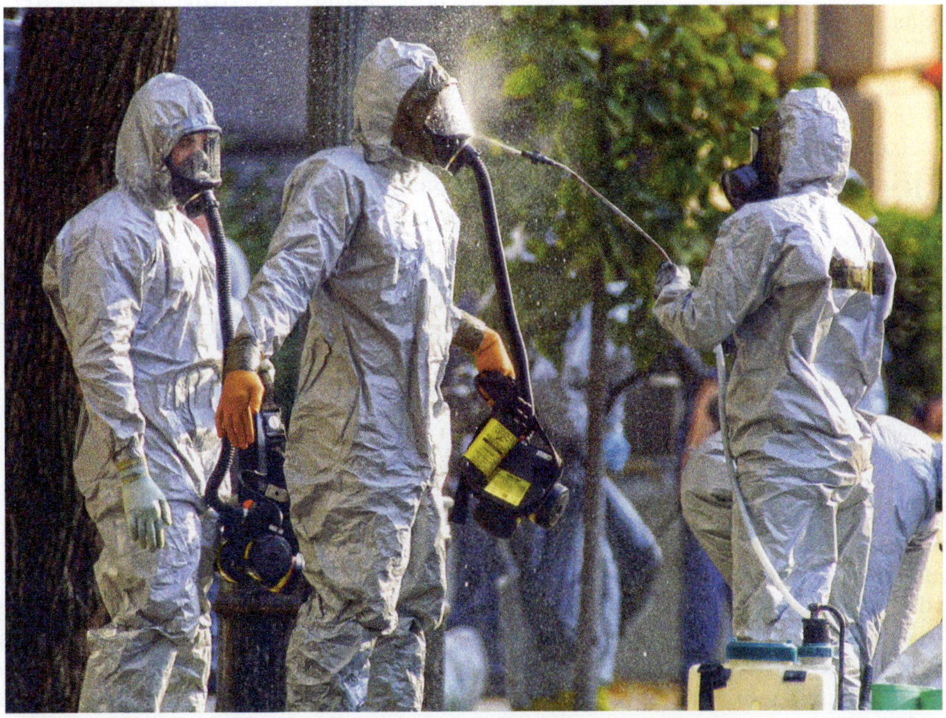

Hazardous materials workers investigate the Longworth House Office Building in Washington, D.C., during the anthrax scare of 2001. In September and October of that year, 22 individuals were exposed to anthrax spores after opening letters sent by a bioterrorist. Five of them died. *© Alex Wong/Staff/Getty Images*

WORDS TO KNOW

BIOMODULATOR Short for biologic response modulator. An agent that modifies some characteristic of the immune system, which may help in the fight against infection.

PATHOGEN A disease-causing agent, such as a bacterium, a virus, a fungus, or another microorganism.

QUARANTINE The practice of separating from the general population people who have been exposed to an infectious agent but have not yet developed symptoms. In the United States, this can be done voluntarily or involuntarily by the authority of states and the federal Centers for Disease Control and Prevention.

RING VACCINATION The vaccination of all susceptible people in an area surrounding a case of an infectious disease. Because vaccination makes people immune to the disease, the hope is that the disease will not spread from the known case to other people. Ring vaccination was used in eliminating the smallpox virus.

TOXIN A poison produced by a living organism.

ing the episode. This is in keeping with the pattern of effective terror tactics in which expenditures of time, effort, and funds can be minimal but impact on the target population is maximized.

History and Scientific Foundations

Since 2001 most defensive activity against bioterrorism threats has been focused on preventing or combating known "Class A" threats, which include organisms that cause anthrax, plague, smallpox, tularemia, and viral hemorrhagic fevers, as well as botulinum toxin. In 2004 funds to develop new drugs and vaccines were budgeted under Project BioShield, which is directed by the US Department of Homeland Security (DHS) and the US Department of Health and Human Services (HHS).

The three aims of Project BioShield were purchasing needed countermeasures (antibiotics, antitoxins, etc.), facilitating research and development under the US (NIH/NIAID), and setting guidelines for the use of medical countermeasures in a public health emergency.

As a multiagency initiative, Project BioShield's mission included defining and setting priorities for public health emergency medical countermeasures; performing research, development, and procurement activities on prioritized requirements; and setting deployment and best-practice strategies for medical countermeasures stored in the Strategic National Stockpile (SNS). Project BioShield thus established a substantial, long-term budget to provide incentives for pharmaceutical and other industries to meet US government requirements for the development of critical medical countermeasures for the public.

In 2014 the activity reporting and medical countermeasure procurement functions of Project Bioshield were transferred by Congress to the Biomedical Advanced Research and Development Authority (BARDA). Bioterrorism agents are essentially identical to biological warfare agents. Such agents may be classified operationally, as deadly or incapacitating agents, and as agents with or without the potential for secondary transmission (the ability to spread disease from one person affected by bioterrorism to another who was not exposed during the attack). Bioterrorism agents can also be classified according to their intended target, as when they are intended to sicken or kill people, animals, or vegetation such as crops, and according to type, including replicating pathogens, toxins, or biomodulators. Bioterrorism agents are classified as chemical, biological, radiological, and nuclear agents. Replicating pathogens and toxins are recognized as among the greatest current threats. BARDA supports state-of-the-art development and procurement of drugs, vaccines, and other products in all these categories that are considered to be critical for public health security through its programs. BARDA's federal agency partners that perform the various functions described above include the US Centers for Disease Control and Prevention (CDC), the HHS, the US Department of Defense (DOD), the DHS, the NIH, and the US Food and Drug Administration (FDA).

In 2014 BARDA added to the SNS quantities of Anthrasil® (anthrax immunoglobulin [AIG]); Ebola medical countermeasures, including therapeutics and vaccine candidates in response to the West African Ebola epidemic; and Amgen's Neupogen® (filgrastim), an immune system booster with a new indication for Acute Radiation Syndrome (ARS), in which the immune system is decimated by a radiation source that might be placed by terrorists in a populated area. Large quantities of other products added to the SNS included Raxibacumab®, another postexposure anthrax prophylactic agent; botulinum antitoxin; smallpox vaccine; and smallpox antiviral drug (ST-246).

Applications and Research

Smallpox

The World Health Organization (WHO) has worked globally since 2003 to "improve awareness and assist countries in building up their preparedness" against bioterror attacks. Although the anthrax attacks in the United States are the only known bioterrorism attack since 2001, former WHO director-general Gro Harlem Brundtland (1939–) delivered an address on "General Bioterrorism and Military Health Risks" at the G20

Health Ministers Forum during the World Economic Forum in Davos, Switzerland, in January 2003 in which she emphasized that combatting and preventing bioterror attacks was not just an issue for the United States. She went on to say that "disease surveillance and control has immediate civilian benefits, since it improves protection against all disease outbreaks, whatever the cause." Although many pathogens could be used to attack populations worldwide, only a few, including the smallpox virus, could cause illness or panic that could overwhelm existing medical and public health systems. WHO authorizes two laboratories in the world to maintain stores of smallpox virus for research purposes, and authorities fear additional smallpox virus may be hidden away in laboratories other than the two WHO-designated repositories.

A new outbreak of smallpox could spread rapidly. The CDC strategy for controlling a new outbreak of smallpox incorporates principles that were used 30 to 40 years ago in eradicating the disease and have proven their effectiveness. They are based on knowledge that smallpox is mostly transmitted by close, face-to-face contact with infected individuals, while only a few cases could be transmitted by dry or aerosolized particles in close proximity to persons with the disease. New cases develop two weeks after exposure and take another two weeks to progress to pustules and scabs, giving a newly aware medical community some time to respond.

Smallpox vaccine is a live-virus vaccine composed of vaccinia virus, which induces antibodies that also protect against smallpox. Smallpox vaccine production ceased in the early 1980s, and current supplies of smallpox vaccine are limited. Large quantities of a new vaccine manufactured using cell cultures have been available since 2014 under the BARDA program.

After several years of considering mass vaccination as an alternative, the CDC has settled on a ring vaccination strategy (vaccinating all susceptible people in an area surrounding a case of an infectious disease) to combat a new smallpox outbreak. This includes the isolation of confirmed and suspected smallpox cases with tracing, vaccination, and close surveillance of contacts to these cases, as well as vaccination of the household contacts of the smallpox cases. Ring vaccination takes advantage of the relatively low infectivity of smallpox and focuses currently scarce vaccine resources where they will do the most good. Ring vaccination also works to minimize adverse events, including rare deaths that could occur during indiscriminate mass vaccination.

The smallpox vaccine is no longer publicly available because smallpox has been eliminated and no longer exists in nature. Nevertheless, the CDC has stockpiled enough smallpox vaccine to vaccinate everyone in the United States if a smallpox epidemic were to break out as a result of bioterrorism.

The antiviral drug tecovirimat has been shown to be effective against the virus that causes smallpox in laboratory tests. In the laboratory this drug was effective in animal testing on diseases similar to smallpox. Although tecovirimat has not been tested in people sick with smallpox, it has been administered to healthy volunteers. The results of these tests indicated that it is safe for humans and causes only mild side effects. The CDC now stockpiles tecovirimat in the SNS.

Two other antiviral drugs, cidofovir and brincidofovir, have also been shown to be effective against the virus that causes smallpox in laboratory tests. In the laboratory these drugs were effective in animal testing on diseases similar to smallpox. Although cidofovir and brincidofovir have not been tested in smallpox victims, they have been administered to healthy volunteers and in patients with other viral illnesses. These preliminary results indicate that brincidofovir may cause fewer side effects than cidofovir, which can damage kidneys.

It is not known whether a smallpox victim would respond to treatment with these drugs because they were not tested in people sick with smallpox. Nonetheless, treatment with these antivirals may be attempted if there ever is a smallpox outbreak.

Anthrax

Anthrax is an infectious disease caused by a spore-forming bacterium, the spores of which are persistent and hard to break down in the environment. This makes anthrax a persistent public health threat in spite of available treatment with familiar drugs.

There are three forms of anthrax infection: skin, gastrointestinal, and inhalational. The FDA has determined that the mortality rates from anthrax vary according to exposure. Death rates are approximately 20 percent for cutaneous (skin) anthrax without antibiotics and 25 to 75 percent for gastrointestinal anthrax. Inhalation anthrax has a fatality rate that may exceed 80 percent. Inhalation anthrax occurs when spores are inhaled and infect the lungs. The treatments for all types of anthrax are the antibiotics ciprofloxacin, tetracycline drugs such as doxycycline, and some types of penicillin.

The anthrax vaccine is primarily given to people in the military and is only recommended for individuals considered to be at high risk of contracting the disease, such as scientists who handle anthrax bacteria. Current government efforts are focused on encouraging the development of new anthrax vaccines intended to prevent inhalational anthrax before and after exposure. The emergency response to anthrax consists of administration of antibiotics and spore cleanup by workers using personal protective equipment. Unvaccinated, exposed people and remediation workers begin taking preventive antibiotics at the time of their exposure and continue to take them for at least 60 days.

The stockpiling of Anthrasil® is another preventive measure employed by the CDC. The stockpiles are maintained so that they can be used in the event of an anthrax outbreak. This would involve injecting antibodies into patients that are infected with the anthrax bacillus. These antibodies have been shown to be effective against naturally occurring anthrax infections and are produced by the immune systems of infected people and other animals when they fight off an anthrax infection.

Antitoxins that neutralize the toxins the anthrax bacillus produces when anthrax spores are activated in a host's body can also be employed to reduce the severity of an anthrax infection in conjunction with antibiotic treatment.

The CDC collaborates with other federal agencies and local health departments to prepare for potential anthrax attacks. The agency sponsors conferences to coordinate local emergency operations. It provides funding and guidance for health departments to strengthen responses to public health crises. The CDC offers anthrax emergency response training for the public health community and health care providers. It regulates the possession, use, and transfer of biological agents and toxins. The CDC also promotes best-preparedness practices and helps to set up laboratories capable of quickly conducting tests for suspected anthrax. Finally, the CDC ensures that health care providers have the necessary medicine and supplies and provides guidance for the protection of health care providers and emergency responders in the case of an anthrax epidemic.

Plague

Plague is caused by the bacterium *Yersinia pestis.* Bubonic plague is the most common type of naturally occurring plague and is transmitted through the bite of an infected flea or exposure through a cut. Symptoms of bubonic plague include headache, fever, chills, and swollen, tender lymph nodes. If untreated with common antibiotics, bubonic plague may result in death. Untreated plague has a high fatality rate and has been among the greatest pestilences in history. The most notorious and deadly outbreak of plague was "The Black Death," which took several forms and caused the death of 60 percent of Europe's population.

In pneumonic plague the lungs are infected with the plague bacterium. People with pneumonic plague can transmit plague to other people, whereas bubonic plague cannot be spread from person to person. Antibiotics approved by the FDA to treat plague are streptomycin, doxycycline, and other tetracycline drugs. The public health response to pneumonic plague would be similar to that of anthrax, with the addition of quarantines that could impact sizable crowded geographic areas.

In recent years some terrorist organizations such as al-Qaeda have been reported to have an interest in using plague as a bioweapon. A 2009 report stated that an offshoot of al-Qaeda in Algeria tried to use plague in terrorist operations there in an effort that backfired and inadvertently resulted in the deaths of al-Qaeda fighters.

In the late 1990s Osama bin Laden (1957–2011), the founder of al-Qaeda, set up chemical and biological weapons laboratories in Afghanistan that were discovered by Allied forces during the US-led invasion of that country. According to the US Central Intelligence Agency, bin Laden stocked them with anthrax, plague, and botulinum toxins and hired experts from Ukraine and Russia to train his people to "conduct attacks with toxic chemicals or biological toxins." In 2008 an al-Qaeda operative posted instructions online on how to use plague in terror attacks.

■ Impacts and Issues

The response to the 2001 anthrax attacks has been extensively analyzed as researchers attempt to model the optimal response to future attacks. The 2001 attacks were small-scale events, affecting relatively few people in restricted geographic areas. In a recent study of a small-scale attack, Veterans Health Administration researchers conducted a cost-effectiveness analysis using a simulation model to determine the optimal response strategy for a small-scale anthrax attack against US Postal Service distribution centers in a large metropolitan area. (A cost-effectiveness analysis compares the relative effectiveness of two or more alternatives in view of their costs and attempts to determine the best value for the money.) The study compared three different strategies: (1) pre-attack vaccination of all US distribution center postal workers, (2) postattack antibiotic therapy followed by vaccination of exposed personnel, and (3) postattack antibiotic therapy without vaccination of exposed personnel. The results showed that postattack antibiotic therapy and vaccination of exposed postal workers is the most cost-effective response compared with postattack antibiotic therapy alone. This was because of the greater prevention of death and disease when postattack vaccination was combined with antibiotics. Pre-attack vaccination of all distribution center workers is less effective and more costly than the other two strategies. This is because vaccinating all postal employees would be expensive, the immunity conferred by the current vaccine is not perfect or always permanent, and the time between vaccination and an anthrax attack is indeterminate.

Some commentators have decried the resources and energy being poured into bioterrorism defense. According to this perspective, bioterrorism preparedness programs have wasted public health resources with little evidence of benefit. For example, several deaths and many serious illnesses have resulted from the smallpox vaccination program, but there is no clear evidence that any threat of smallpox exposure has existed since the eradication of the disease. Even the anthrax attacks were linked to secret US military laboratories; without these laboratories the attacks probably would not have been possible. The huge effort to prepare the country against bioterrorist threats is seen by some critics as a great distraction from the need to allocate public health resources to address other health needs and has been conducted at the expense of some vital programs.

Nevertheless, the anthrax attacks did demonstrate the havoc that individuals could wreak with sufficient determination, access to pathogens, and laboratory resources. As public protection will always be a primary responsibility of government, leaving the population unprepared for the eventuality of bioterrorism is not an option in the post-9/11 world. Accordingly, the Center for Law and the Public's Health at Georgetown and Johns Hopkins universities drafted the Model State Emergency Health Powers Act (MSEHPA, or Model Act) at the request of the CDC. The Model Act provides states with the powers needed to detect and contain either bioterrorism or a naturally occurring disease outbreak. To this extent, bioterrorism preparedness appears in sync with more conventional public health preparedness. Legislative bills based on the MSEHPA have been introduced in most states. This legislative effort has uncovered problems of state law obsolescence, inconsistency, and inadequacy. Most current state laws provide inadequate public protection whether a disease outbreak would be natural or intentional. They often date back to the early 20th century and predate the immense changes in public health science over the past half century.

The Model Act is structured to support five basic public health functions to be facilitated by law: (1) preparedness, including comprehensive planning for a public health emergency; (2) surveillance, including measures to detect and track public health emergencies; (3) management of property, including ensuring adequate availability of vaccines, pharmaceuticals, and hospitals, as well as providing power to abate hazards to the public's health; (4) protection of persons, including powers to compel vaccination, testing, treatment, isolation, and quarantine when clearly necessary; and (5) communication, including providing clear and authoritative information to the public. The act is also based on a legal framework to protect personal rights.

Use of Spectroscopy in Identifying Pathogens

Traditional detection of pathogens such as bacteria and viruses involves blood testing in which potential pathogens in a tissue sample from an infected patient are cultured in the laboratory and various stains and reagents are made to react with proteins of the pathogen's outer membrane. This is a slow and labor-intensive process. A new technique of rapidly identifying bacteria such as anthrax—called desorption electrospray ionization, which was developed by Graham Cooks at Purdue University—could be used for homeland security. This technique enables the fast "fingerprinting" bacteria using mass spectrometry (an instrumental method for identifying the chemical constitution of a substance). The analysis of bacteria and other microorganisms usually takes several hours. The spectrographic technique ionizes molecules outside of the spectrometer's vacuum chamber. Ionized molecules can then be manipulated, detected, and analyzed using electromagnetic fields. This technique is extremely sensitive, capable of detecting one-billionth of a gram of a particular bacterium and identifying its subspecies, which is the level of accuracy required for detecting and monitoring infectious microorganisms. The technology can determine the subspecies and collect other information by observing the pattern of the pathogen's outer membrane proteins and creates a sort of fingerprint as revealed by mass spectrometry. Such accuracy and timeliness makes the technology particularly apt for detecting bioterrorism agents, as word of an intentionally caused outbreak would need to be spread very soon after the appearance of suspected cases in order to prevent rapid transmission of the pathogen.

Involving the General Public in Preparedness

The public health emergency responses being created by the CDC to a bioterrorist attack focus mainly on readying emergency and medical workers to cope with infection transmission, panic, and decontamination. There has been considerable refinement in terms of how agencies and response personnel should coordinate their efforts. The CDC has oriented some of its bioterrorism emergency instructions on its website to the general public, developing a brochure and a website titled "Are You Prepared?" It provides specific instructions to individuals at risk in a public health emergency, whether or not it is related to bioterrorism. This instruction is being disseminated to local health departments, which can spread the information to communities. The instructions direct the public to "Get a Kit" (emergency supplies and personal response instructions developed by the CDC), provides instructions on how to "Make a Plan" that improves chances of survival in various types of emergencies, and offers additional help in keeping up with the latest information pertaining to such emergencies ("Be Informed"). Promising new research on detection technologies, vaccines, and medicines to prevent or combat infections is now being funded under BARDA.

Most bioterrorism policy discussion and response planning has been conducted among experts and has not involved much public participation. The capacity of the public to take an active role and even to lead in the response to bioterrorism is often discounted, and some policy makers have assumed that local populations would get in the way of an effective response. This bias is based on fears of mass panic and social disorder. While no one knows exactly how a population will react to an extraordinary act of bioterrorism, experience with natural and technological disasters and disease outbreaks indicates that the public response would be generally effective and adaptive collective action. Therefore, the public is a partner in the medical and public health response. Failure to involve the public in planning could hamper effective management of an epidemic and increase the likelihood of social breakdown. Ultimately, actions taken by nonprofessional individuals and groups could end up having the greatest impact on the outcome of a bioterrorism attack. Guidelines suggested by the CDC for integrating the public into bioterrorism response planning include (1) treating the public as a capable ally in the response to an epidemic, (2) enlisting civic organizations in practical public health activities, (3) anticipating needs for home-based patient care and infection control, (4) investing in public outreach and communication strategies, and (5) ensuring that planning reflects the values and priorities of affected populations.

PRIMARY SOURCE

Biodefense R&D: Anticipating Future Threats, Establishing a Strategic Environment

SOURCE: *Smith, Bradley T., Thomas V. Inglesby, and Tara O'Toole. "Biodefense R&D: Anticipating Future Threats, Establishing a Strategic Environment."* Biosecurity & Bioterrorism *1, no. 3 (2003): 193–202.*

INTRODUCTION: *Following the September 11, 2001, terror attacks on the United States, renewed scrutiny was focused on the possibility of a biomedical attack. In the following excerpt from a journal article, the authors argue for a greater role for the biomedical research community in defense efforts against bioterrorism. Bradley T. Smith, PhD, is a fellow, Thomas V. Inglesby, MD, is deputy director, and Tara O'Toole, MD, MPH, is director, all at the Johns Hopkins Center for Civilian Biodefense Strategies in Baltimore, Maryland.*

INTRODUCTION

The ultimate objective of the U.S. civilian biodefense strategy should be to eliminate the possibility of massively lethal bioterrorist attacks. A central pillar of this strategy must be an ambitious and aggressive scientific research, development, and production (R&D&P) program that delivers the diagnostic technologies, medicines, and vaccines needed to counter the range of bioweapons agents that might be used against the nation. A successful biodefense strategy must take account of the rapidly expanding spectrum of bioweapons agents and means of delivery made possible by 21st century advances in bioscientific knowledge and biotechnology. Meeting this challenge will require the engagement of America's extraordinary scientific talent and investments of financial and political capital on a scale far beyond that now committed or contemplated. The purpose of this article is to provide a brief analysis of the current biomedical R&D&P environment and to offer recommendations for the establishment of a national biodefense strategy that could significantly diminish the suffering and loss that would accompany bioterrorist attacks. In the longer term, a robust biodefense R&D&P effort, if coupled to substantial improvements in medical and public health systems, could conceivably render biological weapons ineffective as agents of mass lethality.

THE PROBLEM: 20th AND 21st CENTURY BIOWEAPONS

The advantage is now firmly with those who would seek to deploy offensive bioweapons; the state of biodefense is relatively weak. Following the terrorist attacks of 2001, the National Institute of Allergy and Infectious Diseases (NIAID) at the National Institutes of Health (NIH) received $1.7 billion to fund biodefense research projects. NIAID has since established a "roadmap" describing the scientific research needed to devise new "countermeasures" (i.e., diagnostic technologies, therapeutic drugs, and vaccines) for the pathogens thought to be the bioweapons agents of greatest concern. Much of the NIAID roadmap has, appropriately, focused on developing countermeasures for the six CDC Category A bioweapons threats (anthrax, smallpox, plague, botulism, tularemia, and the viral hemorrhagic fevers) for which there are striking gaps in available countermeasures ..., and a selection of other bioweapons threats on the CDC's Category B and C lists (collectively termed "20th century bioweapons" in this article).

Growing numbers of people in the scientific community now recognize that looming just ahead is a far more daunting array of potential engineered bioweapon agents (collectively termed "21st century bioweapons" in this article). The life sciences are at the beginning of a revolutionary period. Scientific understanding of living systems and how to manipulate them is expanding exponentially, fueled by advances in computerization, the global dispersion of bioscientific expertise as well as biological databases, and substantial economic investment in biomedical and agricultural research and product development.

A prime example of these powerful advances was the identification in 2001 of the approximately 40,000 genes in the human genome. Scientists are rapidly learning how to translate this genomic "parts list" into a sophisticated understanding of how specific genes control human biological systems in the body. Such discoveries will bring great benefit to humankind, but they will also allow the development of a new constellation of powerful 21st century bioweapons.

There are already countless portents of the coming power of bioscience and how it will propel bioweapons developments. Scientists have shown that it is possible to create strains of the bacterium that causes anthrax to be resistant to the most powerful existing antibiotics. They have demonstrated the capacity to make viruses that can overcome vaccine-induced immunity. Viruses can be genetically modified to increase their ability to kill infected cells, or to become capable of attacking entirely new target species. Viruses and bacteria can be manipulated in ways that make them better able to survive environmental stress and to be disseminated over distances in the air as weapons. Technologies already exist that could be used to protect pathogens from detection or destruction by the human immune system. These are only a small sample of the developments ahead on the bioscience landscape.

The "dual use" aspect of bioscience does not pertain only to specific, isolated technological applications, as is the case in nuclear weapons work. Rather, it is biological knowledge itself that is the source of the power that can be applied toward beneficent or malevolent ends. The knowledge needed to engineer a more lethal viral or bacterial bioweapon is essentially the same as that needed to understand how that virus or bacteria causes disease and how to create an effective vaccine against it. The distinction between good biology and its "dark side" lies only in intent and application. With rare exception, it will be very difficult to sequester new bioscientific knowledge that might be applied to building biological weapons without simultaneously harming beneficial biomedical research and essential biodefense R&D&P.

Given the size, momentum, and global dissemination of the bioscientific enterprise and the great demand for the medical and agricultural products being created, the rapid global advance of bioscience is essentially unstoppable. A successful biodefense R&D&P strategy must accept that the growth and international diffusion of bio-scientific knowledge and technologies will continue at a phenomenal pace and must seek to leverage these powerful forces against the bioterrorist threat. ...

CONCLUSION

The full power of the nation's biomedical research, development, and production enterprise is not yet engaged in biodefense, and given the current environment, funding levels, priorities, and lack of clear vision for the biodefense R&D&P program, large numbers of the best biomedical scientists are unlikely to engage. Current biodefense initiatives, when compared to other U.S. government efforts to address top national security threats, suggest that the U.S. government either does not yet understand the grave nature and scope of the bioterrorist threat or is not prepared to commit fully to a robust biodefense research, development, and production effort. This must change if the nation is to counter the coming bioweapons threat and set the course to eliminate bioweapons as weapons of mass lethality.

Editor's note: Referenced citations omitted.

See Also *Public Health and Infectious Disease; War and Infectious Disease*

BIBLIOGRAPHY

Books

Fong, I. W., and Kenneth Alibek, eds. *Bioterrorism and Infectious Agents: A New Dilemma for the 21st Century.* New York: Springer, 2005.

Vargo, Marc E. *The Weaponizing of Biology: Bioterrorism, Biocrime and Biohacking.* Jefferson, NC: McFarland, 2017.

Periodicals

Cohen, Hillel W., Robert M. Gould, and Victor W. Sidel. "The Pitfalls of Bioterrorism Preparedness: The Anthrax and Smallpox Experiences." *American Journal of Public Health* 94 (October 2004): 1667–1671.

Evans, Sam Weiss. "Biosecurity Governance for the Real World." *Issues in Science and Technology* 33, no. 1 (2016): 84–88.

Noble, Ronald K. "Keeping Science in the Right Hands: Policing the New Biological Frontier." *Foreign Affairs* 92, no. 6 (November/December 2013): 47–53.

Schneeman, A., and M. Manchester. "Anti-Toxin Antibodies in Prophylaxis and Treatment of Inhalation Anthrax." *Future Microbiolgy* 4, no. 1 (2009): 35–43.

Websites

"Are You Prepared?" Centers for Disease Control and Prevention, 2017. https://www.cdc.gov/phpr/areyouprepared/ (accessed January 15, 2018).

"Biomedical Advanced Research and Development Authority (BARDA)." US Department of Health and Human Services. https://www.medicalcountermeasures.gov/barda/ (accessed January 7, 2018).

"Bioterrorism." Centers for Disease Control and Prevention. https://www.cdc.gov/anthrax/bioterrorism/index.html (accessed January 7, 2018).

Brundtland, Gro Harlem. "Bioterrorism and Military Health Risks." World Health Organization. http://www.who.int/dg/brundtland/speeches/2003/DAVOS/en/ (accessed January 15, 2018).

Maginnis, Robert. "Al Qaeda and the Plague." Human Events, January 23, 2009. http://humanevents.com/2009/01/23/alqaeda-and-the-plague/ (accessed January 15, 2018).

Mauroni, Al. "We Don't Need Another National Biodefense Strategy." Modern War Institute, August 1, 2017. https://mwi.usma.edu/dont-need-another-national-biodefense-strategy/ (accessed January 7, 2018).

"Project BioShield Annual Report to Congress." US Department of Health and Human Services, 2016. https://www.medicalcountermeasures.gov/barda/cbrn/project-bioshield-overview/project-bioshield-annual-report.aspx (accessed January 7, 2018).

Kenneth T. LaPensee

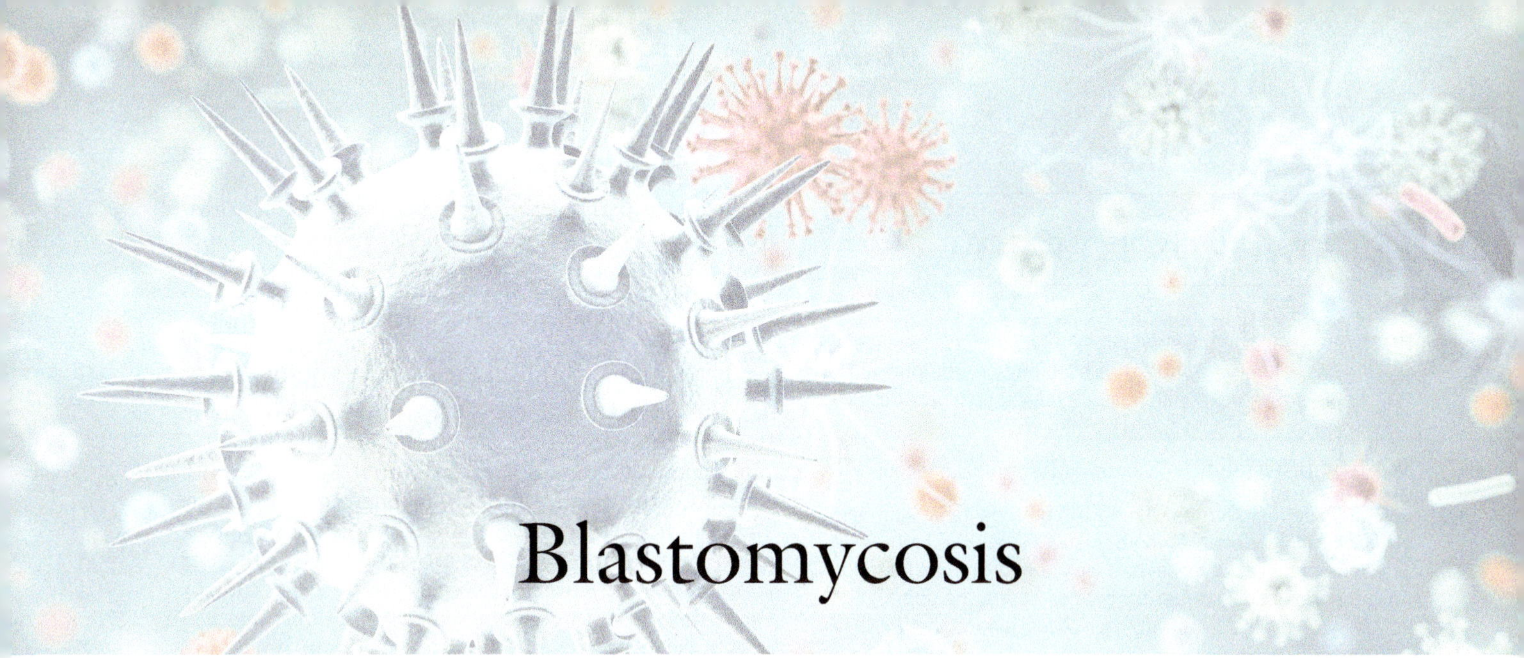

Blastomycosis

■ Introduction

Blastomycosis is a rare fungal infection caused by inhaling the fungal organism *Blastomyces dermatitidis* through the nose or mouth. The organism is usually found in habitats containing wood and soil. It lives commonly as a mold in warm, sandy soils located near water and within moist soil full of decomposing organic matter. The infection is restricted to humans, dogs, and other mammals in portions of North America. Human symptoms of the infection are similar to the influenza-like disease of the lungs called histoplasmosis (also called Darling's disease). Rarely, persons with blastomycosis develop chronic pulmonary infection or widespread disseminated infection, which can be fatal.

When found in a host, *Blastomyces dermatitidis* lives as yeast. Because it lives as mold outside a host and as yeast inside, it is called a biphasic organism. Blastomycosis is commonly misdiagnosed as valley fever (coccidioidomycosis), Lyme disease, or other viral infections.

■ Disease History, Characteristics, and Transmission

The first description of blastomycosis came in 1876 from French biologist Philippe Edouard Leon Van Tieghem (1839–1914). Later, in 1894, American dermatologist Thomas Gilchrist (1862–1927), from the University of Maryland School of Medicine, described

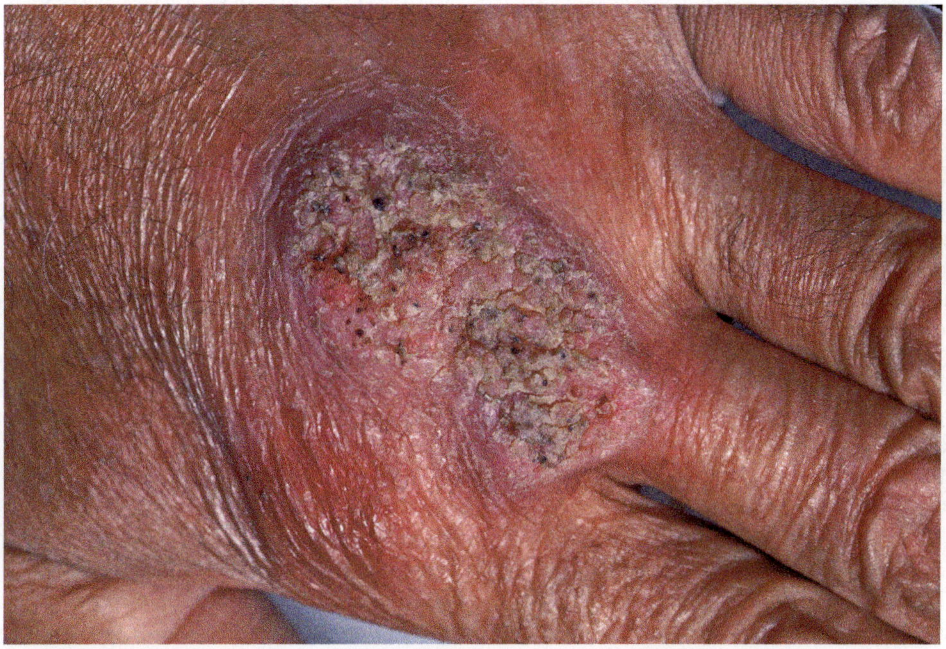

A typical blastomycosis skin lesion is shown here. © *Scott Camazine/Science Source*

WORDS TO KNOW

HOST An organism that serves as the habitat for a parasite or possibly for a symbiont. A host may provide nutrition to the parasite or symbiont, or it may simply provide a place in which to live.

MYCOTIC DISEASE A disease caused by fungal infection.

SPORE A dormant form assumed by some bacteria, such as anthrax, that enables the bacterium to survive high temperatures, dryness, and lack of nourishment for long periods of time. Under proper conditions, the spore may revert to the actively multiplying form of the bacteria.

it more thoroughly. Gilchrist isolated and proved the cause of the human infection. Because of this, it is often called Gilchrist's disease or Gilchrist's mycosis. It is also sometimes called Chicago disease and North American blastomycosis.

Transmission of the fungus is by inhalation of airborne spores after contaminated soil has been disturbed. Forestry workers as well as campers, hunters, and farmers located near wooded sites are at increased risk. People with compromised immune systems also are at high risk. Animals, including pets, are susceptible to blastomycosis infection. However, blastomycosis is not contagious, either between people or between animals and people.

According to the Centers for Disease Control and Prevention Division of Bacterial and Mycotic Diseases, symptoms occur in about 50 to 70 percent of all cases. Common symptoms, which sometimes parallel symptoms of influenza (flu), include a nonproductive cough, fever, chills, headache, and pain or stiffness in muscles or joints. When it resembles bacterial pneumonia, symptoms include high fever, chills, a productive cough with brown or bloody-looking sputum, and chest pain of the lungs. When it looks like tuberculosis or lung cancer, symptoms include a low-grade fever, productive cough, night sweats, and weight loss. Other symptoms can include shortness of breath, sweating, exhaustion, overall discomfort and ill feeling, rash, skin and bone lesions, and problems with the bladder, kidney, ovaries, prostate, and testes.

Once the infection is inside the lungs, it grows rapidly, becoming noticeable in the blood, brain, bone, lymphatic system, skin, and genital and urinary systems. The incubation period is generally 3 to 15 weeks. No symptoms occur in about one-third to one-half of infections. The death rate from the infection is about 5 percent.

Scope and Distribution

Blastomycosis is concentrated in parts of North America, especially in the central-southern, midwestern, and southeastern parts of the United States and the northwestern part of Ontario in Canada. Infection is more frequent in the basin areas around the Ohio River and Mississippi River and in the areas surrounding the Great Lakes. The region with the highest rates of infection is northern Wisconsin, where some counties report 10 to 40 cases per 100,000 people each year. In other endemic North American areas, blastomycosis occurs in about one to two people out of 100,000.

Some cases are reported in Central America, South America, and Africa. Although anyone can contract the infection, it more commonly affects people with compromised immune systems. Males are more likely to become infected than are females. According to the 2014 study by Diana Khuu and her colleagues in *Emerging Infectious Diseases*, older people, Native Americans, African Americans, and young people of Asian origin are at an elevated risk of dying from infection. This study also found that death occurs more frequently in regions where blastomycosis is endemic—namely, the American South and Midwest. Overall, however, death occurs rarely.

Treatment and Prevention

No blastomycosis vaccine has been developed, and infection cannot otherwise be prevented. To reduce risk of infection, the CDC recommends that people at risk for infection, such as those who live in endemic areas and have compromised immune systems, refrain from disrupting soil, which may contain *Blastomyces dermatitidis* spores.

If blastomycosis is contracted and identified, the diagnosis can be confirmed with cellular and tissue tests, such as the KOH test. The KOH test is a procedure performed with a microscope that uses potassium hydroxide (KOH) to dissolve skin tissue and reveal fungal cells. Other diagnostic tests employed may include chest X-rays to show nodule growth or pneumonia; skin, organ, or tissue biopsies; and blood and sputum cultures. When other tests fail, a urine antigen test usually identifies the disease.

Blastomycosis in the lungs does not always require drug treatment to eliminate it. However, when the infection spreads outside the lungs or has become severe within the lungs, amphotericin B (such as Abelcet® and Fungisome®), itraconazole (such as Sporanox®), or other antifungal medicines may be prescribed orally or intravenously. Amphotericin B is usually reserved for severe cases. While it is more effective than other antifungals, it also is more toxic. Periodic follow-up by a physician is recommended to detect any recurrences. Cure rates are high; however, treatment often takes many weeks or months.

People with minor irritations of the skin and lungs usually recover without suffering permanent problems. Major complications—such as large abscesses, relapses, or recurrences of the disease and negative side effects of drugs—can lead to complications. If patients do not recover, they may develop chronic lung infection or widespread infection of the bones, skin, and genitourinary tract. On occasion, the fungus affects the meninges, the protective covering of the brain and spinal column. If left untreated, severe cases can progress rapidly and eventually cause death.

■ Impacts and Issues

According to various studies, reports of blastomycosis are on the rise in various parts of the United States, including in Indiana and Vermont. However, it is difficult to know whether—and, if so, how—growing numbers of reports correspond to true rates of infection, as blastomycosis has not been accurately and reliably reported by the medical community in the past. This is largely due to the fact that national reporting is not required in Canada and the United States and that its occurrence has been restricted to North America. Some observers have called for blastomycosis to be added to the CDC's list of reportable disease, which would require doctors and laboratories to notify the agency of confirmed infections. As of early 2018, however, this had not occurred.

Inconsistencies in reporting mean that epidemiologists still do not completely understand rates of blastomycosis and the ways in which infection is transmitted. Lack of information about the disease is primarily due to the difficulty in isolating the causative organism from its natural environment.

Most medical practitioners consider blastomycosis to be an important mycotic disease. According to the editors in the November 14, 2000, edition of the *Canadian Medical Association Journal* (*CMAJ*), its prevalence may be more extensive than previously thought. The editors of *CMAJ* suggest that physicians include it in the potential diagnoses of unexplained granulomatous pulmonary (relating to the lungs) disease and cutaneous (relating to the skin) disease.

In the early 21st century, a number of uncertainties still surround the origins, characteristics, causes, and other important medical facts of blastomycosis. A greater understanding of the epidemiology of this disease will allow it to be more effectively combated in the future.

PRIMARY SOURCE

This Man Thought He Had the Flu. Months Later, He Could Barely Eat or Talk

SOURCE: *Loney, Sydney. "This Man Thought He Had the Flu. Months Later, He Could Barely Eat or Talk."* Reader's Digest. *https://www.rd.com/health/conditions/blastomycosis-flu-symptoms/ (accessed January 26, 2018).*

INTRODUCTION: *This article from* Reader's Digest *describes a Canadian man's infection with blastomycosis and how that infection was identified and treated.*

The patient: Ted*, a public sector worker in his late 40s

The symptoms: Low-grade fever, persistent cough and fatigue

The doctor: Dr. Neil Shear, head of dermatology at Sunnybrook Health Sciences Center in Toronto, Canada

For three weeks last February, Ted struggled to banish what he thought was a nasty flu bug. He had a dry cough, a fever of 100.4 degrees F and a feeling of fatigue that eight hours of sleep—and over-the-counter cold medications—couldn't fix....

Finally, fed up with feeling lousy, Ted went to his family doctor, who discovered puzzling sores the size of small warts inside his mouth and nose and referred him to the internal medicine clinic at Sunnybrook Hospital in Toronto. The physician there suspected vasculitis, inflammation in the veins and arteries that often presents with fatigue, coughing and skin sores.

It was now April, three months after Ted started feeling sick, and his health quickly deteriorated: his cough worsened and he was so tired he could barely make it through his workday. He'd also lost his typically healthy appetite and was dropping weight. More troubling: the lesions in his mouth and nose were getting larger, and had spread to his throat.

Ted was referred to an oral surgeon, who biopsied the lesions in his mouth. The results were read as granulomatous vasculitis, aligning with the internist's earlier suspicions. This variant typically involves the upper respiratory tract—an X-ray revealed a fuzzy shadow in Ted's lungs. The disease affects about one in 25,000 people, often in their 40s and 50s, and may lead to heart disease and kidney damage. While the condition can be very serious, when it's diagnosed and treated promptly, the current survival rate is about 90 percent.

Unfortunately, two weeks of taking corticosteroids to control inflammation and suppress his immune system didn't relieve Ted's symptoms. The lesions had spread to the skin on his arms, legs and torso, and the abscesses in his mouth and throat made it difficult to eat or talk. By this point, it had been almost six months since the onset of his illness, and Ted had lost hope of ever getting better. Because the sores on his body were so disfiguring, he was referred to dermatologist Dr. Neil Shear....

Shear took one look at the patient and knew he didn't have vasculitis. "Once you see a condition like this, you don't forget it," he says. What Shear saw was blastomycosis, an airborne fungal infection that originates from mold that grows in damp soil and decomposing leaves. It's found in the U.S. and Canada, as well as parts of India and Africa, and affects people (and animals) who breathe in the spores, though not everyone who's exposed will develop the infection.

Flu-like symptoms typically appear one to three months after a person inhales the fungus. Once the microorganisms enter the lungs, they transform into a yeast that spreads through the bloodstream. "Eventually, the patient would have been on a ventilator and likely would have died," Shear says.

Blastomycosis is uncommon in many regions, and Ted is still unsure where he picked up the illness. According to the Centers for Disease Control and Prevention, yearly incidence rates in the U.S. are approximately one to two cases for every 100,000 people. Shear says the infection is often misdiagnosed because it so closely resembles the flu. When reviewing biopsy results, it's helpful to know what to look for, he says....

In Ted's case, the fungal elements were noted but weren't perceived as being significant. "It can take a little extra detective work."

Fortunately, the condition is treatable. Although Shear performed a second biopsy and fungal culture, he didn't wait for the results to start a regimen. He promptly prescribed a high dose of antifungal medication two times a day for a month. "After a week, the patient started getting better," Shear says. Today, Ted has fully recovered.

**Name changed to protect patient privacy*

SEE ALSO *Coccidioidomycosis; Histoplasmosis; Mycotic Disease*

BIBLIOGRAPHY

Books

Al-Doory, Yousef, and Arthur F. DiSalvo, eds. *Blastomycosis.* New York: Plenum Medical, 1992.

Sobel, Jack D. *Contemporary Diagnosis and Management of Fungal Infections.* Longboat Key, FL: Handbooks in Health Care, 2009.

Periodicals

Bradsher, Robert W., Jr. "The Endemic Mimic: Blastomycosis an Illness Often Misdiagnosed." *Transactions of the American Clinical and Climatological Association* 125 (2014): 188–203.

Carlos W. G., et al. "Blastomycosis in Indiana: Digging Up More Cases." *Chest* 138, no. 6 (2010): 1377–1382.

Khuu, Diana, et al. "Blastomycosis Mortality Rates, United States, 1990–2010." *Emerging Infectious Diseases* 20, no. 11 (2014): 1789–1794. This article can also be found online at https://wwwnc.cdc.gov/eid/article/20/11/13-1175_article (accessed January 26, 2018).

Kiatsimkul, Porntip. "Increasing Incidence of Blastomycosis Infection in Vermont." Supplement, *Open Forum Infectious Diseases* 4 (2017): S84–S85. This article can also be found online at https://www.ncbi.nlm.nih.gov/pmc/articles/PMC5631645/ (accessed January 25, 2018).

Lester, Robert S., et al. "Novel Cases of Blastomycosis Acquired in Toronto, Ontario." *Canadian Medical Association Journal* 163 (November 14, 2000): 1309–1312.

Ross, John J., and Douglas N. Keeling. "Cutaneous Blastomycosis in New Brunswick: Case Report." *Canadian Medical Association Journal* 163 (November 14, 2000): 1303–1305.

Websites

"About Blastomycosis." Minnesota Department of Health. http://www.health.state.mn.us/divs/idepc/diseases/blastomycosis/basics.html (accessed January 25, 2018).

"Blastomycosis." Centers for Disease Control and Prevention, January 26, 2017. https://www.cdc.gov/fungal/diseases/blastomycosis/index.html (accessed January 25, 2018).

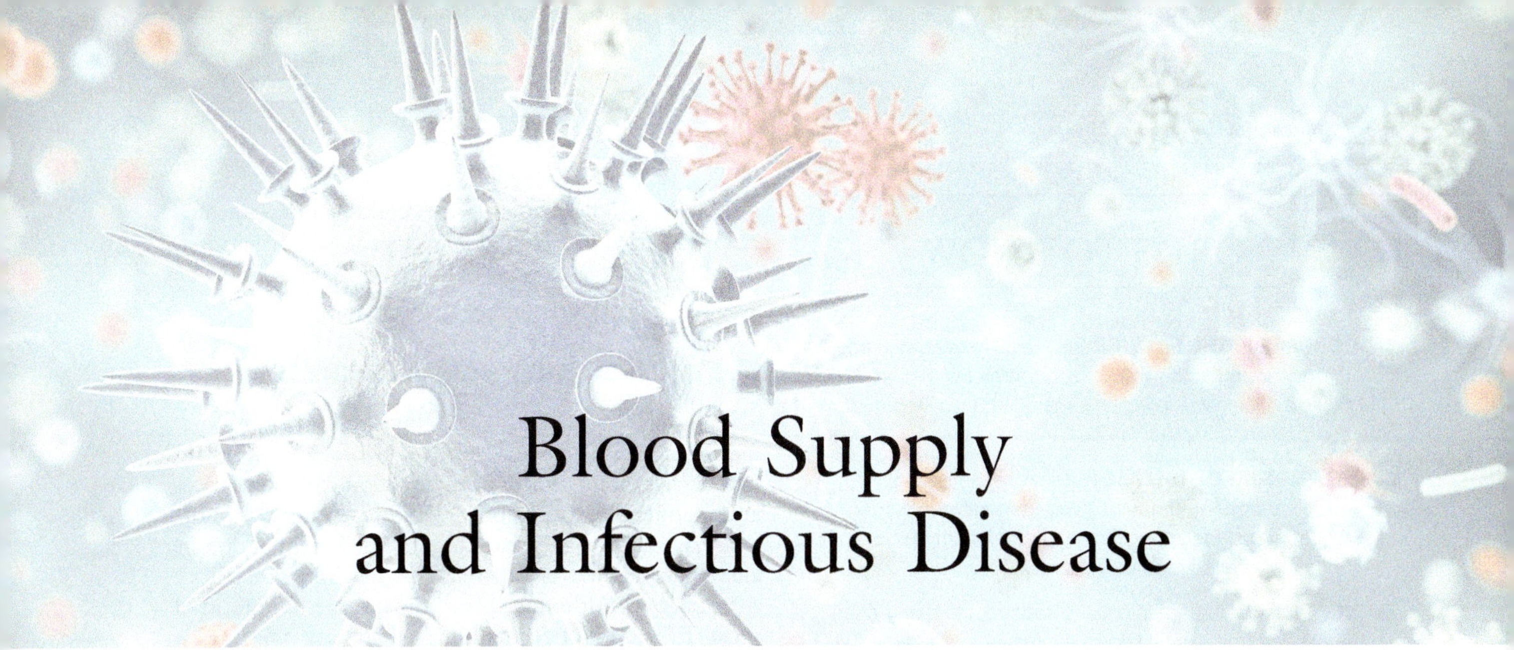

Blood Supply and Infectious Disease

Introduction

According to the US Centers for Disease Control and Prevention (CDC), there are more than 9.5 million blood donors in the United States and an estimated 5 million patients who receive blood annually, resulting in a total of 14.6 million transfusions per year. In the United States and Europe, the blood supply is safer than ever before due to screening of donors and use of blood screening tests. Although there is a low risk of transmission of life-threatening transfusion-transmissible illnesses (TTIs) for the vast majority of people in the United States and Europe, the medical benefits of blood transfusion or blood products now outweigh the risk from infection. However, this is not the case in many developing countries, where lack of resources and infrastructure mean that donors and donated blood may not be screened as carefully.

History and Scientific Foundations

The US Centers for Disease Control and Prevention reported the first few cases of human immunodeficiency virus (HIV) in 1981. Prior to more stringent blood safety measures and more sensitive tests, HIV from infected blood donors made its way into blood products.

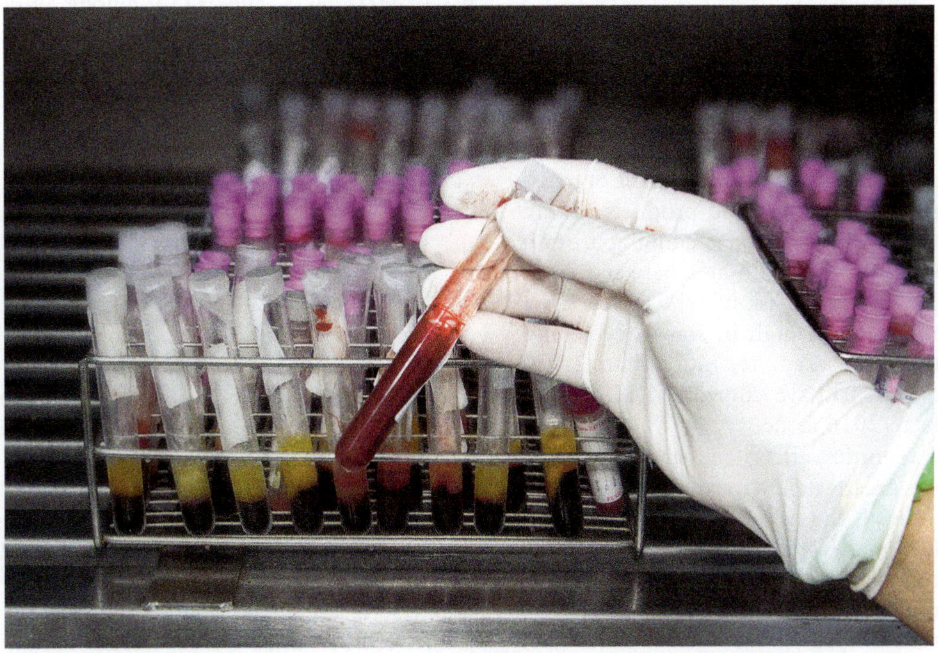

In the United States all donated blood must pass a screening for HIV, HBV, HCV, human T-lymphotropic virus, and syphilis before it can be used in a transfusion. *© Prakaymas vitchitchalao/Alamy Stock Photo*

WORDS TO KNOW

BLOODBORNE PATHOGENS Disease-causing agents carried or transported in the blood. Bloodborne infections are those in which the infectious agent is transmitted from one person to another via contaminated blood.

CREUTZFELDT-JAKOB DISEASE (CJD) A transmissible, rapidly progressing, fatal neurodegenerative disorder related to bovine spongiform encephalopathy (BSE), commonly called mad cow disease.

PRIONS Proteins that are infectious. Indeed, the name *prion* is derived from "proteinaceous infectious particles." The discovery of prions and confirmation of their infectious nature overturned a central dogma that infections were caused only by intact organisms, particularly microorganisms such as bacteria, fungi, parasites, or viruses. Because prions lack genetic material, the prevailing attitude was that a protein could not cause disease.

TRANSFUSION-TRANSMISSIBLE INFECTIONS Any infection that can be transmitted to a person by a blood transfusion (the addition of stored whole blood or blood fractions to a person's own blood). Some diseases that can be transmitted in this way are AIDS, hepatitis B, hepatitis C, syphilis, malaria, and Chagas disease.

People with hemophilia, a blood clotting disorder, were at especially high risk due to frequent transfusions of factor VIII (a blood clotting factor) derived from pooled blood donations. According to the CDC, as of December 2001, an estimated 14,262 people in the United States had been diagnosed with HIV or acquired immunodeficiency syndrome (AIDS) as a result of transfusing contaminated blood or blood products. There were no reports of HIV infection stemming from a blood transfusion in the United States between 2008 and early 2018. However, the risk of HIV infection via blood transfusion remained high in some developing countries. In India, for example, more than 2,000 people were reported to have contracted HIV from blood transfusions in 2016 alone.

In developed countries, efforts and strategies in the 21st century have greatly helped reduce transfusion-associated risks. Indeed, the risk of being infected by a contaminated blood unit is significantly lower than the risk in the 1980s. A considerable portion of this improvement is due to the introduction of nucleic acid testing (NAT), which directly detects the pathogenic organism rather than relying solely on measuring pathogen-specific antibody responses in the donor. NAT was introduced in the developed world in the late 20th and early 21st century. As of 2017 around 33 countries in the world had implemented NAT for HIV and around 27 countries for hepatitis B virus (HBV).

■ Applications and Research

To minimize the risk of TTIs, the World Health Organization (WHO) has developed a twofold approach to blood safety. First, for regular donations, blood services are encouraged to use only voluntary, unpaid donors who have a low risk of carrying a TTI. Potential donors answer a detailed health-related questionnaire before the donation. Although this eliminates the likelihood of most TTIs, WHO recommends mandatory testing of donated blood for HIV-1 and 2, hepatitis B and C (HCV), and syphilis. Screening of donations for other infections, such as those causing malaria or Chagas disease, should be based on geographical location where these diseases are prevalent.

According to the CDC, donated blood in the United States is also tested for bacterial contamination, human T-lymphotropic virus 1 and 2 (HTLV-1 and 2), and West Nile virus. NAT is conducted for HCV, HIV-1 and 2, and West Nile virus.

According to the Joint United Kingdom (UK) Blood Transfusion and Tissue Transplantation Services Professional Advisory Committee, the UK Department of Health requires donated blood to be tested for HIV, HBV, HCV, HTLV-1 and 2, and syphilis. HIV-1 and 2, as well as HCV, are tested with NAT. These measures for improving the safety of the UK blood supply have reduced the residual risk of HIV, HCV, and HTLV among all donations to below 1 per 1 million donations and that of hepatitis B to close to 1 per 300,000 donations.

According to the American Red Cross, the risk of contracting HIV from donated blood is 1 in 2 million. The odds of getting hepatitis B from donated blood is about 1 in 300,000, and the risk with hepatitis C is 1 in 1.5 million. The risk of getting West Nile virus from a blood transfusion is approximately 1 in 350,000.

■ Impacts and Issues

Much as when HIV took the world by surprise in the late 20th century, there is always the possibility of a new infection that might threaten the blood supply. In the 21st century, concern grew over variant Creutzfeldt-Jakob disease (vCJD), a rare, fatal brain disease that was first identified in the United Kingdom in 1995. As of February 2015, 3 out of a total of 229 cases worldwide were traced to contaminated blood.

As of 2017 there was no test for the prion protein, which is the infective agent in vCJD. Therefore, donations cannot be screened. Prions also cannot be destroyed using current techniques for inactivating pathogens in the blood

PERSONAL AND SOCIAL RESPONSIBILITY

Blood donation is the process by which a blood donor voluntarily gives blood that will be securely stored at a designated place, often called a blood bank, for some future use, often for a blood transfusion. People sometimes donate blood for themselves, particularly when they are scheduled for surgery.

Transfusion is the medical process of transferring whole blood or blood components from one person (donor) to another (recipient) to restore lost blood, improve clotting time, and improve the ability of the blood to deliver oxygen to the body's tissues. Whole blood is used exactly as it was received from the donor. Blood components are parts of whole blood, such as red blood cells (RBCs), plasma, platelets, clotting factors, immunoglobulins, and white blood cells. Using blood components is a more efficient way to use the blood supply because blood that has been processed, or fractionated, into components can be used to treat more than one person.

On average, one pint of blood components is used for three patients. Transfusions have saved countless people around the world. Each year in the United States, about 4.5 million people are in need of blood transfusions.

supply. The American Red Cross is dealing with the threat that vCJD could pose to the US blood supply by disqualifying potential donors who have received blood donations in the United Kingdom after 1980.

Meanwhile, the safety of blood continues to be a global issue. Many developing countries have not yet adopted WHO rules. Family or paid donors, known to carry a higher risk of TTIs, account for more than 50 percent of blood donated in developing countries. The populations in these countries are also at risk from the use of untested blood in transfusions. WHO has several projects underway aimed at building and supporting the blood supply around the world so that everyone has access to safe transfusions and blood products.

Despite the potential for disease transmission through transfused blood, the safety of the blood supply in the United States continues to improve and as of 2017 was at the highest level it had ever been. As known threats continue to be managed, however, new challenges will continue to arise. Careful donor selection, vigilant screening, "lookback" programs (procedures to trace the distribution of blood from a donor who later tests positive for an infectious disease), inactivation of pathogens, and efforts to develop new techniques for screening and inactivation will be required to make blood products, and thus blood transfusions, safe.

SEE ALSO *Bloodborne Pathogens; Hepatitis B; Hepatitis C; HIV*

BIBLIOGRAPHY

Books

Barbara, John A. J., Fiona A. M. Regan, and Marcela Contreras, eds. *Transfusion Microbiology.* Cambridge, UK: Cambridge University Press, 2008.

Osaro, Erharbor. *Blood Transfusion Services in Sub Saharan Africa: Challenges and Constraints.* Bloomington, IN: AuthorHouse, 2012.

Periodicals

Hans, Rekha, and Neelam Marwhara. "Nucleic Acid Testing—Benefits and Constraints." *Asian Journal of Transfusion Science* 8, no. 1 (January–June 2014): 2–3. This article can also be found online at https://www.ncbi.nlm.nih.gov/pmc/articles/PMC3943139/ (accessed February 12, 2018).

Kralievits, Katherine E., et al. "The Global Blood Supply: A Literature Review." *Lancet* 385 (April 27, 2015). This article can also be found online at http://www.thelancet.com/journals/lancet/article/PIIS0140–6736(15)60823–6/fulltext (accessed February 12, 2018).

Landro, Laura. "The Rising Risk of a Contaminated Blood Supply." *Wall Street Journal* (September 27, 2015). This article can also be found online at https://www.wsj.com/articles/the-rising-risk-of-a-contaminated-blood-supply-1443407428 (accessed February 12, 2018).

Nunez, Christina. "Mad Cow Disease Still Menaces U.K. Blood Supply." *National Geographic* (February 16, 2015). This article can also be found online at https://news.nationalgeographic.com/news/2015/02/150215-mad-cow-disease-vcjd-blood-supply-health/ (accessed February 12, 2018).

Websites

"Blood Safety and Availability." World Health Organization, June 2017. http://www.who.int/mediacentre/factsheets/fs279/en/ (accessed February 12, 2018).

"Blood Safety Basics." Centers for Disease Control and Prevention, January 31, 2013. https://www.cdc.gov/bloodsafety/basics.html (accessed February 12, 2018).

Koerth-Baker, Maggie. "To Keep the Blood Supply Safe, Screening Blood Is More Important Than Banning Donors." FiveThirtyEight, June 16, 2016. https://fivethirtyeight.com/features/to-keep-the-blood-supply-safe-screening-blood-is-more-important-than-banning-donors/ (accessed February 12, 2018).

"Risks and Complications." American Red Cross. https://www.redcrossblood.org/learn-about-blood/blood-transfusions/risks-complications (accessed February 12, 2018).

Susan Aldridge
Malini Vashishtha

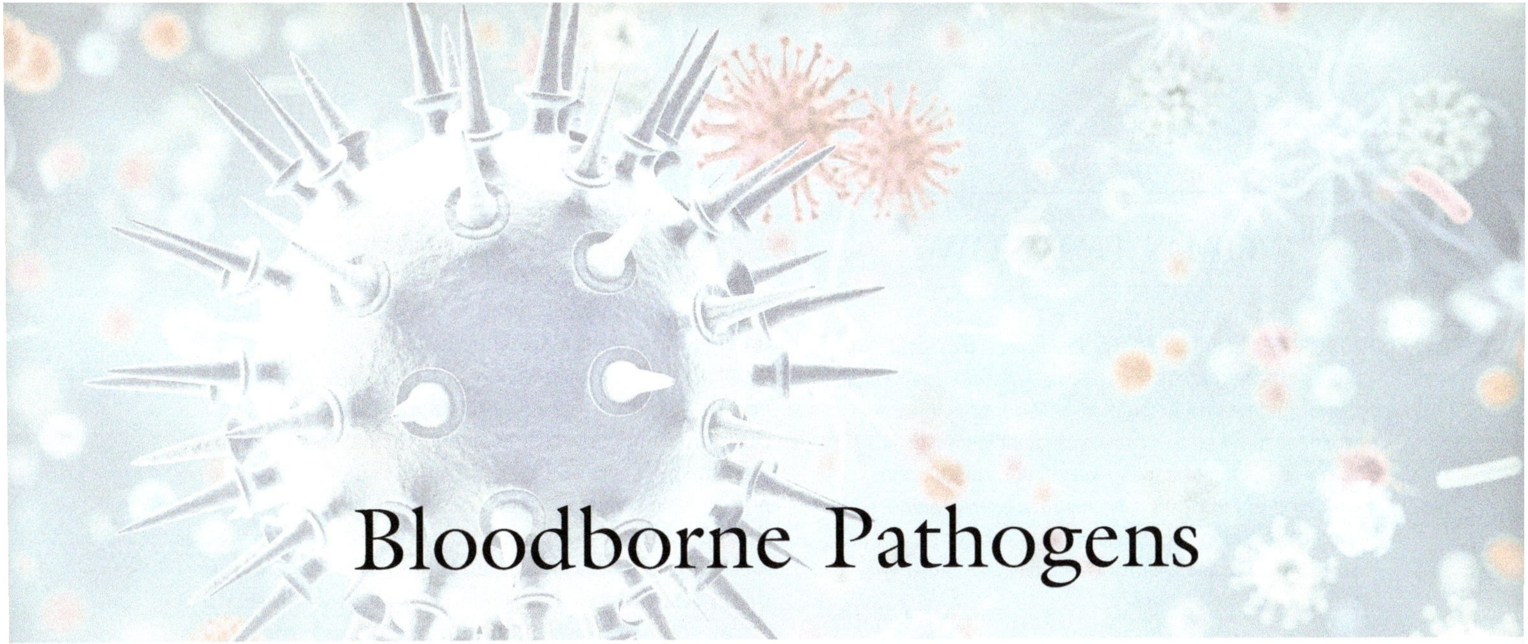

Bloodborne Pathogens

■ Introduction

Bloodborne pathogens are microscopic, disease-causing organisms present in the blood of humans with certain infections. Bloodborne pathogens can infect humans who come in contact with infected blood. The three major bloodborne pathogens are hepatitis B virus (HBV), hepatitis C virus (HCV), and human immunodeficiency virus (HIV), although other diseases such as malaria, brucellosis, and syphilis can also be transmitted via exposure to infected blood.

Health care workers, including doctors, dentists, and nurses, can become exposed through needlestick injuries (NSIs), which occur if they are accidentally pricked with a needle that has been used on an infected person. Drug addicts/users who share needles can also become infected with bloodborne pathogens. This is a major route of transmitting HCV. Reducing the risk from bloodborne pathogens depends on people following the strict precautions laid down by the US Occupational Safety and Health Administration (OSHA) and equivalent organizations in other countries.

■ History and Scientific Foundations

When HIV was identified in the early 1980s, it soon became clear that transmission through infected blood was a real possibility. Thousands of people with the blood clotting disorder hemophilia became infected with HIV because of their dependence on blood products. Now that blood and donors are screened in many countries and the World Health Organization (WHO) has endeavored to make this a global practice, this route of exposure to HIV and the two other major bloodborne pathogens (HBV and HCV) has become less significant.

However, there is still a risk of transmission of bloodborne pathogens to those who become exposed to infected blood, either through their occupation or through their lifestyle. For health care workers, a major risk of exposure comes from NSI, which occurs if a health care worker is accidentally pricked with a needle that has been used to

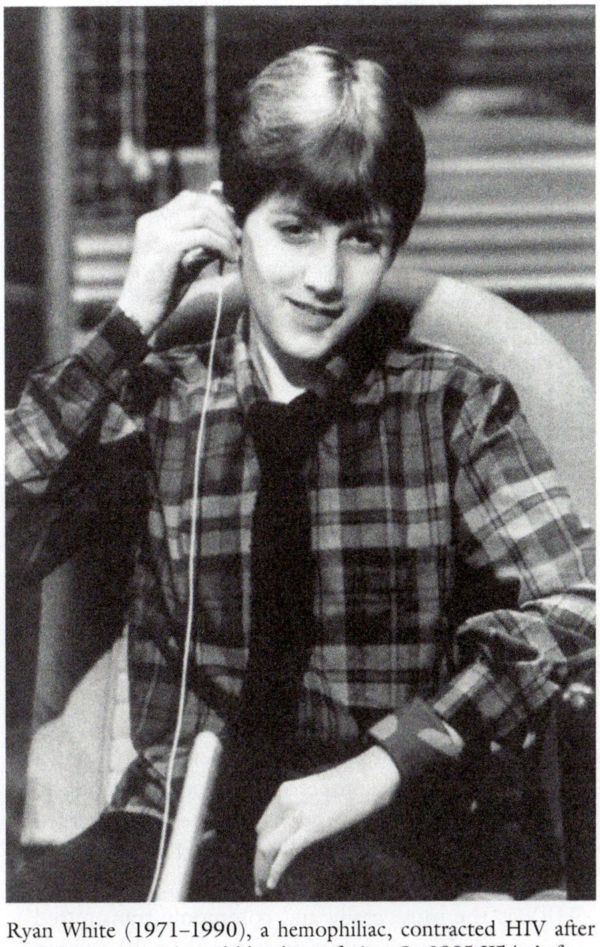

Ryan White (1971–1990), a hemophiliac, contracted HIV after receiving a contaminated blood transfusion. In 1985 White's family won a legal battle that allowed him to continue attending school despite his infection. *© AP Images/BRUNO MOSCONI*

WORDS TO KNOW

BLOODBORNE Via the blood. For example, bloodborne pathogens are pathogens (disease-causing agents) carried or transported in the blood. Bloodborne infections are those in which the infectious agent is transmitted from one person to another via contaminated blood. Infections of the blood can occur as a result of the spread of an ongoing infection caused by bacteria such as *Yersinia pestis*, *Haemophilus influenzae*, and *Staphylococcus aureus*.

NEEDLESTICK INJURY (NSI) Any accidental breakage or puncture of the skin by an unsterilized medical needle (syringe). Health care providers are particularly at risk for needlestick injuries, which may transmit disease, because of the large number of needles they handle.

PATHOGEN A disease-causing agent, such as a bacterium, a virus, a fungus, or another microorganism.

POSTEXPOSURE PROPHYLAXIS Treatment with drugs immediately after exposure to an infectious microorganism. The aim of this approach is to prevent an infection from becoming established.

STANDARD PRECAUTIONS The safety measures taken to prevent the transmission of disease-causing bacteria. These measures include proper handwashing; wearing gloves, goggles, and other protective clothing; proper handling of needles; and sterilization of equipment.

inject or draw blood from an infected person. An NSI can occur during the procedure or during disposal of the needle. A similar risk exists from cuts occurring from sharp surgical instruments, such as scalpels, that have been contaminated with infected blood. Instruments that can cause this kind of injury are generally known as sharps.

Splashes of infected blood to the eye, nose, mouth, or skin also carry a risk. Bloodborne infections are more common in low-income countries where unsafe practices such as repeated use of needles exist. In some highly populated regions in poor countries, health care facilities are known to reuse needles without proper sterilization. According to a 1999 study, bloodborne infections can often be prevented in such settings by using more recent and effective oral drugs.

HBV is the most easily and commonly transmitted bloodborne pathogen, infecting more than 20 million people around the world annually according to the US Centers for Disease Control and Prevention (CDC). The CDC indicates that the risk of a health care worker contracting HBV through a single needlestick or cut exposure ranges from 6 to 30 percent. However, if health care personnel are immunized against HBV, the chances of contracting the virus is almost eliminated.

HCV is the second-most common bloodborne pathogen worldwide, infecting about 2 million people each year through contaminated injections. In the year 2000 there was an outbreak of HCV through unsafe injections reported in Egypt. For HIV the risk of becoming infected through an NSI is about 1 in 300, although the risk is higher when a person with advanced AIDS is the source of the infected blood. Deep injections and instruments that are obviously contaminated with blood also carry a higher risk of infection. The risk following HIV-infected blood splashes is around 1 in 1,000. There have been no documented cases of HIV transmission from exposure of intact skin to infected blood.

■ Applications and Research

Commonsense precautions, such as protecting the hands, eyes, and mouth when dealing with blood from patients potentially infected with HBV, HCV, and HIV, can go a long way to reducing the risk of transmission of these bloodborne pathogens. It is also important to use properly trained staff (phlebotomists) to take blood samples. Simply reducing the number of times needles are used on patients or for injections, the number of times catheters are placed, and the number of times blood samples are taken also reduces the risk of transmitting bloodborne pathogens by cutting down on the number of occasions on which accidents can take place.

Science and technology have also contributed to reducing the risk of transmission of bloodborne pathogens. For instance, the CDC notes that the annual number of HBV infections has decreased more than 90 percent since the introduction of the vaccine in 1982. Unfortunately, there are no such vaccines against HCV or HIV, although research is ongoing as of 2018. The development of vaccines against HCV faces many scientific challenges, but the effort continues.

Due to enormous variation in the virus envelope protein, it has been difficult to develop a vaccine against HIV. A trial of one such vaccine, RV144, used a combination of two vaccines given in four doses. The trial showed positive results, with a 31.2 percent lower infection rate in the group receiving the vaccine versus the control group not receiving the vaccine. Although these results are not adequate for regulatory approvals, the study has been important in understanding the way forward in HIV vaccine research.

BLOODBORNE INFECTIONS TRANSMITTED THROUGH BARBER SHOPS

The practice of men going to neighborhood barber shops for a shave or haircut has raised the level of risk in contracting hepatitis B virus (HBV) and hepatitis C virus (HCV) infections in Asian and Middle Eastern countries. This is due to the multiple reuse of razors and nondisposable instruments.

A study from Japan indicated that razor shaving is associated with significant risk of HCV infection among hospital patients. Another study in Pakistan showed the rate of HCV transmission via used razor blades and syringes was higher than that of sexual transmission. Even in some European countries, such as Italy and Turkey, spread of viral hepatitis through razor shaving has been reported.

Educating barbers on maintaining hygiene and using single-use, disposable blades will largely benefit communities and towns where this practice is prevalent.

■ Impacts and Issues

Due to lack of reporting, epidemiological studies do not correctly estimate the global burden of bloodborne infections transmitted through unsafe injections. A mathematical model developed in 1999 by researchers and published in *Bulletin of the World Health Organization* to give regional estimates of bloodborne pathogens suggested that each year injection-related infection probably accounts for 8 million to 16 million HBV infections, 2.3 million to 4.7 million HCV infections, and 80,000 to 160,000 HIV infections.

In 1991 OSHA issued the Bloodborne Pathogens Standard, which was updated in 2001. This law encompasses the standard requirements for employers to implement in the worksite and the precautions to be taken by health care workers. Basically, all people receiving care are considered potentially contaminated with bloodborne pathogens unless proven otherwise. Therefore, using protective measures to avoid contact with blood is now standard procedure for health care workers.

Prevention of exposure involves physical protection of the worker with gloves, masks, and eye shields during surgery or other procedures where there is potential for contact with blood. Safe devices such as retractable or sheathed needles must be used when taking blood, and any NSIs must be reported and followed up. Protection from infection depends on all those who may be at risk taking this code seriously and following it before, during, and after handling blood from potential sources of bloodborne pathogen risk.

The advent of safer devices, such as needleless injectors, has also been an important advancement in preventing NSIs. OSHA reports that there has been a reduction in NSIs due to introduction of better medical devices that reduce the risk of needlesticks and injuries due to sharps. For injection drug users at risk of bloodborne infections, especially HCV, education in harm reduction and needle exchange schemes may reduce the incidence of new infections. However, it is difficult to document this, as there is often a lengthy time lag between exposure and evidence of infection.

SEE ALSO *Blood Supply and Infectious Disease; Hepatitis B; Hepatitis C; HIV; Infection Control and Asepsis; Standard Precautions*

BIBLIOGRAPHY

Books

Bartlett, J. G. "Occupational Exposure to Human Immunodeficiency Virus and Other Bloodborne Pathogens." In *Current Surgical Therapy*, edited by John Cameron and Andrew Cameron. Philadelphia: Elsevier Saunders, 2016.

Periodicals

Alter, M. J. "Epidemiology of Hepatitis C in the West." *Seminars in Liver Disease* 15, no. 1 (1995): 5–14.

Frank, C., et al. "The Role of Parenteral Antischistosomal Therapy in the Spread of Hepatitis C Virus in Egypt." *Lancet* 355 (2000): 887–891.

Hauri, A. M., G. L. Armstrong, and Y. J. Hutin. "The Global Burden of Disease Attributable to Contaminated Injections Given in Health Care Settings." *International Journal of STD and AIDS* 15 (2004): 7–16.

Kane, A., et al. "Transmission of Hepatitis B, Hepatitis C and Human Immunodeficiency Viruses through Unsafe Injections in the Developing World: Model-Based Regional Estimates." *Bulletin of the World Health Organization* 77, no. 10 (1999): 801–807.

Khan, Gulfaraz, et al. "Risk of Blood-Borne Infections in Barber Shops." *Journal of Infection and Public Health* 3 (2010): 88–89.

Simonsen, L., et al. "Unsafe Injections in the Developing World and Transmission of Bloodborne Pathogens." *Bulletin of the World Health Organization* 77, no. 10 (1999): 789–800.

Websites

"Exposure to Blood: What Healthcare Personnel Need to Know." Centers for Disease Control and Prevention, July 2003. https://www.cdc.gov/hai/pdfs/bbp/exp_to_blood.pdf (accessed February 23, 2018).

Highleyman, Liz. "Hepatitis C Vaccine Shows Progress but Scientific Barriers Remain." World Hepatitis Alliance, September 12, 2016. http://www.worldhepatitisalliance.org/latest-news/infohep/3084554/hepatitis-c-vaccine-development-shows-progress-scientific-barriers-remain (accessed February 26, 2018).

"HIV Vaccine Development." World Health Organization. http://www.who.int/immunization/research/development/hiv_vaccdev/en/ (accessed February 26, 2018).

"OSHA Fact Sheet: OSHA's Bloodborne Pathogens Standard." United States Department of Labor, Occupational Safety and Health Administration, January 2011. https://www.osha.gov/OshDoc/data_BloodborneFacts/bbfact01.pdf (accessed February 25, 2018).

"Preventing the Spread of Bloodborne Pathogens." American National Red Cross, 2011. http://www.in.gov/isdh/files/BBP_American_Red_Cross_Fact_Sheet_xps(1).pdf (accessed February 23, 2018).

"Revision to OSHA's Bloodborne Pathogens Standard." United States Department of Labor, Occupational Safety and Health Administration, April 2001. https://www.osha.gov/needlesticks/needlefact.html (accessed February 23, 2018).

Susan Aldridge
Kausalya Santhanam

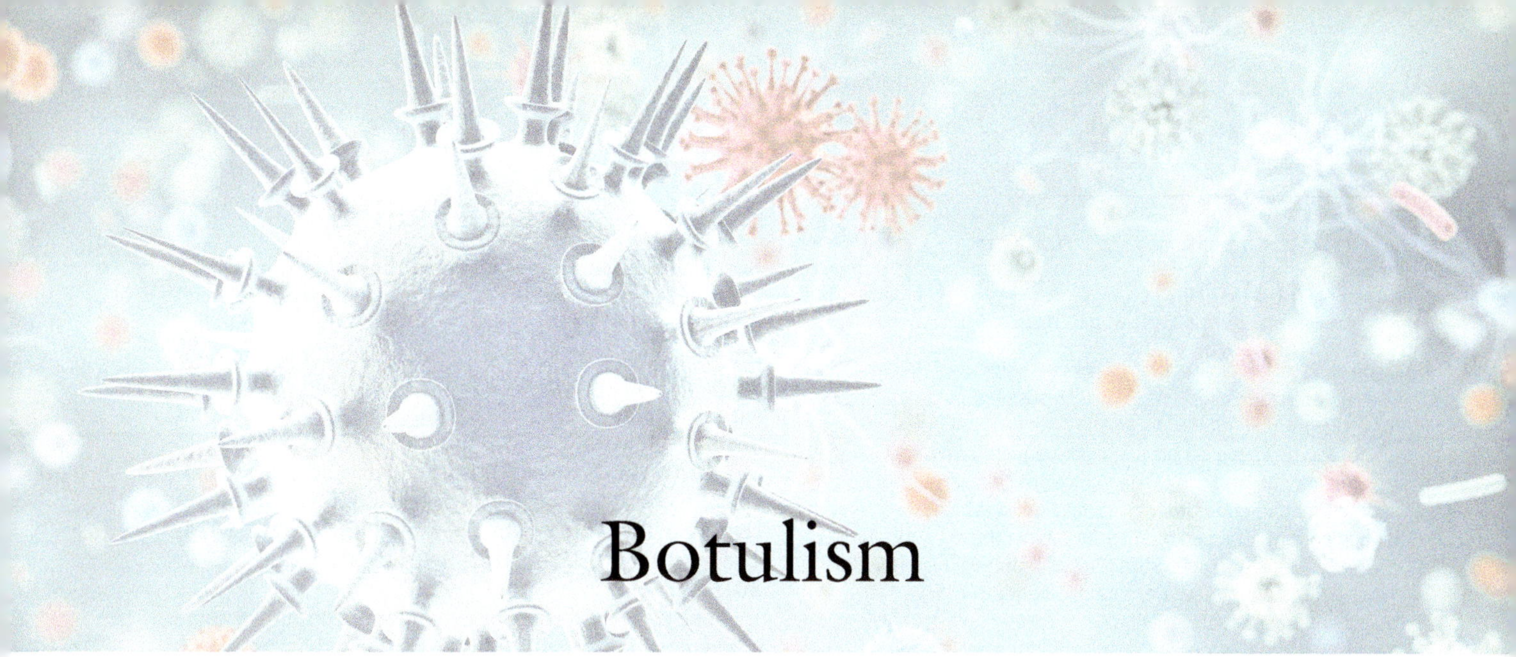

Botulism

Introduction

Botulism is a disease that is caused by a bacterial toxin. The toxin is one of seven (types A–G) made and released by the bacterium *Clostridium botulinum.* Botulism toxin types A, B, E, and F cause botulism in humans. Another bacterium, *Clostridium baratii*, can also produce a disease-causing toxin, but this bacterium is rarely encountered, thus it is responsible for far fewer cases of botulism than is *C. botulinum.*

Botulism toxins are powerful neurotoxins; they affect nerves and can produce paralysis. One microgram of toxin—a millionth of a gram—can kill a person. Paralysis from botulism affects the functioning of organs and tissues, and, when botulism is fatal, death is usually the result of failure of the respiratory muscles.

Disease History, Characteristics, and Transmission

Botulism was first described in 1735 in an illness outbreak that was traced to the consumption of contaminated German sausage. Indeed, the word botulism was derived from the Latin word *botulus*, meaning sausage.

C. botulinum bacteria are commonly found in soil. They can be present on vegetables and other food grown in soil and can be eaten if the food is not completely washed free of bacteria. Fortunately, under these conditions where oxygen is present, the bacteria do not produce the toxin and so are harmless when eaten. Botulism is not a contagious disease—it cannot be spread from person to person. Rarely, botulism occurs as the result of a wound infected with *C. botulinum.*

The toxin is produced when the bacterium grows in the absence of oxygen. Growth of the bacteria in, for example, the low-oxygen and slightly acidic environment (the bacteria cannot grow above pH 5) of some canned foods is associated with the production of gas. Cans can bulge due to the buildup of the gas; bulging cans should be discarded. With food-borne botulism, growth of the bacteria in the food may occur but is not mandatory for developing botulism, as the presence of the toxin alone is sufficient to cause illness. Because the toxin causes the illness, food-borne botulism is often described as a food intoxication.

In rare cases botulism can also be caused by an infection of *C. botulinum* in an open wound. Growth of the bacteria deep in the tissues leads to the production of the toxin, which then spreads via the bloodstream.

Symptoms of botulism are produced when the toxin enters the bloodstream. The toxin blocks the production of the neurotransmitter acetylcholine, a chemical that bridges the physical gap between nerve cells and aids in the transmission of impulses from nerve to nerve. As nerves are affected and paralysis occurs, a person has difficulty seeing, talking, and swallowing and can become nauseous.

C. botulinum is one of a few types of bacteria that can produce spores. A spore is a form of the bacterium that is nongrowing but can persist in that form for a long time and in conditions of excess heat, dryness, and other harsh environments that would kill the normally growing cell. The spore form allows the organism to survive inhospitable

WORDS TO KNOW

NEUROTOXIN A poison that interferes with nerve function, usually by affecting the flow of ions through the cell membrane.

SPORE A dormant form assumed by some bacteria, such as anthrax, that enables the bacterium to survive high temperatures, dryness, and lack of nourishment for long periods of time. Under proper conditions, the spore may revert to the actively multiplying form of the bacteria.

BOTULINUM TOXIN AS A BIOLOGICAL WEAPON

According to the Centers for Disease Control and Prevention, aerosolized botulinum toxin is a possible mechanism for a bioterrorism attack. As of 2017 inhalational botulism could not, however, be clinically differentiated from the naturally occurring forms. The symptoms that develop are similar to those of naturally occurring botulism. The inhalation form of infection may be suspected by a medical professional based on the patient's medical history. What factors might assist or complicate the definitive determination of such an attack?

Key clinical or epidemiological factors assisting the determination of an intentional attack:

- Inhalational botulism does not occur naturally.
- Botulism is not transmissible from person to person.
- Indications of intentional release of aerosolized botulinum toxin might include an unusual geographic clustering of illness (e.g., persons who attended the same public event or gathering).
- Symptoms begin within six hours to two weeks after exposure (often within 12 to 36 hours).

conditions. When conditions improve, such as in canned food or inside the body, the bacteria can resume growth, division, and toxin production.

Scope and Distribution

Botulism is a fairly rare illness. In the United States, for example, fewer than 200 cases have been reported each year since the 1990s. Most cases are due to the improper canning of foods at home. The US Centers for Disease Control and Prevention (CDC), in partnership with state and District of Columbia health agencies, has been keeping track of the number of cases since 1973 as part of the National Botulism Surveillance System. There were 199 confirmed cases in 2015 (the most recent year for which data are available), 161 in 2014, 153 in 2013, 160 in 2012, 140 in 2011, and 112 in 2010.

The different forms of the botulism toxin display some differences in their geography. In the United States, type A botulism toxin, which is the most severe, occurs most often in western regions, particularly in the Rocky Mountains. Type B toxin, whose symptoms tend to be less severe, is more common in the eastern United States. Type E toxin is found more in the bacteria that live in freshwater sediments. The reasons for this distribution are not clear.

Treatment and Prevention

Diagnosis of botulism is complicated by the fact that the disease is infrequently seen. A physician may have little experience in dealing with the illness. In its early stages botulism has symptoms that are similar to those of other ailments, such as Guillain-Barré syndrome and stroke. Both of these considerations sometimes lead to a delayed diagnosis of botulism.

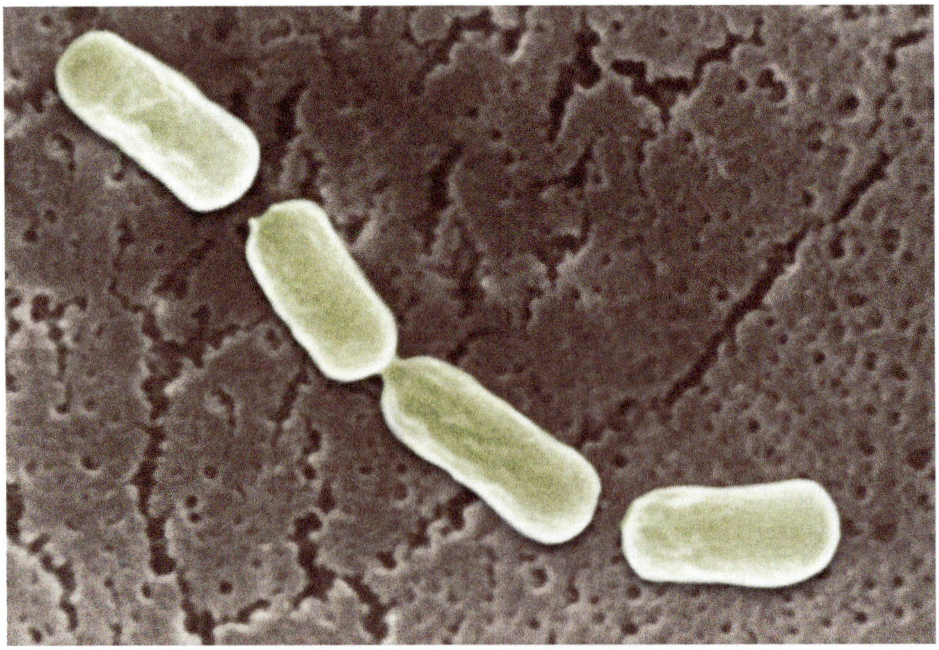

Clostridium botulinum, the bacterium responsible for botulism, is seen under an electron microscope. © *BSIP/UIG/Getty Images*

Diagnosis involves the detection of toxin in the infected person's blood, which can be accomplished using specific immune components, or antibodies. An antibody to the specific botulism toxin will react with the toxin, producing a visible clump of material. Sometimes living bacteria can be recovered from the infected person's feces.

Treatment for botulism often involves the administration of an antibody-containing antitoxin that blocks the binding of the toxin to the nerve cells. With time, paralysis fades. However, recovery can take many weeks. If botulism is suspected soon after exposure to the bacteria, the stomach contents can be emptied to remove potentially contaminated undigested food. When lung muscles have been affected, a patient may need mechanical assistance in breathing.

There was no vaccine for botulism licensed by the US Food and Drug Administration (FDA) as of 2017. That year a combined vaccine for influenza and botulism was being evaluated.

Impacts and Issues

In the 1800s botulism was frequently a death sentence—one out of every two people who became ill with it died. According to the CDC, there were no deaths (out of 199 confirmed cases of botulism) in 2015 and two deaths (out of 161 confirmed cases) in 2014. In contrast to some other diseases that take a disproportionate toll on underdeveloped countries, botulism is more prevalent in developed regions, particularly where food is processed, canned, and sold.

Botulism does have significance in its potential as a bioterrorist threat. During World War II (1939–1945) several nations, including the United States and Canada, experimented with the development of botulism toxin–based weapons. Sprays that contained the spore form of *C. botulinum* were developed and tested. The idea was that inhalation of the spores would lead to resumed growth of the bacteria and production of the lethal neurotoxin. The sprays were never used in battle.

Botulinum toxin A is exploited cosmetically as a means of lessening wrinkles. Injection of Botox relaxes muscles, which can produce a more youthful appearance. *Worldwide Facial Injectables Market Drivers, Opportunities, Trends, and Forecasts: 2017–2023*, a June 2017 report issued by Dublin firm Research and Markets, documented just over 7 million injections of Botox globally in 2016. Botulinum toxin A has also shown promise in lessening dystonia (muscle spasms) that occurs in cerebral palsy and in treating crossed eyes (strabismus).

In 1976 a form of botulism was recognized in infants in the United States that stemmed from babies ingesting *C. botulinum* spores, which colonized their intestinal tract (an infant's intestinal tract is less acidic than that of an adult) and eventually produced botulinum toxin. Evidence indicated that honey was linked with both the reservoir of the bacteria and the resulting disease. Honey-linked infant botulism has since been reported in other countries, prompting recommendations from the American Academy of Pediatrics for all infants less than 12 months of age not to receive foods containing honey. As of 2017 this recommendation remained in effect.

Because botulism is a rare occurrence, the CDC maintains a central supply of antitoxin against botulism. State health departments consult with the CDC for release of the antitoxin when a case has been reported to them. Fast action is essential because the antitoxin reduces the severity of the symptoms only if given early.

When a food source of botulism is discovered, the FDA issues a class 1 recall of the product. Class 1 recalls are reserved for dangerous or defective products that could cause serious health problems or death; these recalls involve communication between the FDA, the manufacturer or supplier, and the public to remove the product from the market or remove the food source from the food supply. An FDA recall took place in mid-December 2016, when a species of fish sold by one outlet was found to be contaminated with *C. botulinum.*

SEE ALSO *Bacterial Disease; Food-Borne Disease and Food Safety*

BIBLIOGRAPHY

Books

Research and Markets. *Worldwide Facial Injectables Market Drivers, Opportunities, Trends, and Forecasts: 2017–2023.* Dublin: Research and Markets, 2017.

Ryan, Jeffrey. *Biosecurity and Bioterrorism: Containing and Preventing Biological Threats.* New York: Butterworth-Heinemann, 2016.

Tortora, Gerard J., Berell R. Funke, and Christine L. Case. *Microbiology: An Introduction.* Boston: Pearson, 2016.

Periodicals

Ramachandran, Prashanth, et al. "Adult Food Borne Botulism in Australia: The Only 2 Cases from the Last 15 Years." *Journal of Clinical Neuroscience* 41 (2017): 86–87.

Yan, Yongyong, et al. "A Combinatory Mucosal Vaccine against Influenza and Botulism." *Journal of Immunology* 196, no. 1 Supplement (May 1, 2016): 145–158.

Websites

"Botulism." Centers for Disease Control and Prevention. https://www.cdc.gov/botulism/resources.html (accessed December 3, 2017).

"Botulism." US Food and Drug Administration. https://www.foodsafety.gov/poisoning/causes/bacteriaviruses/botulism/index.html (accessed November 14, 2017).

Brian Hoyle

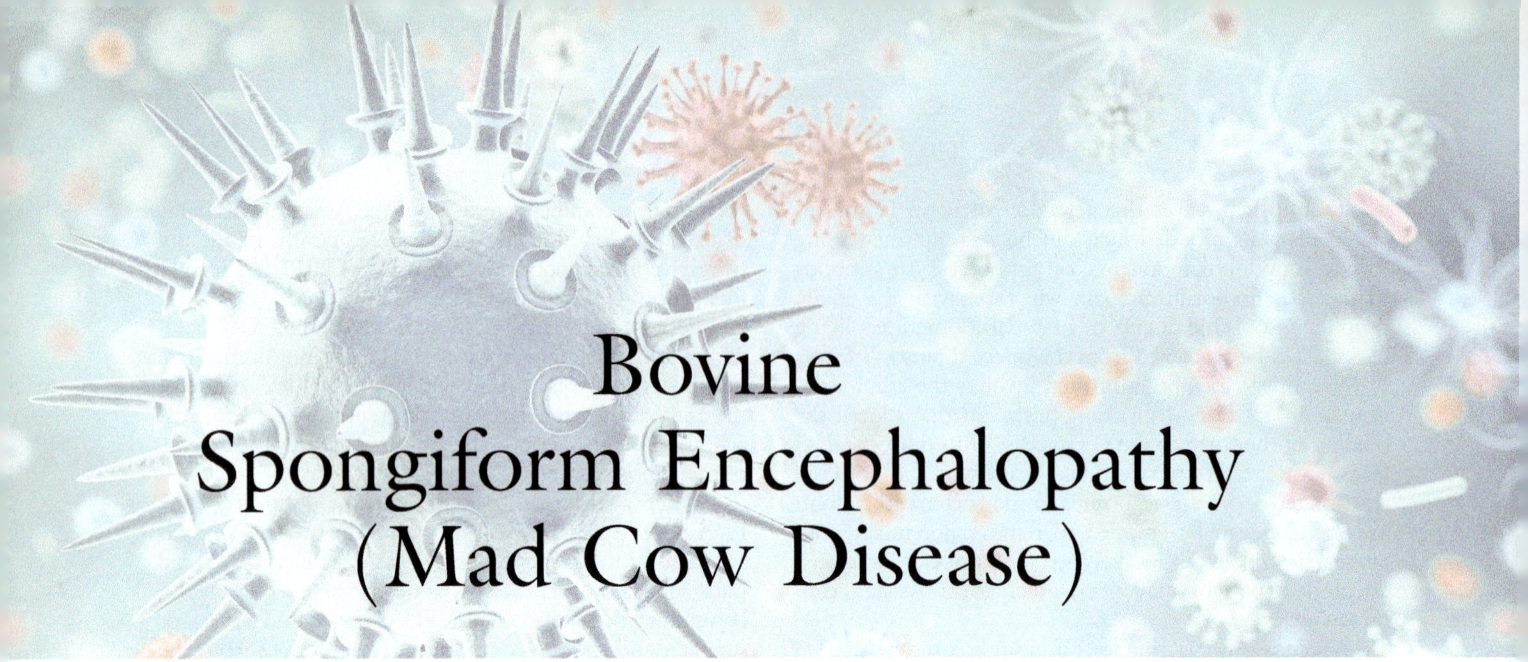

Bovine Spongiform Encephalopathy (Mad Cow Disease)

■ Introduction

Bovine spongiform encephalopathy (BSE) is a progressive infection of the brain and nervous system found in cattle. It is often known as mad cow disease because of the way affected animals stagger. There is much evidence that BSE can be transmitted from cattle to humans via the consumption of infected beef, resulting in an invariably fatal brain disorder called variant Creutzfeldt-Jakob disease (vCJD). An epidemic of BSE in the United Kingdom in the 1980s and 1990s has been linked to several cases of the human form of vCJD, mainly among younger people. The impact of BSE on Britain's farmers and beef industry was severe, as countries rushed to boycott imports of meat that might have come from infected cows. Although the BSE epidemic largely died away, cases still appear occasionally around the world. Meanwhile, many scientific questions on how BSE is transmitted remain unanswered.

WORDS TO KNOW

ENCEPHALOPATHY Any abnormality in the structure or function of the brain.

PRIONS Proteins that are infectious. Indeed, the name *prion* is derived from "proteinaceous infectious particles." The discovery of prions and confirmation of their infectious nature overturned a central dogma that infections were caused only by intact organisms, particularly microorganisms such as bacteria, fungi, parasites, or viruses. Because prions lack genetic material, the prevailing attitude was that a protein could not cause disease.

TRANSMISSION The movement of pathogens, or microorganisms that cause disease in humans and other species, to a human or other host. Transmission can occur in a number of ways, depending on the microorganism.

ZOONOSES Diseases of microbiological origin that can be transmitted from animals to people. The causes of the diseases can be bacteria, viruses, parasites, or fungi.

■ Disease History, Characteristics, and Transmission

BSE is a relatively new disease of cattle that was first identified in the United Kingdom in 1986. It proved to be one of a group of diseases called the transmissible spongiform encephalopathies (TSEs). On postmortem examination with a light microscope, the brain tissue of an animal with a TSE shows a characteristic spongy appearance because the pathology of the disease creates holes within the brain tissue, hence the term *spongiform.*

TSEs affect other animals, including humans. For instance, scrapie, a TSE found in sheep, has been known since the 18th century and is found at a low level in many parts of the world. The name comes from the tendency of animals with the disease to scrape their fleece against trees and bushes. TSEs have also been found in mink (transmissible mink encephalopathy) and in mule, deer, and elk (chronic wasting disease). CJD is the most significant TSE in humans. It is rare, usually occurring at a rate of around one per million of the population. The cases that arose from exposure to BSE in the United Kingdom from the mid-1990s represent a new form of CJD.

BSE occurs in adult animals of both sexes. The incubation period (the time lag from exposure to the appearance of symptoms) is usually measured in years. Therefore, the disease is rarely seen in young animals, even though they may be infected. Animals with BSE exhibit abnormalities of movement and posture, as well as changes in mental state that an experienced vet or farmer would be able to detect. The disease lasts for several weeks and is invariably both progressive and fatal.

TSEs can be transmitted from one animal to another. However, there is a species barrier, which means that transmission within species is more likely than transmission between species. For instance, there are no known instances of scrapie being transmitted to humans.

It is widely but not universally accepted that BSE arose in cattle from exposure to feed derived from sheep infected with scrapie. Adding protein from the carcasses of ruminants (sheep and cows) to animal feed is a long-established practice. The United Kingdom BSE Inquiry, which was set up to identify the underlying causes of the BSE epidemic, concluded that changes in the way the feed was processed probably allowed infectious material to survive and infect the cattle consuming it. From the time the BSE epidemic first took hold, there were fears that the disease might be transmitted to humans through exposure to meat and meat products (such as hamburgers) from infected animals. These fears were realized with the announcement of the first case of vCJD in 1996.

However, it has been hard to prove for certain that exposure to BSE causes vCJD. This is because the infective agent in TSEs is an unusual entity known as a prion. Research on infected tissue has shown that prions are not destroyed by either heat, which would destroy bacteria, or ultraviolet light, which would destroy viruses. Prions are an abnormal form of a protein normally found in the brain. When it infects the brain, the prion corrupts the normal prion protein molecules. These newly formed abnormal prion protein molecules go on to corrupt further normal prion molecules, beginning a cascade effect. The accumulation of more and more abnormal prion molecules triggers the brain damage that produces the symptoms of TSEs.

Scope and Distribution

Through the end of 2015, more than 184,500 cases of BSI were confirmed in over 35,000 herds of cattle in the United Kingdom, according to the US Centers for Disease Control and Prevention (CDC). The epidemic in the United Kingdom peaked in January 1993 at almost 1,000 new cases a week but then fell sharply. In 2010 there were only 11 cases and in 2015 only two cases.

Although BSE has reached epidemic levels only in the United Kingdom, it has affected other countries too. The World Organisation for Animal Health (OiE) collects data on BSE. Although as of 2017 there were no cases to date in Australia, New Zealand, Africa, and much of Asia, there had been several in European countries such as France, Germany, Ireland, and Portugal. As of July 2017 there were 25 confirmed cases of BSE in North America, including 20 in Canada and 5 in the United States.

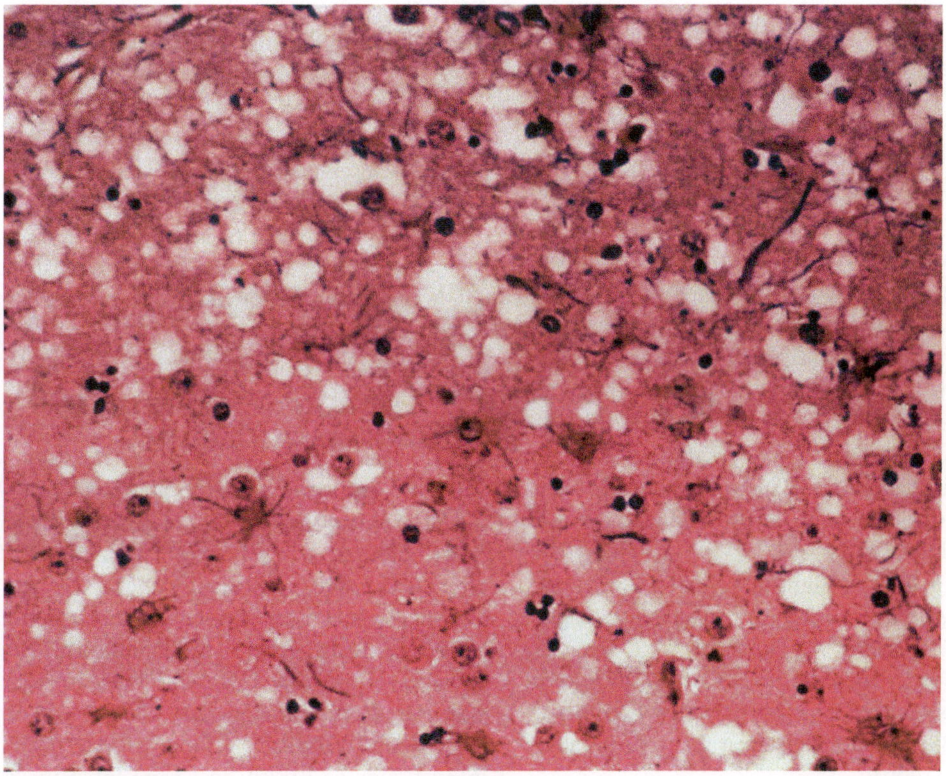

Bovine spongiform encephalopathy, or mad cow disease, causes microscopic holes to form in the brain of an infected cow. These holes give brain tissue a spongelike appearance when viewed under a microscope. *© CDC/Science Source*

EFFECTIVE RULES AND REGULATIONS

Variant CJD (vCJD) is the human form of bovine spongiform encephalopathy (BSE) disease, which emerged in Britain in the mid-1990s. The vCJD outbreak echoed the emergence in the 1950s of a strange and invariably fatal condition called kuru (meaning "trembling with fear") among the Fore people of New Guinea. After years of living among the group, American doctor Carleton Gajdusek (1923–2008), who went on to win the Nobel Prize for Medicine or Physiology in 1976, concluded that the disease was transmitted in the ritualistic eating of the brains of the deceased, a Fore funeral custom. He suspected that one of these brains, at least, must have belonged to someone with sporadic or familial CJD. There were some striking parallels between the emergence of vCJD and its links with the earlier epidemic of BSE, or mad cow disease, one of the transmissible spongiform encephalopathies (TSEs) found in cattle. The latter prompted a public enquiry to investigate the cause of the outbreak.

The inquiry confirmed that vCJD is, indeed, the human form of BSE. The inquiry concluded that infected material, either from sheep infected with scrapie (a sheep TSE) or from BSE-infected cattle, was incorporated into cattle feed. Further, it was found that changes in the processing of carcasses used for animal feed were likely the cause of this contamination. Fortunately, the epidemic, though tragic for the victims and their families, was limited by steps such as the wholesale slaughtering of infected cattle and a ban on imports of British beef.

The inquiry led to a variety of developments. For example, to restore public confidence, the Food Standards Agency was set up in the United Kingdom to advise on food safety issues. Regulatory authorities moved toward eliminating animal products from the manufacture of medicines and other items destined for human consumption. The BSE inquiry also led to changes in the supply of blood and blood products in an attempt to screen out donors that are unknowingly carrying vCJD.

Treatment and Prevention

There is no treatment for BSE, but much has been done to prevent its spread, both to other cattle in a herd and to humans. The government of the United Kingdom has introduced a number of measures to keep BSE under control. In July 1988 it imposed a ban on feeding cattle with potentially infected material. This measure kept animals that were not already infected from becoming infected and has been adopted in many countries, including those who are currently BSE-free. This measure alone made a major contribution to halting the growth of the UK BSE epidemic. However, because BSE has a long incubation time, there was a lag between introducing the ban and a fall in the number of cases. Thus, the number of cases continued to rise after 1988, despite the ban. In 1997 the United Kingdom also began a selective cull, slaughtering those animals that were at risk of contracting BSE. This further reduced the risk of the spread of infection.

The spread of BSE to humans has been limited by restricting imports of meat and meat products that might be infected. In 1996 cattle over 30 months old were no longer allowed to enter the food chain. Instead, they were incinerated after slaughter. This ban has now been lifted and replaced by BSE testing. Only meat that tests negative can enter the food supply.

Because animal feed containing meat and bone meal is thought to be a source of the spread of BSE among cattle, the UK Food Standards Agency enforces the following controls, which as of 2017 remained in force throughout Europe:

- a prohibition on the use of mammalian protein in feed to ruminant animals
- a prohibition on the incorporation of mammalian meat and bone meal in any farmed livestock feed (except processed animal protein in aquaculture feed)
- a ban, except in tightly defined circumstances, on mammalian meat and bone meal material on premises where livestock feed is used, produced, or stored

Impacts and Issues

The BSE epidemic hit British farmers and the United Kingdom meat industry hard. In 1996 the UK government admitted a link between BSE and vCJD. Shortly afterward France and many other European countries announced a ban on imports of British beef and related products. South Africa, Singapore, and South Korea soon joined in. The UK Meat and Livestock Commission stated that the bans had caused half of the country's slaughterhouse workers to lose their jobs. The import bans of British beef were lifted in 2001, as the BSE epidemic began to die down. But it has taken many years for British beef sales to begin to recover, both at home and abroad. These circumstances resulted in the British beef industry seeking new markets. In August 2017 an export deal for UK beef products worth £34 million was secured by the UK Agricultural and Horticultural Development Board (AHDB) with the Philippines.

In 1998 a public inquiry into BSE and vCJD began to stop such a catastrophe from happening again. People in Britain and elsewhere are now more aware of safety issues around food, wanting to know where their food comes from and what is in it. In 2000 the UK government set up the Food Standards Agency, a department that looks after public health and consumer interests with respect to food. This was a response to public distrust generated by the way the government was seen to have handled the BSE crisis. Formerly, food and agriculture had been the responsibility of the same department, which many felt marginalized the interests of the consumer.

BSE has substantial economic impact. During the 1990s outbreak of BSE in the United Kingdom, hundreds of animals were destroyed. Quarantined farms and slaughterhouses lost business. New regulations governing cattle feed and BSE testing programs proved expensive to implement. However, in most nations where BSE is detected, the most significant economic impact is the loss of revenue from the export of beef products. Beginning in 2001 several nations restricted the import of American beef products, concerned that the US beef industry lacked sufficient testing and identification methods for BSE. In 2003, when the US Department of Agriculture announced that BSE had been discovered in one cow in Washington state, approximately 60 nations temporarily banned the import of US beef. The infected cow was later traced to a herd in Canada, but the discovery of BSE in the North American herd resulted in approximately $4.7 billion in beef industry losses that year.

On July 18, 2017, the US Department of Agriculture (USDA) announced the confirmation of the fifth US case of BSE, in an 11-year-old cow in Alabama found during the USDA's regular program of surveillance. This was an atypical form of BSE that spontaneously occurs in older cattle. The cow was not destined to be slaughtered and therefore was not considered a threat to human health. The OiE recognized the United States as having negligible risk for BSE.

SEE ALSO *Creutzfeldt-Jakob Disease-nv; Prion Disease; Zoonoses*

BIBLIOGRAPHY

Periodicals

Ducrot, Christian, et al. "Modelling BSE Trend over Time in Europe, a Risk Assessment Perspective." *European Journal of Epidemiology* 25, no. 6 (2010): 411–419.

Websites

"All about BSE (Mad Cow Disease)." US Food and Drug Administration. https://www.fda.gov/animalveterinary/resourcesforyou/animalhealthliteracy/ucm136222.htm (accessed January 29, 2017).

"Bovine Spongiform Encephalopathy (BSE), or Mad Cow Disease." Centers for Disease Control and Prevention, August 9, 2017. https://www.cdc.gov/prions/bse/index.html (accessed January 29, 2017).

"BSE: Frequently Asked Questions." Department for Environment, Food and Rural Affairs, October 3, 2006. http://webarchive.nationalarchives.gov.uk/20080908074619/http://www.defra.gov.uk/animalh/bse/faq.html (accessed January 29, 2017).

"BSE and Other Transmissible Spongiform Encephalopathies." Food Standards Agency, September 28, 2015. https://www.food.gov.uk/science/bse-and-other-transmissible-spongiform-encephalopathies (accessed January 29, 2017).

"BSE Situation in the World and Annual Incidence Rate (1989–31/12/2016)." World Organisation for Animal Health, December 31, 2016. http://www.oie.int/en/animal-health-in-the-world/bse-specific-data (accessed January 29, 2017).

"New Export Market Opens for UK Beef." Agricultural and Horticultural Development Board, August 9, 2017. http://beefandlamb.ahdb.org.uk/wp-content/uploads/2017/08/090817-Export-release.pdf (accessed January 20, 2017).

"USDA Detects a Case of Atypical Bovine Spongiform Encephalopathy in Alabama." US Food and Drug Administration, July 18, 2017. https://www.aphis.usda.gov/aphis/newsroom/stakeholder-info/sa_by_date/sa-2017/sa-07/bse-alabama (accessed January 29, 2017).

Susan Aldridge
Anna Marie E. Roos

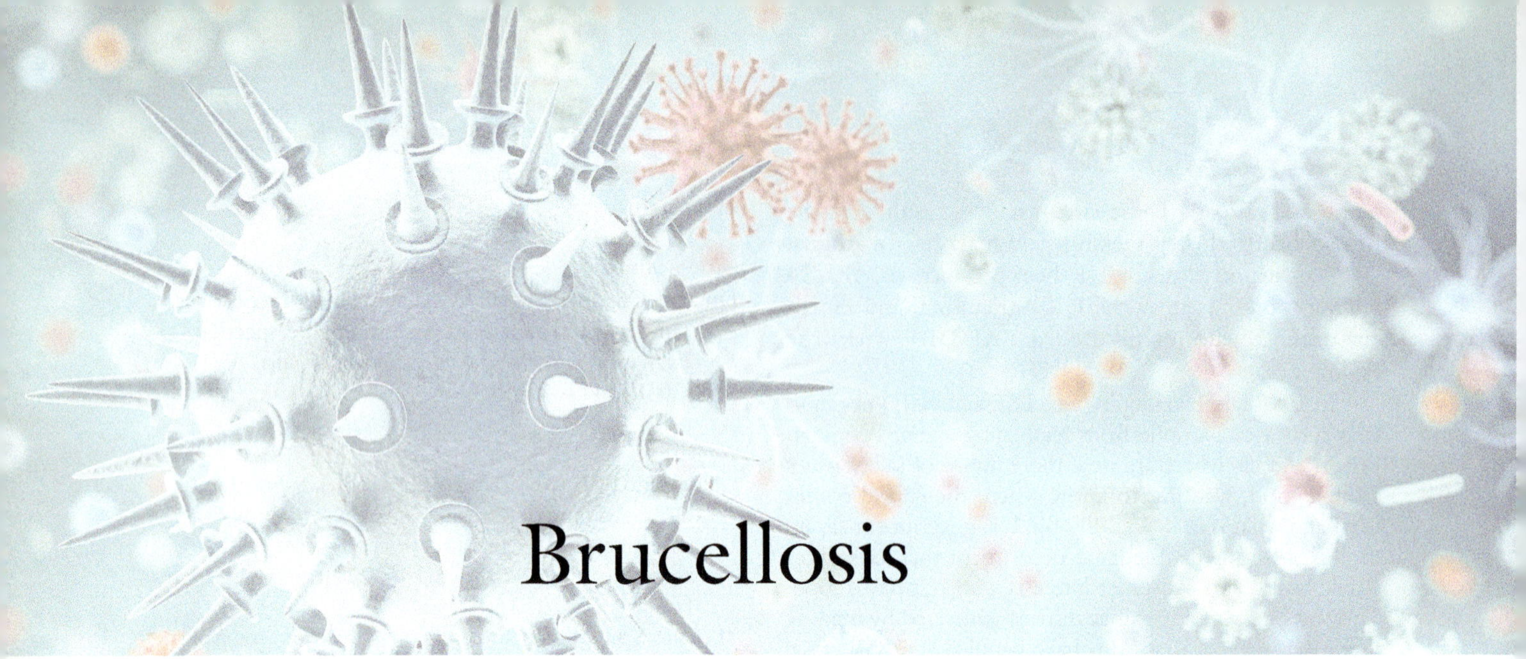

Brucellosis

Introduction

Brucellosis (broo-sell-OH-sis) is a disease that is caused by a variety of bacteria in the genus *Brucella.* Swine, cattle, and sheep can be directly infected by brucellosis. Humans can develop brucellosis indirectly by contact with infected animals (brucellosis is a zoonotic infection) or by consuming milk or dairy products that are contaminated with the bacteria.

Animals born and raised in the United States must be vaccinated against brucellosis, which helps protect both the livestock and humans most at risk of being secondarily infected. However, because vaccination programs are not in effect in every country, monitoring of imported livestock is necessary to prevent introducing brucellosis into a population of animals.

WORDS TO KNOW

CULL The selection, often for destruction, of a part of an animal population. Often done just to reduce numbers, a widespread cull was carried out during the epidemic of bovine spongiform encephalopathy (BSE), or mad cow disease, in the United Kingdom during the 1980s.

NOTIFIABLE DISEASES Diseases that the law requires must be reported to health officials when diagnosed, including active tuberculosis and several sexually transmitted diseases; also called reportable diseases.

ZOONOTIC A disease that can be transmitted between animals and humans. Examples of zoonotic diseases are anthrax, plague, and Q fever.

Disease History, Characteristics, and Transmission

Brucellosis was named after David Bruce (1855–1931), a researcher who isolated the organism in 1887 from five sick British soldiers stationed on the island of Malta. The designation of brucellosis as Malta fever recognizes this origin, as well as the 1905 description of human brucellosis cases in Malta traced to *Brucella*-contaminated unpasteurized milk. The disease is also known as undulant fever because the fever tends to increase and decrease with time. Brucellosis dates back much further than these formal descriptions. Descriptions from the time of the Greek physician and philosopher Hippocrates (c. 460 BCE–370 BCE) are thought to refer to brucellosis.

A number of different species of the bacterium are responsible for the disease in various livestock. *Brucella melitensis* infects goats and sheep; *B. suis* infects pigs and caribou; *B. abortus* causes the disease in cattle, bison, and elk; *B. ovis* also infects sheep; and *B. canis* causes the disease in dogs.

Brucella bacteria are shaped somewhat like footballs. Many disease-causing bacteria have capsules, but *Brucella* lack this outer coating. A capsule can help shield a bacterium from host defenses such as antibodies. Because it lacks a capsule, *Brucella* would be exposed to the body's defenses if not for its method of infection. The bacteria cause infection by entering host cells. Within host cells, the bacteria are shielded and able to grow and multiply.

B. melitensis, *B. abortus*, and *B. suis* are capable of causing brucellosis in humans. *B. canis* is not transmitted to humans. *B. ovis* causes brucellosis in sheep but not in humans. Humans acquire the infection indirectly, usually by handling infected animals or even a carcass. If a person has a cut or an abrasion on the skin, especially on the hands, the bacteria easily gain access to the bloodstream. However, entry is possible even in the absence of a wound because the bacteria can invade skin cells and reach the bloodstream. Another route of infection is via contaminated moist soil and hay. In these environments the bacteria can remain alive and capable of infection for months. People may also be infected by drinking unpasteurized milk or eating cheese or ice cream that has been made from unpasteurized milk. The organism can also be inhaled and the bacteria spread to the bloodstream following invasion of lung cells.

Person-to-person spread via breastfeeding and during sex can occur but is rare. It is possible that the transplantation of contaminated tissue could cause brucellosis.

When the bacteria enter the bloodstream, they migrate to lymph nodes. Normally, lymph nodes such as those located in the neck and the armpit function to destroy invading bacteria and viruses. However, *Brucella* circumvents this and invades the lymph node cells. From there the bacteria can spread to the spleen, bone marrow, and liver. Tissue irritation and organ damage can occur. In severe cases, the lining of the heart can be infected.

The time from exposure to the appearance of symptoms is usually around three weeks. Symptoms include general feelings of weakness and tiredness, muscle pain, chills, and fever. The fever and chills can subside and recur during the illness. Brucellosis is fatal in about 10 percent of cases, usually because of heart infection.

■ Scope and Distribution

The prevalence of human brucellosis is related to the prevalence of the infection in domestic and wild animal populations. In countries such as the United States and Canada, where stringent monitoring and infection control measures are in place and where longtime vaccination programs have been operating, brucellosis in both livestock and humans is rare. Culling (slaughtering) of infected animals in some North American wild elk and bison populations has been carried out to ensure that the infection does not spread from the wild populations to livestock.

Infection is most common in those who come into frequent contact with domestic and wild animals, including veterinarians, cattle ranchers, and workers in slaughterhouses. In the United States there are about 100 human brucellosis cases per year, representing one out of every 3 million Americans. Data from the US Centers for Disease Control and Prevention (CDC), as part of the National Notifiable Diseases Surveillance System established in 1993, report 115 cases in 2010 (the most current data available), 115 cases in 2009, 80 cases in 2008, 139 in 2007, and 124 in 2006.

Brucellosis is more frequent in countries where agriculture involves more people in closer contact with unvaccinated livestock and where infection control precautions are not as stringent. Areas considered to be high risk as of 2012 (the most recent year with data available) according to the CDC were the Mediterranean, Mexico, South and Central America, Eastern Europe, Asia, Africa, the Caribbean, and the Middle East.

Age and race do not influence the occurrence of brucellosis. In developing countries where mostly women

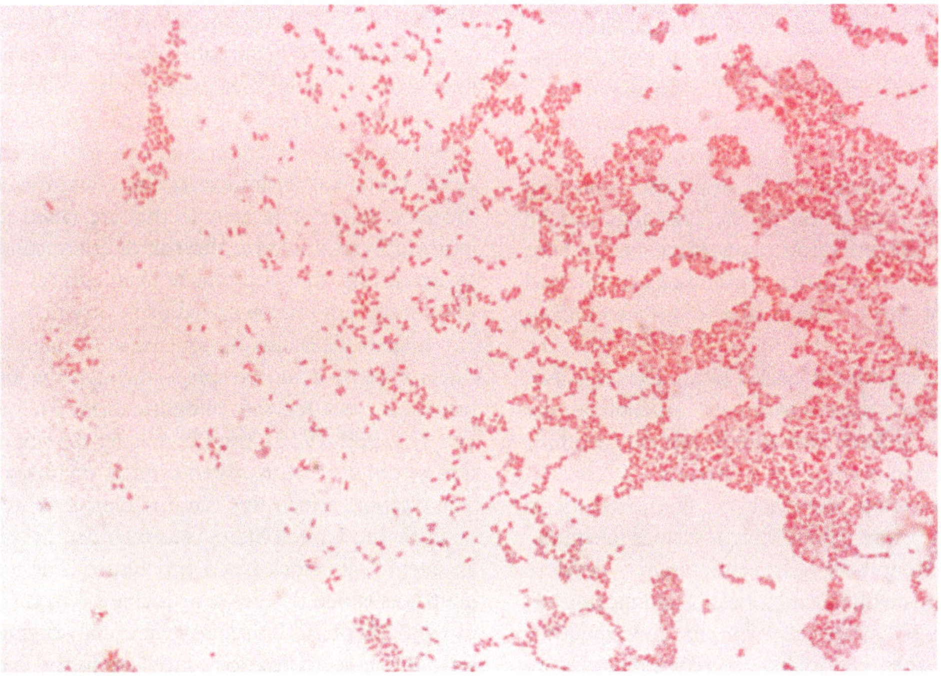

The bacterium *Brucella melitensis* is seen in a Gram stain, which researchers use to identify bacteria. *Brucella melitensis* causes the zoonotic disease brucellosis. © Smith Collection/Gado/Getty Images

PERSONAL RESPONSIBILITY AND PROTECTION

According to the Centers for Disease Control and Prevention (CDC), "person-to-person spread of brucellosis is extremely rare. Infected mothers who are breast-feeding may transmit the infection to their infants. Sexual transmission has also been reported. While uncommon, transmission may also occur via tissue transplantation or blood transfusions."

To prevent infection, the CDC recommends that travelers avoid consuming undercooked meat and unpasteurized dairy products. Further, the CDC advises that "people who handle animal tissues (such as hunters and animal herdsmen) should protect themselves by using rubber gloves, goggles, [and] gowns or aprons."

As of 2017 there was no vaccine available for humans.

tend livestock, the disease is initially more prevalent in women. In developing countries where mostly men tend livestock, the situation is reversed.

■ Treatment and Prevention

Brucellosis is suspected based on the symptoms and a history of contact with animals. Confirmation of the infection relies on the recovery of the bacteria from blood samples, bone marrow, or liver tissue. The confirmation step can take months because *Brucella* grows slowly during laboratory culture. The culture process also poses a hazard for lab personnel, who may be exposed to the bacteria during the incubation period. A quicker means of detecting the bacteria is by the presence of antibodies produced against the infecting bacteria. Antibody production by the host may not be efficient because the infection takes place inside host cells, but commercially available antibodies can be used to test blood for the presence of the corresponding bacterial component.

Human brucellosis that is caused by *B. abortus* is usually mild and may not require treatment. In contrast, the disease caused by *B. melitensis* and *B. suis* can produce severe, prolonged symptoms if not treated.

People who develop brucellosis are first cared for to control symptoms before complications, such as inflammation of the lining around the heart (endocarditis), develop. Treatment typically involves antibiotics, including doxycycline, gentamicin, streptomycin, rifampin, and trimethoprim-sulfamethoxazole. For adults, different antibiotics are given orally and by injection for several weeks. Intramuscular injections are necessary to allow the antibiotic to penetrate the host cells to reach the site of infection. The choice of treatment depends on the physician's assessment of whether the infection needs to be controlled very quickly, such as in patients with endocarditis, and on whether a patient is allergic to an antibiotic that might be used.

Prevention in animals, but not humans, is possible because of vaccines. Typically, vaccination of animals is the norm. Control of the disease in animals controls the disease in humans. In fact, two vaccine formulations used for animals contain live but weakened bacteria and are capable of causing brucellosis if accidentally given to a person.

Multiple episodes of brucellosis among laboratory workers have been reported in the past, mostly from inhaling the bacteria in the confined space of a laboratory. To prevent exposure in the laboratory, scientists study the bacteria using biosafety level 3 precautions, including wearing gowns and gloves and performing tests under a biosafety cabinet.

■ Impacts and Issues

In North America brucellosis is prevalent in wild elk and bison herds. Trap-and-slaughter campaigns of affected animals have been undertaken in Montana and in Wood Buffalo National Park, which straddles the Canadian provinces of Alberta and British Columbia. Ironically, Wood Buffalo National Park was created in the 1920s to protect the declining bison population. The culls, which have been controversial, are aimed at keeping cattle and swine herds free of brucellosis.

While brucellosis in commercial livestock is unusual in North America, the continent is at risk if infected animals or food products are imported. Preventive measures include the vaccination of all animals that are raised for food. An individual can minimize the risk of contracting brucellosis by not eating animal products from suspect countries and not consuming unpasteurized dairy products.

Brucellosis is also recognized as a potential biological threat because it can be spread through the air. There is a historical basis for this categorization. Following World War II (1939–1945), the US military developed a weapon that would disperse *B. abortus* and *B. suis* upon detonation. The weapon, which was the first biological weapon developed by the United States, was intended in part to cripple an enemy's livestock-based agriculture. The weapons program was ended by President Richard Nixon (1913–1994) in 1967. As of 2017 scientists were still working to develop a rapid diagnostic test for brucellosis in the event of a suspected biological attack, and brucellosis remained among the list of nationally notifiable diseases.

See Also *Animal Importation; Bacterial Disease; Bioterrorism; Public Health and Infectious Disease; Zoonoses*

BIBLIOGRAPHY

Books

Animal and Plant Health Inspection Service. *Brucellosis: Questions and Answers (Classic Reprint).* London: Forgotten Books, 2017.

Madkour, M. Monir. *Brucellosis.* Oxford, UK: Butterworth-Heinemann, 2014.

Periodicals

Chakravarthy, Kalyana, et al. "Paediatric Brucellosis: A Case Series from a Tertiary Care Center in Karnataka." *Indian Journal of Applied Research* 7, no. 6 (2017): 738–739.

Websites

"Brucellosis." Centers for Disease Control and Prevention. https://www.cdc.gov/brucellosis/index.html (accessed November 14, 2017).

Brian Hoyle

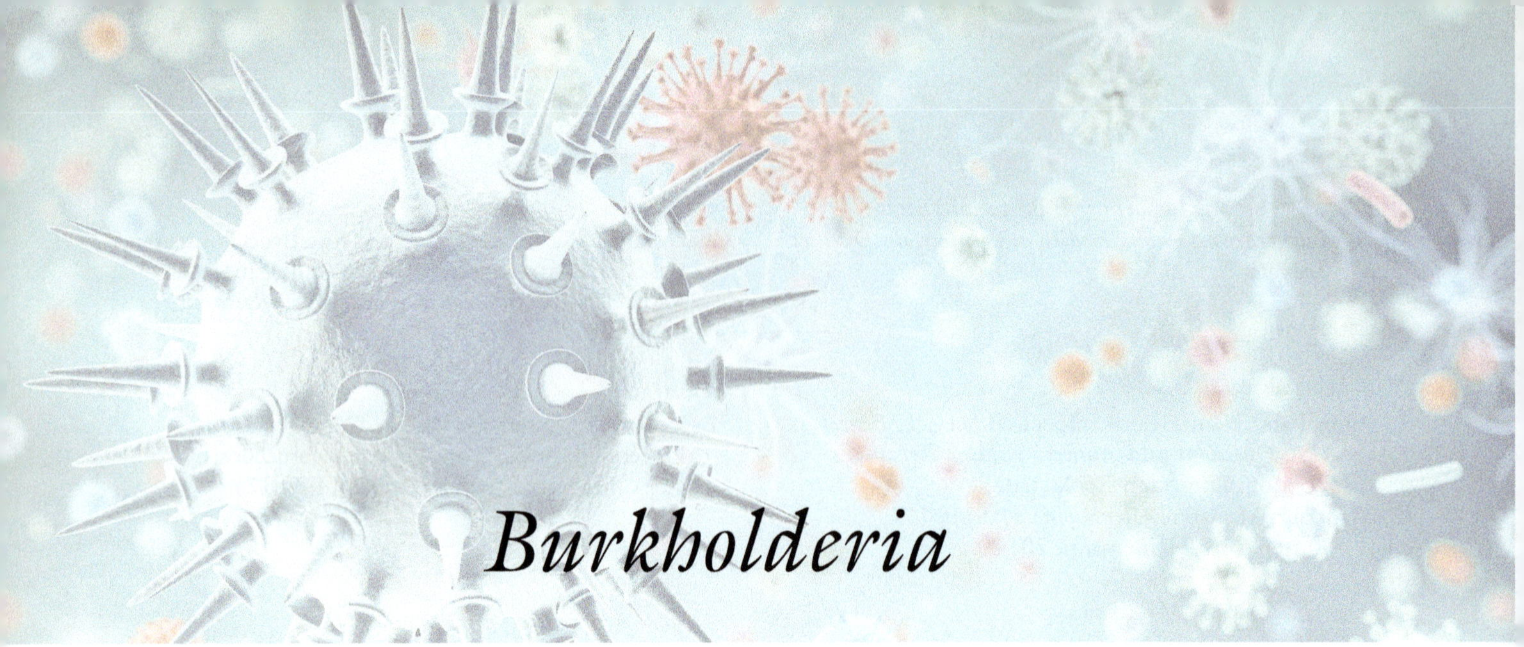

Burkholderia

Introduction

Burkholderia is a genus of bacteria. Several species of *Burkholderia* can cause illness in humans and animals. *Burkholderia cepacia* can cause a lung infection in people who have cystic fibrosis. *B. pseudomallei* causes melioidosis, an infection of the blood that can result in pain and tissue destruction at different sites in the body. *B. mallei* causes glanders, a respiratory illness that occurs primarily in horses, mules, and donkeys and can be transmitted to humans. Glanders infection is often lethal in people.

By 2017 infections such as melioidosis had reached epidemic levels in various regions of the world, including Thailand, Vietnam, and northern Australia. The respiratory infection caused by *B. cepacia* is a major health threat in those with cystic fibrosis. Adding to the concern about *Burkholderia*, several species are worrisome because of their documented use as biological warfare agents.

WORDS TO KNOW

ANTIBIOTIC RESISTANCE The ability of bacteria to resist the actions of antibiotic drugs.

BIOLOGICAL WARFARE As defined by the United Nations, the use of any living organism, such as a bacterium or virus, or an infective component, such as a toxin, to cause disease or death in humans, animals, or plants. In contrast to bioterrorism, biological warfare is the state-sanctioned use of biological weapons on an opposing military force or civilian population.

COLONIZE To persist and grow at a given location as a microorganism.

ZOONOSES Diseases of microbiological origin that can be transmitted from animals to people. The causes of the diseases can be bacteria, viruses, parasites, or fungi.

Disease History, Characteristics, and Transmission

B. cepacia was discovered in the 1940s by Cornell University researcher Walter Burkholder (1891–1983) during an investigation into a disease outbreak in New York state. By the 1980s the organism was recognized as being able to colonize and form an infection in the lungs of people with cystic fibrosis. At this point the infection was regarded as being minor, compared to that caused by *Pseudomonas aeruginosa*. Indeed, at first the organism was not recognized as a unique genus and was called *Pseudomonas cepacia*. However, only a decade later the uniqueness and seriousness of *B. cepacia* in cystic fibrosis had been recognized.

The lung infection caused by *B. cepacia* can become chronic. Over years, or even decades, the infection will alternately become severe, leading to difficulty in breathing, or less severe, when it is managed more effectively by antibiotics and other forms of therapy. The lung infection is not contagious.

Glanders is another lung infection that, in contrast, can be spread from person to person by coughing. If not treated the infection can be lethal within days. A less invasive form of the infection can require months from which to fully recover.

As of 2017 glanders was not a significant health concern in North America and Europe, as imported livestock are monitored for the disease. No naturally occurring cases had been reported in the United States since the 1940s. However, cases continued to be reported sporadically in Africa, Asia, the Middle East, Central America, and South America.

Melioidosis is a third *Burkholderia*-mediated disease that is caused by *B. pseudomallei.* It is also a disease of the respiratory tract. Indeed, it displays symptoms that are similar to glanders. However, melioidosis and glanders differ in how they are acquired.

Melioidosis is prevalent in tropical climates. For example, by 2017 the disease had been endemic (frequently present year-round) for decades in the Southeast Asian countries of Cambodia, Thailand, Vietnam, Laos, Malaysia, and Myanmar and was prevalent in northern Australia. The disease was also present but less prevalent in the South Pacific, India, Africa, and the Middle East.

Melioidosis occurs elsewhere in the world but only sporadically. Cases have been reported from Mexico, Ecuador, Panama, Haiti, Brazil, Peru, and in the US states of Hawaii and Georgia. Between 2008 and 2013 there were 37 confirmed cases of melioidosis in the United States. The majority (64 percent) involved people who had been traveling in areas where melioidosis was prevalent.

Many animals are susceptible to melioidosis, including horses, sheep, cattle, goats, dogs, and cats. A zoonosis, the disease can be transferred from the infected animals to humans. In addition, the disease can be spread from person to person by drinking contaminated water or by coming into contact with contaminated water in a crop field.

Melioidosis can occur in the respiratory tract only or, if the blood becomes infected, can become more widespread in the body. The symptoms of fever, muscle or bone ache, headache, and weight loss may appear in only a few days or may take years to become evident.

Scope and Distribution

Burkholderia are common environmental organisms and are found in many areas of the world.

Some types of *Burkholderia* infections are at epidemic proportions in tropical regions and are less common, but nevertheless present, elsewhere in the world. The distribution of *B. cepacia* is global. It is a health threat in persons with cystic fibrosis worldwide.

Treatment and Prevention

Melioidosis is diagnosed by isolating the organism from the blood, urine, or sputum or from sores on the skin. The illness is treated using antibiotics. As of 2017 there was no vaccine for melioidosis. Prevention consists of minimizing contact with potential sources of the organism.

B. cepacia lung infections and glanders are treated using appropriate antibiotics and, in the case of cystic fibrosis, other treatments designed to lessen the clogging of the lungs with the overproduced mucous.

As with other bacteria capable of causing disease, resistance to antibiotics has become a problem with *Burkholderia*. Resistance to a group of antibiotics called beta-lactam antibiotics is still rare (less than 1 percent of more than 4,000 disease-causing isolates of *B. pseudomallei*). However, once antibiotic resistance appears, in general, it will become more common over time if the resistance is a survival advantage to the bacteria. Another form of antibiotic resistance that relies on the pumping out

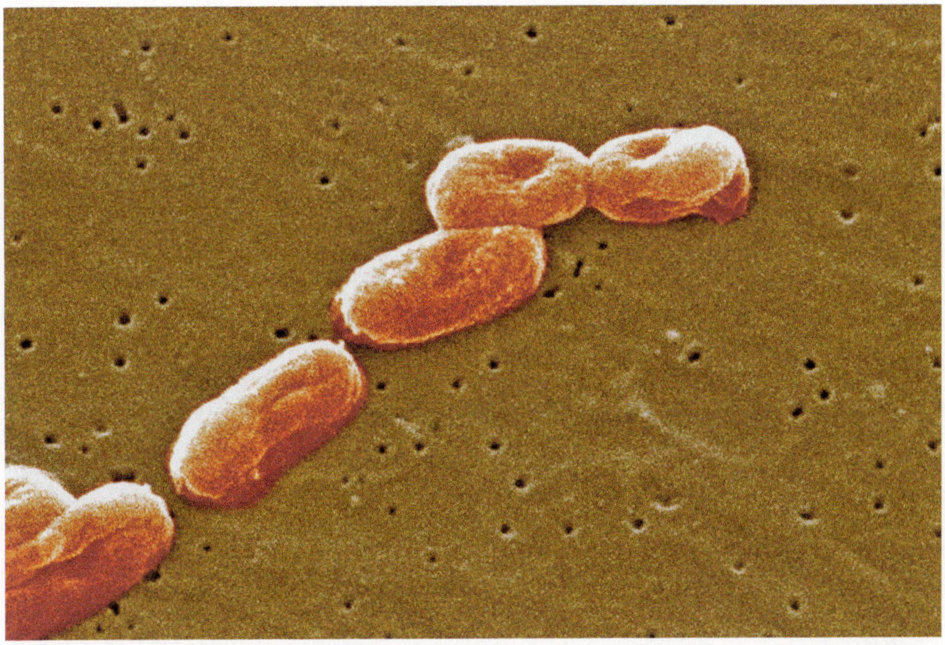

The bacterium *Burkholderia cepacia* is seen under magnification. © BSIP/UIG/Getty Images

BIOLOGICAL WEAPON THREATS

B. mallei and *B. pseudomallei* are considered potential biological weapons. Horses and other animals used in the transport of troops and military gear were deliberately infected with glanders during World War I (1914–1918), and it was used by the Japanese to infect prisoners during World War II (1939–1945).

of antibiotics from the bacteria is more common, as is resistance due to the changed arrangement of the bacterial surface, which can prevent the antibiotic from binding to the surface.

The problem of antibiotic resistance in a species of *Burkholderia* called *B. cepacia* is an especial concern for people with cystic fibrosis or those whose immune system is not working properly. Infections with *B. cepacia* in these people can be severe.

■ Impacts and Issues

Melioidosis is an important disease in some tropical regions of the world. The more persistent form of the illness can be debilitating, disrupting family life and making it impossible for a person to work.

B. cepacia is an important disease-causing organism for millions of people who have cystic fibrosis. The lung infection can persist for decades, and the long-term attempts by the host's immune system to destroy the infection can progressively damage the lungs to such an extent that survival is threatened.

B. cepacia lung infections also can progressively lessen lung function. Additionally, the attempts to eradicate the infection using antibiotics can be less than effective, which can result in the development of bacteria that are resistant to the antibiotics being used. This can make subsequent treatment more difficult and, as more potent antibiotics may be necessary, increasingly expensive.

B. mallei and *B. pseudomallei* are considered potential biological weapons. Both organisms can be resistant to a variety of antibiotics, which can make it more difficult to treat the infections they cause. Also, because they can infect both livestock and humans, they have been exploited during wartime.

Some species of *Burkholderia* are beneficial. In particular, *B. cepacia* and *B. fungorum* are able to degrade certain pesticides that otherwise tend to persist in the environment and cause ecological damage. This environmental benefit comes with the risk that those exposed to, for example, sprays containing the organisms could be at risk of developing illness. However, under controlled conditions of use, *Burkholderia* can be useful in reducing pesticide contamination.

See Also *Bacterial Disease; Bioterrorism; Glanders (Melioidosis); Opportunistic Infection*

BIBLIOGRAPHY

Books

Coenye, Tom, and Eshwar Mahenthiralingam, eds. *Burkholderia: From Genomes to Function.* Norfolk, UK: Caister Academic Press, 2014.

Ryan, Jeffrey R. *Biosecurity and Bioterrorism: Containing and Preventing Biological Threats.* 2nd ed. Amsterdam: Elsevier/Butterworth-Heinemann, 2016.

Periodicals

Limmathurotsakul, Direk, et al. "Predicted Global Distribution of *Burkholderia pseudomallei* and Burden of Melioidosis." *Nature Microbiology* 1, no. 1 (2016): 15008.

Mazer, Dale M., et al. "*In vitro* Activity of Ceftolozane-Tazobactam and Other Antimicrobial Agents against *Burkholderia cepacia* Complex and *Burkholderia gladioli.*" *Antimicrobial Agents and Chemotherapy* 61, no. 9 (2017).

Rhodes, Katherine A., and Herbert P. Schweizer. "Antibiotic Resistance of *Burkholderia* Species." *Drug Resistance Update* 28, no. 8 (2017): 82–90.

Websites

"Melioidosis." Centers for Disease Control and Prevention. https://www.cdc.gov/melioidosis/index.html (accessed November 14, 2017).

Brian Hoyle

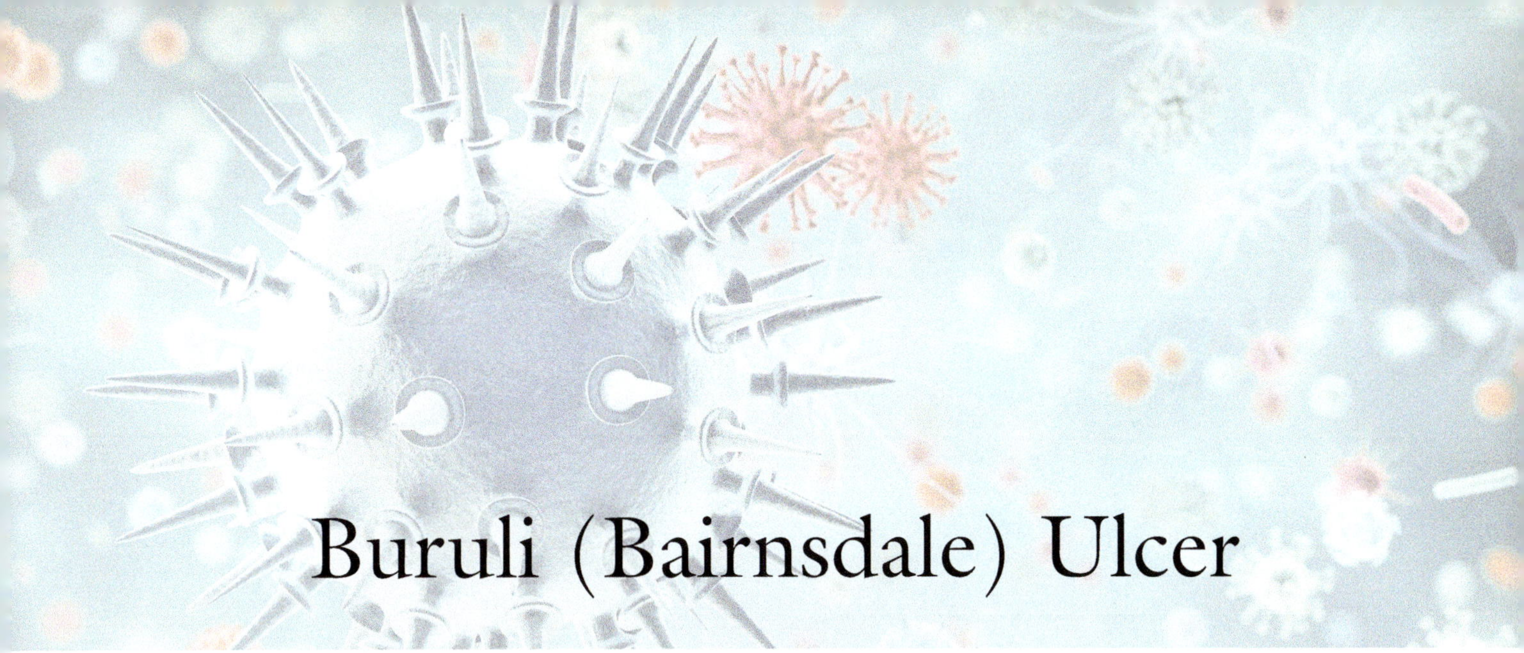

Buruli (Bairnsdale) Ulcer

Introduction

Buruli ulcer, also called Bairnsdale ulcer, is a chronic, infectious disease caused by the bacterium *Mycobacterium ulceranus*. This bacterium is a member of the family *Mycobacteriaceae*, the same family that includes the bacteria responsible for tuberculosis and leprosy.

Infection from the disease leads to deformation and destruction of blood vessels, nerves, soft skin tissues, and, occasionally, bones. Large ulcers often form on the body, usually on the legs or arms. The name *Buruli* is often associated with the infection because of its widespread incidence during the 1960s in Buruli County (now Nakasongola District) of Uganda. Although the majority of cases have been reported in Africa, the disease is also endemic in Australia. Medical professionals have had difficulty containing the disease, in part due to uncertainty about how precisely it is transmitted to humans.

Disease History, Characteristics, and Transmission

European explorers in Africa first identified and described infections consistent with Buruli ulcer in the late 19th century. Scottish explorer James Augustus Grant (1827–1892) described experiencing symptoms consistent with the disease in his book *A Walk across Africa*, which he published in 1864. During an expedition Grant described his infected leg as being stiff and swollen and, later, as discharging bodily fluids. His account is considered the first factual description of the disease. In 1897 British physician Sir Albert Cook (1870–1951) described patients infected with the disease in the Ugandan capital of Kampala and attributed the infection to *M. ulceranus*. In the 1930s the disease was reported in the Bairnsdale district of southeastern Australia, earning the illness its alternative name of Bairnsdale ulcer. Australian physician Sir Peter McCallum (1885–1974) connected cases of the disease in Victoria to *M. ulceranus* in 1948.

The *M. ulceranus* bacterium is commonly found during flooding in still or slow-moving water sources, such as

WORDS TO KNOW

BACTERIOLOGICAL STRAIN A bacterial subclass of a particular tribe and genus.

ENDEMIC Present in a particular area or among a particular group of people.

HISTOPATHOLOGY The study of diseased tissues. A synonym for histopathology is pathologic histology.

LESION The tissue disruption or the loss of function caused by a particular disease process.

MYCOBACTERIA A genus of bacteria that contains the bacteria that causes leprosy and tuberculosis. The bacteria have unusual cell walls that are harder to dissolve than the cell walls of other bacteria.

PCR (POLYMERASE CHAIN REACTION) A widely used technique in molecular biology involving the amplification of specific sequences of genomic DNA.

TOXIN A poison produced by a living organism.

ULCER An open sore on the inside or outside of the body that is accompanied by disintegration or necrosis of the surrounding tissue.

ZOONOTIC A disease that can be transmitted between animals and humans. Examples of zoonotic diseases are anthrax, plague, and Q fever.

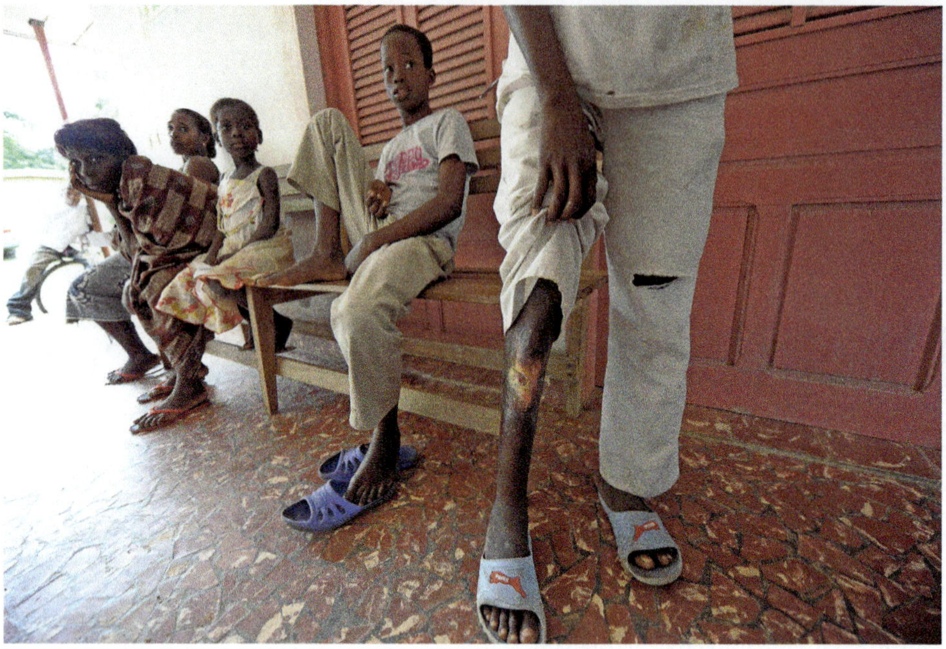

A man with Buruli ulcer on his leg in Africa's Ivory Coast. There are around 30,000 cases of Buruli ulcer disease in the country. © ISSOUF SANOGO/AFP/Getty Images

swamps, ponds, and lakes, and in small aquatic animals, such as insects. Humans are infected by contact with insects or with contaminated materials from water sources. Scientists have not yet determined the mode of transmission, although evidence suggests that Buruli ulcer may be a zoonotic infection that is transmitted by possums and mosquitos, among other possible hosts and vectors.

According to the World Health Organization (WHO), infections occur in all ages and genders; however, most infections occur in children under 15 years of age, probably because they spend more time swimming in bodies of water.

Infection usually begins as a nodule within subcutaneous fat (the pre-ulcerative stage). Eventually, fat cells die due to exposure to countless numbers of mycobacteria (any rod-shaped bacteria of genus *Mycobacterium*). The infection can also occur as a skin ulceration—a pimple, or nodule, on the skin. In both cases the infection is usually painless and without fever.

Later larger lesions develop on the skin (the ulcerative stage). The infection may heal on its own, but more commonly the disease slowly progresses with more ulcers and resultant scarring. As much as 15 percent of the body can eventually be covered with ulcers. As this happens destructive and dangerous toxins called mycolactone attack the immune system and destroy skin, tissues, and bones. According to WHO, scarring of the skin can create permanent disabilities: most commonly, restricted movement of limbs.

The disease primarily affects the limbs but also can occur on other exposed areas. WHO states that about 90 percent of lesions occur on the limbs, with almost 60 percent occurring on the lower limbs. Buruli ulcers do not occur on the hands or feet of adults. In children the disease can occur anywhere. A painful form of the disease produces fever and severe swelling of limbs. The infection in this case can occur anytime, including after being wounded and incurring more serious physical traumas. Patients who suffer from this form and who are not treated early often suffer long-term disabilities, such as impaired joint movement and disfiguring cosmetic problems.

Scope and Distribution

Historically, Buruli ulcer has occurred in more than 30 countries, primarily those with subtropical and tropical climates. These countries are in central and western Africa (such as Benin, Cameroon, the Democratic Republic of the Congo, Ghana, the Ivory Coast, Liberia, Nigeria, Uganda, and Zaire), Central and South America, the western Pacific (including Australia and New Guinea), and Southeast Asia. In the early 21st century, the disease is becoming more frequent in developing countries, specifically in the countries of western Africa. Worldwide, Buruli ulcer is the third-most-common mycobacterial disease after tuberculosis and leprosy. (In some parts of Africa, Buruli ulcer is more common than leprosy.)

Treatment and Prevention

Diagnosis of Buruli ulcer is usually made from the ulcer that appears in an infected area. Tests performed to confirm a diagnosis of Buruli ulcer include polymerase chain reaction (PCR, a technique that copies a specific deoxyribonucleic acid [DNA] sequence); Ziehl-Neelsen stain (a bacteriological stain that identifies mycobacteria); a culture of *M. ulceranus* (ulcer or tissue biopsies); and histopathology (tissue biopsies).

The treatment of Buruli ulcer usually involves surgical removal of the lesion. Surgical treatment that occurs in later stages of the infection may require long-term care with extensive skin grafting. In addition, surgery to remove necrotic tissue, repair skin defects, and correct deformities is often necessary for patients with Buruli ulcer. While surgical treatment is normally successful, especially when performed early in the infection, it is also expensive, invasive, and difficult to access in the impoverished and poorly served areas where infections are most common. This has led to a growing effort to find drug treatments for infection. In a series of studies published between 2004 and 2017, researchers demonstrated the effectiveness of treating Buruli ulcers with rifampicin, streptomycin, and clarithromycin, which are typically used to treat tuberculosis. As a result, since 2006, treatment of patients infected with Buruli ulcer has involved a combination of both surgery and antibiotic chemotherapy.

In 2013 WHO began a clinical trial in Benin and Ghana that sought to identify a method for treating Buruli ulcer that relied entirely on drug therapy without need for surgical intervention. As of early 2018, these trials were ongoing. WHO has also been leading an effort since 2016 to develop new methods of detecting the mycolactone toxins more rapidly, using a method known as fluorescent thin-layer chromatography.

Although scientists have tested the effectiveness of the anti-tuberculosis bacille Calmette-Guérin (BCG) vaccination for preventing Buruli ulcer, such research indicates that this kind of vaccine is not effective. The authors of the 2015 article "Effectiveness of Routine BCG Vaccination on Buruli Ulcer Disease: A Case-Control Study in the Democratic Republic of Congo, Ghana and Togo" tested BCG vaccination in the Democratic Republic of the Congo, Ghana, and Togo between 2010 and 2013 and "did not observe significant evidence of a protective effect of routine BCG vaccination."

Impacts and Issues

For much of the 20th century, health officials largely ignored Buruli ulcer disease, even as significant efforts were made to combat similar tropical diseases such as leprosy and tuberculosis. This began to change in 1998 when WHO launched the Global Buruli Ulcer Initiative (GBUI), which devoted significant resources to reducing infections and treating infected patients. Six years later, in 2004, the World Health Assembly resolved to improve the research, detection, and control of Buruli ulcer. This resolution called upon the international community "(1) to cooperate directly with countries in which the disease is endemic in order to strengthen

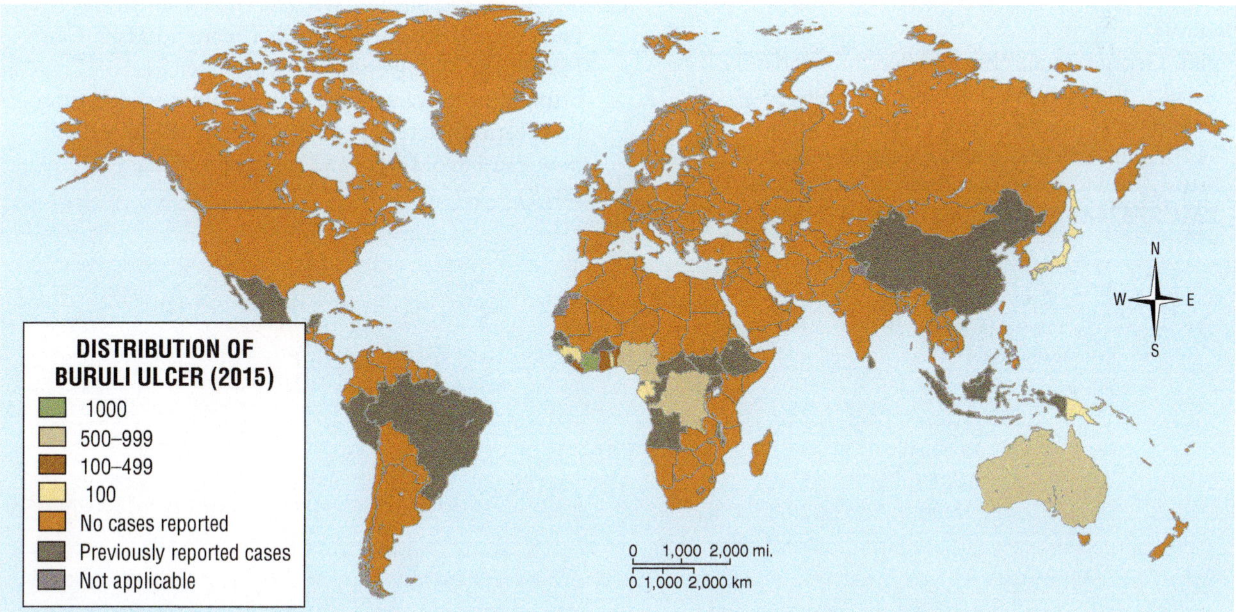

SOURCE: Adapted from "Distribution of Buruli Ulcer, Worldwide, 2015." World Health Organization. 2016. Available from: http://gamapserver.who.int/mapLibrary/Files/Maps/Buruli_2015.png?ua=1

control and research activities, (2) to develop partnerships and to foster collaboration with organizations and programmes involved in health-system development in order to ensure that effective interventions can reach all those in need; (3) to provide support to the Global Buruli Ulcer Initiative."

Although Buruli ulcer disease is found around the world, there is limited awareness about the infection, among both health workers and the general public in areas where infections are most prevalent. As a result, only limited reporting of the disease occurs. This lack of reporting, in turn, has limited efforts to combat infection.

In February 2007 a team of researchers lead by Australian scientist Tim Stinear published the entire genome sequence of *M. ulceranus.* Such insight about the disease and its causes, along with an increase of outbreaks in the developed world (including a rise in cases in Victoria, Australia, beginning in 2016) are likely to stimulate more research into diagnostic tests, drug treatments, and vaccines.

See Also *Bacterial Disease; Emerging Infectious Diseases; Tropical Infectious Diseases; World Health Organization (WHO)*

BIBLIOGRAPHY

Books

Cohen, Jonathan, William G. Powderly, and Steven M. Opal, eds. *Infectious Diseases.* Amsterdam: Elsevier, 2017.

Gyapong, John, and Boakye Boatin, eds. *Neglected Tropical Diseases—Sub-Saharan Africa.* New York: Springer, 2016.

Periodicals

Amofah, George, et al. "Buruli Ulcer in Ghana: Results of a National Case Search." *Emerging Infectious Diseases* 8, no. 2 (February 2002): 167–170. This article can also be found online at https://www.ncbi.nlm.nih.gov/pmc/articles/PMC2732443/ (accessed January 17, 2018).

Matthews, Melissa. "Buruli Ulcer: Will the Flesh-Eating Bacteria Spreading through Australia Come to the U.S.?" *Newsweek* (September 22, 2017). This article can also be found online at http://www.newsweek.com/buruli-ulcer-australia-flesh-eating-bacteria-come-us-669684 (accessed January 17, 2018).

Merritt, Richard W., et al. "Ecology and Transmission of Buruli Ulcer Disease: A Systematic Review." *PLOS Neglected Tropical Diseases* (December 4, 2010). This article can also be found online at http://journals.plos.org/plosntds/article?id=10.1371/journal.pntd.0000911 (accessed January 17, 2018).

Phillips, Richard Odame. "Effectiveness of Routine BCG Vaccination on Buruli Ulcer Disease: A Case-Control Study in the Democratic Republic of Congo, Ghana and Togo." *PLOS Neglected Tropical Diseases* (January 8, 2015). This article can also be found online at http://journals.plos.org/plosntds/article?id=10.1371/journal.pntd.0003457 (accessed January 26, 2018).

Websites

"Buruli Ulcer." Centers for Disease Control and Prevention, January 26, 2015. https://www.cdc.gov/buruli-ulcer/index.html (accessed January 17, 2018).

"Buruli Ulcer." World Health Organization. http://www.who.int/buruli/en/ (accessed January 17, 2018).

Cheng, Allen. "Explainer: What Is the Flesh-eating Bacterium that Causes Buruli Ulcer and How Can I Avoid It?" Conversation, September 21, 2017. http://theconversation.com/explainer-what-is-the-flesh-eating-bacterium-that-causes-buruli-ulcer-and-how-can-i-avoid-it-84432 (accessed January 17, 2018).

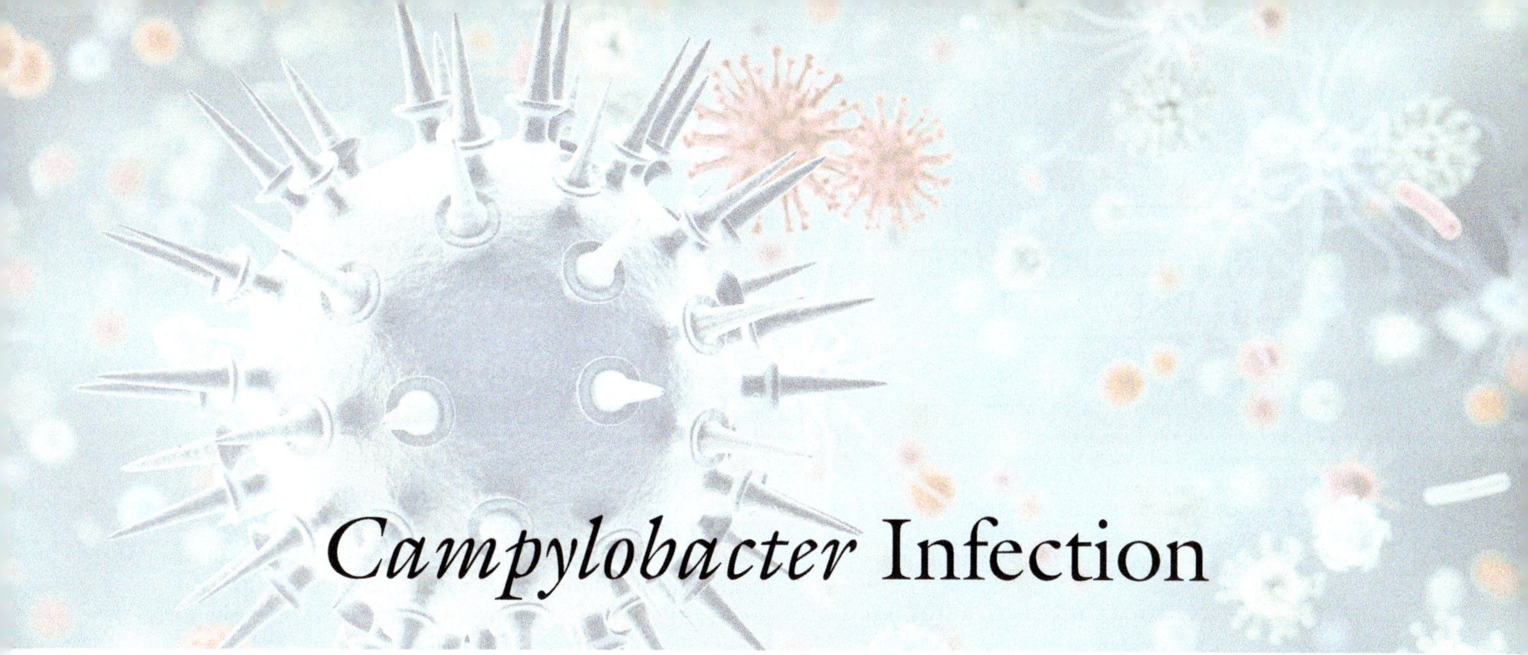

Campylobacter Infection

Introduction

Campylobacteriosis is the infection caused by bacteria in the genus *Campylobacter*. The infection, which occurs in the intestinal tract of humans, causes abdominal pain and diarrhea. The US Centers for Disease Control and Prevention (CDC) estimates that there are 1.3 million cases of campylobacteriosis annually in the United States. According to 2017 statistics from the CDC, *Campylobacter jejuni* is responsible for more bacterial diarrhea in the United States than any other bacteria, and an estimated 14 percent of all diarrhea worldwide is caused by campylobacteriosis. Other species of concern are *C. fetus*, *C. lari*, *C. upsaliensis*, and *C. hyointestinalis*. The first three also cause diarrhea, and *C. hyointestinalis* can cause illness in people with a weakened immune system.

Campylobacter infections typically result from eating contaminated food or drinking contaminated water. The bacteria need time to grow to numbers that produce the symptoms of the infection; this usually takes two to five days after the contaminated food or water has been ingested.

Disease History, Characteristics, and Transmission

Researchers have known for decades that *Campylobacter* bacteria are pathogenic—that is, they are capable of causing illness. For example, the capability of the bacteria to cause disease in animals has been known since the first decade of the 20th century. However, the identification of *Campylobacter* bacteria as human pathogens only took place in the 1980s.

According to the CDC, the rate of *Campylobacter* infections each year is about 14 cases per 100,000 people, which, given the 2017 US population of 323.1 million, translates to an estimated 45,234 cases each year. Considering that the symptoms of nausea, fever, abdominal cramps, vomiting, and diarrhea are likely often not reported (or, if they are, the underlying disease is not diagnosed), the actual number of cases is no doubt higher. Indeed, the CDC estimates that infections in the United States number in the millions each year.

The symptoms of *Campylobacter* infections are not usually life-threatening in the developed world, where the level of health and sanitary conditions are better than in underdeveloped and developing countries. Most people who become infected recover in about a week without the need for medical aid. Still, even in developed countries, severe *Campylobacter* infections occur, producing bloody diarrhea (the result of damage to intestinal cells). Some people can have abdominal cramps for several months after an infection. The fluid loss from the diarrhea can dehydrate a person if enough fluids are not taken in; in severe cases that require hospitalization, the fluid may need to be supplied intravenously. Very rarely, a high fever that accompanies an infection will trigger a seizure. In an estimated one case in every 1,000, *Campylobacter* infection contributes to Guillain-Barré syndrome, a neurological disorder in which a person's own immune system attacks the nerves, produc-

WORDS TO KNOW

MYCOTIC Having to do with or caused by a fungus. Any medical condition caused by a fungus is a mycotic condition, also called a mycosis.

PATHOGEN A disease-causing agent, such as a bacteria, virus, fungus, or other microorganism.

ZOONOTIC A disease that can be transmitted between animals and humans. Examples of zoonotic diseases are anthrax, plague, and Q fever.

PERSONAL RESPONSIBILITY AND PREVENTION

The Mycotic Disease Branch of the US Centers for Disease Control and Prevention (CDC) recommends the following tips for preventing campylobacteriosis:

- Cook all poultry products thoroughly. Make sure that the meat is cooked throughout (no longer pink), any juices run clear, and the inside is cooked to 170°F (77°C) for breast meat and 180°F (82°C) for thigh meat.
- If you are served undercooked poultry in a restaurant, send it back for further cooking.
- Wash hands with soap after handling raw foods of animal origin and before touching anything else.

Prevent cross-contamination in the kitchen:

- Use separate cutting boards for foods of animal origin and other foods. Carefully clean all cutting boards, countertops, and utensils with soap and hot water after preparing raw food of animal origin.
- Avoid consuming unpasteurized milk and untreated surface water.
- Make sure that persons with diarrhea, especially children, wash their hands carefully and frequently with soap to reduce the risk of spreading the infection.
- Wash hands with soap after having contact with pet feces.

ing paralysis. Also, an estimated 5 percent to 20 percent of people who experience *Campylobacter* infections develop irritable bowel syndrome for a short time, and up to 5 percent develop arthritis.

■ Scope and Distribution

Campylobacter infections are an example of a zoonotic illness or disease, one that is transmitted to humans by animals or animal products. This is because *Campylobacter* is a natural resident in the intestinal tracts of creatures including swine, cattle, dogs, shellfish, and poultry. The animals harbor the bacteria without any ill effect. The bacteria also naturally inhabit the soil.

■ Treatment and Prevention

Campylobacter is readily susceptible to fairly conventional antibiotics. Treatment is not routinely given because symptoms usually ease within a few days.

Preventing infection from the ingestion of contaminated food or water is a greater challenge. Poultry is an important source of the infection. Over 50 percent of raw chicken is contaminated with *Campylobacter*. During slaughter the bird's intestinal contents (including *Campylobacter*) can contaminate the carcass. If the chicken is undercooked, the bacteria can survive and can cause an infection after the meat is ingested. Fortunately, the bacteria do

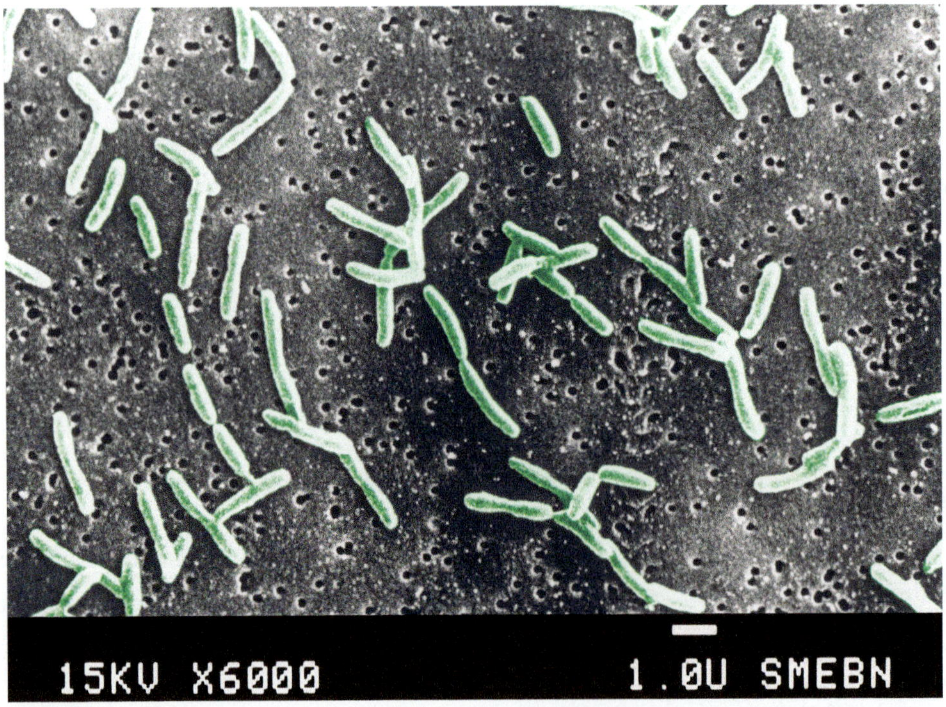

The bacterium *Campylobacter jejuni* is seen under magnification. Species of the *Campylobacter* genus of bacteria are responsible for the intestinal infection campylobacteriosis. *© BSIP/UIG/Getty Images*

not tolerate temperatures that are even slightly above room temperature (approximately 68°F [20°C]). Proper cooking of food kills the bacteria. Washing a cutting board after exposure to poultry, refrigerating raw meat and poultry, and thawing meat and poultry in the refrigerator or microwave help prevent the transfer of *Campylobacter* to other foods.

■ Impacts and Issues

Research into *Campylobacter* infections consists primarily of genetic studies that are aimed at detecting genes of particular importance in the infection process. It is hoped that this knowledge will lead to strategies to block the infection or to rapidly detect the presence of the bacteria on food products. One example of the latter approach is the incorporation of a detection system into food packaging. The presence of living bacteria is evident as a color change in an indicator strip in the packaging.

The US Department of Agriculture carries out research on how to prevent *Campylobacter* infection from poultry. The CDC and other organizations maintain surveillance programs that help determine how often *Campylobacter* disease occurs and track factors that favor development of the infection.

In 1982 the CDC began a national *Campylobacter* surveillance program. The program was revised in 1996 to further identify risk factors. In 2005 the Food and Drug Administration (FDA) revised its Model Food Code in an effort to reduce the risk of exposure to contaminated chicken. As of 2017 the revised items remained in effect in the latest revision, which was issued in 2013. Exposure is not only risky and costly to those infected, including food service employees and consumers, but can also potentially ruin or severely affect business and earnings for a commercial food establishment.

As with other pathogenic bacteria, researchers work to discover or manufacture antibiotics that are more adept at killing the bacteria without promoting the development of resistance to the antibiotic by the target bacteria.

See Also *Food-Borne Disease and Food Safety*

BIBLIOGRAPHY

Books

Klein, Günter. *Campylobacter: Features, Detection, and Prevention of Foodborne Disease*. New York: Academic Press, 2016.

Tang, John Y. H. *Campylobacter—An Overview*. Saarbrücken, Germany: Lambert Academic Publishing, 2016.

Periodicals

Denis, Martine, et al. "No Clear Differences between Organic and Conventional Pig Farms in the Genetic Diversity or Virulence of *Campylobacter coli* Isolates." *Frontiers in Microbiology* 6 (2017).

Vacca, Irene. "Bacterial Pathogenesis: *Campylobacter* Follows the Clues." *Nature Reviews Microbiology* 15 (May 2017): 381.

Websites

"*Campylobacter* (Campylobacteriosis)." Centers for Disease Control and Prevention. https://www.cdc.gov/campylobacter/index.html (accessed November 14, 2017).

Brian Hoyle

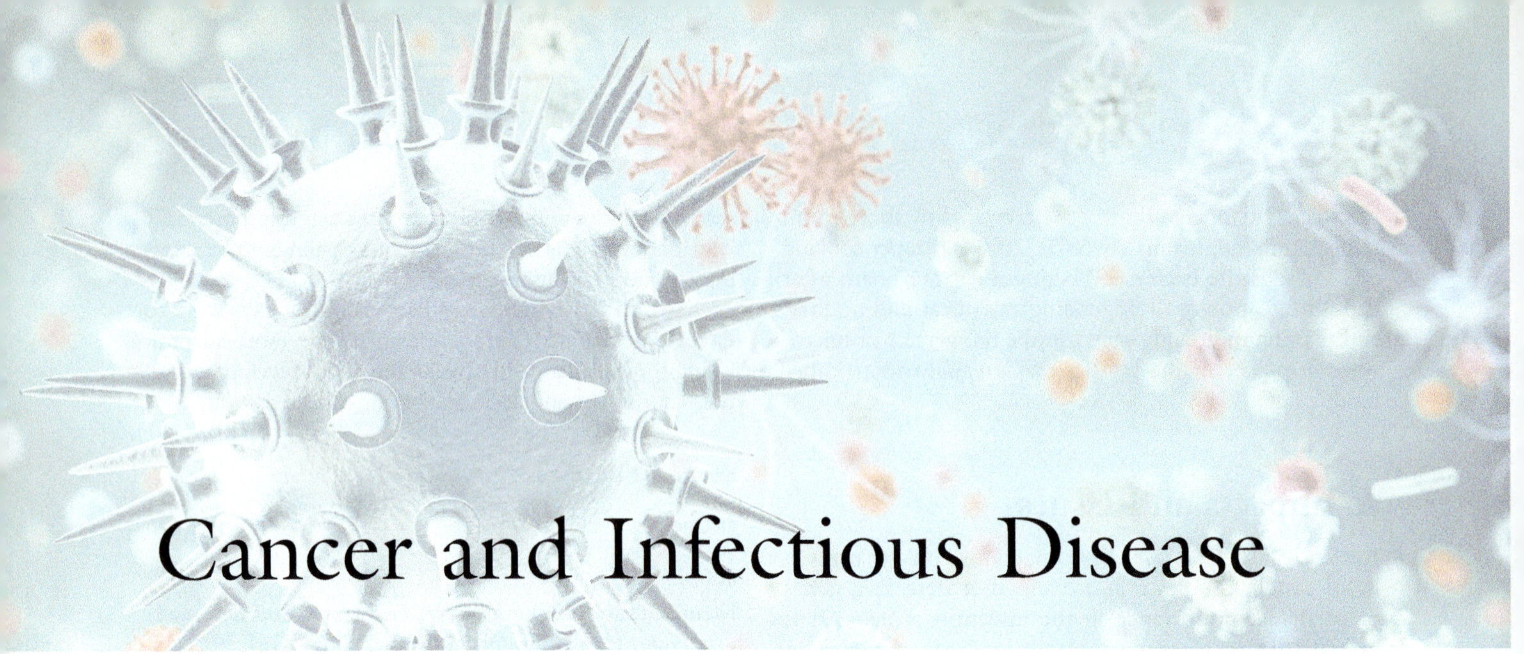

Cancer and Infectious Disease

Introduction

Cancer is not considered an infectious disease. Yet there is an important link between some infectious agents and certain cancers. Research has shown that chronic infection with certain viruses, bacteria, and even parasites can increase the risk of contracting cancers. For example, human papillomavirus (HPV) is the leading cause of cervical cancer, and chronic hepatitis B virus or hepatitis C virus infection may develop into liver cancer. Viruses have a number of ways of triggering changes in cells that can cause them to divide uncontrollably, leading to formation of a tumor.

WORDS TO KNOW

CARCINOGEN Any biological, chemical, or physical substance or agent that can cause cancer. There are more than 100 types of cancer, which can be distinguished by the type of cell or organ that is affected, the treatment plan employed, and the cause of the cancer. Most commonly discussed carcinogens come from chemical sources artificially produced by humans, such as the pesticide DDT (dichlorodiphenyltrichloroethane), asbestos, and the carcinogens produced when tobacco is smoked.

RETROVIRUS Viruses in which the genetic material consists of ribonucleic acid (RNA) instead of the usual deoxyribonucleic acid (DNA). Retroviruses produce an enzyme known as reverse transcriptase that can transform RNA into DNA, which can then be permanently integrated into the DNA of the infected host cells.

Globally, it is estimated that risk of cancers due to infectious agents is about 16 percent. The recognition that infection can play a role in cancer has lead to new approaches for prevention and treatment. For instance, vaccination against HPV is now given to girls and young women because there is good evidence that it protects against cervical cancer in later life.

History and Scientific Foundations

It has long been known that certain viruses can cause cancer in animals. Danish researchers Wilhelm Ellermann and Oluf Bang discovered a virus that spreads leukemia among chickens in 1908. Then, in 1911, Peyton Rous (1879–1970) of the Rockefeller Institute in New York identified a virus responsible for sarcoma (a cancer of a connective tissue, such as bone or cartilage) in chickens. By the 1930s it was recognized that viruses played a role in several animal cancers. However, the significance of Rous's work for human cancer was not appreciated for many years; he was finally awarded a Nobel Prize in Physiology or Medicine in 1966.

The first discovery of a human cancer virus came from research carried out in Uganda in the 1950s by the Irish surgeon Denis Burkitt (1911–1993). He discovered a type of cancer of the jaw that affected young children. The dis ease became known as Burkitt's lymphoma, and it is still the most common tumor among African children. Tumor samples were analyzed by Anthony Epstein (1921–) in London, who discovered the presence of a new type of herpes virus, named Epstein–Barr virus (EBV).

It is well known that cancer develops in multiple stages over a long period of time. There are many risk factors that work in tandem, aided by genetic changes, environmental factors, daily habits (e.g., smoking), and, in many cases, exposure to infectious agents such as viruses. Because viruses can replicate only in a host, they transfer the viral genes into the host. This can alter the host cells, causing them to divide more rapidly and lead to the formation of a tumor.

As of early 2018, it had been established that two types of herpes virus may cause cancer: (1) the EBV (or HHV-4) associated with nasopharyngeal carcinoma and some forms of lymphoma, including Burkitt's lymphoma and Hodgkin's lymphoma, and (2) the human herpesvirus HHV-8, which has a role in causing Kaposi's sarcoma (KS).

The human papillomaviruses (HPVs) are a large group of viruses that can cause warts on the skin, mouth, and genitals. HPV infection is common among people who are sexually active, and certain strains are well established as causative agents of cervical cancer. Most women who have cervical cancer show signs of infection with one of these strains. Hepatitis B virus (HBV) and hepatitis C virus (HCV) may cause chronic viral hepatitis, an infection of the liver that is linked to an increased risk of hepatocellular (liver) cancer.

The human immunodeficiency virus (HIV) does not, in itself, cause cancer. However, HIV does increase the risk of contracting other infections and thus is associated with malignancies such as KS, non-Hodgkin lymphoma, and anal and cervical cancer. Indeed, it was the appearance of KS among homosexual men in the United States in the early 1980s that first alerted the medical community to the existence of HIV. Before the emergence of HIV, KS was rare in the West, although it was known in central Africa and the Middle East. HHV-8 is isolated from most KS tumors. Meanwhile, the human T-lymphotrophic virus (HTLV-1) is associated with a blood cancer called adult T-cell leukemia (ATL). Like HIV, HTLV-1 is a retrovirus: a type of virus whose genetic material is made of RNA rather than DNA. Both HIV and HTLV-1 are related to retroviruses known to cause leukemia in animals.

Finally, infection with the bacterium *Helicobacter pylori* increases the risk of stomach cancer. *H. pylori* is unusual because it can survive the acid conditions of the stomach. Infection causes inflammation of the stomach lining, increasing the risk of both stomach ulcers and stomach cancer. About half of the world's population have *H. pylori* infection. Infection with *H. pylori* is believed to be a risk factor for causing stomach cancer as the bacterium triggers cell proliferation, a key marker for cancer.

Among parasites, *Schistosoma haematobium* (causative agent of schistosomiasis) is associated with bladder cancer. Evidence also indicates that *S. japonicum* may cause colorectal cancer. The worm's eggs cause inflammation, which serves as a trigger for the development of cancer.

VACCINES FOR HPV AND HBV

Infections with human papillomavirus (HPV) lead to cervical cancer and anal cancer and, to a lesser extent, to oropharyngeal,, vaginal, vulvar, and penile cancer. As of 2018 there were three approved vaccines for prevention against HPV in the United States: Gardasil, Gardasil 9, and Cervarix. Gardasil and Gardasil 9 are used for prevention of related cancers in males (ages 9 to 15) and females (ages 9 to 26). Cervarix is used only in females for prevention against cervical cancer. However, accessibility and affordability of these vaccines are still a major concern in lower-income countries.

For hepatitis B virus (HBV) infections that cause liver cancer, multiple vaccines are available. Energix-B and Recombivax HB are used across all age groups and render protection against HBV infection, while Twinrix protects against HBV and hepatitis A virus. In the United States, Pediarix vaccine is now routinely given to infants shortly after birth for protection against HBV, poliovirus, pertussis, tetanus, and diphtheria (caused by bacteria).

■ Applications and Research

Viruses and bacteria can raise the risk of cancer in various ways. They can cause chronic inflammation of the tissue they infect. Or, like HIV, they may suppress immunity and allow cancer-causing viruses to take hold. Immune suppression after an organ transplant is an important cause of HBV-associated lymphoma, for example. Some viruses can invade cells directly and alter their genetic machinery, disrupting normal control over cell division. But infection is only ever one link in a chain of events leading to tumor formation. Other factors, such as smoking, diet, or genetic disposition, may be equally important. The chain may be broken using a vaccine, which prevents infection, or by an antibiotic, which eliminates it.

Research in cancer vaccines falls into two categories: (1) preventive (also known as prophylactic) vaccines that prevent cancer development, and (2) therapeutic vaccines that treat the existing tumor. Preventive vaccines to control HPV and hepatitis B virus are approved and available in the United States.

The possibility that the role of infection in cancer may be even wider is being investigated. For example, there is evidence that infection with *Chlamydia trachoma* could increase the risk of cervical cancer, and a related species, *Chlamydia psittaci*, could be linked to a rare cancer of the eyes known as mucosa-associated lymphoid tissue lymphoma. A monkey virus called SV40 has been linked to mesothelioma, a cancer of the lining of the chest wall, in which asbestos exposure is another risk factor. Researchers in England have even suggested that common infections contracted either in the womb or during childhood may lead to clusters of childhood cancers that have previously been attributed to other environmental factors.

■ Impacts and Issues

Most viruses and bacteria are not known to be a risk factor for cancer, and cancer is not, in itself, contagious. Moreover, the majority of people infected with agents known to be carcinogenic will not actually contract cancer; the presence of one or more other risk factors is necessary for cancer to develop.

Cervical cancer is the most commonly diagnosed cancer occurring in women, leading to an estimated 266,000 deaths globally. Persistent HPV infections are responsible for nearly all cases of cervical cancers, pressing the need for vaccinating the susceptible population against the virus. The World Health Organization (WHO) recommends two doses of HPV vaccination for girls between 9 and 14 years old in countries where cervical cancer is a serious concern. In the United States and Western Europe, there are low incidences of cervical cancer due to decades-long implementation of screening and treatment programs, whereas in sub-Saharan Africa, Latin America, and the Caribbean, prevention efforts are far from thorough. For screening of HPV infection, pap smears are the most preferred and effective testing method.

Chronic HBV infection remains asymptomatic for many years in an affected person and can lead to cirrhosis (liver damage) and liver cancer. According to the CDC, in 2016 1.4 million people in the United States were infected with HBV, and about 2,000 deaths occur each year due to related complications, such as liver cancer. Vaccines for both the adult and pediatric populations are available for use against HBV in the United States.

With nearly 500,000 new cases of cervical cancer globally and more than half of cases leading to death in lower-income countries, the affordability of HPV vaccines is a cause for concern. Although programs exist to try to get vaccines to the world's most impoverished populations, the price of Gardasil and Cervarix continue to remain out of reach for some countries. The Bill & Melinda Gates Foundation, along with the Program for Appropriate Technology in Health (PATH) and other organizations, have set up the Alliance for Cervical Cancer Prevention to address prevention in developing countries.

See Also *Epstein-Barr Virus; Helicobacter pylori; Hepatitis B; Hepatitis C; HPV (Human Papillomavirus) Infection*

BIBLIOGRAPHY

Books

Cohen, J. I. "Herpesviruses." In *Cancer Medicine*, edited by Waun Ki Hong, et al. Shelton, CT: People's Medical, 2010.

Mustacchi, Piero. "Parasites." In *Cancer Medicine*, edited by Waun Ki Hong, et al. Shelton, CT: People's Medical, 2010.

Wilson, Walter R., and Merle A. Sande. *Current Diagnosis & Treatment in Infectious Diseases.* New York: McGraw Hill, 2001.

Periodicals

Boseley, Sarah. "Can You Catch Cancer?" *Guardian* (January 24, 2006). This article can also be found online at https://www.theguardian.com/society/2006/jan/24/cancercare.health (accessed January 26, 2018).

Clendinen, C., et al. "Manufacturing Costs of HPV Vaccines for Developing Countries." *Vaccine* 34, no. 48 (November 2016): 5984–5989.

De Martel C., et al. "Global Burden of Cancers Attributable to Infections in 2008: A Review and Synthetic Analysis." *Lancet Oncology* 13, no. 6 (June 2012): 607–615.

Khalifa, Mohammed Mahdy, Radwa Raed Sharaf, and Ramy Karim Aziz. "*Helicobacter pylori*: A Poor Man's Gut Pathogen?" *Gut Pathogens* 2, no. 2 (2010).

Senkomago, Virginia. "CDC Activities for Improving Implementation of Human Papillomavirus Vaccination, Cervical Cancer Screening, and Surveillance Worldwide." Global Health Security Supplement 23 (December 2017). This article can also be found online at https://wwwnc.cdc.gov/eid/article/23/13/17–0603_article (accessed January 26, 2018).

Websites

"Cancer Vaccines." National Cancer Institute, December 18, 2015. https://www.cancer.gov/about-cancer/causes-prevention/vaccines-fact-sheet (accessed January 26, 2018).

Georges, Helen. "Alliance for Cervical Cancer Prevention Receives $50 Million Gift from Bill and Melinda Gates." Bill & Melinda Gates Foundation. https://www.gatesfoundation.org/Media-Center/Press-Releases/1999/09/Alliance-for-Cervical-Cancer-Prevention (accessed January 26, 2018).

"Hepatitis B VIS." Centers for Disease Control and Prevention, October 18, 2016. https://www.cdc.gov/vaccines/hcp/vis/vis-statements/hep-b.html (accessed January 26, 2018).

Parsonnet, Julie. "Infectious Disease: A Surprising Cause of Cancer." *Stanford Medicine Newsletter*, Spring 2008. http://stanfordmedicine.org/communitynews/2008spring/infectiousdisease.html (accessed January 26, 2018).

Susan Aldridge
Kausalya Santhanam

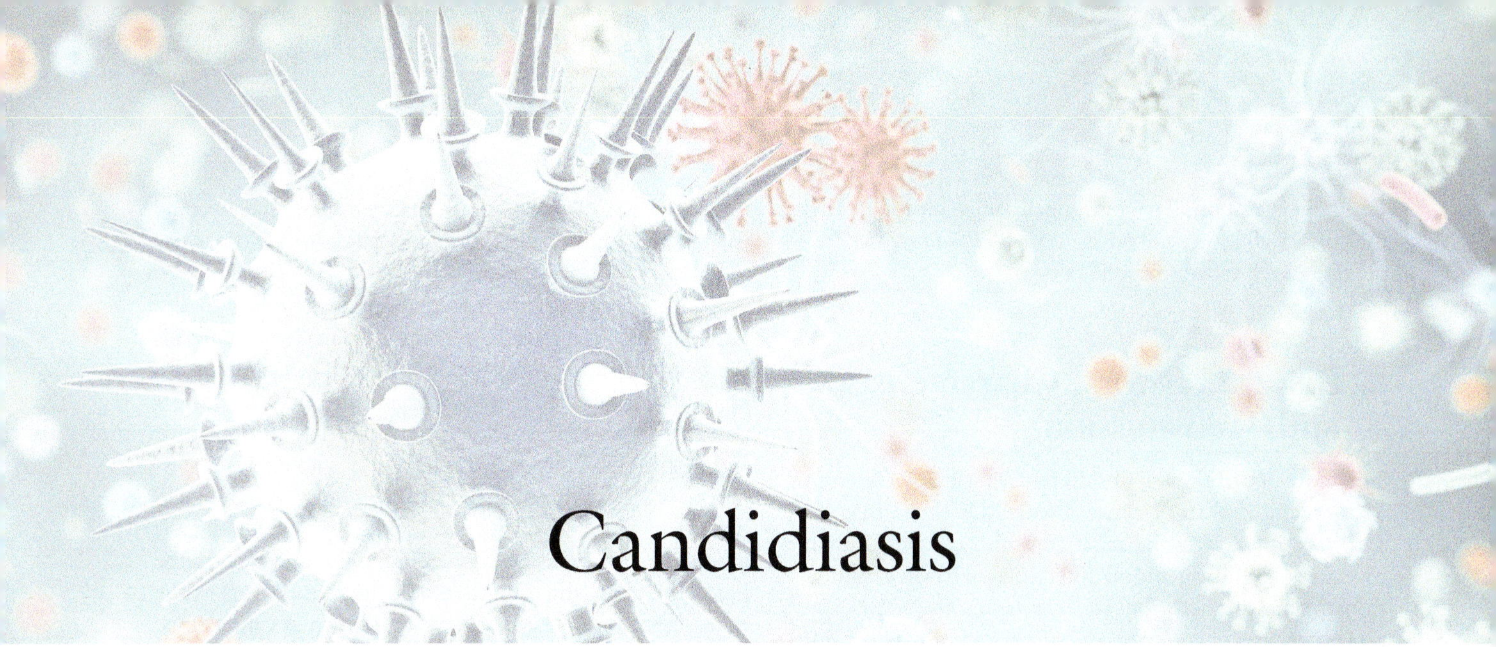

Candidiasis

Introduction

Candidiasis (can-di-DYE-a-sis) is a fungal infection caused by the genus *Candida*, with *Candida albicans* being the major cause of disease in humans. *Candida*, the major fungal component of human flora, is a closely related species of yeast that occurs naturally on the skin and in the gastrointestinal and urinary tracts. If a person's flora remains in a healthy balance with their human host, then they do not cause disease.

Candida is an opportunistic pathogen and, under certain factors, such as antibiotic use or a weakened immune system, may upset this balance and lead to infection. A 2013 report by the US Centers for Disease Control and Prevention (CDC) lists candidiasis as the fourth major cause of hospital-acquired systemic infection, and mortality rates can reach as high as 60 percent depending on the type of infection and method of treatment. Candidiasis ranges from mild to severe and even life-threatening clinical conditions, depending on the location of the infection. Infection due to *C. albicans* may manifest as a superficial infection, such as oral and vaginal candidiasis, or a life-threatening systemic infection that affects the bloodstream.

WORDS TO KNOW

ENZYME Molecules that act as critical catalysts in biological systems. Catalysts are substances that increase the rate of chemical reactions without being consumed in the reaction. Without enzymes, many reactions would require higher levels of energy and higher temperatures than exist in biological systems. Enzymes are proteins that possess specific binding sites for other molecules (substrates). A series of weak binding interactions allows enzymes to accelerate reaction rates. Enzyme kinetics is the study of enzymatic reactions and mechanisms. Enzyme inhibitor studies have allowed researchers to develop therapies for the treatment of diseases, including AIDS.

FLORA In microbiology, the collective microorganisms that normally inhabit an organism or system. Human intestines, for example, contain bacteria that aid in digestion and are considered normal flora.

INTERTRIGO A skin rash, often occurring in obese people on parts of the body symmetrically opposite each other. Sometimes called eczema intertrigo, it is caused by irritation of skin trapped under hanging folds of flesh such as pendulous breasts.

MYCOTIC DISEASE A disease caused by fungal infection.

NOSOCOMIAL INFECTION An infection that is acquired in a hospital. More precisely, the US Centers for Disease Control and Prevention (CDC) in Atlanta, Georgia, defines a nosocomial infection as a localized infection or an infection that is widely spread throughout the body that results from an adverse reaction to an infectious microorganism or toxin that was not present at the time of admission to the hospital.

PATHOGEN A disease-causing agent, such as a bacterium, a virus, a fungus, or another microorganism.

VIRULENCE The ability of a disease organism to cause disease. A more virulent organism is more infective and liable to produce more serious disease.

Candidiasis responds to antifungal drugs, although they must be carefully prescribed, as some *Candida* species have developed resistance to specific drugs.

■ Disease History, Characteristics, and Transmission

There are more than 150 different species of *Candida*. Most of these do not cause disease. Of those that do, *Candida albicans* is the most common cause of human mycoses, including blood infections. However, infections from so-called non-*albicans Candida* (NAC) species, such as *C. glabrata* and *C. krusei*, are becoming more common. *C. albicans* is distinguished from NAC species under microscope by the appearance of tiny cylindrical projections, called germ tubes, that appear within two to four hours of incubating a sample under investigation.

Most *Candida* species remain a part of the normal flora of the body. However, they are also recovered from hospital equipment such as respirators, air-conditioning vents, and countertops, thus acting as a source of hospital-acquired infection. Certain *Candida* species are also equipped with a set of virulence factors that help them cause disease.

When the immune system is healthy and the skin and mucous membranes of the gastrointestinal and vaginal tract are intact, the existence of *Candida* will not cause any health problems. However, when immunity is compromised due to other conditions, then *Candida* may become pathogenic, causing infection and leading to various types of illness.

Colonization of the mucocutaneous surfaces of the body (such as the mouth, genitals, or skin) by *Candida* is the first step in the process of infection. The oral infection of *Candida* is called oral candidiasis and may also affect part of the pharynx (cavity behind the nose and mouth) and esophagus. Vulvovaginal candidiasis is another manifestation of *Candida* infection affecting approximately 75 percent of women during their lifetime. Invasive candidiasis is a third type of infection, wherein the fungi may enter the heart, the brain, the eyes, the bones, and other parts of the body. Infection of the bloodstream, known as candidemia, is a common infection noted in hospitalized patients.

One of the most important factors causing candidiasis is weakened immunity, which occurs in patients suffering from human immunodeficiency virus (HIV) or acquired immunodeficiency syndrome (AIDS), after cancer chemotherapy (which depletes the white cells that fight infection), and after bone marrow or organ transplantation. Patients having transplants must take medication to stop rejection of the new organ for the rest of their lives. Unfortunately, this also impairs their immune systems and puts them at increased risk of infection, including candidiasis. Other causes of candidiasis include antibiotic use, which can alter the balance of the intestinal flora; the contraceptive pill; pregnancy; old age; malnutrition; and diabetes. In hospitals the use of intravenous and urinary catheters, which are tubes inserted into the body to deliver fluids and medication and drain the bladder, respectively, often lead to inva-

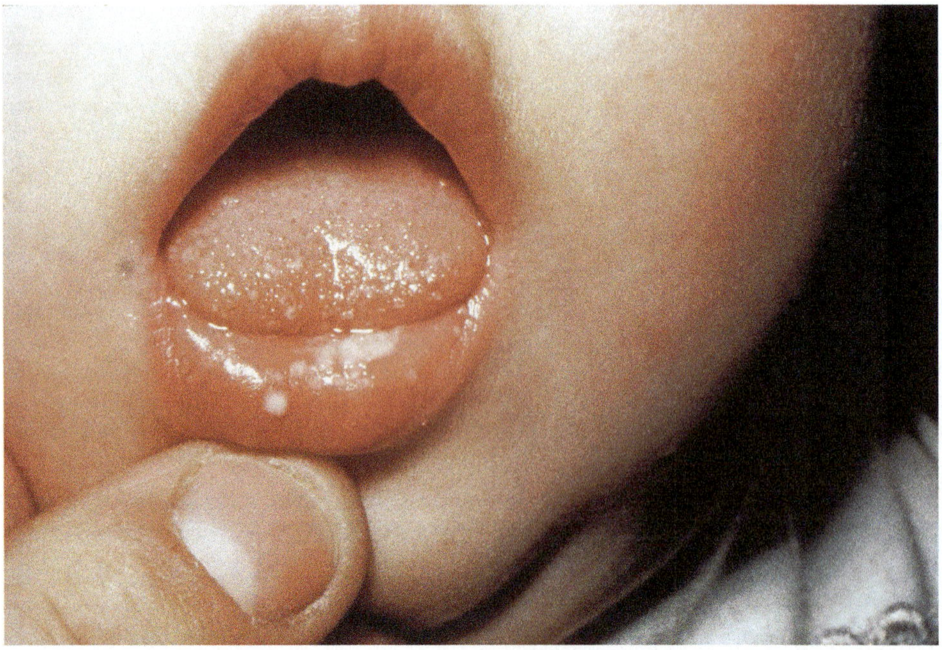

This picture shows a typical case of oral candidiasis. Candidiasis is the most common form of fungal infection. *© John Watney/Science Source*

sive candidiasis. *Candida* infection in newborn infants may develop into a severe form of candidiasis in babies with low birth weight or conditions such as necrotizing enterocolitis (death of cells in the intestine).

■ Scope and Distribution

The most common sites of candidiasis are the mouth, esophagus, skin, vagina, and bloodstream. Oral and esophageal candidiasis are often also known as thrush or oropharyngeal candidiasis (OPC). According to a 2002 study, oral candidiasis is the world's most common form of fungal infection, with 45 to 65 percent of children and 30 to 45 percent of adults being asymptomatic carriers of *C. albicans.* Oral thrush is common among people with weakened immunity, especially those with HIV/AIDS, who have an OPC prevalence of 80 to 95 percent. It causes white patches on the tongue and inside the mouth and may be associated with soreness and a burning sensation. Some people also have difficulty swallowing and experience pain, nausea, and vomiting.

Vulvovaginal candidiasis is also common, affecting three-quarters of all women at some stage in their lives. It causes genital itching and burning, with or without a "cottage cheese"-like discharge. Candidiasis can occur when the normal acidity of the vagina changes or with hormonal changes, both of which can encourage the overgrowth of *Candida.* Risk factors include pregnancy, diabetes, use of broad-spectrum antibiotics, and steroid medications. Men can get a form of the disease—genital candidiasis, which causes an itchy rash on the penis. However, transmission of thrush through sexual intercourse is rare; most infections are endogenous.

Candidiasis of the skin is sometimes called intertrigo and produces a rash in warm, moist areas such as the armpit, the groin, and under the breast. Diaper rash is often a form of candidiasis that affects babies in the area where the diaper comes into contact with the skin. Sometimes, especially in people with HIV/AIDS, candidiasis may also affect the nails.

Oral, esophageal, vaginal, and skin candidiasis can all clear up with antifungal treatment, with no lasting effects on health, although they may recur. They may cause some discomfort, even pain, but are relatively mild infections even though the patient may be suffering from serious disease, such as HIV/AIDS or diabetes, which is the primary reason for candidiasis to develop.

Invasive candidiasis, however, can be serious or life-threatening. It occurs when *Candida* invades the bloodstream, and it is dangerous because it may then spread throughout the body, reaching the liver, kidneys, spleen, and other organs. Patients with cancer, depletion of white cells from cancer treatment, or major burns are at risk, as are those who have had organ transplants, abdominal surgery, or broad-spectrum antibiotics. Patients with catheters are also at risk of invasive candidiasis. The death rate from invasive candidiasis can be as high as 60 percent. Therefore, if *Candida* is found in a blood culture from a patient, especially if he or she has a fever, it can be assumed that candidiasis may be spreading through the whole body, and prompt treatment is essential.

REAL-WORLD RISKS

Recent data indicates the emergence of *Candida auris*, a fungal pathogen first isolated in 2009, as an important species of *Candida* that is causing serious problems around the world. It is considered a serious global health threat mainly for the following reasons:

- It is resistant to multiple antifungal agents that are known to treat other *Candida* infections.
- Diagnosis is difficult, leading to misidentification, which further leads to mismanagement of the infection.
- It has caused outbreaks in health care settings, raising serious concern about the need to identify the organism quickly.

■ Treatment and Prevention

Candida species are a part of the normal flora of human gastrointestinal and urinary tracts and hence cannot be avoided or eliminated from the body. Therefore, prevention depends on maintaining proper immune function and limiting risk factors such as open wounds or weakened mucosal barriers (layers of mucus in the gut that prevent against infection) due to long-term use of broad-spectrum antibiotics, which can disrupt beneficial microbiota in the intestines. Other risk factors include diabetes, a prolonged stay in an intensive care unit, presence of a catheter in the body, long-term corticosteroid treatment, abdominal surgery, and old age. Newborns with low birth weight and necrotizing enterocolitis are also at greater risk of developing *Candida* infection.

An early, effective, and rapid treatment regimen of antifungal drugs is used to treat invasive candidiasis to ensure early clearance of yeast. The main antifungal drugs used in the treatment for candidiasis are amphotericin B, fluconazole, and nystatin. Antifungal drugs can be applied either topically, as a cream or powder, or orally, as a tablet. Vaginal thrush can be treated with antifungal suppositories inserted into the vagina. As of 2018 there were several new drugs being tested by researchers.

For invasive candidiasis, a five-point management is suggested: (1) administer an antifungal agent that will rapidly and effectively clear the infection; (2) remove the source of infection (e.g., catheter or any infected device); (3) modify treatment according to species and susceptibility e.g., voriconazole is suggested for *C. krusei* or

C. glabrate, which are resistant to fluconazole); (4) assess efficacy of treatment using a laboratory blood culture test; and (5) check spread of infection to other organs, including the kidneys, liver, spleen, bones, and central nervous system.

■ Impacts and Issues

Infections acquired in hospitals, also known as nosocomial infections, are an increasing public health problem. Those affected are often already very sick, with weakened immune systems, and are unable to fight an infection the way a healthy person would. In addition, many organisms that cause nosocomial infections are becoming resistant to antibiotics, so treatment may be ineffective. The CDC estimates that 46,000 cases of nosocomial bloodstream infection of *Candida* are reported in the United States each year and carry a mortality rate of approximately 30 percent, though other studies have shown mortality rates as high as 60 percent. However, these incidences and the distribution of *Candida* species causing invasive infection vary substantially by geographic location (*C. glabrate* is more prevalent in the United States, Europe, and Australia, for example, while *C. albicans* is more common in Africa and Latin America) and patient population. Even if a patient survives, hospital stays are prolonged, which involves significant extra health care costs. Once found, *Candida* may spread to all areas of a hospital. An aging population, the more frequent use of invasive therapies involving catheters, and the overuse of antibiotics are among the contributing factors to the spread of *Candida* infection.

SEE ALSO *Mycotic Disease; Nosocomial (Health Care–Associated) Infections*

BIBLIOGRAPHY

Books

Bennett, John E., Raphael Dolin, and Martin J. Blaser. *Mandell, Douglas, and Bennett's Infectious Disease Essentials.* Philadelphia: Elsevier, 2017.

Bennett, John E., Raphael Dolin, and Martin J. Blaser, eds. *Mandell, Douglas, and Bennett's Principles and Practice of Infectious Diseases.* 8th ed. Philadelphia: Elsevier, 2015.

Calderone, Richard A. Candida *and Candidiasis.* Washington, DC: ASM, 2012.

Calderone, Richard A., and Ronald Cihlar, eds. Candida *Species: Methods and Protocols.* New York: Humana, 2015.

Periodicals

Akpan, A., and R. Morgan. "Oral Candidiasis." *Postgraduate Medical Journal* 78, no. 922 (2002): 455–459. This article can also be found available online at http://pmj.bmj.com/content/78/922/455 (accessed January 25, 2018).

Chowdhary, Anuradha, Cheshta Sharma, and Jacques F. Meis "*Candida auris*: A Rapidly Emerging Cause of Hospital-Acquired Multidrug-Resistant Fungal Infections Globally." *PLOS Pathogens* 13, no. 5 (2017). This article can also be found online at http://journals.plos.org/plospathogens/article?id=10.1371/journal.ppat.1006290 (accessed January 25, 2018).

Cleveland, Angela Ahlquist, et al. "Declining Incidence of Candidemia and the Shifting Epidemiology of *Candida* Resistance in Two US Metropolitan Areas, 2008–2013: Results from Population-Based Surveillance." *PLOS ONE* (March 30, 2015). This article can also be found online at http://journals.plos.org/plosone/article?id=10.1371/journal.pone.0120452 (accessed January 25, 2018).

Kullberg, Bart Jan, and Maiken C. Arendrup. "Invasive Candidiasis." *New England Journal of Medicine* 373 (2015): 1445–1456.

Lamoth, Frederic, et al. "Changes in the Epidemiological Landscape of Invasive Candidiasis." *Journal of Antimicrobial Chemotherapy* 73 (January 2018): i4–i13.

Pappas, P. G., et al. "Clinical Practice Guideline for the Management of Candidiasis: 2016 Update by the Infectious Diseases Society of America." *Clinical Infectious Diseases* 62, no. 4 (2016): e1–e50.

Whitney, Laura C., and Tihana Bicanic. "Treatment Principles for *Candida* and *Cryptococcus*." *Cold Spring Harbor Perspectives in Medicine* 5, no. 6 (2014): 1–12.

Websites

"Antibiotic Resistance Threats in the United States, 2013." Centers for Disease Control and Prevention, April 10, 2017. https://www.cdc.gov/drugresistance/threat-report-2013/index.html (accessed January 23, 2018).

"Fungal Diseases: Candidiasis." Centers for Disease Control and Prevention, August 7, 2015. https://www.cdc.gov/fungal/diseases/candidiasis/index.html(accessed January 23, 2018).

"The Unexpected and Troubling Rise of *Candida auris*." Medscape, August 24, 2017. https://www.medscape.com/viewarticle/884470?src=par_cdc_stm_mscpedt&faf=1 (accessed January 23, 2017).

"Vulvovaginal Candidiasis." Centers for Disease Control and Prevention, June 4, 2015. https://www.cdc.gov/std/tg2015/candidiasis.htm (accessed January 23, 2018).

Susan Aldridge
Kausalya Santhanam

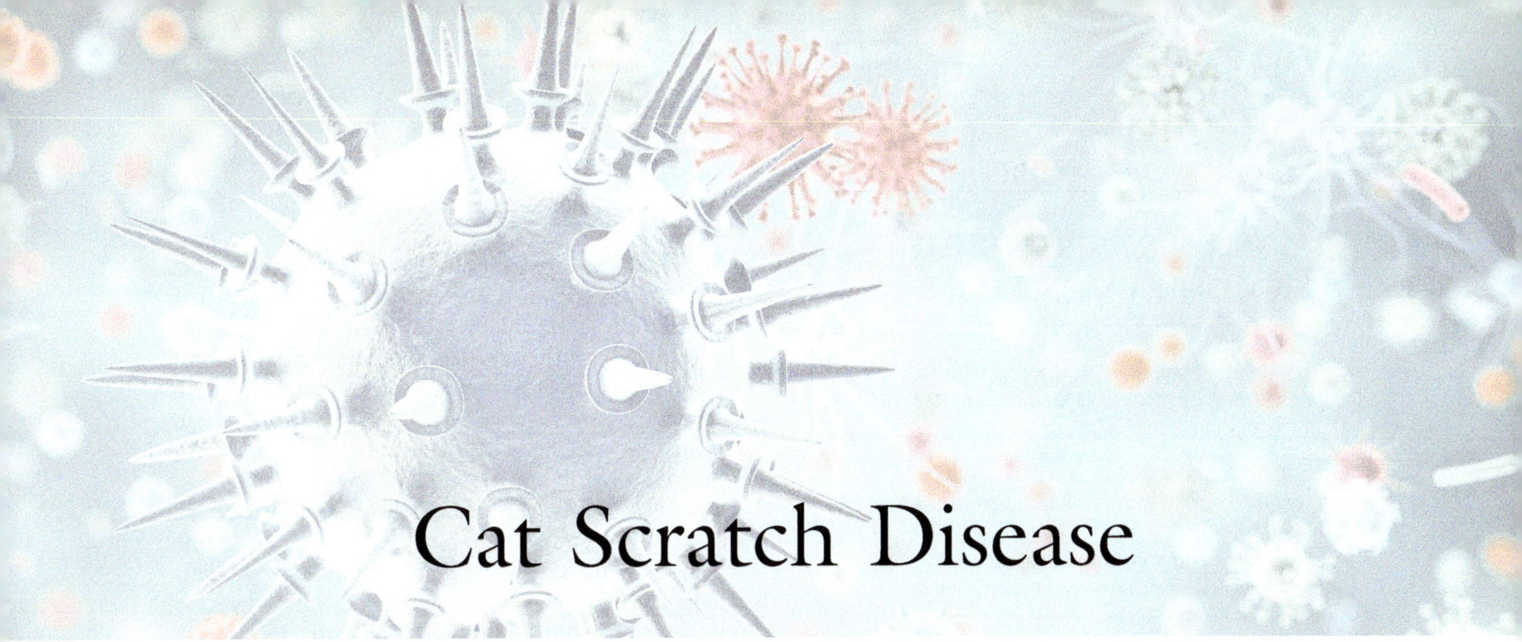

Cat Scratch Disease

Introduction

Cat scratch disease is an infection caused by the bacterium *Bartonella henselae.* It is most often transmitted to humans through a bite or scratch from a cat.

Disease History, Characteristics, and Transmission

Cat scratch disease was first described in 1889. Recognition that the cat is important in the spread of the disease came in 1931, but the bacterium responsible for cat scratch disease was not identified until 1985. This bacterium was initially identified as *Rochalimaea henselae* (the bacterium that causes the disease trench fever) but was later reclassified as *Bartonella henselae.* It took so long to identify *B. henselae* as the cause of cat scratch disease because the bacterium is difficult to grow in artificial lab media. It has specific nutrient requirements, and it grows slowly in the laboratory even in the presence of the appropriate food sources.

The first sign of cat scratch disease is a mild infection or swelling at the site of the bite or scratch. Red, raised, and round areas of the skin can be present. Often, this injury does not receive much attention because it is minor, but if the injured area is not cleaned, the bacteria can enter the bloodstream. Characteristics of the resulting infection that can develop at the site of the bite or scratch up to two weeks later include soreness at the wound site (which may take days to develop), expansion of the wound site and production of pus, swelling of the lymph nodes near the wound (generally those in the underarm and neck) to an inch or more in size, loss of appetite, headache, moderate fever, bone and joint pain, rash, sore throat, and a feeling of persistent weakness.

A domestic cat can carry the bacteria in its saliva but not display any symptoms of infection (a process called colonization), making it impossible for those who handle the cat to know that it can infect them. For many people, there is no need to worry, because the body's immune system can successfully fight off the infection. However, if a person is immunocompromised (the immune system is not functioning efficiently), cat scratch disease can develop. A compromised immune system is sometimes a natural result of the aging process or can arise as the result of a disease that affects the immune system, such as infection with human immunodeficiency virus (HIV). The immune system also may be suppressed deliberately in patients who have received an organ transplant to avoid rejection of the transplanted organ. Some immunocompromised individuals can develop more severe symptoms, including infections of the spleen, liver, lungs, and eyes, when they contract cat scratch disease.

Cat scratch disease cannot be passed from person to person, and it usually does not require medical treatment. Once a person has had this infection, he or she is immune to the bacterium for life.

Scope and Distribution

About 40 percent of domestic cats will carry *B. henselae* at some time in their lives. The bacteria tend to be as-

WORDS TO KNOW

COLONIZATION The process of occupation and increase in number of microorganisms at a specific site.

IMMUNOCOMPROMISED Having an immune system with reduced ability to recognize and respond to the presence of foreign material.

ZOONOTIC A disease that can be transmitted between animals and humans. Examples of zoonotic diseases are anthrax, plague, and Q fever.

PERSONAL RESPONSIBILITY AND PREVENTION

The US Centers for Disease Control and Prevention's Healthy Pets Healthy People published guidelines to reduce the risk of cat scratch disease:

- Avoid "rough play" with cats, especially kittens. This includes any activity that may lead to cat scratches and bites.
- Wash cat bites and scratches immediately and thoroughly with running water and soap.
- Do not allow cats to lick open wounds.
- Control fleas.
- If you develop an infection (with pus and pronounced swelling) where you were scratched or bitten by a cat or you develop symptoms, including fever, headache, swollen lymph nodes, and fatigue, contact your physician.

sociated with younger cats, especially those who have fleas in their fur, and with wild (feral) cats.

In the United States cat scratch disease develops in approximately one out of every 10,000 people. Most cases involve people under the age of 21, with many of these being children who have been scratched or bitten by their family cat during play with the pet.

Treatment and Prevention

Cat scratch disease is typically diagnosed by the detection of swollen lymph nodes when the individual has been bitten or scratched by a cat. The infection tends to be resolved without treatment. However, immunocompromised patients may require treatment with antibiotics. If necessary, the swollen lymph nodes can be drained by inserting a needle into the node and withdrawing the fluid.

Bartonella can be detected using the polymerase chain reaction (PCR) test. As of 2017 this test was in clinical use.

The risk of cat scratch disease is minimized by properly handling cats. Anyone who is scratched or bitten by a cat should wash the wound with soap and water to disinfect the area. Because cats can harbor the bacteria in their saliva, they should not be allowed to lick a person's face or a cut. Treating cats to reduce flea infestations is also a wise preventive strategy.

Impacts and Issues

As of 2017 there were an estimated 74 million pet cats in the United States. This creates ample opportunity for the spread of cat scratch disease. For most people, the consequences of the disease are not serious, and the disease does not require medical treatment. However, for about 10 percent of people who contract cat scratch disease, the result can be more serious, with consequences such as altered mental state, loss of vision, and even pneumonia.

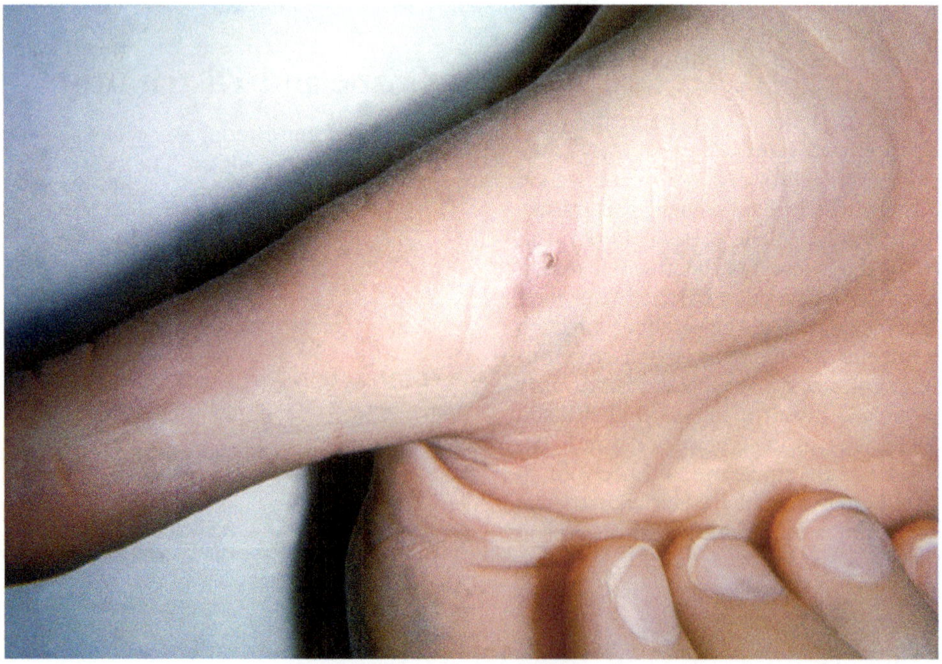

This hand shows a cat-scratch disease lesion. The disease is transmitted to humans by the bite or scratch of a cat. © *Smith Collection/Gado/Getty Images*

Cat scratch disease is seasonal. More than 90 percent of cases occur in the fall and early winter. This may be because many kittens are born during the summer, and the population of new kittens has been infested with bacterium-carrying fleas by the fall. In more northern climates, the cooler months of the year usually bring people into closer contact with their house cats. In both cases treating pets for fleas and handwashing after petting cats or kittens will reduce the chances of contracting the disease.

In addition to its close association with cat bites and scratches, cat scratch disease has been linked to the bites of dogs and even monkeys. Because monkeys are linked to the disease, zoo staff and some veterinarians are at risk for the disease in western countries, and larger populations are at risk in developing countries where monkeys and humans come into contact.

SEE ALSO *Bacterial Disease; Vector-Borne Disease; Zoonoses*

BIBLIOGRAPHY

Books

Kudva, Indira T., et al. *Virulence Mechanisms of Bacterial Pathogens.* Washington, DC: American Society for Microbiology, 2016.

Tortora, Gerard J., Berdell R. Funke, and Christine L. Case. *Microbiology: An Introduction.* Boston: Pearson, 2016.

Periodicals

Curi, Andre L., and Rim Kahloun. "Cat-Scratch Disease." *Emerging Infectious Uveitis* (June 2017): 57–63.

Hobson, C., et al. "Detection of Bartonella in Cat Scratch Disease Using a Single-Step PCR Assay Kit." *Journal of Medical Microbiology* 66 (2017).

Nelson, Christina A., Shubhayu Saha, and Paul S. Mead. "Cat-Scratch Disease in the United States, 2005–2013." *Emerging Infectious Diseases* 22, no. 10 (2016): 1741–1746.

Websites

"Bartonella Infection (Cat Scratch Disease, Trench Fever, and Carrión's Disease)." Centers for Disease Control and Prevention. https://www.cdc.gov/bartonella/index.html (accessed November 14, 2017).

Brian Hoyle

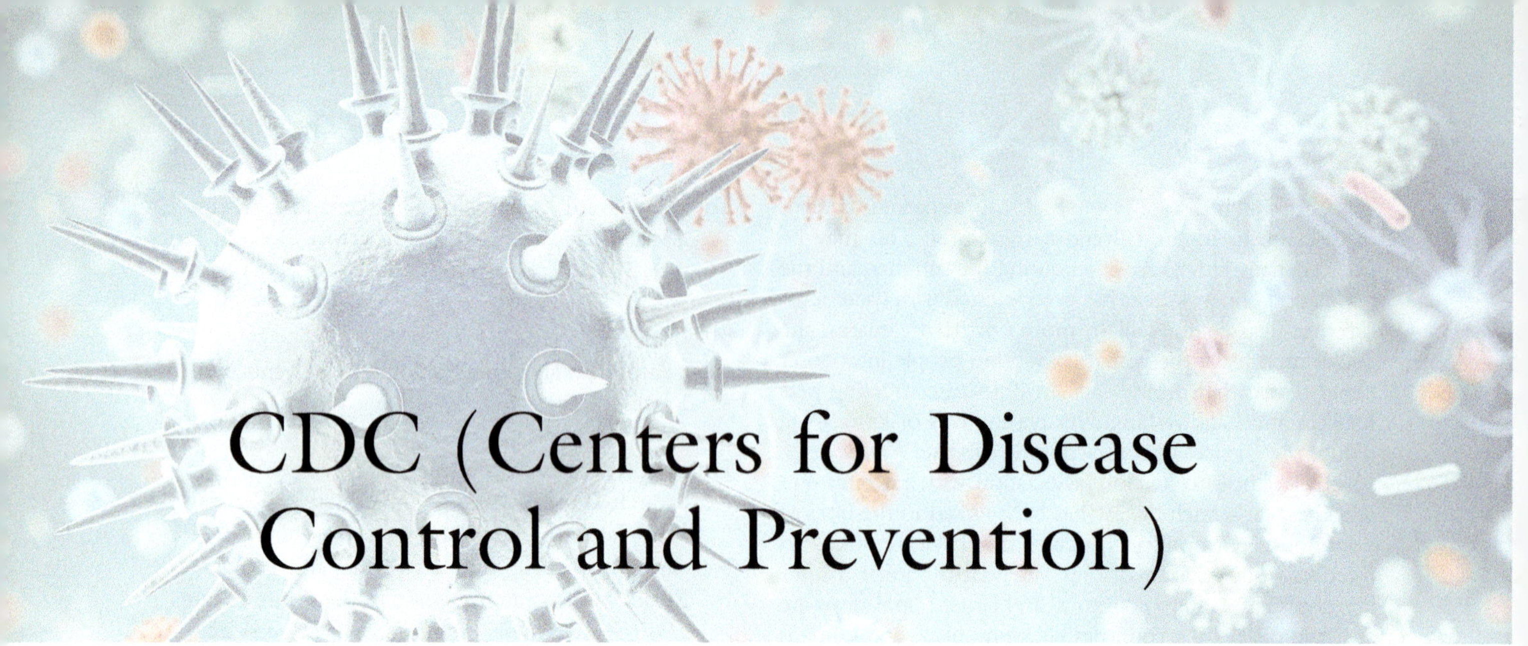

CDC (Centers for Disease Control and Prevention)

Introduction

The Centers for Disease Control and Prevention (CDC) is part of the US federal government's Department of Health and Human Services. The CDC is headquartered in Atlanta, Georgia. The organization's efforts are geared to protect the health and safety of the public by controlling and preventing diseases, along with disabilities and injuries. By maintaining viable relationships with state health departments and other related organizations, the CDC researches all aspects of diseases, along with developing and applying disease prevention and control, environmental health, and health education activities for all citizens of the United States. As the organization states, it deals with "most deadly germs in the world" to identify and counter health threats within the United States and abroad. Its researchers are continually developing and reviewing guidelines to protect all Americans.

The CDC also participates in international infectious disease research and response. In all, the CDC partners with more than 1,600 organizations and more than 130 countries. The organization is also a founding member of the International Association of National Public Health Institutes, a group of government agencies working to prevent diseases around the world.

With more than 15,000 employees in nearly 150 positions, the staff of the CDC includes biologists, behavioral and social scientists, physicians, veterinarians, microbiologists, chemists, economists, engineers, epidemiologists, statisticians, and various other scientists and support personnel. With an average annual budget of over $13 billion, the CDC has the strength and ability to protect Americans from health-related problems.

The CDC's headquarters coordinates its operations across the United States and Puerto Rico. Supporting those activities are centers, institutes, and offices. The CDC has

Centers for Disease Control and Prevention (CDC) Timeline

1946	National Communicable Disease Center (NCDC), the precursor to the CDC, is formed.
1957	NCDC establishes influenza surveillance unit during the 1957 flu pandemic.
1966	NCDC announces measles eradication campaign.
1969	NCDC launches national rubella immunization campaign.
1970	NCDC renamed Center for Disease Control (CDC).
1974	CDC begins developing health curriculum for use in schools.
1981	CDC publishes report on first cases of acquired immuno-deficiency syndrome (AIDS).
1982	CDC begins international campaign to eliminate dracunculiasis (Guinea worm disease).
1992	CDC is renamed Centers for Disease Control and Prevention to better reflect its mission.
1994	CDC certifies polio eradication in the Americas.
1999	CDC launches the National Pharmaceutical Stockpile to ensure emergency health security.
2001	CDC investigates first US case of anthrax since 1976.
2004	CDC announces rubella eradication in the United States.
2006	CDC responds to a mumps outbreak in the Midwest.
2009	CDC identifies the H1N1 influenza virus and responds to the ensuing pandemic.
2014	CDC activates Emergency Operations Center to respond to outbreak of Ebola in Africa.
2016	CDC responds to Zika virus outbreak.

SOURCE: US Centers for Disease Control and Prevention

WORDS TO KNOW

BIOSAFETY LABORATORY A laboratory that deals with all aspects of potentially infectious agents or biohazards.

BIOSAFETY LEVEL 4 FACILITY A specialized biosafety laboratory that deals with dangerous or exotic infectious agents or biohazards that are considered high risks for spreading life-threatening diseases, either because the disease is spread through aerosols or because there is no therapy or vaccine to counter the disease.

EPIDEMIC An outbreak of an illness or disease in which the number of individual cases significantly exceeds the usual or expected number of cases in any given population.

EPIDEMIOLOGY The study of various factors that influence the occurrence, distribution, prevention, and control of disease, injury, and other health-related events in a defined human population. By the application of various analytical techniques, including mathematical analysis of the data, the probable cause of an infectious outbreak can be pinpointed.

ERADICATE To get rid of; the permanent reduction to zero of global incidence of a particular infection.

LEGIONNAIRES' DISEASE A type of pneumonia caused by *Legionella* bacteria. The bacterial species responsible for Legionnaires' disease is *L. pneumophila.* Major symptoms include fever, chills, muscle aches, and a cough that is initially nonproductive. Definitive diagnosis relies on specific laboratory tests for the bacteria, bacterial antigens, or antibodies produced by the body's immune system. As with other types of pneumonia, Legionnaires' disease poses the greatest threat to people who are elderly, ill, or immunocompromised.

OUTBREAK The appearance of new cases of a disease in numbers greater than the established incidence rate or the appearance of even one case of an emergent or rare disease in an area.

PANDEMIC An epidemic that occurs in more than one country or population simultaneously. *Pandemic* means "all the people."

SEPSIS A bacterial infection in the bloodstream or body tissues. Sepsis is a very broad term covering the presence of many types of microscopic disease-causing organisms. It is also called bacteremia. Closely related terms include septicemia and septic syndrome.

VACCINATION The inoculation, or use of vaccines, to prevent specific diseases within humans and animals by producing immunity to such diseases. It is the introduction of weakened or dead viruses or microorganisms into the body to create immunity by the production of specific antibodies.

VECTOR Any agent that carries and transmits parasites and diseases. Also, an organism or a chemical used to transport a gene into a new host cell.

personnel actively working in over 25 countries. Its mission statement declares that the "CDC works 24/7 to protect America from health, safety, and security threats, both foreign and in the US. Whether diseases start at home or abroad, are chronic or acute, curable or preventable, human error or deliberate attack, CDC fights disease and supports communities and citizens to do the same."

History and Scientific Foundations

The CDC was established on July 1, 1946, in Atlanta, Georgia, under its original name, the Communicable Disease Center. At that time it had fewer than 400 employees. Its founder was US public health official Joseph Walter Mountin (1891–1952).

The organization was established out of the Office of Malaria Control in War Areas, a US military agency that was active during World War II (1939–1945). By taking over the military office, the CDC gained access to over 600 military bases and related establishments to combat mosquitoes carrying malaria, which was still prevalent in the southern United States. The fledgling organization also worked with typhus and other infectious diseases.

The agency hired engineers, entomologists (scientists who study insects), and physicians to research and develop ways to combat infectious health problems. These professionals fought mosquito-carrying malaria with the use of the insecticide DDT (dichlorodiphenyltrichloroethane), which is now restricted in the United States and in many other countries because it was found to endanger wildlife and damage the environment. Before DDT was restricted, the organization sprayed millions of homes to combat malaria.

By 1947 Mountin was promoting the Communicable Disease Center as an effective organization to pursue additional public health issues such as birth defects, chronic diseases, communicable diseases, health statistics, injuries, occupational health concerns, and toxic chemical exposure.

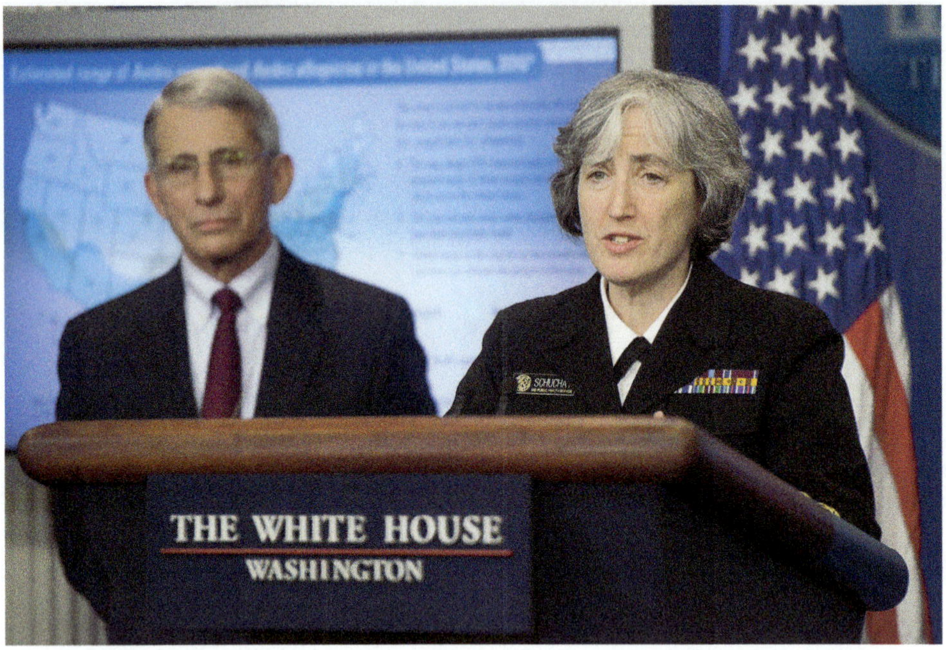

Dr. Anne Schuchat of the Centers for Disease Control and Prevention (CDC) speaks about the Zika virus in April 2016. She is joined by Dr. Anthony Fauci of the National Institutes of Health. The CDC plays an important role in keeping the public informed about health issues. © SAUL LOEB/AFP/Getty Images

The organization expanded its operations when 15 acres (6 hectares) of Emory University land in Atlanta was donated by Robert Woodruff (1889–1985), chairman of the board of the Coca-Cola Company. The campus included two Biosafety Level 4 laboratories and other scientific facilities. Branches were established in Morgantown, West Virginia; Cincinnati, Ohio; Fort Collins, Colorado; and locations overseas.

Over the next 60 years, the organization expanded its expertise in the control and prevention of diseases. In 1970 its name was changed to the Center for Disease Control to include its work with communicable diseases such as acquired immunodeficiency syndrome (AIDS), chronic diseases such as cancer and heart disease, emerging diseases, birth defects such as those caused by lead poisoning, occupational illnesses and disabilities, injury control, workplace hazards, blood supply, environmental health threats, and bioterrorism.

In 1980, with expansion of the organizational structure, the organization's name was changed yet again to the Centers for Disease Control. Twelve years later, in 1992, its current name was adopted: the Centers for Disease Control and Prevention. The US Congress requested that the organization maintain the initials CDC.

In 2006, on the 60th anniversary of being established, the CDC was internationally recognized as one of the leading national public health organizations in the world. It continues to conduct research and investigations geared toward improving the health of people and responding to health emergencies.

In the 2010s the organization focused on five essential health areas: supporting local and state health departments, improving health policies, implementing measures to reduce the leading causes of death, improving epidemiology and surveillance, and improving global health conditions. As an example, in 2016 the CDC activated its Emergency Operations Center (EOC) to counter the Zika virus, which is spread by the mosquito species *Aedes aegypti* and *Aedes albopictus.*

The CDC also developed a Strategic Framework for fiscal years 2016–2020. It consists of three strategic priorities: "(1) Improve health security at home and around the world; (2) Better prevent the leading causes of illness, injury, disability, and death; and (3) Strengthen public health and healthcare collaboration." Health security is deemed of high importance for the CDC because of the ability of diseases to spread rapidly. For instance, the CDC states that easily dispersed foodborne illnesses, which sicken about 48 million people each year, cost over $15.5 billion annually to the US economy. The CDC works diligently to find better, faster, and more cost-effective means to fight such health-security problems.

The top three causes of death in the United States —cardiovascular disease, stroke, and cancer—are responsible for over 50 percent of all deaths in the country. The top 10 causes account for almost 75 percent of all deaths. For these reasons the CDC is dedicated to improving health and health care for all Americans while reducing the severity and amount of illness, injury, disability, and death.

The CDC is also improving its ability to collaborate with other public health and health care organizations. For example, as of 2015 *Vital Signs*, a monthly report initiated in 2010, had the technical ability to reach 6.6 million people. Each issue contains informative articles on breast cancer screening, alcohol use, human immunodeficiency virus (HIV) testing, cardiovascular disease, foodborne disease, and many other health-related subjects.

Vaccination programs for US children are an essential part of the CDC's fight to improve health in the country. In all the CDC is involved with about half of all childhood vaccination programs in the United States. With such coordination, each vaccination saves $3 to $10 in direct/indirect costs for each $1 spent. In yet another example of the benefits gained from CDC collaboration with communities, statistics show that the Tips From Former Smokers® (Tips®) campaign has helped at least 400,000 smokers quit since 2012.

Applications and Research

The CDC provides health information to various sectors of the US economy. Working with state and local organizations, the CDC collects and analyzes data to detect disease outbreaks and health threats, researches effective measures for disease and injury control and prevention, and identifies risk factors and causes of diseases and injuries. Along with actively protecting health and safety, the CDC provides information to individuals making personal health decisions and organizations making professional decisions affecting larger populations.

In general, the CDC conducts research both in the field and in the laboratory. Several CDC offices maintain field response teams to aid in the identification and surveillance of infectious diseases. International health agencies may request CDC assistance in identifying or studying disease outbreaks.

The operational hierarchy of the CDC begins with the Office of the Director and continues with the National Institute for Occupational Safety and Health and the Center for Global Health. The Office of the Director manages CDC activities by providing overall direction to its medical and scientific programs and by furnishing assessments of general management activities. The National Institute for Occupational Safety and Health, which joined the CDC in 1973, ensures safety and health for all people in the workplace. Research into preventing workplace accidents and exposures and improving the health and safety of workers is primarily accomplished through its National Occupational Research Agenda, which was created in 1996. Personnel at the Center for Global Health work to accomplish their six-part objective:

- Coordinate and execute the CDC's global health strategy.
- Partner with various organizations in providing strong public health programs and helping countries promote ownership and sustainability with regard to health.
- Help the US government and world organizations in meeting health goals.
- Promote and strengthen CDC programs that concentrate on major causes of mortality, morbidity, and disability.
- Develop and apply information to meet health goals.
- Strengthen health systems.

Five offices concentrate on specific areas of concern for the CDC:

- Office of Public Health Preparedness and Response
- Office for State, Tribal, Local, and Territorial Support
- Offices of Infectious Diseases
- Office of Noncommunicable Diseases, Injury, and Environmental Health
- Office of Public Health Scientific Services

The Office of Public Health Preparedness and Response (OPHPR) takes charge of health emergencies in the United States and works with its partners to deal with health catastrophes in other parts of the world. Whether the emergency is a chemical or radiological release, natural disaster, or pandemic, the OPHPR is prepared at a moment's notice to respond to any type or size of health problem. Within the OPHPR are four divisions: Division of Emergency Operations, Division of State and Local Readiness, Division of Strategic National Stockpile, and Division of Select Agents and Toxins. The Division of Strategic National Stockpile, as an example, manages the Strategic National Stockpile, which is a comprehensive repository of pharmaceuticals and medical supplies deemed necessary to protect the citizens of the United States if multiple large-scale public emergencies occur, after local and state supplies have been depleted.

The Office for State, Tribal, Local, and Territorial Support (OSTLTS) is an essential part of the CDC's role in helping all types of health agencies in the country's public health system. The CDC uses the OSTLTS as its communications source with health officials and personnel at state, tribal, local, and territorial levels, along with government officials dealing with health-related matters. For instance, the OSTLTS manages the Preventive Health and Health Services Block Grant for all 50 states and the District of Columbia, eight US territories, and two Native American tribes. Its only division, the Division of Public Health Performance Improvement, is targeted to improve the performance of the public health system. It contains the Applied Systems Evaluation and Research Branch and the Health Department and Systems Development Branch.

The Office of Infectious Diseases (OID) is tasked with creating and improving policies, programs, and science with respect to infectious diseases in the United States and around the world. Three infectious disease national centers support these activities: the National Center for Emerging and Zoonotic Infectious Diseases; National Center for HIV/AIDS, Viral Hepatitis, STD, and TB Prevention; and National Center for Immunization and Respiratory Diseases. In response to the increasing global incidence of HIV/AIDS and reemerging tuberculosis (TB), the CDC's National Center for HIV/AIDS, Viral Hepatitis, STD, and TB Prevention focuses on initiatives involving control, disability, intervention, prevention, and research to combat TB and sexually transmitted infections (STIs), including HIV/AIDS. Center research efforts help to improve treatment and education programs, as well as to advance vaccine development.

The Office of Noncommunicable Diseases, Injury, and Environmental Health (ONDIEH) consists of four national centers: the National Center on Birth Defects and Developmental Disabilities, National Center for Chronic Disease Prevention and Health Promotion, National Center for Environmental Health/Agency for Toxic Substances and Disease Registry, and National Center for Injury Prevention and Control. The National Center on Birth Defects and Developmental Disabilities is dedicated to saving the lives of those who cannot take care of themselves (babies, children, and those living with disabilities). To accomplish this important task, the center concentrates on the prevention of birth defects through medical research, comprehension of developmental disabilities, protection of those with blood disorders, and improvement in those with health disabilities.

The National Center for Chronic Disease Prevention and Health Promotion is also responsible for preventing chronic diseases. It does this by working with states and communities to implement effective strategies to prevent chronic diseases and promote healthy lifestyles. The National Center for Environmental Health coordinates a national plan to reduce untimely deaths and to prevent the spread of avoidable illnesses and disabilities caused by nonoccupational, noninfectious environmental scenarios. In coordination with the National Center for Environmental Health, the Agency for Toxic Substances and Disease Registry is geared toward protecting people from human-made and natural hazardous substances. The National Center for Injury Prevention and Control deals with the consequences of violence and injuries, such as those from homicides and vehicle accidents.

The Office of Public Health Scientific Services (OPHSS) is dedicated to improving the general environment at the CDC with regard to its surveillance capabilities, along with parallel capabilities within the US public health system. As such, the OPHSS emphasizes the use of strict science policies and standards. The OPHSS provides guidance to the National Center for Health Statistics and the Center for Surveillance, Epidemiology, and Laboratory Services. The mission statement for the National Center for Health Statistics states that it will provide relevant and timely statistics to coordinate activities pertinent to all Americans' health. Among its duties are providing accurate information to the country's health community, training personnel in the public health field, improving the effectiveness and efficiency of CDC programs, providing strong laboratory systems within the country, and modernizing tracking systems used by the public health sector.

The CDC also publishes several journals intended to relay information throughout the international public health community. *Emerging Infectious Diseases* is published monthly online and in limited print. The open-access journal compiles articles and announcements on infectious diseases worldwide. *Morbidity and Mortality Weekly Report*, commonly known as *MMWR*, collects and publishes reports from state public health agencies. Because *MMWR* is the primary CDC health publication, the journal is commonly called "the voice of the CDC." Most readers of *MMWR* are health care professionals, such as physicians and nurses, public health practitioners, medical researchers and educators, scientists, and laboratorians. Both publications foster communication and share up-to-date information among various health organizations.

The CDC has its main biosafety level 4 laboratories in the United States in its Special Pathogens Branch. A biosafety level 4 laboratory is one of a select few laboratories whose scientists and technicians are allowed to work with dangerous and unusual agents that have the highest potential for individual health risks and life-threatening diseases. This is the highest level of biosafety laboratory in the world. The only other biosafety level 4 sites are at the State Research Center of Virology and Biotechnology in Koltsovo, Russia.

Another important task taken on by the CDC is being the only repository of smallpox in the United States. Smallpox is a highly contagious disease that is contracted only by humans. It is caused by two virus variants: *Variola major* and *Variola minor*.

The CDC is also vigilant with respect to early recognition and expedient treatment of sepsis, a dangerous, sometimes life-threatening, reaction to infection. More than 250,000 Americans die from sepsis each year. Worldwide, sepsis claims over 1.5 million lives annually. In August 2017 the CDC introduced Get Ahead of Sepsis, an educational program aimed at protecting Americans from the extremely harmful effects of sepsis. The program emphasizes understanding the symptoms of sepsis and seeking immediate medical care when infections do not heal or get worse over time.

The CDC participates in several international efforts to identify, research, and respond to infectious disease. For example, the CDC's international outreach includes participation in the Integrated Disease Surveillance and Response (IDSR) program. IDSR seeks to strengthen local public health surveillance of and response to infectious disease outbreaks. The program's goals also include increasing communication between various health agencies, sharing accurate and timely information about outbreaks, and collecting samples and utilizing laboratory research to assist further disease surveillance.

Following increased concern about how fast viruses can spread around the world, many international organizations have stepped up their actions to prepare for pandemics. In the United States, the CDC maintains a comprehensive website that details the multiple facets of preparing and planning for such emergencies. Among the pandemic concerns, influenza is especially troublesome because it can spread quickly and often uncontrollably. The CDC maintains constant vigilance of seasonal influenza, along with other variations that circulate among animals and humans alike. There are three basic types of flu virus, termed influenza A, B, and C. Influenza A viruses are the most common. The CDC labels four types (A, B, C, and D) of influenza A viruses, which may then be further divided into different subtypes, strains, or lineages. In 2018 influenza A viruses posed an increased risk for initiating a pandemic. Networks and programs, such as the IDSR, are set up among domestic and international health partners to monitor and analyze potential infections and outbreaks. The use of the internet by the CDC and its partners has become an integral part of such analysis.

Impacts and Issues

The CDC has made dramatic impacts on the health of US citizens throughout its existence. Two important CDC accomplishments have been identifying the causes of toxic shock syndrome (TSS, a rare disease in which *Staphylococcus aureus* bacteria infect human skin, oral cavities, and vaginal tissue) and Legionnaires' disease (a serious type of pneumonia caused by the bacterium *Legionella pneumophila* that was first recognized in July 1976 at an American Legion convention in Philadelphia).

In 2014 the CDC, along with one of its main partners, the World Health Organization (WHO), led a health battle against the spread of Ebola virus in West Africa. The effort is considered to have been the largest mobilization of CDC personnel. In all, approximately 4,000 people worked on communications, infection control, research, and various other essential duties. Of those, 1,400 people were stationed on the ground in West Africa. Because of this concerted effort, the CDC was able to stop the spread of Ebola.

In 2015 a Zika virus outbreak began in Brazil and then spread quickly in North and South America, the Pacific islands, Asia, and Africa. In the United States, the CDC's Emergency Operations Center was elevated to its highest activation status in early February 2016 to fight the disease. Zika is caused by infection from the mosquito species *Aedes aegypti* and *Aedes albopictus*. The center of the US outbreak was in southern Florida, particularly the Miami-Dade County area. The precautionary "red" and "yellow" designations and travel alerts were removed between December 2016 and June 2017 after the CDC concluded that its safety requirements had been met.

As of 2018 the CDC continued its work to find solutions for many global health threats, from malaria to HIV/AIDS. It is committed to education and outreach efforts promoting food and water safety, sanitation, nutrition, wellness, and personal hygiene as means of fighting infectious disease.

The CDC's broad international experience and close relations with other public health agencies also aid the fight against infectious diseases within the United States. The CDC is currently participating in WHO's Global Alliance for Vaccines and Immunization (GAVI) initiatives to identify the sources of disease in developing nations, as well as to increase development of and access to vaccines and therapeutic medications. The CDC's commitment to GAVI includes assisting in disease identification, control, elimination, and eradication efforts through field and laboratory research. It also participates in GAVI research programs on microbial resistance, antibiotic usage, and pandemic influenza preparedness planning.

The CDC is also working on the Global Health Security Agenda. Its Division of Global Health Protection (DGHP) is leading the way for strengthening the world's fight to minimize the spread of infectious diseases worldwide. The CDC states that an outbreak can originate in a remote village and spread to a major city within 36 hours. To prevent this from happening, the DGHP is working with its partners to build strong international health capacities. With such a concerted effort, outbreaks can likely be contained within a country's borders to avoid worldwide epidemics. The CDC states that such efforts have proven valuable in stopping outbreaks of Ebola in Nigeria (2014), poliomyelitis (commonly called polio) in Mali (2015), yellow fever (also called yellow plague) in Angola (2015–2016), and Avian influenza (avian flu) in Cameroon (2016).

SEE ALSO *Avian Influenza; Bacterial Disease; Ebola; Emerging Infectious Diseases; Globalization and Infectious Disease; Legionnaires' Disease (Legionellosis); Pandemic Preparedness; Smallpox; Smallpox Eradication and Storage; Toxic Shock; Travel and Infectious Disease; World Health Organization (WHO)*

BIBLIOGRAPHY

Books

Adams, Vincanne, ed. *Metrics: What Counts in Global Health.* Durham, NC: Duke University Press, 2016.

Bartlett, Karen. *The Health of Nations: The Campaign to End Polio and Eradicate Epidemic Diseases.* London: Oneworld, 2017.

Birn, Anne-Emanuelle, Yogan Pillay, and Timothy H. Holtz. *Textbook of Global Health.* Oxford, UK; New York: Oxford University Press, 2017.

Enemark, Christian. *Biosecurity Dilemmas: Dreaded Diseases, Ethical Responses, and the Health of Nations.* Washington, DC: Georgetown University Press, 2017.

Osterholm, Michael T., and Mark Olshaker. *Deadliest Enemy: Our War Against Killer Germs.* New York: Little, Brown and Company, 2017.

Rushton, Simon, and Jeremy Youde, ed. *Routledge Handbook of Global Health Security.* London; New York: Routledge, 2014.

Skolnik, Richard. *Global Health 101.* Burlington, MA: Jones & Bartlett, 2016.

Periodicals

Polgreen, Philip M., et al. "Using Internet Searches for Influenza Surveillance." *Clinical Infectious Diseases* 47, no. 11 (December 1, 2008): 1442–1448. This article can also be found online at https://academic.oup.com/cid/article/47/11/1443/282247 (accessed January 26, 2018).

Websites

"CDC Updates Guidance Related to Local Zika Transmission in Miami-Dade County, Florida." Centers for Disease Control and Prevention. https://www.cdc.gov/media/releases/2016/p1019-zika-florida-update.html (accessed January 25, 2018).

"CDC Urges Early Recognition, Prompt Treatment of Sepsis." Centers for Disease Control and Prevention. https://www.cdc.gov/media/releases/2017/p0831-sepsis-recognition-treatment.html (accessed January 25, 2018).

"Emergency Preparedness and Response." Centers for Disease Control and Prevention. https://emergency.cdc.gov/planning/index.asp (accessed January 31, 2018).

"Keeping You Safe 24–7." Centers for Disease Control and Prevention. https://www.cdc.gov/about/24–7/index.html (accessed January 25, 2018).

"Types of Influenza Viruses." Centers for Disease Control and Prevention. https://www.cdc.gov/flu/about/viruses/types.htm (accessed January 25, 2018).

"What We Do: Prepare Countries to Prevent, Detect, and Respond to Global Health Threats." Centers for Disease Control and Prevention. https://www.cdc.gov/globalhealth/healthprotection/ghs/about.html (accessed January 25, 2018).

William Arthur Atkins

Chagas Disease

Introduction

Chagas (SHA-gus) disease, also known as American trypanosomiasis, is caused by infection with the parasite *Trypanosoma cruzi*. The disease is transmitted by insects from an animal reservoir to a human or another animal host. Chagas disease occurs mostly in Latin America and is endemic (occurs naturally in a region) to rural areas in Mexico, Central America, and South America, where some 8 million people were infected with the disease as of 2017, according to the Centers for Disease Control and Prevention (CDC). However, through migration and other mass movements of people, the disease has been spread all over the world, including to the United States. Because parasites can be transmitted via the bloodstream, another mode of infection is via exposure to infected blood. This is the main mode of infection in non-endemic countries.

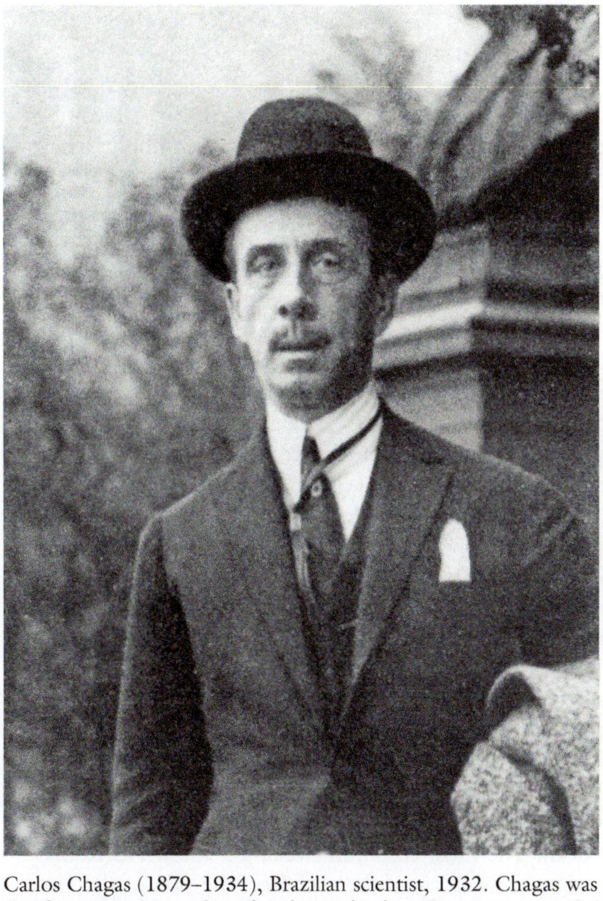

Carlos Chagas (1879–1934), Brazilian scientist, 1932. Chagas was the first scientist to describe the cycle that *Trypanosoma cruzi* traverses before infecting humans. © Wellcome Images/Science Source

Chagas disease, which causes severe heart disease in about one-third of people infected with *T. cruzi*, is best prevented through avoidance of insects that may be infected or through preventing infection from contaminated blood. For those who do get infected, two drug treatments have long been available in much of Latin America: nifurtimox, which was first introduced in 1965, and benznidazole, first introduced in 1971. The drugs were long unavailable in the United States (although the CDC had offered them in special cases to infected patients); in 2017, however, the Food and Drug Administration (FDA) granted approval to benznidazole in response to increasing rates of *T. cruzi* infection in the United States. Despite this FDA approval, the drug was still not available in US pharmacies as of early 2018. (Also, as the side effects for the drugs increase with age, the FDA only approved the drug's use for children ages 2 to 12.)

Disease History, Characteristics, and Transmission

Brazilian physician Carlos Chagas (1879–1934) is credited with first identifying in 1909 what would become known as Chagas disease. However, as Arthur Goldhammer notes in his introduction to François Delaporte's *Chagas Disease: History of a Continent's Scourge*, Chagas's description of the disease conflated it "with other endemic conditions" and did not "clinically

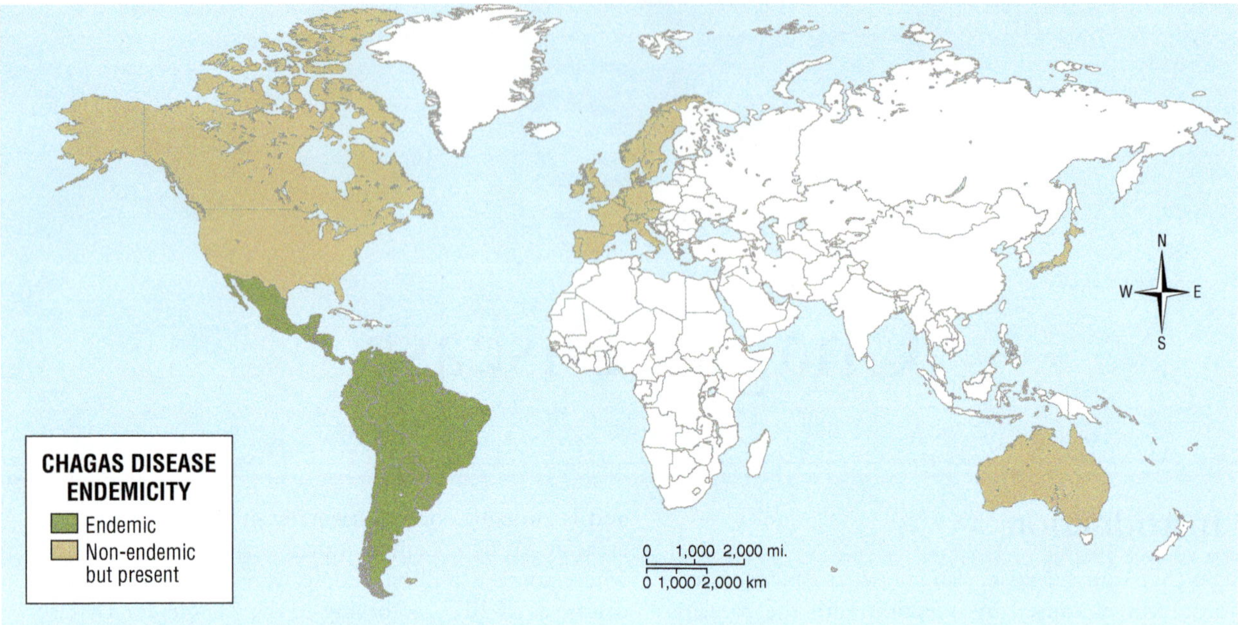

SOURCE: Drugs for Neglected Diseases initiative (DNDi)

specify the disease." According to Goldhammer, the "clinically recognizable and discrete entity known as American trypanosomiasis," or Chagas disease, was not identified until 1935, when Argentinian physician Cecilio Romaña (1899–1997) described the swelling of the eyelids that is correlated with infection. This symptom became known as Romana's sign.

Chagas disease is caused by the parasite *Trypanosoma cruzi*, which is transmitted to animals and humans by the insect vector *Triatoma infestans* (also known as triatomine bugs or, more commonly, kissing bugs due to their propensity to bite people near their lips while they sleep). While such bugs are endemic to Latin America, they have begun to move northward into the United States. According to the CDC, kissing bugs could be found in 28 US states as of 2015. Many of these states were located in the southern United States, but *Triatoma infestans* have also been identified in northern states, including Pennsylvania.

Human infection usually occurs in one of two ways: when parasites in the feces of insects enter the body by ingestion or through the skin or, less commonly, when parasites are passed from an infected bloodstream into an uninfected bloodstream.

In endemic areas contact with an insect vector is the source of most infections. When blood-sucking insects feed on infected animals, they become infected with the parasites. These insects then bite another animal or human and leave behind feces. These feces are usually rubbed into the open bite wound or into mucous membranes, such as those in the eyes or mouth, when the animal or human scratches the area. The parasite enters the bloodstream of the host and infects tissue cells.

Transmission can also occur when blood from an infected person is introduced into an uninfected person. Such infections can occur during blood transfusions, between mothers and babies, during organ transplants, and from blood exposure in laboratories.

Chagas disease is characterized by acute and chronic stages, both of which can be symptom free. Though the acute phase tends to have no symptoms, some people experience fever, fatigue, body aches, headaches, rashes, diarrhea, vomiting, and loss of appetite during this phase. Swelling can also occur in areas where the parasite entered the body. The most common swelling is known as Romana's sign—a swelling of the eyelid on the side of the face closest to the site of the parasite's entry. Symptoms usually fade, although infection persists if untreated.

WORDS TO KNOW

ARTHROPOD A member of the largest single animal phylum, consisting of organisms with segmented bodies, jointed legs or wings, and exoskeletons. Includes insects and spiders.

ENDEMIC Present in a particular area or among a particular group of people.

VECTOR Any agent that carries and transmits parasites and diseases. Also, an organism or a chemical used to transport a gene into a new host cell.

The chronic phase usually occurs many years after infection; most people, however, never develop this stage of the disease. According to the CDC, between 20 and 30 percent of people infected with *T. cruzi* "develop debilitating and sometimes life-threatening medical problems over the course of their lives." The most common chronic problems are cardiac, including an enlarged heart, heart failure, altered heart rate, or cardiac arrest, and intestinal, such as an enlarged esophagus or colon, which causes problems with eating or passing stool.

■ Scope and Distribution

Because Chagas disease can be transmitted by infected blood as well as by insect vectors, it can exist outside endemic areas. However, vector-borne infections of Chagas disease generally occur only in endemic areas from the southern United States to southern Argentina. Rural areas in Mexico, Central America, and South America are the principle locations of vector-borne infections.

The human populations at highest risk for developing Chagas disease are low-income people living in rural areas. Housing is often of poor quality and provides ideal habitats for insects carrying the disease. For example, rural areas in Central and South America, where houses are often built of mud, adobe, or thatch, have a high incidence of infection. It is estimated that as many as 11 million people in Mexico, Central America, and South America are infected with Chagas disease.

As populations have begun to make large-scale migrations, Chagas disease has spread from rural areas into previously uninfected areas. This has increased its global distribution and given rise to other modes of infection, resulting in a need to adopt new infection-control strategies. Countries into which the disease is introduced must take steps to identify infected persons to prevent the spread of the disease. Any activities that involve potential mixing of blood, such as transfusions, require stringent monitoring.

■ Treatment and Prevention

Chagas disease can be effectively treated with medication during the acute stages of infection. The drugs most commonly used to treat Chagas disease are benznidazole and nifurtimox. These are antiparasitic drugs aimed at killing the parasite. However, they are toxic and must be taken under medical supervision because they may cause adverse side effects. Benznidazole is considered the less toxic of the two drugs and requires fewer doses to be effective. As a result, it is more commonly prescribed than nifurtimox. Chemotherapy can also be used in an attempt to remove the parasite, although this treatment is not 100 percent effective.

Treatment during the chronic stages of Chagas disease focuses on controlling the effects of the disease, such as cardiac and intestinal complications. This may include insertion of a pacemaker, to control the heart's rhythm and to prevent chronic heart failure, or surgery on enlarged organs, such as the esophagus or colon. Organ transplants are also sometimes performed to replace damaged organs.

As there is no vaccine or drug available to prevent infection, prevention efforts focus on avoiding parasite transmission. In terms of vector-borne infection, avoiding rural areas in which the disease is likely to exist or treating houses, clothes, and bodies with insect repellants may prevent contact with a vector. Feces-contaminated food can also carry the parasite, making careful handling and preparation of food, plus an awareness of whether insects have been near it, necessary.

Bloodborne transmission of Chagas disease can also occur. Therefore, medical procedures such as blood transfusions and organ transplants require strict screening to prevent transmission of the parasite. In addition, mothers infected with Chagas disease can potentially pass the parasite to babies while breastfeeding, if the skin around the nipple is broken. Avoiding breastfeeding when the nipples have broken skin can prevent infection.

■ Impacts and Issues

Large-scale population movements have led to an increased risk of Chagas disease in areas outside Latin America where the disease is not endemic. In non-endemic areas, the disease is largely spread by infected blood, making strict screening of the blood supply imperative. However, some countries do not perform routine tests for Chagas disease in their blood banks; thus, the risk of infection is high in those countries. The World Health Organization ranks the infection rate for Chagas disease from Latin American blood banks higher than human immunodeficiency virus (HIV), hepatitis B, and hepatitis C.

T. cruzi, the parasite that causes Chagas disease, has also been discovered in wild animals in some American states. This discovery suggests that wild reservoirs of this parasite may exist in the United States, raising the possibility of an outbreak of vector-borne infections if insects feeding on these wild animals come in contact with humans.

While growing cases of—and concerns about—Chagas disease in the United States led the FDA to grant limited approval of benznidazole in 2017, many observers expressed concerns that the FDA license the drug under a priority review voucher, which is "sometimes called a 'golden ticket' by people in the pharmaceutical industry, because the vouchers can be used for the speedy review of a subsequent drug candidate, or bought and sold to help companies leapfrog rivals in getting a drug to market," according to a 2017 NPR article on the FDA's actions. In response to such fears, the nonprofit organization Drugs for Neglected Diseases Initiative helped a for-profit drug company gain approval for benznidazole in exchange for agreeing to sell it at a reasonable price to patients.

Transmission between a vector and human is less likely to occur in densely vegetated habitats, such as rain forests, or in urban areas. However, regions in which habitat is thinned out and the abundance of fauna is reduced while the human population increases are hotspots for an outbreak of Chagas disease. In these areas a decrease in the abundance of animals drives the vector insects to seek a new food source, and the growing human population provides a ready target. Deforestation of the Amazon and other areas of tropical rain forest in Central and South America may create just such hotspots, and more people may be infected with Chagas disease as a result.

SEE ALSO *Arthropod-Borne Disease; Blood Supply and Infectious Disease; Bloodborne Pathogens; Economic Development and Disease; Host and Vector; Immigration and Infectious Disease; Parasitic Diseases; Vector-Borne Disease; Zoonoses*

BIBLIOGRAPHY

Books

Delaporte, François. *Chagas Disease: History of a Continent's Scourge*. Translated by Arthur Goldhammer. New York: Fordham University Press, 2012.

Telleria, Jenny, and Michel Tibayrenc, eds. *American Trypanosomiasis, Chagas Disease: One Hundred Years of Research*. Amsterdam: Elsevier, 2017.

Periodicals

Aufderheide, Arthur C., et al. "A 9,000-year Record of Chagas' Disease." *Proceedings of the National Academy of Sciences of the United States of America* 101, no. 7 (February 2004): 2034–2039.

Frazer, Jennifer. "Bed Bugs, Kissing Bugs Linked to Deadly Chagas Disease in U.S." *Scientific American* (December 10, 2014). This article can also be found online at https://www.scientificamerican.com/article/bed-bugs-kissing-bugs-linked-to-deadly-chagas-disease-in-u-s/ (accessed January 18, 2017).

Smith, Jennie Erin. "America's War on the Kissing Bug." *New Yorker* (November 20, 2015). This article can also be found online at https://www.newyorker.com/tech/elements/americas-war-on-the-kissing-bug-and-chagas-disease (accessed January 18, 2017).

Websites

"Chagas Disease (American trypanosomiasis)." World Health Organization, March 2017. http://www.who.int/mediacentre/factsheets/fs340/en/ (accessed January 18, 2017).

Columbus, Courtney. "Drug for 'Neglected' Chagas Disease Gains FDA Approval Amid Price Worries." NPR, September 10, 2017. https://www.npr.org/sections/health-shots/2017/09/10/547351794/drug-for-neglected-chagas-disease-gains-fda-approval-amid-price-worries (accessed January 18, 2017).

"Parasites—American Trypanosomiasis (also known as Chagas Disease)." Centers for Disease Control and Prevention, May 24, 2016. https://www.cdc.gov/parasites/chagas/ (accessed January 18, 2017).

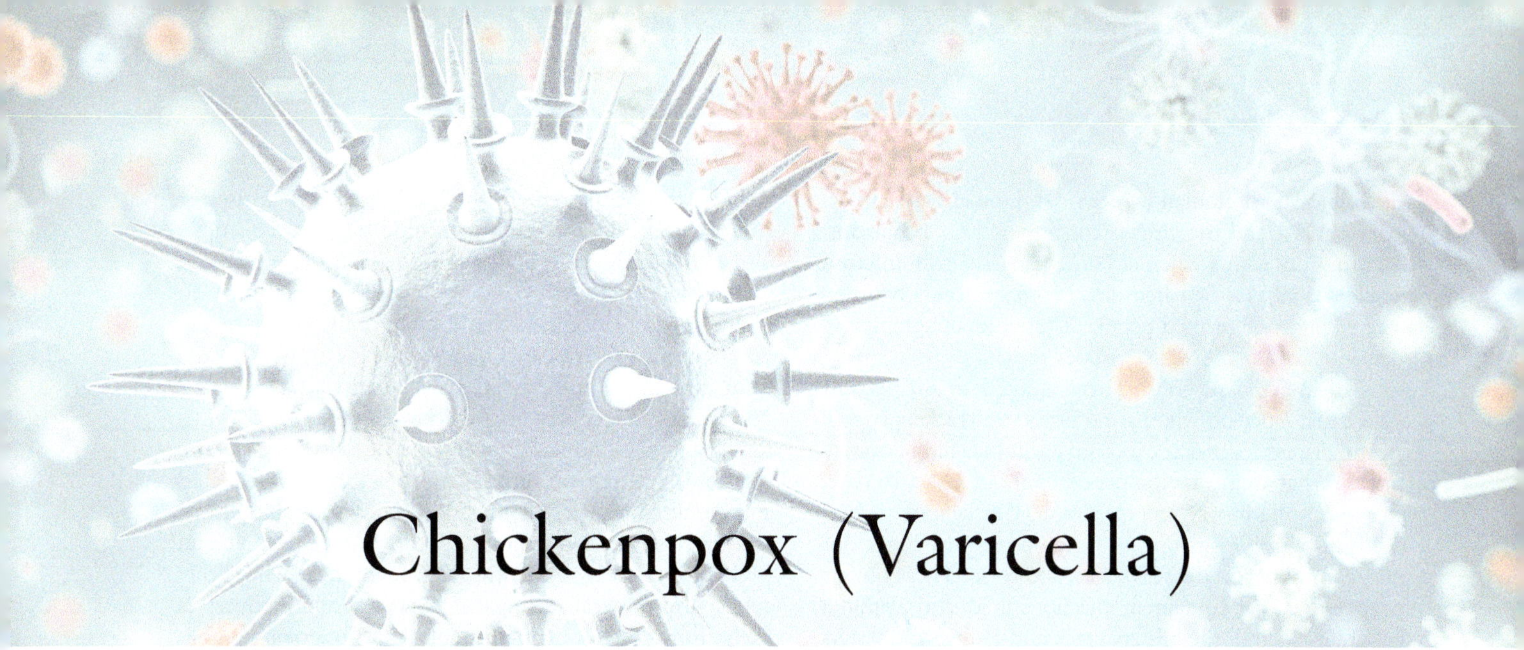

Chickenpox (Varicella)

Introduction

Varicella, commonly known as chickenpox, is a viral disease primarily of children, although it can infect any nonimmune person. Infection is caused by the varicella-zoster virus (VZV), which is stored in human hosts and is transmitted by direct contact as well as by inhalation of contaminated airborne particles. Infection with this virus results in the formation of an itchy rash that is sometimes accompanied by a fever. Treatment usually centers on alleviating the symptoms of the infection—namely, the rash and fever—rather than on the virus itself. Antiviral medication may be administered in severe cases. Complications such as bacterial infections, brain infections, viral pneumonia, and even death occur rarely. Following recovery from chickenpox, the virus remains in the body and can be reactivated (usually in old age), causing a new disease called herpes zoster, commonly referred to as shingles.

Chickenpox is a worldwide disease, and most people who have not been vaccinated will develop it by adulthood. Immunity develops after vaccine or the infection. The chickenpox vaccine available is 90 percent effective after two doses. If a vaccinated person develops chickenpox, the vaccination appears to lessen the severity of infection.

Children develop chickenpox most frequently, although adults can contract the disease. Adults tend to have more severe infections. High-risk groups for infection include those with compromised immune systems, newborns, and pregnant women. Individuals in these groups are also unable to use the vaccine due to the risk of developing the disease from the vaccine.

Disease History, Characteristics, and Transmission

Chickenpox has existed for centuries. Originally, doctors were aware of the disease without knowing its cause. Similarities between chickenpox and smallpox, a deadly disease that no longer occurs in humans, made it hard for practitioners to differentiate between the two. The first description of chickenpox on record was made by Italian scientist Giovanni Filippo (1510–1580) during the 1500s. Subsequently, English physician Richard Morton (1637–1698) identified the disease in the 1600s, as did English physician William Heberden (1710–1801) in the 1700s. Heberden first demonstrated that chickenpox and smallpox are different diseases.

Chickenpox is a viral disease that arises when humans become infected with the varicella-zoster virus (VZV),

WORDS TO KNOW

IMMUNOCOMPROMISED A reduction in the ability of the immune system to recognize and respond to the presence of foreign material.

POSTHERPETIC NEURALGIA Neuralgia is pain arising in a nerve that is not the result of any injury. Postherpetic neuralgia is neuralgia experienced after infection with a herpesvirus, namely *Herpes simplex* or *Herpes zoster*.

VACCINE A substance that is introduced to stimulate antibody production and thus provide immunity to a particular disease.

VARICELLA-ZOSTER IMMUNE GLOBULIN (VZIG) A preparation that can give people temporary protection against chickenpox after exposure to the varicella virus. It is used for children and adults who are at risk of complications of the disease or who are susceptible to infection because they have weakened immunity.

VESICLE A membrane-bound sphere that contains a variety of substances in cells.

which is a type of human herpes virus. Humans are a reservoir for VZV, and the virus is contagious among humans. Transmission occurs when airborne particles from infected people are inhaled or when direct contact occurs between infected and noninfected people. Therefore, coughing and sneezing spreads the virus, as does touching the open lesions of infected persons. There is a 70 to 80 percent chance that a person who has no history of chickenpox will get the disease following exposure to an infected person.

VZV has an incubation period of about 14 to 16 days, after which the first symptoms appear. Chickenpox is characterized by the formation of itchy blisters that break out most commonly on the scalp, face, and torso. These blisters form vesicles that contain an infectious fluid, and, within a day of developing, the blisters break and crust over. Blisters tend to continually form over a period of five to seven days, and the outbreak is over when all sores have formed a crust. Scratching the blisters may cause scarring. Accompanying symptoms include fever, headache, and fatigue.

A person is contagious approximately one to two days prior to the rash developing, and he or she remains contagious until all the blisters have crusted over. Since the incubation period is two to three weeks, a person may be unaware that he or she has contracted the disease until weeks after contact with an infected person.

While most cases of chickenpox are not considered serious and while recovery is likely, the disease can potentially be fatal. Children are the least at-risk age group for complications. Complications include bacterial infections under the skin, within bones and tissue, in the lungs, and in the blood. The virus can also cause complications directly, such as encephalitis and pneumonia. Prior to the development of a vaccine, approximately 100 people died from chickenpox in the United States every year.

Following recovery from chickenpox, the varicella virus remains in the body and settles among nerve fibers. The virus tends to remain dormant, but it can be reactivated and result in a different infection, known as shingles or zoster. This infection generally occurs in older people and is characterized by a painful rash, fever, headache, body aches, and general feelings of illness. While recovery is likely from shingles, many patients suffer ongoing complications: in particular, postherpetic neuralgia. Postherpetic neuralgia is nerve pain that arises most likely as a result of the virus becoming active within the nerve fibers and damaging them. This pain can vary from mild to severe and may be present for only three months or chronically. In general, people do not suffer a second case of chickenpox, but there have been some exceptions.

■ Scope and Distribution

Chickenpox is a worldwide virus. People who live in temperate regions tend to be likelier to contract the

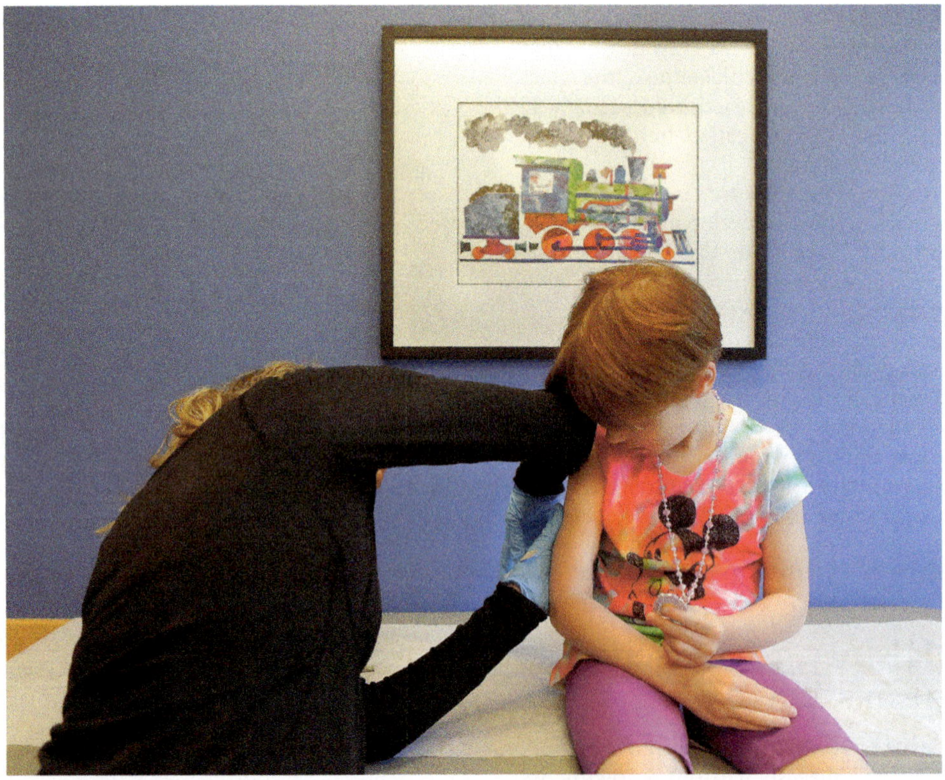

A child in Portland, Maine, receives a chickenpox vaccine. In the United States vaccination prevents around 3.5 million cases of chickenpox per year. *© Gregory Rec/Portland Press Herald/Getty Images*

disease at a younger age than people who live in the tropics. In temperate regions chickenpox is prevalent in winter and spring. In the tropics it is prevalent in cool, dry seasons. According to a 2015 statement by the World Health Organization (WHO), "the epidemiology of the disease differs between temperate and tropical climates. The reasons for the differences are poorly understood and may relate to properties of VZV (known to be sensitive to heat), climate, population density and risk of exposure (e.g., attendance at childcare facility or school or the number of siblings in the household)."

Before the development of the chickenpox vaccine in 1995, the disease's prevalence within society was so high that by adulthood almost all people had contracted the disease. Although children still contract the highest number of cases, anyone who comes in contact with an infected person and has not previously had the disease is at risk of becoming infected. WHO conservatively estimates that each year about 4.2 million people across the globe are hospitalized and 4,200 people die from chickenpox. In the United States, approximately 350,000 cases of chickenpox are reported annually (down from 4 million cases prior to the development of the vaccine). Despite vaccinations, about 20 people die from chickenpox each year in the United States (down from about 100 deaths each year prior to the vaccine).

When children of school age contract the virus, they are required to stay home from school until they are no longer contagious. However, due to the high infectiousness of this disease, outbreaks are hard to prevent, and, despite policies that keep infected children at home, outbreaks are likely to occur.

Adults also contract the virus, although the number of adult cases is much lower than the number of cases among children. Despite this, prior to the release of a vaccine in the United States, half of all fatalities were adults. This statistic highlights the fact that adults tend to develop more severe cases of chickenpox.

There are also groups of high-risk people within society. These include immunocompromised people, pregnant women, newborn babies, and health care workers. Immunocompromised people include cancer and AIDS patients, as well as transplant recipients. Their immune systems are less able to fight off infection, making them more likely to contract the virus. Chickenpox infection during pregnancy may result in complications with fetal development. These complications may include growth retardation, such as underdevelopment of limbs and lack of growth in some parts of the brain. In addition, a chickenpox infection during pregnancy may lead to miscarriage, premature labor, or infection of the fetus with the virus. Newborn babies have an increased fatality rate if they contract the disease and do not receive treatment. Health care workers and people taking care of sick family members are also at risk of contracting the virus.

The development of a second bout of chickenpox is rare and does not seem to be predetermined by any condition. However, the occurrence of shingles tends to be more likely in people 50 or older and in immunocompromised people. Shingles is not as common as chickenpox but still has an annual rate of 1 million cases annually in the United States. Of these, approximately 10 to 13 will develop postherpetic neuralgia. However, shingles does not spread from person to person but arises in people who already have the varicella-zoster virus in their bodies. And, although shingles can cause chickenpox in noninfected people, it is not as contagious as chickenpox and usually requires contact with the blister fluid in order for transmission to occur. The Centers for Disease Control and Prevention (CDC) recommends that healthy people who are 50 or older get two doses of the shingles vaccine Shingrix. The doses should be spaced two to six months apart. Shingrix was approved by the US Food and Drug Administration in 2017 and replaced the vaccine Zostavax, which was in use since 2006, as the recommended shingles vaccine.

Treatment and Prevention

Most cases of chickenpox do not require treatment for recovery to occur. In general, treatment is provided for the symptoms, namely the fever and rash. Fever is treated with nonaspirin medications, such as acetaminophen, because aspirin is linked with the development of Reye's syndrome in children. The rash is generally treated with calamine lotion, cool compresses, or oatmeal baths to alleviate the itching.

However, in some cases more specific treatment is employed. Antiviral medication may be given to adults or to children at risk of developing a serious illness. In addition, bacterial infections may arise when blisters are scratched and opened, and antibacterial medication may be necessary. Bacterial infections can be prevented by avoiding scratching the blisters and keeping them clean.

After infection with the chickenpox virus, most patients have a lifelong immunity to the disease. This reduces their chances of contracting the virus again, but it does not keep them from developing shingles. Newborn babies receive immunity from immune mothers, but this immunity lasts only for the first few months of their lives.

A vaccine is available to prevent chickenpox. The vaccine was developed in Japan and the United States. The United States was the first country to implement a nationwide vaccination program, in 1995. Other countries that offer the chickenpox vaccine include Australia, China, Germany, Israel, Italy, Spain, Taiwan, Turkey, and Uruguay. WHO recommends that countries that are able to vaccinate 80 percent or more of their population should use the vaccine; in practice, this means that primarily wealthier, industrialized countries have chickenpox vaccination programs, although there are also noneconomic reasons behind countries not vaccinating. Great Britain, for example,

SOCIAL AND PERSONAL RESPONSIBILITY

One of the best ways to avoid contracting or transmitting chickenpox is to get vaccinated. The Centers for Disease Control and Prevention (CDC) summarizes how the epidemiology of chickenpox changed after the introduction of a vaccine, noting, "Chickenpox used to be very common in the United States. In the early 1990s, an average of 4 million people got varicella, 10,500 to 13,000 were hospitalized (range, 8,000 to 18,000), and 100 to 150 died each year. In the 1990s, the highest rate of varicella was reported in preschool-aged children.

"Chickenpox vaccine became available in the United States in 1995. In 2014, 91% of children 19 to 35 months old in the United States had received one dose of varicella vaccine, varying from 83% to 95% by state. Among adolescents 13 to 17 years of age without a prior history of disease, 95% had received 1 dose of varicella vaccine, and 81% had received 2 doses of the vaccine. Eighty-five percent of adolescents had either a history of varicella disease or received 2 doses of varicella vaccine.

"Each year, more than 3.5 million cases of varicella, 9,000 hospitalizations, and 100 deaths are prevented by varicella vaccination in the United States."

does not include the chickenpox vaccine in its routine youth vaccinations, citing that exposure to children with chickenpox gives nearby adults a boost of defense against shingles.

Each country has its own vaccination recommendations regarding chickenpox. In the United States, it is recommended that children under 13 years old receive two doses of the vaccine—one dose between the ages of 12 and 15 months and the second dose between four and six years. This vaccination schedule was approved in June 2006. Prior to that only one vaccination against chickenpox was given. One dose of the vaccine did reduce the number and size of chickenpox outbreaks, but outbreaks still occurred, so the CDC began recommending two vaccinations instead of one. Those 13 and older who have never had chickenpox or been vaccinated against it require two doses of the vaccine administered at least four weeks apart. Adults who are not immune to chickenpox may benefit from two doses of the vaccine if they have come into contact with someone with the disease. Some people develop chickenpox after being vaccinated, but they tend to have very mild cases of the disease. Vaccination is recommended for almost everyone who has not had chickenpox, with the exceptions noted below.

Because of the risk that they may develop the disease as a result of the vaccination, some individuals should not be vaccinated against chickenpox, including newborns, people with cancer, people with immune problems, people taking drugs that suppress the immune system, and pregnant women. However, if a person in one of these categories is exposed to the virus, they can receive a temporary protective vaccine known as varicella-zoster immune globulin (VZIG). VZIG acts to prevent the development of the disease or to modify the disease after exposure. The protection conferred by VZIG is only short term, and the treatment is expensive. As a result, it is only administered to people at high risk of developing severe chickenpox when they are exposed to the virus.

During an outbreak of the disease, transmission can be minimized by separating those infected from others and by limiting the duration of any contact that must occur between infected and noninfected individuals. Because chickenpox is highly contagious, anyone who is not immune to the disease should avoid inhaling contaminated air and touching open lesions on infected people. Protection from shingles patients is less difficult due to the fact that transmission occurs via contact with rash fluid only. If these rashes are well covered, risk of transmission is greatly reduced.

Impacts and Issues

Despite the introduction of an effective vaccine, many people are still not vaccinated against chickenpox for a number of reasons. In developing countries there are many diseases with high rates of morbidity and mortality that can be prevented by vaccination. Vaccination against chickenpox may not be as high a priority as vaccinations against other diseases, especially when funding is limited and the health care delivery system is overburdened.

In countries where the vaccine is affordable, generally available, and of significant benefit to the public health, many still avoid getting vaccinated. People may remain unvaccinated voluntarily because of misconceptions surrounding the seriousness of this disease. Many people are under the impression that chickenpox is a relatively mild virus that all people will encounter and recover from during their lives. However, complications and deaths occur from chickenpox infections, even in healthy individuals. Prior to the vaccine being made available in the United States, 100 people or more died annually from this disease, and some 10,000 people were hospitalized. These people were not all high-risk patients; rather, most were healthy individuals. Vaccination appears to be a more cost-effective option for many populations as the costs of preventing cases of chickenpox often outweigh the costs of combating an outbreak and treating those who contract the disease.

The introduction of the chickenpox vaccine has changed the epidemiology of the disease areas where vaccination rates are high. Most of the studies of the disease's changing epidemiology come from the United States, where vaccination for chickenpox is almost ubiquitous. Numerous US studies have shown that the vaccine (both one-dose and two-dose administrations) has dramatically reduced the number of people who contract chickenpox each year.

A 2008 study published in the *Journal of Infectious Diseases* showed that one dose of chickenpox vaccine reduced chickenpox incidence by about 90 percent. The authors noted, however, that, even in areas with "high vaccine coverage," chickenpox incidence still occurred; this was because one dose of the vaccine was only 80 to 85 percent effective. A 2013 report published in *Pediatrics* showed that, in a study in California and Pennsylvania, two doses of the vaccine were far more effective than one dose. The authors found that "declines in [chickenpox] incidence across all ages, including infants who are not eligible for varicella vaccination, and adults, in whom vaccination levels are low, provide evidence of the benefit of high levels of immunity in the population." An international meta-analysis published in *Pediatrics* in 2016 confirmed the above findings and also found that, "within the first decade after vaccination, 1 dose of varicella vaccine was moderately effective at preventing all varicella (81%) and highly effective at preventing combined moderate and severe varicella (98%)." Meanwhile, they showed two doses of the vaccine protected against virtually all chickenpox.

There is evidence that the chickenpox vaccine is preventing children and adolescents from developing shingles (a rare occurrence among young people, although a possibility). It remains unclear if the chickenpox vaccine will prevent shingles later in life.

See Also *AIDS (Acquired Immunodeficiency Syndrome); Cancer and Infectious Disease; Childhood Infectious Diseases, Immunization Impacts; HIV; Meningitis, Viral; Shingles (Herpes Zoster) Infection; Smallpox; Vaccines and Vaccine Development; Viral Disease*

BIBLIOGRAPHY

Books

Bennett, John E., Raphael Dolin, and Martin J. Blaser. *Mandell, Douglas, and Bennett's Principles and Practice of Infectious Diseases.* Philadelphia: Elsevier/Saunders, 2015.

Periodicals

Bialek, S. R., et al. "Impact of a Routine Two-Dose Varicella Vaccination Program on Varicella Epidemiology." *Pediatrics* 132, no. 5 (November 2013): e1134–1140. This article can also be found online at https://www.ncbi.nlm.nih.gov/pubmed/24101763 (accessed February 1, 2018).

Guris, Dalya, et al. "Changing Varicella Epidemiology in Active Surveillance Sites—United States, 1995–2005." *Journal of Infectious Diseases* 197, supplement no. 2 (March 1, 2008): S71–S75. This article can also be found online at https://academic.oup.com/jid/article/197/Supplement_2/S71/848964 (accessed January 31, 2018).

Marin, Mona, et al. "Global Varicella Vaccine Effectiveness: A Meta-Analysis." *Pediatrics* (February 2016). This article can also be found online at http://pediatrics.aappublications.org/content/early/2016/02/14/peds.2015-3741 (accessed January 31, 2018).

Websites

"Chickenpox (Varicella)." Centers for Disease Control and Prevention, July 1, 2016. https://www.cdc.gov/chickenpox/ (accessed January 31, 2018).

"Chickenpox Vaccine FAQs." National Health Service, March 31, 2016. https://www.nhs.uk/conditions/vaccinations/chickenpox-vaccine-questions-answers/ (accessed February 1, 2018).

"Monitoring the Impact of Varicella Vaccination." Centers for Disease Control and Prevention, July 1, 2016. https://www.cdc.gov/chickenpox/surveillance/monitoring-varicella.html (accessed February 15, 2018).

Moyer, Melinda Wenner. "What to Do If You Get Invited to a Chickenpox Party." *Slate*, November 15, 2013. http://www.slate.com/articles/double_x/the_kids/2013/11/chickenpox_vaccine_is_it_really_necessary.html (accessed February 1, 2018).

"Shingles." Centers for Disease Control and Prevention, January 30, 2018. https://www.cdc.gov/shingles/ (accessed February 1, 2018).

"Varicella." World Health Organization, April 4, 2015. http://www.who.int/immunization/diseases/varicella/en/ (accessed February 1, 2018).

"Varicella and Herpes Zoster Vaccination Position Paper." World Health Organization, June 2014. http://www.who.int/immunization/position_papers/WHO_pp_varicella_herpes_zoster_june2014_summary.pdf?ua=1 (accessed February 1, 2018).

"Weekly Epidemiological Record." World Health Organization, June 10, 2014. http://www.who.int/wer/2014/wer8925.pdf?ua=1 (accessed February 1, 2018).

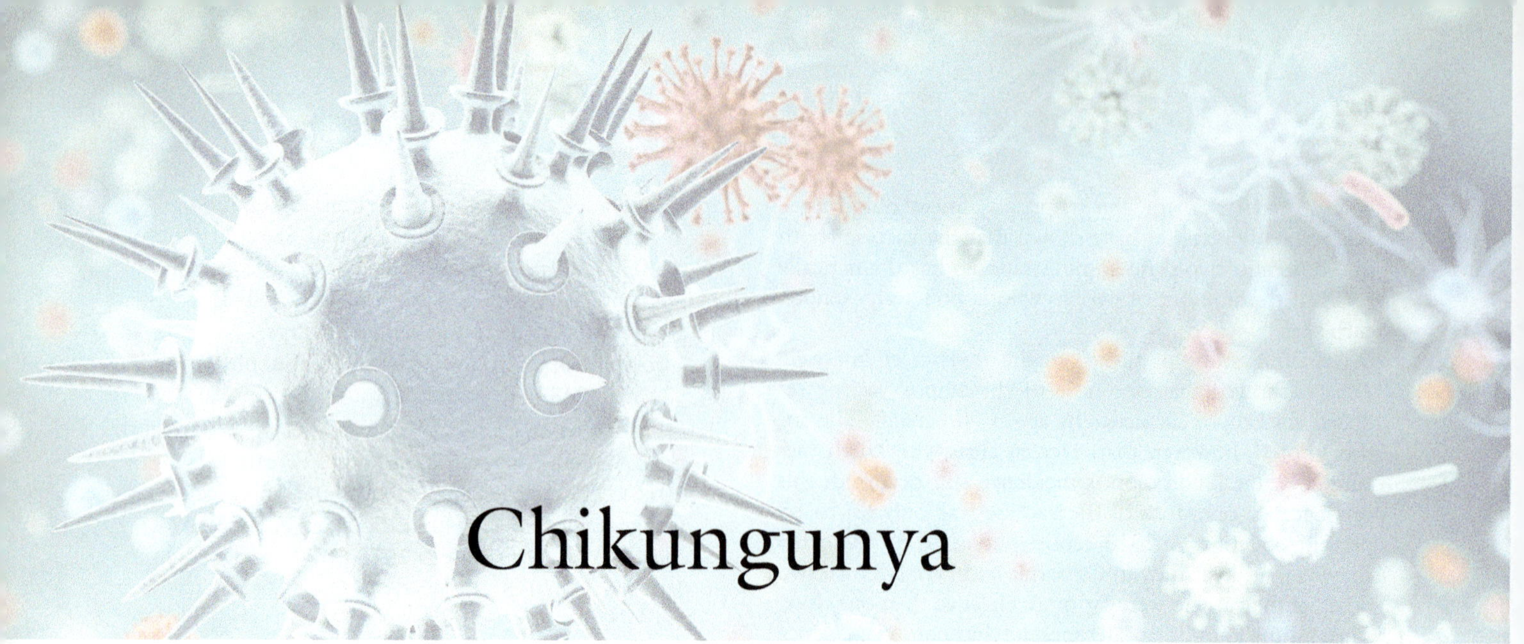

Chikungunya

Introduction

Chikungunya (chick-un-GUNE-ya) is an arthropod-borne virus transmitted to humans via mosquito bite. Transmission of the disease predominantly occurs in regions within India, Africa, Southeast Asia, the Philippines, and the Caribbean. However, since 2000 infections have occurred worldwide, both as the result of travelers contracting chikungunya in endemic regions, as well as new and unexpected outbreaks in areas not typically affected by the disease.

Infection usually results in a range of symptoms, including fever, aches, joint pain, nausea, vomiting, and chills. However, a full recovery is common following treatment involving rest, fluids, and drugs for fever or joint pains. There have been a large number of outbreaks in the early 21st century, particularly in India and groups of islands in the Indian Ocean in the years 2004 to 2007, in a coastal village in Italy in 2007, and in the Americas beginning in December 2013. Because of these outbreaks, the World Health Organization (WHO) considers chikungunya an important reemergent disease.

There is no vaccine available to protect against infection with the chikungunya virus; therefore, the best prevention method is avoidance of mosquitoes. This is achieved by using insect repellants, wearing long-sleeved clothing, using mosquito nets, and removing stagnant water where mosquitoes can breed.

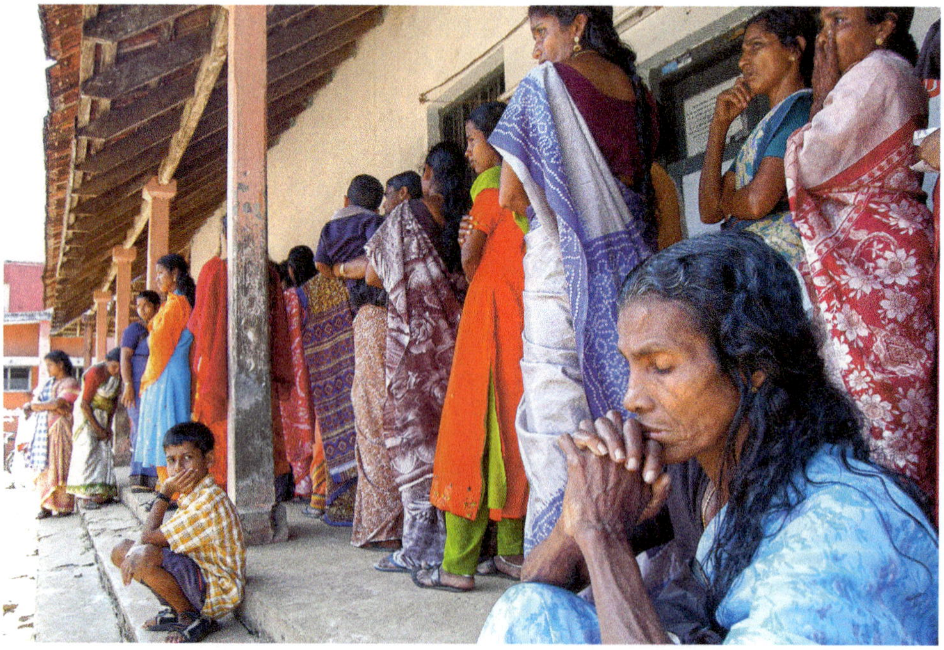

A woman prays while patients receive medical treatment for chikungunya. In 2006 the government in the southern Indian state of Kerala implemented a public health program designed to educate people about the mosquito-borne virus. © *AP Images/Anonymous*

Disease History, Characteristics, and Transmission

Chikungunya virus infection was first described during the 1950s by scientists Marion Robinson and W. H. R. Lumsden (1914–2002). The first known outbreak occurred during 1952 in Africa, and the first outbreak in India was in 1963 in Calcutta. The name *chikungunya* is derived from the Makonde language of East Africa and means "that which bends up," a reference to the stooped posture witnessed in those suffering from the debilitating joint pain associated with the disease.

This virus is from the family Togoviridae and the genus *Alphavirus*. Infection is transmitted to humans via a bite from mosquitoes in the genus *Aedes*. These mosquitoes are also responsible for the transmission of dengue and yellow fever. Mosquitoes pick up the infection when they feed on infected people or nonhuman primates. Infection is not thought to be transmitted directly from person to person. However, 38 cases of transmission from mother to baby at birth were recorded during a 2005 to 2006 outbreak on the island of Réunion, and many similar cases were described during the late 2013 outbreak in the Americas.

Chikungunya manifests itself in humans 1 to 12 days (usually about a week) after being bitten by the infected mosquito. Most cases result in a range of symptoms, although there have been some asymptomatic cases. The most common symptoms are fever, headache, joint pain, swelling of joints, arthritis of the joints, chills, nausea, and vomiting. A rash may also occur; in rare cases, bleeding and hemorrhaging result. Acute fever usually lasts from a few days to two weeks, and some people with chikungunya experience prolonged fatigue. The symptoms of chikungunya are similar to dengue fever, and, as a result, the disease is sometimes misdiagnosed. Lifelong immunity is thought to occur following chikungunya infection.

Scope and Distribution

Chikungunya first appeared in Africa in 1952 and was first discovered in India 10 years later. The virus is distributed around Africa and Asia. Outbreaks have traditionally been reported in India, Africa, Southeast Asia, the Philippines, and the Caribbean. In the 21st century, however, there have been several outbreaks in Europe and the Americas, raising new concerns about the expansion of chikungunya endemicity to the Western Hemisphere.

In 2005 there was a reemergence of chikungunya in India, with 180,000 cases reported between 2005 and 2007. In early 2005 an outbreak occurred in the Comoro Islands. Since this outbreak other islands in the Indian Ocean have reported infections. On the island of Réunion, chikungunya infection was first identified in March 2005, with 300,000 cases identified by August 2006. Among the other islands in the Indian Ocean, 300,000 suspected cases were reported before May 2006.

By 2007 chikungunya had reached the European mainland, with 217 confirmed cases reported in northeastern Italy and 254 cases by March 2015. Another outbreak with 11 confirmed cases was reported in Montpellier, France, in October 2014.

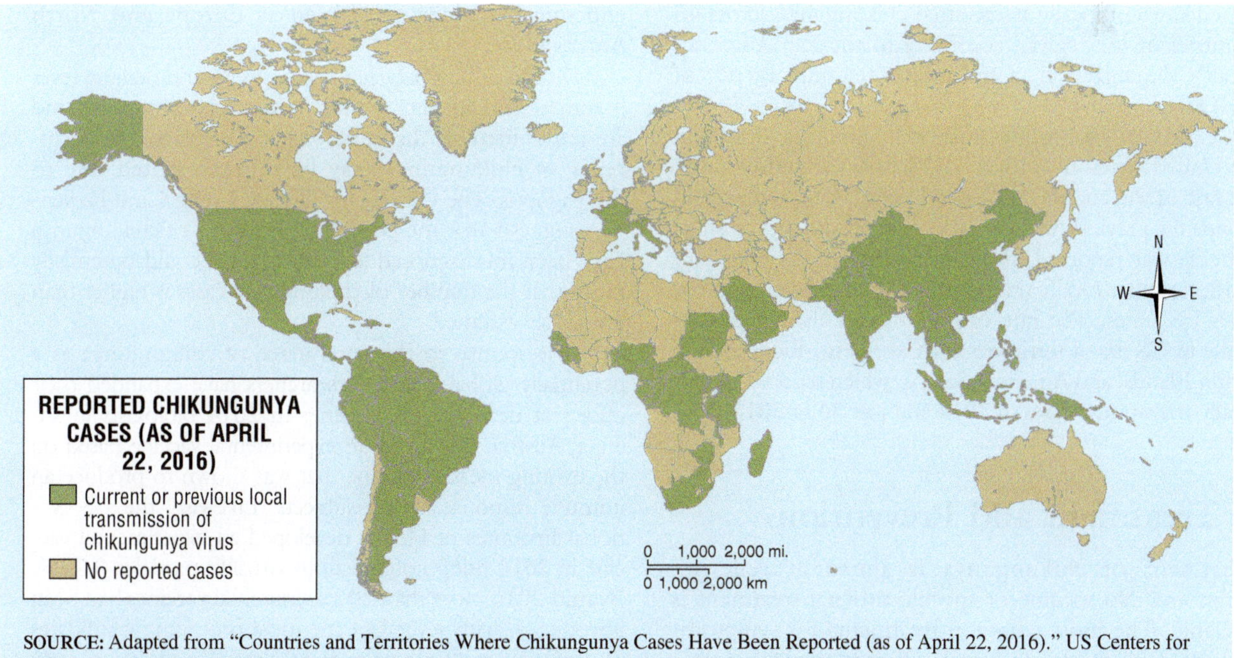

SOURCE: Adapted from "Countries and Territories Where Chikungunya Cases Have Been Reported (as of April 22, 2016)." US Centers for Disease Control and Prevention. 2016. Available from: https://www.cdc.gov/chikungunya/geo/index.html

WORDS TO KNOW

ARTHROPOD-BORNE DISEASE A disease caused by one of a phylum of organisms characterized by exoskeletons and segmented bodies.

ENDEMIC Present in a particular area or among a particular group of people.

NOTIFIABLE DISEASE A disease that the law requires be reported to health officials when diagnosed. Also called a reportable disease.

REEMERGING DISEASE Many diseases once thought to be controlled are reappearing to infect humans again. These are known as reemerging diseases because they have not been common for a long period of time and are starting to appear again among large population groups.

VECTOR Any agent that carries and transmits parasites and diseases. Also, an organism or a chemical used to transport a gene into a new host cell.

In December 2013 an outbreak of chikungunya was reported in the Caribbean island of St. Martin, marking the first local transmission (caused by mosquitoes native to the region rather than imported by travelers) in the Americas. The disease spread rapidly throughout the region, and by the end of 2017 there had been more than 2.2 million suspected cases and more than 300,000 confirmed cases of locally transmitted chikungunya across 45 countries in the region, according to the Pan American Health Organization, a specialized regional agency of WHO.

Chikungunya became a nationally notifiable disease in the United States in 2015 after 12 locally transmitted cases, the first in the continental United States, were reported in Florida the previous year. In 2015 only one locally transmitted case was reported, this time in Texas. As of January 2018, no other locally transmitted cases had been reported from US states. The rate of transmission also fell significantly in US island territories such as Puerto Rico, the US Virgin Islands, and American Samoa, which reported 4,659 locally transmitted cases in 2014 and just 36 in 2017.

■ Treatment and Prevention

Treatment of chikungunya is aimed at relieving symptoms. No vaccine or specific antiviral treatment is available. The most common treatments for symptoms include rest, fluids, and anti-inflammatory/analgesic drugs such as ibuprofen, naproxen, acetaminophen, or paracetamol. These treatments help relieve fever, aches, joint pain, and arthritis. In most cases people recover fully from chikungunya, often in a few days. However, in rare cases joint pain can persist or prolonged fatigue may be experienced. Death is unlikely, although there are a few reported deaths related to bleeding from this infection. Some deaths appear to be the result of using aspirin to treat symptoms, which may be linked with bleeding in people with chikungunya.

As this infection is primarily transmitted via mosquitoes, the best prevention method is to avoid the bite of infected mosquitoes. This can be achieved by eliminating mosquito breeding grounds, such as stagnant water bodies; using insect repellants on the body and clothing; using mosquito nets; and wearing long-sleeved clothing. In addition, to prevent infection from being spread to more mosquitoes, the above prevention methods should be used by infected people as well.

■ Impacts and Issues

Although chikungunya transmission has historically been confined to a few endemic countries, several outbreaks in the 21st century have shown the possibility of the risk for large geographic expansion of endemic areas of the disease. The distribution of one chikungunya disease vector, the mosquito *Aedes aegypti*, is almost worldwide, and another vector, *Aedes albopictus*, has been the source of several outbreaks in Europe since 2007. Because *Aedes albopictus* is better suited to survive in temperate regions than *Aedes aegypti*, disease researchers worry about its ability to make chikungunya endemic in colder areas such as Europe and North America.

Distinguishing between chikungunya and dengue fever is sometimes difficult, as they have similar symptoms and are transmitted via the same vector. Therefore, the occurrence of chikungunya may be misrepresented due to misdiagnosis. The Centers for Disease Control and Prevention suggests that the possibility that cases of chikungunya have been misdiagnosed as dengue fever could potentially mean that the number of chikungunya cases is higher than previously assumed.

In response to the emergence of chikungunya as a potentially global disease, researchers have expanded their efforts at developing a vaccine. In 2014 biologists in Vienna, Austria, developed an experimental vaccine based on the existing measles vaccine that was shown to produce an immune response in test subjects. Likewise, the US National Institutes of Health developed an experimental vaccine in 2014 using noninfectious viruslike particles (VLPs). By mid-2016 more than 20 experimental vaccines had been introduced, with several of the most promising candidates undergoing multiple rounds of clinical trials as of early 2018.

SEE ALSO *Arthropod-Borne Disease; Dengue and Dengue Hemorrhagic Fever; Mosquito-Borne Diseases; Travel and Infectious Disease; Vector-Borne Disease; Yellow Fever*

BIBLIOGRAPHY

Books

Okeoma, Chioma M., ed. *Chikungunya Virus: Advances in Biology, Pathogenesis, and Treatment.* Cham, Switzerland: Springer, 2016.

Periodicals

Sahadeo, N. S. D., et al. "Understanding the Evolution and Spread of Chikungunya Virus in the Americas Using Complete Genome Sequences." *Virus Evolution* 3, no. 1 (January 2017). This article can also be found online at https://academic.oup.com/ve/article/3/1/vex010/3792090 (accessed January 31, 2018).

Shragai, Talya, et al. "Zika and Chikungunya: Mosquito-Borne Viruses in a Changing World." *Annals of the New York Academy of Sciences* 1399 (July 2017): 61–77. This article can also be found online at http://onlinelibrary.wiley.com/doi/10.1111/nyas.13306/full (accessed January 31, 2018).

Smalley, Claire, et al. "Status of Research and Development of Vaccines for Chikungunya." *Vaccine* 34, no. 26 (June 2016): 2976–2981. This article can also be found online at https://www.sciencedirect.com/science/article/pii/S0264410X16300731 (accessed January 31, 2018).

Websites

"Chikungunya." Pan American Health Organization. http://www.paho.org/hq/index.php?Itemid=40931 (accessed January 31, 2018).

"Chikungunya." World Health Organization, April 2017. http://www.who.int/mediacentre/factsheets/fs327/en/ (accessed January 31, 2018).

"Chikungunya Virus." Centers for Disease Control and Prevention, August 29, 2017. https://www.cdc.gov/chikungunya/index.html (accessed January 31, 2018).

Locke, Susannah. "The Painful, Mosquito-Borne Chikungunya Virus Has Reached the US." *Vox*, July 19, 2014. https://www.vox.com/2014/7/19/5916249/chikungunya-fever-virus-caribbean-florida-disease-symptoms-explained (accessed January 31, 2018).

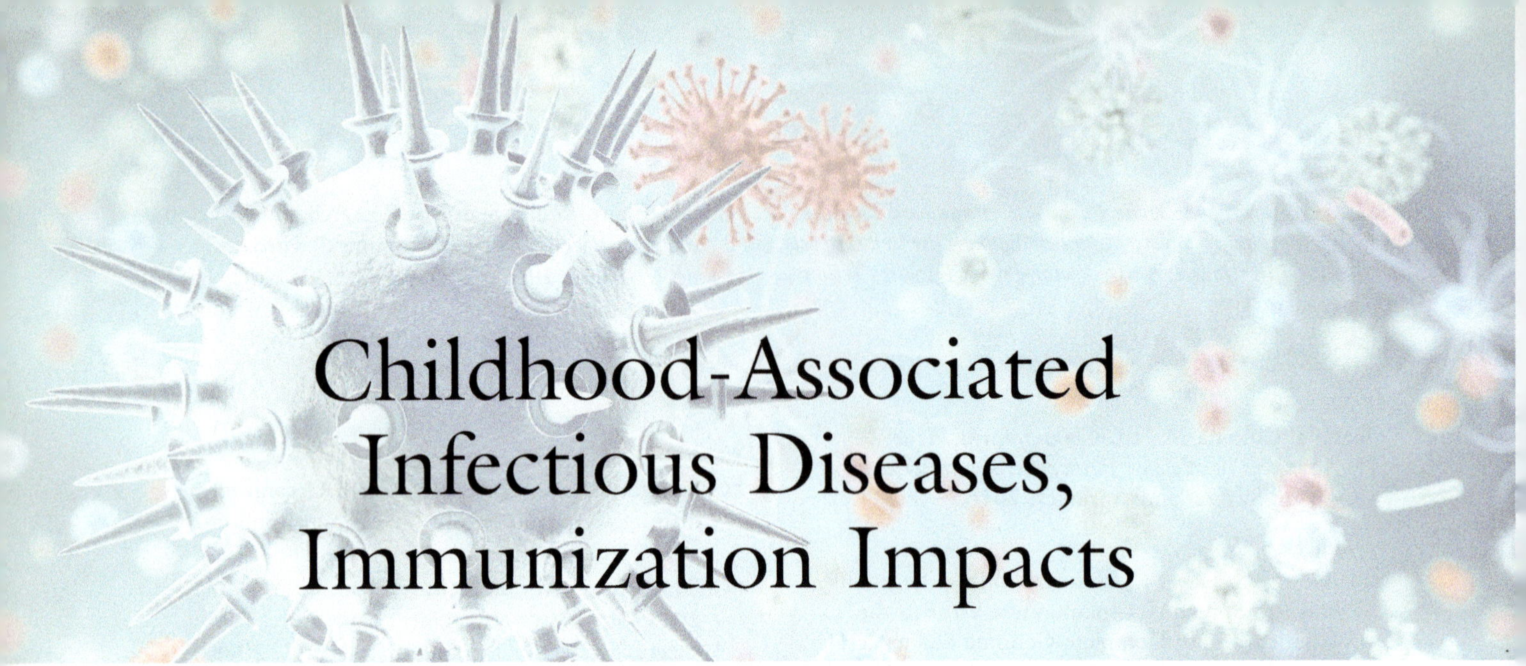

Childhood-Associated Infectious Diseases, Immunization Impacts

Introduction

In the early 20th century, nearly one-third of all deaths occurred among children less than five years old, and infectious diseases such as pneumonia, tuberculosis, diphtheria, diarrhea, and enteritis accounted for more than half of all fatalities. In the 21st century, children in the United States are routinely vaccinated against many infectious diseases. According to the Centers for Disease Control and Prevention (CDC), strategic vaccination campaigns have virtually eliminated many previously common childhood diseases in the United States. There has been an almost 100 percent reduction in mortality due to smallpox, diphtheria, tetanus, and polio in the last century. Similar successes have occurred throughout the developed world. However, vaccination rates remain low in many developing countries, leaving a large percentage of the world's children exposed to potentially deadly diseases.

WORDS TO KNOW

ENDEMIC Present in a particular area or among a particular group of people.

HERD IMMUNITY A resistance to disease that occurs in a population when a proportion of them have been immunized against it. The theory is that it is less likely that an infectious disease will spread in a group where some individuals are unlikely to contract it.

MORTALITY The condition of being susceptible to death. The term *mortality* comes from the Latin word *mors*, which means death. Mortality can also refer to the rate of deaths caused by an illness or injury (e.g., "Rabies has a high mortality rate").

VACCINATION The inoculation, or use of vaccines, to prevent specific diseases within humans and animals by producing immunity to such diseases. It is the introduction of weakened or dead viruses or microorganisms into the body to create immunity by the production of specific antibodies.

History and Policy Response

The primary cause of infant and child deaths throughout recorded history has been infectious disease. For centuries futile attempts were made to control infections by bloodletting, purging, use of leeches, or treatment with various mixtures of herbs and poisons. However, diseases such as smallpox caused millions of deaths even in the 20th century.

In 1798 English physician Edward Jenner (1749–1823) proved the effectiveness of vaccination as a strategy in preventing smallpox. Using the techniques developed early in the 19th century, vaccines for diphtheria, pertussis, tuberculosis, and tetanus were added into the medical arsenal in the 1920s. Despite the relative crude nature of the early vaccines, they provided effective control of many diseases, and further refinement in vaccine design reduced side effects and other reactions.

In 1949, after the World Health Organization (WHO) was established, efforts were initiated to eradicate infectious diseases. Nations around the globe began widespread immunization programs in the mid- to late 20th century. Polio virus, which can cause paralysis and even death in 1 percent of patients, has been nearly eliminated in most of the world. The first polio vaccine was an inactivated polio virus developed by Jonas Salk (1914–1995) in 1955. The oral polio vaccine developed by Albert Sabin (1906–1993) came into commercial use in 1961. A successful vaccination campaign eliminated polio from North America in 1991. As of 2018 only three countries still have polio in circulation: Afghanistan, Pakistan, and Nigeria.

Efforts to eradicate smallpox began during the World Health Assembly in 1958 by Soviet scientist Victor Zhadanov (1914–1987), who had had success containing the disease in Soviet Russia. Zhadanov's expertise in freeze-drying the virus allowed for large-scale production and distribution of the smallpox vaccine to remote corners of Asia and Africa. In 1956 WHO, in conjunction with national governments, began an immunization program to eradicate smallpox from the world. However, in 1966 smallpox was still prevalent in 31 countries. With a boost in financial support, the campaign was intensified, and in 1977 health officials in Somalia reported the last natural case of smallpox. WHO officially declared victory over smallpox in 1979. According to the United Nations Children's Fund (UNICEF), eradication of smallpox is saving approximately 5 million lives annually, and, since Jenner's first vaccines, nearly 9 million lives have been saved due to vaccination.

In 1962 the Vaccination Assistance Act (Section 317 of the Public Health Service Act) was passed to provide federal support toward financing and administering a complete series of childhood vaccines. The Expanded Program on Immunization begun in 1974 by WHO provides similar support worldwide for childhood vaccination.

Most often active immunization is used to protect against infectious diseases. In active immunization, a vaccine, which may be purified toxins, specific bacterial or viral proteins, or weakened infectious organisms, is injected into a person. This induces protective immunity, which may last a lifetime. Most vaccines need booster shots to maintain the lifelong immunity. For instance, it is recommended that tetanus shots be given every 10 years to reactivate the immunity against the tetanus-causing bacteria.

While only smallpox has been eradicated worldwide, immunization programs have virtually eliminated tetanus, diphtheria, measles, mumps, rubella, and *Haemophilus influenzae* type B meningitis from the United States. These successes derive from the practices of giving vaccines to many children early in life. In many countries school immunization laws facilitate active immunization of children against a core group of diseases prior to school entry. While the specific vaccinations vary from country to country, recommended routine immunizations by WHO for children include diphtheria, *Haemophilus influenzae* type b, rubella, measles, polio, tetanus, pertussis, hepatitis B, pneumococcus, rotavirus, human papillomavirus (HPV), and tuberculosis. Additionally, children may receive vaccination against meningitis, typhoid, cholera, hepatitis A, and yellow fever in countries where the diseases are endemic.

Impacts and Issues

Success in defeating infectious diseases depends on obtaining and sustaining high rates of immunization in children. No vaccine is 100 percent effective. Even if every child received vaccinations against all diseases, some would remain susceptible. A phenomenon called "herd immunity" helps to protect those children who remain susceptible after vaccination. Diseases do not spread effectively if most children are protected and even if a few are not.

Immunization of children is extremely cost effective. In the United States, every $1 invested saves between $2 and $27 in medical costs to treat infectious diseases. In developing countries every $1 invested in vaccinations saves nearly $16 in health care costs. In addition, the vaccines widely used as of 2018 produce few side effects or reactions.

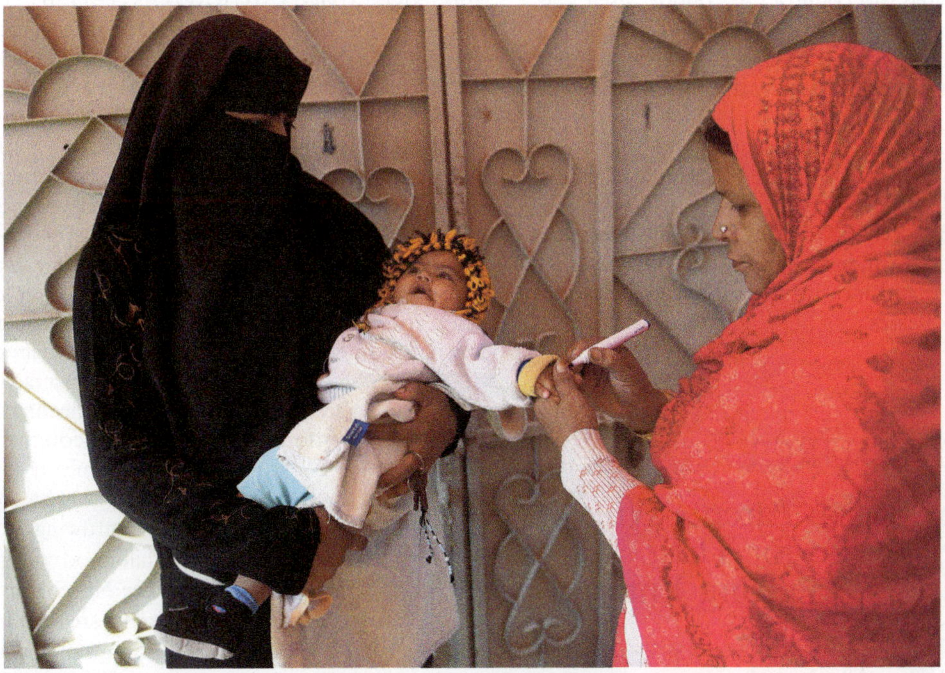

A health care worker marks an infant's finger after administering a polio vaccine in Pakistan in 2016. Polio remains endemic in the country. © RIZWAN TABASSUM/AFP/Getty Images

Immunization programs do save lives, yet major efforts remain. According to WHO, an estimated 19.5 million children worldwide are either unvaccinated or not fully vaccinated against diphtheria, tetanus, and pertussis (DTP). In 2015 alone the estimated number of deaths due to measles was 134,200. Global vaccination coverage for these four diseases could save nearly 2 to 3 million lives.

Likewise, rotavirus causes the most common type of diarrheal disease worldwide. According to estimates from the CDC, since 2008 vaccination in the United States by a new rotavirus vaccine has resulted in a 63 to 94 percent decline in rotavirus gastroenteritis hospital visits, saving nearly $1 billion annually. Yet high costs have prevented widespread use of rotavirus vaccines in countries such as India, where one WHO study estimated that routine vaccination with rotavirus vaccination could prevent about 4 percent of deaths among children younger than five.

In developed countries, while vaccination has eliminated or reduced incidence of most deadly childhood infections, there has still been a resurgence of some of these diseases. This is mainly because some parents choose not to get their children immunized because of fears that vaccines may cause autism. One of the reasons given by parents is the possible neurotoxic effect of mercury in the preservative used in certain vaccine preparations. In the United States, several recent outbreaks of measles, varicella, pertussis, pneumococcal disease, and *Haemophilus influenzae* have been attributed to vaccine refusal. While a number of parents continue to express concern about a link between autism and vaccines, this connection has been debunked on the basis of several studies.

Rates of vaccination in developed countries may reduce in the future because so few people get sick from diseases such as polio or diphtheria. However, until a disease is completely eliminated, no country can consider itself safe. In this age of frequent air travel, infectious diseases can reach across continents, and, if the percentage of immune individuals in a population declines, the risk of epidemics increases greatly.

Compared to the early 20th century, the practice of immunization has reduced the burden of infectious disease worldwide. Children have benefited the most, with millions more children surviving to adulthood. The challenges for the 21st century include maintaining the progress, expanding the scope, and moving toward eventual eradication of infectious diseases.

PRIMARY SOURCE

Bucking the Herd: Parents Who Refuse Vaccination for Their Children May Be Putting Entire Communities at Risk

SOURCE: *Allen, Arthur. "Bucking the Heard: Parents Who Refuse Vaccination for Their Children May Be Putting Entire Communities at Risk."* Atlantic *(September 2002). This article can also be found online at https://www.theatlantic.com/magazine/archive/2002/09/bucking-the-herd/302556/ (accessed February 21, 2018).*

INTRODUCTION: *In the following article in the* Atlantic, *Arthur Allen relates the story of a community in Colorado that has experienced outbreaks of pertussis (whooping cough) and other preventable diseases after parents chose not to vaccinate their children according to state recommendations. As most of a population becomes vaccinated, a herd-immunity effect provides some protection to those who are unvaccinated. As Allen relates, this herd immunity is not enough to prevent outbreaks of infectious disease. Allen, a Washington-based journalist, is also the author of* Vaccine: The Controversial Story of Medicine's Greatest Lifesaver *(2007).*

Boulder, Colorado, a university town of 96,000, lies in a sequestered valley on the western edge of the Great Plains. Both geographically and culturally it is a place apart. Ralph Nader won more than 10 percent of Boulder's vote in the most recent presidential election. Natural-food groceries outnumber Safeways; chiropractors' offices line the main drag; and the city council recently declared that dog owners would henceforth be referred to as "dog guardians." A popular bumper sticker reads, WELCOME TO BOULDER, 20 SQUARE MILES SURROUNDED BY REALITY. Boulder is, in short, an experiment-oriented city.

A particularly interesting experiment, from a public-health perspective, has taken shape at the Shining Mountain Waldorf School, a campus of one-story wooden buildings set amid cottonwood and willow trees hard by the foothills of the Rockies. By their parents' choosing, nearly half of the 292 students at Shining Mountain have received only a few, and in some cases none, of the twenty-one childhood vaccinations mandated by Colorado state law in accordance with federal guidelines. The shunning of one of the vaccines, against diphtheria, tetanus, and pertussis, has resulted in a revival of whooping cough, the illness that occurs when colonies of the bacteria *Bordetella pertussis* attach to the lining of the upper respiratory passages, releasing toxins that cause inflammation and a spasmodic cough. The high-pitched whoop is a symptom heard mainly in younger children; it's the sound of a desperate attempt to breathe.

Shining Mountain exemplifies a growing movement in American life: the challenge to childhood vaccination. According to a survey published in the November 2000 issue of *Pediatrics*, one fourth of all parents are skeptical of some or all of the standard vaccines. Some states grant exemptions to the law so that parents can refuse vaccinations for their children. In Colorado parents who don't want their children vaccinated have only to sign a card stating as much. In Oregon the rate of religious exemptions—which are granted to all parents who choose not to have their children immunized for philosophical reasons—tripled, from 0.9 percent in the 1996–1997 school year to 2.7 percent in 2001.

Those skeptical of vaccines have various reasons. Some believe that vaccines are responsible for otherwise unexplained increases in conditions such as autism, asthma, and multiple sclerosis. Others, including the conservative activist Phyllis Schlafly, see government attempts to track and enforce immunization as an intrusion on privacy. Still others—parents whose recollections of their own bouts of chickenpox or measles are bathed in nostalgia—argue that the elimination of traditional childhood illnesses is an attack on childhood itself. The parents at Shining Mountain are influenced by the philosophy of Rudolf Steiner, a turn-of-the-century Austrian philosopher who founded the Waldorf movement. Steiner (who was not a medical doctor) believed that children's spirits benefited from being tempered in the fires of a good inflammation.

The critics have concluded that the dangers of vaccination outweigh the risks of vaccine-preventable disease. Like all medical interventions, vaccination entails some risk, although the extent and gravity of potential side effects are matters of debate. For example, febrile seizures occur in roughly one in 10,000 children—perhaps 1,000 a year in the United States—who receive the current whooping-cough vaccine. Such seizures rarely, if ever, lead to permanent brain damage, however, and in any case febrile seizures are triggered just as easily by a run-of-the-mill infection as by a vaccine. Suspicions that mercury preservatives used in vaccines inflicted neurological damage on children are worrisome but unproved (mercury has largely been phased out of vaccines over the past three years).

To some extent vaccination is a victim of its own success. Owing to vaccination campaigns, smallpox no longer exists in man, and polio has been driven from the Western Hemisphere. Measles, diphtheria, and invasive hemophilus bacterial disease (such as meningitis) are rare in the United States, and even whooping cough is unusual enough that few parents consider it a threat. All these diseases, with the exception of smallpox, still infest various corners of the world, but in most of the United States even those who have not been vaccinated against them, or in whom the vaccine is not effective, are protected, because most of the people we meet have been vaccinated. Epidemiologists call this phenomenon "herd immunity": the more vaccinated sheep there are, the safer an unvaccinated one is. When vaccination rates drop, disease returns.

Precisely at what point herd immunity fails is difficult to calculate, but there is ample evidence that it does. Since the collapse of the Soviet public-health system diphtheria has returned to Russia with a vengeance, killing thousands. Sweden suspended vaccination against whooping cough from 1979 to 1996 while testing a new vaccine. In a study of the moratorium period that was published in 1993, Swedish physicians found that 60 percent of the country's children got whooping cough before they were ten. However, close medical monitoring kept the death rate from whooping cough at about one per year during that period.

SEE ALSO *Developing Nations and Drug Delivery; Immune Response to Infection; Polio Eradication Campaign*

BIBLIOGRAPHY

Books

Myers, Martin G., and Diego Pineda. *Do Vaccines Cause That?!: A Guide to Evaluating Vaccine Safety Concerns.* Galveston, TX: Immunizations for Public Health, 2008.

Offit, Paul A. *Vaccinated: One Man's Quest to Defeat the World's Deadliest Diseases.* New York: Collins, 2007.

Oshinsky, David M. *Polio: An American Story.* New York: Oxford University Press, 2005.

Payne, Daniel C., and Umesh D. Parashar. "Chapter 13: Rotavirus." In *Manual for the Surveillance of Vaccine-Preventable Diseases.* Atlanta: Centers for Disease Control and Prevention, 1996. This chapter can also be found online at https://www.cdc.gov/vaccines/pubs/surv-manual/chpt13-rotavirus.html (accessed February 13, 2018).

Periodicals

Doherty, Mark, et al. "Vaccine Impact: Benefits for Human Health." *Vaccine* 34, no. 52 (December 20, 2016): 6707–6714. This article can also be found online at https://www.sciencedirect.com/science/article/pii/S0264410X16309434 (accessed February 13, 2018).

Feldstein, Leora R., et al. "Global Routine Vaccination Coverage, 2016." *Morbidity and Mortality Weekly Report* 66, no. 45 (November 17, 2017): 1252–1255. This article can also be found online at https://www.cdc.gov/mmwr/volumes/66/wr/mm6645a3.htm (accessed February 13, 2018).

Maron, Dina Fine. "How to Get More Parents to Vaccinate Their Kids." *Scientific American* (February 19, 2015). This article can also be found online at https://www.scientificamerican.com/article/how-to-get-more-parents-to-vaccinate-their-kids/ (accessed February 13, 2018).

Morris, Shaun K. et al. "Rotavirus Mortality in India: Estimates Based on a Nationally Representative Survey of Diarrhoeal Deaths." *Bulletin of the World Health Organization* 90 (2012): 720–727. This article can also be found online at http://www.who.int/bulletin/volumes/90/10/12-101873/en/ (accessed February 13, 2018).

Ozawa, Sachiko, et al. "Return on Investment from Childhood Immunization in Low- and Middle-Income Countries, 2011–20." *Health Affairs* 35, no. 2 (February 2016).

Websites

Breene, Keith. "7 Deadly Diseases the World Has (Almost) Eliminated." World Economic Forum, May 26, 2017. https://www.weforum.org/agenda/2017/05/7-deadly-diseases-the-world-has-almost-eradicated/ (accessed February 13, 2018).

Collins, Francis. "Resurgence of Measles, Pertussis Fueled by Vaccine Refusals." Directors Blog, National Institutes of Health, March 22, 2016. https://directorsblog.nih.gov/2016/03/22/resurgence-of-measles-pertussis-fueled-by-vaccine-refusals/ (accessed February 13, 2018).

"Global Health Observatory (GHO) Data: Vaccination Coverage." World Health Organization. http://www.who.int/gho/immunization/en/ (accessed February 13, 2018).

"Immunization Coverage." World Health Organization, January 2018. http://www.who.int/mediacentre/factsheets/fs378/en/ (accessed February 13, 2018).

"Vaccine-Preventable Diseases, Immunizations, and MMWR—1961–2011" https://www.cdc.gov/mmwr/preview/mmwrhtml/su6004a9.htm

"Vaccines and Immunizations." Centers for Disease Control and Prevention, February 8, 2017. https://www.cdc.gov/vaccines/index.html (accessed February 13, 2018).

Lloyd Scott Clements
Malini Vashishtha

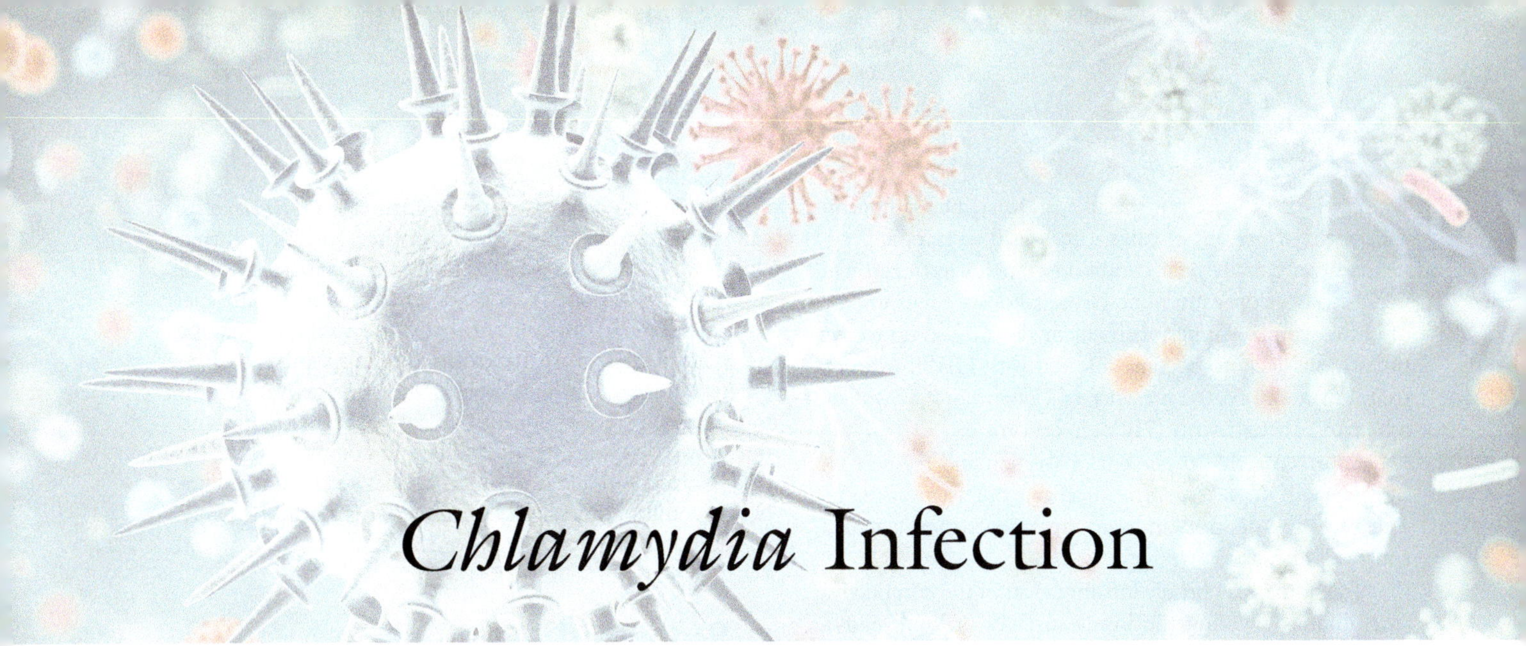

Chlamydia Infection

Introduction

Chlamydia trachomatis is the most common cause of sexually transmitted infection (STI) around the world, with about 131 million new cases each year among people ages 15 to 49. Because most cases produce no symptoms, people often do not realize they are infected, and they go on to infect others.

Chlamydia can have serious consequences for a woman's reproductive health and often leads to infertility. Certain strains of *C. trachomatis* cause an eye disease called trachoma. According to reports from the World Health Organization (WHO), the disease is prevalent in more than 42 countries across the globe, with 1.9 million cases of infectious blindness in the developing world. In addition, *C. psittaci* is a *Chlamydia* species carried by birds that occasionally infects humans, resulting in an unusual form of pneumonia. The other important *Chlamydia* species is *C. pneumoniae*, which infects approximately half of the world's population and sometimes causes upper and lower respiratory tract infections. All of these infections can be treated successfully with antibiotics, but many people go undiagnosed or do not have access to treatment.

Disease History, Characteristics, and Transmission

The three main *Chlamydia* species are among the world's most prevalent microbial pathogens and are a significant cause of ill health. *C. trachomatis* exhibits two phases in the life cycle in an extracellular infectious form: an elementary body and an intracellular noninfectious reticulate body. The reticulate body is a replicative form of the organism, which is eventually released from the host cell and infects adjacent host cells.

C. trachomatis infects the genital tract and often produces no symptoms, though women may report a burning sensation during urination and a vaginal discharge. *C. trachomatis* is responsible for most cases of nongonococcal urethritis in men. The disease may remain asymptomatic in 40 to 96 percent of men, and symptoms may vary from a discharge from the penis to an itching or burning sensation to an inflammation of the epididymides and testes.

Chlamydia infection, if left untreated, can cause extensive damage to the female reproductive system, leading to pelvic inflammatory disease (PID) and infertility in 26 percent of women with persistent infection. The signs and

WORDS TO KNOW

ENZYME-LINKED IMMUNOSORBENT ASSAY (ELISA) A technique used to detect antibodies or infectious agents in a sample. The procedure involves interactions via serial binding to a solid surface, usually a polystyrene multiwell plate. The result is a colored product that correlates to the amount of analyte present in the original sample.

FOMITE An object or a surface to which infectious microorganisms such as bacteria or viruses can adhere and be transmitted. Papers, clothing, dishes, and other objects can all act as fomites. Transmission is often by touch.

PATHOGEN A disease-causing agent, such as a bacterium, a virus, a fungus, or another microorganism.

SEXUALLY TRANSMITTED INFECTION (STI) Infections that vary in their susceptibility to treatment, their signs and symptoms, and the consequences if they are left untreated. Some are caused by bacteria. These usually can be treated and cured. Others are caused by viruses and can typically be treated but not cured.

symptoms of PID are not specific. PID may be asymptomatic, or in 10 percent of cases it may lead to ectopic pregnancy, a potentially fatal condition where a fertilized egg begins to develop within one of the fallopian tubes instead of in the womb. Women with chlamydia are also up to five times more likely to become infected with HIV if exposed to it. Furthermore, the presence of *Chlamydia* may worsen a human papillomavirus (HPV) infection.

Approximately 70 percent of women and 50 percent of men with *C. trachomatis* infections are asymptomatic. Because they do not undergo treatment, they act as a source of infection.

Trachoma is a chronic inflammation of the conjunctiva (membranes covering the inside surfaces of the eyelids), the white of the eye, and the cornea. The infection leads to blindness through scarring of these tissues. *C. trachomatis* eye infection is spread by contact, direct or indirect, through fomites, hands, bedding, flies, and contaminated towels.

C. psittaci causes pneumonia that exhibits gradual onset over one to two weeks, with severe headache and cough that may result in spitting up blood. *C. pneumoniae* is spread through respiratory droplets and causes a range of infections, including sinusitis, pharyngitis (throat infection), bronchitis, and pneumonia. It is responsible for up to 12 percent of cases of community-acquired pneumonia.

C. trachomatis is transmitted from person to person through genital, oral, or anal sexual intercourse and can affect anyone who is sexually active. Young women are especially at risk because the infection is more likely to take hold where the cervix is not fully matured. *C. trachomatis* can also be transmitted from mother to child during childbirth. Newborns exposed to *C. trachomatis* from their mother's cervix may develop conjunctivitis or pneumonia. The strains of *C. trachomatis* that cause trachoma may be transmitted by shaking hands or handling fomites such as sheets, crockery, clothing, books, and papers. Trachoma is more common in conditions of poor hygiene and overcrowding. It is often found in arid countries where access to water is limited. Reinfection between family members is common. Finally, *C. pneumoniae* is spread by hand-to-hand contact or by coughs or sneezes.

Scope and Distribution

Each year an estimated 131 million cases of *Chlamydia* infection are reported globally, making it the most prevalent sexually transmitted infection. Three strains of *C. trachomatis* cause lymphogranuloma venereum (LGV) and trachoma (eye infection). LGV is a genital ulcer disease caused by an invasive strain. It occurs in developing countries. In the 21st century there have been several outbreaks of LGV. In particular, it has become a cause for concern among men who have sex with other men.

In the United States, according to the US Centers for Disease Control and Prevention (CDC), nearly 1,598,354 chlamydial infections were reported in 2016, corresponding to 497 cases per 100,000 people. The true number is probably much greater because many people are unaware

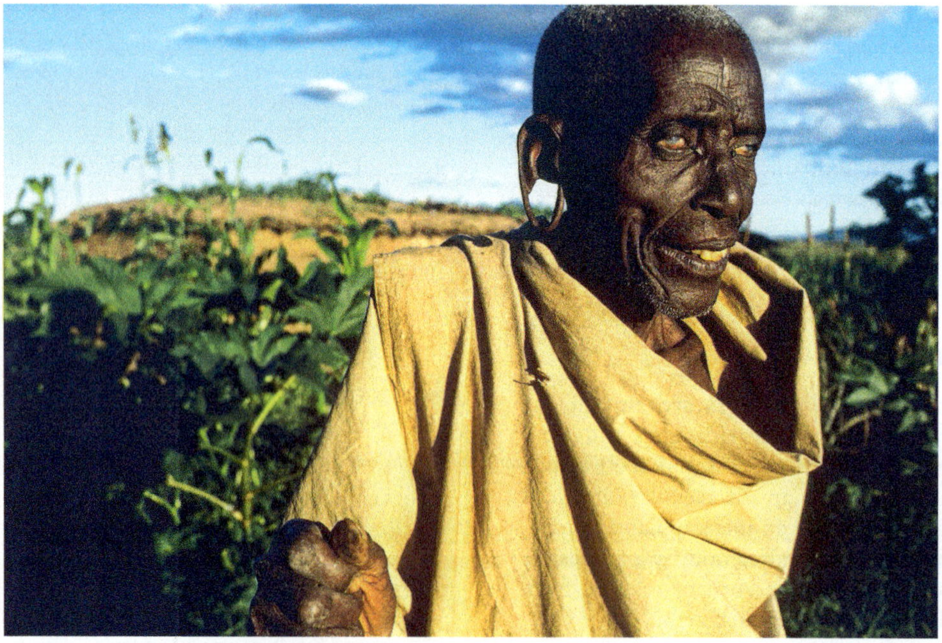

This Tanzanian man was blinded by trachoma, an eye disease caused by *Chlamydia trachomatis.* Unlike other forms of chlamydia infection, which are spread by sexual contact, trachoma is spread by contact with fluids from the eyes or nose of an infected person. © *Joe McNally/Getty Images*

they are infected. Chlamydia occurs in approximately 40 to 60 percent of cases of male nongonococcal urethritis, with a high prevalence of asymptomatic males who serve as a reservoir of infection, and is a leading cause of infertility in women.

Adolescent and young adults aged 15 to 24 years are the most frequently affected group. Each year there are 1,804 cases per 100,000 people among 15- to 19-year-olds and 2,484.6 cases per 100,000 among 20- to 24-year-olds. Prevalence of chlamydia is high compared to that of other bacterial STIs due to the high rate of asymptomatic infection and repeat infection after single-dose therapy.

■ Treatment and Prevention

Treatment of chlamydia was once straightforward, with antibiotics such as tetracyclines, macrolides, or fluoroquinolones. However, increasing resistance to tetracyclines and macrolides has caused concern. Broad-spectrum antibiotics are used to treat acute PID, which covers *C. trachomatis, N. gonorrhoeae*, and anaerobic bacteria. In refractory cases, surgery is also used to drain the abscess or hydrosalpinx (a fallopian tube that is filled with fluid). A variety of antibiotic regimens have been used to address marked geographical variation and resistance patterns of bacterial pathogens, but generally the treatment involves multiple agents to cover *C. trachomatis.*

WHO and the CDC recommend azithromycin and doxycycline as first-line drugs for the treatment of chlamydia. Patients with PID should be monitored until clinical signs of improvement appear.

The sexual partners of those infected should also be tested and treated, if necessary, to prevent reinfection. Moreover, people with chlamydia should abstain from sexual intercourse until treatment is completed. Condom use provides some protection against transmission of the bacterium.

Highly sensitive and quick assays such as nucleic acid amplification tests (NAATs) have been developed for accurate diagnosis and screening of chlamydia. Screening is an important part of monitoring the prevalence of chlamydia. Many countries have adopted screening programs. The CDC recommends annual screening for all sexually active women age 25 or younger. Older women with risk factors, such as a new sex partner or multiple sex partners, are often advised to have an annual screening as well, as should all pregnant women.

According to WHO, a vaccine against *C. trachomatis* that is administered prior to adolescence and remains effective through the childbearing years is the best way to halt the toll of the infection globally. As of 2017 there were several such vaccines being developed, some of which were at the stage of clinical trials.

ADVANCES IN DIAGNOSIS

Tremendous developments in the diagnosis of chlamydia have been made in the 21st century. The microbe can be diagnosed by cell culture, direct immunofluorescence assay (DFA), enzyme-linked immunosorbent assay (ELISA), and the nucleic acid amplification test (NAAT). The high sensitivity and specificity of NAAT makes it the most recommended for diagnosis. The patient sample for this test can be urine in men or vulvovaginal, cervical, or urethral swabs in women. This noninvasive method of specimen collection has made the collection process convenient at the local, primary level of care.

■ Impacts and Issues

The greatest impact of sexually transmitted *C. trachomatis* is the silent nature of the infection. Three-quarters of those infected are unaware of the fact because they have no symptoms. This means they can infect others and continue to do so until the disease is diagnosed. For women the damage that untreated chlamydia inflicts on the reproductive system is also silent. Over one-third of women with untreated chlamydia develop PID and can lose fertility, often without even being aware of the reason why. Screening is important so that infection can be dealt with before permanent damage to the uterus, fallopian tubes, and surrounding tissue develops.

The control of chlamydia and other sexually transmitted infections involves education aimed at reducing risky sexual behaviors. Both sexual abstinence and having sexual intercourse only with a partner who is not infected are effective ways of avoiding infection with *C. trachomatis.* International health officials attempt to offer advice and present facts about sexual behaviors and their link to STIs such as chlamydia in a nonjudgmental manner, taking into account cultural differences in differing populations.

The impact of *C. trachomatis* in developing countries has important social and economic implications. Loss of vision from trachoma often starts in midlife, although the infection may be present much earlier. It is also two to three times more common among women, probably because women generally spend greater time in close contact with small children, who are the main reservoir of infection. Middle-aged women often make an important contribution to the family income, so disability in this group has a severe economic impact.

See Also *Chlamydia pneumoniae*; Psittacosis; Sexually Transmitted Infections; Trachoma

BIBLIOGRAPHY

Books

Wilson, Walter, and Merle A. Sande. *Current Diagnosis & Treatment in Infectious Diseases.* New York: McGraw-Hill, 2001.

Periodicals

Savaris, R. F., et al. "Antibiotic Therapy for Pelvic Inflammatory Disease." *Cochrane Database of Systematic Reviews* 4 (April 2017): CD010285.

Websites

"Chlamydia." Centers for Disease Control and Prevention, September 26, 2017. https://www.cdc.gov/std/stats16/chlamydia.htm (accessed January 24, 2018).

"Chlamydia—CDC Fact Sheet (Detailed)." Centers for Disease Control and Prevention, September 26, 2017. https://www.cdc.gov/std/chlamydia/stdfact-chlamydia-detailed.htm (accessed January 25, 2018).

"Global Incidence and Prevalence of Selected Curable Sexually Transmitted Infections—2008." World Health Organization, 2012. http://apps.who.int/iris/bitstream/10665/75181/1/9789241503839_eng.pdf (accessed January 25, 2018).

Susan Aldridge
Kausalya Santhanam

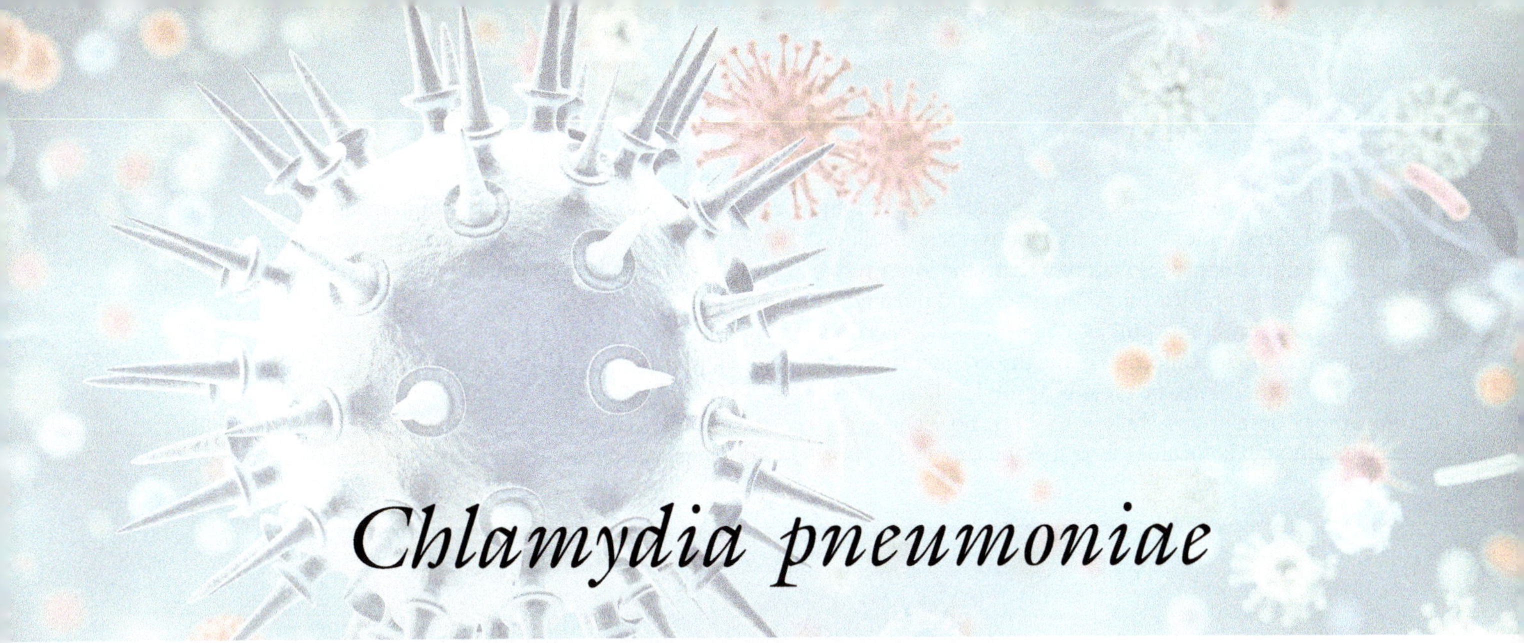

Chlamydia pneumoniae

■ Introduction

Chlamydia pneumoniae (also *Chlamydophila pneumoniae*) is a bacterium that is capable of causing upper and lower respiratory tract infections, which range from mild to severe to life-threatening. As the name suggests, the most common infection associated with *C. pneumoniae* is pneumonia, a potentially fatal lung infection. In addition to causing pneumonia and other respiratory infections, such as bronchitis, research shows that *C. pneumoniae* infection may have a long-term impact on other aspects of patient health, including playing a role in the development of heart disease and disorders of the central nervous system.

C. pneumoniae is commonly found in humans. However, it does not cause any obvious health problems in most people, making it difficult for researchers to precisely determine how many people are infected with the bacteria. Though some researchers describe it as ubiquitous, the Centers for Disease Control and Prevention (CDC) estimates that 300,000 infections occur annually in the United States, while also acknowledging that "the true size of the health problem is unknown and likely underestimated." Once symptoms of *C. pneumoniae* begin to be expressed, they can be treated with antibiotics. Most often, however, *C. pneumoniae* infections are self-limiting, meaning they do not require treatment for symptoms to be resolved.

■ Disease History, Characteristics, and Transmission

C. pneumoniae was first isolated in 1965 in Taiwan. However, it was not until 1983, in the US state of Washington, that it was first identified as a distinct species of *Chlamydia*. (Despite the similar names, *Chlamydia pneumoniae* is not part of the sexually transmitted disease of *Chlamydia trachomatis*.) More than 15 years later, in 1999, scientists suggest reclassifying and renaming the bacteria *Chlamydophila pneumoniae* to accord with a proposed new naming convention for the family of bacteria *Chlamyadiaceae*, to which *C. pneumoniae* belongs. This new nomenclature was not universally accepted, however, and *C. pneumoniae* has since been known interchangeably as both *Chlamydia pneumoniae* and *Chlamydophila pneumoniae*.

Transmission of *C. pneumoniae* occurs via exposure to the aerosols created by coughing and sneezing. While exposure can occur in brief interactions, such as when shaking hands with an infected person who has coughed into his or her hand, transmission of *C. pneumoniae* typically involves more extended periods of exposure, making transmission more common between people who live or work together.

After transmission it typically takes three to four weeks for symptoms of *C. pneumoniae* infection to develop—if they ever do. Such symptoms are typically mild. A person infected with a mild case of *C. pneumoniae* will develop a

WORDS TO KNOW

AEROSOL Particles of liquid or solid dispersed as a suspension in gas.

COMMUNITY-ACQUIRED INFECTION An infection that develops outside of a hospital, in the general community. It differs from hospital-acquired infections in that those infected are typically in better health than hospitalized people.

NOTIFIABLE DISEASE A disease that the law requires must be reported to health officials when diagnosed; also called a reportable disease.

PATHOGEN A disease-causing agent, such as a bacterium, a virus, a fungus, or another microorganism.

runny nose, sore throat, cough, or low-grade fever, among other cold-like symptoms. In more serious cases, the illness spreads from the upper respiratory tract to the lower respiratory tract, infecting the lungs. Bronchitis and pneumonia are the most common forms of *C. pneumoniae* infection. Sinusitis, pharyngitis (infection of the throat), and laryngitis (infection of the larynx or voice box) are less likely. Pneumonia may develop gradually with fever, hoarseness, and cough, although sometimes fever may be absent. *C. pneumoniae* may also make asthma symptoms worse. The symptoms of *C. pneumoniae* infection vary, depending on the extent of the infection, but can persist for weeks after they first present.

■ Scope and Distribution

C. pneumoniae infection is relatively common. Unlike influenza, *C. pneumoniae* is not seasonal in nature and

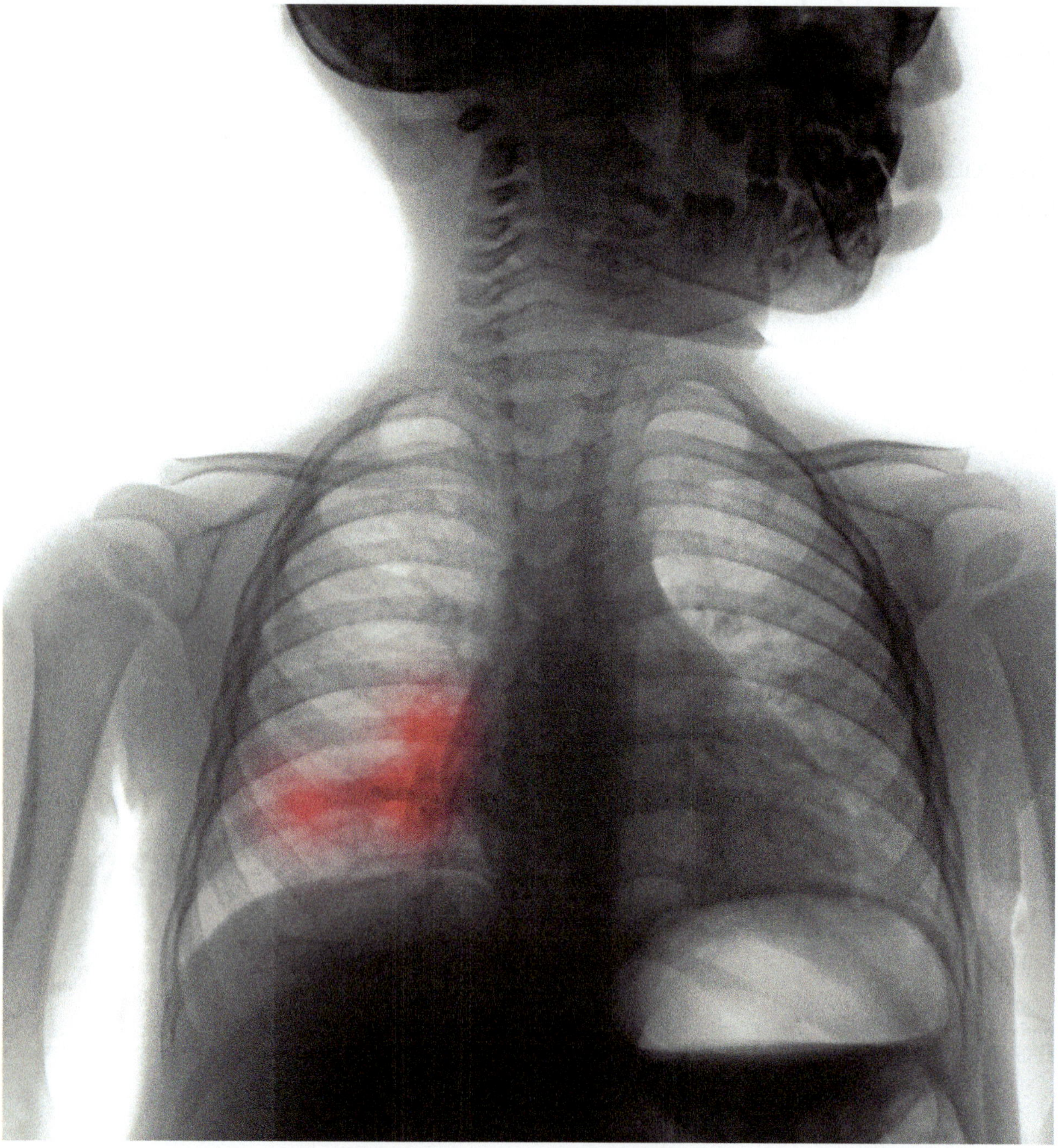

This chest X-ray of a child shows a typical case of right middle lobe pneumonia. *Chlamydia pneumonia* bacteria are responsible for 6 to 12 percent of cases of community-acquired pneumonia. © *Scott Camazine/Science Source*

does not peak in the winter months. Rather, research suggests that rates of infection rise and fall over approximately four-year periods but little is understood about the factors that cause these peaks of infection.

Due to its tendency to be transmitted over periods of prolonged exposure, *C. pneumoniae* infections occur most commonly in nursing homes, prisons, schools, and other residential settings. Initial infection occurs most commonly in young adults and school-age children, whereas older adults are more susceptible to reinfection and are most at risk for pneumonia and other severe complications from *C. pneumoniae* infection. Research indicates *C. pneumoniae* accounts for approximately 4 to 10 percent of all community-acquired pneumonia (CAP)—that is, as the name suggests, pneumonia acquired in community rather than medical settings, where pneumonia infection is more common.

Treatment and Prevention

Most often *C. pneumoniae* infection is self-limiting, meaning it does not require treatment for symptoms to be resolved. However, when mild symptoms persist or develop into more severe symptoms, such as lung infection, treatment of *C. pneumoniae* may include antibiotics. Macrolides are typically used first, with tetracycline prescribed in cases of severe respiratory infection. In some instances a two-course treatment may be required. Like all infections spread by hand-to-hand contact or aerosol exposure, the best approach to prevention is frequent and thorough handwashing. Though no *C. pneumoniae* vaccine exists, a doctor may prescribe preventative antibiotics in certain cases where a person is at a high risk both of infection and of developing severe symptoms.

Impacts and Issues

C. pneumoniae is a significant contributor to CAP, which is a "leading infectious cause of hospitalization and death among U.S. adults," according to a 2015 article in the *New England Journal of Medicine*. The authors of this study found that bacterial pathogens—of which *C. pneumoniae* is one—were found in 14 percent of the adult patients studied at hospitals in Chicago and Nashville. While the percentage of patients with *C. pneumoniae* was not identified and the extent of the bacteria's prevalence is not known, it is among the various causes of pneumonia, which was the eighth-leading cause of death in the United States as of 2017.

Research suggests that *C. pneumoniae* may have other consequences for health as well. Various studies have investigated the relationship between *C. pneumoniae* and asthma, with many of these studies suggesting that the presence of these bacteria exacerbates patient asthma. Research also suggests that *C. pneumoniae* can lead to worsening of chronic obstructive pulmonary disease (COPD), a condition that creates difficulty in patients' breathing, but overall results are unclear. Research has also investigated possible connections between *C. pneumoniae* and neurological disorders such as multiple sclerosis and Alzheimer's disease, but no definitive links have been identified.

Atherosclerotic plaques are fatty deposits that are found lining the inner walls of the coronary and carotid arteries, the vessels serving the heart and brain, of those with heart disease. *C. pneumoniae* infection has been located within these plaques, possibly because the bacterium can infect many of the cells that make up the deposits. Research shows that *C. pneumoniae* may aid in creating the inflammation and immune reaction within blood vessel walls that contribute to heart attacks, strokes, and other forms of coronary heart disease. However, there is no definitive evidence that a *C. pneumoniae* infection actually causes heart disease, merely that it is associated with it. There have been several clinical trials aimed at testing whether antibiotics can prevent heart disease by wiping out *C. pneumoniae* infection. As of early 2018, it appeared that antibiotic therapy does not reduce overall mortality from heart disease or the overall rate of heart attack or stroke. The potential role of *C. pneumoniae* in heart disease continues to be explored, while significantly and for the first time, evidence points to an infectious agent as a risk factor for the number-one killer in the United States.

In general, much remains to be understood about *C. pneumoniae*. According to the authors of a 2009 article in *Clinical Microbiology and Infection*, "there is a clear need for further well-designed studies to determine both the importance of *C. pneumoniae* involvement in human diseases and the usefulness of antibiotic treatment."

SEE ALSO *Chlamydia Infection; Pneumonia; Psittacosis*

BIBLIOGRAPHY

Books

Gates, Robert H. *Infectious Disease Secrets.* Philadelphia: Hanley & Beltus, 2003.

Wilson, Walter R., and Merle A. Sande. *Current Diagnosis & Treatment in Infectious Diseases.* New York: McGraw Hill, 2001.

Periodicals

Andraws, R., J. S. Berger, and D. L. Brown. "Effects of Antibiotic Therapy on Outcomes of Patients with Coronary Artery Disease: A Meta-Analysis of Randomized Controlled Trials." *Journal of the American Medical Association* 293, no. 21 (2005): 2641–2647.

Blasi, F., P. Tarsia, and S. Aliberti. "*Chlamydophila pneumoniae.*" *Clinical Microbiology and Infection* 15, no. 1 (2009): 29–35. This article can also be found online at http://onlinelibrary.wiley.com/doi/10.1111/j.1469-0691.2008.02130.x/full (accessed January 29, 2018).

Jain, Seema, et al. "Community-Acquired Pneumonia Requiring Hospitalization among U.S. Adults." *New England Journal of Medicine* 373 (July 30, 2015): 415–427. This article can also be found online at http://www.nejm.org/doi/full/10.1056/NEJMoa1500245 (accessed February 15, 2018).

Kuo, Cho-Chou, et al. "*Chlamydia pneumoniae* (TWAR)." *Clinical Microbiology Reviews* 8, no. 4 (1995): 451–461. This article can also be found online at http://cmr.asm.org/content/8/4/451.long (accessed January 26, 2018).

Witte, L., D. Droemann, K. Dalhoff, and J. Rupp. "*Chlamydia pneumoniae* Is Frequently Detected in the Blood after Acute Lung Infection." *European Respiratory Journal* 37 (2011): 712–714. This article can also be found online at http://erj.ersjournals.com/content/37/3/712 (accessed January 26, 2018).

Zhou, Min, et al. "Effects of Chlamydia Pneumonia Infection on Progression of Coronary Heart Disease in Elderly Patients." *Biomedical Research* 28, no. 7 (2017). This article can also be found online at http://www.alliedacademies.org/articles/effects-of-chlamydia-pneumonia-infection-on-progression-of-coronary-heart-disease-in-elderly-patients.html (accessed January 26, 2018).

Websites

"*Chlamydia pneumoniae* Infection." Centers for Disease Control and Prevention, September 26, 2016. https://www.cdc.gov/pneumonia/atypical/cpneumoniae/index.html (accessed January 26, 2018).

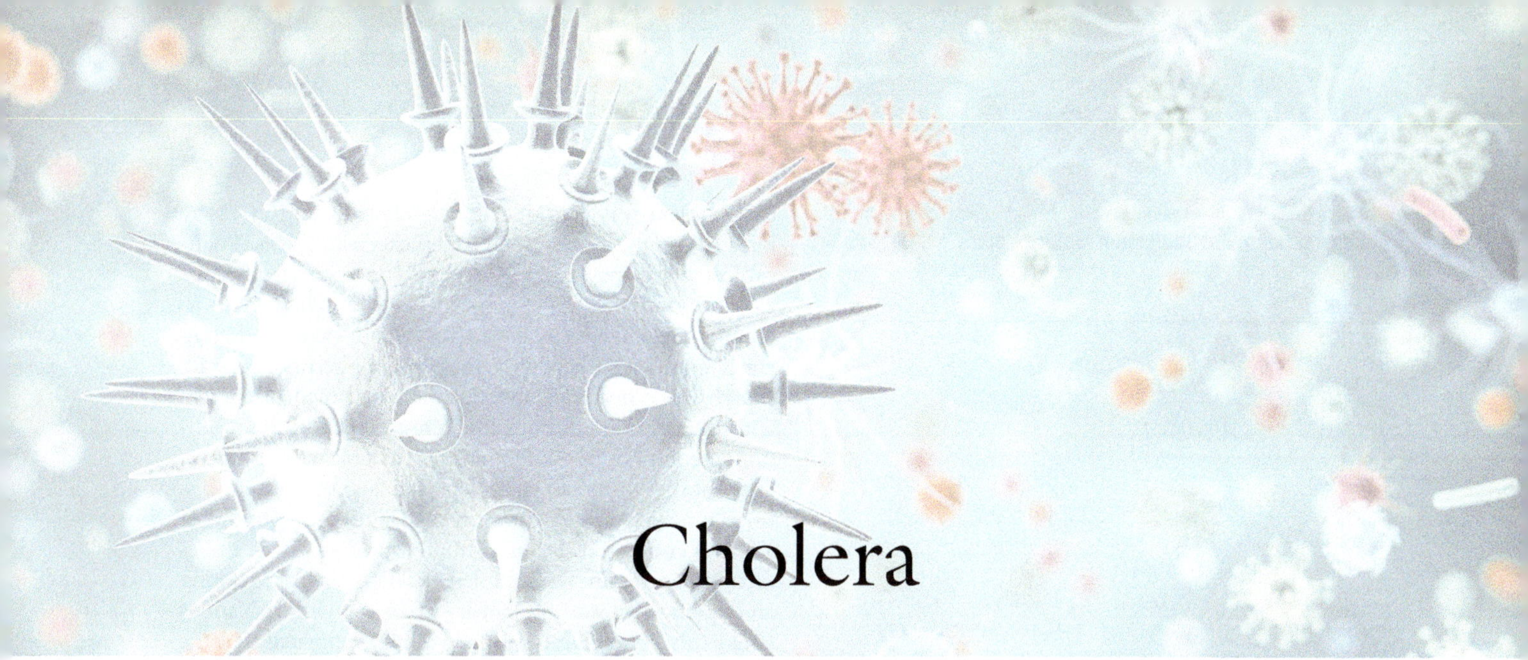

Cholera

Introduction

Cholera, sometimes called Asiatic cholera or epidemic cholera, is a disease with roots in antiquity that remains a global threat. Cholera is an acute intestinal infection caused by the bacterium *Vibrio cholerae.* It can cause rapid dehydration of the body, which can be fatal. Cholera is transmitted by contaminated food and water and is endemic in countries where there is inadequate access to clean water. Treatment of cholera is simple and relies on restoring fluids lost by the body. However, even this simple treatment may not be available to patients in very poor countries. The best approach to preventing cholera lies in better sanitation—improving public health through adequate sewage disposal and cleaning up the water supply. In many less developed countries, this is a difficult challenge to meet because it requires political stability and increased investment in the national infrastructure.

Disease History, Characteristics, and Transmission

V. cholerae belongs to the *Vibrio* genus of Gram-negative bacteria. Gram-negative refers to the way in which a bacterium absorbs visualizing stains under a microscope for identification purposes. *Vibrio* species prefer marine environments and grow best in the presence of salt. They are one of the most common organisms in the surface waters of the world.

V. cholerae includes nearly 139 serotypes (intimately related microorganisms distinguished by the number and type of antigen [protein] molecules on their cell surfaces). Most cholera infections are caused by the *V. cholerae* 01 serotype, but others have been found in specific outbreaks or epidemics. For instance, the *El Tor* serotype was first isolated in the quarantine station of the same name in Sinai in 1906 and was linked to an outbreak among pilgrims returning from Mecca. It seemed to survive far longer than the 01 serotype, which was killed by 15 minutes of heating. In 1992 the 0139 serotype was first identified in Chennai, India, and was responsible for outbreaks in Bangladesh and Thailand the following year. The disease-causing serotypes of *V. cholerae* produces a potent toxin that affects the mucosal lining of the small intestine, causing severe diarrhea with very rapid onset.

Most people infected with *V. cholerae* do not actually become ill, although the bacterium is present in their feces for 7 to 14 days, which means they could transmit the disease to others. The incubation period of *V. cholerae* ranges from just a few hours to five days. In most cases, the illness is difficult to distinguish from other diarrheal diseases. In severe cholera, however, the diarrhea is copious —the patient may lose more than a quart (liter) of fluid every hour. The stools of cholera patients have been described to resemble rice water (clear but flecked with mucus). The diarrhea may be accompanied by vomiting, but pain and fever are minimal and certainly not as severe as the diarrhea.

Through a combination of diarrhea and vomiting, the patient may enter a state of shock due to massive fluid loss

WORDS TO KNOW

ELECTROLYTES Compounds that ionize in a solution; electrolytes dissolved in the blood play an important role in maintaining the proper functioning of the body.

ENDEMIC Present in a particular area or among a particular group of people.

FECAL-ORAL ROUTE The transmission of minute particles of fecal material from one organism (human or animal) to the mouth of another organism.

Access to Improved Sanitation (Select Countries, 2015)

Countries	Percentages
Niger	11
Chad	12
Eritrea	16
Uganda	19
Democratic Republic of the Congo	29
Nigeria	29
Afghanistan	32
India	40
Rwanda	62
Guatemala	64
Russian Federation	72
China	77
Vietnam	78
Romania	79
Mexico	85
Iraq	86
Iran (Islamic Republic of)	90
Tonga	91
Cuba	93
Ukraine	96
United Arab Emirates	98
Canada	100
United States of America	100

SOURCE: World Bank

and electrolyte imbalance, suffering seizures, kidney failure, heart rhythm abnormalities, and unconsciousness. Death from dehydration and shock may occur within hours. As a result, cholera is always considered a medical emergency, and, indeed, it is one of the most rapidly fatal illnesses ever known. Left untreated, severe cholera has a death rate of 30 to 50 percent; when treated promptly, mortality falls to less than 1 percent.

Transmission of *V. cholerae* is through the fecal-oral route and usually spreads by consumption of, or contact with, contaminated food and water. *V. cholerae* is hard to avoid in places where sanitation is poor and access to clean water for drinking or washing is limited or nonexistent. Imported foodstuffs are only a rare cause of cholera, and the risk can be greatly reduced through high standards of food-handling hygiene.

■ Scope and Distribution

Cholera affects many countries around the world. According to the World Health Organization (WHO), there were 132,121 cases of cholera reported in 2016, resulting in 2,420 deaths. The number of cholera cases in Africa and Asia has been steadily decreasing since 2011, helping to bring down the number of global cases.

Although the burden of cholera is greatest in Africa and South Asia, there have been some outbreaks in other areas in the last few years. There was a big spike in the number of cholera cases in 2010 in Haiti after a catastrophic earthquake struck the region. It is widely believed that cholera was introduced into Haiti during 2010 by infected United Nations (UN) peacekeeping forces. Political instability and resulting sanitary conditions further fueled the outbreak. Efforts by the UN in aiding Haiti to combat the cholera epidemic have been meager, and cholera is now a resurgent disease spreading across Haiti. By March 2017 nearly 10,000 Haitians had died of cholera and several hundred thousand were sickened in the neighboring countries of the Dominican Republic and Cuba.

Another outbreak of cholera, the largest in recent history, was ongoing as of early 2018 in the country of Yemen. The outbreak was attributed to destruction of Yemeni infrastructure by Saudi-led coalition air strikes during an ongoing civil war. By January 2018 the United Nations Children's Fund (UNICEF) and WHO estimated that the number of cases in this outbreak exceeded 1 million with 2,241 deaths.

In 2015 a total of 172,454 cases and 1,304 deaths were reported to WHO by 42 countries worldwide. This number may not reflect the actual incidence of the disease, which may be much higher. Underreporting could be due to lack of adequate diagnosis, inadequate surveillance, and fear of economic losses due to decreased tourism in these areas.

According to WHO, nearly 1.3 billion people were at risk of cholera in endemic countries as of 2018. As with many infectious diseases, children are at a higher risk of getting sick with cholera and dying as a result of the disease. In crowded cities such as Kolkata and Jakarta, the incidence of cholera has been estimated to be between 1.2 and 6.2 of 1,000 children between the ages of two and four.

■ Treatment and Prevention

The most important treatment for cholera is fluid and electrolyte (salt) replacement to treat the losses caused by diarrhea and vomiting. Oral rehydration fluid, containing glucose and salt dissolved in water, is the most convenient form of this treatment. Eighty percent of all cases of cholera can be treated in this way, and the treatment needs to be continued until the diarrhea stops. Intravenous administration of rehydration fluid sometimes may be necessary. In countries where oral rehydration fluid is not available, water in which rice has been boiled provides a good alternative. According to WHO guidelines, if antibiotic treatment is needed, doxycycline is the first treatment choice, as it has been shown to shorten the duration of the disease. Ampicillin is a suitable alternative for children and pregnant women. Ciprofloxacin and azithromycin are alternatives in cases of doxycycline resistance. Drug resistance is frequently seen in cholera endemic areas and can make the treatment of cholera much more difficult.

Clean water and effective sanitation are the most effective preventive measures against cholera. Chlorination of water, boiling of water in households, and the construction and maintenance of latrines are basic measures that can help achieve these goals. High standards of personal hygiene and food preparation can also reduce the spread of the disease. Accurate and ongoing surveillance of outbreaks and epidemics can help reduce the toll from cholera.

In 2016 the US Food and Drug Administration (FDA) approved a single-dose oral cholera vaccine called Vaxchora. This vaccine is made up of live, weakened cholera bacteria and can be given to adults 18 to 64 years of age. This vaccine is recommended for people who are traveling to an area with endemic cholera or with a cholera epidemic. Vaxchora has been shown to reduce the severity of diarrhea by nearly 90 percent at 10 days after vaccination, and the protection persists for nearly three months after vaccination. Two other oral inactivated cholera vaccines are available. These are prequalified by WHO. However, they are not approved in the United States by the FDA.

According to WHO, since 2013 nearly 15 million doses of oral cholera vaccine have been used in mass vaccination campaigns. These campaigns have been undertaken in areas experiencing an outbreak and in areas of higher vulnerability to a cholera epidemic.

■ Impacts and Issues

Cholera is one of the great killers of all time. The characteristic symptoms of the disease were described by the Greek physician Hippocrates (c. 460 BCE–c. 357 BCE), and the disease is also mentioned by early Indian and Chinese writers. Epidemic cholera was first described in 1563 by Garcia del Huerto, a Portuguese physician working in Goa, India. The original "home" of cholera appears to be the Gangetic plains and delta in northern India and Bangladesh. From here it spread along trade routes, although for many centuries the disease was generally confined to India. Beginning in the 19th century, cholera began to spread around the world as trade expanded. Between 1817 and 1923, there were six pandemics. It was the second pandemic, beginning in 1824, that brought cholera to England (1831), North America (1832), and the Caribbean and Latin America (1833).

The seventh pandemic of cholera, caused by the *El Tor* serotype, began in 1961 and affected the Far East, although most of Europe was spared. During the 1980s outbreaks of cholera were common in refugee camps and city slums in famine and war-stricken countries such as Ethiopia and Sudan. The disease, carried by the *El Tor* serotype, returned to the Western Hemisphere in the early 1990s, beginning in Peru (where it had been absent for over 100 years) and spreading outward through Latin America. In 1992 a large epidemic in Bangladesh was attributed to the newly identified 0139 serotype.

The rapid onset and high mortality of cholera brought great fear to populations during the 19th century as it affected many areas for the first time. Many people thought the cause of cholera, and other diseases, was "miasma" or "bad air." Therefore, the standard treatment was to burn huge bonfires to cleanse the air. However, some blamed cholera on low morals and drunkenness. The belief that "cleanliness is next to godliness" at least led to the begin-

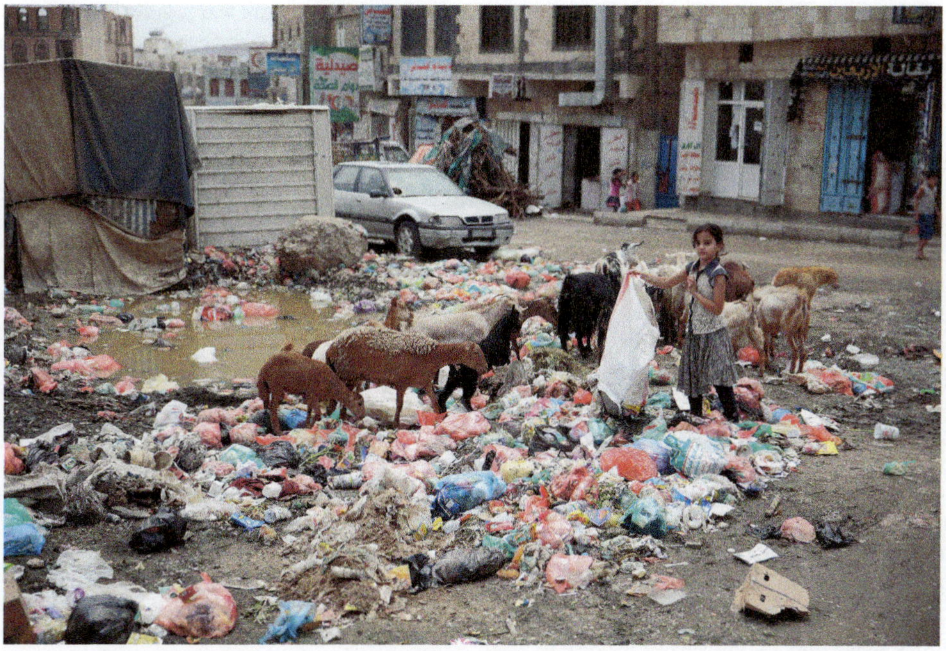

A girl picks over items at a garbage dump in Sanaa, Yemen. Yemen's civil war (2015–) created unsanitary conditions that precipitated the 21st century's most severe cholera outbreak. The outbreak killed over 2,000 people between fall 2016 and spring 2017. *© AP Images/Hani Mohammed*

nings of an interest in public health in England and America. Social reformers began to campaign for piped water, drains, and proper sewage disposal. Although these changes took many years to bring about, they eventually made a significant contribution toward cutting the death toll from cholera and many other infectious diseases.

It was the English physician John Snow (1813–1858) who suggested that contaminated water, rather than bad air, caused the transmission of cholera. He carried out a scientific investigation during the 1848 epidemic in London, which became the subject of his classic work, "On the Mode of Communication of Cholera." In August 1854 there was a fresh outbreak of cholera in and around Broad Street, near Snow's home. He suggested removing the handle from the Broad Street public water pump because he suspected it was the source of the outbreak. After the handle was removed, there were no more major cholera outbreaks in London.

Snow accepted the germ theory of disease, put forward by Louis Pasteur (1822–1895) and Robert Koch (1843–1910). In 1882 Koch discovered the bacillus that causes tuberculosis—also a major killer—and the following year, working in Egypt, he identified *V. cholerae* as the cause of cholera.

Thanks to Snow, Koch, and other researchers, cholera is a well-understood disease in scientific and clinical terms. The causative agents have been discovered, an effective cure is known, and there are vaccines against the disease. Its continuing prevalence is not due to a lack of scientific understanding or effective treatment and prevention options but to the economic and political factors in many countries that affect their level of development. According to WHO and its Global Task Force on Cholera Control (GTFCC), improvements in sanitation and access to clean water represent the only sustainable approach to cholera prevention and control. These factors are more important than drugs to treat the disease or vaccines to protect against it. In areas of the world afflicted by poverty or war (or both), high standards of public health are too often hard to achieve and sustain.

The response to cholera is often reactive—that is, dealing with an outbreak or epidemic once it has occurred. Fighting the threat of cholera requires a multidisciplinary approach involving a country's agriculture, water, health, and education sectors. Investment in infrastructure, including construction of water and sewage treatment plants, is key to improving public health. Long-term planning is needed so attention can be given not just to responding to cholera when it happens but also to prevention and surveillance. There is a need for far more openness and transparency on surveillance and reporting. Some countries fear that reporting a cholera outbreak will lead to travel and trade restrictions that will hurt their economy.

Because the above goals may be difficult to achieve in many countries, especially in urban slums and in crisis situations, the use of oral cholera vaccines as a complementary management tool is becoming more popular. For example, from 2002 to 2003, a mass vaccination campaign—the first in an endemic setting—was carried out in Beira, Mozambique, where there are yearly outbreaks. Vaccinated people were shown to have a high level of protection from cholera. Other mass vaccinations have been carried out in emergency settings, such as in Darfur in Sudan in 2004 and Haiti in 2016. These campaigns are challenging because they are costly and hard to implement, but WHO regards the experience gained as encouraging.

Cholera often is a seasonal disease, occurring each year during the rainy season. For example, in Bangladesh, where it is endemic, rates of cholera increase after the monsoons. This is related to an increase in the growth of algae during the rainy season in the watery environment inhabited by *V. cholerae*. The algae and bacteria form a mutually beneficial relationship, which allows the bacteria to survive indefinitely in contaminated water. Cholera is also associated with floods and cyclones and often spreads in times of war, especially in refugee camps, because upheaval and overcrowding cause the breakdown of basic facilities, such as water supply. For example, about 45,000 people died of cholera in refugee camps during the war in Rwanda in 1994. Likewise, more than 1 million refugees in Nigeria were considered at risk of cholera in late 2017 as outbreaks occurred among groups fleeing violence by the jihadist group Boko Haram.

The GTFCC has been considering how to improve the use of vaccination as a control tool. It is looking for ways to identify the populations most at risk and protocols for proper use of vaccines in complex emergency settings. Many countries are making significant efforts to control the spread of cholera. For example, there was an outbreak of more than 5,000 cases in Nigeria in 2017, including 61 deaths, but this outbreak was rapidly brought under control because the Nigerian government, in partnership with WHO and other international aid groups, was able to mount an effective emergency response. However, there are also increasing numbers of vulnerable people living in unsanitary conditions as a result of war, environmental degradation, and wealth inequality, leaving large swaths of the world at risk of a rapid and devastating outbreak of the disease.

PRIMARY SOURCE

Sick City

SOURCE: *Shapin, Steven. "Sick City."* New Yorker *(November 6, 2006).*

INTRODUCTION: *Sometimes the fear of disease can be as captivating as the reality. Although rare in industrialized nations for more than a century, cholera still raises a powerful and feared specter, especially following disasters that devastate local sanitation resources. The essay below reflects on the fear of widespread cholera following Hurricane Katrina's landfall along the Mississippi Gulf Coast and the devastation of New Orleans by flooding after levee breaks. The author, Steven Shapin, is Franklin L. Ford Professor of the History of Science at Harvard University. Shapin previously served as professor of sociology at the University of California, San Diego, and at Edinburgh University. He is a frequent contributor to the* New Yorker *magazine.*

After Katrina, cholera. On August 31, 2005—two days after the hurricane made landfall—the Bush Administration's Health and Human Services Secretary warned, "We are gravely concerned about the potential for cholera, typhoid, and dehydrating diseases that could come as a result of the stagnant water and other conditions." Around the world, newspapers and other media evoked the spectre of cholera in the United States, the world's hygienic superpower. A newspaper in Columbus, Ohio, reported that New Orleans was a cesspool of "enough cholera germs to wipe out Los Angeles." And a paper in Tennessee, where some New Orleans refugees had arrived, whipped up fear among the locals with the headline "KATRINA EVACUEE DIAGNOSED WITH CHOLERA."

There was to be no outbreak of cholera in New Orleans, nor among the residents who fled. Despite raw sewage and decomposing bodies floating in the toxic brew that drowned the city, cholera was never likely to happen: there was little evidence that the specific bacteria that cause cholera were present. But the point had been made: Katrina had reduced a great American city to Third World conditions. Twenty-first-century America had had a cholera scare.

Cholera is a horrific illness. The onset of the disease is typically quick and spectacular; you can be healthy one moment and dead within hours. The disease, left untreated, has a fatality rate that can reach fifty per cent. The first sign that you have it is a sudden and explosive watery diarrhea, classically described as "rice-water stool," resembling the water in which rice has been rinsed and sometimes having a fishy smell. White specks floating in the stool are bits of lining from the small intestine. As a result of water loss —vomiting often accompanies diarrhea, and as much as a litre of water may be lost per hour—your eyes become sunken; your body is racked with agonizing cramps; the skin becomes leathery; lips and face turn blue; blood pressure drops; heartbeat becomes irregular; the amount of oxygen reaching your cells diminishes. Once you enter hypovolemic shock, death can follow within minutes. A mid-nineteenth-century English newspaper report described cholera victims who were "one minute warm, palpitating, human organisms—the next a sort of galvanized corpse, with icy breath, stopped pulse, and blood congealed—blue, shrivelled up, convulsed." Through it all, and until the very last stages, is the added horror of full consciousness. You are aware of what's happening: "the mind within remains untouched and clear,—shining strangely through the glazed eyes ... a spirit, looking out in terror from a corpse."

You may know precisely what is going to happen to you because cholera is an epidemic disease, and unless you are fortunate enough to be the first victim you have probably seen many others die of it, possibly members of your own family, since the disease often affects households en bloc. Once cholera begins, it can spread with terrifying speed. Residents of cities in its path used to track cholera's approach in the daily papers, panic growing as nearby cities were struck. Those who have the means to flee do, and the refugees cause panic in the places to which they've fled. Writing from Paris during the 1831–32 epidemic, the poet Heinrich Heine said that it "was as if the end of the world had come." The people fell on the victims "like beasts, like maniacs."

Cholera is now remarkably easy to treat: the key is to quickly provide victims with large amounts of fluids and electrolytes. That simple regime can reduce the fatality rate to less than one per cent. In 2004, there were only five cases of cholera reported to the Centers for Disease Control, four of which were acquired outside the U.S., and none of which proved fatal. Epidemic cholera is now almost exclusively a Third World illness—often appearing in the wake of civil wars and natural disasters—and it is a major killer only in places lacking the infrastructure for effective emergency treatment. Within the last several years, there has been cholera in Angola, Sudan (including Darfur), the Democratic Republic of the Congo, and an arc of West African countries from Senegal to Niger. In the early nineteen-nineties, there were more than a million cases in Latin America, mass deaths from cholera among the refugees from Rwandan genocide in 1994, and regular outbreaks in India and Bangladesh, especially after floods. The World Health Organization calls cholera "one of the key indicators of social development." Its presence is a sure sign that people are not living with civilized amenities.

Of course, this is a state that continues to elude much of the world—including all those underdeveloped countries which are currently experiencing what epidemiologists call the Seventh Pandemic. The problem is no longer an incorrect understanding of the cause: around the world, people have known for more than a century what you have to do to prevent cholera. Rather, cholera persists because of infrastructural inadequacies that arise from such social and political circumstances as the Third World's foreign-debt burdens, inequitable world-trade regimes, local failures of urban planning, corruption, crime, and incompetence. Victorian London illustrates how much could be done with bad science; the continuing existence of cholera in the Third World shows that even good science is impotent without the resources, the institutions, and the will to act.

SEE ALSO *Public Health and Infectious Disease; Sanitation; War and Infectious Disease; Waterborne Disease*

BIBLIOGRAPHY

Books

Hamlin, Christopher. *Cholera: The Biography*. Oxford, UK: Oxford University Press, 2009.

Ramamurthy, T., and S. K. Bhattacharya, eds. *Epidemiological and Molecular Aspects on Cholera*. New York: Springer, 2011.

Periodicals

Allana, Alia. "How War Created the Cholera Epidemic in Yemen." *New York Times* (November 12, 2017). This article can also be found online at https://www.nytimes.com/2017/11/12/opinion/cholera-war-yemen.html (accessed February 12, 2018).

"Cholera Vaccines: WHO Position Paper, August 2017." *World Health Organization Weekly Epidemiological Record* 92, no. 34 (August 25, 2017): 477–500. This article can also be found online at http://apps.who.int/iris/bitstream/10665/258763/1/WER9234.pdf?ua=1 (accessed February 12, 2018).

Harmon, Katherine. "Why Is Cholera Spreading in Haiti Now?" *Scientific American* October 25, 2010. This article can also be found online at https://www.scientificamerican.com/article/cholera-outbreak-haiti/ (accessed February 12, 2018).

Websites

"Cholera." World Health Organization. http://www.who.int/gho/epidemic_diseases/cholera/en/ (accessed February 12, 2018).

"Cholera—Vibrio Holerae Infection." Centers for Disease Control and Prevention, October 27, 2014. https://www.cdc.gov/cholera/index.html (accessed February 12, 2018).

Dewan, Angela, and Henrik Pettersson. "Cholera Outbreak Hits Record 1 Million." CNN, December 21, 2017. https://www.cnn.com/2017/12/21/health/yemen-cholera-intl/index.html (accessed February 12, 2018).

"John Snow." University of California, Los Angeles, School of Public Health, Department of Epidemiology. http://www.ph.ucla.edu/epi/snow.html (accessed February 12, 2018).

Susan Aldridge
Malini Vashishtha

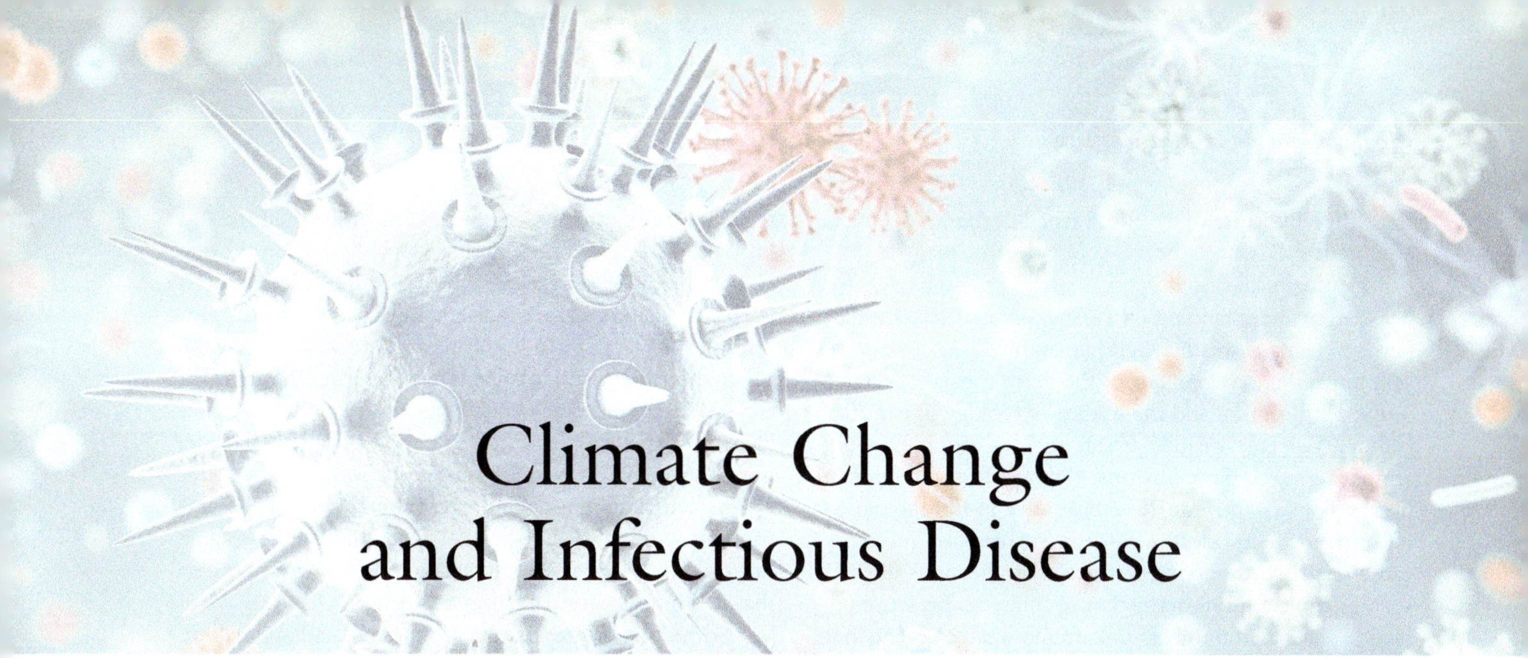

Climate Change and Infectious Disease

■ Introduction

Climate change is any change in the weather pattern over a given area that lasts longer than a single season. It may be local or worldwide. It may mean higher or lower than average temperatures, higher or lower than average rainfall, more or less frequent storms, or other shifts. Climate change can take place on a time scale of a few years, such as the El Niño climate oscillation, which recurs every three to eight years. Or it can be long term and nonreversible, such as the global climate change caused by burning of fossil fuels and unsustainable agricultural practices.

Climate change can interact in complex ways with infectious disease. It may encourage or discourage the growth of mosquitoes or other animals that spread disease, change the seasonal availability of hosts for pathogens, stimulate the evolution of new pathogens, or change temperatures or precipitation rates to make it more difficult to raise food or obtain clean drinking water. Scientists forecast that the global prevalence of some infectious diseases will increase in years to come if human-caused climate change continues unabated.

■ History and Scientific Foundations

The connection between climate and disease has long been suspected. More than 2,000 years ago, Greek physician Hippocrates (c. 460 BCE–c. 375 BCE) taught that weather was related to epidemics of infectious disease. In trying to understand such epidemics, doctors should, he said, have "due regard to the seasons of the year, and the diseases which they produce, and to the states of the wind peculiar to each country and the qualities of its waters." In the 17th century, English naturalist Robert Plot (1640–1696) wrote that, if humans could make weather observations over widely separated parts of the world at one time, they might "in

WORDS TO KNOW

ASYMPTOMATIC A state in which an individual does not exhibit or experience symptoms of a disease.

ECOLOGY The study of the relationships among communities of living things.

EPIDEMIC From the Greek *epidemic*, meaning "prevalent among the people," it is most commonly used to describe an outbreak of an illness or a disease in which the number of individual cases significantly exceeds the usual or expected number of cases in any given population.

GERM THEORY OF DISEASE A fundamental tenet of medicine that states that microorganisms, which are too small to be seen without the aid of a microscope, can invade the body and cause disease.

PATHOGEN A disease-causing agent, such as a bacterium, a virus, a fungus, or another microorganism.

PREVALENCE The actual number of cases of disease or injury that exist in a population.

REEMERGING DISEASE Many diseases once thought to be controlled are reappearing to infect humans again. These are known as reemerging diseases because they have not been common for a long period of time and are starting to appear again among large population groups.

VECTOR Any agent that carries and transmits parasites and diseases. Also, an organism or a chemical used to transport a gene into a new host cell.

time thereby learn to be forewarned certainly of divers emergencies (such as heats, colds, deaths, plagues, and other epidemical distempers)."

Better understanding of the complicated relationships between climate, weather, and human health has been possible since the development of the germ theory of disease in the 19th century and the science of ecology in the 20th century. Extreme weather events such as drought, flood, and heat waves have obvious, direct effects on human health. For example, the 2003 heat wave in Europe caused more than 70,000 deaths. Such events can also indirectly cause death by triggering outbreaks of infectious diseases such as cholera. Long-term climate shifts can be accompanied by increased numbers of extreme weather events but can also change the infectious disease picture in less obvious ways. Scientists in the 21st century are increasingly concerned with these subtle, long-term relationships between global climate change and infectious disease.

Global climate change is the shifting of climate and weather patterns throughout the world. Scientists have measured faster melting of glaciers and ice caps, rising sea levels, warmer winters, and hotter summers. The years 1998 to 2017 contained 10 of the hottest years on record. During that time sea levels rose at an average rate of 0.12 inches (3.4 millimeters) per year. Rainfall has increased in some parts of the world and decreased in others.

Global climate change has occurred naturally many times in the history of Earth. However, the phrase "global climate change" is most often used to refer to changes caused by human beings. Humans cause climate change by releasing gases into the atmosphere from agriculture and burning fossil fuels. These gases, especially carbon dioxide (CO_2), methane (CH_4), and nitrous oxide (NO), absorb infrared radiation (heat) radiated by Earth's surface, preventing the planet from losing heat to space. In effect, the atmosphere acts like a blanket wrapped around Earth. Increased greenhouse gas concentrations make it a warmer blanket. The atmospheric concentration of carbon dioxide, the most significant greenhouse gas, has increased by about 35 percent since the beginning of the Industrial Revolution in the mid-1700s. Scientists who study climate agree not only that global climate change is occurring but also that it is mostly caused by human activity.

Some of climate change's predicted effects include warmer weather, hotter and more frequent heat waves, more frequent and more violent weather events such as hurricanes, and increased or decreased precipitation depending on location. These changes affect the environmental pathways by which organisms contaminate food and drinking water supplies. They also affect human activities and how and where people live. These changes in turn can affect the prevalence of diseases borne by water, insects, and rodents. Diseases such as human immunodeficiency virus (HIV)/acquired immunodeficiency syndrome (AIDS), which involve organisms that are usually transmitted directly from person to person, are usually less likely to be affected by climate change. Disease organisms that spend a significant part of their life cycle outside the human body, such as the malaria parasite, are most likely to be affected by climate change.

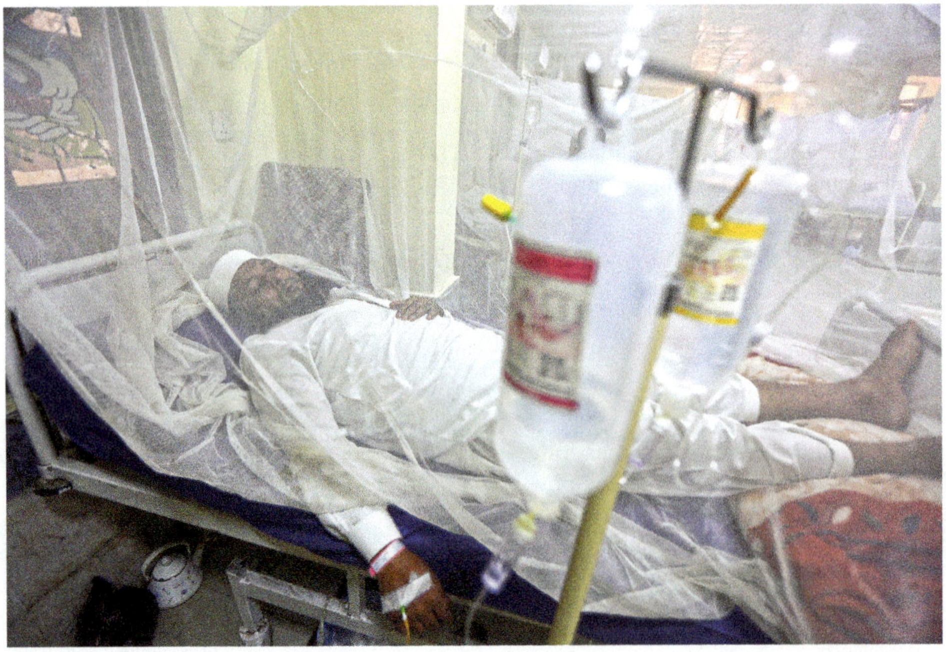

A patient suffers from dengue fever in Peshawar, Pakistan. Climate change, which allows mosquitoes to thrive in a wider range of areas around the world, has contributed to escalating rates of dengue fever since 1990. *© AP Images/Muhammad Sajjad*

Research

That global warming might someday be caused by human-released greenhouse gases was first proposed in 1890 by Swedish scientist Svante Arrhenius (1859–1927). The idea was revived by American physicist Stephen Schneider (1945–2010), among others, in the mid-1970s. By the 1990s climate scientists were in broad agreement that global warming is real and is primarily caused by humans. This view has been supported by on-the-ground weather and temperature observations and by satellite measurements of Earth's heat output.

As the reality of global climate change became clearer in the 1990s, scientists saw that it might have implications for infectious disease, especially diseases that are waterborne and vector-borne (transmitted through vectors such as insects). Malaria, a vector-borne disease that kills between 1 million and 3 million people per year, was studied intensively. Both the malaria parasite and the mosquitoes that transmit it to humans are affected by temperature. Mosquito populations are also affected by rainfall. Mosquitoes require stagnant water in which to breed. In general, increases in rainfall tend to mean more mosquitoes. Multiple studies have predicted that the mosquito that carries malaria will spread in to colder regions, thus allowing mosquitoes to transmit the disease in previously unaffected areas.

Impacts and Issues

Uncertainties

It is difficult to accurately predict the impact of climate change on human health for two reasons. First, forecasting climate change is difficult, especially over specific areas. Such forecasts can only be made using computer models, and these predictions always carry some level of uncertainty when the system being modeled is as complex as the weather. Predictions of average global effects (or continent-wide effects) are less uncertain but also less useful in predicting the effects of climate change on infectious diseases.

Second, infectious disease patterns depend not only on climate but also on human population size, population density, poverty, government prevention policies, and medical advances. For example, spending money to provide village water pumps in some African villages could tend to decrease disease from waterborne organisms and might offset some or all the negative effects—that is, those effects relating to waterborne disease of decreased rainfall. The development of a cheap, effective vaccine for malaria could also alter predictions of malaria's future prevalence. In 2017 there was a vaccine for malaria in the final stages of clinical trials, with pilot programs occurring in Ghana, Kenya, and Malawi in 2018.

Certain large-scale issues, however, are not in doubt. For example, extreme weather events such as severe hurricanes are predicted by climate models to become more common, and such events can cause outbreaks of infectious disease. In 1998, for example, Hurricane Mitch dropped 6 feet (1.8 meters) of rain over much of Central America. Besides the 11,000 people killed directly by flooding, there were 30,000 cases of malaria and 1,000 cases of dengue fever in Honduras in the aftermath of the rains. In India, during monsoon season, torrential rains trigger almost yearly outbreaks of malaria and dengue fever, among other diseases such as leptospirosis, a bacterial disease spread by the urine of infected animals, particularly rats. During the 2015 monsoon, for instance, 15,867 people in Delhi contracted dengue fever, and 60 died.

Some of the infectious disease effects of climate change are likely to involve drinking water. As of 2017 lack of clean drinking water, or water free of significant quantities of microbes, toxins, and parasites, was already one of the worst health problems in the world. At that time around 2 billion people had drinking water that was contaminated with feces. It has been estimated that diarrhea caused by waterborne microorganisms kills 842,000 people per year, and adequate sanitation could prevent the deaths of 361,000 children under five years old. The World Health Organization (WHO) predicts that climate change will cause 48,000 deaths from diarrhea between 2030 and 2050.

Climate change may cause food instability and undernutrition, which in turn may make some people more susceptible to some infectious diseases. The editors of the medical journal the *Lancet* wrote in December 2017 that "undernutrition has been identified as the greatest effect of climate change on health. Undernutrition is a leading risk factor for lower respiratory tract infections, and influences the severity of infections such as measles and diarrhoeal diseases. The complex and interconnected nature of infection and climate change needs to be appreciated, and understood."

Malaria, West Nile Virus, and Lyme Disease

About half of the world's population is vulnerable to infection by malaria. Malaria is a worsening problem due to the movement of people into malarial areas, destruction of forests, the evolution of resistance to pesticides by mosquitoes and to antimalarial drugs by malaria parasites, and the breakdown of public health facilities in some poor countries. Human-caused climate change is also contributing to the increasing prevalence of malaria and is likely to become a more important factor as time progresses.

Warmer temperatures can cause mosquitoes to mature more rapidly, breed over a longer season, and bite more often. Warmer climates can also speed the growth of malaria parasites in the insect's digestive system. Extreme weather events caused by climate change, which give rise to excessive rainfall and humidity, can also encourage the proliferation of mosquitos and thus the spread of malaria among humans. In Africa and Latin America, malaria is spreading to higher elevations in mountainous regions as the climate at those altitudes warms. Projects such as the Lubombo Spatial Development Initiative in South Africa, Mozambique, and Swaziland that use house-to-house insecticide spraying, systematic surveillance to detect malaria outbreaks, and improved medical care can greatly reduce malaria infection and death rates.

HIV/AIDS is sometimes cited as a disease that is unlikely to be affected by climate change. However, in 2007 researchers reported that infection with malaria tends to increase the viral load of people with HIV/AIDS, making it easier to transmit HIV to a sexual partner. Moreover, AIDS can help malaria spread by weakening the immune system and making it more likely that a person will catch malaria. As malaria will likely become more widespread because of climate change, the HIV/AIDS pandemic may be amplified.

West Nile virus claims fewer lives than many other infectious diseases but has received widespread publicity in North America due to its sudden reemergence in 1999 and subsequent rapid spread. The virus probably evolved about 1,000 years ago and was first identified in 1937. Outbreaks of West Nile have occurred since 1990 in Eastern Europe, Africa, and North America. Infection with the virus is most often asymptomatic. But in a minority of cases, it causes a debilitating or fatal infection of the central nervous system. The disease occurs throughout the continental United States.

Lyme disease is a bacterial disease transmitted to humans by the bites of ticks, a type of blood-sucking insect. Lyme disease is found in North America, Europe, China, and Japan. Although rarely fatal, it can be severely debilitating. Ticks require wild populations of deer and mice to thrive and to pass Lyme disease to human beings. Colder temperatures limit the tick's survival away from the mammal host, over 90 percent of the tick's life cycle. In the United States regrowth of forests in formerly agricultural areas has been the primary culprit in the increase of tick populations and the spread of Lyme disease. But scientists predict that climate change will play an increasing role in spreading Lyme disease. Warmer climates allow for larger tick populations and tend to spread Lyme disease to areas formerly protected by cold winters.

Mitigation

There is ongoing controversy over how to respond to climate change. Because change is already occurring, adaptation (changes in human practices in response to the effects of changing climate, including new infectious disease challenges) is also occurring. Many countries have agreed to mitigate climate change by stabilizing the amount of greenhouse gases in the atmosphere.

In 2015 almost every country in the world signed the Paris climate agreement, although the United States backed out of the agreement two years later. Signatory nations pledged to reduce their fossil fuel emissions to mitigate climate change and its associated environmental effects. The agreement encouraged countries to move away from fossil fuels toward greener forms of energy, such as wind and solar power, among others. However, even if signatory nations can meet the emissions targets laid out in the agreement, WHO predicted that climate change–related health care costs will range between $2 billion and $4 billion each year, beginning in 2030.

PRIMARY SOURCE

Climate Change May Accelerate Infectious Disease Outbreaks, Say Researchers: Study of Natural Disaster in Ecuador Showed 12-Fold Increase in Zika Cases

SOURCE: *"Climate Change May Accelerate Infectious Disease Outbreaks, Say Researchers: Study of Natural Disaster in Ecuador Showed 12-Fold Increase in Zika Cases."* Science Daily *(October 12, 2017). This article can also be found online at https://www.sciencedaily.com/releases/2017/10/171012122835.htm (accessed March 2, 2018).*

INTRODUCTION: *A 2017 study showed that Zika virus spread extremely quickly among humans after a major earthquake occurred in Ecuador in 2016 during the height of the Zika epidemic in the Americas. Researchers from the University of Colorado Anschutz Medical Campus proposed that climate change caused an exceptionally strong El Niño weather pattern that, in turn, caused increased rainfall in Ecuador. The increased rainfall allowed mosquitoes that carried Zika to flourish. Because the earthquake destroyed shelters, many people were forced to sleep outside and spend time outdoors, where they were susceptible to bites from Zika-infected mosquitos. Ultimately, the researchers argued, climate change, coupled with a natural disaster, caused a situation in which an infectious disease present in a mosquito population to spread more easily than usual.*

Aside from inflicting devastating natural disasters on often vulnerable communities, climate change can also spur outbreaks of infectious diseases like Zika, malaria and dengue fever, according to a new study by researchers at the University of Colorado Anschutz Medical Campus.

"Climate change presents complex and wide-reaching threats to human health," said Cecilia Sorensen, MD, lead author of the study and the Living Closer Foundation Fellow in Climate and Health Policy at CU Anschutz. "It can amplify and unmask ecological and socio-political weaknesses and increase the risk of adverse health outcomes in socially vulnerable regions."

When natural disasters strike such places, she said, the climatic conditions may make the public health crisis significantly worse.

The researchers said these vulnerabilities can happen anywhere. After Hurricane Katrina hit New Orleans, cases of West Nile disease doubled the next year. Climate change in Africa appears to be increasing cases of malaria. And the recent destruction in Houston, Florida and Puerto Rico due to hurricanes may usher in more infectious diseases in the years ahead.

The study focused specifically on a magnitude 7.7 earthquake that struck coastal Ecuador in April 2016, coinciding with an exceptionally strong El Niño event. El Niños are associated with heavy rainfall and warmer air temperatures. They are also linked to outbreaks of dengue fever.

Sorensen, a clinical instructor in emergency medicine at CU Anschutz, was in Ecuador with her co-authors working with the Walking Palms Global Initiative. They were operating a mobile health clinic after the disaster.

"We were seeing all of these viral symptoms in the wake of the quake," she said. "We noticed a huge spike in Zika cases where the earthquake occurred. Prior to this, there were only a handful of Zika cases in the whole country." In fact, the researchers found the number of Zika cases had increased 12-fold in the quake zone.

Zika virus is transmitted by mosquitos. Symptoms are usually mild but the infection can cause major abnormalities and even death in a developing fetus.

Warmer temperatures and increased rainfall from the El Niño, along with a devastated infrastructure and an influx of people into larger cities, likely caused the spike in Zika cases, Sorensen said.

"We saw so many people affected by the earthquake that were sleeping outside without any shelter from mosquitoes, so we were worrying that the region's changing climate could facilitate the spread of diseases," she said. "Natural disasters can create a niche for emerging diseases to come out and affect more people."

Sorensen's team reviewed the existing research on the link between short-term climate changes and disease transmission. They applied those findings to explain the role of the earthquake and El Niño in the Zika outbreak.

The researchers suggest El Niño created ideal conditions for Zika-carrying mosquitos to breed and make more copies of the Zika virus. The warmer temperatures and increased rainfall from El Niño have previously been associated with a higher likelihood of dengue outbreaks. Warmer temperatures can also accelerate viral replication in mosquitoes and influence mosquitos' development and breeding habits.

At the same time, the El Niño event brought warmer sea-surface temperatures, which have been shown to correlate with outbreaks of mosquito-transmitted diseases. Estimates from remote sensing data in coastal Ecuador show that sea-surface temperatures were higher than average from 2014–2016.

The team also believes an increase in water scarcity after the earthquake indirectly benefited mosquito development. The quake damaged municipal water systems, forcing people to store water in open containers outside their homes. These served as additional habitats for mosquito larvae.

The new findings could be used by governments to identify and protect vulnerable communities before natural disasters happen, Sorensen said.

"One idea is to develop disease models that can use existing climate models to predict where these vectors will show up due to climate variability," she said. "Applying these new models to areas that have pre-existing social vulnerabilities could identify susceptible regions, allowing us to direct healthcare resources there ahead of time."

SEE ALSO *Dengue and Dengue Hemorrhagic Fever; Lyme Disease; Malaria; Reemerging Infectious Diseases*

BIBLIOGRAPHY

Books

Leal, Filho W., Ulisses M. Azeiteiro, and Fátima Alves, eds. *Climate Change and Health: Improving Resilience and Reducing Risks.* Cham, Switzerland: Springer, 2016.

Periodicals

"Climate Change: The Role of the Infectious Disease Community." *Lancet Infectious Diseases* 17, no. 12 (December 2017): 1219. This article can also be found online at http://www.thelancet.com/journals/laninf/article/PIIS1473-3099(17)30645-X/fulltext (accessed March 2, 2018).

Robine, J. M., et al. "Death Toll Exceeded 70,000 in Europe during the Summer of 2003." *Comptes rendus Biologies* 331, no. 2 (February 2008): 171–178. This article can also be found online at https://www.ncbi.nlm.nih.gov/pubmed/18241810 (accessed March 2, 2018).

Saxena, Astha. "Delhi Hit by Dengue and Malaria Outbreaks as Monsoon Rains Boost Mosquito Numbers." *Daily Mail India* (July 18, 2017). This article can also be found online at http://www.dailymail.co.uk/indiahome/indianews/article-3696319/Delhi-hit-dengue-malaria-outbreaks-monsoon-rains-boost-mosquito-numbers.html (accessed March 2, 2018).

Websites

"Climate Change and Health." World Health Organization, July 2017. http://www.who.int/mediacentre/factsheets/fs266/en/ (accessed March 2, 2018).

"Climate Effects on Health." Centers for Disease Control and Prevention, July 26, 2016. https://www.cdc.gov/climateandhealth/effects/default.htm (accessed March 2, 2018).

"Drinking-Water." World Health Organization, July 2017. http://www.who.int/mediacentre/factsheets/fs391/en/ (accessed March 2, 2018).

Lindsey, Rebecca. "Climate Change: Global Sea Level." Climate.gov, September 11, 2017. https://www.climate.gov/news-features/understanding-climate/climate-change-global-sea-level (accessed March 2, 2018).

"The 10 Hottest Global Years on Record." Climate Central, January 18, 2018. http://www.climatecentral.org/gallery/graphics/the-10-hottest-global-years-on-record (accessed March 2, 2018).

Larry Gilman
Claire Skinner

Clostridium difficile Infection

Introduction

Clostridium difficile is an anaerobic, spore-forming bacterium that can produce toxins that cause stomachache, diarrhea, inflammation of the colon, and organ failure. In the elderly or in those with weakened immunity, *C. difficile* infection may prove fatal. Though *C. difficile* is naturally present in two-thirds of infants and 3 percent of adults, it does not usually cause problems in children or healthy adults. However, under certain conditions *C. difficile* proliferates, leading to the onset of symptoms of varying severity. Sick people, especially if they are on long-term antibiotic treatment, are especially vulnerable to *C. difficile* infections. Since the identification of a new and more virulent strain of *C. difficile* at the turn of the 21st century, efforts to combat infection have redoubled.

In 2013 the US Centers for Disease Control and Prevention (CDC) named *C. difficile* one of the three most urgent drug-resistant threats to the United States due to its pervasiveness, the excess medical cost it creates, and its deadliness. The CDC estimated the annual cost of *C. difficile* infections to be $4.8 billion. The growing prevalence,

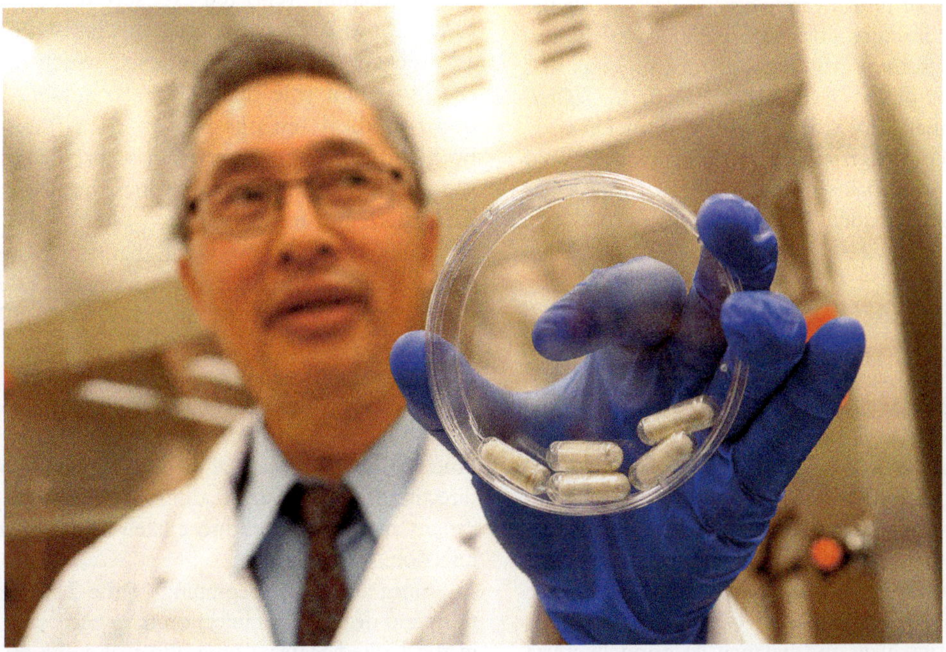

An infectious disease specialist with a container of stool pills in gel capsules. Patients suffering from *Clostridium difficile* infection often receive potent antibiotic treatments that leave their gut flora out of balance and susceptible to future infections. Recent studies show that regiments of stool pills from healthy donors can help patients maintain a healthy balance of gut flora. © AP Images/The Canadian Press/Jeff McIntosh

WORDS TO KNOW

ANAEROBIC BACTERIA Bacteria that grow without oxygen, also called anaerobic bacteria or anaerobes. Anaerobic bacteria can infect deep wounds, deep tissues, and internal organs where there is little oxygen. These infections are characterized by abscess formation, foul-smelling pus, and tissue destruction.

NORMAL FLORA The bacteria that normally inhabit some part of the body, such as the mouth or intestines, are normal flora. Normal flora are essential to health.

NOSOCOMIAL INFECTION An infection that is acquired in a hospital. More precisely, the US Centers for Disease Control and Prevention (CDC) in Atlanta, Georgia, defines a nosocomial infection as a localized infection or an infection that is widely spread throughout the body that results from an adverse reaction to an infectious microorganism or toxin that was not present at the time of admission to the hospital.

TOXIN A poison that is produced by a living organism.

cost, and virulence of *C. difficile* has led to various efforts to track down the cause of infections. Although poor hygiene on the part of health care workers—lack of regular handwashing, for instance—has been identified as the underlying cause of some outbreaks, evidence suggests that there may also be dietary factors that lead to *C. difficile* infections. A January 2018 article in the journal *Nature* presented evidence that growing *C. difficile* is likely related to consumption of trehalose, a naturally occurring sugar used with increasing frequency in food products.

Disease History, Characteristics, and Transmission

The characteristics of *C. difficile* infection vary widely. Often, an individual will harbor *C. difficile* bacterium in his or her gut for a prolonged period of time with no symptoms. In addition, levels of the naturally occurring bacterium tend to decline as a person ages. Although the factors that cause the bacteria to proliferate are not entirely understood, researchers have identified the use of antibiotics as a major cause of *C. difficile* infections because antibiotics alter the balance of good bacteria that helps keep *C. difficile* and other potentially harmful bacterium in check.

As *C. difficile* bacterium multiplies, it tends to cause colitis, an inflammation of the lining of the large intestine. Symptoms include watery diarrhea, loss of appetite, nausea, and abdominal pain and tenderness. In severe cases infection can cause more pronounced conditions, such as perforation of the colon, which leads to fever, vomiting, nausea, and stomach pain; peritonitis, an inflammation of the lining of the abdomen and its organs; or septicemia, a serious and potentially fatal blood infection. Symptoms can start during antibiotic treatment or weeks after it has ended. Nearly all antibiotics can result in *C. difficile* infection. More severe *C. difficile* infections occur in patients who are elderly or who are already dealing with medical conditions.

C. difficile bacteria are found in feces, and people can spread infection if they touch items or surfaces that are contaminated and then touch their mouth or eyes. *C. difficile* also forms spores that can survive for long periods on surfaces and clothes, so reinfection is common.

Scope and Distribution

In 2015 the CDC released a study of *C. difficile* infections in the United States over the course of 2011. According to this study, an estimated 500,000 *C. difficile* infections occurred annually. Of these, an estimated two-thirds were associated with inpatient stays in medical facilities, most often nursing homes and hospitals. Although approximately 150,000 infections occurred in people who "had no documented inpatient health care exposure," a separate study found that 82 percent of this population "reported exposure to outpatient health care settings such as doctor's or dentist's offices in the 12 weeks before their diagnosis." Such data point to the important role that hospitals, nursing homes, and other medical settings play in *C. difficile* infections, both through the transmission of bacteria and through the seeming overuse of antibiotics that allow the *C. difficile* bacterium to multiply.

The CDC study also found that people over the age of 65 were most vulnerable to the more severe effects of *C. difficile* infection. According to the CDC, 80 percent of those who died from infection in 2011 were in this age group, and 1 out of 11 people over 65 died within 30 days of being diagnosed with infection. Overall, approximately 29,000 cases of infection proved fatal within this 30-day time period. About half of these deaths could be attributed directly to *C. difficile.* In addition, evidence suggests Caucasians and women are more likely to contract *C. difficile* infection.

Since about the beginning of the 21st century, infections and deaths from infection have been on a marked rise in the United States, suggesting that some other factor or factors may be leading to increased incidence of *C. difficile* infection. Researchers have speculated that diet may contribute to *C. difficile* growth. A 2018 study linked increased consumption of a sugar known as trehalose to increased rates of *C. difficile* infection.

Treatment and Prevention

When treating *C. difficile* infection, physicians seek to restore the balance of the intestinal flora. The first step typically involves discontinuing the antibiotic that has triggered the condition. If this is not possible or is unsuccessful, further antibiotic treatment is used to get the infection under control. Vancomycin, metronidazole, and fidaxomicin are the three antibiotics most commonly prescribed for *C. difficile*. Although the FDA has not approved metronidazole for the treatment of *C. difficile*, physicians sometimes prescribe it in cases of mild initial infections. It is not used in cases of severe infection or for repeated reinfection. Reinfection occurs in about one of five patients who experience an initial *C. difficile* infection, and repeated reinfection occurs in a smaller subset of patients. When infection recurs multiple times, physicians may conduct a fecal transplant, in which stool from a noninfected person is moved to the patient's colon. Although such transplants have shown some promise in dealing with difficult cases of recurring *C. difficile* infection, more research is required to demonstrate the safety and efficacy of this treatment.

Diarrhea often leads to dehydration, so it is also important to restore fluids and salts when treating infection. Nonantibiotic treatment may sometimes be used to restore the intestinal flora. These may include *Lactobacillus* (as found in bioactive yogurts) and the yeast *Saccharomyces boulardii*.

Anyone infected with *C. difficile* can spread the infection to others, whether or not they have become ill themselves. Transmission can be prevented by washing hands with soap and water, especially after using the bathroom and before eating. Surfaces in bathrooms, kitchens, and other areas should be kept clean with detergent and disinfectant on a regular basis. Research also suggests that people at risk of infection during an outbreak in an inpatient medical setting, such as a hospital or a nursing home, can reduce the risk of infection by eliminating or reducing the amount of trehalose in their diet.

Impacts and Issues

C. difficile infection highlights the potential dangers of long-term broad-spectrum antibiotic treatment. Although these drugs can play a valuable role in bringing infectious diseases under control, they can also upset the natural balance of the normal intestinal flora (bacteria that do not normally cause disease or that serve a beneficial purpose and regularly inhabit the intestines). This sets the scene for the emergence of *C. difficile*, which may cause the patient a more serious health problem than that for which the antibiotic was initially prescribed. That is why physicians avoid routine prescription of broad-spectrum antibiotics, especially over the long term among the elderly.

According to a 2015 CDC report, reducing the use of antibiotics linked to *C. difficile* infections in hospitals by 30 percent led deadly infection to decline by at least 25 percent in patients who were or had been hospitalized recently. Studies published in 2004 and 2012 in England and Canada, respectively, support the notion that improved prescribing of antibiotics can reduce *C. difficile* infections. One study of English patients showed that *C. difficile* infections declined 60 percent after the implementation of changes in how antibiotics were prescribed. Although antibiotics play an important role in how infections emerge and are treated, other important factors contribute to *C. difficile* infections and outbreaks.

Beginning in 2001 and continuing through 2005, new and more virulent (and more antibiotic-resistant) forms of *C. difficile* emerged in Canada, the United States, and parts of Europe. People who contracted these new strains included those not previously identified as at risk for the infection, including nonhospitalized people, children, people not taking antibiotics, and one pregnant woman. In addition to infecting a wider range of people, this new strain of bacteria led to "a dramatic increase in deaths related to *C. difficile*," according to a 2017 *Nature* article by Jimmy D. Ballard. As this strain has spread globally since 2005, scientists have been working to identify it, understand why it emerged, and figure out how to combat it.

That research has found various new strains of *C. difficile*, many of which can be traced to a certain *C. difficile* bacteria known as ribotype 027 (or RT027). A second, related strain known as ribotype 078 (or RT078) has also been identified as emerging since the growth in *C. difficile* began in 2001. In a 2018 article in *Nature*, the authors argued that "the implementation of trehalose as a food additive into the human diet, shortly before the emergence of these two epidemic lineages [RT027 and RT078], helped select for their emergence and contributed to hypervirulence."

PRIMARY SOURCE

Food additive to blame for C. *difficile* epidemic

SOURCE: *Hewings-Martin, Yella. "Food Additive to Blame for C. difficile Epidemic." Medical News Today, January 4, 2018. https://www.medicalnewstoday.com/articles/320520.php (accessed January 31, 2018).*

INTRODUCTION: *This article from* Medical News Today *describes new research that shows that the simple sugar trehalose is the likely cause of the* C. difficile *epidemic.*

When *Clostridium difficile* infections rear their ugly head, patients are at serious risk. But no one knows what is behind the soaring number of infections. New research puts a food additive at the heart of the epidemic.

Clostridium difficile is a bacterium capable of causing life-threatening diarrhea, colitis, toxic megacolon, organ failure, and death.

According to the Centers for Disease Control and Prevention (CDC), *C. difficile* is currently "the most common microbial cause of healthcare-associated infections in U.S. hospitals and costs up to $4.8 billion each year."

In fact, *C. difficile* causes half a million infections and kills 15,000 people each year, the majority of whom are seniors. Yet these numbers used to be much lower.

Exactly why the past 20 years have seen a rising epidemic of *C. difficile* infections has remained a mystery—until now.

Writing in the journal *Nature* recently, researchers from Baylor College of Medicine in Houston, TX, and colleagues at the University of Oregon in Eugene, Leiden Medical Center in the Netherlands, and the Wellcome Trust Sanger Institute in Hinxton, United Kingdom, might have located the missing piece in the puzzle.

They point the finger squarely at a food additive, the simple sugar trehalose, which is widely used by the food industry.

The Rise of *C. difficile*

The turn of the century saw the emergence of epidemic strains of *C. difficile*, explains Jimmy D. Ballard—a professor in the Department of Microbiology and Immunology at the University of Oklahoma in Oklahoma City—in an accompanying article in the journal *Nature*.

Prof. Ballard explains that most of these strains originated from a single source: a type of *C. difficile* known as ribotype 027 (RT027), which spread from the U.S., Canada, and Europe around the world.

In 2013, the CDC classed the threat level of *C. difficile* as urgent, putting the bug in the top 3 of 18 drug-resistant microbes—well above tuberculosis and MRSA.

Robert A. Britton—who is a professor of molecular virology and microbiology at Baylor College of Medicine—and his team have been on the hunt for the answer for a number of years.

Prof. Britton pointed me in the direction of a study that the team published back in 2014, which showed that RT027 can outcompete other *C. difficile* strains in laboratory and animal models.

Based on this work, they decided to delve deeper to get to the bottom of what gives RT027 this advantage.

Hunt for the Missing Link

"To begin to ask this question we screened [around] 200 sugars and other carbon sources for their ability to support growth of RT027 strains better than other ribotypes," Prof. Britton explained.

"Through this screen," he continued, "we found that RT027 and a second hypervirulent, epidemic ribotype (ribotype 078) were able to grow on low concentrations of trehalose that do not support the growth of other *C. difficile* strains."

Trehalose is a naturally occurring sugar. It is a disaccharide, meaning that it is made up of two individual sugar molecules—in this case glucose. Trehalose can be found in fungi, algae, and other plants. The food industry uses the sugar to improve the texture and stability of food products.

Prof. Britton explains in his article that the use of trehalose was somewhat limited before the turn of the century; it cost approximately $7,000 to produce just 1 kilogram.

However, the discovery of an enzymatic process that allows trehalose to be extracted from corn starch brought this number down to just $3 per kilogram.

"Granted [the] 'generally recognized as safe' status by the U.S. Food and Drug Administration [FDA] in 2000 and approved for use in food in Europe in 2001," Prof. Britton reports, "reported expected usage ranges from concentrations of 2 percent to 11.25 percent for foods including pasta, ground beef, and ice cream."

Connecting the Dots

Prof. Britton and his team put the two strains of *C. difficile* to the test in order to find out what gives them the edge over other *C. difficile* strains when it comes to trehalose metabolism.

Interestingly, RT027 and RT078 achieve this in different ways. The RT027 strain has one mutation in a protein that normally represses the trehalose-metabolizing enzyme phosphotrehalase. This mutation switches off the repressor protein, allowing RT027 to use low levels of trehalose.

On the flipside, RT078 has four extra genes that support trehalose metabolism and allow it to grow much better in environments with low levels of trehalose than other strains.

Commenting on the results, Prof. Britton told me that "the most surprising finding of this work is that a dietary additive impacted the emergence of epidemic strains of *C. difficile* that have caused increased morbidity and mortality."

"The other surprise," he added, "is the fact that trehalose appears to directly increase the virulence of *C. difficile*." In fact, the team's research shows that while trehalose does not necessarily increase the number of RT027 bacteria, it does allow the bugs to produce significantly more bacterial toxins, which are responsible for the gut-wrenching symptoms that many patients experience.

But how much trehalose would I need to consume to allow these potentially deadly bugs to take a foothold in my gut?

In the study, the scientists tested fluid collected from the small intestine of three volunteers who consume a normal diet. The results revealed that there was enough trehalose to support the growth of RT027 but not other strains of *C. difficile*.

Does this mean that I should be looking to reduce my trehalose consumption?

The 'Unexpected Culprit'

I asked Prof. Britton whether he thought that the use of trehalose in food will be restricted based on these data. He didn't think so.

"What this work does suggest is that if a hospital or long-term nursing care facility has an outbreak of *C. difficile* caused by a RT027 or RT078 strain, then patients' diets should be modified to restrict trehalose consumption," he suggested instead.

The biggest group of people at risk of *C. difficile* infection are over 65, and particularly those who are taking antibiotics and find themselves in a healthcare setting such as a hospital.

For the rest of the population, *C. difficile* poses less of a threat. However, the CDC are very clear in their objective that "preventing *C. difficile* is a national priority."

Prof. Britton and his colleagues are certainly doing their bit. "We are working now to understand how trehalose increases disease severity of *C. difficile* strains that can metabolize low concentrations of trehalose," he told me.

"We are also screening," he continued, "emerging *C. difficile* strains from hospitals for their ability to consume trehalose and other dietary sugars to further investigate the link between the diet and *C. difficile* infection."

While there are many questions still to be answered by the scientists, the link between trehalose and *C. difficile* is part of an emerging theme showing that our diet seems to play an increasingly crucial role in how our gut microbes behave in sickness and health.

SEE ALSO *Antibiotic Resistance; Nosocomial (Health Care–Associated) Infections; Resistant Organisms; Vancomycin-Resistant Enterococci*

BIBLIOGRAPHY

Books

O'Neal, Christopher, Raf Rizk, and Marianne Khalil. Clostridium difficile: *A Patient's Guide.* Tustin, CA: Inner Workings, 2011.

Wilcox, Mark H., ed. Clostridium difficile *Infection: Infectious Disease Clinics of North America.* London: Elsevier Health Sciences, 2015.

Wilson, Walter R., and Merle A. Sande. *Current Diagnosis & Treatment in Infectious Diseases.* New York: McGraw Hill, 2001

Periodicals

Ballard, Jimmy D. "Pathogens Boosted by Food Additive." *Nature* (December 21, 2017). This article can also be found online at https://www.nature.com/articles/d41586-017-08775-4 (accessed February 1, 2018).

Collins, J., et al. "Dietary Trehalose Enhances Virulence of Epidemic *Clostridium difficile.*" *Nature* 553 (2018): 291–294. This article can also be found online at https://www.nature.com/articles/nature25178 (accessed February 1, 2018).

Websites

"*C. Difficile* Infection." American College of Gastroenterology, July 2016. http://patients.gi.org/topics/c-difficile-infection/ (accessed January 31, 2018).

"*Clostridium difficile* Infection Information for Patients." Centers for Disease Control and Prevention, February 24, 2015. https://www.cdc.gov/hai/organisms/cdiff/cdiff-patient.html (accessed January 31, 2018).

"*Clostridium difficile* Infections." MedlinePlus, October 20, 2017. https://medlineplus.gov/clostridiumdifficileinfections.htmlhttps://medlineplus.gov/clostridiumdifficileinfections.html (accessed January 31, 2018).

Hewings-Martin, Yella. "Food Additive to Blame for *C. difficile* Epidemic." Medical News Today, January 4, 2018. https://www.medicalnewstoday.com/articles/320520.php (accessed January 31, 2018).

"Nearly Half a Million Americans Suffered from *Clostridium difficile* Infections in a Single Year." Centers for Disease Control and Prevention, February 25, 2015. https://www.cdc.gov/media/releases/2015/p0225-clostridium-difficile.html (accessed January 31, 2018).

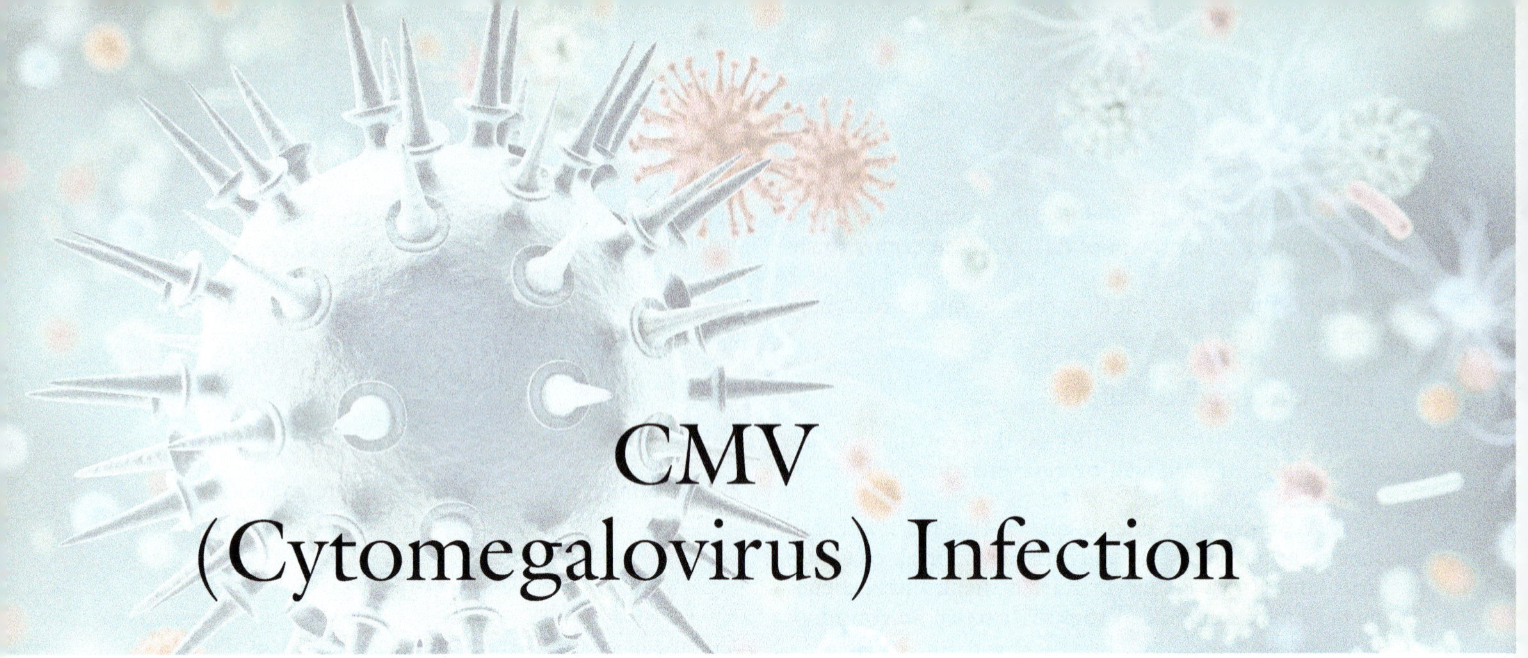

CMV (Cytomegalovirus) Infection

Introduction

Cytomegalovirus (si-to-MEG-a-lo-vi-rus), or CMV, is among the most common viruses infecting human beings. In healthy people it rarely causes any symptoms. However, it is of concern in people who have weakened immunity, such as organ transplant recipients and those with human immunodeficiency virus (HIV) or acquired immunodeficiency syndrome (AIDS). In addition, some babies born with CMV infection, transmitted in the womb, may suffer from severe health problems.

CMV belongs to the herpes family of viruses, all of which exist as viral particles of around 200 nanometers in diameter, consisting of a protein exterior enclosing a molecule of double-stranded deoxyribonucleic acid (DNA). Other significant herpes viruses include the herpes simplex viruses, varicella-zoster virus (which causes chickenpox), and Epstein-Barr virus. CMV may lie dormant in white blood cells for many years, but the infection can be reactivated at any time. CMV cannot be eliminated, but symptoms of active infection can be treated with antiviral drugs. Efforts to create a preventive vaccine were ongoing as of 2018.

Disease History, Characteristics, and Transmission

CMV infects a variety of cell types, including neurons, smooth muscle cells, and fibroblasts, which are found in skin and connective tissue. In most people the infection lies dormant. However, some people may experience symptoms similar to those of mononucleosis, including fever, swollen glands, fatigue, and sore throat. In fact, in some cases, CMV may lead to mononucleosis. Because the symptoms of mononucleosis mimic those of many other conditions, it can be difficult to determine that CMV is responsible.

For people with weakened immunity, including those with HIV/AIDS or organ transplant recipients, CMV can become a serious problem because the immune system is unable to keep the virus in check. This group may experience complications such as retinitis (an eye infection that can lead to blindness) and problems with the digestive and nervous systems. CMV may also cause potentially fatal pneumonia among organ transplant recipients because they

WORDS TO KNOW

ANTIBODIES Proteins found in the blood that help fight against foreign substances called antigens. Antigens, which are usually proteins or polysaccharides, stimulate the immune system to produce antibodies, or Y-shaped immunoglobulins. The antibodies inactivate the antigen and help remove it from the body. While antigens can be the source of infections from pathogenic bacteria and viruses, organic molecules detrimental to the body from internal or environmental sources also act as antigens. Genetic engineering and the use of various mutational mechanisms allow the construction of a vast array of antibodies (each with a unique genetic sequence).

CONGENITAL Existing at the time of birth.

FIBROBLAST A cell type that gives rise to connective tissue.

HORIZONTAL TRANSMISSION The transmission of a disease-causing microorganism from one person to another, unrelated person by direct or indirect contact.

IMMUNOSUPPRESSION A reduction of the ability of the immune system to recognize and respond to the presence of foreign material.

SHED To cast off or release. In medicine, the release of eggs or live organisms from an individual infected with parasites is often referred to as shedding.

take immunosuppressant drugs to protect the new organ. Another group at risk of CMV infection includes newborns, who may become infected in the womb. Congenital CMV infection can lead to many problems, including deafness and intellectual disability, some of which may not become apparent until the child gets older.

Transmission of CMV is by contact with infected body fluids such as blood, semen, vaginal fluid, tears, urine, and saliva. The infection is not spread by casual contact. A woman can transmit CMV to her unborn child through the placenta while he or she is still in the womb, by exposure to cervical fluids during childbirth, or through breast milk. Infected children shed the virus in urine and other fluids for years and may transmit the infection horizontally to other children and adult caregivers in a nursery group setting.

Scope and Distribution

The US Centers for Disease Control and Prevention (CDC) estimates that almost one-third of children in the United States are infected with CMV by the time they reach five years of age. More than half of all Americans are infected by the time they reach 40. Worldwide, rates of CMV infection vary. Countries such as the United States that have rates of infection between 50 and 70 percent are considered to have relatively low prevalence of CMV, whereas countries with infection rates of about 70 percent are considered to have high prevalence. Countries with a high prevalence of CMV include Brazil, India, and South Africa.

According to a 2011 article in *Clinical and Vaccine Immunology*, an estimated 0.7 percent of babies are born with CMV infections worldwide. This study also found that between 15 and 20 percent of infected infants suffer from permanent disability resulting from congenital CMV infection. A 2013 article in *Clinical Microbiology Reviews* noted that "human cytomegalovirus (CMV) is a leading cause of congenital infections worldwide."

CMV infection is widespread but is generally contained by the immune system. However, if the immune system begins to break down, infection will take hold, which is why HIV/AIDS patients and organ transplant recipients are at risk of infection, as they are from many other normally harmless microbes, such as *Candida*. Evidence also suggests that the children of HIV-positive mothers are more likely to have congenital CMV infection, even if the mother is undergoing antiretroviral therapy.

Treatment and Prevention

CMV does not respond to the antiviral drug acyclovir but is sensitive to a closely related drug called ganciclovir, which has been shown to reduce the complications of CMV-induced mortality among immunosuppressed people. Foscarnet, cidofovir, and valganciclovir are other antiviral drugs used in the treatment of CMV. Preemptive antiviral treatment is recommended for transplant

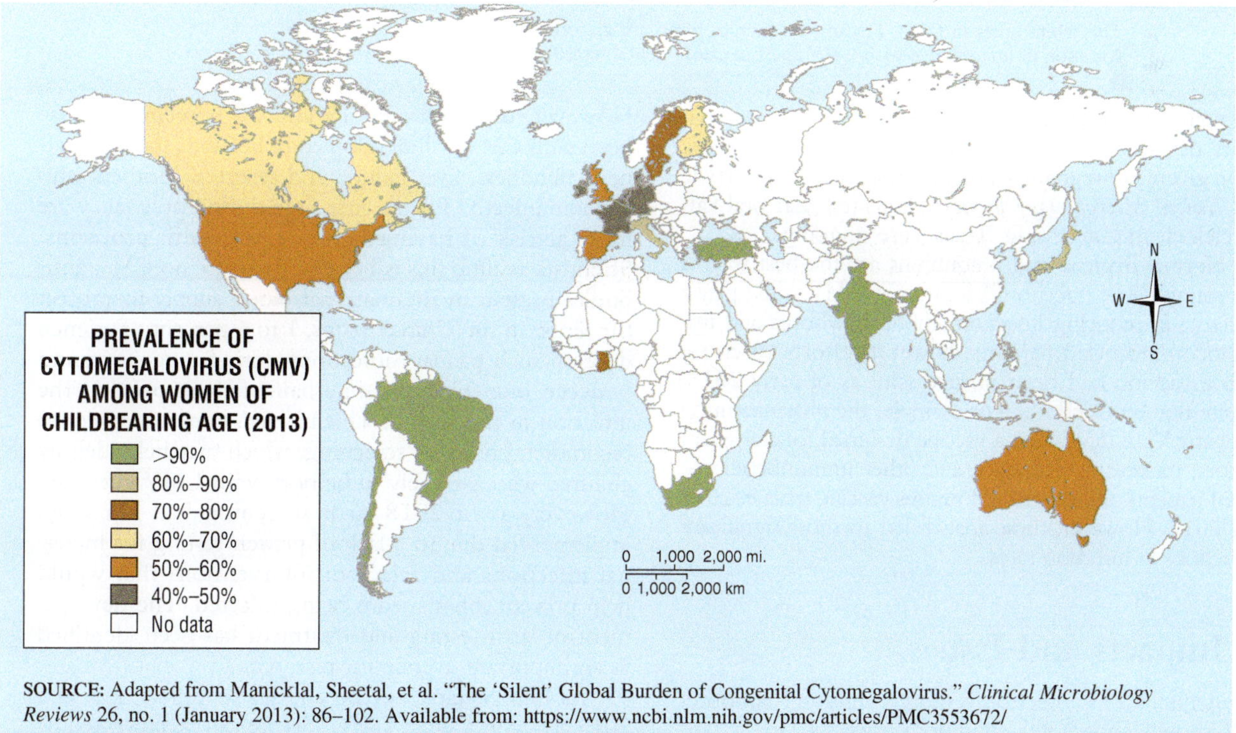

SOURCE: Adapted from Manicklal, Sheetal, et al. "The 'Silent' Global Burden of Congenital Cytomegalovirus." *Clinical Microbiology Reviews* 26, no. 1 (January 2013): 86–102. Available from: https://www.ncbi.nlm.nih.gov/pmc/articles/PMC3553672/

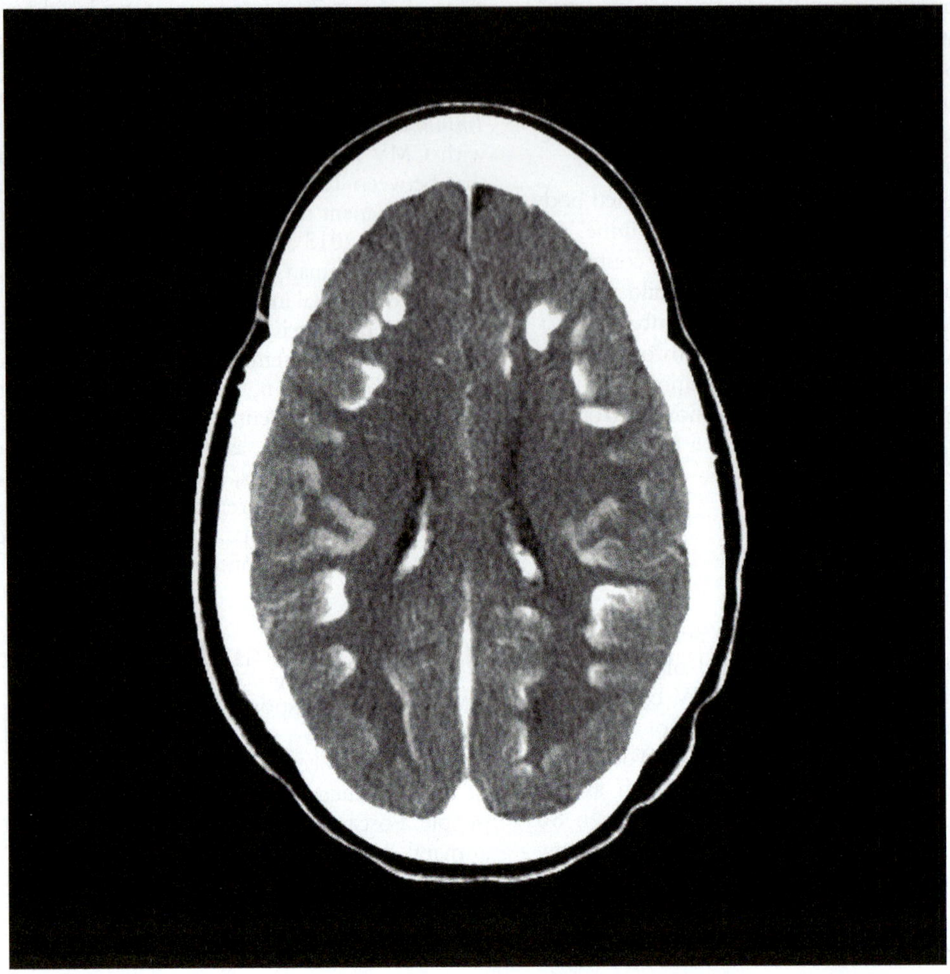

The white areas in this CT scan of a human brain are abnormal calcifications. Such calcifications are common in infants born with CMV and can cause mental retardation. *© Living Art Enterprises/Science Source*

recipients, as between 30 and 75 percent of these patients develop CMV infection. Ganciclovir is too toxic to be given to pregnant women, however, a 2013 article in *Clinical Microbiology Reviews* indicated that oral valganciclovir might be safe. Trials were ongoing.

Normal hygiene and precautions are the best way of preventing CMV infection. Vaccines for CMV could play a vital role in reducing infection among newborns and immunocompromised patients, however, efforts to create such a vaccine had been unsuccessful as of early 2018, despite numerous efforts. For example, the pharmaceutical company Vical developed a vaccine designed for transplant donors, transplant recipients, and other immunocompromised patients and conducted various vaccine trials in 2016 and 2017. However, these trials failed to show significant reductions in infection rates.

■ Impacts and Issues

Congenital CMV infection is more common than other well-known congenital conditions such as Down syndrome, fetal alcohol syndrome, and neural tube defects. However, only between 15 and 20 percent of those born with CMV will develop complications such as deafness, blindness, liver failure, and seizures. Mothers who become infected for the first time during pregnancy are most at risk of having babies with health problems. Scientists assume this is because there are no CMV antibodies present in the maternal blood supply to protect the fetus. In the United States, 1 to 4 percent of women develop such primary infections during pregnancy, and between one-third and one-half of these pass on the infection in the womb. This has led some observers to recommend prenatal screening, which may help identify children who are likely to be born with CMV infection. However, as of 2018 such screening had not been implemented due to a lack of proven testing for maternal infections and a lack of interventions that would help prevent infants from being infected. The development of such testing and treatment has been identified as an important avenue for research.

As Luiz Sergio Azevedo and his coauthors note in a 2015 article in *Clinics*, CMV "disease can be prevented by prophylaxis (the administration of antiviral drugs to all or to a subgroup of patients who are at higher risk of viral replication) or by preemptive therapy (the early diagnosis of viral replication before development of the disease and prescription of antiviral treatment to prevent the appearance of clinical disease)." Although both prophylaxis and preemptive therapy have been shown to be safe and effective, Azevedo and his coauthors note that no consensus on which therapy is preferable has yet been reached. In fact, some transplant centers use both methods to reduce risk of infection.

The most effective means of reducing CMV infection would likely be a vaccine. Although the development of such a vaccine has proven difficult, research and development were ongoing as of early 2018. In a 2016 survey of ongoing CMV vaccine-development efforts published in *Journal of Virus Eradication*, Mark R. Schleiss noted that "a vaccine against congenital CMV infection would have the greatest public health impact and cost-effectiveness," due to severity of congenital infections. Schleiss also observed that there is an "increased interest in developing and testing potential candidates" due to some promising data about the potential for an effective vaccine to be developed.

See Also *AIDS (Acquired Immunodeficiency Syndrome; Antiviral Drugs; Chickenpox (Varicella); Epstein-Barr Virus; Herpes Simplex 1 Virus; Herpes Simplex 2 Virus; HIV; Shingles (Herpes Zoster) Infection*

BIBLIOGRAPHY

Books

Guibert, Hervé. *Cytomegalovirus: A Hospitalization Diary*. Translated by Clara Orban. New York: Fordham University Press, 2016.

Shenk, Thomas E., and Mark F. Stinski, eds. *Human Cytomegalovirus*. Berlin: Springer Berlin, 2014.

Periodicals

Azevedo, Luiz Sergio, et al. "Cytomegalovirus Infection in Transplant Recipients." *Clinics* 70, no. 7 (2015:; 515–523. This article can also be found online at https://www.ncbi.nlm.nih.gov/pmc/articles/PMC4496754/ (accessed February 5, 2018).

Dollard, Sheila C., et al. "National Prevalence Estimates for Cytomegalovirus IgM and IgG Avidity and Association between High IgM Antibody Titer and Low IgG Avidity." *Clinical and Vaccine Immunology* 18, no. 11 (2011): 1895–1899.

Manicklal, Sheetal, et al. "The 'Silent' Global Burden of Congenital Cytomegalovirus." *Clinical Microbiology Reviews* 26, no. 1 (2013): 86–102. This article can also be found online at https://www.ncbi.nlm.nih.gov/pmc/articles/PMC3553672/ (accessed February 5, 2018).

Rychman, Brent J., et al. "Human Cytomegalovirus Entry into Epithelial and Endothelial Cells Depends on Genes UL128 to UL150 and Occurs by Endocytosis and Low-pH Fusion." *Journal of Virology* 80, no. 2 (2006): 710–722. This article can also be found online at http://jvi.asm.org/content/80/2/710.full (accessed February 5, 2018).

Schleiss, Mark R. "Cytomegalovirus Vaccines under Clinical Development." *Journal of Virus Eradication* 2, no. 4 (2016): 198–207. This article can also be found online at https://www.ncbi.nlm.nih.gov/pmc/articles/PMC5075346/ (accessed February 13, 2018).

Websites

"Cytomegalovirus (CMV) and Congenital CMV Infection." Centers for Disease Control and Prevention, June 5, 2017. https://www.cdc.gov/cmv/index.html (accessed February 2, 2018).

"$8.9 Million Collaborative Grant to Understand How Dangerous Virus 'Hides' to Attack Another Day." EurekAlert, January 23, 2018. https://www.eurekalert.org/pub_releases/2018-01/uoah-cg012318.php (accessed February 2, 2018).

Liu, Angus. "Vical's Astellas-Partnered CMV Vaccine Falls Short Again, This Time in Stem Cell Transplant Recipients." FiercePharma, January 22, 2018. https://www.fiercepharma.com/vaccines/vical-s-astellas-partnered-cmv-vaccine-failed-phase-3 (accessed February 2, 2018).

Nordqvist, Christian. "Everything You Need to Know about Cytomegalovirus." Medical News Today, January 11, 2018. https://www.medicalnewstoday.com/articles/173811.php (accessed February 2, 2018).

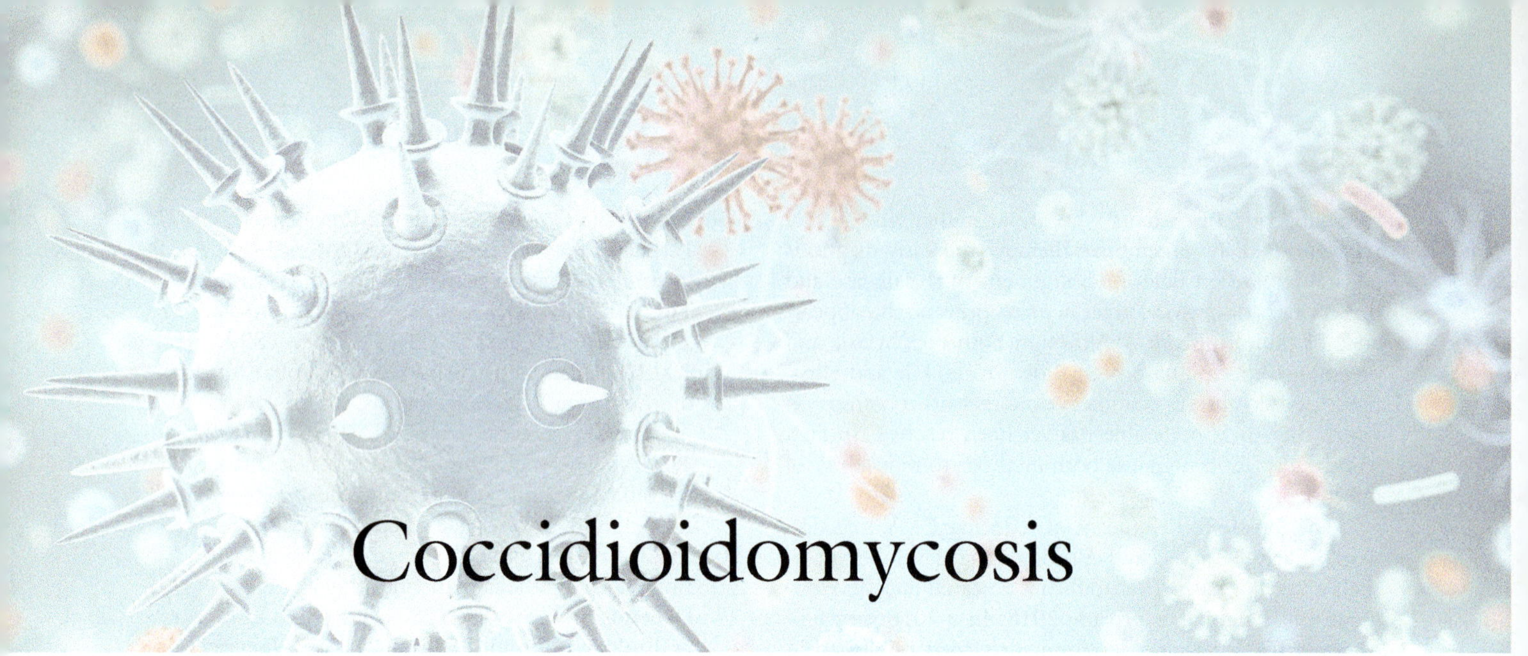

Coccidioidomycosis

Introduction

Coccidioidomycosis, commonly known as valley fever and also called simply cocci, is a fungal disease caused by the spores (tiny seeds) of the fungi *Coccidioides immitis* and *C. posadasii*, which have only slight differences. The fungi are classified as dimorphic, meaning that they exist both as mold and as yeast. *C. immitis* is found in infected soil in California, while *C. posadasii* is endemic to the Sonoran climates of the southwestern United States, northwestern Mexico, and other isolated areas within the Western Hemisphere. Over the course of the early 21st century, cases of valley fever have risen sharply in the American Southwest, with rates of infection reaching epidemic proportions in parts of Arizona and California.

The rise in coccidioidomycosis infection has been attributed to an increase in construction, which involves disturbing soil containing *C. immitis* and *C. posadasii* spores that people subsequently inhale. In many cases the disease causes no symptoms in the infected person. Symptoms of valley fever, when they are present, are similar to those of influenza, including fever, fatigue, and headaches. While these symptoms usually self-resolve, about 5 to 10 percent of people with coccidioidomycosis experience symptoms that persist beyond the usual period of a few weeks or months. In cases of severe valley fever, patients may develop lasting problems with their lungs or, less often, with their skin, bones and joints, or central nervous system. The most serious cases of coccidioidomycosis occur when spores infect the meninges, the protective membranes covering the brain and spinal column. Cases of cocci meningitis are often fatal.

As the incidence and severity of coccidioidomycosis have increased, medical professionals have developed methods of diagnosing infections with greater accuracy. While this has helped improve the tracking of infections, epidemiologists suspect that coccidioidomycosis remains underreported.

WORDS TO KNOW

ACUTE INFECTION An infection of rapid onset and of short duration that either resolves or becomes chronic.

CHRONIC Chronic infections persist for prolonged periods of time—months or even years—in the host. This lengthy persistence is due to a number of factors, which can include masking of the disease-causing agent (e.g., bacteria) from the immune system, invasion of host cells, and the establishment of an infection that is resistant to antibacterial agents.

DIMORPHIC The occurrence of two different shapes or color forms within the species, usually occurring as sexual dimorphism between the males and females.

ENDEMIC Present in a particular area or among a particular group of people.

IMMUNOCOMPROMISED Having an immune system with reduced ability to recognize and respond to the presence of foreign material.

Disease History, Characteristics, and Transmission

Coccidioidomycosis was first described in 1892 in Argentina. A year later a similar infection was reported in San Francisco. In 1905 physician William Ophüls published an article summarizing what was then known about what he deemed "coccidioidal granuloma," which has since come to be known as coccidioidomycosis. As the southwestern United States became increasingly populated and developed over the course of the 20th century, reports of coccidioidomycosis increased, as did medical insight about its causes, characteristics, transmission, and treatment.

The disease occurs in acute, chronic, and disseminated forms. Acute coccidioidomycosis is rare, with few or no symptoms. According to the National Institutes of Health, only about 3 percent of people contract the acute form. For those who do experience symptoms, the incubation period typically lasts 7 to 21 days. Symptoms tend to resemble those of the flu in mild cases of coccidioidomycosis and pneumonia in more severe cases.

In mild cases symptoms can include cough, headache, fever, skin rash (on the lower legs), and muscle and joint pain and stiffness. In more severe cases, symptoms include chest pain, chills, night sweats, neck or shoulder stiffness, blood-tinged sputum, loss of appetite and weight loss, wheezing, changes in behavior, joint swelling (ankles, feet, legs), arthritis, and light sensitivity. According to the US Centers for Disease Control and Prevention (CDC), approximately three-quarters of people with coccidioidomycosis experience symptoms that cause them to miss work or school. Some cases resolve on their own and are not treated medically. However, in 40 percent of cases, people with coccidioidomycosis are hospitalized, according to the CDC.

With chronic infection, the fungus enters internal tissues and organs, such as the meninges, joints, heart, and bone. It can also produce neurologic damage and tumors. People with compromised immune systems are especially affected by the chronic form of the disease. Coccidioidomycosis is not always recognized upon examination, but it does show up as nodules or cavities in the lungs. If diagnosis takes years, these lung abscesses can rupture. The chronic form occurs in 5 to 10 percent of infected patients.

Disseminated coccidioidomycosis is the least common form of the disease, occurring in less than 1 percent of patients. Disseminated coccidioidomycosis occurs when spores spread to the lungs, bones (ankles, knees, feet, pelvis, wrists), organs (adrenal glands, gastrointestinal tract, liver, thyroid), meninges, brain, skin, and heart. Meningitis is the most serious complication that can result from coccidioidomycosis, and it is usually fatal.

Transmission almost always occurs by inhalation of airborne dust containing the fungal spores. The fungus can also be contracted through the skin from infected soil, but this is rare. When they travel into the lungs, the spores grow into spherical cells called spherules. The spherules enlarge, divide, and explode into numerous particles about 2 to 5 micrometers (1 micrometer equals 1 millionth of a meter) in size. While the spores typically remain in the respiratory system, they move to other parts of the body in cases of disseminated coccidioidomycosis.

Coccidioides spores grow in soil and are dispersed by wind. Dispersal typically occurs after soil is disturbed by artificial means (such as through farming, excavation, or construction) or by natural events (including earthquakes and dust storms). Black and Filipino people are at higher risk than people in other ethnic groups. People over 60 years of age, people with diabetes, women in the third

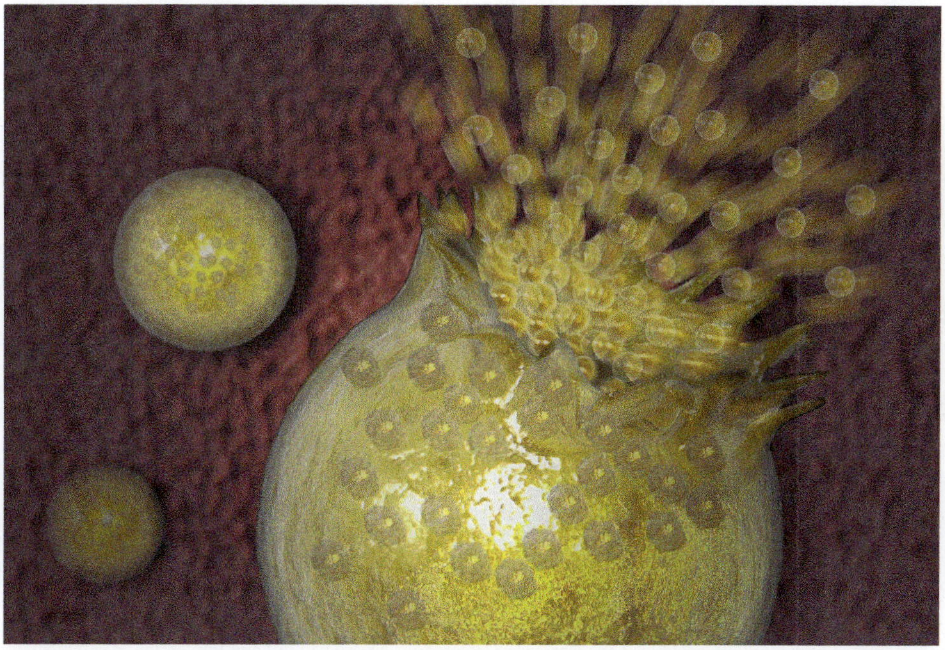

In chronic cases nodules of coccidioidomycosis can grow undetected in the lungs for years before bursting and further spreading the fungal disease. © *Carol and Mike Werner/Science Source*

trimester of pregnancy, and immunocompromised individuals, including those with HIV and organ-transplant recipients, are also at higher risk.

Scope and Distribution

Coccidioides occurs only in the Western Hemisphere, as far north as Washington state and as far south as Argentina, where *Coccidioides* spores can be found growing in areas with alkaline soils, hot summers, and annual rainfalls of 5 to 20 inches (13 to 50 centimeters). Evidence suggests *C. immitis* is restricted to California, where coccidioidomycosis is prevalent and on the rise. The San Joaquin Valley, which is located in the central part of the state, is a particular hot spot for infections. *C. posadasii* is found elsewhere, in semiarid and desert regions of the southwestern and western United States (specifically Arizona, Nevada, New Mexico, Texas, Utah, and Washington), the northern part of Mexico, and parts of Central and South America, including Argentina, Brazil, Colombia, Guatemala, Honduras, Paraguay, and Venezuela.

Beginning in the mid-1990s, epidemiologists noticed a spike in cases of coccidioidomycosis in the American Southwest. According to a 2013 article in the CDC's *Morbidity and Mortality Weekly Report*, "The incidence of reported coccidioidomycosis increased substantially during this period [of 1998–2011], from 5.3 per 100,000 population in the endemic area (Arizona, California, Nevada, New Mexico, and Utah) in 1998 to 42.6 per 100,000 in 2011." As of 2014 there were approximately 150,000 reported cases of coccidioidomycosis in the United States. Some two-thirds of cases occur in Arizona, where it is the second-most-reported disease.

Treatment and Prevention

Diagnosis can be made in a variety of ways, including recovery of *Coccidioides immitis* from cultures and smears of sputum or other body fluid; blood tests showing the body's reaction to fungal presence; skin tests (such as the Spherulin skin test); tissue biopsy; chest X-ray; and CT scan. The reliability of each method, however, may vary depending on the disease stage.

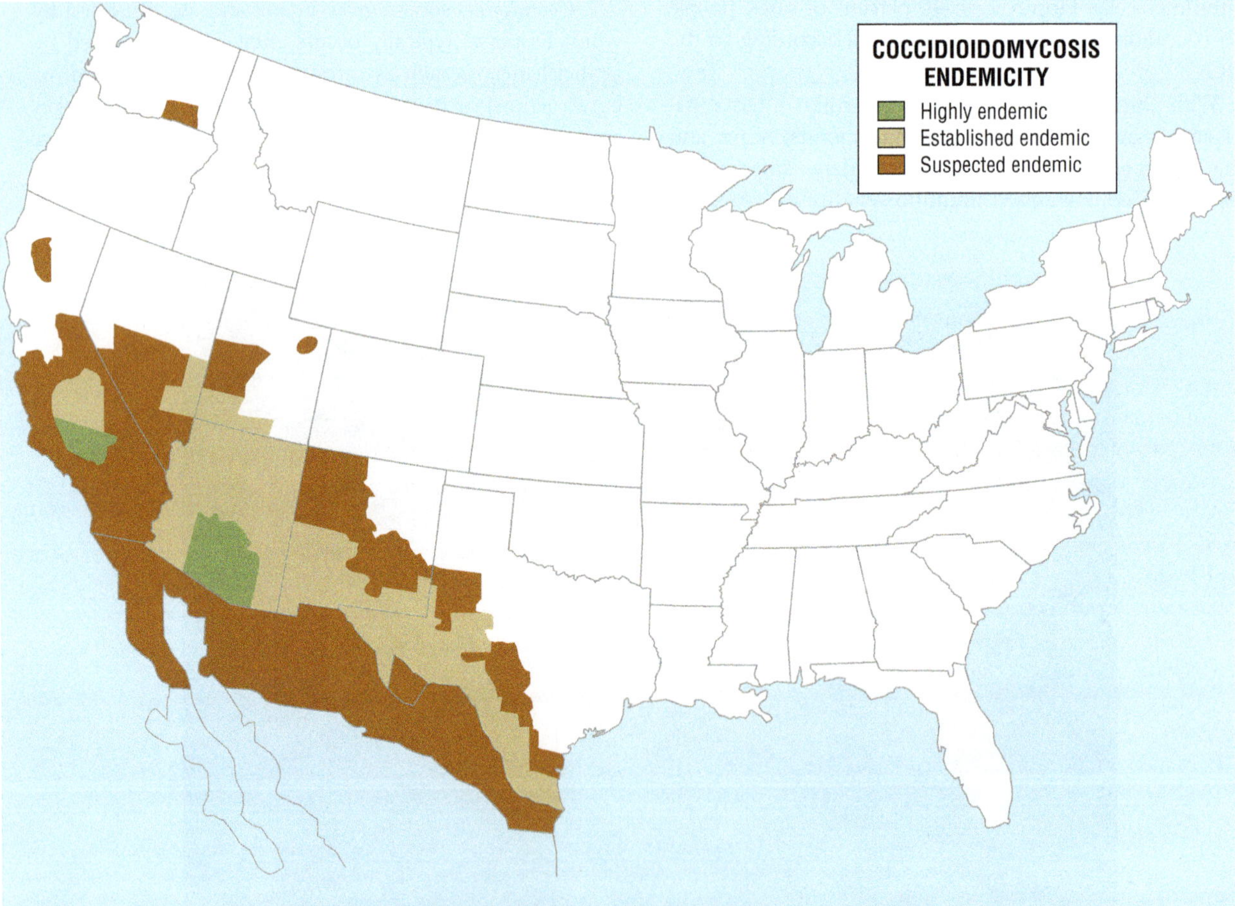

SOURCE: Adapted from "Areas Endemic for Coccidioidomycosis." US Centers for Disease Control and Prevention. Available from: https://www.cdc.gov/fungal/images/coccidio-distributionmap-300px.jpg

Chest X-rays are used to find lung abnormalities, but the specific disease causing the abnormalities is difficult to identify from the X-ray alone.

Coccidioidomycosis is often self-limiting within a matter of weeks or months, and physicians often allow the disease to run its course without treatment. However, patients with flulike symptoms are sometimes given antifungal medicines, which can limit the dissemination of spores as well as the severity of symptoms. Patients who are at elevated risk of developing severe coccidioidomycosis are more likely to receive medication to combat infection. Amphotericin B, fluconazole, itraconazole, and ketoconazole are among the antifungal medications prescribed to treat coccidioidomycosis. One-year treatments are common, but patients with the acute form usually recover completely. Severe cases of disseminated coccidioidomycosis may require surgery to excise affected tissue. Cocci meningitis can require shunts to funnel antifungals to the brain. Relapses are more likely with chronic or severe forms of coccidioidomycosis.

■ Impacts and Issues

While physicians and researchers have sought and tested a variety of methods for treating and preventing coccidioidomycosis since the disease was first identified in the late 19th century, the disease remains almost impossible to control and difficult to treat. As the areas where *Coccidioides* is endemic have become increasingly developed and densely settled, especially in California and the American Southwest, rates of infection have increased. Epidemiologists largely attribute this rise in incidence to new construction, which requires digging up and otherwise unsettling soils that contain *Coccidioides* spores, and to denser populations, which mean that these spores are more likely to be inhaled. Climate change, which may have led to improved conditions for the fungus to grow, has also been suspected to be a cause of the rise in infection.

One of the earliest spikes in coccidioidomycosis occurred in 1977 in California's San Joaquin Valley, when a massive dust storm spread dirt containing *Coccidioides* spores and led to over 100 reported case of the disease and six deaths from it in Sacramento County. In the previous two decades, the greatest number of reported cases in the county in a year was six. While this was an early sign that coccidioidomycosis rates were on the rise, it was not until the mid-1990s that public health officials began to note a sustained growth in incidence. Between 1998 and 2011, the CDC noted that reported cases increased approximately eightfold: "During 1998–2011, a total of 111,717 coccidioidomycosis cases were reported to CDC from 28 states and the District of Columbia: 66% from Arizona, 31% from California, 1% from other endemic states, and <1% from nonendemic states." Since this report was issued, cases of coccidioidomycosis have continued to rise and to become increasingly concentrated in Arizona and California. In 2016 alone California experienced a 71 percent increase from the year before, to 5,358 reported cases. Arizona has even higher rates of infection, with 7,622 reported cases in 2015.

As infection rates have continued to rise, public health officials in Arizona and California have pursued a number of initiatives designed to educate people about the dangers of the disease. An ongoing campaign in Arizona is aimed at educating the medical community to consider coccidioidomycosis whenever anyone seeks medical treatment for flu or pneumonia symptoms in regions where coccidioidomycosis is endemic. The University of Arizona is also tracking the outbreak and, as of 2018, is studying the effectiveness of a new drug, nikkomycin Z, that has shown potential to cure the disease when tested in mice. Nikkomycin Z was also briefly tested in humans in 2017, but the high cost of manufacturing the medication led to a stall in the clinical trial. As of January 2018, six bills had been introduced in the California legislature. These bills included provisions that would require mandatory training on valley fever for health professionals, codify data collection and reporting of the disease, and require physicians to perform specified blood tests for the disease in Kern County, where rates of infection are highest. According to an article in the *Bakersfield Californian*, "Never before has as much legislation been introduced to target the disease, which has historically received little attention politically despite the toll it takes on impacted communities."

SEE ALSO *Airborne Precautions; Colds (Rhinitis); Influenza; Mycotic Disease; Pneumonia*

BIBLIOGRAPHY

Books

Kumar, Vinay, Abul Abbas, and Nelson Fausto. *Robbins and Cotran Pathologic Basis of Disease.* 7th ed. Philadelphia: Saunders, 2004.

Ryan, Kenneth J., and C. George Ray. *Sherris Medical Microbiology: An Introduction to Infectious Diseases.* 4th ed. New York: McGraw-Hill, 2003.

Periodicals

Galgiani, John N., et al. "Coccidioidomycosis." *Clinical Infectious Diseases,* 41, no. 9 (2005): 1217–1223. This article can also be found online at https://doi.org/10.1086/496991 (accessed February 6, 2018).

Goodyear, Dana. "Death Dust." *New Yorker* (January 20, 2014). This article can also be found online at https://www.newyorker.com/magazine/2014/01/20/death-dust (accessed February 6, 2018).

Hector, Richard F., and Rafael Laniado-Laborin. "Coccidioidomycosis—A Fungal Disease of the Americas." *PloS Medicine* (January 25, 2005). This article can also be found online at https://doi.org/10.1371/journal.pmed.0020002 (accessed February 6, 2018).

Pierce, Harold. "Unprecedented Six Bills Introduced within Days of Each Other to Address Valley Fever." *Bakersfield Californian* (January 16, 2018). This article can also be found online at http://www.bakersfield.com/news/unprecedented-six-bills-introduced-within-days-of-each-other-to/article_fe783238-fb2f-11e7-a3ce-03cfff6cb9ff.html (accessed February 6, 2018).

Websites

"Coccidioidomycosis." American Lung Association. http://www.lung.org/lung-health-and-diseases/lung-disease-lookup/coccidioidomycosis/ (accessed February 6, 2018).

"Coccidioidomycosis." Center for Food Security and Public Health. http://www.cfsph.iastate.edu/Factsheets/pdfs/coccidioidomycosis.pdf (accessed February 6, 2018).

"Valley Fever (Coccidioidomycosis)." Centers for Disease Control and Prevention. https://www.cdc.gov/fungal/diseases/coccidioidomycosis/index.html (accessed February 6, 2018).

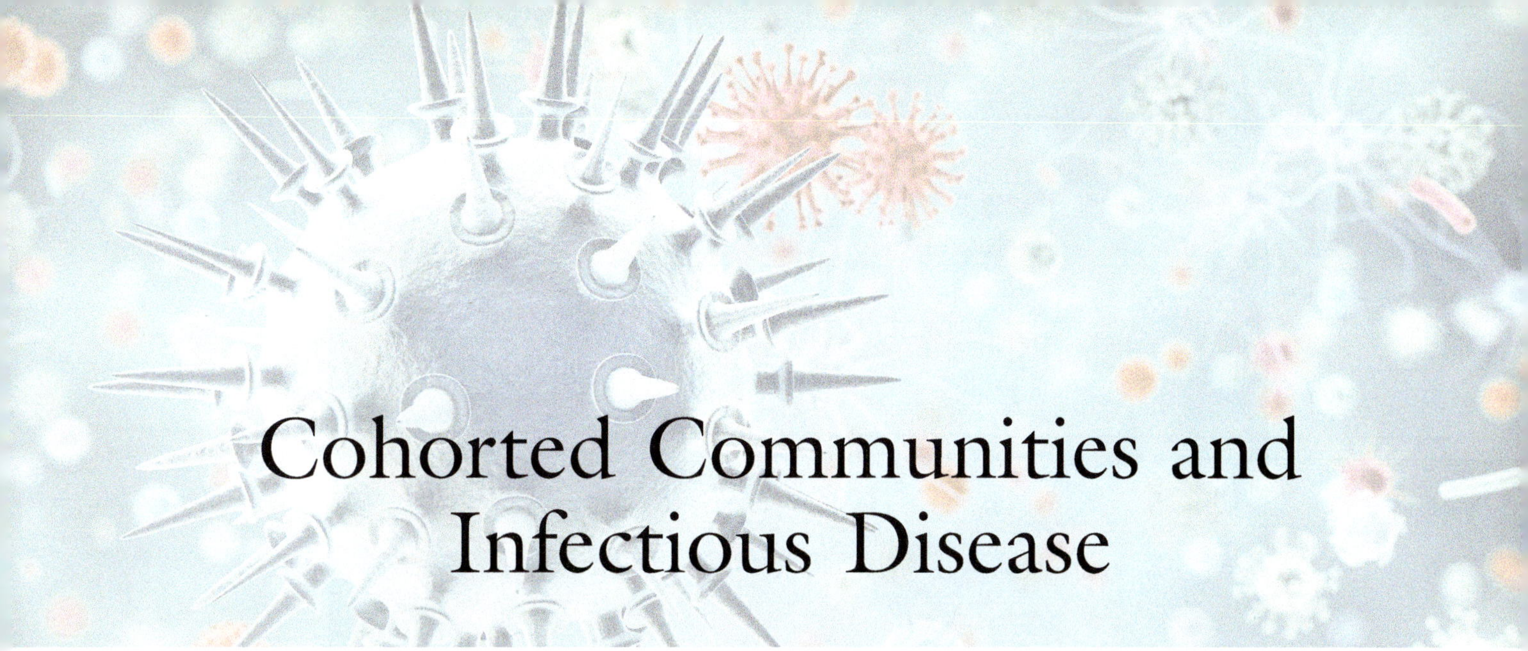

Cohorted Communities and Infectious Disease

■ Introduction

Living in close proximity to others is a strong risk factor for the transmission of many diseases, including tuberculosis (TB), pneumonia, and influenza. That is why infections tend to spread among cohorted communities —that is, large groups of people who occupy the same living space and tend to share, or come into contact with, items that could transmit infection.

The types of diseases transmitted in cohorted communities vary depending on the characteristics of the group. However, three situations pose specific public health problems. College students living in dormitories may be more vulnerable to meningitis, an infection of the lining of the brain. People in prison, both inmates and staff, may be exposed to a number of infections, including human immunodeficiency virus (HIV) and TB. Finally, the elderly residents of nursing homes run a high risk of urinary and gastrointestinal infections, as well as pneumonia.

■ History and Scientific Foundations

Close contact between individuals in overcrowded dwellings has always been a factor in the transmission of disease. In modern societies people generally have more personal space, but there are still situations when they may be at risk of infection because they find themselves in close proximity to others. College students have also become a focus for concern. At colleges and universities, thousands of students may live together in shared residence halls or dormitories. Although most students are young and healthy, these conditions put them at risk of two infections in particular—mononucleosis (sometimes known as glandular fever) and bacterial meningitis.

Mononucleosis is spread through saliva (that is why it is sometimes known as the "kissing disease"), so close physical contact between individuals and sharing items such as drinking glasses will increase the risk. Mononucleosis is characterized by sore throat, fever, and extreme fatigue; there is no cure other than prolonged rest, which will interrupt studies. Bacterial meningitis, an inflammation of the meninges, which are the membranes covering the brain and spinal cord, is a far more serious condition. In students the cause of meningitis is usually *Neisseria meningitides*, which is present in the normal flora—or natural bacterial community—of the nose and mouth. It has long been known that meningitis is transmitted more readily among closed or crowded populations and that meningitis outbreaks on college campuses occur with some regularity. Meningitis gives rise to high fever, severe headache, and stiff neck; untreated, the mortality rate can be as high as 70

WORDS TO KNOW

COHORT A group of people (or any species) sharing a common characteristic. Cohorts are identified and grouped in cohort studies to determine the frequency of diseases or the kinds of disease outcomes over time.

ISOLATION AND QUARANTINE Public health authorities rely on isolation and quarantine as two important tools among the many they use to fight disease outbreaks. Isolation is the practice of keeping a disease victim away from other people, sometimes by treating them in their homes or by the use of elaborate isolation systems in hospitals. Quarantine separates people who have been exposed to a disease but have not yet developed symptoms from the general population. Both isolation and quarantine can be entered voluntarily by patients when public health authorities request them, or they can be compelled by state governments or by the federal Centers for Disease Control and Prevention.

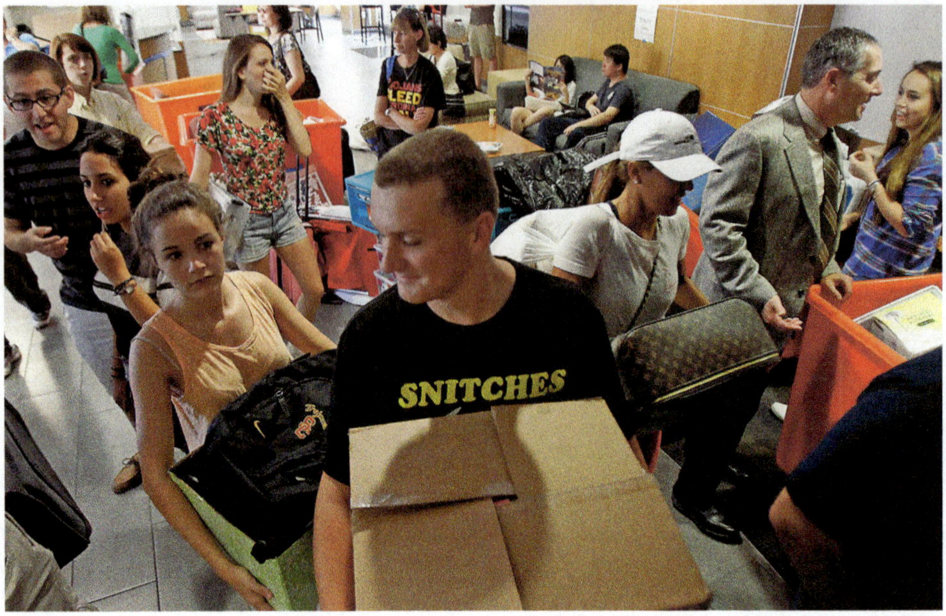

Pictured here are University of Southern California freshmen moving into their residence halls. University students often live in crowded dormitories where they are at increased risk of contracting mononucleosis and meningitis. *© Luis Sinco/Los Angeles Times/Getty Images*

percent. To combat outbreaks of meningitis, some universities have instituted awareness programs to teach students about the signs and symptoms of the disease.

Prison inmates face a quite different spectrum of infection risk from overcrowding, with bloodborne viruses (BBVs), including HIV and viral hepatitis, being the main concern. A high proportion of prison entrants have a history of drug use and may continue to use drugs in prison where clean needles and other drug preparation equipment are likely unavailable. Unsafe sex, coupled with sexual assault and rape, increases the risk of transmission of BBVs in prison. Tattooing with makeshift and unclean needles is also a transmission route of BBVs in prisons. Standards of hygiene within prison may be low, which encourages the spread of all infectious diseases, including TB.

Elderly residents of many nursing homes have been found to be at risk of several infections, including pneumonia, TB, and diarrheal diseases, some of which are antibiotic resistant. Older people are more at risk of infection because they may have other chronic illnesses and their immune systems tend to be weaker and less able to resist an infection. Standards of hygiene may be lower in the presence of residents who are incontinent or who have dementia, thus increasing the likelihood of outbreaks of infectious disease.

SOCIAL AND PERSONAL RESPONSIBILITY

People who live in close quarters, especially adolescents and college students, are at a greater risk of contracting meningitis than the larger population. To reduce cases of meningitis, the Centers for Disease Control and Prevention states that adolescents should receive a meningitis vaccine at the age of 11 or 12 followed by a booster vaccination between the ages of 16 and 23.

■ Applications and Research

According to the World Health Organization, as of 2018 the estimated global HIV prevalence among prisoners was 3 percent. Research reveals case reports of transmission through sharing injecting equipment and sexual activity.

Meanwhile, research on nursing homes suggests influenza, which can be fatal in the elderly, is the most common cause of infectious outbreak. Reactivation of old TB infection is also common. Norwalk, rotavirus, and *Clostridium difficile* account for many outbreaks of gastrointestinal infection among nursing homes.

■ Impacts and Issues

There are many ways in which the spread of infection in cohorted communities can be prevented. Hygiene, both personal and institutional, should be paramount, whether the setting is a college dorm, a daycare center, a prison, or a nursing home. Programs that provide condoms and syringes have been found to decrease HIV and other BBV transmission among at-risk populations. Screening of potential entrants to prisons and nursing homes for relevant infections such as HIV or TB can help identify those at risk and give treatment where appropriate. The CDC also recommends that freshmen entering dorms receive vaccination against meningitis.

Cohorting is also used to prevent the spread of infection under some conditions. Physicians, especially those who specialize in treating children, often provide separate waiting areas in their offices to separate sick patients from those without symptoms. Hospitals often cohort patients with like infections into semiprivate rooms. During a large-scale epidemic of infectious disease, community health officials have plans to both cohort infected persons (such as in the severe acute respiratory syndrome [SARS] outbreak in Singapore in 2003, where all suspected SARS cases were taken to one hospital for evaluation and care) and to suspend natural cohorting that could encourage disease spread (including temporarily closing schools).

SEE ALSO *Hepatitis B; Hepatitis C; HIV; Isolation and Quarantine; Meningitis, Bacterial*

BIBLIOGRAPHY

Books

Bennett, John E., Raphael Dolin, and Martin J. Blaser. *Mandell, Douglas, and Bennett's Principles and Practice of Infectious Diseases.* 8th ed. Philadelphia: Elsevier/Saunders, 2015.

Periodicals

Beachum, Lateshia. "Prisons around the World Are Reservoirs of Infectious Disease." *Washington Post* (July 20, 2016). This article can also be found online at https://www.washingtonpost.com/news/to-your-health/wp/2016/07/20/prisons-around-the-world-are-reservoirs-of-infectious-disease/?utm_term=.5633ed12c8ea (accessed February 9, 2018).

Bick, Joseph A. "Infection Control in Jails and Prisons." *Clinical Infectious Diseases* 45, no. 8 (October 15, 2007): 1047–1055. This article can also be found online at https://academic.oup.com/cid/article/45/8/1047/344842 (accessed February 9, 2018).

Dolan, Kate, et al. "Global Burden of HIV, Viral Hepatitis, and Tuberculosis in Prisoners and Detainees." *Lancet* 388, no. 10049 (September 10, 2016): 1089–1102. This article can also be found online at http://www.thelancet.com/journals/lancet/article/PIIS0140-6736(16)30466-4/fulltext (accessed February 9, 2018).

Websites

"Behind Bars II: Substance Abuse and America's Prison Population." National Center on Addiction and Substance Abuse at Columbia University, February 2010. https://www.centeronaddiction.org/addiction-research/reports/behind-bars-ii-substance-abuse-and-america%E2%80%99s-prison-population (accessed February 9, 2018).

"Correctional Health." Centers for Disease Control and Prevention, May 13, 2016. https://www.cdc.gov/correctionalhealth/ (accessed February 9, 2018).

"Meningitis." Centers for Disease Control and Prevention, April 10, 2017. https://www.cdc.gov/meningitis/index.html (accessed February 9, 2018).

"Nursing Homes and Assisted Living (Long-Term Care Facilities [LTCFs])." Centers for Disease Control and Prevention, February 28, 2018. https://www.cdc.gov/longtermcare/ (accessed February 9, 2018).

Singh, Maanvi. "Why College Campuses Get Hit by Meningitis Outbreaks." NPR, November 19, 2013. https://www.npr.org/sections/health-shots/2013/11/19/246178160/why-college-campuses-get-hit-by-meningitis-outbreaks (accessed February 9, 2018).

Susan Aldridge
Claire Skinner

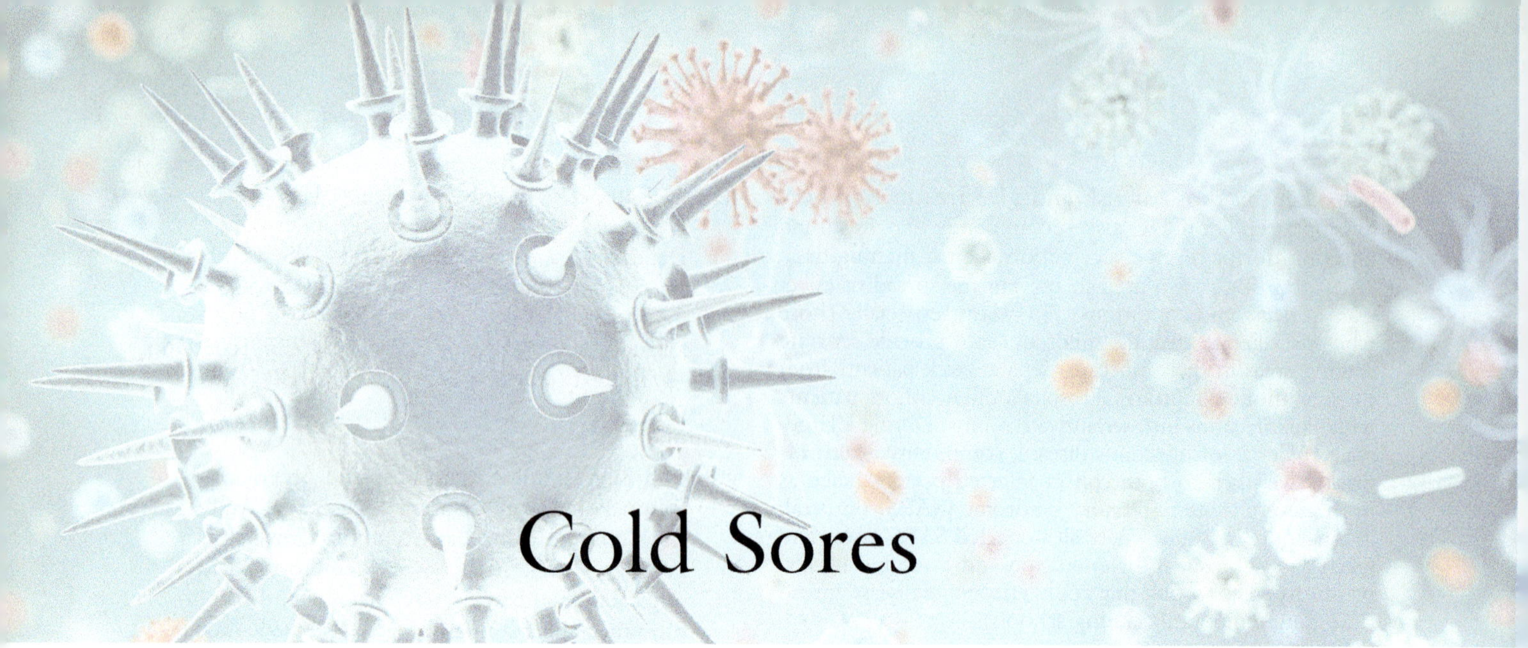

Cold Sores

Introduction

Cold sores, also commonly known as fever blisters, are caused by an infection with herpes simplex 1 virus (HSV-1). An estimated 95 percent of all people have been exposed to the virus. The infection causes one or more fluid-filled blisters in the tissues of the mouth or around the nose. After the initial outbreak, the virus lies dormant in the skin and surrounding nerve tissue and is reactivated from time to time, most often due to colds, influenza, too much sun, or stress. Why the virus causes outbreaks at different times is not completely understood. During an outbreak the fluid within the blisters and the skin around the ulcer contain high levels of HSV-1 and so are highly contagious until the ulcer is healed. Frequent handwashing and avoiding direct contact with others minimize the risk of spreading HSV-1. Some antiviral medications may shorten the course of the cold sore if given early in the outbreak.

Editor's note: Infrequently, HSV-1 is also responsible for eye infections and other skin infections. A small percentage of genital herpes cases are also caused by HSV-1. More information about cold sores is found in the article about their causative agent, the herpes simplex 1 virus.

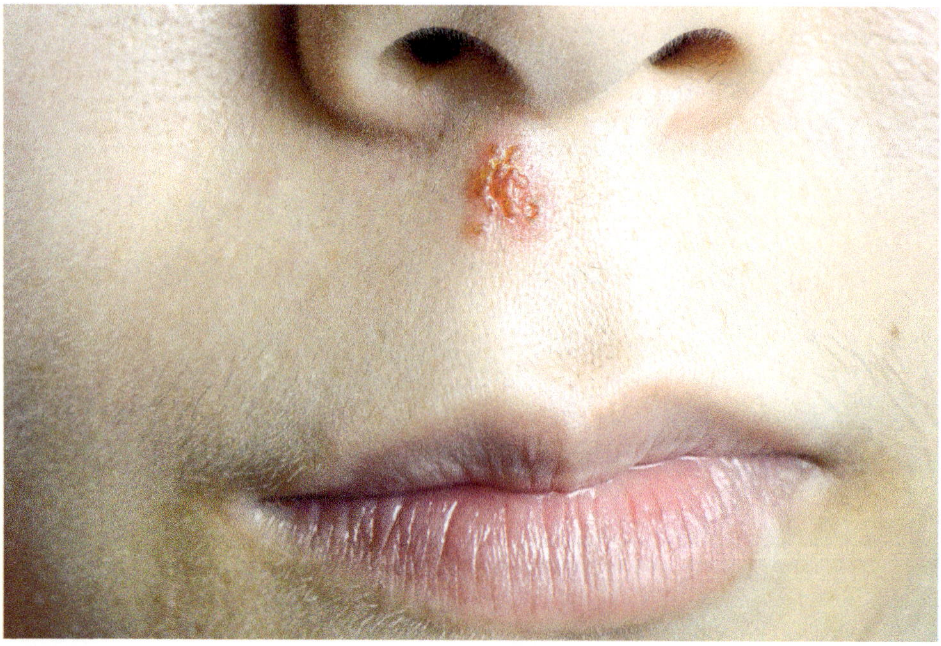

Cold sores on the lips and face are usually caused by the herpes simplex virus type 1, also known as HSV-1 or oral herpes. Between 50 and 80 percent of the US population has oral herpes. *© Pan Xunbin/ Science Source*

SEE ALSO *Herpes Simplex 1 Virus*

BIBLIOGRAPHY

Books

Diefenbach, Russell J., and Cornel Fraedel, eds. *Herpes Simplex Virus: Methods and Protocols.* New York: Springer, 2016.

Periodicals

Jordan, Vanessa. "Cochrane Corner: Preventing Cold Sores: Do Antivirals Work?" *Journal of Primary Health Care* 7, no. 4 (2015): 348.

Kennedy, Peter G. E., et al. "A Comparison of Herpes Simplex Virus Type 1 and Varicella-Zoster Virus Latency and Reactivation." *Journal of General Virology* 96 (2015): 1581–1602.

Websites

"Cold Sore." Mayo Clinic, May 15, 2015. https://www.mayoclinic.org/diseases-conditions/cold-sore/symptoms-causes/syc-20371017 (accessed December 6, 2017).

"Cold Sores: Overview." American Academy of Dermatology Association. https://www.aad.org/public/diseases/contagious-skin-diseases/cold-sores> (accessed December 6, 2017).

Laura J. Cataldo

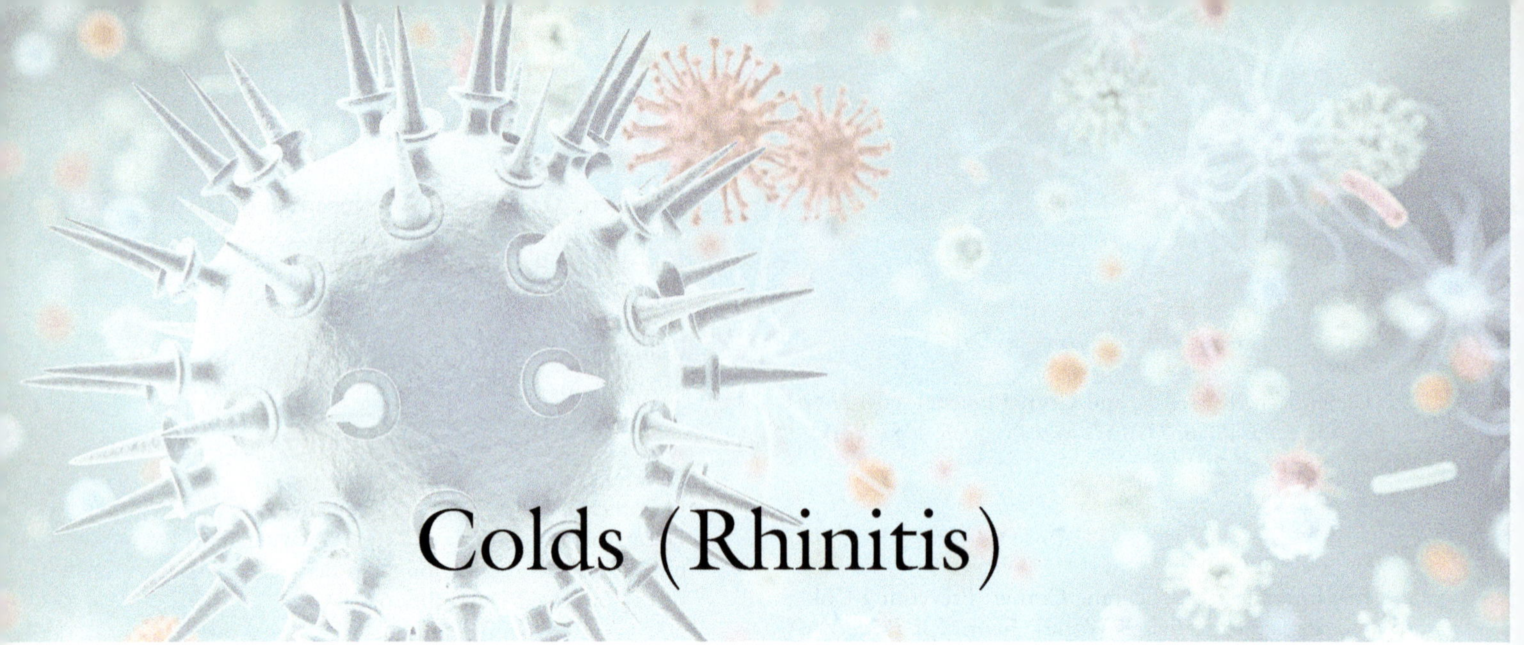

Colds (Rhinitis)

Introduction

The common cold, or rhinitis, is a viral infection of the upper respiratory tract, which includes the linings of the sinuses (cavities in the head behind the nose and eyes), throat, and pharynx. The word *rhinitis* means inflammation of the nose. The common cold is indeed common, being the infectious disease most often caught by human beings. Cold symptoms include runny nose, sore throat, tiredness, and sometimes coughing or sneezing. The common cold is never fatal in people with normal immune systems. The viruses that cause colds exist in a great variety of slightly different forms, and, although a person cannot catch the same cold twice —that is, be reinfected by exactly the same cold virus —there are always other colds to be caught. There is no vaccine for the common cold for the same reason. Because a cold is a viral infection, antibiotics do not affect it.

WORDS TO KNOW

ANTIGEN A substance, usually a protein or polysaccharide, that stimulates the immune system to produce antibodies. While antigens can be the source of infections from pathogenic bacteria and viruses, organic molecules detrimental to the body from internal or environmental sources also act as antigens.

COLONIZATION The process of occupation and increase in number of microorganisms at a specific site.

MENINGITIS An inflammation of the meninges, the three layers of protective membranes that line the spinal cord and the brain. Meningitis can occur when there is an infection near the brain or spinal cord, such as a respiratory infection in the sinuses, the mastoids, or the cavities around the ear. Disease organisms can also travel to the meninges through the bloodstream. The first signs may be a severe headache and neck stiffness followed by fever, vomiting, a rash, and, then, convulsions leading to loss of consciousness. Meningitis generally involves two types: nonbacterial meningitis, or aseptic meningitis, and bacterial meningitis, or purulent meningitis.

RECEPTOR Protein molecules on a cell's surface that act as a "signal receiver" and allow communication between cells.

Disease History, Characteristics, and Transmission

Most colds are caused by an adenovirus or a coronavirus. The only other animals that can be infected by these viruses are the few primates most closely related to humans, including chimpanzees. Colds have been known throughout recorded history. Egyptian drawings dating to the 1st century depict a nose and a symbol representing nasal drainage. Premodern European doctors thought colds were caused by an imbalance of the four humors (blood, yellow bile, black bile, and phlegm). The existence of disease-causing microorganisms was not known until the 1800s, and viruses were not known until the 1890s.

Even after the discovery of viruses, for many years doctors mistakenly thought colds were caused by bacteria. The viral nature of colds was discovered in the early 20th century when German researcher Walter M. Kruse (1928–) showed that colds could be transmitted by nose secretions passed through a filter having holes too small for bacteria to pass through. The actual viruses causing most colds were isolated and grown in culture in laboratories in the 1950s and 1960s.

Cold symptoms include stuffy nose, runny nose, mild fever and chills, tiredness, sore throat, cough, impairment of smell and taste, and hoarseness of voice. The average duration of a cold is 7.4 days; mild colds last only 2 to 3 days, and about 25 percent of colds last about 14 days. Symptoms are not caused directly by the virus interfering with body functions but by the body's defensive response to the virus. When cells in the respiratory tract are infected, substances called inflammatory mediators are released by the body. These cause small blood vessels to widen, which makes tissue swell. They also increase mucus secretion, stimulate pain-sensing nerve fibers, and activate cough and sneeze reflexes. The body eventually clears itself of a cold by learning to identify specific molecules, or antigens, which exist only on the surface of the particular cold virus causing that cold. Immune system cells can then attack anything in the body that bears these antigens. The antigens on each cold virus are slightly different, which is why the body has to learn from scratch how to fight every new cold.

About 1 to 5 percent of colds are complicated by acute bacterial sinusitis, a bacterial infection of the sinuses that can have serious side effects, including eye infection and meningitis. Unlike cold viruses, the bacteria that cause bacterial sinusitis can be killed using antibiotics.

Mild cases of influenza (flu) resemble colds; more severe cases cause the usual cold symptoms but also muscle aches, fever, and a more severe cough. However, influenza is a distinct disease from the common cold.

Colds are usually contracted when cold-virus particles are picked up by touching a person with a cold or a surface contaminated with the cold virus. Cold-virus particles are then often transferred to the nostrils or eyes, again by touch. A virus can be inhaled into the nostrils and deposited in the back of the adenoid area (behind the soft palate at the back of the mouth). Virus particles in the eyes are transported down into the nasal passages and then to the adenoid area. There they colonize cells, which is why many colds begin with a sore throat. Some colds may be transmitted by airborne mucus particles ejected by sneezing. As few as 1 to 30 virus particles introduced into the nose can reliably produce an infection.

Cold viruses colonize cells by attaching to a molecular structure on the surface of the cell called a receptor (specifically, the ICAM-1 receptor). After attachment, the virus is absorbed into the cell, where it tricks the cell into manufacturing more of the virus. Eventually the cell produces so much virus that it ruptures, releasing many new virus particles. The cycle of virus reproduction takes about 8 to 12 hours. Cold symptoms begin about 10 hours after infection, and symptoms peak between 36 and 72 hours after infection.

■ Scope and Distribution

Colds afflict all countries, climates, and social classes. Typically adults suffer 1 to 4 colds per year, and children suffer 6 to 10.

Despite a widespread assumption that exposure to cold temperatures causes colds, populations living in colder climates do not get more colds. A 2005 experiment at Cardiff University in Wales counted cold symptoms reported by groups who either underwent controlled chilling of the feet or did not. Those subjects whose feet had been chilled

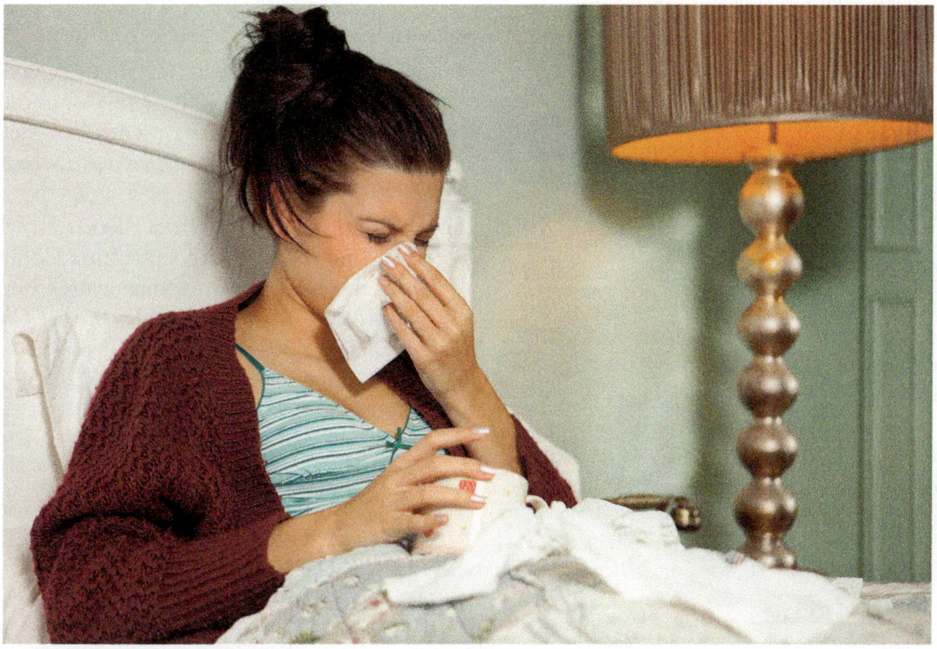

A woman suffers from symptoms of the common cold, or rhinitis, including muscle aches, cough, and runny nose. *© Image Source/Getty Images*

REAL-WORLD RISKS

The National Institute of Allergy and Infectious Diseases (NIAID) asserted that research data does not support the popular linkage of colds to cold weather or the development of the common cold from a person becoming either chilled or overheated. The NIAID reported that data developed by researchers find that "these conditions have little or no effect on the development or severity of a cold. Nor is susceptibility apparently related to factors such as exercise, diet, or enlarged tonsils or adenoids. On the other hand, research suggests that psychological stress, allergic disorders affecting the nasal passages or pharynx (throat), and menstrual cycles may have an impact on a person's susceptibility to colds."

showed a higher rate of symptoms. However, the study has been criticized for not verifying whether experimental subjects who reported symptoms actually had colds. There is no scientific consensus that being chilled increases one's chance of catching a cold.

■ Treatment and Prevention

There is no effective treatment for the common cold. Contradictory evidence exists for the effectiveness of herbal treatments, zinc gluconate, and vitamin C, but there is no scientific agreement that any of these substances decrease one's chances of catching a cold, the length of a cold, or the severity of a cold. Cold treatment primarily targets the symptoms of the infection. Cold medicines often include antihistamines to reduce mucus production, pain relievers, cough suppressants, and alcohol and other drugs to induce sounder sleep.

Experimental antiviral drugs have shown some ability to combat the common cold, but scientists question whether the use of these drugs is appropriate, given the harmlessness of the common cold and the high cost and possible risks of antiviral drugs.

Colds can be prevented by following good hygiene practices. Four basic steps are recommended by disease-transmission specialists: washing hands, avoiding close contact with people who have colds (or, if you have a cold, avoiding close contact with uninfected persons), covering up when sneezing or nose-blowing, and, for health care professionals, wearing masks and clean gloves.

■ Impacts and Issues

There are at least 500 million colds per year in the US population of about 300 million people, causing about 20 million lost workdays for adults and 22 million lost school days for children. The direct costs of colds, including purchase of cold remedies, are $17 billion per year in the United States; indirect costs, including lost productivity, are $22.5 billion. Lost workdays are a far more significant hardship for people in nonprofessional, unskilled, or service-sector jobs that entitle the worker to few or no paid sick days.

In 2006 research at the Mayo Clinic indicated that some viruses that cause colds, picornaviruses, may damage the brain, causing cumulative loss of memory over a lifetime. The researchers reported, "Our findings suggest that picornavirus infections throughout the lifetime of an individual may chip away at the cognitive [thinking ability] reserve, increasing the likelihood of detectable cognitive impairments as the individual ages." There is no proof that picornavirus-caused colds do cause memory loss in human beings, but this is an active area of research.

SEE ALSO *Handwashing*

BIBLIOGRAPHY

Books

Estenson, Joseph. *Chronic Sinusitis.* Washington, DC: Capitol Hill, 2015.

Haddad, S. F. *X-Plain Hand Washing—Preventing Infections.* Coralville, IA: Patient Education Institute, 2016.

Zuckerman, Jane N., Gary W. Brunette, and Peter A. Leggat. *Essential Travel Medicine.* New York: Wiley-Blackwell, 2015.

Periodicals

Hemilä, Harri, et al. "Zinc Acetate Lozenges May Improve the Recovery Rate of Common Cold Patients: An Individual Patient Data Meta-Analysis." *Open Forum Infectious Diseases* 4 (2017): 59.

Klimek, Ludger, et al. "Factors Associated with Efficacy of an Ibuprofen/Pseudoephedrine Combination Drug in Pharmacy Customers with Common Cold Symptoms." *International Journal of Clinical Practice* 71 (2017): e12907.

Starling, Shimona. "Viral Infection: Competing Membrane Proteins Regulate Picornavirus Genome Delivery." *Nature Reviews Microbiology* 15 (2017): 132–133.

Stein, Richard A. "Hopes and Challenges for the Common Cold." *International Journal of Clinical Practice* 71 (2017): e12921.

Zumla, Alimuddin, et al. "Rapid Point of Care Diagnostic Tests for Viral and Bacterial Respiratory Tract Infections—Needs, Advances, and Future Prospects." *Lancet* 14 (2014): 1123–1135.

Websites

"Common Cold." Mayo Clinic, 2017. https://www.mayoclinic.org/diseases-conditions/common-cold/symptoms-causes/syc-20351605 (accessed December 6, 2017).

"Common Cold." MedlinePlus, 2017. https://medlineplus.gov/commoncold.html (accessed January 5, 2018).

"Common Cold." PubMed Health, 2017. https://www.ncbi.nlm.nih.gov/pubmedhealth/PMHT0024671/ (accessed December 6, 2017).

Díaz, Herminio R. Hernández. "The Common Cold." Pan American Health Organization. http://www.paho.org/English/AD/DPC/CD/AIEPI-1-3.9.pdf (accessed December 6, 2017).

Laura J. Cataldo

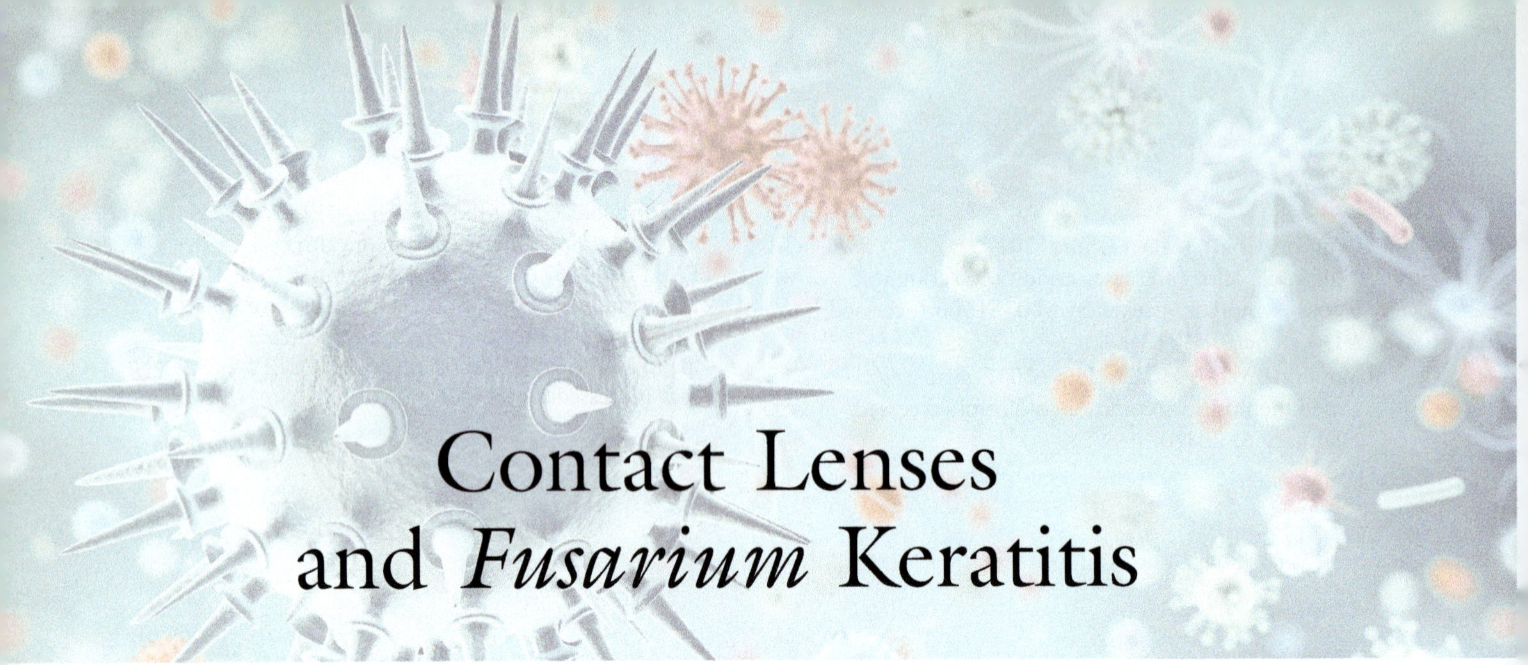

Contact Lenses and *Fusarium* Keratitis

■ Introduction

Fusarium is a type of fungus that is commonly found in soil and on plants. In a 2005 outbreak of disease caused by *Fusarium*, the fungus was identified in contact lens cleaning solution, through which it was transferred to the inner surface of a contact lens during the cleaning process. When the lens was worn, fungal growth caused an inflammation of the wearer's cornea, the outermost layer of the eye. Corneal inflammation is generally termed keratitis. In the case of this fungal infection, the inflammation is called *Fusarium* keratitis.

Until the first decade of the 21st century, *Fusarium* keratitis was more common in agriculture-intensive regions, such as Florida, than in more populated areas. In 2006 a wider investigation of the 2005 outbreak by the US Centers for Disease Control and Prevention (CDC) identified cases in 33 states and one territory.

The symptoms of *Fusarium* keratitis in contact lens wearers include blurred vision and a red or swollen eye. These symptoms do not improve when the contact lens is removed because fungal growth takes place in or on the cornea. Treatment typically involves antifungal drugs, such as natamycin and amphotericin B, which can be irritating and even toxic in high doses. In extreme cases removal of the cornea and transplantation of another cornea is performed.

WORDS TO KNOW

ANTIFUNGAL Antifungals (also called antifungal drugs) are medicines used to fight fungal infections. They are of two kinds, systemic and topical. Systemic antifungal drugs are medicines taken by mouth or by injection to treat infections caused by a fungus. Topical antifungal drugs are medicines applied to the skin to treat skin infections caused by a fungus.

KERATITIS Keratitis, sometimes called corneal ulcers, is an inflammation of the cornea, the transparent membrane that covers the colored part of the eye (iris) and pupil of the eye.

RESISTANT BACTERIA Resistant bacteria are microbes that have lost their sensitivity to one or more antibiotic drugs through mutation.

■ History and Scientific Foundations

Until 2005 *Fusarium* keratitis was a rare disease. This is because sources of the fungus, particularly soil and plants, rarely come in contact with the eyes. However, in 2005 a case of *Fusarium* keratitis was diagnosed in the United States in a person who did not have a history of recent corneal damage caused by contact with a plant or soil. The infection was subsequently linked to a wider outbreak and traced to contaminated contact lens cleaning solution.

Analysis of the data implicated a particular brand of contact lens solution (ReNu with MoistureLoc). The source of the fungal contamination was not determined because the fungus was not isolated from the production factory, storage warehouse, filtered samples of cleaning solutions, or unopened solution bottles from the same production runs. Nonetheless, sales of the product were stopped by parent company Bausch & Lomb, which subsequently issued a recall of the product.

■ Applications and Research

Fusarium keratitis research is focused on understanding the scope of the problem. Whether *Fusarium* keratitis is mainly an infrequent contamination of lens cleaning solution during manufacture or is a more widespread problem involving improper hygiene on the part of the user is not clear. Improved lens cleaners continue to be investigated with the goal of developing a cleaner that is lethal to microbes but is safe for the user if cleaner residue remains on the lens.

Precautions that people can observe include handwashing before handling contact lenses, taking lenses out prior to sleeping, and avoiding wearing lenses while showering or during recreational activity in a pool or hot tub.

The advent of molecular techniques of microorganism detection has aided the diagnosis of *Fusarium* keratitis. Advances in a technique that can quickly obtain many copies of a gene(s) of interest and the use of antibodies to *Fusarium* are being exploited to develop a rapid detection test for the fungus. As of 2017 the fungus was identified by culturing a scraping of cells from the cornea, but this process could take up to a week to yield a result.

Real-World Risks

Eye infections can be caused by viral, bacterial, and fungal microorganisms. These organisms do not cause infections solely in the eye. Rather, eye infections tend to occur as infections disseminate, or spread, in the body. The cornea, the clear front part of the eye through which light passes, is subject to many infections and to injury from exposure and from foreign objects. Infection and injury cause keratitis, an inflammation of the cornea. Tissue loss that results from the inflammation produces an ulcer. The ulcer can either be centrally located, thus greatly affecting vision, or peripherally located. As of 2017 there were an estimated 30,000 to 75,000 cases of bacterial corneal ulcers in the United States each year.

■ Impacts and Issues

Each year in the United States, about one out of every 20 contact lens wearer develops a lens-related eye complication. Almost all (99 percent) of contact lens wearers will experience an eye problem during the time they use contact lenses. Some of these complications, including *Fusarium* keratitis, can threaten vision permanently.

One factor that may play a role in the survival of the *Fusarium* fungus in contact lens cleaning solution is the surface growth of the organism. Some microorganisms, including fungi and bacteria, become very resistant to a variety of agents when the organisms grow attached to a nonliving or living surface. Unattached organisms are usually readily killed by antibiotic agents. The increased hardiness of attached organisms involves changes in their growth following attachment. These changes can be the result of genetic adaptation, with the activity of some genes being enhanced by attachment while other genes become less active.

Until the early 21st century, contact lens keratitis usually involved bacterial infections, predominantly caused by bacteria common in the environment or on the surface of the skin. Fungal keratitis caused by organisms such as *Fusarium* was typically caused by accidental contact of plant material with the eye, especially in people whose immune systems are functioning inefficiently as a consequence of illness or drug therapy. Common routes of transmission included rubbing an eye with soil-laden fingers, sustaining injury to the eye by a thorn, or plant material coming in contact with the eye during harvesting. The association of *Fusarium* keratitis with contact lenses developed after the 2005 outbreak and may reflect the growing popularity of these lenses, particularly lenses that are non-disposable and are repeatedly cleaned.

Fusarium keratitis is an example of how improper hygiene or contaminated lens cleaners can cause illness. Even a properly cleaned lens can become contaminated if, after handling soil or plant materials, hands have not been thoroughly washed. Repeated use of lens cleaning solution can also cause contamination. Fresh solution should be used for each cleaning. According to the American Optometric Association, other useful precautions are wiping the lenses before storing them in the lens case and replacing the lens case every few months.

Fungal keratitis is a growing concern because extended-wear contact lenses are becoming increasingly popular. These extended-wear lenses remain in contact with the cornea for a longer period of time than conventional non-disposable lenses, and they are cleaned less often. With the convenience of extended wear can come a relaxed vigilance concerning lens hygiene.

SEE ALSO *Contact Precautions; Mycotic Disease*

BIBLIOGRAPHY

Books

Gipe, Abigail. *Keratitis: Essentials in Ophthalmology.* New York: Hayle Medical, 2017.

Tabbara, Khalid, Ahmed M. M. Abu El-Asrar, and Moncef Khairallah. *Ocular Infections.* New York: Springer, 2016.

Periodicals

Cope, Jennifer R., et al. "Contact Lens Wearer Demographics and Risk Behaviors for Contact Lens-Related Eye Infections—United States, 2014." *Morbidity and Mortality Weekly Report* 64, no. 32 (2015): 865–870.

Cope, Jennifer R., et al. "Risk Behaviors for Contact Lens-Related Eye Infections among Adults and Adolescents—United States, 2016." *Morbidity and Mortality Weekly Report* 66, no. 32 (2017): 841–845.

Websites

"Basics of Fungal Keratitis." Centers for Disease Control and Prevention. https://www.cdc.gov/contactlenses/fungal-keratitis.html (accessed November 14, 2017).

Brian Hoyle

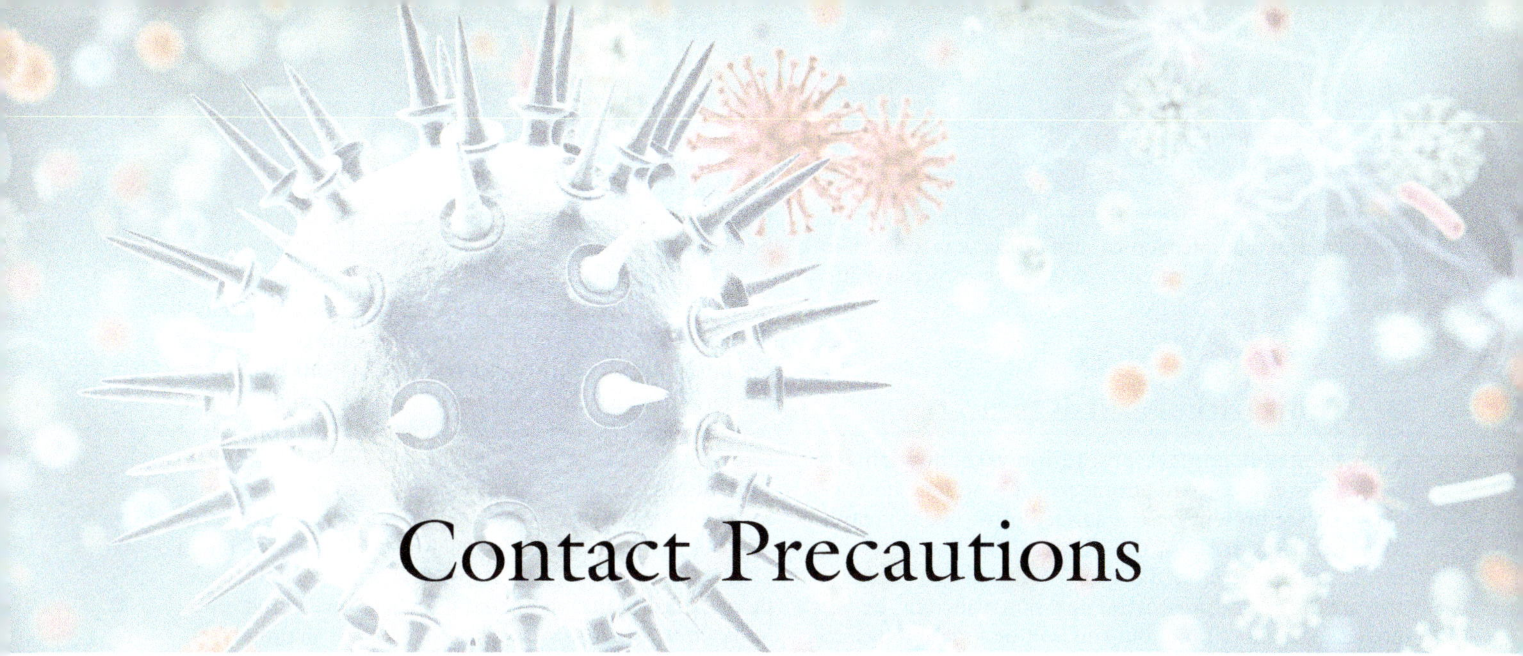

Contact Precautions

■ Introduction

Contact precautions are a series of procedures designed to minimize the transmission of infectious organisms by direct or indirect contact with infected patients or their environments. Along with standard precautions, which assume all body fluids and tissues are potentially infected with harmful microorganisms, contact precautions require the use of protective equipment such as disposable gowns, gloves, and masks when exposure to a patient's body fluids is anticipated. Contact precautions are often used with patients who have wound or skin infections.

A series of contact precautions has been formulated by the US Centers for Disease Control and Prevention (CDC) and are intended to minimize the risk of the direct or indirect transfer of disease-causing (pathogenic) microorganisms. Direct-contact transmission involves person-to-person contact such as when a patient is touched by a health care provider. Indirect transfer involves contact with items that have been in contact with an infected person and that have become contaminated. These items, or fomites, include clothing, towels, and utensils. A fomite may be only transiently contaminated by an infectious microbe, or the pathogen may actually colonize the object.

■ History and Scientific Foundations

It has been known for centuries that infection and hygiene are connected. More than 2,000 years ago, Hippocrates, who laid the groundwork for modern-day medical practices, observed that physicians' cleanliness affected their patients' health. Centuries later Joseph Lister (1827–1912) demonstrated in the mid-19th century that spraying a disinfectant over a patient's wound during an operation reduced postoperative complications and death considerably. These improvements were subsequently attributed to the protection of the wound from airborne microbes.

Microorganisms are readily transferred from one location to another via surfaces. The surface can be living, such as the skin of someone's hand, or nonliving, such as a piece of equipment or clothing. Care must be taken to ensure that contact with a patient involves surfaces that are free of disease-causing (pathogenic) microorganisms.

In 1996 the CDC and the Hospital Infection Control Practices Advisory Committee (HICPAC) established contact precautions as part of the *Guideline for Isolation Procedures in Hospitals*, precautions that were still in use as of 2017. Periodically the guidelines are reviewed and, if necessary, revised. In 2007 the revision, *Guideline for Isolation Precautions: Preventing Transmission of Infectious Agents in Healthcare Settings*, was released. The guidelines stress the importance of integrating isolation-control procedures and

WORDS TO KNOW

ANTIBIOTIC RESISTANCE The ability of bacteria to resist the actions of antibiotic drugs.

FOMITE An object or a surface to which an infectious microorganism such as bacteria or viruses can adhere and be transmitted. Transmission is often by touch.

PATHOGENIC Causing or capable of causing disease.

STANDARD PRECAUTIONS The safety measures taken to prevent the transmission of disease-causing bacteria. These measures include proper handwashing; wearing gloves, goggles, and other protective clothing; proper handling of needles; and sterilization of equipment.

of hospital staff recognizing the need for such procedures. It also ensures that infection-control expertise is available in each hospital and that infection control is incorporated into building design.

■ Applications and Research

A fundamental contact precaution is handwashing. Proper washing with an antimicrobial soap will kill bacteria that are present on the surface of the skin, including normal residents of the skin such as *Staphylococcus aureus* and bacteria in the genus *Streptococcus.* Bacteria that are normally present on the skin will only be removed for a short time, but this will be long enough to protect patients. The physical act of washing, with the friction of skin rubbing against skin, helps remove viruses if it is done for long enough. A few seconds of handwashing before surgery is dangerous because it may not be enough time to kill or remove the bacteria but could make them more easily transferred when another surface is touched. More time spent in handwashing can save a life. When using soap and water, a 30-second scrub of the hands is usually sufficient.

The CDC guidelines specify that handwashing be accomplished before and after contact with a patient and, if gloves are worn, as the final action after the gloves have been properly disposed of.

Fresh gloves need to be put on when coming into contact with a patient for the first time. If various locations are to be touched on a patient, then the order should be from the least to the most contaminated, which minimizes transfer of microbes to a relatively clean site. Gloves should be disposed of in a container designed for that purpose.

The high death rate following surgery that was the norm in the early decades of the 19th century was traced to the habit of physicians of wearing the same blood-soaked operating gowns during their rounds from patient to patient. Essentially, the physician was incubating each patient in turn with the collective microbial population that was adhering to the gown. To be an effective safety measure, disposable gloves, masks, and gowns are worn prior to seeing a patient and discarded in a designated container after seeing the patient. Containers should be available in each patient ward so that the used protective clothing can be discarded in that room and not elsewhere on the hospital floor. This reduces the likelihood of transferring an infection from one room to another.

Another CDC-mandated contact precaution is to limit patient transport in the hospital as much as possible. A patient requiring contact precautions should only be moved when necessary, such as to an operating theater or X-ray room. Then transport should be done to minimize contact with other patients. For example, a patient should not be moved into a hallway and kept there for a period of time before being transported to the final destination. Rather, transport should be direct and prompt. The more a patient is moved, the more the chance that an infection can be transferred from that patient to others.

When contact precautions are used, medical equipment such as blood pressure monitors, stethoscopes, or poles that hold intravenous solutions are dedicated solely to one patient and are not shared. When contact precautions are discontinued, the equipment is cleaned and disin-

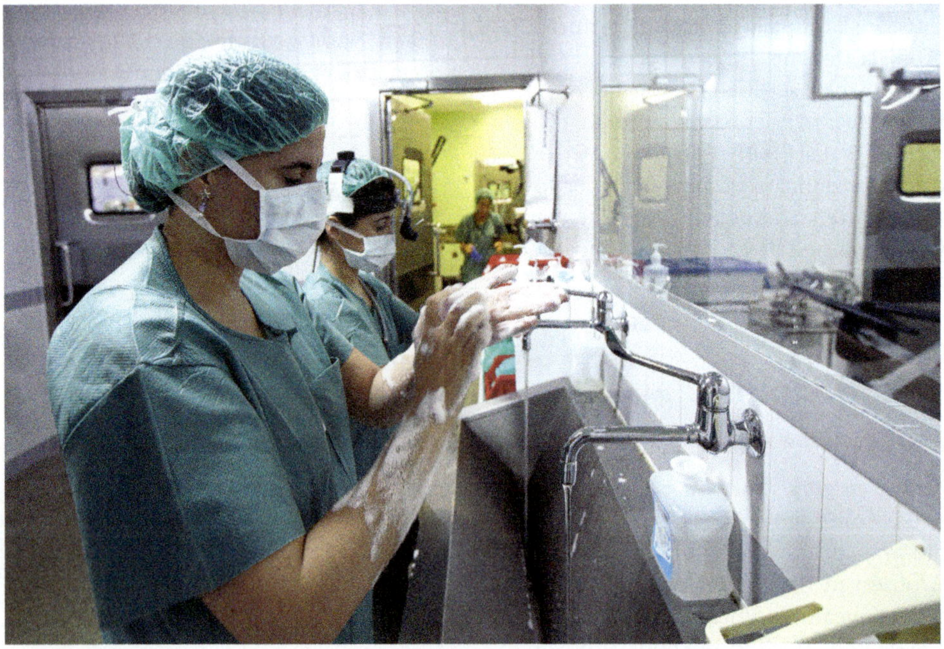

Surgeons wearing protective clothing wash hands at Hospital Donostia in San Sebastian, Spain. Handwashing and protective clothing are two of the most common contact precautions used by health care professionals to limit the spread of infectious organisms. *© Javier Larrea/Getty Images*

fected before being used on another patient. Standards for the cleaning and disinfection of equipment, and for monitoring the success of these decontamination procedures, exist and must be followed. In addition, records of equipment cleaning and maintenance must be kept, which makes it easier to investigate the source of a disease outbreak.

Impacts and Issues

In 1850 surgery was almost a death sentence. The cause of this dismal record was the inadvertent contamination of the patient by people whose task it was to ensure their care and recovery. Since then precautions that minimize patient exposure to dangerous microbes has vastly improved the quality of health care.

Nonetheless, problems remain. The spread of antibiotic-resistant bacteria such as methicillin-resistant *S. aureus* (MRSA), vancomycin-resistant *S. aureus*, and carbapenem-resistant Enterobacteriaceae in hospital wards shows that person-to-person transfer is still a reality. Part of this problem has been inadequate handwashing by health care providers. The use of alcohol-based hand sanitizers, which are effective after only a few seconds of exposure on the skin, is helping to encourage more compliance with handwashing by busy health care staff, as is increased patient awareness of the importance of proper hygiene.

Contact precautions such as handwashing and wearing protective clothing are also important when dealing with a patient with a disease caused by antibiotic-resistant bacteria such as MRSA and bacteria that have developed resistance to the antibiotic vancomycin. Improper contact precautions can allow the bacteria to spread to both fellow patients and health care workers.

PRIMARY SOURCE

Safe Management of Patients with Ebola Virus Disease (EVD) in U.S. Hospitals

SOURCE: *"Safe Management of Patients with Ebola Virus Disease (EVD) in U.S. Hospitals." Centers for Disease Control and Prevention, July 11, 2016. https://www.jointcommission.org/assets/1/6/Safe_Management_of_Patients_with_Ebola_Virus_Disease_(EVD)_in_U.S._Hospitals_FAQ.pdf (accessed January 5, 2018).*

INTRODUCTION: *Following the confirmation of four Ebola cases in the United States in 2014, the US Centers for Disease Control and Prevention (CDC) announced guidelines for managing care of Ebola patients in US hospitals. These guidelines emphasize the important role of contact precautions when caring for patients infected with the virus and discuss why these precautions differ from those implemented in other countries.*

If a patient in a U.S. hospital is identified to have suspected or confirmed EVD, what infection control precautions should be put into place? If a patient in a U.S. hospital is suspected or known to have Ebola virus disease, healthcare teams should follow standard, contact, and droplet precautions, including the following recommendations:

- **Isolate the patient:** Patients should be isolated in a single patient room (containing a private bathroom) with the door closed.
- **Wear appropriate PPE:** Healthcare providers entering the patient's room should wear: gloves, gown (fluid resistant or impermeable), eye protection (goggles or face shield), and a facemask. Additional protective equipment might be required in certain situations (e.g., copious amounts of blood, other body fluids, vomit, or feces present in the environment), including but not limited to double gloving, disposable shoe covers, and leg coverings.
- **Restrict visitors:** Avoid entry of visitors into the patient's room. Exceptions may be considered on a case by case basis for those who are essential for the patient's wellbeing. A logbook should be kept to document all persons entering the patient's room. See CDC's infection control guidance on procedures for monitoring, managing, and training of visitors.
- **Avoid aerosol-generating procedures:** Avoid aerosol-generating procedures. If performing these procedures, PPE should include respiratory protection (N95 or higher filtering facepiece respirator) and the procedure should be performed in an airborne infection isolation room.
- **Implement environmental infection control measures:** Diligent environmental cleaning and disinfection and safe handling of potentially contaminated materials is of paramount importance, as blood, sweat, vomit, feces, urine and other body secretions representing potentially-infectious materials should be done following hospital protocols.

Why do responders in Africa wear so much personal protective equipment (that can include full body suits) for this Ebola outbreak when CDC says hospitals here could safely manage the care of an Ebola patient without a full body suit?

There are important differences between providing care or performing public health tasks in Africa versus in a U.S. hospital.

In field medical settings, additional PPE may be necessary to protect healthcare workers. In some places in Africa, workers may not have the ability to prepare for potential exposures. For example, in some places, care may be provided in clinics with limited resources (e.g., no running water, no climate control, no floors, inadequate medical supplies), and workers could be in those areas for several hours with a number of Ebola infected patients. Additionally, certain job responsibilities and tasks, such as attending to dead bodies, may also require different PPE than what is used when providing care for infected patients in a hospital.

SEE ALSO *Airborne Precautions; Handwashing; Infection Control and Asepsis; Nosocomial (Health Care–Associated) Infections; Standard Precautions*

BIBLIOGRAPHY

Books

Amer, Fatma. *Hospital Infection Control, Part 1.* 3rd ed. Saarbrücken, Germany: Noor, 2017.

Saint, Sanjay, and Sarah Krein. *Preventing Hospital Infections: Real-World Problems, Realistic Solutions.* Oxford. UK: Oxford University Press, 2014.

Periodicals

Fox, Cherie, et al. "Use of a Patient Hand Hygiene Protocol to Reduce Hospital-Acquired Infections and Improve Nurses' Hand Washing." *American Journal of Critical Care* 24 (2015): 216–224.

Seibert, Grace, et al. "What Do Visitors Know and How Do They Feel about Contact Precautions?" *American Journal of Infection Control* 45 (2017).

Websites

"Transmission-Based Precautions." Centers for Disease Control and Prevention. https://www.cdc.gov/infectioncontrol/basics/transmission-based-precautions.html (accessed December 4, 2017).

Brian Hoyle

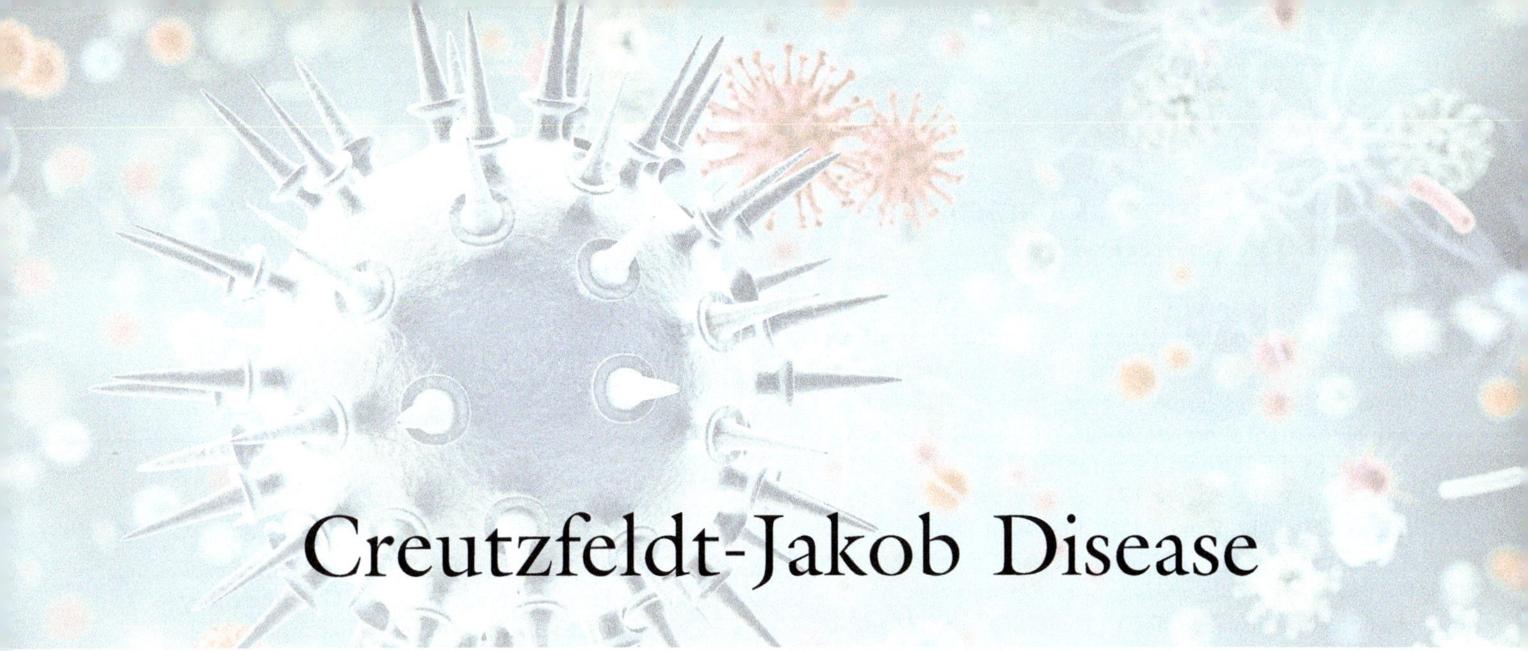

Creutzfeldt-Jakob Disease

■ Introduction

Creutzfeldt-Jakob Disease (CJD) is a rare and invariably fatal brain disorder. It belongs to a group of diseases called transmissible spongiform encephalopathies (TSEs). It affects both humans and animals, leading to the appearance of tiny holes within the brain tissue, giving it a spongy appearance. In 1996 several cases of a new form of CJD were reported in the United Kingdom. Because the new form differed in many ways from the so-called classical form of the disease, it was named variant CJD (vCJD, also known as new variant CJD, or CJD-nv). Between 1996 and 2015, around 200 cases of vCJD were reported around the world.

The cause of vCJD appears to be exposure to bovine spongiform encephalopathy (also known as mad cow disease), a TSE of cattle, through the consumption of beef. Control of bovine spongiform encephalopathy (BSE) has led to a dramatic fall in the number of cases of vCJD. However, there is still a risk that the disease could be transmitted through blood donated by an infected, but asymptomatic, individual.

WORDS TO KNOW

ATAXIA An unsteadiness in walking or standing that is associated with brain diseases such as kuru or Creutzfeldt-Jakob disease.

CADAVER The body of a deceased human, especially one designated for scientific dissection or other research.

DEMENTIA A progressive deterioration and eventual loss of mental ability that is severe enough to interfere with normal activities of daily living, lasts more than six months, has not been present since birth, and is not associated with a loss or alteration of consciousness. From the Latin word *dement* (meaning "away mind"), dementia is a group of symptoms caused by gradual death of brain cells. It is usually caused by degeneration in the cerebral cortex, the part of the brain responsible for thoughts, memories, actions, and personality. Death of brain cells in this region leads to the cognitive impairment that characterizes dementia.

ENCEPHALOPATHY Any abnormality in the structure or function of the brain.

HUMAN GROWTH HORMONE A protein that is made and released from the pituitary gland, which increases growth and manufacture of new cells.

PRIONS Proteins that are infectious. Indeed, the name *prion* is derived from "proteinaceous infectious particles." The discovery of prions and confirmation of their infectious nature overturned a central dogma that infections were caused only by intact organisms, particularly microorganisms such as bacteria, fungi, parasites, or viruses. Because prions lack genetic material, the prevailing attitude was that a protein could not cause disease.

SPONGIFORM The clinical name for the appearance of brain tissue affected by prion diseases, such as Creutzfeldt-Jakob disease or bovine spongiform encephalopathy (mad cow disease). The disease process leads to the formation of tiny holes in brain tissue, giving it a spongy appearance.

Disease History, Characteristics, and Transmission

The classical form of CJD has been known since the early years of the 20th century. A rare disease, it affects around one in a million worldwide. In the United States, which was home to approximately 323 million people in 2016, there are about 300 cases per year. According to the European Centre for Disease Prevention and Control, there were 174 cases of definite or probable vCJD in the United Kingdom as of January 2015. About 15 percent of classical cases are inherited, while the rest are sporadic, arising for no obvious reason. The classical form usually affects people over age 50 and is marked by ataxia (unsteadiness on the feet), dementia (a sharp decline in mental performance), blurred vision, and slurred speech. The majority of patients with classical CJD die within six months of the onset of symptoms. vCJD, on the other hand, has been found largely among teenagers and young adults, although there have been cases in older people. It begins with psychiatric symptoms, such as anxiety and depression, and persistent pain and odd sensations in the face and limbs. Later, ataxia and sudden jerky movements set in, along with progressive dementia. The course of vCJD is longer, with death usually occurring around a year after the onset of symptoms. There are also significant differences in brain imaging, electroencephalogram (a test used to measure brain activity), and pathology data between classical and vCJD.

The infective agent in all TSEs, including CJD, is neither a bacterium or a virus but a prion, which is best described as an infectious protein. A prion is an abnormally shaped version of a protein that occurs naturally in the brain. When the normal prion protein comes into contact with the abnormal version, it is converted into the abnormal version and can go on to corrupt other normal prion protein molecules. This cascade of damage then spreads throughout the brain. In sporadic cases of CJD, there may be a spontaneous change of a normal prion protein molecule into the abnormal form; no risk factors for this are known, however. In inherited CJD, there are mutations in the gene for prion protein that may render a person more susceptible to prion infection.

All reported cases of vCJD have involved individuals who have spent time in a country affected by BSE, which provides at least indirect evidence for the mode of transmission: consumption of BSE-contaminated beef. Meanwhile, there have been a few cases of so-called iatrogenic (an illness that is inadvertently introduced by a medical professional during treatment or examination) CJD. In such

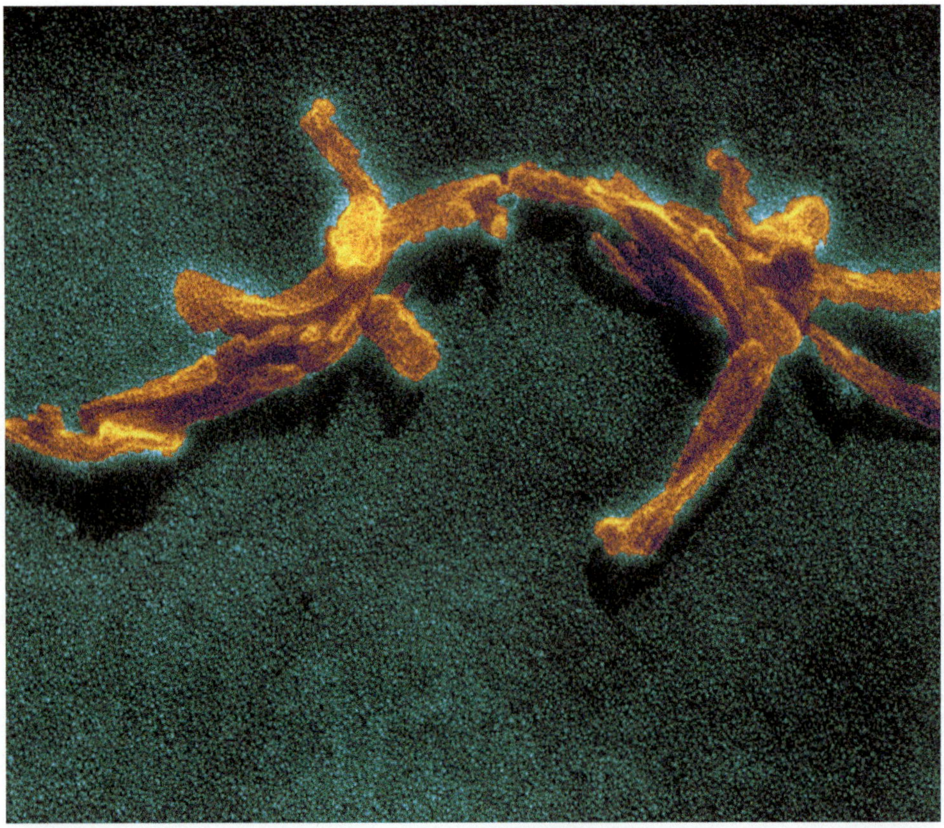

Color-enhanced electron micrograph of prions. Prions are infectious protein molecules that cause Creutzfeldt-Jakob disease and other nervous system diseases. *© Eye of Science/Science Source*

US Creutzfeldt-Jakob Disease Deaths (2000–2016)

Year	Deaths (approximate)	Year	Deaths (approximate)
2000	238	2009	353
2001	259	2010	396
2002	260	2011	409
2003	284	2012	380
2004	279	2013	478
2005	296	2014	441
2006	290	2015	481
2007	330	2016	492
2008	352		

SOURCE: Adapted from "Creutzfeldt-Jakob Disease Deaths and Age-Adjusted Death Rate, United States, 1979–2016." US Centers for Disease Control and Prevention. December 22, 2017. Available from: https://www.cdc.gov/prions/cjd/occurrence-transmission.html

cases, the disease is transmitted from one person to another through contaminated human growth hormone (which used to be extracted from the pituitary glands of human cadavers) or instruments used in brain surgery. There have also been three cases of vCJD arising among recipients of blood from an asymptomatic donor who later developed the disease. However, there have been no cases of direct person-to-person transmission of vCJD.

■ Scope and Distribution

Most of the cases of vCJD have occurred in the United Kingdom. As of December 2017 there had been 178 primary cases (contracted, presumably, through contaminated beef). Recent research suggests that blood may be a efficient carrier of vCJD. In 2008 the UK Health Protection Agency carried out an anonymized survey of 100,000 tonsil samples to determine how many people were potentially incubating vCJD. Sixteen positive cases were discovered, a prevalence rate of about 1 in 2,000 in the United Kingdom. Because the relationship between infection in the lymphoid system and the brain is not clear, several of these individuals may be silent carriers who will not develop vCJD. Though many scientists believe the incubation period for vCJD is a decade, this is still a matter of debate. Kuru, a human TSE discovered in Papua New Guinea in the 1950s, can have an incubation period of up to 40 years. Without knowing more about the details of how vCJD is transmitted, it is impossible to say how many more cases of vCJD may occur.

■ Treatment and Prevention

There is no proven cure for any form of CJD, and treatment is palliative (aimed at reducing symptoms). Some evidence suggests that pentosan polysulphate, a semisynthetic chemical derived from shavings of beech wood, given as an injection into the brain, could prolong survival. As such, the UK Medical Research Council (MRC) is analyzing data on a number of patients who have received this treatment. However, the MRC's Prion Clinic reported that "it cannot be concluded that the treatment has had a beneficial effect, because it was impossible to make direct comparison with similar but untreated patients. It is also very difficult to determine exactly when the disease starts and this obviously affects the estimation of survival time." One report suggests that flupirtine can improve cognition in CJD, but it does not appear to prolong survival. There is substantial evidence for the effectiveness and safety of antibody treatments, which bind to prions, and investigation of their effectiveness continues in laboratory mice.

There are a number of drugs that can relieve symptoms and make the patient more comfortable, such as valproate and clonazepam for jerking movements. Eventually, all patients with CJD will require 24-hour nursing care, as they will lose the ability to do anything for themselves.

Prevention of vCJD depends on elimination of exposure to BSE-contaminated beef. A number of measures have been adopted in the United Kingdom and elsewhere to this end. There remains the possibility that people could become infected through CJD-contaminated blood and blood products. Those who have received blood from an infected donor in the United Kingdom have been banned from giving blood. In the United States, there are restrictions on people who have resided in the United Kingdom acting as blood donors, in case they are incubating vCJD.

■ Impacts and Issues

In 1986 BSE appeared in cattle in the United Kingdom. Researchers identified cattle feed containing remnants of slaughtered cows, especially parts of the brain and nervous system, as the likely culprit of the disease. The UK government banned the use of cattle remnants in feed. In 1992 the incidence of BSE in UK cattle peaked, with 36,700 confirmed, about 1 percent of the UK cattle herd. Despite the epidemic of mad cow disease, consumers were assured that British beef products were safe to eat. In 1996 researchers identified BSE-contaminated beef as the probable cause of vCJD in humans.

The link between BSE and vCJD had widespread social and economic effects. The UK cattle heard was culled of possibly infected animals, resulting in losses to herders. As the emergence of vCJD received global media attention, consumption of beef within the United Kingdom dropped dramatically, possibly as much as 40 percent in 1996 and 1997. The meat slaughtering and packing industry was scrutinized, revealing slaughtering practices that carried the possibility of BSE-tainted nervous system tissue entering ground beef. Other European nations temporarily banned the import of UK beef products and began to evaluate their own herds for BSE. By 2005 BSE had been found in Europe, Asia, North America, and the Falkland Islands, a British territory off the coast of Argentina. The vCJD epidemic peaked in the United Kingdom in 2000. There have been 178 deaths there since May 1990. France has had the second-highest number of vCJD cases. In the United States, there have been four cases. Worldwide, there have been 201 cases of vCJD in 11 countries.

For decades inherited or "classic" cases of CJD had affected only people who made a particular form of the normal prion protein, the "M," or methionine amino acid, type at position 129 on the protein chain. In 2017, however, a case was confirmed in someone with a mix of genes for not only the "M" type but also a "V," or valine amino acid, type. This may mean that a new wave of cases was misdiagnosed and could potentially become manifest in the UK population.

The vCJD epidemic also prompted fears about the safety of the international supply of human blood, plasma, tissues, and organs. Many nations excluded, or continue to exclude, donors who resided for several months in parts of Europe and the United Kingdom between 1980 and 2000. People who received transfusions or organ or tissue transplants in the United Kingdom are also excluded as potential donors in several countries. The three cases of transfusion-associated vCJD in the United Kingdom came from a pool of 23 recipients of blood from the infected donor. Because the term of incubation for vCJD remains unknown, others who received the contaminated blood remain at risk. A prototype blood test for vCJD has been developed by the prion unit at the MRC in the United Kingdom.

CJD, including vCJD, is still a rare disease and one that is poorly understood. Although US researcher Stanley Prusiner (1942–) was awarded the 1997 Nobel Prize in Medicine or Physiology for his work on prions, there is still much to be learned about how these unconventional infective agents work. For example, the routes of transmission of prion diseases are not yet well established. Adding to the difficulty of making an unambiguous diagnosis, most neurologists have never seen a case of CJD even when symptoms are present. The disease, like other TSEs, may be present without symptoms for many years, putting people at risk of infection. However, ongoing research aims to better understand all forms of CJD and other prion-transmitted diseases.

SEE ALSO *Blood Supply and Infectious Disease; Bovine Spongiform Encephalopathy (Mad Cow Disease); Kuru*

BIBLIOGRAPHY

Books

Koata, Gina. *Mercies in Disguise: A Story of Hope, a Family's Genetic Destiny, and the Science That Rescued Them.* New York: St. Martin's, 2017.

Ridley, Rosalind M., and Harry F. Baker. *Fatal Protein: The Story of CJD, BSE, and Other Prion Diseases.* New York: Oxford University Press, 1998.

Periodicals

Callaway, Ewen. "One in 2,000 UK People Might carry vCJD Proteins." *Nature* (October 15, 2013). This article can also be found online at https://www.nature.com/news/one-in-2-000-uk-people-might-carry-vcjd-proteins-1.13962 (accessed January 29, 2018).

MacKenzie, Debora. "Many More People Could Still Die from Mad Cow Disease in the UK." *New Scientist* (January 18, 2017). This article can also be found online at https://www.newscientist.com/article/2118418-many-more-people-could-still-die-from-mad-cow-disease-in-the-uk/ (accessed January 29, 2018).

Websites

"Creutzfeldt-Jakob Disease: Diagnosis." National Health Service (NHS), January 21, 2015. https://www.nhs.uk/conditions/creutzfeldt-jakob-disease-cjd/diagnosis/ (accessed January 29, 2018).

"Creutzfeldt-Jakob Disease Fact Sheet. National Institute of Neurological Disorders and Stroke, May 10, 2017. https://www.ninds.nih.gov/Disorders/Patient-Caregiver-Education/Fact-Sheets/Creutzfeldt-Jakob-Disease-Fact-Sheet (accessed January 29, 2018).

"Creutzfeldt-Jakob Disease Surveillance in the UK." National CJD Research and Surveillance Unit, University of Edinburgh, 2016. https://www.cjd.ed.ac.uk/sites/default/files/report25.pdf (accessed January 29, 2018).

"Drug Treatments." Medical Research Council Prion Unit, 2018. http://www.prion.ucl.ac.uk/clinic-services/research/drug-treatments (accessed January 29, 2018).

"European Creutzfeldt-Jakob Disease Surveillance Network (EuroCJD)." European Centre for Disease Prevention and Control. https://ecdc.europa.eu/en/about-us/partnerships-and-networks/disease-and-laboratory-networks/european-creutzfeldt-jakob (accessed February 1, 2018).

"Variant Creutzfeldt-Jakob Disease (vCJD)." Centers for Disease Control and Prevention, February 6, 2015. https://www.cdc.gov/prions/vcjd/index.html (accessed January 29, 2018).

Susan Aldridge
Anna Marie E. Roos

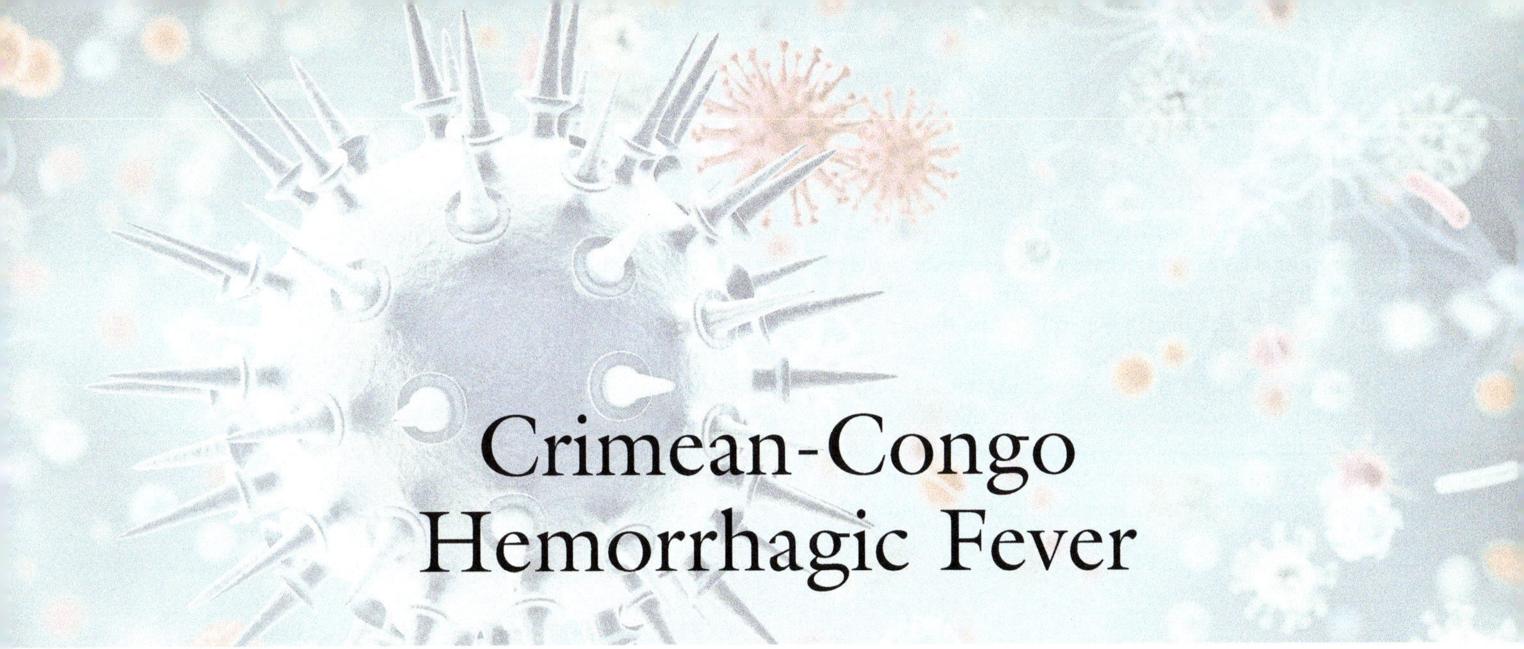

Crimean-Congo Hemorrhagic Fever

■ Introduction

Crimean-Congo hemorrhagic fever (CCHF) is a viral disease caused by infection from a tick-borne virus. The virus that causes CCHF is contained within *Nairovirus*, a member of related pathogenic (disease-causing) viruses within the Bunyaviridae family.

All nairoviruses are transmitted by the bite of argasid (soft) or isodid (hard) ticks. However, only a few of these ticks have proven to cause human infections. According to the World Health Organization (WHO) and the Centers for Disease Control and Prevention (CDC), the tick of the *Hyalomma* genus is most capable of serving as the vector for the disease, especially in small vertebrates on which immature ticks feed.

CCHF is an infectious disease that is capable of being transmitted by ticks between domesticated and wild animals, from animals to humans, and from humans to animals. Common animals infected are cattle, sheep, goats, and hares. Humans are infected through contact with the blood of an infected animal or tick. Approximately one-third of humans who contract Crimean-Congo hemorrhagic fever die as a result of the illness.

■ Disease History, Characteristics, and Transmission

CCHF was documented in Russia in the 12th century. However, the first accurate description came from the Crimea region of the former USSR in 1944 and 1945. It was at that time called Crimean hemorrhagic fever. In 1969 it was realized that the pathogen causing the fever was also the illness identified in 1956 in what is now Kisangani, Democratic Republic of Congo. It was therefore renamed Crimean-Congo hemorrhagic fever.

CCHF is an arthropod-borne illness. Small vertebrates on which immature ticks feed seem to serve as the primary means of spreading the virus. Infected female ticks pass the disease into their eggs, which develop into infected immature ticks. Mature ticks carry the virus to larger animals, such as large vertebrates, who can become intermediate hosts. CCHF transmission to humans occurs when people butcher or eat infected livestock and when health workers become exposed to infected blood. Animals do not show clinical signs of the illness, making it difficult for humans to identify and avoid potential carriers of CCHF.

After a tick bite, the incubation period in humans is about one to three days but can take up to nine days. After contact with infected blood or tissue, the incubation period is

WORDS TO KNOW

ARTHROPOD A member of the largest single animal phylum, consisting of organisms with segmented bodies, jointed legs or wings, and exoskeletons. This includes insects and spiders.

HEMORRHAGIC FEVER A high fever caused by viral infection that features a high volume of bleeding. The bleeding is caused by the formation of tiny blood clots throughout the bloodstream. These blood clots, also called microthrombi, deplete platelets and fibrinogen in the bloodstream. When bleeding begins, the factors needed for the clotting of the blood are scarce. Thus, uncontrolled bleeding (hemorrhage) ensues.

INTERMEDIATE HOST An organism infected by a parasite while the parasite is in a developmental, not sexually mature form.

VECTOR Any agent that carries and transmits parasites and diseases. Also, an organism or a chemical used to transport a gene into a new host cell.

usually five to six days, with a maximum of 13 days. Influenza-like symptoms occur suddenly. In most cases these symptoms last for about one week. However, signs of bleeding appear 75 percent of the time in cases lasting longer than one week. Death occurs in up to 40 percent of cases, according to the WHO.

Symptoms include high fever, aching muscles, dizziness, neck pain, backache, stomach pain, headache, sore eyes, and light sensitivity. Later, nosebleeds, red eyes, flushed face, red throat, bruising, bloody urine, vomiting, black stools, skin rash, and diarrhea occur. Still later, abdominal pain occurs, along with mental confusion and mood swings.

Scope and Distribution

The disease is primarily found in places where *Hyalomma* ticks, including *H. marginatum, H. rufipes, H. anatolicum*, and *H. asiaticum*, are found. Biting midges of the *Culicoides* species can also be vectors. As of 2011 epidemiologists identified approximately 5,000 cases of CCHF in some 140 outbreaks in more than 30 countries. While human CCHF infections are most commonly reported in Central Asia, the Middle East, and North Africa, the scope of infections has expanded since CCHF was first identified in Crimea and the Congo in the mid-20th century. A growing number of CCHF infections have been identified as far afield as Turkey, South Africa, and the Indian subcontinent. In Spain in 2016 two cases of people contracting the disease locally alarmed and confounded epidemiologists. According to a 2017 NPR story, "This was the first time the disease had shown up in Western Europe in two people who had not traveled to an area where the fever is endemic." Although researchers suggested the disease may have been carried to Spain via birds or livestock infected with *Nairovirus*-carrying *Hyalomma* ticks, no definite source of the infection had been identified as of early 2018.

Most cases occur in domesticated and wild animals. Small mammals carry the disease, especially the Middle-African hedgehog, multimammate rat, and European hare. Domestic animals, such as sheep, goats, and cattle, also carry the tick. Most birds do not become infected, except ostriches.

CCHF occurs less frequently in humans. Groups most likely to become infected are slaughterhouse workers, veterinarians, surgeons and other medical workers, animal herders, and agricultural workers. Widespread infections in medical facilities have occurred due to improper sterilization of equipment, reuse of injection needles, and supply contamination. Travelers are at risk in countries where CCHF is present.

Treatment and Prevention

Diagnosis includes: serological test (to find antibodies in serum); immunohistochemical staining (to find viral antigen in tissue); microscopic examination (to find viral RNA [ribonucleic acid] sequence in blood or tissue); polymerase chain reaction (PCR) technique (to detect viral genome); and enzyme-linked immunosor-

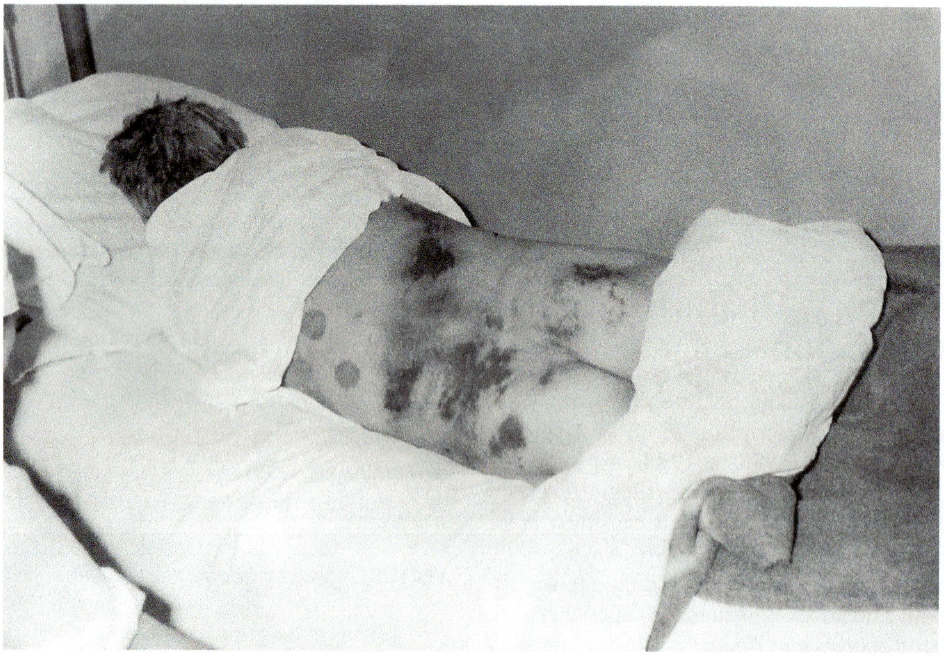

A patient suffering from Crimean-Congo hemorrhagic hever, 1969. The bruising shown here is a common symptom of the disease. *© Smith Collection/Gado/Getty Images*

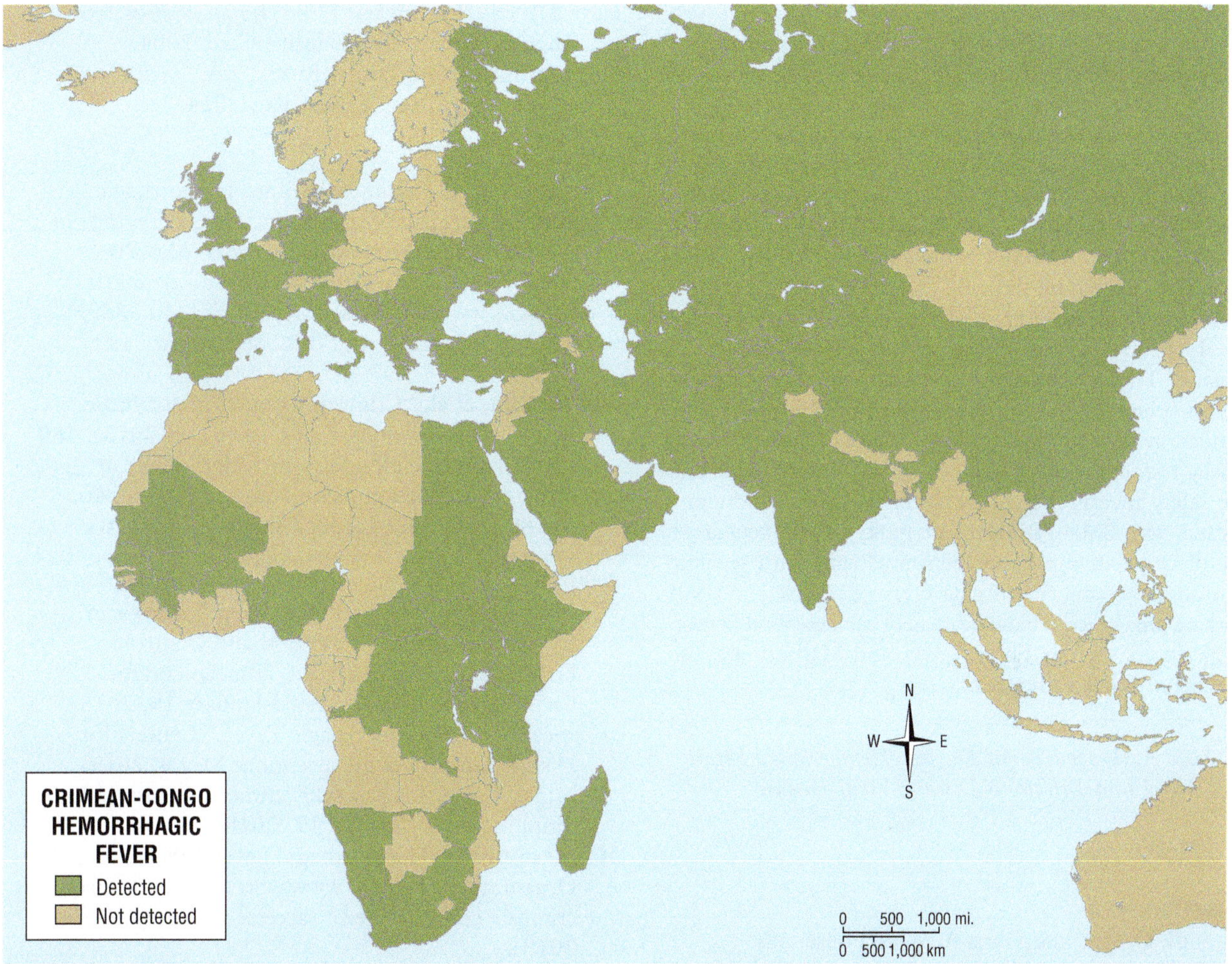

bent assay (ELISA) technique (to detect immunoglobulin-G and immunoglobulin-M antibodies in serum).

Oral and intravenous treatment involves the antiviral drug ribavirin (Copegus®, Ribasphere®, Virazole®). Ribavirin has been seemingly effective during actual outbreaks, although scientific studies have not supported that conclusion.

Treatment is generally supportive and based on the symptom's type and degree of severity. Fluid balance, electrolyte levels, and secondary infections are carefully monitored. Fatality rates in hospitalized patients range widely, depending on infection severity, care quality, and other variables.

CCHF is commonly prevented by governments that require de-ticking of farm animals. Insect repellents (containing DEET (N,N-diethyl-meta-toluamide), acaricides (chemicals intended to kill ticks), appropriate clothing (gloves and clothing treated with permethrin), and body inspections help prevent the disease. People living in endemic areas are advised to avoid contact with blood and fluids of infected livestock and humans, to avoid areas where tick vectors are abundant, and to regularly examine clothing and skin for ticks.

While an "inactivated, mouse brain-derived vaccine against CCHF has been developed and used on a small scale in Eastern Europe," according to WHO in 2013, this vaccine has not been proven to be safe and effective and is not widely available for human use. In 2017 the Turkish health minister announced that scientists from the nation's health ministry were nearing completion of a CCHF vaccine. Turkey had 10,000 reported cases of CCHF as of 2015. As of early 2018, however, no vaccine had been approved for use in Turkey or elsewhere.

■ Impacts and Issues

Crimean-Congo hemorrhagic fever is one of the world's most severe arthropod-borne diseases. It has a mortality rate of up to 40 percent. CCHF is a growing public health problem in an increasing number of places. Because of this, numerous health agencies and researchers have identified the need for increased knowledge about CCHF.

In a 2017 article for *Frontiers in Cellular and Infection Microbiology*, Anna Papa, Katerina Tsergouli, Katerina Tsioka, and Ali Mirazimi noted that a greater understanding of how, at a cellular level, the viruses that cause CCHF move from ticks to humans and other animals will help unlock new ways of treating and preventing infections. Study of the virus that causes CCHF is limited, however, by the need for high-level containment to study it.

Crimean-Congo hemorrhagic fever's causative agent, the *Nairovirus*, is classified as a biosafety level 4 (BSL4) pathogen by the CDC. Scientists study BSL4 pathogens, which are mostly viruses, in specialized facilities designed to contain them. All BSL4 pathogens have the capacity to cause life-threatening diseases, and no effective vaccine is readily available to prevent them. As of 2017 there were 10 BSL4 facilities in the United States, as well as one in Canada. There were eight BSL4 labs in the European Union (plus one in Switzerland) as of 2013, with more planned in that continent as well. Access to BSL4 labs is usually restricted to essential personnel. Among the extensive safety measures used by scientists when conducting research with BSL4 pathogens are multi-containment areas, one-piece positive pressure personnel suits with separate ventilation systems, negative air pressure rooms, and a safe working area called a biological safety cabinet. Viral hemorrhagic fevers such as Ebola, Lassa, and Marburg are also considered BSL4 pathogens.

See Also *Arthropod-Borne Disease; Hemorrhagic Fevers; Travel and Infectious Disease; Viral Disease*

BIBLIOGRAPHY

Books

Ergonul, Onder, and Chris A. Whitehouse, eds. *Crimean-Congo Hemorrhagic Fever: A Global Perspective.* New York: Springer, 2010.

Farb, Daniel. *Bioterrorism Hemorrhagic Viruses.* Los Angeles: University of Health Care, 2004.

Singh, Sunit K., and Daniel Ruzek, eds. *Viral Hemorrhagic Fevers.* New York: CRC, 2014.

Periodicals

Papa, Anna, et al. "Crimean-Congo Hemorrhagic Fever: Tick-Host-Virus Interactions." *Frontiers in Cellular and Infection Microbiology* (May 26, 2017). This article can also be found online at https://www.frontiersin.org/articles/10.3389/fcimb.2017.00213/full (accessed January 19, 2018).

Shayan, Sara, et al. "Crimean-Congo Hemorrhagic Fever." *Laboratory Medicine* 46, no. 3 (2015): 180–189. This article can also be found online at https://academic.oup.com/labmed/article/46/3/180/2657762 (accessed January 19, 2018).

Websites

"Crimean-Congo Haemorrhagic Fever." European Center for Disease Prevention and Control. https://ecdc.europa.eu/en/crimean-congo-haemorrhagic-fever (accessed January 19, 2018).

"Crimean-Congo Hemorrhagic Fever." Centers for Disease Control and Prevention, May 9, 2015. https://www.cdc.gov/vhf/crimean-congo/index.html (accessed January 19, 2018).

"Crimean-Congo Haemorrhagic Fever." World Health Organization. http://www.who.int/csr/disease/crimean_congoHF/en/ (accessed January 19, 2018).

Brian Hoyle

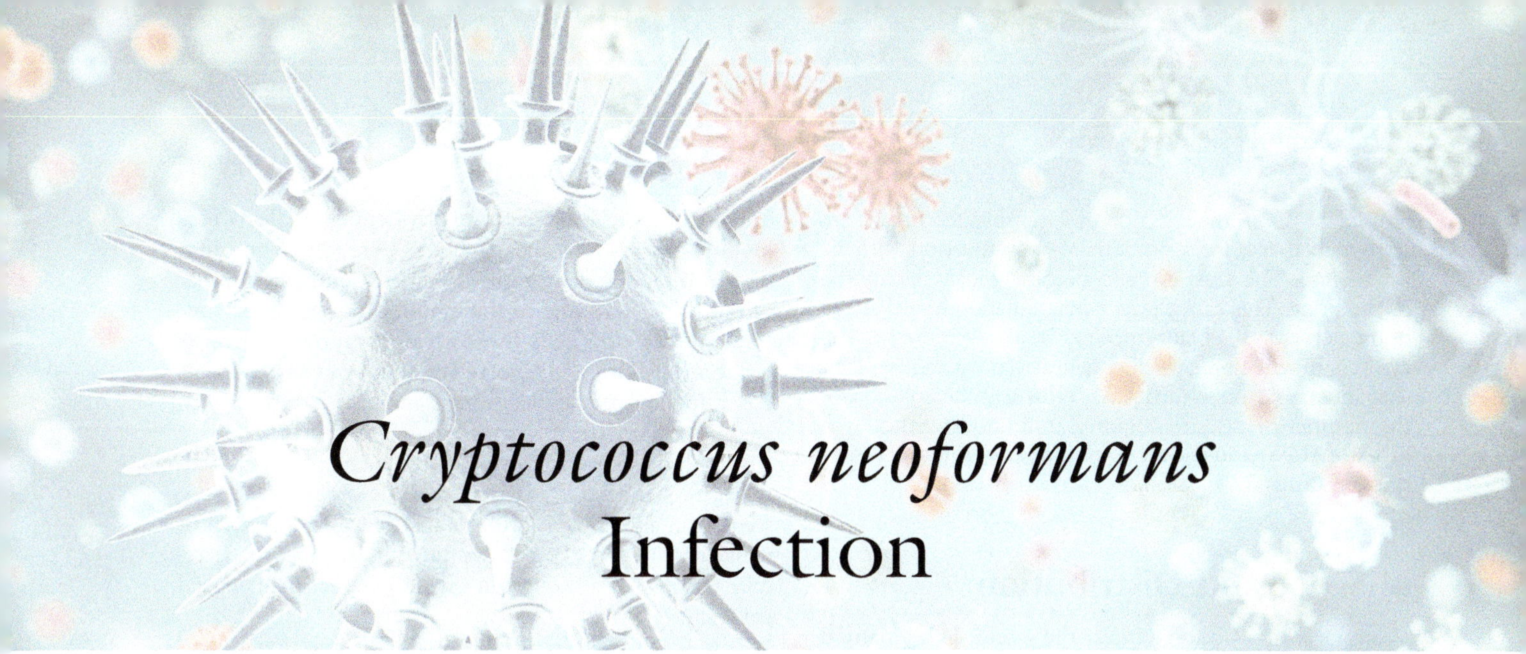

Cryptococcus neoformans Infection

Introduction

Cryptococcus neoformans is a yeast that is the sole species of the genus *Cryptococcus*- capable of causing mycotic (fungal) disease. There are three versions of *C. neoformans* based on differences in the capsule that surrounds the yeast, the use of various sugars as nutrients, and the shape of the environmentally resilient structures (spores) that can be produced by the yeast. *C. neoformans* variety *neoformans* causes most of the cryptococcal infections in humans.

Disease History, Characteristics, and Transmission

C. neoformans causes cryptococcosis. The infection begins in the lungs following the inhalation of the microorganism, particularly the small form of *C. neoformans* called a basidiospore. These spores are smaller than the growing (vegetative) form of the yeast and thus can penetrate deeper into the very small air passages (alveoli) of the lung. In the warm and moist conditions of the lung, the basidiospores can increase in size, and normal growth of the yeast can resume.

When the yeast begins to grow, a capsule that is usually only minimally produced by the spores is exuberantly produced. Like the capsule produced by some bacteria, the capsule of *C. neoformans* is made of sugars. The capsule helps shield the yeast from the immune response of the host, in particular the engulfing (phagocytosis) and breakdown of the yeast by a type of immune cell called a macrophage.

C. neoformans is equipped with enzymes known as proteases, which degrade proteins, as well as enzymes that destroy phospholipids. Both proteins and phospholipids are important components of the cell wall that surrounds cells. This causes the destruction of host cells, which makes it easier for *C. neoformans* to enter the host cells and to invade tissue.

Evidence from laboratory studies indicates that *C. neoformans* is not only capable of evading the host's immune response but may also actively impair the response. This would explain the observation that people who survive a bout of cryptococcal meningitis can continue to have a malfunctioning immune system.

Most commonly, *C. neoformans* causes the form of meningitis called cryptococcal meningitis. (Meningitis can also be caused by bacteria or viruses.) People who are immunocompromised (whose immune system is not functioning properly due to infection with, for example, the human immunodeficiency virus [HIV] or deliberate sup-

WORDS TO KNOW

BASIDIOSPORE A fungal spore of the class Basidomycetes. Basidomycetes are classified under the Fungi kingdom in the phylum Mycota (i.e., Basidomycota or Basidiomycota), class Mycetes (i.e., Basidomycetes or Basidiomycetes). Fungi are frequently parasites that decompose organic material from their hosts, such as those growing on rotten wood, although some may cause serious plant diseases such as smuts (Ustomycetes) and rusts (Teliomycetes). Some live in a symbiotic relationship with plant roots (Mycorrhizae). A cell type termed basidium is responsible for sexual spore formation in Basidomycetes through nuclear fusion followed by meiosis, thus forming haploid basidiospores.

IMMUNOCOMPROMISED Having an immune system with reduced ability to recognize and respond to the presence of foreign material.

MYCOTIC Having to do with or caused by a fungus. Any medical condition caused by a fungus is a mycotic condition, also called a mycosis.

pression to lessen the rejection of a transplanted organ) are at particular risk for a potentially fatal infection with *C. neoformans.* The yeast can also become widely distributed in the body. This can produce inflammation and damage of the nerves in the brain (meningitis) and infections of the eye (conjunctivitis), ear (otitis), heart (myocarditis), liver (hepatitis), and bone (arthritis). Prior to the explosion of the number of cases of acquired immunodeficiency syndrome (AIDS) and the more routine use of immunosuppressant drugs, *C. neoformans* infections were rare.

■ Scope and Distribution

C. neoformans is found all over the world. It is a natural inhabitant of some plants, fruits, and birds such as pigeons and chickens. The microbe is often transferred to humans via bird feces. As the feces dry, the yeast spores can be wafted into the air to be subsequently inhaled.

■ Treatment and Prevention

Treatment for cryptococcal meningitis usually includes antifungal drugs such as fluconazole. Often, a compound called amphotericin B is also administered. These can also be given in combination. The combination strategy uses amphotericin along with fluconazole for two weeks followed by fluconazole alone for at least 10 weeks. Treatment is usually done intravenously, which produces a higher concentration of the drug throughout the body. This is important because the infection can quickly become widespread. Treatment side effects may include fever, chills, headache, nausea with vomiting, diarrhea, kidney damage, and a decrease in the number of red blood cells due to the inhibition of bone marrow. Fewer red blood cells means less oxygen, and iron is capable of being transported throughout the body, a condition called anemia. Also, some people can have an allergic reaction to the drug.

Both drugs are available as liposome preparations, with the drug packaged inside spheres made of lipid. The liposomes can also contain proteins that recognize target proteins in the patient. This allows the drug to be more specifically targeted to a site within the body rather than applied generally.

Prospects for recovery are good if the infection is identified and treated while it is still confined to the lungs. However, spread of the infection beyond the lungs, especially to the central nervous system, is a serious complication and can threaten the life of someone who is immunocompromised.

■ Impacts and Issues

The prevalence of cryptococcal illness in the Pacific Northwest region of the United States and on Vancouver Island on Canada's west coast has been increasing since the late 20th century. Researchers from the US Centers for Disease Control and Prevention (CDC) and Health Canada who have been studying the illnesses have concluded that the increasingly temperate climate of the region favors the expansion of the yeast into a

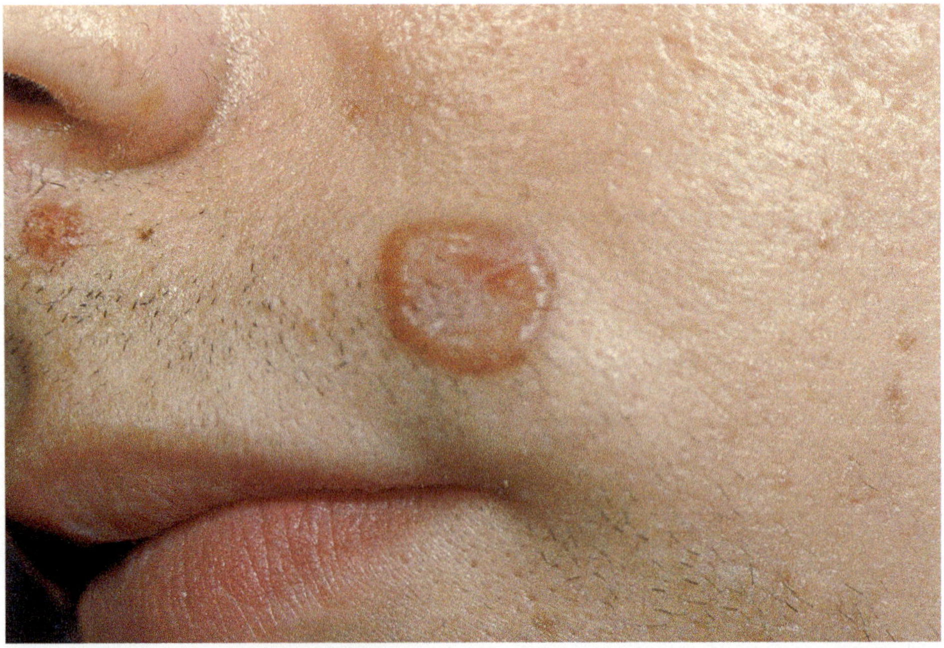

Some cases of cryptococcosis develop skin changes such as rashes, nodules, pustules, and ulcers. *© BSIP/ UIG Via Getty Images*

Estimated Yearly Cases of HIV-Related Cryptococcal Meningitis

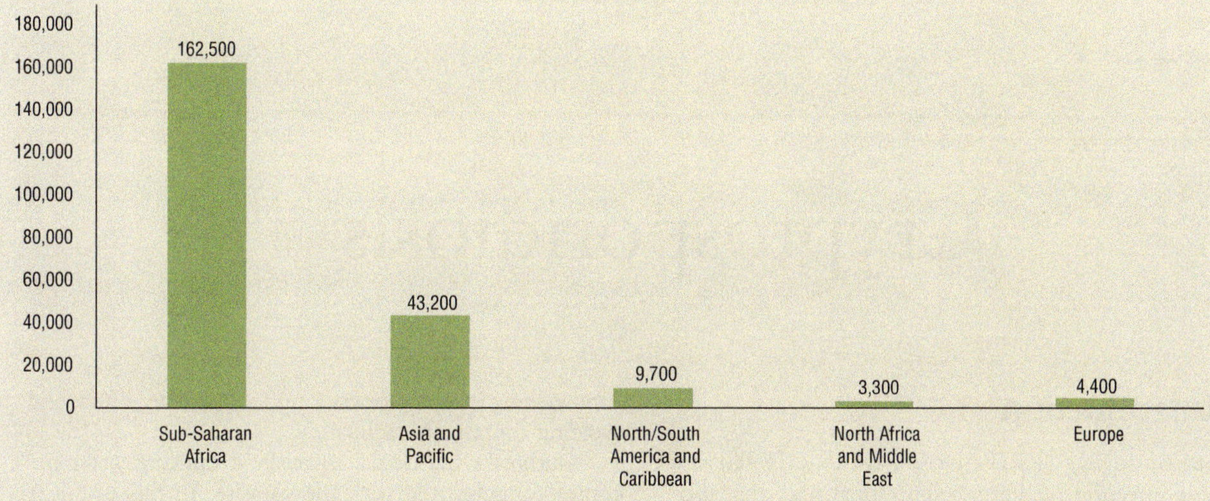

SOURCE: "*C. neoformans* Infection Statistics." Centers for Disease Control and Prevention. 2015. Available from: https://www.cdc.gov /fungal/diseases/cryptococcosisneoformans/statistics.html

region that it formerly did not occupy. With regions of the world expected to warm over the next century, the geographic range of *C. neoformans* may increase.

Cryptococcosis is the most common fungal infection of the central nervous system in HIV-positive people and is the main manifestation of AIDS in about two-thirds of those who are HIV positive. As of 2017 there was no prevention strategy.

SEE ALSO *AIDS (Acquired Immunodeficiency Syndrome); Mycotic Disease; Opportunistic Infection*

BIBLIOGRAPHY

Books

Quammen, David. *The Chimp and the River: How AIDS Emerged from an African Forest.* New York: Norton, 2015.

Whiteside, Alan. *HIV and AIDS: A Very Short Introduction.* 2nd ed. Oxford, UK: Oxford University Press, 2016.

Periodicals

Desjardins, Christopher A., et al. "Population Genetics and the Evolution of Virulence in the Fungal Pathogen *Cryptococcus neoformans.*" *Genome Research* 27 (2015): 1207–1219.

Grossman, Nina T., and Arturo Casadevall. "Physiological Differences in *Cryptococcus neoformans* Strains *in vitro* versus *in vivo* and Their Effects on Antifungal Susceptibility." *Antimicrobial Agents and Chemotherapy* 61 (2017): e02108–e02116.

Websites

"*C. neoformans* Infection." Centers for Disease Control and Prevention. https://www.cdc.gov/fungal/diseases/cryptococcosis-neoformans/index.html (accessed November 15, 2017).

Brian Hoyle

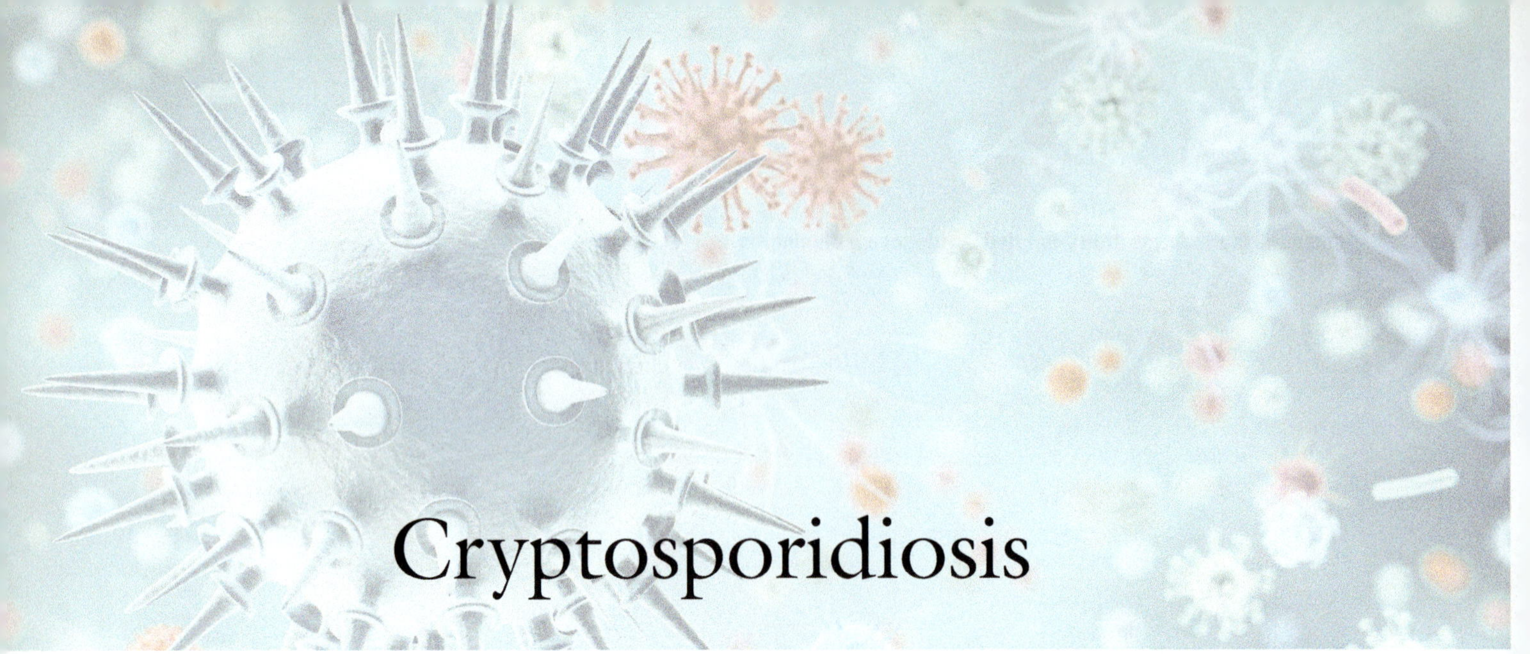

Cryptosporidiosis

Introduction

Cryptosporidiosis (KRIP-toe-spo-rid-ee-OH-sis) is a parasitic infection of the gastrointestinal tract that usually results in diarrhea. It occurs when the parasite *Cryptosporidium* is ingested due to contact between the mouth and fecal material containing the parasite. In addition to humans, more than 45 species of animals, including common farm animals, can become infected with *Cryptosporidium*.

There is often no treatment administered in otherwise healthy individuals following diagnosis, although fluid replacement may be necessary following severe diarrhea. Symptoms last around two weeks, and the disease is transmissible even in the absence of symptoms. Infection can be prevented by adhering to hygienic regimens including handwashing, washing or cooking food, boiling water, and avoiding contact with animals.

Outbreaks can occur, especially if drinking water becomes contaminated with the parasite. In this case it is necessary to filter or boil water to prevent infection.

WORDS TO KNOW

FECAL-ORAL ROUTE The spread of disease through the transmission of minute particles of fecal material from one organism to the mouth of another. This can occur by drinking contaminated water; eating food exposed to animal or human feces, such as food from plants watered with unclean water; or preparing food without practicing proper hygiene.

PREVALENCE The actual number of cases of disease (or injury) that exist in a population.

WATERBORNE DISEASE Diseases that are caused by exposure to contaminated water. The exposure can occur by drinking the water or having the water come in contact with the body. Examples of waterborne diseases are cholera and typhoid fever.

Disease History, Characteristics, and Transmission

Cryptosporidiosis was first diagnosed in humans in 1976 after a three-year-old girl suffering from vomiting and diarrhea was found to be infected with the parasite *Cryptosporidium*. The girl's digestive tract contained large amounts of gas in the colon and large amounts of fluid in the small and large bowel, and on further examination the parasite was found within her digestive tract. Since the initial diagnosis, multiple outbreaks have occurred in the United States, including one significant outbreak transmitted through the Milwaukee, Wisconsin, public water system in 1993, when 403,000 people became infected. In November 2010 45 percent of the residents of Östersund, Sweden, or approximately 27,000 people, fell ill from an outbreak of cryptosporidiosis transmitted through the public water supply.

Cryptosporidiosis occurs after ingestion of the parasite *Cryptosporidium*. This parasite is a one-celled, ball-shaped organism that affects the digestive, biliary, and respiratory systems of other organisms. The parasite lays oocytes, which are egglike structures covered in a protective shell. Oocytes leave an infected organism's body via fecal matter. Oocytes can remain viable for two to six months in a moist environment. Due to their protective outer covering, they are highly resistant to chemical disinfectant. Therefore, these parasites are potentially highly infectious.

Ingestion of infected fecal matter results in transmission of the parasite to a new organism. Ingestion of fecal matter occurs when the mouth comes in direct contact with fecal matter or when it comes in contact with something that has touched fecal matter. This is most commonly due to not washing hands after using the toilet, handling infected animals, not washing food or not cooking food thoroughly, and drinking contaminated water. In addition, swimming pools and spas are common places for infection to occur due to the moist environment and the resistance of the parasite to chemicals, including pool chlorine. In May 2017 the Centers for Disease Control and Prevention (CDC) warned of a sharp rise in the number of cryptosporidiosis outbreaks in the United States linked to contaminated pool water, from 16 cases in 2014 to 32 in 2016.

■ Scope and Distribution

Cryptosporidiosis is widespread within the United States and is also present worldwide. Outbreaks have occurred in more than 50 countries on six continents. The US Food and Drug Administration (FDA) estimates that about 80 percent of the US population has had cryptosporidiosis, and its prevalence is about 2 percent in North America and Europe. The incidence is much higher in developing regions or in areas that lack proper sanitary facilities and water treatment options, reaching as high as 10 percent in parts of Africa, Asia, and Australia. It is often difficult to calculate the true incidence of *Cryptosporidium* infection, however, because many cases go unreported. The people most commonly infected by cryptosporidiosis are children younger than two years of age, animal handlers, health care workers, and travelers. People most at risk of suffering long-term, or even fatal, cases of cryptosporidiosis are those with weak immune systems. Young children are at risk due to the likelihood of them placing infected objects into their mouth or not washing their hands after using the toilet.

Animal handlers come into contact with animals on a daily basis. If hygienic procedures such as handwashing and washing clothes are not undertaken, transmission can occur between the animals and humans. Animals that can be infected include a range of common farm animals such as cattle and sheep, as well as common pets such as cats, dogs, birds, and fish.

Health care workers usually come into contact with fecal matter on a daily basis, which could potentially result in them becoming infected, particularly if they are caring for patients infected with cryptosporidiosis. To avoid infection, health care workers use contact precautions, including handwashing and wearing gloves when anticipating contact with potentially infected feces. People taking care of children may also be exposed to infection during diaper changing, as they are likely to come into contact with fecal matter.

Travelers are at risk as they may travel through areas with differing levels of hygiene in terms of food preparation and water standards. Lower standards may result in food and water harboring the parasite.

People with weak immune systems are most at risk of suffering prolonged or severe symptoms of cryptosporidiosis. People with human immunodeficiency virus (HIV)/acquired immunodeficiency syndrome (AIDS), organ transplant recipients, and those who were born with weakened immune systems are more likely to develop complications from cryptosporidiosis, including severe dehydration and lung infection (pulmonary cryptosporidiosis) that can lead to death.

■ Treatment and Prevention

The most common symptoms of cryptosporidiosis in humans are diarrhea, stomach cramps, nausea, vomiting, slight fever, and weight loss. These symptoms usually appear between 2 and 10 days after infection and last up to two weeks, sometimes occurring sporadically during that time. Following recovery, relapses may occur. In some cases symptoms are not present. However, the infection is still contagious and can be passed on to other humans.

There is no standard cure for cryptosporidiosis, and the symptoms usually disappear after about two weeks. In

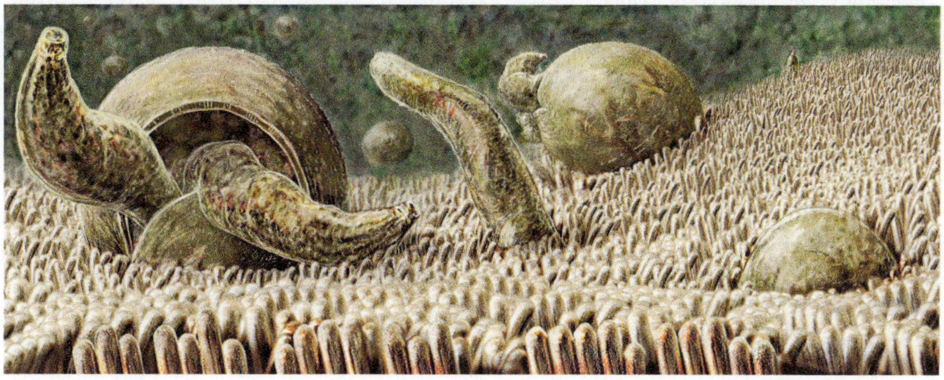

An artist's rendering of *Cryptosporidium* protozoans incubating on an intestinal wall. The round shapes are oocysts, which hatch the wormlike sporozoites that cause cryptosporidiosis infection. *© Russell Kightley/Science Source*

Filtering Water to Prevent Cryptosporidiosis

Advertising on water filters can be deceptive. The Centers for Disease Control and Prevention, National Center for Infectious Diseases, Division of Parasitic Diseases, offers the following guidance about messages on packaging.

Likely to Filter out *Cryptosporidium parvum*

Reverse osmosis (with or without NSF 53 or NSF 58 labeling)
Absolute pore size of 1 micron or smaller (with or without NSF 53 or NSF 58 labeling)
Tested and certified by NSF/ANSI Standard 53 or NSF/ANSI Standard 58 for cyst removal
Tested and certified by NSF/ANSI Standard 53 NSF/ANSI Standard 58 for cyst reduction

Unlikely to Filter out *Cryptosporidium parvum*

Nominal pore size of 1 micron or smaller
1-micron filter
Effective against *Giardia*
Effective against parasites
Carbon filter
Water purifier
EPA approved—Caution: EPA does not approve or test filters.
EPA registered—Caution: EPA does not register filters for *Cryptosporidium parvum* removal.
Activated carbon
Removes chlorine
Ultraviolet light
Pentiodide resins
Water softener
Chlorinated

SOURCE: "*Cryptosporidium* (Crypto) and Drinking Water from Private Wells." Centers for Disease Control and Prevention, National Center for Infectious Diseases, Division of Parasitic Diseases. July 1, 2015. Available from: https://www.cdc.gov/healthywater/drinking/private/wells/disease/cryptosporidium.html

2002 the FDA approved nitazoxanide for treatment of the diarrhea associated with cryptosporidiosis in children under 11 who were otherwise healthy. In 2004 the FDA extended this approval to treatment of older children and adults. Some people also receive relief from antibiotics and from common antidiarrheal and antivomiting medicines. For people with HIV, antiretroviral therapy, often used in conjunction with nitazoxanide, has been shown to substantially reduce the risk of death associated with cryptosporidiosis. To prevent dehydration, fluid and electrolyte replacement may be necessary in some cases. Therefore, people with *Cryptosporidium* infection are encouraged to increase their water intake and to watch for signs of dehydration, such as dry mouth, headaches, fatigue, joint aches, and decreased skin elasticity.

To prevent contracting cryptosporidiosis, contact with fecal matter should be avoided. This can be achieved by washing hands after handling soil, after toileting, or after handling animals. To avoid infection via food, washing with uninfected water or cooking it thoroughly will remove or kill the parasite. Water is a major source of infection due to the parasite's protective covering against chemicals. Boiling infected water for at least one minute will kill the parasite, and filtering it through filters small enough to prevent the parasite passing will remove the parasite. This water can then be used for drinking, washing food, and making ice. Health officials also recommend that infected people stay away from public places, especially public swimming areas, while exhibiting cryptosporidiosis symptoms and for two weeks after experiencing diarrhea to prevent possible infection of other people.

In 2010 the CDC launched CryptoNet, a system for analyzing the deoxyribonucleic acid (DNA) fingerprint of *Cryptosporidium* parasites and for comparing data on the causes of outbreaks. As of 2017 the program had helped the CDC identify nearly 30 genetic subtypes of the germ and was being used to track the spread of various subtypes in the United States and to develop strategies for preventing future outbreaks.

■ Impacts and Issues

Cryptosporidiosis has the potential to spread rapidly and affect many people in a short time, and infection of a community's drinking source puts the whole community at risk. Before 2001 water treatment in many locations in the United States did not remove the parasite, as chemical treatment usually did not kill it and filters were too large to prevent it from passing. The outbreak in Milwaukee in 1993 resulted in more than 400,000 reported cases and remains the single largest outbreak of waterborne disease reported in the United States. More than 100 people, mostly people with HIV/AIDS and the elderly, died during the outbreak. The estimated monetary costs of the outbreak spiraled to over $95 million, including $30 million of direct medical care costs and $60 million attributed to lost productivity in the Milwaukee workplace. As a result of this outbreak, the US Environmental Protection Agency (EPA) mandated that major US water systems (those relying on surface water sources, such as rivers or lakes, and serving more than 10,000 people) implement new EPA standards by 2001 that strengthened control over microbial contaminants, including *Cryptosporidium.* More stringent requirements covering all water systems regardless of size were put in place beginning in 2006, and a second round of monitoring began in 2015 to determine the treatment needs for water systems at higher risk of *Cryptosporidium* infection. The EPA estimated that full compliance with the updated guidelines would eliminate up to 1,459,000 cases of cryptosporidiosis and save up to 314 lives per year.

People with compromised immune systems are often advised to take extra precautions with their drinking water to prevent *Cryptosporidium* infection, including boiling it, installing point-of-use filters that remove particles 1 micrometer or less in diameter, or drinking bottled water from protected well or protected spring water sources. In 2008 a number of public health organizations, including WHO, the US Agency for International Development (USAID), and the World Bank, issued a call for increased focus on water filtration rather than chlorination in developing regions with high rates of HIV infection. This focus included sub-Saharan Africa, which had approximately 25 million people living with HIV/AIDS in 2017.

Malnourished children can also be at elevated risk of death from cryptosporidiosis. The Global Enteric Multicenter Study (GEMS), a major study of childhood diarrheal diseases in developing regions conducted from 2007 to 2011, found that *Cryptosporidium* was the second-leading cause of moderate or severe diarrhea among infants (rotavirus was the leading cause) and that children ages 12 to 23 months with cryptosporidiosis had mortality rates more than twice as high as those who were not infected.

Cryptosporidiosis disease is a major cause of diarrhea worldwide. Due to differing food- and water-quality controls around the world, this disease has a large impact on travelers who are unfamiliar with a region's water quality. Travelers are often advised to consider the following precautions to prevent infection: bringing water to a full boil for one minute, avoiding undercooked food, handling or peeling raw food such as fruit themselves, avoiding swimming in freshwater rivers and lakes, and carrying bottled water when unsure of an area's water quality.

SEE ALSO *AIDS Acquired Immunodeficiency Syndrome; Contact Precautions; Gastroenteritis (Common Causes); Handwashing; HIV; Parasitic Diseases; Travel and Infectious Disease; Waterborne Disease*

BIBLIOGRAPHY

Books

Bennett, John E., Raphael Dolin, and Martin J. Blaser. *Mandell, Douglas, and Bennett's Principles and Practice of Infectious Diseases.* Philadelphia: Elsevier, 2015.

Ortega-Pierres, Guadalupe. *Giardia and Cryptosporidium: From Molecules to Disease.* Wallingford, UK: CABI, 2009.

Periodicals

Miyamoto, Yukiko, and Lars Eckmann. "Drug Development against the Major Diarrhea-Causing Parasites of the Small Intestine, *Cryptosporidium* and *Giardia.*" *Frontiers in Microbiology* 6 (2015): 1208. This article can also be found online at https://www.frontiersin.org/articles/10.3389/fmicb.2015.01208/full (accessed January 16, 2018).

Peletz, Rachel, et al. "Preventing Cryptosporidiosis: The Need for Safe Drinking Water." *Bulletin of the World Health Organization* 91, no. 4 (2013): 237–312. This article can also be found online at http://www.who.int/bulletin/volumes/91/4/13-119990/en/ (accessed January 16, 2018).

Shrivastava, Arpit Kumar, et al. "Revisiting the Global Problem of Cryptosporidiosis and Recommendations." *Tropical Parasitology* 7, no. 1 (2017): 8–17. This article can also be found online at https://www.ncbi.nlm.nih.gov/pmc/articles/PMC5369280/ (accessed January 16, 2018).

Squire, Sylvia Afriyie, and Una Ryan. "*Cryptosporidium* and *Giardia* in Africa: Current and Future Challenges." *Parasites & Vectors* 10, no. 1 (2017): 195. This article can also be found online at https://parasitesandvectors.biomedcentral.com/articles/10.1186/s13071-017-2111-y#Sec8 (accessed January 16, 2018).

Websites

"Crypto Outbreaks Linked to Swimming Have Doubled Since 2014." CDC Newsroom, May 18, 2017. https://www.cdc.gov/media/releases/2017/p0518-cryptosporidium-outbreaks.html (accessed January 16, 2018).

"Cryptosporidiosis." European Centre for Disease Prevention and Control. https://ecdc.europa.eu/en/cryptosporidiosis (accessed January 16, 2018).

"Global Enteric Multicenter Study (GEMS)." University of Maryland School of Medicine. http://www.medschool.umaryland.edu/GEMS/ (accessed January 16, 2018).

"Parasites—Cryptosporidium (Also Known as 'Crypto')." Centers for Disease Control and Prevention, April 1, 2015. https://www.cdc.gov/parasites/crypto/index.html (accessed January 16, 2018).

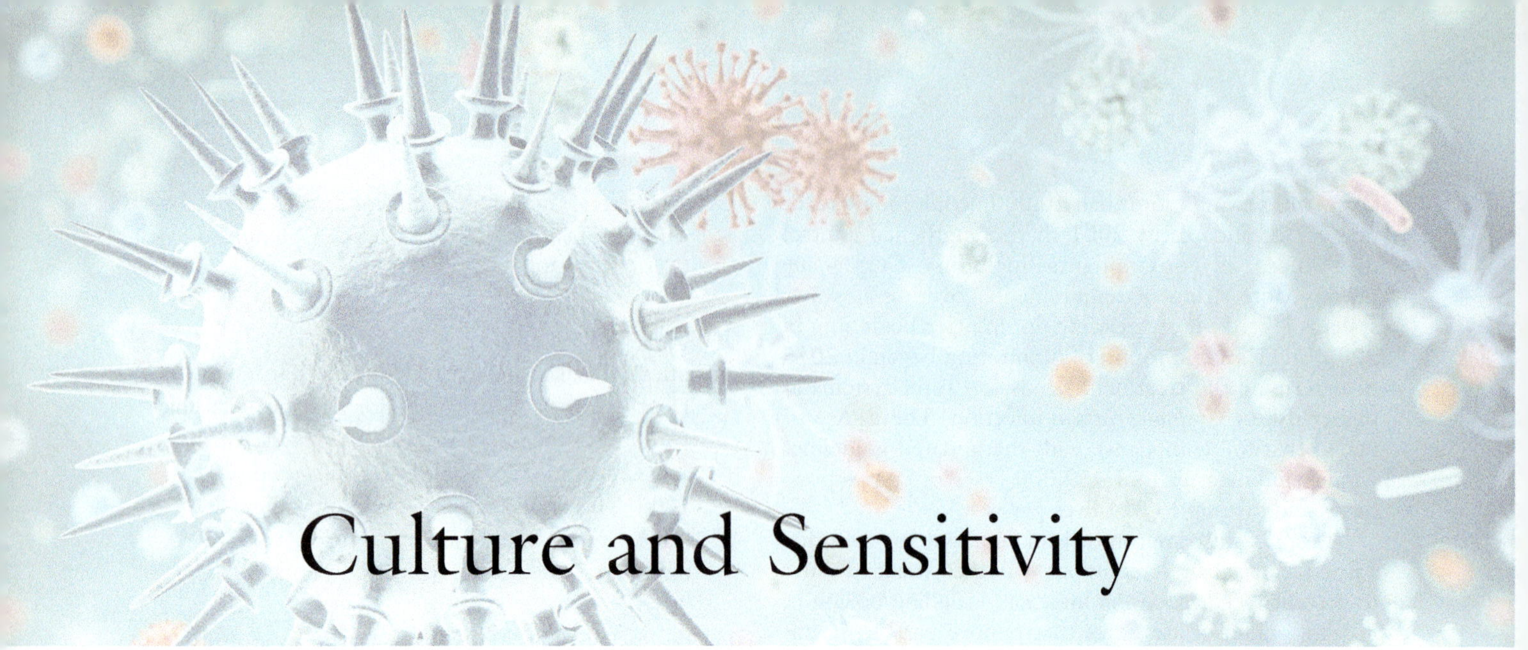

Culture and Sensitivity

Introduction

Culture and sensitivity in microbiology refers to laboratory techniques that allow a disease-causing microorganism to be identified and that determine which antibiotics are sensitive to (effective against) the identified microorganism.

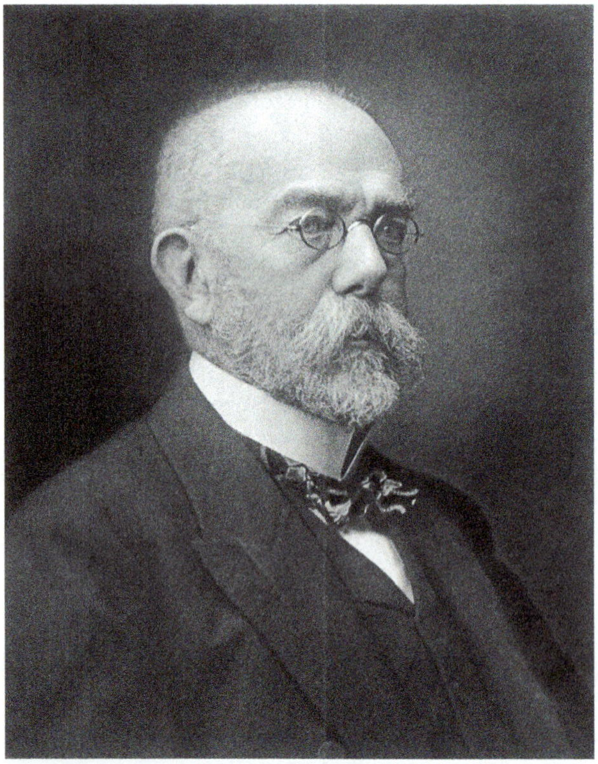

Robert Koch (1843–1910), German scientist. Koch developed a technique for identifying and growing specific bacterial cultures. He used this technique to isolate *Bacillus anthracis*, the bacteria responsible for tuberculosis. At the time tuberculosis was a serious threat responsible for around 14 percent of all European deaths. Often credited as the founder of bacteriology, Koch was awarded the Nobel Prize in Physiology in 1905. *© NLM/Science Source*

Physicians must consider numerous important factors when deciding how to appropriately treat infectious disease. Broad patient-specific factors include the natural history of the infection and the strength of the patient's immune system. If antibiotic treatment of the disease is suitable, as in the case of bacterial, certain fungal, and some other microbial diseases, the type of antibiotics used may depend on ease of absorption, metabolism, ability to reach the infection site, and other factors such as the prevalence of bacterial strains that are resistant to commonly used antibiotics. Microbe culturing and susceptibility testing offers information to help make appropriate decisions. The availability of such information from laboratory testing can provide lifesaving assistance to doctors, but it can also result in excessive reliance on testing when a simpler, broader approach to treatment (e.g., empiric treatment, or starting with broader-spectrum antibiotics without culturing) may be more efficient.

History and Scientific Foundations

Most of the techniques of culturing microbes were developed in the mid- to late 1800s by Robert Koch (1843–1895), Paul Ehrlich (1854–1915), and Hans Christian Gram (1853–1938). Using some of these techniques, Louis Pasteur (1822–1895) developed the foundations of the modern science of infectious disease. Koch, a German physician, perfected a technique to distinguish different types of bacteria and grow pure cultures of these bacterial types, and in the process he founded the science of bacteriology. He formalized the approach of determining whether a particular microbe caused a given disease in a set of rules now known as Koch's Postulates (1882), which supported the concept that a disease is caused by a specific microbe:

- The agent of an infectious disease must be present in every case of the disease.

WORDS TO KNOW

ANTIBIOTIC RESISTANCE The ability of bacteria to resist the actions of antibiotic drugs.

ANTIBIOTIC SENSITIVITY The susceptibility of a bacterium to an antibiotic. Bacteria can be killed by some types of antibiotics and not be affected by other types. Different types of bacteria exhibit different patterns of antibiotic sensitivity.

BROAD-SPECTRUM ANTIBIOTICS Drugs that kill a wide range of bacteria rather than just those from a specific family. For example, amoxicillin is a broad-spectrum antibiotic that is used against many common illnesses such as ear infections.

COHORTING The practice of grouping people with similar infections or symptoms together to reduce transmission to others.

GRAM-NEGATIVE BACTERIA Bacteria whose cell walls are composed of an inner and outer membrane that are separated from one another by a region called the periplasm. The periplasm also contains a thin but rigid layer called the peptidoglycan.

GRAM-POSITIVE BACTERIA All types of bacteria identified and classified as a group that retain crystal-violet dye during Gram's method of staining.

INPATIENT A patient who is admitted to a hospital or clinic for treatment, typically requiring the patient to stay overnight.

MINIMAL INHIBITORY CONCENTRATION (MIC) The lowest level of an antibiotic that prevents growth of the particular type of bacteria in a liquid food source after a certain amount of time. Growth is detected by clouding of the food source. The MIC is the lowest concentration of the antibiotic at which no cloudiness occurs.

OUTPATIENT A person who receives health care services without being admitted to a hospital or clinic for an overnight stay.

SEPSIS A bacterial infection in the bloodstream or body tissues. Sepsis is a very broad term covering the presence of many types of microscopic disease-causing organisms. It is also called bacteremia. Closely related terms include septicemia and septic syndrome.

- The agent must be isolated from the host and grown *in vitro* (pure culture) for several generations.
- The disease must be reproduced when a pure culture of the agent is inoculated into a healthy susceptible host.
- The same agent must be recovered once again from the experimentally infected host.

Koch developed a solid medium for bacterial growth using gelatin, which was later modified by other scientists to include a seaweed called agar to keep the medium solid at room temperature. German bacteriologist Richard Julius Petri (1852–1921) developed the Petri dish, a glass dish still in use to help foster optimal bacterial growth.

In 1877 Koch also developed a technique for dry-fixing thin films of bacterial culture on glass slides, staining them with aniline dyes, and recording the microscopic images on film. Dry-fixing continues to be a standard procedure in identifying various bacterial cultures. Different types of media are optimal for specific types of bacteria, and identification of a specific pathogen can still be a matter of clinical experience and judgment.

Microbe staining techniques were developed in 1839 by German scientist Christian Gottfried Ehrenberg (1795–1876). These staining techniques depended on two properties of stains: chromogenicity (inclusion of groups of atoms that are color-forming) and the ability to dissociate into positively charged ions (cations) and negatively charged ions (anions). For example, when methylene blue dye is added to water, it dissociates into a chloride anion and a methylene blue cation, which is visible in solution and makes methylene blue a "cation dye." Another common dye, eosin, dissociates into a sodium cation and a visible eosin anion and is an anion dye. Anionic dyes such as eosin interact with the cationic portions of the bacterial protein being identified, while the converse happens with cationic dyes.

Ehrlich invented the precursor technique to Gram staining bacteria using methylene blue dye. This technique made it possible to distinguish between different types of blood cells, which enabled the diagnosis of numerous blood diseases. In 1882 Ehrlich published his method of staining the tubercle bacillus. Ehrlich's method laid the foundations for subsequent modifications that are still in contemporary use.

The Gram stain, developed in 1884 and named after discoverer Hans Christian Gram, is in a different category from ionic stains. This technique involves first staining bacteria with gentian violet dye, washing the stained bacteria with iodine solution, and then washing it with ethyl alcohol. For "Gram-negative" bacteria, the second and

REAL-WORLD RISKS

The medical dangers and escalating health care costs associated with antimicrobial resistance led to the formation of a special interagency task force charged with developing effective plans to combat the problem. Formed in 1999, the Interagency Task Force on Antimicrobial Resistance is cochaired by the Centers for Disease Control and Prevention, the Food and Drug Administration, and the National Institutes of Health, and it also includes the Agency for Healthcare Research and Quality, the Centers for Medicare and Medicaid Services (formerly the Health Care Financing Administration), the Department of Agriculture, the Department of Defense, the Department of Veterans Affairs, the Environmental Protection Agency, and the Health Resources and Services Administration.

One of the top priorities of the task force is to "conduct a public health education campaign to promote appropriate antimicrobial use as a national health priority."

third steps wash away the dye, while "Gram-positive" bacteria remain colored after being washed with iodine and alcohol. The final step is to stain the Gram-negative bacteria with a reddish-pink dye that does not stain the Gram-positive bacteria. The Gram-positive bacteria will thus have violet structural features under a microscope, while the Gram-negative bacteria will have pinkish structural features. Whether a bacterium is Gram-positive or Gram-negative is often an indicator of whether the bacteria can be destroyed using a particular antibiotic.

Many antibiotics can kill Gram-positive bacteria, while Gram-negative bacteria resist common antibiotics. Gram-negative bacteria have an extra layer of polysaccharides, proteins, and phospholipids, which blocks many antibiotics from reaching the peptidoglycan cell wall. For example, penicillin works by attacking the cell wall but is prevented from doing so by this extra layer, making the bacteria penicillin-resistant.

The susceptibility methods used by clinical laboratories include the Kirby-Bauer disc diffusion susceptibility test, the macrotube dilution susceptibility test, and the microtube dilution test. In the Kirby-Bauer test, discs containing antibiotics are placed over an agar plate inoculated with the organism. The size of the zone of inhibition indicates whether the organism is sensitive or resistant to the antibiotic at the level normally used (doses). Laboratories report antibiotic sensitivities as "Susceptible," "Intermediate," or "Resistant," as defined by the National Committee on Clinical Laboratory Standards (NCCLS).

The minimal inhibitory concentration (MIC) is the lowest concentration of the antibiotic (mcg/ml) that will inhibit bacterial growth in vitro and is correlated with the concentration of the antibiotic achievable in blood. The MIC is traditionally determined using the macrotube dilution technique, in which a standard inoculum is tested against serial dilutions of a particular antibiotic—a time-consuming process. A newer technique uses tiny wells in an automated plastic susceptibility card. The wells are injected with standard dilutions of antimicrobial agents by the manufacturer. The laboratory adds a standard concentration of the organism to the card, and the organism is automatically dispersed to all of the wells. After an incubation period of 12 to 24 hours, the card is machine-read for bacterial growth at hourly intervals, and a growth curve for the isolate is calculated for each antibiotic on the card. The antibiotics are grouped according to whether the organism being tested is Gram-positive or Gram-negative, and the antibiotics for the Gram-negative isolate are further grouped according to whether they can be used in an inpatient or outpatient setting, depending on whether the patient is in the process of being admitted to or discharged from the hospital.

Depending on MIC results, physicians may change the dosage of a particular antibiotic to be used in treatment or choose a different antibiotic to treat the infection. For example, a blood-borne *Escherichia coli* infection tested with ampicillin may have a MIC of 2 mcg/ml (sensitive), multiplied by two to four times, gives 4 to 8 mcg/ml as a potential peak level of the antibiotic in the blood, which is considerably less than an intravenous representative dose from the patient of 47 mcg/ml. Thus, ampicillin would be expected to provide adequate therapy for the patient.

In a different example of a leg wound tested with ampicillin, a higher MIC of 16 mcg/ml would be correlated with a 32 to 64 mcg/ml peak blood concentration, which could fall over the range of the representative intravenous dose of 47 mcg/ml of bacteria from the patient. Furthermore, because the patient has a leg wound, so the infection is in tissue rather than blood, the concentration of antibiotics in tissue will be lower than in blood. In this case the physician would consider a higher ampicillin dose or a different antibiotic for treatment.

■ Impacts and Issues

Culturing and MIC testing are possible for most, but not all, types of bacteria-caused diseases. Infections for which cultures generally cannot be obtained include ear infections, sinusitis, and bronchitis, along with viral infections. For such infections there is a considerable risk of overprescribing antibiotic treatments that are likely to be inappropriate and ineffective, and there are increasing calls for the distribution of procedures and new guidelines to address this issue.

Molecular biology has contributed new tools enabling microbiologists to identify minute genetic variations within species of microbes, even within microbial strains. This has profoundly altered the capabilities of microbiology, which was becoming constrained by reliance on old-style laboratory methods.

Molecular techniques have progressed to a level of sophistication in which typing, distinguishing between strains of the same species, has value in specialized fields, such as epidemiology and pharmaceutical development. The methods and equipment to assist with identifying species and types are commercially available for many applications, although they are more commonly used for research than for individual patient diagnosis.

Identification methods employing microbial colony and cell morphology, Gram stain and other staining features, nutritional and physical conditions for growth, metabolic features, and pathogenicity have been advanced so that even small laboratories can rapidly identify species isolates using simple traditional test procedures.

Tests related to microbial metabolism and other features such as fermentation have been packaged into easy-to-use kits. Many automated systems come with internal databases against which test isolates can be compared for accurate identification. These kits and systems can often provide reliable results within 24 to 48 hours and save diagnostic materials and technician time. They have largely replaced manual tests on individual isolates.

Traditional microbial identification methods focus on observable organism structure and function, or phenotypic microbial characteristics, which are the products of gene expression. Examining the microbial genome itself makes it possible to identify a species using genotypic characteristics. For instance, bacterial species can often be detected by sequencing sections of their ribosomal DNA.

The timing and choice of antibiotics can be important in treating older adults. For example, in sepsis most research suggests that starting with broad-spectrum antibiotics without culturing is beneficial because deaths and long hospital stays are reduced if the initial antibiotic treatment attacks and reduces the infectious agent. Delaying therapy initiation by four or more hours after hospital admission, as could happen with long laboratory testing, is associated with higher mortality. However, up to 75 percent of antibiotic use in long-term care may be inappropriate, so strict minimum criteria for initiating antibiotic treatment should be set.

The emergence of resistant bacteria has led to a reliance on fluoroquinolones, a class of antibiotics, for relatively routine infections such as community-acquired pneumonia (CAP) in spite of the potential for adverse effects. Overutilization has, in turn, given rise to increasing fluoroquinolone resistance in some geographic regions. Infectious Disease Society of America (IDSA) guidelines advise keeping newer fluoroquinolones that are active against *S. pneumoniae* in reserve while using other antibiotics such as an advanced-generation cephalosporin (e.g., ceftriaxone or ceftaroline) as initial therapy.

This example demonstrates the vicious circle that arises from physicians' reliance on specialized antibiotics that show *in vivo* (in the body) potency against given infections when treatment with broad-spectrum antibiotics would provide faster treatment yet would not lead to resistance to the specialized antibiotics.

Furthermore, overreliance on antibiotics in long-term care facilities and in hospitals can cause health care workers to disregard simple infection control activities such as handwashing, isolation and cohorting of infected patients, skin testing for tuberculosis, and immunization to prevent infection with resistant organisms in the first place.

Invasive devices such as catheters and ventilators, as well as surgical procedures and the insertion of central intravenous (IV) lines to treat patients and to help them recover, can give rise to such health care–associated infections (HAIs) as central line–associated bloodstream infections, catheter-associated urinary tract infections, and ventilator-associated pneumonia. Infections that occur at surgery sites are known as surgical site infections. The CDC has a program to monitor and prevent HAIs, which are a major patient safety threat.

See Also *Antibacterial Drugs; Bacterial Disease; Resistant Organisms; Vancomycin-Resistant Enterococci*

BIBLIOGRAPHY

Books

Ryan, Kenneth J., and C. George Ray. *Sherris Medical Microbiology.* 6th ed. New York: McGraw-Hill Medical, 2014.

Washington, John A. "Principles of Diagnosis." In *Medical Microbiology*, edited by Samuel Baron. 4th ed. Galveston: University of Texas Medical Branch at Galveston, 1996. This article can also be found online at http://www.ncbi.nlm.nih.gov/books/bv.fcgi?rid=mmed.section.5451 (accessed January 26, 2018).

Periodicals

Xu, Y., et al. "Monitoring of the Bacterial and Fungal Biodiversity and Dynamics during Massa Medicata Fermentata Fermentation." *Applied Microbiology and Biotechnology* 97, no. 22 (2013): 9647–9655.

Websites

"Microbial Identification and Strain Typing Using Molecular Techniques." Rapidmicrobiology. http://www.rapidmicrobiology.com/test-method/molecular-techniques-for-microbial-identification-and-typing/ (accessed February 1, 2018).

"A Public Health Action Plan to Combat Antimicrobial Resistance." Centers for Disease Control and Prevention. https://www.cdc.gov/drugresistance/actionplan/aractionplan.pdf (accessed January 21, 2018).

"Types of Healthcare-Associated Infections." Centers for Disease Control and Prevention. https://www.cdc.gov/hai/infectiontypes.html (accessed January 21, 2018).

Kenneth T. LaPensee

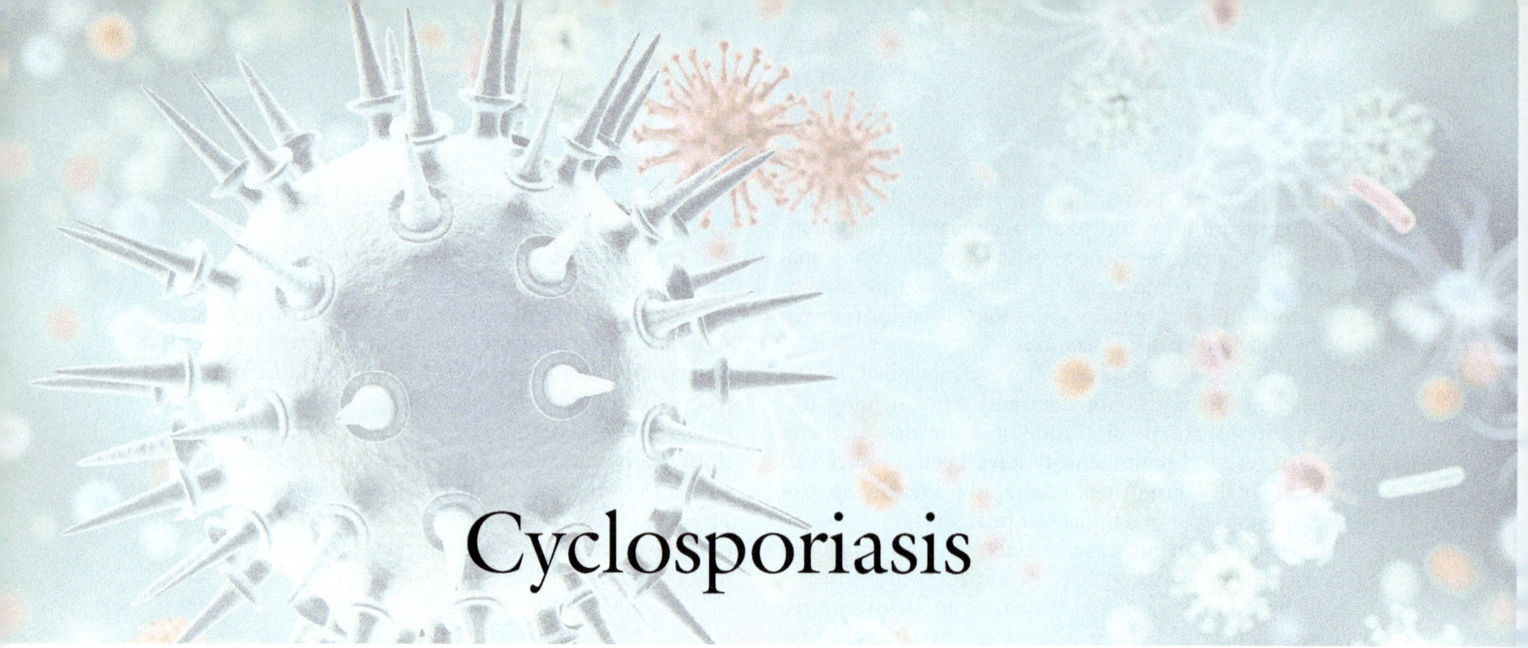

Cyclosporiasis

Introduction

Cyclosporiasis (sigh-clo-spore-EYE-uh-sis), also called Cyclospora, is an infection caused by the pathogenic protozoan *Cyclospora cayetanensis.* The protozoan is a coccidium parasite, or a parasite that infects the gastrointestinal (GI) tract. *Cyclospora* is spread when humans drink water or eat food contaminated with infected feces. However, the protozoan does not become infectious until several days or even a week after being passed in a bowel movement.

In the United States, consumption of produce such as raspberries, cilantro, basil, and snow peas grown outside the country is most frequently associated with outbreaks of *Cyclospora* infection. *Cyclospora* often infect humans and other animals such as moles, myriapods (small, long arthropods such as centipedes), rodents, and vipers (poisonous snakes). Transmission between humans or between animals and humans is unlikely. The primary source of the parasite is unknown. The infection sometimes causes diarrhea in travelers visiting foreign countries.

Distribution of Cyclosporiasis Cases by Continent

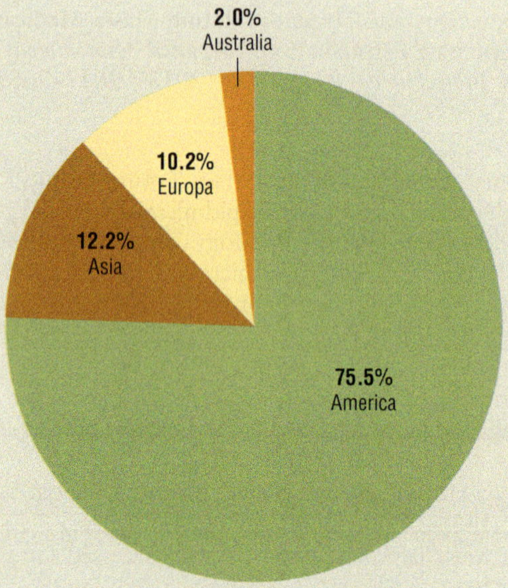

SOURCE: Adapted from "Cyclospora cayetanensis." Global Water Pathogen Project. 2017. Available from: http://www.waterpathogens.org/cyclospora-cayetanensis

Disease History, Characteristics, and Transmission

According to the US Centers for Disease Control and Prevention (CDC), the first human case of *Cyclospora* infection was documented in 1979, although it had been recognized as early as 1977. During the mid-1980s cases were frequently reported. Large outbreaks in the United States and Canada were reported in the 1990s. In the early 21st century outbreaks occurred in North America with increasing frequency.

The first US case occurred in Chicago, Illinois, inside a medical dormitory whose water source became infected. A US epidemic occurred between 1996 and 1997 when basil, lettuce, and raspberries became contaminated. A Canadian epidemic occurred in 1999 when berries became contaminated, and in 2004 a Pennsylvania outbreak was traced to basil and snow peas. In 2005 582 people in Florida contracted *Cyclospora* infections from eating basil imported from Peru. Consumption of cilantro from Mexico was blamed for a series of cyclosporiasis outbreaks in the United States between 2013 and 2015. A major outbreak in 2017 led to more than 1,000 *Cyclospora* infections of people from 40 states. While some of these people may have contracted an infection while traveling abroad, more than half of those diagnosed with cyclosporiasis did not report leaving the country, and the CDC was unable to identify a single source or cause of the rash of infections.

The *Cyclospora cayetanensis* parasite is a one-celled organism. Identification of the parasite requires specialized microscopic inspection, often of multiple stool samples. Transmission occurs when an oocyst (a fertilized sex cell) of *C. cayetanensis* is located within contaminated water that is ingested. It enters the small intestine (bowel) and travels to the mucous membrane (the moist lining inside body passages). The oocyst incubates for approximately one week (with a range from 1 to 14 days). After incubation is complete, the victim begins to experience symptoms of bloating, diarrhea, frequent and sometimes large bowel movements, low-grade fever, muscle aches, and stomach cramps. Other diarrhea-caused symptoms include fatigue, appetite and weight loss, and increased gas. However, some people show no symptoms. If not treated, the illness lasts from several days to a month, sometimes longer. Relapses of the illness often occur.

Although all humans are susceptible to the infection, people in developing countries are most at risk. Death rarely occurs but can result in infected people with immunosuppressed systems. *Cyclospora* affect both sexes and all ages and races equally, though children in developing countries are especially susceptible, as they are often the primary water carriers for their families.

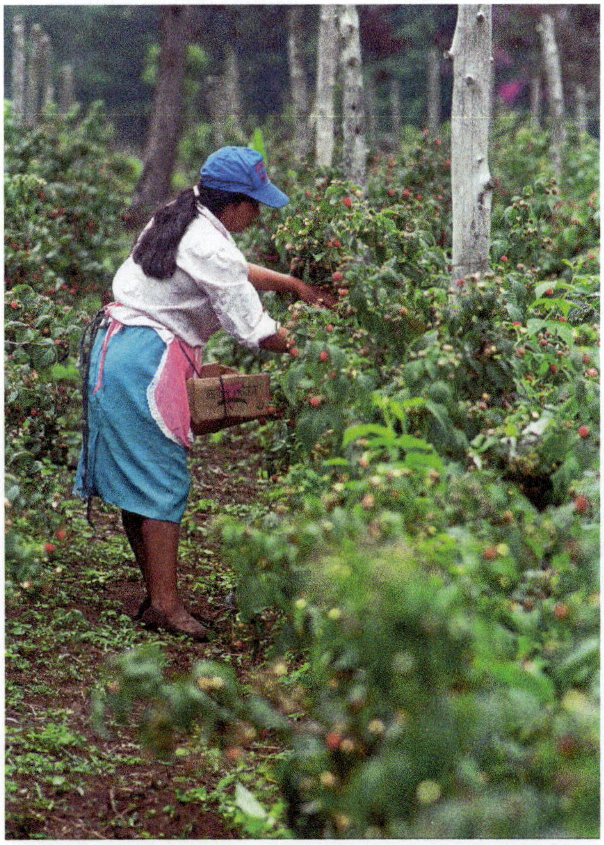

A woman picks raspberries on a farm in Guatemala, 1997. A year earlier, imports of Guatemalan raspberries had contributed to an outbreak of cyclosporiasis in the United States. Scientific investigation of the outbreak proved that *Cyclospora* can be a food-borne pathogen. *© AP Images/MOISES CASTILLO*

WORDS TO KNOW

COCCIDIUM Any single-celled animal (protozoan) belonging to the subclass Coccidia. Some Coccidia species can infest the digestive tract, causing coccidiosis.

ENDEMIC Present in a particular area or among a particular group of people.

FOOD PRESERVATION Any one of a number of techniques used to prevent food from spoiling, such as canning, pickling, drying or freeze-drying, irradiation, pasteurization, smoking, and the addition of chemical additives. Food preservation has become an increasingly important component of the food industry as fewer people eat foods produced on their own lands and as consumers expect to purchase and consume foods that are out of season.

OOCYST A spore phase of certain infectious organisms that can survive for a long time outside the organism and therefore continue to cause infection and resist treatment.

PROTOZOA Single-celled animal-like microscopic organisms that live by taking in food rather than making it by photosynthesis and must live in the presence of water. (Singular: protozoan.) Protozoa are a diverse group of single-celled organisms, with more than 50,000 different types represented. The vast majority are microscopic, many measuring less than 5 one-thousandth of an inch (0.005 millimeters), but some, such as the freshwater Spirostomun, may reach 0.17 inches (3 millimeters) in length, large enough to enable it to be seen with the naked eye.

■ Scope and Distribution

It is possible for the infection to occur anywhere in the world, although it is often found in underdeveloped or developing countries. As of 2017 cyclosporiasis was endemic in Haiti, Nepal, and Peru. It was also reported by people traveling within India, Indonesia, Mexico, Morocco, Pakistan, Puerto Rico, and Southeast Asia. When it occurs in the United States, it happens mostly in the warmer months of late spring and summer.

■ Treatment and Prevention

Diagnosis is often difficult because oocysts in feces and water are difficult to identify. Stool specimens are used in diagnosis. Frequently, several specimens are taken over numerous days. The Epidemiology and Disease Control Program (EDCP) suggests that physicians specifically request a *Cyclospora* test to assure accurate laboratory results. The polymerase chain reaction–based deoxyribonucleic acid (DNA) test and acid-fast staining test are often used.

Treatment involves antibiotics, often in combination, such as trimethoprim and sulfamethoxazole. Traditional antiprotozoan drugs are usually not effective enough to stop the protozoan. People with compromised immune systems and severe diarrhea require additional supportive treatment.

To prevent transmission through food, all fruits and vegetables should be washed before consuming. Hand-washing before handling or eating food removes most of the parasites. Drinking water suspected to be contaminated, especially from rivers, streams, springs, and other untreated waters, should be avoided to prevent cyclosporiasis. Hand-washing after using the toilet and changing diapers also prevents transmission of *Cyclospora.*

■ Impacts and Issues

Cyclosporiasis infection is part of a wider problem: emerging food-borne outbreaks on a national or international scale. Food-borne illnesses such as cyclosporiasis continue to increase in numbers and severity as the world moves rapidly toward a global food market. Contaminated food in one part of the world can lead to an outbreak halfway across the globe in a matter of days.

According to the CDC, better recognition and management of outbreaks of food-borne infections such as those caused by *Cyclospora* are needed. This would entail better coordination and action by federal, state, and local agencies; more comprehensive laboratory diagnostic training; structured development of epidemiologic studies; coordination between affected governments and the media; and early and effective involvement of companies involved in the growing, processing, exporting, importing, transporting, and wholesale and retail sales of foods.

Irradiation, or the use of ionizing radiation for food pasteurization, is one way to reduce bacterial and parasitic causes of food-borne diseases. The CDC and World Health Organization (WHO) and other international groups promote irradiation as a safe and effective method to reduce the risk of infection in globally distributed foods. Nevertheless, some food advocacy groups continue to oppose the use of ionizing radiation.

See Also *Food-Borne Disease and Food Safety; Microorganisms; Travel and Infectious Disease*

BIBLIOGRAPHY

Books

Nguhiu, Purity, and Dorcas Yole. *Intestinal Protozoa: Human Cyclosporiasis, Emerging Foodborne Zoonosis: The African Green Monkey Model.* Saarbrüken, Germany: Noor, 2017.

Periodicals

Abanyie, F., et al. "2013 Multistate Outbreaks of *Cyclospora cayetanensis* Infections Associated with Fresh Produce: Focus on the Texas Investigations." *Epidemiology & Infection* 143, no. 16 (December 2015): 3451–3458.

Neal, David J. "It's a Mysterious Infection. It's on the Rise. Here's How to Recognize It." *Miami Herald* (October 2, 2017). This article can also be found online at http://www.miamiherald.com/news/health-care/article176512621.html (accessed December 18, 2017).

Websites

"Cyclosporiasis (Cyclospora Infection)." Centers for Disease Control and Prevention, July 28, 2016. https://www.cdc.gov/parasites/cyclosporiasis/index.html (accessed December 18, 2017).

"Increase in Reported Cases of *Cyclospora cayetanensis* Infection, United States, Summer 2017." Centers for Disease Control and Prevention Health Alert Network, August 7, 2017. https://emergency.cdc.gov/han/han00405.asp (accessed December 18, 2017).

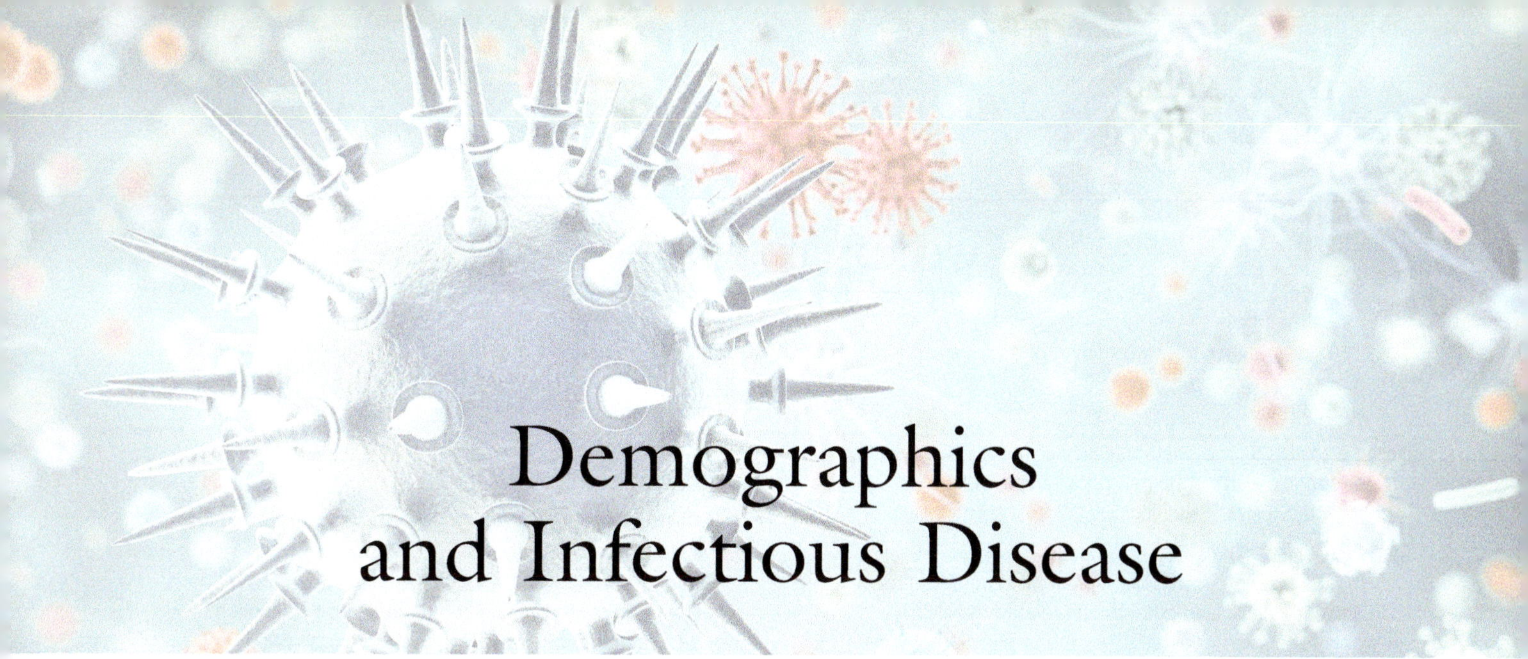

Demographics and Infectious Disease

■ Introduction

Trends in a population's vital statistics, or demographic trends, within nations and across national boundaries have a profound effect on the distribution of infectious disease worldwide. Gender, age, the movement of populations due to economic opportunity or to escape conflict, and the sheer density of population relative to the capacity of local ecosystems, civic infrastructure, and public health resources all influence the infectivity and virulence of infectious diseases. Close quartering of a population such as in refugee camps, prisons, or schools can also affect the outbreak and spread of infectious disease.

■ History and Scientific Foundations

Mass migration of a population to a host nation that has limited resources and is unprepared for the burden of caring for so many vulnerable people, in combination with close quarters and unsanitary conditions, often results in environments that are ripe for the transmission of pathogens. Movement of populations such as migrants or refugees affects the population itself, the populations encountered, and the ecosystem. Each translocated person carries cultural practices, genetic vulnerabilities and resistances to infections, and organisms that have been held at bay by the individual's immunity but lie dormant and are potentially dangerous to previously unexposed persons. In addition, the moving populations unwittingly transport microbes, animals that are disease vectors (transmitters), and other flora and fauna (plants and animals) that are foreign to the destination ecosystems.

One example of demographic factors coming together at once and contributing to disease was the mass exodus of more than a million Kurds from Iraqi villages at the end of the first Gulf War in 1991. With the absence of sanitary facilities and the crowding together of so many people in a weakened condition, contaminated water supplies from human waste quickly gave rise to an epidemic of cholera, as well as other communicable diseases. Beginning in 2003 conflict in the Darfur region of Sudan resulted in the movement of more than 1 million internally displaced people to crowded refugee camps where epidemics of typhoid, hepatitis E, cholera, and meningitis took hold.

Yet another example is that of the flight of 800,000 Rohingya people from Myanmar to Bangladesh. In 2017 there was a Burmese military crackdown on Rohingya insurgents that put many ordinary people in grave danger, causing them to flee across the border. So many Rohingya people (mostly women and children) arrived in Bangladesh that it became the center of the world's fastest-growing refugee crisis. The overcrowded conditions in the Bangladeshi refugee camps resulted in a resurgence of diphtheria, which had been nearly eradicated in the country. In the last two months of 2017, 2,526 suspected cases of diphtheria were reported, with 27 resulting in death. The Rohingya refugees were weakened by malnutrition, poor routine immunization coverage, and limited access to clean water and sanitary toilets, which can increase the risk for diphtheria and other infections.

Even when no mass population movements are taking place, the changing age and sex mix of stable populations over time can affect the spread of infectious disease. In other words, the population of potential disease hosts changes rather than remains stable. These changes affect the patterns of communicable diseases, particularly diseases that are sexually transmitted and that give rise to symptoms in one gender or the other (such as cervical cancer caused by human papillomavirus) or that attack people differentially in different age brackets, such as seasonal influenza, which usually infects older people more often than younger people.

Demographics such as the population density of various age, sex, and ethnic subgroups, along with other statistics that affect patterns of disease, can be made into mathematical models that help scientists map and predict

WORDS TO KNOW

CLUSTER In epidemiology, a grouping of an infectious disease or foodborne illness that occurs very close in time or place.

DEMOGRAPHICS The characteristics of human populations or specific parts of human populations, most often reported through statistics.

EPIDEMIOLOGY The study of various factors that influence the occurrence, distribution, prevention, and control of disease, injury, and other health-related events in a defined human population. By the application of various analytical techniques, including mathematical analysis of the data, the probable cause of an infectious outbreak can be pinpointed.

HERD IMMUNITY A resistance to disease that occurs in a population when a proportion of them have been immunized against it. The theory is that it is less likely that an infectious disease will spread in a group where some individuals are less likely to contract it.

INCIDENCE The number of new cases of a disease or an injury that occur in a population during a specified period of time.

MORBIDITY Both the state of being ill and the severity of the illness. The term *morbidity* comes from the Latin word *morbus*, which means "sick." A serious disease is said to have high morbidity.

MORTALITY The condition of being susceptible to death. The term *mortality* comes from the Latin word *mors*, which means "death." Mortality can also refer to the rate of deaths caused by an illness or injury (e.g., "Rabies has a high mortality rate").

NOSOCOMIAL INFECTION An infection that is acquired in a hospital. More precisely, the US Centers for Disease Control and Prevention (CDC) in Atlanta, Georgia, defines a nosocomial infection as a localized infection or an infection that is widely spread throughout the body that results from an adverse reaction to an infectious microorganism or toxin that was not present at the time of admission to the hospital.

PATHOGEN A disease-causing agent, such as a bacterium, a virus, a fungus, or another microorganism.

PERSISTENCE The length of time a disease remains in a patient. Disease persistence can vary from a few days to life-long.

PREVALENCE The actual number of cases of disease (or injury) that exist in a population.

VIRULENCE The ability of a disease organism to cause disease. A more virulent organism is more infective and liable to produce more serious disease.

infectious disease trends. These models involve various assumptions based on whether people can recover from infections, the rate of disease-related deaths, the development of immunity, and the duration of immunity (whether it is temporary or permanent). These models can also predict infectious disease catastrophes by location. For example, during the 1990s models showed that the persistence of the acquired immunodeficiency syndrome (AIDS) epidemic in many rural African communities reduced the population size to levels below those necessary to maintain the local population of the community. The models showed that AIDS was eliminating adults of reproducing age at a rapid rate. Increases in global AIDS treatment and prevention funding have ameliorated this problem to some extent in the African regions hardest hit by the AIDS epidemic, according to Avert's most recent report on eastern and southern Africa.

The simplest models often assume that the total population size is constant. For short-term outbreaks of a disease, simple disease models used to predict the course of an epidemic assume that the population is fixed and closed and depend only on the disease incidence and prevalence rates, disease duration (persistence), disease death rates, and occurrence of immunity. Models for an endemic disease (one that is naturally occurring in a region such as tuberculosis or malaria) usually assume that births and deaths balance each other so the population size remains unchanged. However, when the disease causes a significant number of deaths, as in the case of AIDS, this assumption is not realistic, and more complicated models assuming variable population are needed to predict the course of the epidemic. These sophisticated models incorporate assumptions about both birth and death rates, which can be influenced by the incidence and prevalence of disease as well as other factors. By the same token, population size influences the rapidity with which a disease is spread, with large, dense populations promoting the rapid spread of disease, and small, dispersed populations inhibiting such spread.

■ Applications and Research

In the early 21st century, war, civil strife, and the breakdown of governance have become the predominant mo-

tivators of mass migration. The global scope of this development has resulted in the largest population of displaced peoples in history. During this period many populations have migrated because of war, civil unrest, ethnic cleansing, and genocide, in addition to reasons related to the economy and natural disasters. As the 20th century ended, about 150 million people (2.5 percent of the global population) were living outside of their country of origin, 10 percent of whom were refugees.

In 2018 nearly 1 in 100 people worldwide have been displaced from their homes, which is, according to the Pew Charitable Trust, "the world's population that has been forcibly displaced since the United Nations High Commissioner for Refugees began collecting data on displaced persons in 1951." The regions with the highest percentages of displaced people are the Middle East (5.6 percent); continental Africa, excluding Egypt, which is considered part of the Middle East (1.6 percent), and Europe (0.7 percent). Population movements resulting from wars or violent conflicts have resulted in epidemiological outbreaks (e.g., cholera and typhoid fever), which arise from population overcrowding, malnutrition, unhygienic conditions, and lack of basic medical services.

The rise of bacterial resistance is another factor that has fundamentally changed the epidemiology of infectious disease. While community-acquired methicillin-resistant *Staphylococcus aureus* (MRSA) is most common in the United States, hospital-acquired MRSA has become the most common pathogen globally. The rates of antibiotic resistance are correlated with use (and overuse or misuse) of common antibiotics.

Seasonality is an important factor in the spread of common infectious diseases that most affect the youngest and oldest demographic groups (schoolchildren and the elderly). Illnesses such as influenza, measles, chickenpox, and pertussis (whooping cough) are all more prevalent at certain times of the year. Seasonality is a particularly important factor in models that predict whether these recurrent infectious diseases will occur in a given year or skip a year. Seasonal changes in disease transmission patterns and the susceptibility of a population to a disease (such as attending school or staying inside in close quarters during the winter) can prevent late-peaking diseases (disease epidemics that take a long time to reach peak infectivity) from spreading widely. When this happens, the remaining population is more susceptible to future epidemics because of a lack of herd immunity.

By analyzing seasonality and how much of the population remains susceptible to a disease, scientists can predict the course of newly emerging and reemerging diseases, such as West Nile virus, that are brought on by seasonal vectors (transmitters) including mosquitoes and migratory birds.

Of course, populations are not distributed uniformly even when they are stable and no significant migration is occurring. Infectious diseases spread in different patterns within a population that is divided into families or other groups than in a population that consists mostly of people who are living alone. A household constitutes a small population cluster, which is in turn composed of members that are resistant to the disease, along with members who are susceptible to the disease. An infectious disease spreads quickly and efficiently within the household, but the outbreak lasts longer if it spreads cluster by cluster or from one household to another.

■ Impacts and Issues

The proportion of children and the elderly in a population is important in the spread of communicable diseases, particularly because both age groups are more likely than the general population to be in close quarters for extended periods in schools and in hospitals or nursing homes. In children, immune functioning is still developing, and they are constantly being exposed to pathogens that are familiar to adults but new to them. At the other end of the demographic scale, aging is associated with increased incidence and severity of many infectious diseases, including nosocomial infections. This increased risk is due to an age-related decline in the body's immune system function. As the average age of the population increases in industrialized nations, the epidemiology, morbidity, mortality, and needs for preventive action against nosocomial infections in the elderly also increase.

When an epidemic of a highly infectious disease is spreading in a community of households, the infection of any member of a household generally results in the infection of all susceptible members of that household. The rapidity of disease spread will thus depend on the household size and the variability of the number of susceptible people per household. If the rate of spread of infection from individual to individual within each household and the spread of infection from household to household are calculated, the rate and pattern of spread of the disease can be put into a mathematical model by public health scientists. This model can be used to calculate the levels of immunity that will be needed to prevent major epidemics in the community. It can also be used to evaluate alternative vaccination strategies that could immunize the same number of individuals.

For a community with households of approximately equal size (as seen in many suburban communities in the United States), random vaccination of individuals is better than immunizing all members of a fraction of households that would amount to the same total number of vaccinated people. On the other hand, when households vary widely in size (as seen in many US urban areas), vaccinating all members of large households can slow down the spread of the epidemic more rapidly than would the vaccination of an equal number of randomly selected individuals. This is because disease transmission within these large households is easier than in the general community. Such epidemic spread models can also be used for a community of households with schools or day care centers. Immunizing every child within the school or day care center will be more effective than randomly immunizing an equal number of children in the community because the schools and day care centers are similar to very large households in which disease spread among many susceptible children is made easy by their close quarters.

Demographic characteristics of populations strongly determine the rate and extent of infectious disease distribution and spread. These demographic characteristics are in turn profoundly influenced by the processes of economic development, globalization, migration, and war. Although population demographics and patterns of infectious disease are in continual flux, they are rarely susceptible to policy-motivated human intervention. Rather, they are all aspects of the evolution of human cultures, which are intimately interconnected with evolving technology and commerce. The tools of epidemiological models that use demographic factors to help forecast the spread of infectious disease will constantly need to be updated as population characteristics change with increasing velocity in the years and decades ahead.

PRIMARY SOURCE

Recommendations for Counteracting Disease Spread through Migration

SOURCE: *Blackburn, Christine Crudo, and Paul E. Lenze Jr. "Forced Migration and the Spread of Infectious Disease: Impact of Syrian Refugee Movements on Disease Prevalence in the European Union." Scowcroft Institute of International Affairs. Texas A&M University, November 2017. http://bush.tamu.edu/scowcroft/papers/blackburn-lenze/Paper%20No.%2010%20Blackburn%20&%20Lenze.pdf (accessed February 5, 2018).*

INTRODUCTION: *Large-scale migrations due to war and political unrest can have significant health impacts on both migrants and the communities that received them. In the following excerpt from a report of the Scowcroft Institute of International Affairs, researchers make recommendations about how best to reduce the impact of infectious diseases following the migration of Syrian refugees to Europe beginning in 2011.*

The mass migration of people from Syria has put significant strain on the European Union. There has been increased economic pressure from supporting thousands of new arrivals, challenges with housing and community integration, and lastly new health issues that stress the public health infrastructure and put the health of citizens and refugees at risk. Many Syrians have traveled long distances, are malnourished, and may not have had appropriate vaccinations or access to any form of health care for long periods of time. We provide three recommendations for addressing the health issues posed by refugees coming into the EU from Syria that we believe can help mitigate the introduction of diseases.

The first recommendation is to provide training of local health care practitioners. Most of the diseases that Syrian refugees are bringing into the EU are not common to Europe, but they are common in Syria. The most common disease coming into the EU from Syria is cutaneous leishmaniasis, but it is not the only one. Educating health care professionals in Europe about the signs, symptoms, and method of transmission for the most common diseases appearing with the movement of Syrian refugees would help clinics to be better prepared to diagnose and treat the diseases when they identify their symptoms. Knowledge about the diseases would help eliminate delay in diagnosis and treatment and eliminating this delay could prevent a large-scale outbreak. If health care professionals are given all the tools they need to fight the new diseases, the threat to the European public and the refugee communities will be greatly reduced.

Our second recommendation is to provide health screening upon entry for those refugees entering the EU through formal channels. These screenings should include a routine medical examination, appropriate vaccinations, and testing for infectious diseases common in Syria. If infectious diseases are identified, the refugee should be started on the proper treatment and contained at the port of entry until the treatment protocol is complete. Once the treatment is complete they will be allowed to be integrated into the community. The purpose of the entry health screenings is to identify and treat diseases before they have an opportunity to spread into the population. European Parliament, the European Council, and the European Commission have all recognised that the health of refugees can no longer be ignored. Both Parliament and the Commission have committed millions of Euros to supporting the healthcare of migrants and have discussed the importance of identifying diseases and other conditions as they enter the EU.

Lastly, because large amounts of Syrian refugees are not entering the EU through formal channels, health outreach must be conducted in refugee communities, regardless of their legal status. Funding should be secured for health care teams to go out into refugee communities on a monthly basis offering free medical care, vaccinations, and infectious disease diagnostic tests. This will help the EU identify diseases that may be circulating in refugee communities and prevent them from finding their way into the larger population. Additionally, it provides refugees who may be afraid to seek health care because of their illegal status, the opportunity to be treated. Health care teams could also offer education and training regarding some of the most common diseases in the communities.

See Also *Economic Development and Infectious Disease; Public Health and Infectious Disease*

BIBLIOGRAPHY

Books

Bustamante, Nirma Dora. "MRSA: A Global Threat." Master's thesis, UT Southwestern Medical School, 2011. This thesis can also be found online at http://www.utsouthwestern.edu/edumedia/edufiles/about_us/admin_offices/global_health/mrsa-bustamante.pdf (accessed February 6, 2018).

Connolly, M. A. *Communicable Disease Control in Emergencies: A Field Manual.* Geneva: World Health Organization, 2005.

Inhorn, Marcia C., and Peter J. Brown, eds. *The Anthropology of Disease: International Health Perspectives.* Hoboken, NJ: Taylor and Francis, 2013.

Jamison, Dean T., et al, eds. *Disease and Mortality in Sub-Saharan Africa.* Washington, DC: World Bank, 2006.

Periodicals

Buckee, Caroline O., Andrew J. Tatem, and Jessica E. Metcalf. "Seasonal Population Movements and the Surveillance and Control of Infectious Diseases." *Trends in Parasitology* 33, no. 1 (January 2017): 10–20.

Hodal, Kate. "Rohingya Children Close to Starvation Amid 'Health Crisis on an Unimaginable Scale.'" *Guardian* (November 10, 2017). This article can also be found online at https://www.theguardian.com/global-development/2017/nov/10/rohingya-kids-starvation-health-crisis-unimaginable-scale-malnutrition-myanmar-bangladesh (accessed February 5, 2018).

Pramodh, Nathaniel. "Limiting the Spread of Communicable Diseases Caused by Human Population Movement." *Journal of Rural and Remote Environmental Health* 2, no. 1 (2003): 23–32. This article can also be found online at http://jrtph.jcu.edu.au/vol/v02nathaniel.pdf (accessed February 5, 2018).

Soto, S. M. "Human Migration and Infectious Diseases." *Clinical Microbiology and Infection* 15, no. 1 (January 2009): 26–28. This article can also be found online at http://onlinelibrary.wiley.com/doi/10.1111/j.1469–0691.2008.02694.x/full (accessed February 6, 2018.)

Stone, Lewi, Ronen Olinky, and Amit Huppert. "Seasonal Dynamics of Recurrent Epidemics." *Nature* (April 2007): 533–536. This article can also be found online at https://www.researchgate.net/publication/6416975_Seasonal_dynamics_of_recurrent_epidemics (accessed February 5, 2018).

Websites

"HIV and AIDS in East and Southern Africa Regional Overview." Avert. https://www.avert.org/professionals/hiv-around-world/sub-saharan-africa/overview (accessed January 27, 2018).

"Key Facts about the World's Refugees." Pew Charitable Trust. http://www.pewresearch.org/fact-tank/2016/10/05/key-facts-about-the-worlds-refugees/ (accessed February 6, 2018).

Sheridan, Jackie. "Diphtheria Outbreak among Rohingya Refugees Enters Third Month." The Disease Daily, January 25, 2018. http://www.healthmap.org/site/diseasedaily/article/diphtheria-outbreak-among-rohingya-refugees-enters-third-month-12518. (accessed January 27, 2018).

Kenneth T. LaPensee

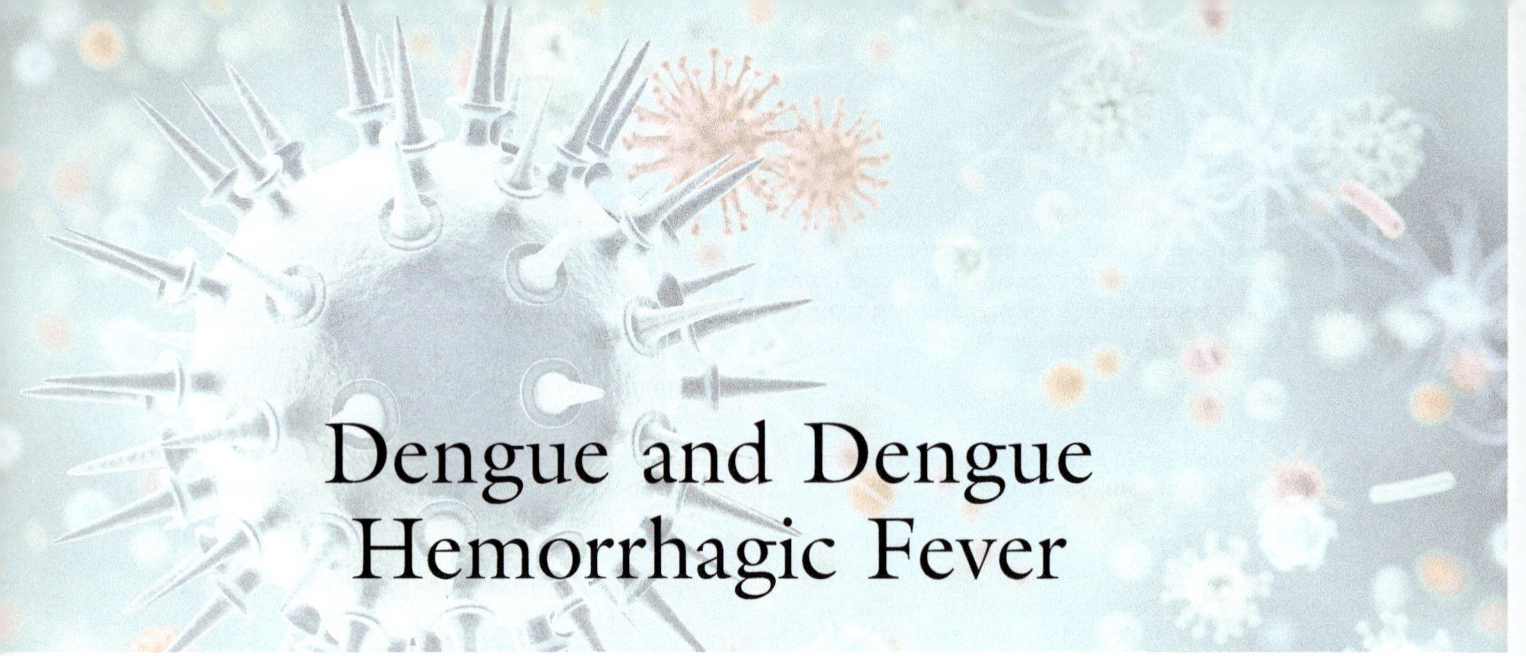

Dengue and Dengue Hemorrhagic Fever

■ Introduction

Dengue (DEN-gay) is an illness that is transmitted to humans by the bite of a mosquito that has the virus in its bloodstream. The disease causes nausea, vomiting, muscle and joint pain, and a characteristic rash. In some people the illness is a more serious and life-threatening infection called dengue hemorrhagic fever.

WORDS TO KNOW

CONJUNCTIVITIS An inflammation or redness of the lining of the white part of the eye and the underside of the eyelid (conjunctiva) that can be caused by infection, allergic reaction, or physical agents such as infrared or ultraviolet light. Conjunctivitis (also called pink eye) is one of the most common eye infections in children and adults in the United States. Luckily, it is also one of the most treatable infections. Because it is so common in the United States and around the world and is often not reported to health organizations, accurate statistics are not available for conjunctivitis.

ENDEMIC Present in a particular area or among a particular group of people.

PANDEMIC An epidemic that occurs in more than one country or population simultaneously. *Pandemic* means "all the people."

SEROTYPES Also called serovars, are classes of microorganisms based on the types of molecules (antigens) that they present on their surfaces. Even a single species may have thousands of serotypes, which may have medically quite distinct behaviors.

SYSTEMIC Any medical condition that affects the whole body (i.e., the whole system).

■ Disease History, Characteristics, and Transmission

Dengue appears to have originated in the Old World. The disease was first reported in the Caribbean–Latin American region (specifically the Virgin Islands) in 1827, presumably imported with African slaves. A second pandemic between 1848 and 1850 involved Cuba and New Orleans. A third pandemic struck the region between 1979 and 1980.

The fact that dengue is not exclusively a "tropical" phenomenon is well illustrated by the American experience with the disease. Dengue was first reported in the United States in 1827 and caused a number of massive outbreaks in Louisiana, Hawaii (50,000 cases in 1903), and Texas (500,000 cases in 1922).

Dengue virus was first isolated in Nigeria between 1964 and 1968. However, surveys suggest that the disease is common in certain areas of western Africa and probably eastern Africa. It is suggested that many cases are misdiagnosed as malaria. Although the disease had been relatively rare in Australia, as many as 800 cases per year were reported there as of 2017.

The World Health Organization (WHO) estimated that about 400 million people were infected as of 2017. However, this estimate may be low. In a 2012 study for *PLOS Neglected Tropical Diseases*, Oliver J. Brady and coauthors estimated that more than 3.9 billion people, about half the world's population, were at risk of infection.

The virus that causes dengue is one of 19 flaviviruses that infect humans. Flaviviruses account for 20 percent of all infectious virus species. Other flaviviruses include the agents of hepatitis C, West Nile fever, Japanese encephalitis, and yellow fever. Only 29 percent of viral diseases are acquired through mosquito bites, but 53 percent of flaviviruses are transmitted in this manner. A variety of mosquito species serve as vectors (transmitters) of flaviviruses that cause dengue, most belonging to the genus *Aedes*. Although dengue is almost exclusively a human disease, natural infection of monkeys has been reported in Asia.

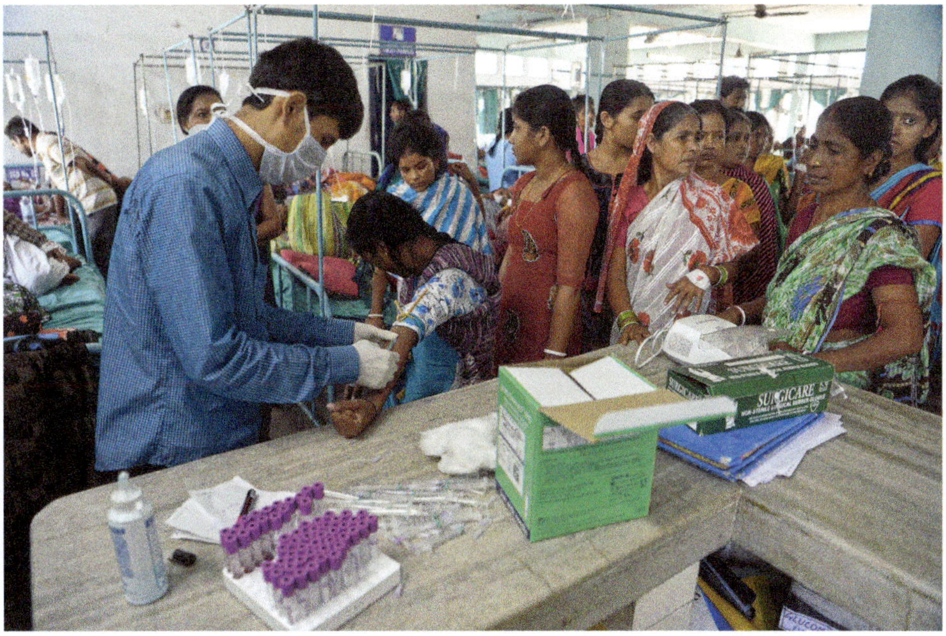

A health care worker collects blood samples in Siliguri, India. Multiple cases of dengue fever were reported in the region in 2017. © DIPTENDU DUTTA/AFP/Getty Images

In most cases dengue is a self-limiting flulike illness. Two to 15 days following a mosquito bite, patients experience fever with varying combinations of headache, retro-orbital (around the eyes) pain, myalgia (muscle aches), arthralgia (joint pain), rash, and leukopenia (low white cell count). Occasionally a saddleback fever pattern is evident, with the fever dropping after a few days and rebounding within 24 hours. The pulse rate is often relatively slow in relation to the degree of fever. Conjunctival redness and sore throat may occur, often with enlargement of regional lymph nodes. A rash appears in as many as 50 percent of persons with dengue, either early in the illness with flushing or mottling or between the second and sixth days as a florid red rash that spreads out from the center of the body. The rash fades after two to three days.

Symptoms generally resolve within two to seven days with no long-term residual effects. However, significant depression may occur and persist for several months.

In a small percentage of people, dengue fever may evolve into a severe and even life-threatening illness such as dengue hemorrhagic fever (DHF) or dengue shock syndrome (DSS). DHF is characterized by initial symptoms of dengue fever, in addition to bleeding tendencies such as petechiae (tiny reddish skin lesions associated with blood vessel injury) or ecchymoses (spontaneous bruises related to blood leakage). In some cases overt bleeding from the nose, mouth, stomach, colon, or other sites occurs. The blood platelet count is low (less than 100,000 per cubic millimeter), and the red blood cell concentration increases due to fluid leakage from the circulatory system. DSS is characterized by the findings of DHF in addition to signs of shock, including low blood pressure, cold clammy skin, and mental obtundation (dullness).

■ Scope and Distribution

As of 2017 dengue was endemic in at least 115 countries, placing an estimated 2.5 to 3.9 billion persons at risk. Each year around 50 million to 100 million people are infected, mostly in Southeast Asia and Latin America, according to WHO. Approximately 30,000 to 50,000 persons die of dengue each year.

Dengue was endemic in more than 100 countries in Africa, the Americas, the eastern Mediterranean, Southeast Asia, and the western Pacific as of 2017. The Americas, Southeast Asia, and the western Pacific were the hardest-hit regions. In 2015 there were more than 2.3 million cases in these regions, with nearly 1,200 deaths.

Large outbreaks have occurred in the early 21st century. In 2012 an outbreak in the Madeira Islands of Portugal sickened more than 2,000 people. A 2015 outbreak in Delhi, India, involved more than 15,000 cases.

Since 2000 most of the 100 or so cases reported annually in the United States have been acquired overseas or by people living in tropical locales such as the US Virgin Islands and Puerto Rico. A 2007 outbreak affected more than 10,000 people in Puerto Rico. A 2005 outbreak in Texas was the largest to date in the continental United States, while a 2015 outbreak in Hawaii caused 181 reported illnesses. Each year between 10 and 40 cases are reported in the southern border area of Texas.

■ Treatment and Prevention

Although few laboratories are equipped to cultivate the dengue virus, a variety of rapid tests are available for diagnosis through identification of the antibodies that

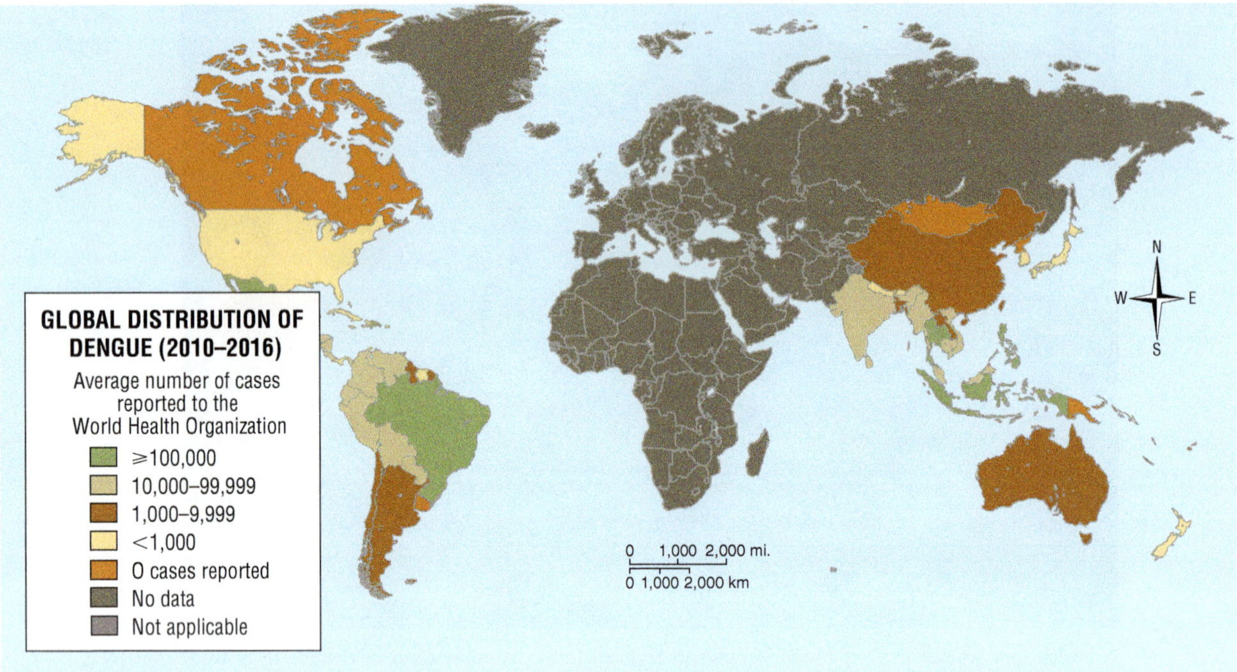

SOURCE: Adapted from "Distribution of Dengue, Worldwide, 2016." World Health Organization. 2016. Available from: http://www.who.int/denguecontrol/epidemiology/en/

appear during the course of illness. A dengue vaccine called Dengvaxia®, made by Sanofi Pasteur, became available for use in early 2016. The vaccine is for people between 9 and 45 years of age and is intended for use in regions where the infection occurs regularly. As of late 2017 other vaccines were being developed.

The controlled release of mosquitoes incapable of breeding could be a means of reducing mosquito populations and therefore transmission of the dengue virus, as has been proven effective for the control of malaria.

Because the major damage to patients with DHF or DSS is related to fluid loss, people with these complications generally respond to intravenous fluid replacement of blood volume. Isolation precautions are not necessary, but steps should be taken to exclude mosquitoes from patient treatment areas in endemic areas.

Impacts and Issues

In the 21st century *Aedes albopictus* (the Asian tiger mosquito) gained prominence as a dengue vector in many parts of the world, largely the result of dissemination of these insects in pools of water that accumulate in automobile tires transported on commercial ships. In addition, the spread of dengue fever is attributed to a rapid rise in the populations of cities in the developing world where dengue vectors thrive due to inadequate water storage and inadequate access to sanitation.

DHF and DSS appear to be related to immunological overreaction in people who develop dengue more than once in their lifetime. There are four serotypes of dengue virus, and sequential outbreaks in the same country may involve more than one serotype. Thus, if a person is infected with dengue type 1 and infected later in life (or during a later trip to a tropical area) with dengue type 2, the immunological experience from the first attack may prime the individual for a severe systemic response to the new infection. As such, anyone who anticipates travel to an endemic country or presents with signs suggestive of DHF or DSS should be questioned regarding previous travel and experience with dengue.

Natural disasters such as hurricanes can cause flooding and disrupt local health care, which makes the affected regions vulnerable to a dengue outbreak. In the aftermath of Hurricane Harvey, which decimated the Houston, Texas, area in late August 2017, there were concerns about a dengue outbreak. But as of December 2017 no outbreak had occurred.

SEE ALSO *Climate Change and Infectious Disease; Host and Vector; Mosquito-Borne Diseases; Tropical Infectious Diseases*

BIBLIOGRAPHY

Books

Greenbaum, Eli. *Emerald Labyrinth: A Scientist's Adventures in the Jungles of the Congo.* Dartmouth, NH: ForeEdge/University Press of New England, 2017.

Gubler, Duana J., et al., eds. *Dengue and Dengue Hemorrhagic Fever*. Boston: CABI, 2014.

Periodicals

Brady, Oliver J., et al. "Refining the Global Spatial Limits of Dengue Virus Transmission by Evidence-Based Consensus." *PLOS Neglected Tropical Diseases* 6, no. 8 (August 7, 2012): e1760. This article can also be found online at http://journals.plos.org/plosntds/article?id=10.1371/journal.pntd.0001760

Feinberg, Mark B., and Rafi Ahmed. "Advancing Dengue Vaccine Development." *Science* 358, no. 6365 (November 17, 2017): 865–866.

Turelli, Michael, and Nicholas H. Barton. "Deploying Dengue-Suppressing *Wolbachia*: Robust Models Predict Slow but Effective Spatial Spread in *Aedes aegypti*." *Theoretical Population Biology* 115 (June 2017): 45–60.

Websites

"Dengue: Epidemiology." Centers for Disease Control and Prevention, June 9, 2014. http://www.cdc.gov/dengue/epidemiology/index.html (accessed December 11, 2017).

"Dengue and Severe Dengue." World Health Organization, April 2017. http://www.who.int/mediacentre/factsheets/fs117/en/ (accessed December 11, 2017).

Stephen A. Berger
Brian Hoyle

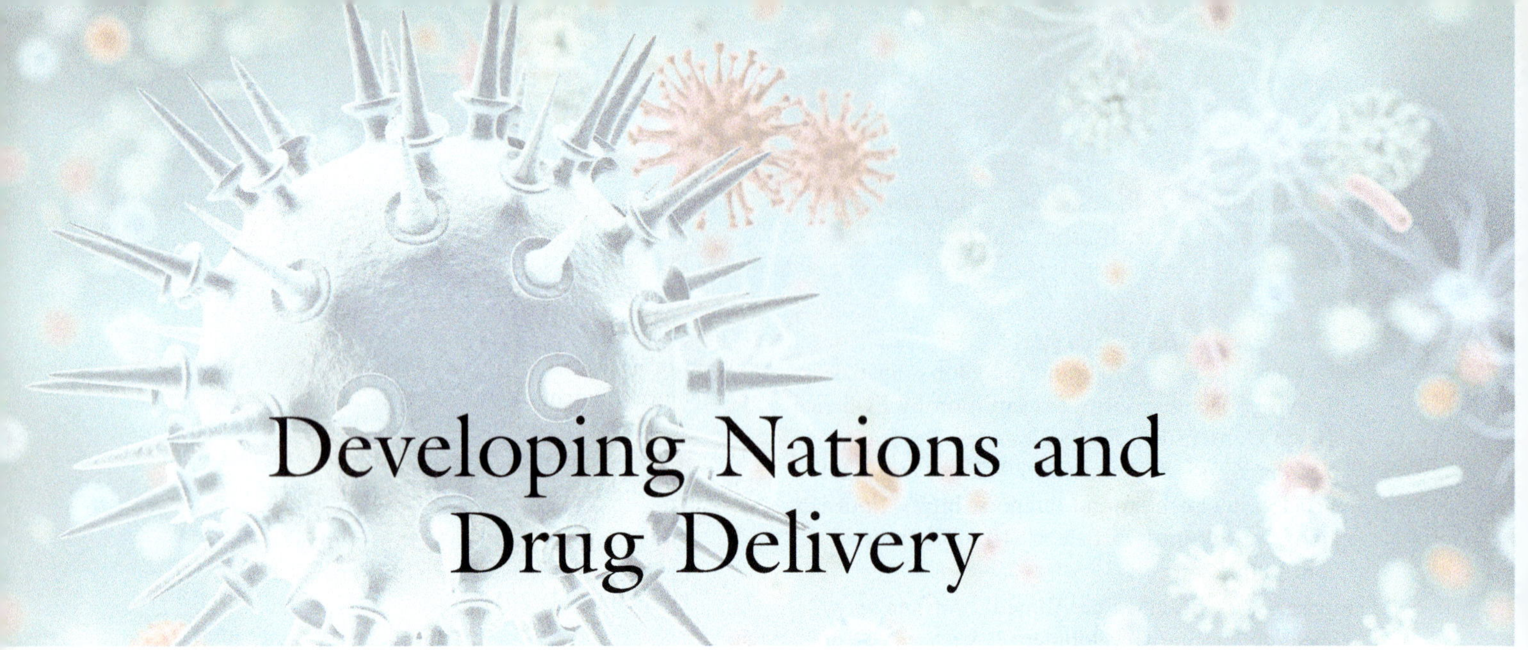

Developing Nations and Drug Delivery

Introduction

In most of the developed world, access to medicines is taken for granted, despite ongoing debate over the price of certain drugs. However, in 2008 around one-third of the world's population still lacked access to essential medicines, such as antibiotics, painkillers, and drugs for infectious diseases such as human immunodeficiency virus (HIV)/acquired immunodeficiency syndrome (AIDS), malaria, and tuberculosis. Even if the drugs are available, people may be unable to afford to pay for them or access them, or they may be of substandard or counterfeit quality or improperly stored.

There have been some concerted efforts to improve the delivery of drugs to developing countries, led by the international humanitarian aid organization Médecins Sans Frontières (MSF; Doctors Without Borders) and the World Health Organization (WHO). Developing countries need not only access to essential medicines but also to know how to use them to gain maximum benefit.

WORDS TO KNOW

ANTIRETROVIRAL (ARV) THERAPY A form of drug therapy that prevents the reproduction of a type of virus called a retrovirus. Human immunodeficiency virus (HIV), which causes acquired immunodeficiency syndrome (AIDS), is a retrovirus. ARV drugs are used to treat HIV infections and keep the virus in check, but they cannot prevent or cure the infection.

PARASITE An organism that lives in or on a host organism and that gets its nourishment from that host. The parasite usually gains all the benefits of this relationship, whereas the host may suffer from various diseases and discomforts or show no signs of the infection. The life cycle of a typical parasite usually includes several developmental stages and morphological changes as the parasite lives and moves through the environment and one or more hosts. Parasites that remain on a host's body surface to feed are called ectoparasites, whereas those that live inside a host's body are called endoparasites. Parasitism is a highly successful biological adaptation. There are more known parasitic species than nonparasitic ones, and parasites affect just about every form of life, including most all animals, plants, and even bacteria.

RESISTANT ORGANISM An organism that has developed the ability to counter something trying to harm it. Within infectious diseases, the organism, such as a bacterium, has developed a resistance to drugs, such as antibiotics.

History and Scientific Foundations

An early example of how to improve drug delivery in developing countries involved a 1989 initiative to treat river blindness (onchocerciasis). The African Program for Onchocerciasis (APOC), which as of early 2018 was a part of the Program for the Elimination of Neglected Diseases in Africa (PENDA), grew out of this and was focused on distribution of the drug ivermectin, which is known to be effective against the disease. The drug is donated by Merck & Co., the company that discovered it. By the end of 2014, the APOC had likely prevented 24.2 million river blindness infections, some 500,000 cases of low vision, and 300,000 cases of blindness.

One major guidance document for drug delivery in developing countries is WHO's Model List of Essential Medicines, which was established in 1977. This helps countries select the appropriate medicines for their public health priorities according to the best scientific evidence on quality, safety, and efficacy. It also provides guidance to the pharmaceutical industry on the global need for medicines.

Applications and Research

WHO also has guidelines on donation of medicines by pharmaceutical companies to ensure the medications meet certain quality standards. Pharmaceutical companies may also make other arrangements to try to improve access to, for example, HIV/AIDS drugs. For instance, they may choose not to take out patent protection in developing countries or not to take action against competitors making generic versions of their drugs.

Two organizations that make major contributions to the delivery of drugs in developing countries are MSF and the International Network for the Rational Use of Drugs (INRUD). In 1999 MSF launched its Campaign for Access to Essential Medicines with the aim of improving the global availability of drugs for the treatment of infectious diseases such as HIV/AIDS, malaria, and tuberculosis, as well as neglected diseases such as Chagas disease, leishmaniasis, and sleeping sickness. The campaign aims to find ways of lowering the price of essential medicines and bring certain inexpensive and effective drugs back into production. The campaign also works to publicly call out pharmaceutical companies for selling drugs at costs that people in developing countries cannot afford.

In 1989 INRUD was established to develop strategies to improve the way drugs are prescribed, dispensed, and used and to address the misuse of scarce resources in developing countries. The network comprises 25 groups, including 20 from Africa, Asia, Latin America, and Eastern Europe, as well as groups from WHO, the Harvard Medical School Department of Ambulatory Care, and other organizations.

Most of the effort in improving drug delivery in developing countries has been focused on the major infectious diseases. With respect to malaria, for instance, MSF has been persuading governments to consider funding the artemisinin-based combination therapy favored by WHO. This will help address the growing problem of chloroquine resistance. Although chloroquine is relatively cheap, it will not be effective in the areas where malaria parasites are resistant. Therefore, there is a need for alternative drugs.

Impacts and Issues

Supplying drugs to developing countries is just one aspect of ensuring universal access to medicine. Education is also needed to teach the best way to use these medicines, and the local infrastructure must be improved to ensure a reliable supply chain. Standardizing the quality of the medicines and their secure storage are also challenges.

In the 21st century many developing countries have policies intended to make essential medicines available to their populations, which is an approach strongly encouraged by WHO. These policies also focus on how to distribute drugs to where they are needed and how the safety of medicines can be guaranteed. Pharmaceutical pricing is a

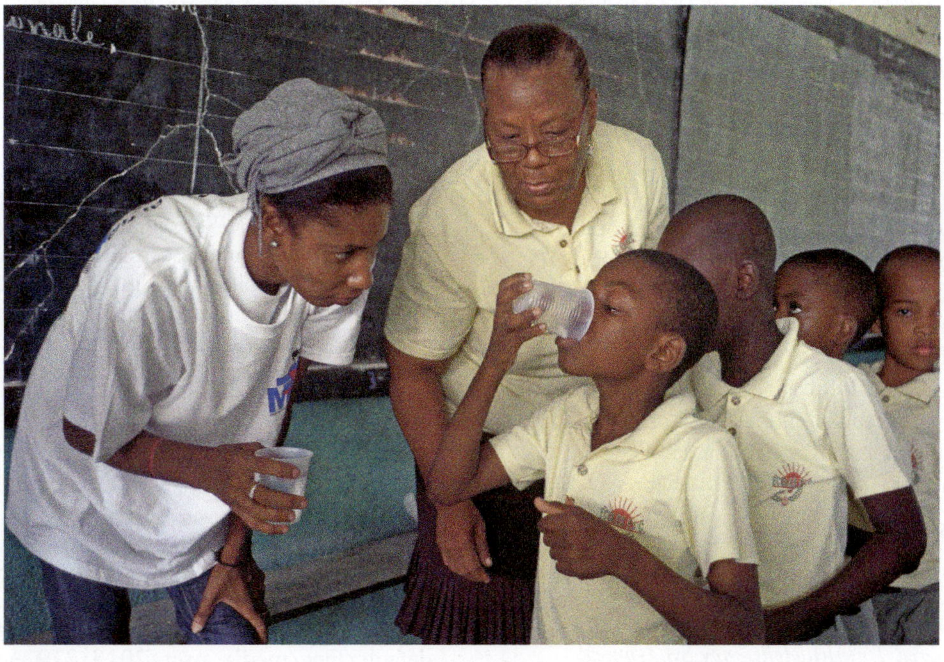

As part of a mass drug administration sponsored by Haiti's public health ministry, elementary school students at L'École Les Frères Clement in the commune of Jacmel line up to take drugs that combat lymphatic filariasis and intestinal worms. *© Maggie Steber/The Washington Post/Getty Images*

ACCESSING ANTIRETROVIRAL DRUGS IN DEVELOPING NATIONS OF EAST AND SOUTHERN AFRICA

Of all the regions in the world, East Africa and southern Africa are the most affected by the HIV/AIDS epidemic. In 2016 19.4 million people living in those regions were HIV positive, or about 7 percent of the population. That year, 420,000 people in those regions died from HIV/AIDS.

Although HIV/AIDS is a serious, ongoing problem in these areas, health care workers, local governments, and international organizations have worked since the introduction of antiretroviral drugs (ARV) in the mid-1990s to connect HIV-positive people with effective and affordable treatment. It is well established that ARV therapy for HIV/AIDS is effective treatment, enabling people to live with the condition rather than almost inevitably dying from it. Therefore, improving access to ARV for patients in developing countries has become a priority.

AVERT, an international HIV/AIDS organization, reported that funding for HIV/AIDS health care services in the region increased by more than 50 percent between 2006 and 2016, despite the 2008–2009 global financial crisis.

Because of such efforts, the number of people on ARV in East Africa and southern Africa doubled between 2006 and 2012, according to the United Nations Joint Programme on HIV/AIDS (UNAIDS). In 2016 UNAIDS also reported that the percentage of people on ARV had increased from 24 percent in 2010 to 54 percent in 2015.

Although more people in East Africa and southern Africa are being treated for HIV/AIDS than ever before, many infected people still do not have access to lifesaving drugs. In general, health care facilities and systems in these countries are underresourced. HIV-positive people who live in rural areas have less access to health care workers and are therefore less likely to be on ART. Stigma surrounding HIV/AIDS prevents some people from seeking care. In addition, women tend to have less access to health care than their male counterparts because of gender inequality.

There have been many challenges involved in trying to get ARVs to those who need them. For instance, there must be a reliable supply chain from the factory where the drug is manufactured to the patient, as the drugs must be taken every day. In many developing countries, transport and communication systems are chronically weak. The funding organizations have been trying to address this by commissioning experts in supply chain management to work in this area.

complex issue. Many companies have not followed Merck's ivermectin example, distributing drugs for free, out of concern for their shareholders' interests. One way around this is for developing countries to establish their own pharmaceutical industries and make cheaper generic copies of essential drugs.

Another problem for developing countries, as well as middle-income ones, is what WHO terms "substandard and falsified medical products." According to WHO, around 10 percent of all drugs sold in developing or middle-income countries are substandard or falsified. Although WHO notes that substandard and falsified medical products affect all people regardless of where they live, it is particularly a problem for people who do not live in wealthy countries. This has a real effect on people's lives. WHO estimates that, if 5 percent of antibiotics given to children to treat pneumonia are substandard or falsified, for example, approximately 37,000 to 85,000 children will die unnecessarily.

See Also *African Sleeping Sickness (Trypanosomiasis); AIDS (Acquired Immunodeficiency Syndrome); Leishmaniasis; Malaria; Médecins Sans Frontières (Doctors Without Borders)*

BIBLIOGRAPHY

Books

Hillery, Anya M., and Kinam Park. *Drug Delivery: Fundamentals and Applications.* 2nd ed. Boca Raton, FL: CRC, 2016.

Periodicals

Ahmadiani, Saeed, and Shekoufeh Nikfar. "Challenges of Access to Medicine and the Responsibility of Pharmaceutical Companies: A Legal Perspective." *DARU Journal of Pharmaceutical Sciences* 24 (2016): 13. This article can also be found online at https://www.ncbi.nlm.nih.gov/pmc/articles/PMC4855755/ (accessed March 1, 2018).

Stevens, Hilde, and Isabelle Huys. "Innovative Approaches to Increase Access to Medicines in Developing Countries." *Frontiers in Medicine* 4 (2017): 218. This article can also be found online at https://www.ncbi.nlm.nih.gov/pmc/articles/PMC5725781/ (accessed March 1, 2018).

Websites

"Access to Antiretroviral Therapy in Africa: Status Report on Progress to the 2015 Targets." UNAIDS, 2013. http://www.unaids.org/sites/default/files/media_asset/20131219_AccessARTAfricaStatusReportProgresstowards2015Targets_en_0.pdf (accessed March 1, 2018).

"African Programme for Onchocerciasis Control (APOC)." World Health Organization. http://www.who.int/apoc/about/en/ (accessed March 1, 2018).

Balasegaram, Manica. "Drugs for the Poor, Drugs for the Rich: Why the Current R&D Model Doesn't Deliver." PLOS Speaking of Medicine Community Blog, February 14, 2014. http://blogs.plos.org/speakingofmedicine/2014/02/14/drugs-poor-drugs-rich-current-rd-model-doesnt-deliver/ (accessed March 1, 2018).

"Essential Medicines." World Health Organization. http://www.who.int/topics/essential_medicines/en/ (accessed March 1, 2018).

"HIV and AIDS in East and Southern Africa Regional Overview." AVERT, March 1, 2018. https://www.avert.org/professionals/hiv-around-world/sub-saharan-africa/overview (accessed March 1, 2018).

Médecins Sans Frontières Access Campaign. https://www.msfaccess.org/ (accessed March 1, 2018).

"17 Million People with Access to Antiretroviral Therapy." World Health Organization, May 31, 2016. http://www.who.int/hiv/mediacentre/news/global-aids-update-2016-news/en/ (accessed March 1, 2018).

"A Study on Public Health and Socioeconomic Impact of Substandard and Falsified Medical Products: Executive Summary." World Health Organization, 2017. http://www.who.int/medicines/regulation/ssffc/publications/SummarySESTUDY-WEB.pdf?ua=1 (accessed March 1, 2018).

Susan Aldridge
Claire Skinner

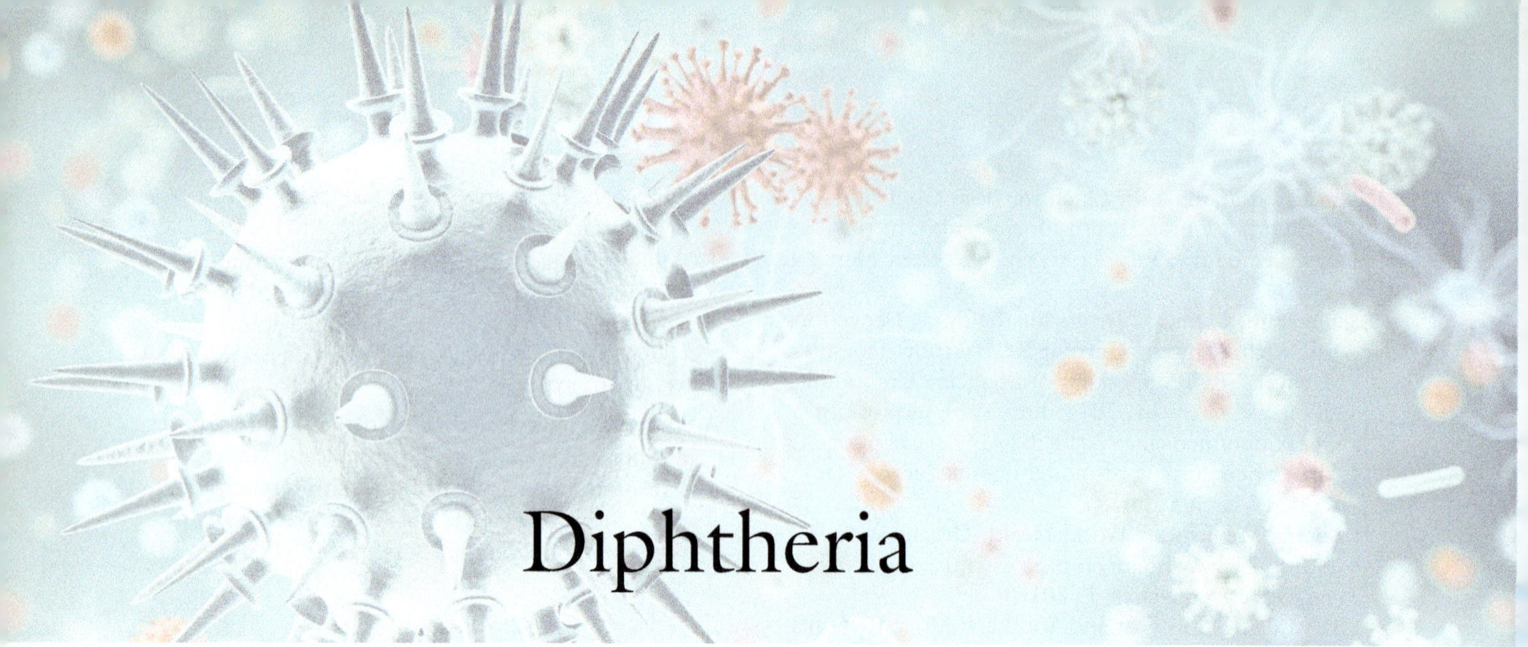

Diphtheria

Introduction

Diphtheria is an acute infectious illness affecting the mucous membranes of the throat and tonsils. In severe cases suffocation may result, and there may be complications involving the heart and nervous system. Diphtheria is caused by the bacterium *Corynebacterium diphtheriae*. Diphtheria was traditionally a major killer, with children being especially susceptible.

The introduction of mass immunization in the 1920s made the disease rare in the industrialized world, including the United States and most other developed countries. However, immunity to diphtheria is lost over time. Those living in stable countries with high standards of public hygiene are unlikely to be at risk. The same cannot be said when health and political systems break down or when childhood immunization is not universal.

For example, the reemergence of diphtheria in the former Soviet Union in the 1990s resulted from a combination of these health and political factors. The reintroduction of mass immunization eventually brought this epidemic under control. However, diphtheria remains a threat in countries where overcrowding, unsanitary conditions, and low levels of immunization are a fact of everyday life.

WORDS TO KNOW

ANTIBODIES Proteins found in the blood that help fight against foreign substances called antigens. Antigens, which are usually proteins or polysaccharides, stimulate the immune system to produce antibodies, or Y-shaped immunoglobulins. The antibodies inactivate the antigen and help remove it from the body. While antigens can be the source of infections from pathogenic bacteria and viruses, organic molecules detrimental to the body from internal or environmental sources also act as antigens. Genetic engineering and the use of various mutational mechanisms allow the construction of a vast array of antibodies (each with a unique genetic sequence).

ANTITOXIN An antidote to a toxin that neutralizes the toxin's poisonous effects.

CUTANEOUS Pertaining to the skin.

REEMERGENCE The reappearance of something that has been absent.

TOXIN A poison that is produced by a living organism.

Disease History, Characteristics, and Transmission

C. diphtheriae is a Gram-positive bacillus. Bacilli are a group of bacteria characterized by their rodlike shape. "Gram-positive" refers to the way certain bacteria absorb stains applied for microscopic study of the organism. Most strains of *C. diphtheriae* produce a potent toxin that is responsible for the complications of diphtheria. There are two forms of the disease: respiratory diphtheria, which is the more common, and cutaneous diphtheria.

The symptoms of respiratory diphtheria include painful tonsillitis or pharyngitis (inflammation of tonsils or throat). The voice may be hoarse, fever is often present, and a nasal discharge is usually noticeable. What distinguishes diphtheria from other throat infections is the presence of a pseudomembrane, a thick, bluish white or gray covering on the throat or tonsils that may develop greenish black patches. The pseudomembrane develops when the *C. diphtheriae* toxin kills cells within the mucous membrane lining the throat and tonsils. The membrane may spread downward and can interfere with breathing, causing difficulty breathing or rapid breathing and eventually, if not treated, paralysis and suffocation. In addition, the neck tends to swell, giving the patient a characteristic "bull neck" appearance.

In 10 to 20 percent of cases, the toxin spreads to the heart and the peripheral nervous system. It can cause myocarditis, an inflammation of the heart muscle and heart valves, which may lead to heart failure in later life. In the nervous system, diphtheria toxin can cause paralysis, which could lead to respiratory failure. Even with prompt treatment, the death rate of respiratory diphtheria is 5 to 10 percent. Diphtheria tends to be more severe in children under the age of five and in adults over 40.

Cutaneous diphtheria, the second form of diphtheria, occurs when the bacterium infects bites or rashes. It is more common in tropical regions, although it can occur in the United States and other developed countries, especially among people living in crowded conditions with a lack of hygiene. Symptoms include redness and swelling of the skin, along with topical pain. Again, a pseudomembrane forms at the site of the infection, and ulcers usually develop on the skin. However, the complications associated with respiratory diphtheria are far less common in the cutaneous form of the disease.

Diphtheria usually is transmitted by contact with droplets from the upper respiratory tract that are propelled into the air by the coughs and sneezes of infected individuals. It is highly infectious. People who are untreated remain infectious for two to three weeks. *C. diphtheriae* can also be spread by contaminated personal and household objects or food.

Scope and Distribution

Diphtheria was a major child killer in the 18th and 19th centuries. In the 21st century, thanks to mass immunization, it is rare in the United States and Western Europe. Before immunization there were 100 to 200 cases of diphtheria per 100,000 of the US population. By 2007 there were only about 0.001 cases per 100,000. In 1942, the year immunization was introduced in the United Kingdom, there were 60,000 cases of diphtheria a year, around 4,000 of which proved fatal. Between 1937 and 1938, diphtheria was second only to pneumonia as a cause of death in childhood. With levels of immunization in the United Kingdom reaching 94 percent in the 21st century, there were only very occasional cases. Several European countries have not seen a single case of diphtheria for many years.

Before the discovery of the vaccine, children were most at risk from diphtheria. Now all ages seem to be at risk, and, although the risk is higher among those who have not been vaccinated, cases occur among those who have had the vaccine too, because immunity appears to decline over time. In the United States, Canada, and many countries in Western Europe, childhood vaccination beginning in the 1930s and 1940s led to a rapid reduction in cases. Where diphtheria occurs, it tends to be in an incompletely vaccinated or unvaccinated person of low socioeconomic status.

Diphtheria is found in temperate climates. As with any highly infectious disease, diphtheria is more commonly found in areas with poor sanitation and overcrowding. The

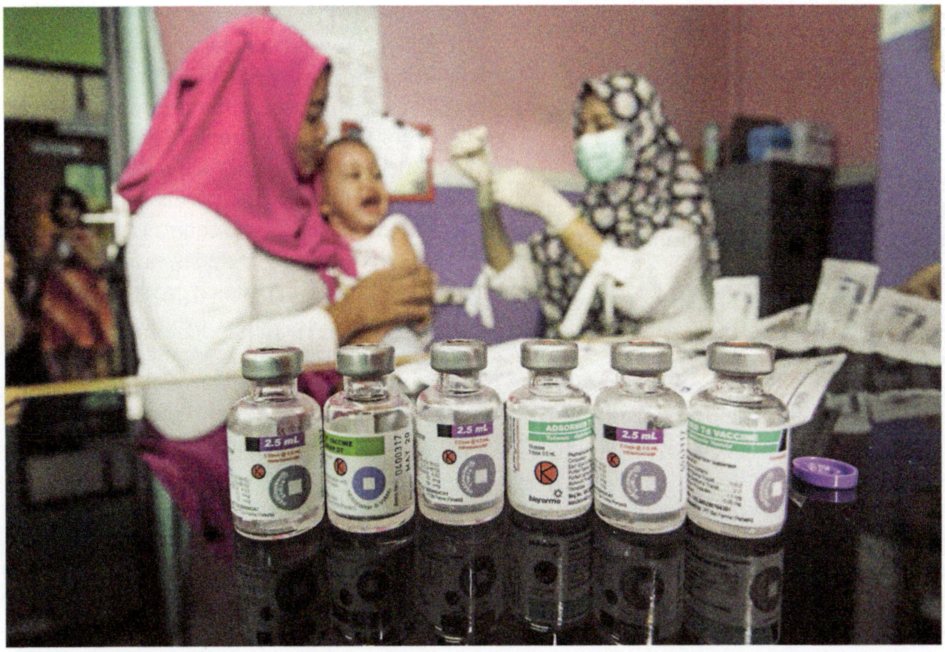

A health officer in Depok, West Java, Indonesia, injects diphtheria immunization to kids at a community health center in response to what the national government deemed an "extraordinary" outbreak of the disease. © *Eko Siswono Toyudho/Anadolu Agency/Getty Images*

REAL-WORLD RISKS

The Centers for Disease Control and Prevention (CDC) states that diphtheria circulation "appears to continue in some settings, even in populations with more than 80% childhood immunization rates. An asymptomatic carrier state can exist even among immune individuals."

Because immunity lessens over time, "a booster dose of vaccine should be administered every 10 years to maintain protective antibody levels. Large populations of older adults may be susceptible to diphtheria, in both developed as well as in developing countries."

disease is endemic in the former Soviet Union, the Indian subcontinent, Southeast Asia, and Latin America. In temperate regions diphtheria is more common in the colder months of the year. In 2000 the World Health Organization (WHO) reported 30,000 cases of diphtheria worldwide, 3,000 of which were fatal.

According to WHO, 7,321 cases were reported worldwide in 2014. However, it was assumed that many cases were not reported. In 2016 WHO reported 7,097 diphtheria cases worldwide. That year 27 percent of all countries had an 80 percent or better immunization rate for diphtheria. According to WHO, the overall fatality rate of diphtheria has remained fairly constant since the 1960s, from 5 to 10 percent of all cases. When considering only children younger than five and adults older than 40, however, the fatality rate climbed to 20 percent.

As of January 2018, WHO reported that worldwide immunizations of vaccine-preventable diseases, including diphtheria, were at 86 percent. The global health organization also indicated that immunizations as a whole prevented about 2 million to 3 million deaths per year. However, the number of deaths could decrease substantially if more infants were vaccinated each year. About 19.5 million infants do not receive basic vaccines annually.

■ Treatment and Prevention

Because diphtheria is so rare in developed countries, it may be difficult for physicians to recognize when it does occur. However, the presence of the pseudomembrane, together with heart rhythm abnormalities linked to the toxin, should alert a physician to the possibility of diphtheria. Ideally, the presence of *C. diphtheriae* should be confirmed in a laboratory (it requires special methods for its identification), but this should not delay the start of treatment. Diphtheria is treated with antitoxin, which neutralizes the toxin before it can do too much damage, and antibiotics. The antitoxin, which causes the pseudomembrane to recede dramatically, has saved the lives of many children since it was discovered in 1888.

Diphtheria antitoxin is prepared from the serum of horses that have been immunized against the disease. It needs to be given within four days of the onset of symptoms. Erythromycin and penicillin are the two most commonly prescribed antibiotics for diphtheria. Hospitalization and isolation are essential when dealing with diphtheria—the latter to prevent others from being exposed to the infection. If breathing is obstructed by the pseudomembrane, a tracheostomy may be needed. This procedure involves cutting an artificial opening in the trachea, or windpipe, and inserting a tube so that the patient can breathe.

Immunization has proven to be the best way to prevent the spread of diphtheria. A toxoid is an inactivated version of a bacterial toxin. It provides an excellent immune response in diseases where bacterial toxins play an important role, such as diphtheria and tetanus.

Most countries use diphtheria toxoid in combination with tetanus toxoid and pertussis (whooping cough) vaccine, also known as DTP vaccine, to protect children. DTP is given by injection. WHO recommends children receive three separate doses of DTP. One vaccination schedule administers the three primary doses at the ages of 6 weeks, 10 weeks, and 14 weeks, with a booster between 18 months and six years of age.

However, there is considerable variation between countries as to the vaccine and vaccination schedule used. For example, in the United States, the Centers for Disease Control and Prevention (CDC) recommends the use of diphtheria, tetanus, and acellular pertussis (DTaP) vaccine rather than DTP as the safer version offering lessened side effects. The formulations vary in terms of the strength of the dose of each vaccine. A capital letter, such as *T*, denotes a full-strength dose, while a lowercase letter, such as *t*, stands for a reduced-strength dose. The *a* in DTaP and other such vaccines stands for *acellular*, a term that means only specific parts of the pertussis bacteria are used rather than the entire cell. Some countries have been using a combination vaccine that includes vaccines against diphtheria, tetanus, pertussis, hepatitis B, and pneumonia.

Besides DTaP, which protects young children, three other vaccines used in the United States are tetanus, diphtheria, and pertussis vaccine for preteenagers, teens, and young adults (Tdap); diphtheria and tetanus vaccine for young children (DT); and tetanus and diphtheria vaccine for preteenagers, teens, and young adults (Td). All three prevent diphtheria and tetanus, but DTaP and Tdap also prevent pertussis. Of the four vaccines, Tdap and Td are used for children and adults seven years of age and older, whereas DTaP and DT are given to children younger than seven years of age.

Parents often worry that a vaccine may harm their child, and this is one reason that vaccine coverage is never universal (some parents always opt out). DTP can cause fever shortly after the child receives an injection, and some complain of pain, redness, and swelling at the injection site. More severe reactions, such as convulsions or shock, occur occasionally. However, for most children, the benefits of DTP far outweigh the risks.

DTP is not usually given after six years of age. Older children and adults are offered Td, and in 2005 Tdap was approved for adolescents and adults in the United States. Booster injections may be needed every 10 years to maintain immunity, where this might be important, such as when traveling to an area where diphtheria is endemic. There is evidence that immunity to diphtheria tends to wane over time.

■ Impacts and Issues

Like cholera, diphtheria has a long history. The disease was first described by the Greek physician Hippocrates (c. 460 BCE–357 BCE), and it was also mentioned in ancient Syrian and Egyptian texts. In 17th-century Spain, epidemic diphtheria was known as "El Garatillo" or "The Strangler." There were also significant epidemics in England in the 1730s and in Western Europe in the second half of the 19th century. Diphtheria was known in the United States from the 18th century and reached epidemic proportions in 1735, often killing entire families. At the start of the 20th century, the disease was still one of the leading causes of death among infants and children. When the first data on diphtheria were gathered in the 1920s, there were around 150,000 cases and 13,000 deaths each year.

In the early 21st century, most physicians in the United States will never see a case of diphtheria. Although diphtheria, like tuberculosis, is highly infectious, it is likely to be endemic in less developed countries where there is poverty, overcrowding, malnutrition, and poor sanitation. Mass immunization is known to be an essential tool in the prevention of diphtheria. However, developing countries tend not to have access to vaccine supplies or the health infrastructure to achieve the WHO's goal of a 95 percent immunization rate.

Diphtheria Outbreaks in Russia and Afghanistan

Diphtheria can still spread and cause significant illness and death, even in a modern society where it had previously been all but eradicated. This was demonstrated by the outbreaks and epidemics of the disease in the former Soviet Union in the 1990s. During the first half of the 20th century, diphtheria rates were high in the Soviet Union. In the 1950s there were around 750,000 cases in Russia alone. When the Communist regime took control, the Soviet Union developed an excellent record on immunization. By 1976 rates of the disease were practically zero in Russia, and eradication was thought to be within reach. However, in 1977 the disease began to make a comeback, with rates increasing in all age groups rather than just among children. Rates peaked in 1984 and declined thereafter, although they never returned to the low of 1976.

American researchers for the CDC argue that the military may have contributed to the spread of diphtheria in the Soviet Union in the 1980s. Military service was universal and led to the housing of recruits, many of whom had not been immunized, in overcrowded conditions. Adult immunity, among those immunized many years earlier, appeared to be declining, accounting for adult cases of diphtheria. The immunization schedule among children was also less intense than before, in part due to a campaign against immunization that found favor in a population increasingly distrustful of its government.

The breakup of the Soviet Union in the late 1980s and early 1990s was the final event that set the stage for a new wave of diphtheria. In 1990 there were more than 1,000 cases reported in St. Petersburg, Kaliningrad, Orlovskaya, and Moscow. The epidemic grew over the next few years, and deaths occurred because of failures in a health care system facing economic crisis.

Diphtheria reached epidemic proportions in urban Russia, Ukraine, and Belarus. In 1993 19,462 cases were reported, 15,211 of which were in Russia, an increase of nearly 300 percent from the previous year. Many of these cases were, again, among adults. This was the first large-scale diphtheria epidemic in a developed country for more than three decades. At the peak of the epidemic, in 1995, there were over 50,000 cases reported in the region, compared to only 24 cases in the rest of Europe.

In 1994 and 1995, WHO, the United Nations Children's Fund (UNICEF), other agencies, and governments in the affected countries undertook massive efforts to vaccinate both children and adults. These efforts began to bring the epidemic under control, resulting in a 60 percent drop in cases by 1996. According to WHO data gathered in 2000, incidence rates of diphtheria in Armenia, Estonia, Lithuania, and Uzbekistan were 0.5 to 1.0 per 100,000 people. In Russia and Tajikistan, rates were as high as 27 to 32 per 100,000. Fatality rates were 2 to 3 percent in Russia and Ukraine and 6 to 10 percent in Armenia, Kazakhstan, Moldova, and Latvia. In Azerbaijan, Georgia, and Turkmenistan, the death rate from diphtheria was 17 to 23 percent. By 2004 the number of cases reported to the WHO European region, which includes the former Soviet Union, was down to 176.

According to the CDC, the outbreak of diphtheria in the former Soviet Union shows that adults can become vulnerable to childhood diseases again when immunization does not confer lifelong immunity. This condition applies in any other country where there is mass immunization against diphtheria. However, there have been no similar epidemics elsewhere in the Western world. It was probably the combination of factors in the Soviet Union at the time that set the scene for the epidemic. Added to the decline in both childhood and adult immunity was the political breakup of the Soviet Union and the formation of several new states.

A WHO report of a diphtheria outbreak in Afghanistan illustrates the factors that increase the risk of the disease. Between June and August 2003, there were 50 cases of diphtheria, including three deaths, in a resettlement camp for internally displaced people in Kandahar. About 75 percent of the patients were between the ages of 5 and 14 years. A mass immunization campaign for the 40,000 residents of the camp was launched in August 2003. The Ministry of Health was assisted by WHO and several other organizations, such as Médecins sans Frontières (Doctors Without Borders) and the Red Cross, in the provision of drugs, antitoxins, and vaccine supplies to help bring the outbreak under control.

Immunization Misconceptions

The CDC recommends that nearly all babies, children, teenagers, and adults in the United States receive a vaccination for diphtheria. Some age-related and health-related situations may necessitate not getting or delaying a diphtheria vaccination.

False claims are often made against vaccines, including those for diphtheria. Some believe vaccines are not safe, while others have philosophic or religious objections to vaccines. Still others point to government interference into their lives when restrictions are imposed relating to immunizations, especially of children. Roberta Kwok, the author of a 2011 article in the journal *Nature*, counters misconceptions about the safety of vaccines: "Vaccines face a tougher safety standard than most pharmaceutical products because they are given to healthy people, often children."

In addition, WHO cites six common misconceptions with immunizations. One is that "vaccines cause many harmful side effects, illnesses, and even death—not to mention possible long-term effects we don't even know about." WHO explains that this misconception is often applied to the DTP vaccine, specifically that it causes sudden infant death syndrome (SIDS). WHO counters this claim by stating, "If you consider that most SIDS deaths occur during the age range when three shots of DTP are given, you would expect DTP shots to precede a fair number of SIDS deaths simply by chance." Therefore, WHO considers it faulty logic to associate DTP vaccines with SIDS deaths. Independent research has also shown that SIDS deaths occur whether or not vaccinations are previously given. Although the benefits of vaccinations far outweigh the risks of not being vaccinated, some risks are present in any vaccine. According to Kwok, vaccinations cause "roughly one case of the disease per 2.4 million doses, often in people with an immune deficiency."

Because of vaccinations, many of the diseases that were common in the past are now rarely seen. WHO concludes by saying, "While any serious injury or death caused by vaccines is too many, it is also clear that the benefits of vaccination greatly outweigh the slight risk, and that many, many more injuries and deaths would occur without vaccinations. In fact, to have a medical intervention as effective as vaccination in preventing disease and not use it would be unconscionable."

See Also *CDC (Centers for Disease Control and Prevention); Childhood-Associated Infectious Diseases, Immunization Impacts; Cholera; Médecins sans Frontières (Doctors Without Borders); World Health Organization (WHO)*

BIBLIOGRAPHY

Books

Blume, Stuart. *Immunization: How Vaccines Became Controversial.* London: Reaktion, 2017.

David, Michael, and Jean-Luc Benoit, eds. *The Infectious Disease Diagnosis: A Case Approach.* Cham, Switzerland: Springer, 2018.

McGuire-Wolfe, Christine. *Foundations of Infection Control and Prevention.* Burlington, MA: Jones & Bartlett Learning, 2018.

Rosner, Lisa. *Vaccination and Its Critics: A Documentary and Reference Guide.* Santa Barbara, CA: Greenwood, 2017.

Tan, Tina Q., John P. Flaherty, and Melvin V. Gerbie. *The Vaccine Handbook: A Practitioner's Guide to Maximizing Use and Efficacy across the Lifespan.* New York: Oxford University Press, 2018.

Periodicals

Kwok, Roberta. "Vaccines: The Real Issues in Vaccine Safety." *Nature* 473 (May 26, 2011): 436–438. This article can also be found online at https://www.nature.com/news/2011/110525/full/473436a.html (accessed February 14, 2018).

Vitek, Charles R., and Melinda Wharton. "Diphtheria in the Former Soviet Union: Reemergence of a Pandemic Disease." *Emerging Infectious Diseases* 4 (October–December 1998). This article can also be found online at https://wwwnc.cdc.gov/eid/article/4/4/98-0404_article (accessed February 14, 2018).

Websites

"Diphtheria." Mayo Clinic, December 8, 2016. https://www.mayoclinic.org/diseases-conditions/diphtheria/symptoms-causes/syc-20351897 (accessed February 14, 2018).

"Diphtheria." Todar's Online Textbook of Bacteriology. http://textbookofbacteriology.net/diphtheria.html (accessed February 14, 2018).

"Diphtheria." World Health Organization. http://www.who.int/topics/diphtheria/en/ (accessed February 14, 2018).

"Diphtheria: Clinicians." Centers for Disease Control and Prevention, January 15, 2016. https://www.cdc.gov/diphtheria/clinicians.html (accessed February 14, 2018).

"Diphtheria, Tetanus, and Whooping Cough Vaccination: What Everyone Should Know." Centers for Disease Control and Prevention, November 22, 2016. https://www.cdc.gov/vaccines/vpd/dtap-tdap-td/public/index.html (accessed February 14, 2018).

"Diphtheria Vaccination." Centers for Disease Control and Prevention, November 22, 2016. https://www.cdc.gov/vaccines/vpd/diphtheria/index.html (accessed February 14, 2018).

"Immunization Coverage." World Health Organization, January 2018. http://www.who.int/mediacentre/factsheets/fs378/en/ (accessed February 14, 2018).

"Immunization, Vaccines and Biologicals: Diphtheria." World Health Organization, August 8, 2017. http://www.who.int/immunization/monitoring_surveillance/burden/diphtheria/en/ (accessed February 14, 2018).

"Six Common Misconceptions about Immunization." World Health Organization. http://www.who.int/vaccine_safety/initiative/detection/immunization_misconceptions/en/index1.html (accessed February 14, 2018).

Susan Aldridge
William Arthur Atkins

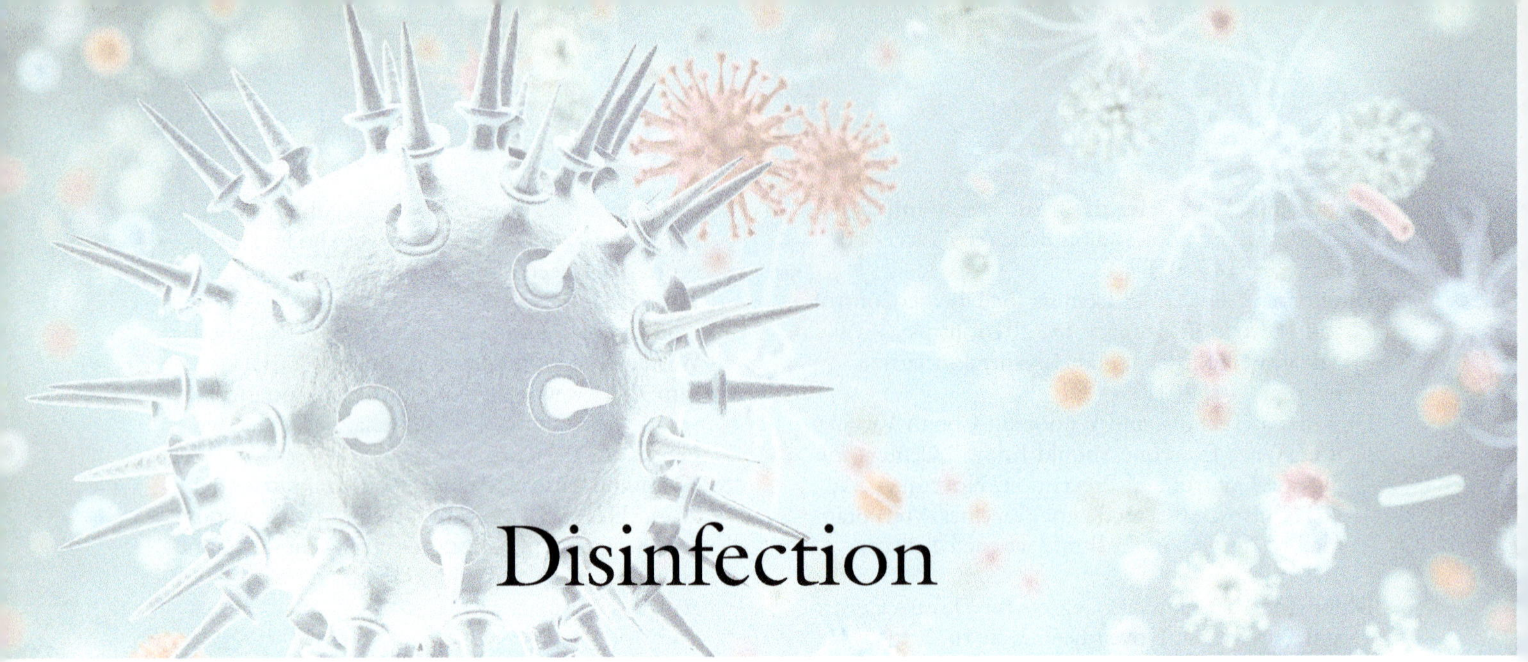

Disinfection

Introduction

Disinfection refers to treatments that reduce to a safe level the number of living microorganisms and viruses. (Viruses are not considered to be alive but can cause disease when they infect a host cell.) Disinfection is not intended to kill all the microbes present, which is a process called sterilization. Still, disinfection is a key component in infection control.

Health care facilities maintain three different levels of disinfection based on patient care levels and the purpose for which equipment and surfaces are used. High-level disinfection destroys all microorganisms on a surface, with the exception of bacterial spores when the spores are present in large numbers. Intermediate-level disinfection kills *Mycobacterium tuberculosis*, most viruses and fungi, and bacteria. However, it does not kill bacterial spores. Low-level disinfection kills most bacteria and certain viruses and fungi but does not reliably kill bacterial spores or the bacteria that cause tuberculosis.

WORDS TO KNOW

BIOFILM A population of microorganisms that forms following the adhesion of bacteria, algae, yeast, or fungi to a surface. These surface growths may be found in natural settings such as on rocks or in streams, as well as in infections such as those that occur on catheters. Microorganisms can colonize living or inert, natural or synthetic surfaces.

HIGH-LEVEL DISINFECTION A process that uses a chemical solution to kill all bacteria, viruses, and other disease-causing agents except for bacterial endospores and prions. High-level disinfection should be distinguished from sterilization, which removes endospores (bacterial structures that are resistant to radiation, drying, lack of food, and other conditions potentially lethal to the bacteria) and prions (misshapen proteins that can cause disease).

INTERMEDIATE-LEVEL DISINFECTION A form of disinfection that kills bacteria, most viruses, and mycobacteria.

LOW-LEVEL DISINFECTION A form of disinfection that kills some viruses and some bacteria.

STERILIZATION The complete killing or elimination of living organisms in the sample being treated. Sterilization is absolute. After the treatment, the sample is either devoid of life or the possibility of life (as from the subsequent germination and growth of bacterial spores), or living organisms are still present or could grow if they were present.

History and Scientific Foundations

Until the middle of the 19th century, surgeries and hospitalization frequently resulted in infections. The importance of personal hygiene and clean clothing had yet to be realized by health care providers. As a result, microbial infections easily spread from patient to patient. French chemist Louis Pasteur (1822–1895) proposed that infections were connected with the presence of microorganisms. This idea prompted English surgeon Joseph Lister (1827–1912) to study microorganisms. Lister became convinced that infections following surgery often involved microorganisms infecting the incision. To minimize this risk, he sprayed a film of carbolic acid over the patient during surgery. The treatment effectively disinfected the wound and helped reduce postsurgical infections. As Lister's findings became accepted, the importance of disinfection to medicine was recognized.

Applications and Research

Disinfection involves the use of a chemical or other type of agent (typically ultraviolet light) to kill microorganisms. These agents are termed disinfectants.

Ultraviolet light disinfects because of the high energy of the waves of light. The energy is sufficient to break the strands of genetic material of the microbes. When many breaks occur in the deoxyribonucleic acid (DNA) or ribonucleic acid (RNA), the damage is lethal, as it cannot be repaired by the microorganism. Ultraviolet light can be used to disinfect liquids of small volume, surfaces, and some types of equipment.

Alcohol is a liquid disinfectant that tends to be used on the skin to achieve short-term disinfection. It kills microbes such as bacteria by dissolving the membrane around the organism. Alcohol may be sprayed on surfaces, and the droplets will kill microbes on contact. Because the alcohol evaporates quickly, however, the spray must be heavily applied to a surface to ensure disinfection. If the alcohol evaporates within a few seconds, the microorganisms may not be exposed long enough to be killed. In the 21st century alcohol-based hand washes are more widely used in hospitals because a busy doctor or nurse need only rub his or her hands for 10 to 15 seconds with an alcohol-based solution to adequately disinfect between patients. Typical disinfectant soaps such as those used in the home require skin contact of 30 seconds or more to be effective.

The compound iodine is another disinfectant. In hospitals, surgical scrubbing is often accomplished using an iodine-containing soap. As with alcohol-based handwashing, the intent is to lower the number of living bacteria on the surface of the skin, although iodine is a more efficient disinfectant than alcohol.

Another liquid disinfectant that remains on a surface much longer is sodium hypochlorite. The active component of the disinfectant is chlorine, which is also the disinfecting agent in household bleach. Water may be treated using chlorine, which is the basis of drinking water chlorination. The concentration of sodium hypochlorite is important. Too much chlorine can dissolve metal surfaces and irritate the cells in the eye and the nose. Medical personnel in the field use a sodium hypochlorite solution (bleach) when investigating outbreaks of diseases that can be spread by contact with infected body fluids, droplets, or contaminated surfaces and when local infrastructure will not support high-tech disinfection methods. For example, during a 2003 outbreak of Ebola in the West Cuvette region of the Democratic Republic of Congo, the US Centers for Disease Control and Prevention (CDC) recommended using household bleach diluted with water in a 1:100 ratio to disinfect areas contaminated with blood and body fluids in a makeshift isolation ward hospital. As of 2017 this strategy is still relevant and recommended.

Surfaces can also be disinfected using compounds that contain a phenol group. A popular example is Lysol®. In a hospital, phenol-based disinfectants are not used in certain cases, such as in an operating theater. This is because some disease-causing bacteria and viruses are resistant to phenol.

Chlorhexidine is a chemical disinfectant that kills fungi and yeast much more effectively than bacteria and viruses. Formaldehyde and glutaraldehyde possess a chemical group called an aldehyde, which is a potent disinfectant. Glutaraldehyde is a general disinfectant, which means it is effective against a wide array of microbes after only a few minutes of contact. Another effective general disinfectant is quaternary ammonium.

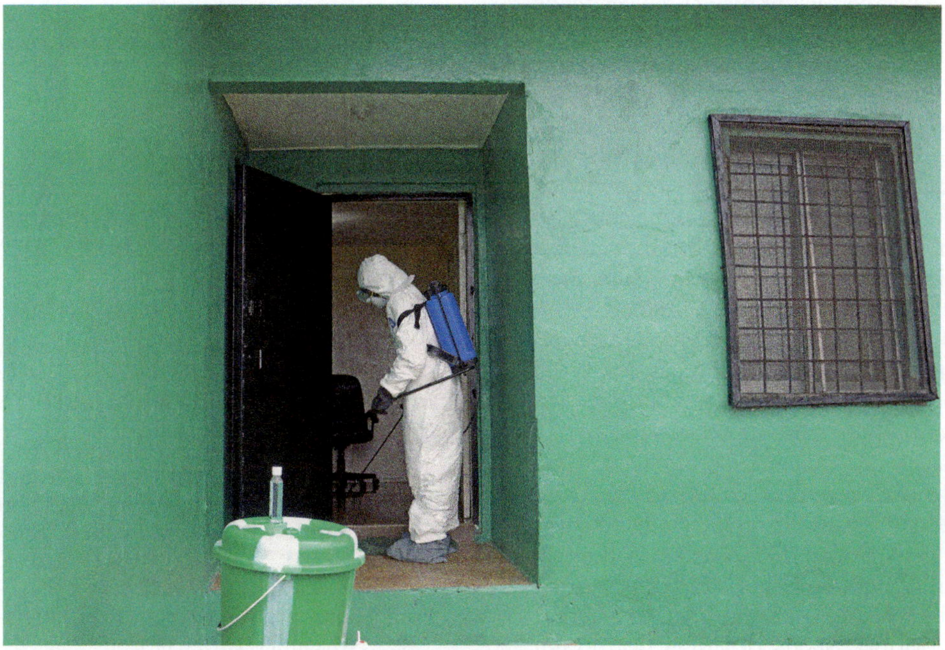

On August 29, 2014, amid an Ebola outbreak in Liberia, a health worker in a protective suit disinfects a house in the capital of Monrovia. © *DOMINIQUE FAGET/AFP/Getty Images*

PERSONAL RESPONSIBILITY AND PROTECTION

Handwashing is an important aspect of disinfection. However, improper handwashing can be dangerous. Particularly harsh soaps, or frequent handwashing (for example, 20 to 30 times a day) can increase the acidity of the skin, which can counteract some of the protective fatty acid secretions. Also, the physical act of washing will shed skin cells. If washing is excessive, the protective microflora will be removed, leaving the newly exposed skin susceptible to colonization by another, potentially harmful microorganism. Health care workers, who scrub their hands frequently, are prone to skin infections and damage.

The disinfection strategy that is selected depends on several factors. These include the surface being disinfected and the intended use of that surface. A doctor's hands, for example, should be disinfected rigorously. A smooth crack- or crevasse-free surface is easier to disinfect and typically requires less time to disinfect than a rougher surface. A rough surface that has niches that microorganisms can fit into is not an appropriate surface to disinfect with a rapidly evaporating spray of alcohol. The surface material is also important. For example, a wooden surface may soak up liquids and reduce the concentration of the disinfectant that acts on the microorganisms.

The number of microorganisms present can determine the type of disinfectant used and how long it should be used for. Higher numbers of microbes usually require a lengthier exposure time to reduce the number of living organisms to a level that is considered safe. How the organisms grow is also important. For example, many disease-causing bacteria can grow in a slime-encased community known as a biofilm. Bacteria are much more resistant to disinfectants when inside a biofilm than when they are dispersed from the biofilm. Bacteria such as *Bacillus anthracis*, the organism that causes anthrax, and *Clostridium botulinum*, a neurotoxin-producing bacterium that can contaminate foods, can form a hardy structure called a spore, which often survives exposure to disinfectants.

Broad-spectrum disinfectants act against a variety of microbes. Glutaraldehyde, sodium hypochlorite, and hydrogen peroxide are examples of broad-spectrum disinfectants. Some disinfectants act on specific microorganisms, while the activity of other disinfectants is in between these extremes. An example is alcohol, which dissolves cell membranes that are made of lipids and is effective against many bacteria and viruses. Spores or viruses that do not have a lipid membrane, however, are not as affected.

■ Impacts and Issues

Disinfectants are a vital defense against infectious disease, especially in the health care, cosmetic, and food service industries. Still, the full benefits of disinfection have yet to be realized. Transfer of infection from patient to patient via the hands of medical personnel and their equipment (such as a stethoscope) still occurs, even though in many cases it could be avoided. Alternatively, overuse of disinfectants may cause microorganisms to develop resistance to disinfectants. For example, if the compound is not applied for an adequate amount of time, resistance may develop. This resistance may make it more difficult to eliminate sources of infection, which allows for their spread.

Wide-scale disinfection of drinking water supplies was one of the most significant public health accomplishments of the 20th century. Outbreaks of waterborne diseases such as typhus and cholera were common in both the United States and abroad before modern disinfection methods were put into place. In the 1990s researchers recognized that, while disinfectants neutralized many pathogens (disease-causing organisms) in water, some disinfectants also reacted with naturally occurring organic and inorganic matter in water sources and municipal water delivery systems. These reactions produced potentially harmful compounds called disinfection byproducts (DBPs). After DBPs were found to cause cancer and adverse reproductive effects in laboratory mice, the Environmental Protection Agency (EPA) set in place in 2001 new regulations to maximize disinfection of drinking water supplies while minimizing public exposure to DBPs. As of 2017 these regulations are contained in the Stage 1 and Stage 2 Disinfectants and Disinfection Byproducts Rules. The regulations especially focus on total trihalomethanes and haloacetic acids.

SEE ALSO *Antimicrobial Soaps; Infection Control and Asepsis*

BIBLIOGRAPHY

Books

Thompson, Clive, Simon Gillespie, and Emma Goslan, eds. *Disinfection By-products in Drinking Water.* Cambridge, UK: Royal Society of Chemistry, 2016.

Periodicals

Unuabonah, Emmanuel I., et al. "Clays for Efficient Disinfection of Bacteria in Waters." *Applied Clay Science* 151 (January 2018): 211–223.

Websites

"Drinking Water Requirements for States and Public Water Systems: Stage 1 and Stage 2 Disinfectants and Disinfection Byproducts Rule." United States Environmental Protection Agency. https://www.epa.gov/dwreginfo/stage-1-and-stage-2-disinfectants-and-disinfection-byproducts-rules (accessed November 15, 2017).

Brian Hoyle

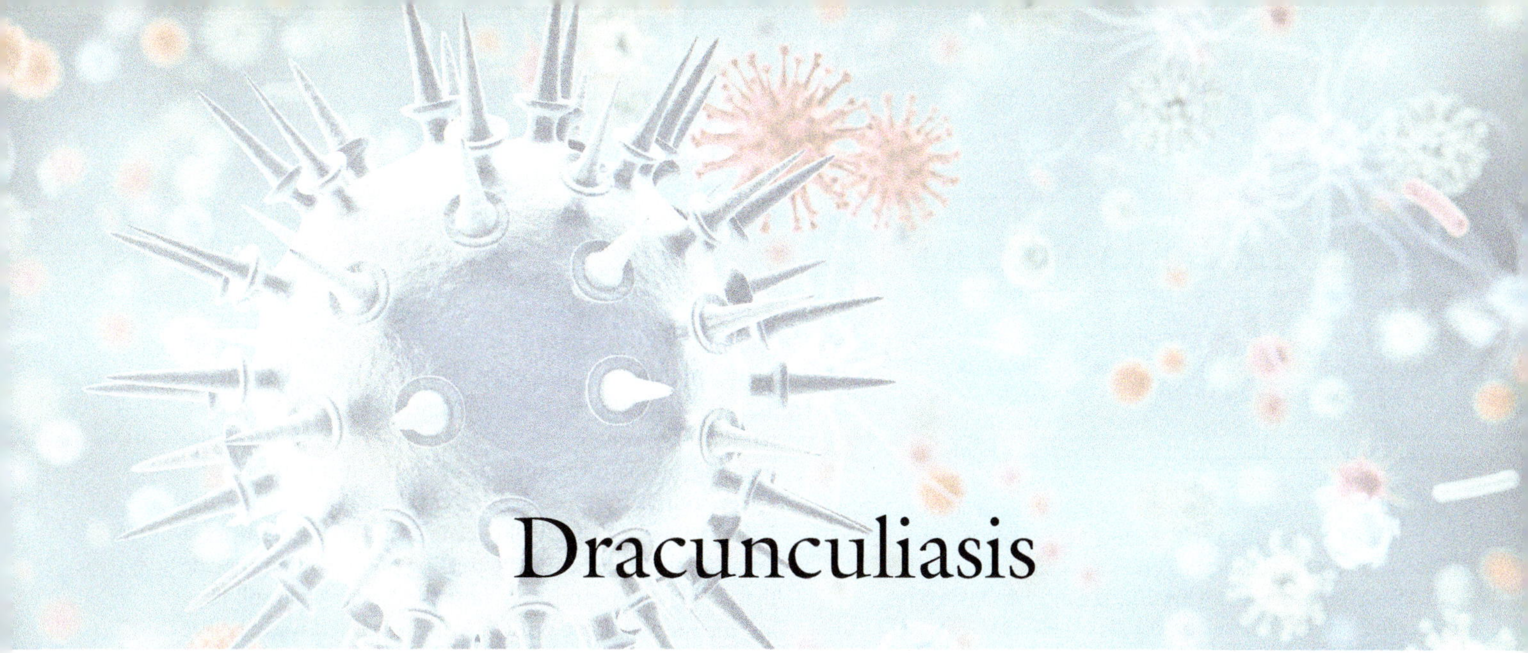

Dracunculiasis

Introduction

Dracunculiasis (dra-KUNK-you-LIE-uh-sis), or guinea worm disease, is a preventable helminth (parasitic worm) infection caused by the large, female roundworm *Dracunculus medinensis.* It is endemic in some African countries, including Sudan, Ghana, and Nigeria, within rural communities without safe drinking water.

The disease occurs when people drink water contaminated with *Dracunculus medinensis* larvae. However, symptoms do not usually manifest until about a year after infection. It is at that stage that the female worm ruptures the skin to release larvae, causing severe pain and discomfort to the infected person. There is no treatment for the infection except to manually remove the worm. However, aggressive efforts to eradicate the disease have proven fruitful. The number of cases was reduced by 99.9 percent between 1986 and 2016. As of 2017 the disease was limited to just three African nations, and researchers were optimistic that it would soon be eradicated.

Disease History, Characteristics, and Transmission

The mode of infection of dracunculiasis was recognized in 1870 when a Russian naturalist noticed the release of larvae from the female worm into a freshwater source. In the 1980s it was found to be endemic throughout Africa, and an eradication initiative was launched.

Symptoms of dracunculiasis do not usually present until around one year after infection, at which time a blister forms at a distal (away from the center) site of the body, such as the lower leg or foot. Some persons may experience allergic-type symptoms such as wheezing, fever, swelling around the eyes, and burning sensations of the skin just before lesion formation. After a few days the blister bursts, and the female worm emerges.

Upon making contact with water, the female worm releases millions of larvae that are ingested by copepods, or water fleas, and subsequently develop into the infective stage. Human infection occurs by drinking contaminated water and ingesting the water fleas. Although the fleas are digested, the larvae survive, migrate to the small intestine, and mate. The females mature to an adult size of up to 39 inches (100 centimeters). The female then migrates to the distal site and the process repeats.

Scope and Distribution

The people most commonly affected by dracunculiasis are those living in rural communities without established water treatment facilities. Due to the mode of transmission, males and females of all ages are vulnerable to infection if exposed to a contaminated water source. In some endemic areas, over half of the infected individuals are children, who are the main water carriers.

Following eradication efforts, the occurrence of dracunculiasis was, by 2006, mostly restricted to remote rural villages in only 12 countries of sub-Saharan Africa. As of November 2017 dracunculiasis was limited to two African nations: Chad and Ethiopia.

WORDS TO KNOW

DISTAL From the same root word as *distant*, the medical word for distant from an agreed-on point of reference. For example, the hand is at the distal end of the arm from the trunk.

HELMINTH A representative of various phyla of wormlike animals.

POTABLE Water that is clean enough to drink safely.

DISEASE ERADICATION

The campaign to eradicate dracunculiasis around the globe is close to reaching its goal. If it succeeds, it will be just the second time that a human disease has been eradicated, and the first since smallpox was eradicated in 1979. It would also be the first time that a parasitic disease was eradicated.

Researchers are optimistic about eradicating the disease for many reasons. Eliminating humans as hosts for guinea worms is likely to lead to the worms' extinction. Moreover, because dracunculiasis cannot be transmitted unless an infected person is symptomatic, screening and education are making it easier to identify and isolate individuals with the disease, preventing contamination of community water sources. Local strategies such as offering rewards to those who notify authorities of new infections, implementing containment measures, and providing simple water filtration devices to residents are all contributing to the vast reduction in new infections and to the optimism that the disease can be eradicated.

Treatment and Prevention

Treatment for dracunculiasis is limited, and there is no definitive medication available to eliminate or prevent infection. The most common method for removing the worm once it has immerged is to gently pull it out a few inches each day. This slow process allows for the complete removal of the worm. Removal may only take a few days, although it generally takes weeks. Analgesics may also be used to reduce swelling and help with pain management.

As dracunculiasis is transmitted only by drinking contaminated water, disease prevention is possible by implementing simple measures. Ensuring the maintenance of a water source free from contamination is vital. Filtering water before drinking is also beneficial. Prevention is most often accomplished either by treating ponds with insecticide that kills the copepods that host the larvae while still leaving the water potable or by filtering untreated water before it is consumed. Both methods break the chain of transmission. It is also essential to prevent people with open guinea worm wounds from swimming or bathing in shared water facilities used for drinking.

Impacts and Issues

Although the mortality rate for dracunculiasis is low, morbidity is a major concern, as the disease often affects entire communities and carries a heavy social and economic burden. People are often bedridden for some time during and following the emergence of the worm and, as such, are unable to contribute to the work within the community. The seasonality of outbreaks

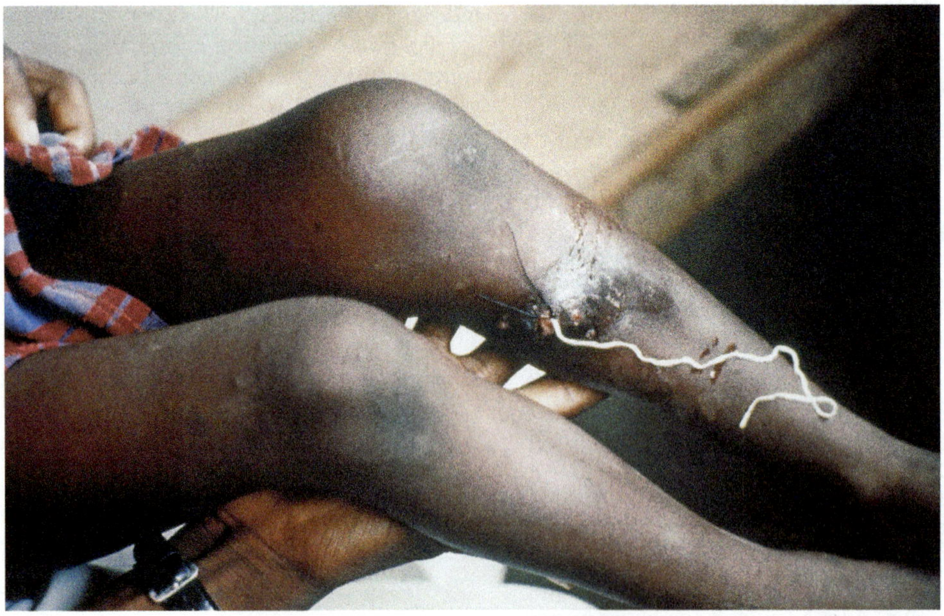

A patient awaits removal of a *Dracunculus medinensis.* More commonly known as guinea worms, this painful nematode can grow up to 31 inches (79 centimeters) in length and cause dracunculiasis. *© Clinical Photography, Central Manchester University Hospitals NHS Foundation Trust, UK/Science Source*

further highlights the impact of disease, whereby emergence often occurs during the peak of the agricultural year, often at harvest time, when the loss of labor is most damaging.

Children of parents infected with dracunculiasis are likelier to suffer from malnutrition than children of uninfected families. With an incapacitated parent, children are often required to assume adult roles within the family that, as a result, may also affect their chances of gaining an education. It is the culmination of these nutritional, social, economic, and educational factors, along with the practicality of possible prevention measures, that has made world health authorities identify dracunculiasis a candidate for eradication.

In 1986 the Carter Center, a nonprofit organization founded by former US president Jimmy Carter (1924–), began a campaign to eliminate guinea worm disease. Working in conjunction with the US Centers for Disease Control and Prevention (CDC), the World Health Organization (WHO), and others, the Carter Center has assisted affected communities in creating educational campaigns to promote the filtration of drinking water and encourage practices that prevent transmission of the disease. At the start of the campaign in 1986, there were roughly 3.5 million cases each year in 21 Asian and African countries. By 1996 the number of cases worldwide had been reduced to around 150,000. By 2006 cases of reported guinea worm disease decreased to about 12,000, and the disease was eliminated from Asia, remaining endemic in only about nine African countries. In 2016 only 25 cases were reported, and these were limited to Chad, South Sudan, and Ethiopia. Between January 1, 2017, and October 31, 2017, there were 26 reported cases: 14 in Chad and 12 in Ethiopia.

SEE ALSO *Helminth Disease; Roundworm (Ascariasis) Infection; Sanitation; Vector-Borne Disease; War and Infectious Disease; Waterborne Disease*

BIBLIOGRAPHY

Books

Hopkins, Donald R., and Ernesto Ruiz-Tiben. "Dracunculiasis (Guinea Worm Disease): Case Study of the Effort to Eradicate Guinea Worm." In *Water and Sanitation-Related Diseases and the Environment: Challenges, Interventions, and Preventive Measures*, edited by Janine M. Selendy, 125–132. Hoboken, NJ: Wiley-Blackwell, 2011.

Periodicals

Fitzpatrick, Christopher, et al. "The Cost-Effectiveness of an Eradication Programme in the End Game: Evidence from Guinea Worm Disease." *PLOS Neglected Tropical Diseases* 11, no. 10 (October 2017): 1–21.

Hopkins, Donald R., et al. "Progress toward Global Eradication of Dracunculiasis, January 2016–June 2017." *Morbidity and Mortality Weekly Report* 66, no. 48 (December 8, 2017): 1327–1331. This article can also be found online at https://www.cdc.gov/mmwr/volumes/66/wr/mm6648a3.htm (accessed January 9, 2018).

Websites

"Dracunculiasis Eradication." World Health Organization. http://www.who.int/dracunculiasis/en/ (accessed November 15, 2017).

"Guinea Worm Case Totals." The Carter Center, November 13, 2017. https://www.cartercenter.org/health/guinea_worm/case-totals.html (accessed November 15, 2017).

Mandt, Rebecca. "The Road to Guinea Worm Eradication: Running the Final Mile." *Science in the News* (blog), December 14, 2015. http://sitn.hms.harvard.edu/flash/2015/the-road-to-guinea-worm-eradication-running-the-final-mile/ (accessed November 15, 2017).

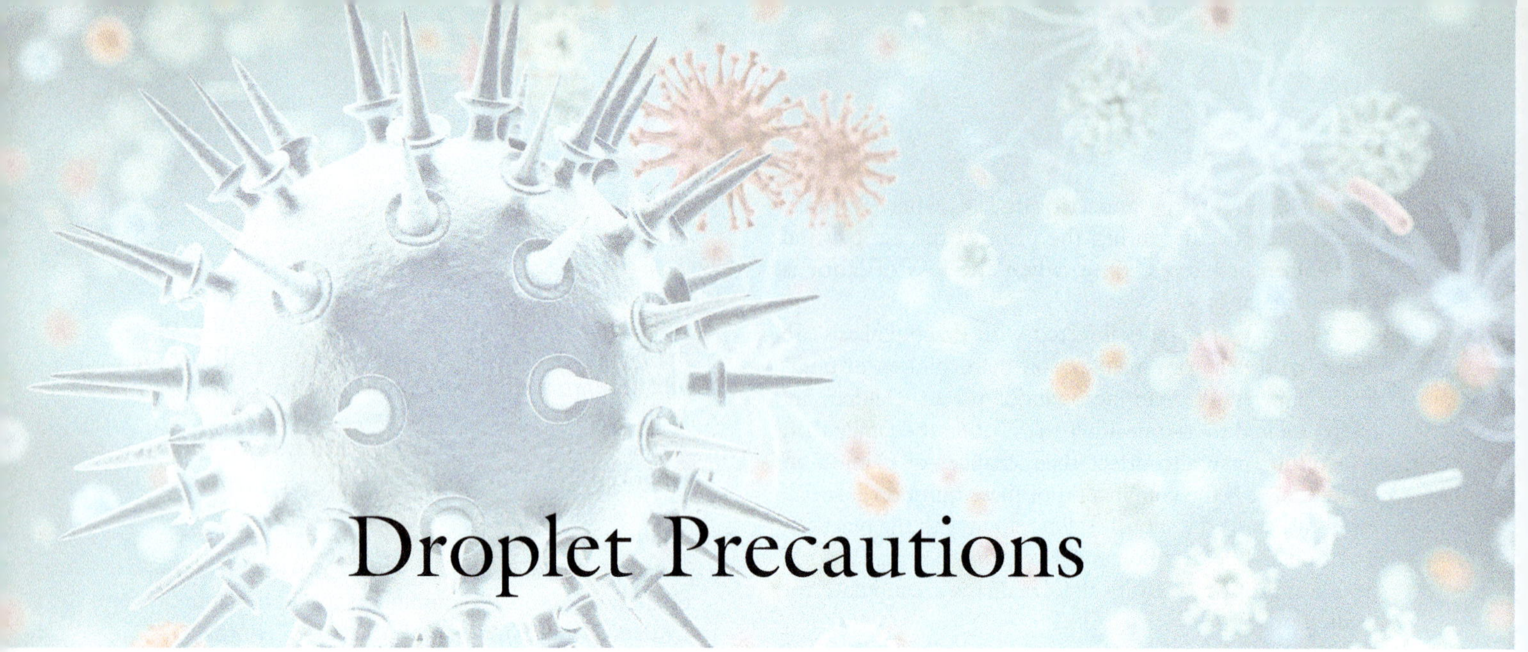

Droplet Precautions

■ Introduction

Droplet precautions are measures that have been developed to limit the airborne spread of microorganisms in droplets that are larger than 5 microns in diameter (a micron is 10^{-6} of a meter, or one-millionth of a meter). These droplets are typically expelled into the air by coughing, sneezing, and even talking.

Droplets that are smaller in diameter are aerosols and, because they may travel greater distances, are governed by the airborne precautions category of infection control.

■ History and Scientific Foundations

The droplet precautions developed by agencies including the US Centers for Disease Control and Prevention (CDC) and issued as guidelines in 1996 are designed to limit the spread of droplets with the cells of the eyes, nose, and mouth. This is important in a hospital, where droplets expelled by someone with an infection could spread the disease to someone else. The guidelines remained in effect as of 2017.

WORDS TO KNOW

AEROSOL Particles of liquid or solid dispersed as a suspension in gas.

CONTACT PRECAUTIONS Actions developed to minimize the transfer of microorganisms by direct physical contact and indirectly by touching a contaminated surface.

DROPLET A drop of water or other fluid that is fewer than 5 microns (a millionth of a meter) in diameter.

Because the droplets are relatively large, they are heavier and tend not to travel as far (less than 3 feet [1 meter]) as aerosolized microorganisms. Thus, droplet precautions are designed to prevent the movement of microorganisms from one person to another who is within about 3 feet (1 meter).

Viral diseases for which droplet precautions are necessary include chickenpox, influenza, measles, German measles, mumps, smallpox, and severe acute respiratory syndrome (SARS). Bacterial diseases requiring these precautions include whooping cough, a form of meningitis, psittacosis, Legionnaire's disease, diphtheria, and pneumonia. In addition, the inhalation of fungi-laden droplets can cause allergic alveolitis, aspergillosis, histoplasmosis, and coccidiodomycosis.

■ Applications and Research

Droplet precautions are a necessary part of a hospital's infection-control strategy. Without such precautions the airborne spread of disease would occur more frequently. These precautions can be initiated by the attending health care providers, including the physician and the nursing staff, and by the person in charge of infection control. The latter usually has the final say in whether precautions will be observed. The use of droplet precautions must be documented in the patient records. This information can be important in tracing the effectiveness of the precautions in controlling the infection and minimizing its spread.

Placing the infected patient in a separate room can be sufficient to prevent the spread of droplet-borne microbes. Specially ventilated rooms are not required, nor does the door to the room need to be closed. If a separate room is not available, then the infected patient should be housed with a patient who has an infection with the same microorganism and no other condition. That way, if the microbe is transferred between the patients via droplets, it will have a negligible influence on either patient's health. Patients' beds should be physically separated by a minimum of 3 feet (1 meter), and visitors should not be allowed within 3 feet (1 meter) of the patient they are visiting.

A face mask should be worn when either a health care provider or a visitor comes in close contact with the infected patient. Standard masks, similar to the type worn by carpenters to prevent inhalation of dust and other construction debris, are sufficient. Ideally the mask should be put on as a person enters the patient's room and should be discarded in a hazardous waste container when the person leaves.

The infected patient should be moved to other areas of the hospital only as is necessary and should wear a mask during the transport. In addition, any visitors who have not been previously exposed to the infection in question should not be allowed to enter the patient's room. Droplet precautions are often used in conjunction with contact precautions (infection control procedures designed to minimize the spread of disease by direct or indirect contact) in hospitals.

Droplet precautions can be discontinued when a patient's symptoms, such as coughing, have disappeared.

How Droplets Spread

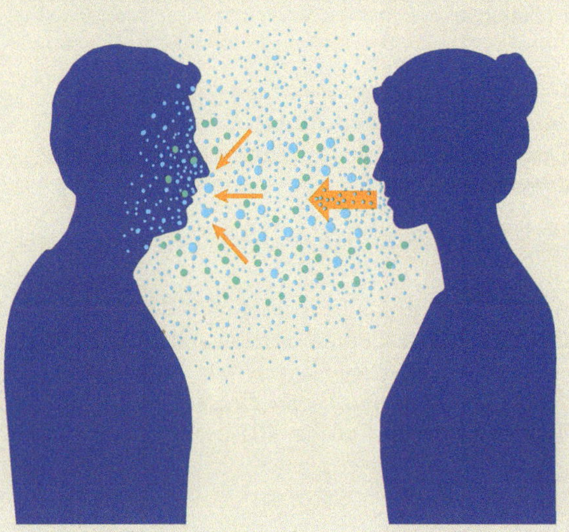

■ Impacts and Issues

Droplet precautions are intended to benefit the patient and medical personnel and to control and contain a disease outbreak. Infections that can be controlled or contained by droplet precautions include those spread by coughing and sneezing (e.g., influenza) and those spread by exposure to contaminated blood and tissue (e.g., Ebola virus). While public awareness of the importance of droplet precautions has increased in the first few decades of the 21st century, challenges remain. This was highlighted during the Ebola outbreak between 2014 and 2016 in some regions in Africa. Part of the reason for the ferocity of the outbreak was a lack of understanding of the disease among those most affected by it. For example, burial customs in many African cultures include an open viewing of the deceased, which potentially exposes mourners to the virus. This practice can amplify the spread of the virus, causing it to affect more people than it otherwise would. Amplification is an important means by which a variety of viral and bacterial diseases can spread. In the case of Ebola and mourning customs, paying respect to a deceased indi-

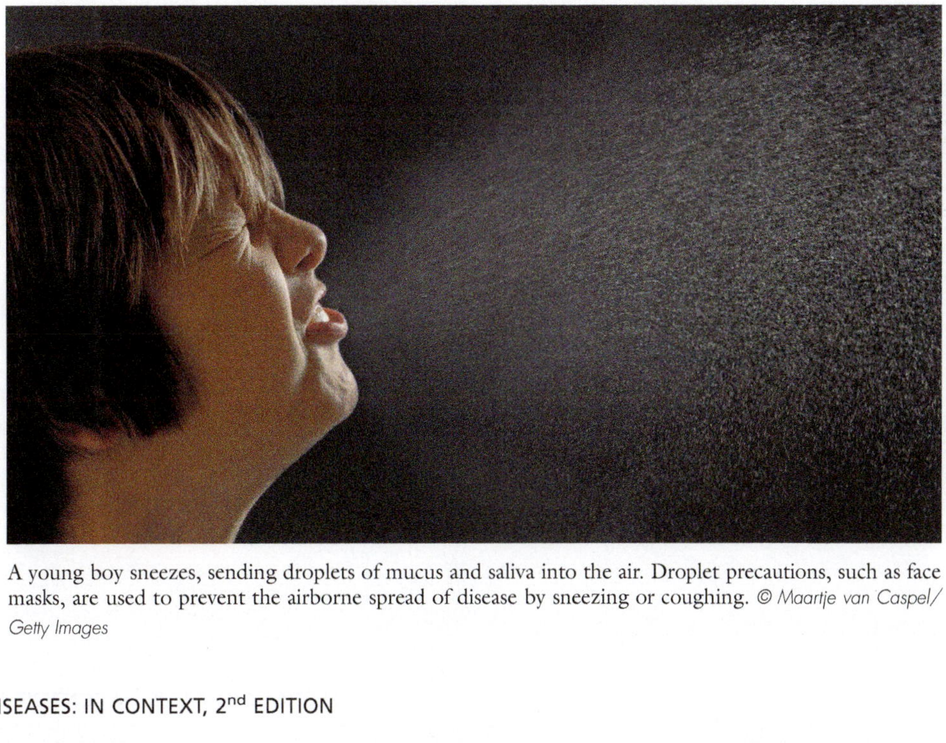

A young boy sneezes, sending droplets of mucus and saliva into the air. Droplet precautions, such as face masks, are used to prevent the airborne spread of disease by sneezing or coughing. *© Maartje van Caspel/ Getty Images*

vidual without touching or viewing the body would minimize the spread of Ebola. Trying to ensure infection control while respecting cultural beliefs can be a great challenge.

See Also *Airborne Precautions; Contact Precautions; Infection Control and Asepsis; Isolation and Quarantine; Nosocomial (Health Care–Associated) Infections*

BIBLIOGRAPHY

Books

Flynn, Laura. *All about Infection Control.* Guelph, ON: Mediscript Communications, 2017.

Miller, Chris H. *Infection Control and Management of Hazardous Materials for the Dental Team.* Toronto: Elsevier Canada, 2017.

Periodicals

Fast, Shannon M., Marta C. González, and Natasha Markuzon. "Cost-Effective Control of Infectious Disease Outbreaks Accounting for Societal Reaction." *PLOS One* 8 (2015): 211–223.

Websites

"Infection Control." Centers for Disease Control and Prevention. https://www.cdc.gov/infectioncontrol/index.html (accessed November 15, 2017).

"Transmission-Based Precautions." Centers for Disease Control and Prevention. https://www.cdc.gov/infectioncontrol/basics/transmission-based-precautions.html (accessed November 15, 2017).

Brian Hoyle

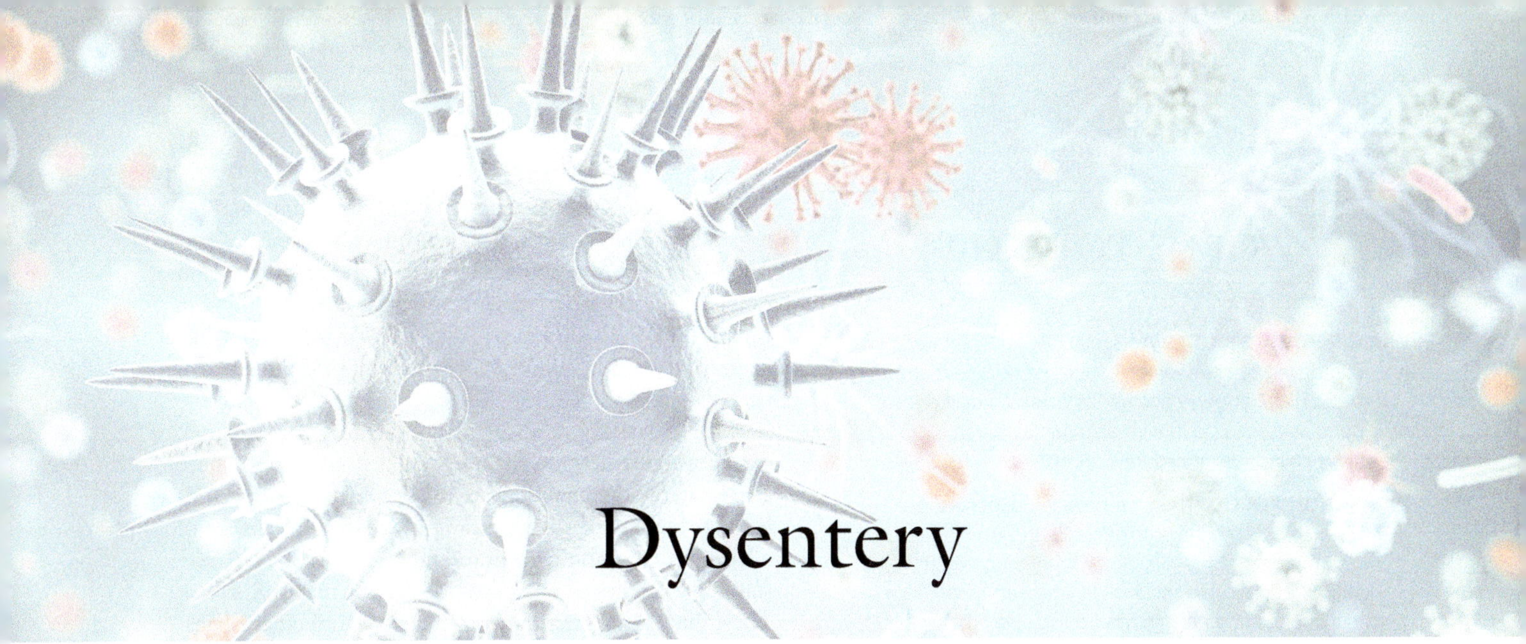

Dysentery

Introduction

Dysentery is an inflammation of the intestines, especially the colon, that leads to abdominal pain and frequent stools. In severe cases, stomach cramps and diarrhea with blood and mucus occur. Dysentery can be caused by bacteria, protozoa, or even noninfectious agents. *Shigella* species are the causative agents in most cases of bacterial dysentery. *Entamoeba histolytica*, a protozoan parasite, is the main cause for amebic dysentery.

Institutional living with minimal facilities and poor sanitary hygiene are major risk factors for dysentery in developing countries. It occurs all around the world, among people of all ages, but children under age five are most susceptible to the infection. Dysentery is sometimes known as travelers' diarrhea because it often affects those who visit developing countries. Although the disease normally clears up without treatment, antibiotics and supportive drugs may be used to get rid of amebic parasites and associated symptoms such as cramps. Prior to the advent of antibiotics and improved sanitation, dysentery could be fatal. It claimed the lives of many famous figures, including King Henry V of England (1387–1422) and Spanish explorer Hernando Cortes (1485–1547).

Disease History, Characteristics, and Transmission

Shigellae are rod-shaped, Gram-negative bacteria 1 to 2 millimeters in diameter, and the four main species responsible for bacterial dysentery are *S. sonnei*, *S. flexneri*, *S. boydii*, and *S. dysenteriae*. Gram-negative refers to the way bacteria interact with the Gram stain when they are prepared for microscopic examination. Infection with *Shigella* is referred to as shigellosis. Amebic dysentery, also called amebiasis, is caused by *Entamoeba histolytica*, a single-celled protozoan parasite.

The incubation period for shigellosis is usually one to three days. For amebic dysentery, the incubation time is much longer, maybe up to one year. Therefore, returning travelers who have acquired microorganisms abroad may not immediately make the connection between infection and symptoms, which may delay diagnosis.

The symptoms of shigellosis and amebic dysentery are similar, the chief one being diarrhea containing blood and mucus. Amebic dysentery is more likely than shigellosis to produce blood. There may also be severe pain in the abdomen, fever, nausea, and vomiting in addition to weight loss and abdominal tenderness. Shigellosis tends to produce a watery diarrhea that progresses to dysentery, especially when *S. dysenteriae* and *S. flexneri* are involved.

Symptoms of dysentery, including the frequency of diarrhea, range from mild to severe. Complications are more likely with *S. dysenteriae* and include sepsis (blood poisoning) and kidney failure. Blood clots may also be seen in the liver and the spleen. Dysentery with severe complications can have a mortality rate of 5 to 20 percent. However, the symptoms in most cases of dysentery last for only a few days, although relapse and chronic infection can also occur.

The fecal-oral route is the most frequent route of transmission for *Shigella* (bacterial) and *entamoeba* (protozoan). Thus, eating or drinking contaminated food or water is a major concern.

In cases of amebic dysentery the amoeba can exist as a cyst, a group of cells surrounded by a wall that can survive the acid of the stomach and progress to the intestines. The cysts can stick to the walls of the colon, causing bleeding ulcers, loss of appetite, and weight loss. The cysts are passed in the feces and can infect others under conditions of poor sanitation. Houseflies may also transfer and deposit the cysts from infected human stool to fruits and vegetables.

Scope and Distribution

Dysentery has long had an impact on human health, but it was not until the 19th century that the cause was determined to be either bacterial or amebic. *Shigella* get their name from Kiyoshi Shiga (1871–1957), who dis-

WORDS TO KNOW

GRAM-NEGATIVE BACTERIA Bacteria whose cell walls are composed of an inner and outer membrane that are separated from one another by a region called the periplasm. The periplasm also contains a thin but rigid layer called the peptidoglycan.

INCUBATION PERIOD The time between exposure to a disease-causing virus or bacteria and the appearance of symptoms of the infection. Depending on the microorganism, the incubation time can range from a few hours, such as with food poisoning due to *Salmonella*, to a decade or more, such as with acquired immunodeficiency syndrome (AIDS).

MORTALITY The condition of being susceptible to death. The term *mortality* comes from the Latin word *mors*, which means "death." Mortality can also refer to the rate of deaths caused by an illness or injury (e.g., "Rabies has a high mortality rate").

PROTOZOA Single-celled, animal-like, microscopic organisms that live by taking in food rather than making it by photosynthesis and must live in the presence of water. (Singular: protozoan.) Protozoa are a diverse group of single-celled organisms, with more than 50,000 different types represented. The vast majority are microscopic, many measuring less than 5 one-thousandth of an inch (0.005 millimeters), but some, such as the freshwater Spirostomun, may reach 0.17 inches (3 millimeters) in length, large enough to enable it to be seen with the naked eye.

RELAPSE A return of symptoms after a patient has apparently recovered from a disease.

SEPSIS A bacterial infection in the bloodstream or body tissues. Sepsis is a very broad term covering the presence of many types of microscopic disease-causing organisms. It is also called bacteremia. Closely related terms include septicemia and septic syndrome.

covered them in 1898. Dysentery has caused massive casualties in conflicts ranging from the Peloponnesian War in 431 BCE to World War II (1939–1945). In the American Civil War (1861–1865), there were nearly 2 million cases of diarrhea, most of which were probably dysentery, resulting in over 44,000 deaths. It has only been with the development of antibiotics that dysentery has ceased to be a major problem in military campaigns.

S. dysenteriae causes most outbreaks of dysentery in developing countries, in the tropics and subtropics, and under conditions of overcrowding or war. Epidemic dysentery in the tropics is more common in the rainy season, perhaps because people tend to spend more time indoors together and sanitation suffers from the abundance of surface water. *S. sonnei* and *S. flexneri* are the most common causes of shigellosis in the United States, England, Europe, Egypt, the Middle East, and Asia. *S. boydii* is found mainly in India and Egypt, although strains of all four species have been found in the United States.

A 2012 study reported that dysentery caused by *S. sonnei* was reemerging in industrialized countries where clean water and sanitation were not concerns. Further studies have highlighted that cleaning up water also gets rid of a harmless common bacterium known as *Plesiomonas shigelloides*, which has an outer coat identical to that of *S. sonnei*. Thus, the natural immunity produced by antibodies against *S. sonnei* is somewhat compromised when the water is cleaner and bereft of *P. shigelloides*, leading to increased *S. sonnei* infection.

Shigellosis is endemic throughout the world but is more common in less developed countries. In Europe, the United States, and other developed regions, shigellosis tends to be a disease found in institutions, including nursery schools, mental health facilities, prisons, and military barracks.

Around 50 million people worldwide are infected with *Entamoeba histolytica*, but fewer than 10 to 20 percent of those infected exhibit any signs of disease. Infection is prevalent in Central and South America, southern and western Africa, Southeast Asia, India, and China. Amebic dysentery is relatively rare in Australia, New Zealand, Canada, the United States, and Europe. However, travelers may become infected abroad. Pregnant women, children, and people in developing nations are most at risk of contracting amebic dysentery.

■ Treatment and Prevention

Most cases of bacterial and amebic dysentery are self-limiting and resolve with rest and consumption of plenty of fluids to replace what is lost from passing watery stool. This is especially important for infants with dysentery because they can become rapidly dehydrated. Sometimes antibiotic treatment, and in rare cases hospitalization for intravenous therapy, may be needed. Antibiotics of choice include beta lactams such as amoxicillin or ampicillin. For persistent amebic dysentery, metronidazole is the medication of choice.

Diagnosis is made by checking the stool sample of the patient for the protozoan parasite (*Entamoeba histolytica*) or its cyst by simple microscopy. Stool culture is necessary for detecting *Shigella*. In cases of liver abscess caused by *E. histolytica*, antibody testing using blood samples confirms the diagnosis.

Good personal hygiene can prevent the transmission of dysentery. This means frequent handwashing, especially

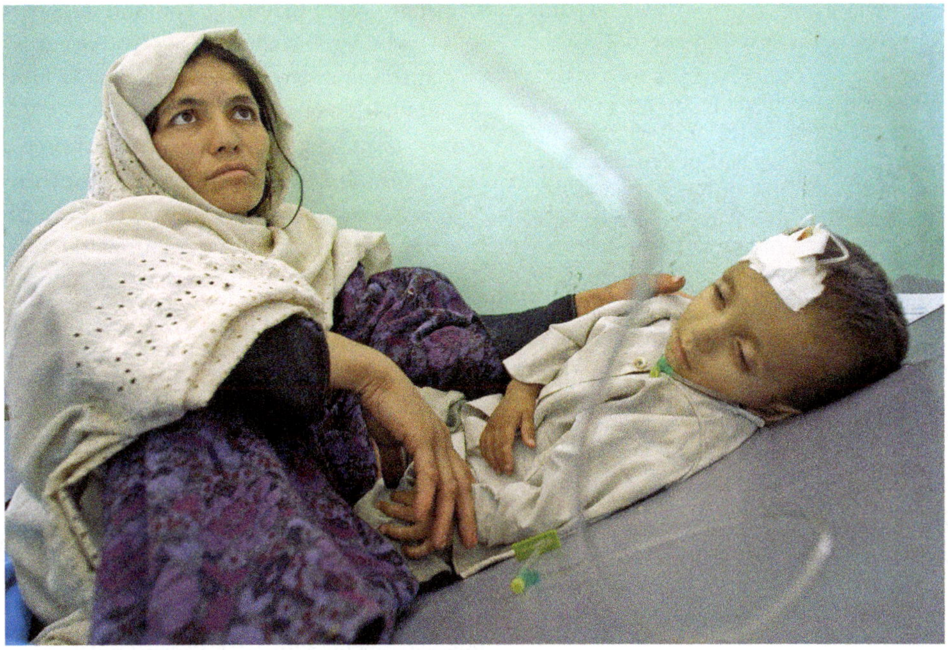

At a children's hospital in Kabul, Afghanistan, a mother watches over her son, who is suffering from dysentery and dehydration. Children are especially susceptible to the deadly effects of dysentery. © *Natalie Behring-Chisholm/Getty Images*

after using the toilet or after contact with someone who is infected with the microorganism, is essential. Hands should also be washed before handling and cooking food, eating, handling infants, and feeding the young or elderly. To avoid spreading infection, personal items such as towels or face cloths should not be shared.

Travelers should avoid drinking tap water in countries known to have poor sanitation and inadequate potable water for consumption. Ice cubes, salad, and uncooked vegetables should also be avoided because these could have been washed in or made with contaminated water.

■ Impacts and Issues

There are approximately 165 million cases of shigellosis worldwide each year. Shigellosis disproportionately affects developing nations. The World Health Organization (WHO) reports 163.2 million annual cases in developing countries, compared to 1.5 million cases in industrialized countries.

Among industrialized nations, the increased popularity of international travel accounts for a significant percentage of dysentery cases. WHO estimates that there are approximately 580,000 reported cases of tourism-related shigellosis annually. The US Centers for Disease Control and Prevention (CDC) and several international health organizations publish infectious disease warnings and medication advisories for travelers. In developing countries dysentery is common due to low standards of hygiene and sanitation. Therefore, personal hygiene, development of adequate sewage disposal, and access to clean drinking water should be a priority to control this important disease globally. In devel-

DISEASE IN DEVELOPING NATIONS

In developing countries rigorous intervention programs have yielded encouraging results. Propagating personal and community hygiene has helped tremendously in reduction of shigellosis. Some positive outcomes include:

- Handwashing with soap resulted in a decrease in secondary infection rates in Bangladesh, and similar results were recorded in Burma.
- The availability of potable water reduced the frequency of *Shigella* infection by 50 percent in Bangladesh.
- Water treatment centers considerably reduced *Shigella* incidence rates in Libya.
- Control of houseflies has also shown positive indications in reducing *Shigella* organisms and related mortality due to diarrheal disease.
- Breastfeeding has resulted in protection against shigellosis in infants up to age three.

While they are beneficial, these interventions need to be consistent, affordable, feasible, and country-specific to yield success in developing countries.

oped countries communal living, oral and anal sex, and travel to or from endemic areas may increase the risk of transmission.

Clean water, sanitation, and hygiene are key areas to be looked into for restricting episodes of dysentery. According to WHO, as of 2015, 71 percent of global population uses "safely managed" (available on premises and free from contamination) drinking water, and 39 percent have access to "safely managed" (excreta disposed appropriately) sanitation. The data provided by WHO further suggest that about 38 percent of health care facilities lack a clean water source, 19 percent have inadequate sanitation, and 35 percent lack water and soap for handwashing. While these aspects clearly need attention, as of 2018 vaccine development was also underway to prevent bacterial dysentery.

SEE ALSO *Amebiasis; Sanitation; Shigellosis; Travel and Infectious Disease; War and Infectious Disease; Water-Borne Disease*

BIBLIOGRAPHY

Books

Ericsson, Charles D., Herbert L. DuPont, and Robert Steffen. *Travelers' Diarrhea*. Hamilton, ON: BC Decker, 2008.

Periodicals

Dans, L. F., and E. G. Martinez. "Amoebic Dysentery." *BMJ Clinical Evidence* (2007): 0918.

Websites

"Amebiasis." Centers for Disease Control and Prevention. https://www.cdc.gov/parasites/amebiasis/(accessed January 16, 2018).

Christian, N. "Everything You Should Know about Dysentery." Medical News Today. https://www.medicalnewstoday.com/articles/171193.php (accessed January 16, 2018).

Cobra, Claudine, and David A. Sack. *The Control of Epidemic Dysentery in Africa: Overview, Recommendations, and Checklists.* Technical Paper No. 37. US Agency for International Development, 1996. http://pdf.usaid.gov/pdf_docs/pnaby890.pdf (accessed January 25, 2018).

"Drinking-water." World Health Organization. http://www.who.int/mediacentre/factsheets/fs391/en/ (accessed January 16, 2018).

"Progress on Drinking Water, Sanitation and Hygiene." World Health Organization Joint Monitoring Programme. http://www.who.int/mediacentre/news/releases/2017/launch-version-report-jmp-water-sanitation-hygiene.pdf (accessed January 17, 2018).

"Shigella—Shigellosis." Centers for Disease Control and Prevention. https://www.cdc.gov/shigella/ (accessed January 16, 2018).

Wellcome Trust Sanger Institute. "Out of Europe: Researchers Look at the Spread of Dysentery from Europe to Industrializing Countries." *ScienceDaily.* https://www.sciencedaily.com/releases/2012/08/120805144818.htm (accessed January 16, 2018).

Susan Aldridge
Kausalya Santhanam

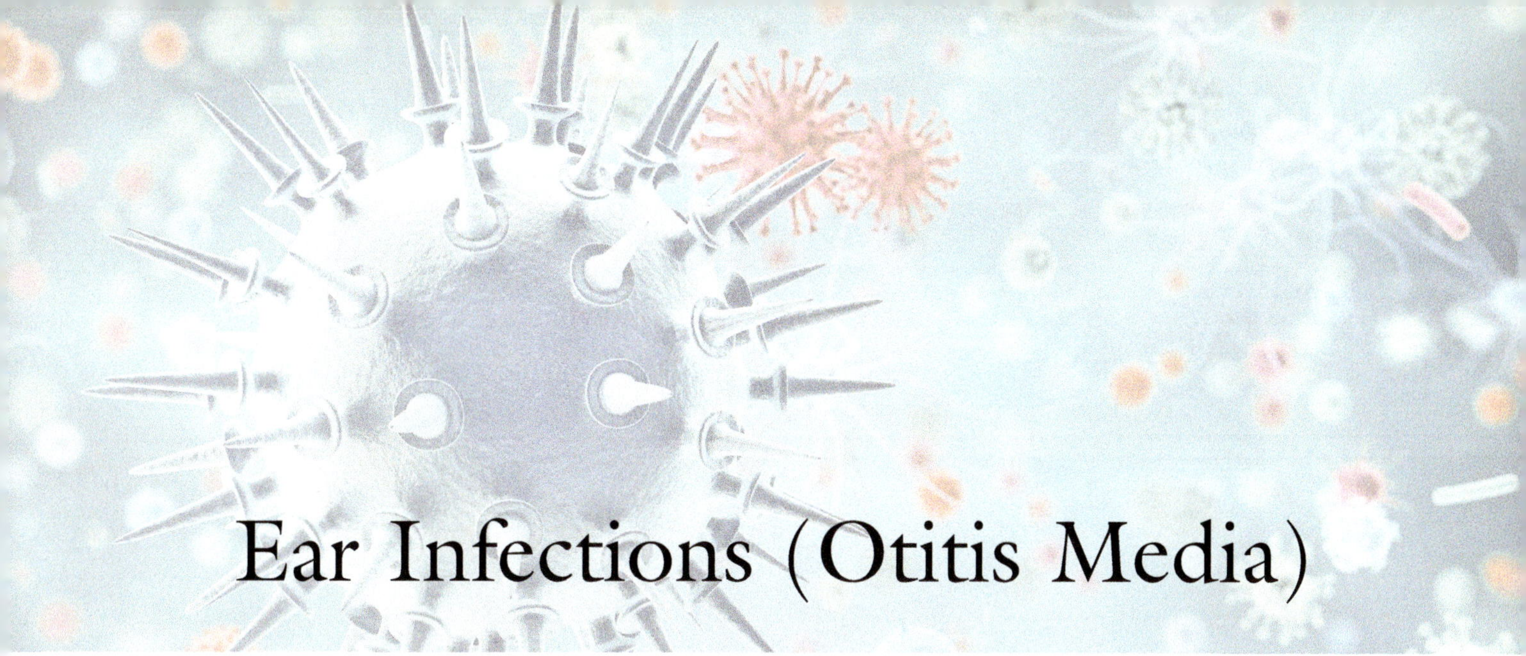

Ear Infections (Otitis Media)

■ Introduction

Otitis media is a recurring bacterial or, occasionally, viral infection of the middle ear. The bacteria most commonly involved are *Streptococcus pneumoniae*, a type of *Haemophilus influenzae*, and *Moraxella catarrhalis*.

■ Disease History, Characteristics, and Transmission

The human ear is composed of three parts—the external (outer) ear, the middle ear, and the inner ear. The outer ear is the visible portion that lies outside of the skull. It functions as a sound trap to route sound waves through a canal to the middle ear. Separating the outer and middle ear is the tympanic membrane or eardrum. In the middle ear an arrangement of three bones passes the sound vibrations to nerve cells that form the inner ear. The eustachian tube connects the middle portion of the ear to the nasal cavity and throat. Normally the eustachian tube acts to equalize the pressure on the two sides of the eardrum. However, when the inflammation associated with otitis media affects the eardrum, the pressure difference on either side of the eardrum can become so great that the eardrum ruptures, a painful complication.

There are several different kinds of otitis media. One type, called acute otitis media, tends to be associated with a runny or stuffy nose and is triggered when the eustachian tube becomes blocked during an upper respiratory infection. In addition to inflammation, pus and fluid accumulate in the middle ear. The infection can also be associated with fever and irritable behavior. Other symptoms include interrupted sleep, tugging at the affected ear, and loss of balance due to the ear blockage. The acute infection tends to be of short duration.

An ear infection that does not display symptoms, including fever and irritable behavior, is known as otitis media with effusion (the infection was known as serous or secretory otitis media). Often, after the acute version of the infection, otitis media with effusion can last longer.

If the infection lasts longer than several weeks, it is referred to as chronic otitis media. The chronic form can involve bacteria growths that have become colonized, or well established, in the ear. These growths are often present as surface-adherent, polysaccharide (slime-enclosed communities called biofilms. Antibiotic treatment will kill some of the bacteria and lessen the infection. However, bacteria deeper within the biofilm survive and can be the cause of a future infection. This is the reason that chronic otitis media can persist for years.

■ Scope and Distribution

In humans episodes of otitis media typically can begin as early as a few months of age. It is a common childhood ailment. Less frequently the infection occurs in

WORDS TO KNOW

ANTIBIOTIC RESISTANCE The ability of bacteria to resist the actions of antibiotic drugs.

BIOFILM A biofilm is a population of microorganisms that forms following the adhesion of bacteria, algae, yeast, or fungi to a surface. These surface growths can be found in natural settings, such as on rocks in streams, and in infections, such as those that occur on catheters. Microorganisms can colonize living and inert natural and synthetic surfaces.

COLONIZATION The process of occupation and increase in number of microorganisms at a specific site.

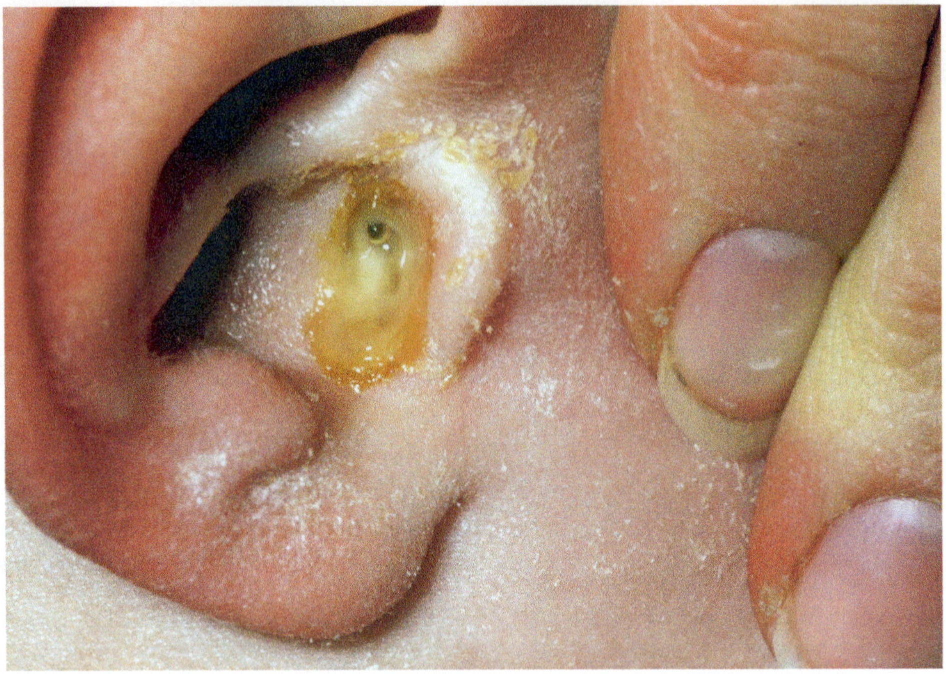

A close-up photograph of the ear of a fourteen-month-old boy shows the effects of otitis media, a recurring bacterial or viral infection of the middle ear that causes inflammation of the eardrum. © Dr P. Marazzi/Science Source

adults. More than 10 million children visit a doctor for treatment of ear infections each year in the United States. As children grow older and the structure of the ear changes, the frequency and incidence of ear infections usually drop. Specifically, as children mature, the eustachian tube becomes more slanted from inside to outside, which allows fluid to drain more easily. In the earlier years of childhood, the eustachian tube can have a more horizontal orientation or can even slant more toward the inside of the ear, which impedes fluid drainage and encourages the development of frequent infections.

Treatment and Prevention

Treatment of otitis media can involve decongestants or antihistamines to help clear the blocked eustachian tube and antibiotics if the bacteria are the cause of the infection (antibiotics are not effective against viruses). Even with antibiotic treatment, an infection may take weeks or months to completely clear, as bacteria within the biofilm are progressively killed. For this reason the full course of antibiotic therapy must be followed. Stopping treatment early, because symptoms diminish or disappear, may allow bacteria to survive. These survivors may develop resistance to the antibiotic that was used, making treatment of the next infection more difficult.

When a chronic infection does not respond to treatment, more drastic action may be necessary. Surgery to install a plastic drainage tube—a procedure called myringotomy—may be performed. Less often surgical removal of infected, swollen adenoids or tonsils may be done. Myringotomy is a common childhood surgery in the United States. The tube is removed later, as the maturing eustachian tube more naturally drains fluid from the middle ear.

Bacterial biofilms have proven to be key factors in chronic otitis media. Researchers continue to examine properties of the biofilms to devise strategies to kill the bacteria. Research to try to clarify why some children are more prone to ear infections than other children and to develop more accurate and rapid means of diagnosing otitis media is also ongoing.

OTITIS MEDIA VS. SWIMMER'S EAR

The Centers for Disease Control and Prevention (CDC) is careful to warn the public that middle ear infection is not the same as swimmer's ear. The CDC states, "If you can wiggle the outer ear without pain or discomfort then your ear condition is probably not swimmer's ear."

Impacts and Issues

Otitis media is the number one reason that parents bring a sick child to a physician. A 2014 study conducted by researchers from Southern Illinois University estimated that annual health care costs due to acute otitis media in the United States was $2.9 billion. The ultimate challenge for researchers of otitis media is to create a vaccine for infants that would prevent the first acute otitis media infection. Several vaccine candidates are at different stages in the testing and approval process, from animal testing to first-phase clinical trials. As of 2017 these efforts were still underway, and there was no vaccine.

Otitis media can be a serious infection, producing chronic diminished hearing ability or permanent hearing loss. Hearing impairment in a child during the years of language acquisition can result in learning and socialization delays, as well as speech disabilities.

As with other chronic bacterial infections, the symptoms associated with chronic ear infections can be less severe and uncomfortable than those of the acute form of the infection. Chronic infections may thus escape detection for long periods of time, potentially leading to serious complications, including permanent damage to the ear and hearing loss.

SEE ALSO *Antibiotic Resistance; Swimmer's Ear and Swimmer's Itch (Cercarial Dermatitis)*

BIBLIOGRAPHY

Books

Friedman, Ellen M., and James P. Barassi. *My Ear Hurts!: A Complete Guide to Understanding and Treating Your Child's Ear Infections.* New York: Simon & Schuster, 2001.

Preciado, Diego. *Otitis Media: State of the Art Concepts and Treatment.* New York: Springer, 2016.

Periodicals

Ahmed, Sameer, Nina L. Shapiro, and Neil Bhattacharyya. "Incremental Health Care Utilization and Costs for Acute Otitis Media in Children." *Laryngoscope* 124, no. 1 (January 2014): 301–305.

Jensen, Ramon Gordon, et al. "Recurrent Otorrhea in Chronic Suppurative Otitis Media: Is Biofilm the Missing Link?" *European Archives of Oto-Rhino-Laryngology* 274, no. 7 (July 2017): 2741–2747.

Van Dyke, Melissa K., et al. "Etiology of Acute Otitis Media in Children Less Than 5 Years of Age: A Pooled Analysis of 10 Similarly Designed Observational Studies?" *Pediatric Infectious Diseases* 36, no. 3 (March 2017): 274–281.

Websites

"Ear Infections in Children." National Institute on Deafness and Other Communication Disorders. https://www.nidcd.nih.gov/health/ear-infections-children (accessed November 15, 2017).

Waseem, Muhammad. "Otitis Media Treatment & Management." Medscape. https://emedicine.medscape.com/article/994656-treatment (accessed November 15, 2017).

Brian Hoyle

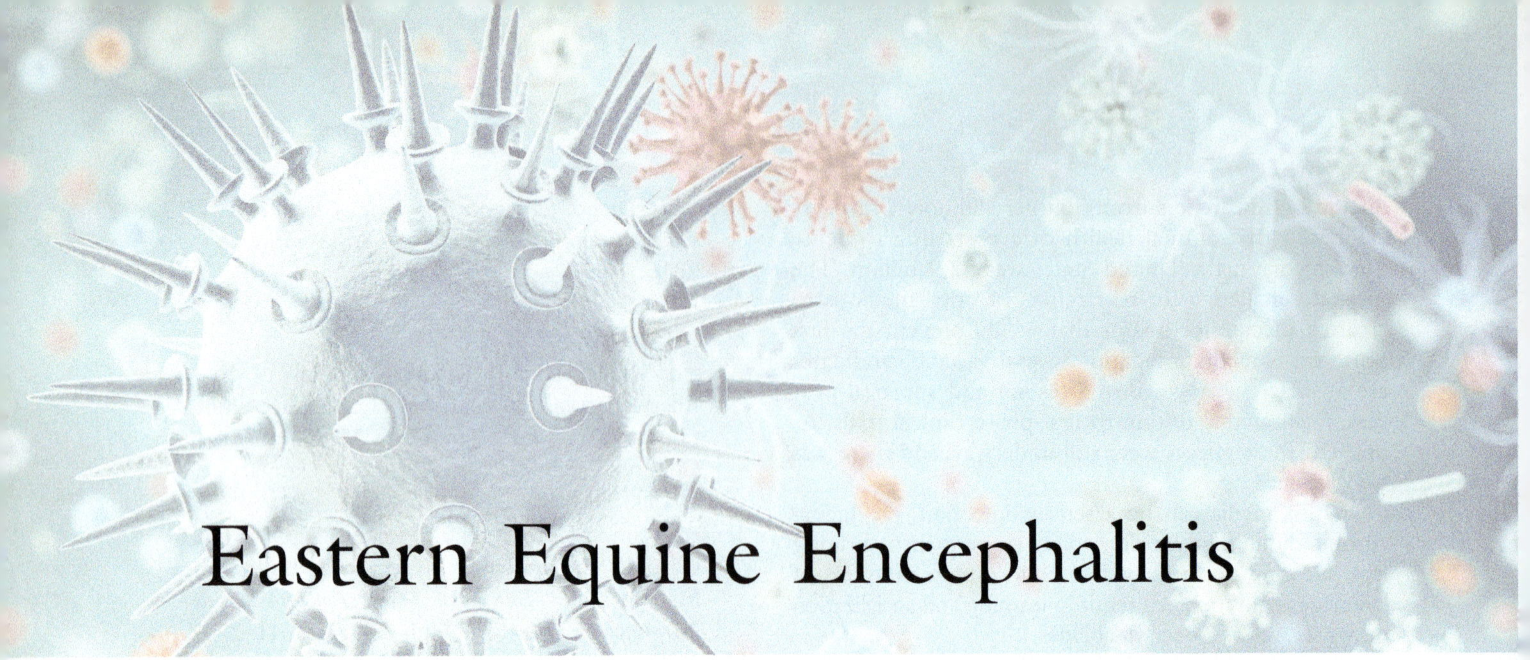

Eastern Equine Encephalitis

Introduction

Eastern equine encephalitis (EEE) is a mosquito-borne virus that infects birds and mammals, including horses and humans. It is a rare disease. According to a 2017 report from the US Centers for Disease Control and Prevention (CDC), an average of seven human cases of EEE occur in the United States each year. These human cases are primarily seen along the East and Gulf coasts. However, the high mortality rate in both humans and horses makes it one of the most serious mosquito-borne diseases.

Transmission of EEE to humans usually occurs from bird reservoir hosts in the late summer months via mosquitoes from the *Aedes* and *Coquillettidia* species. While some cases are asymptomatic, others involve mild to severe symptoms such as fever, headache, and seizures. Severe infections occur when the disease spreads to the central nervous system, which results in permanent neurological damage or death. Although an equine EEE vaccine exists, no vaccine is available for humans, and no drug treatment for the infection is known. Prevention of infection is best achieved by avoiding mosquitoes, either by reducing mosquito populations or wearing protective clothing.

EEE is distributed in North America, Central and South America, and the Caribbean. Increased migration of humans into areas more likely to contain EEE infection raises the potential for exposure to infected mosquitoes and thus increases the risk of infection in humans.

WORDS TO KNOW

ENCEPHALITIS A type of acute brain inflammation, most often due to infection by a virus.

HOST An organism that serves as the habitat for a parasite or possibly for a symbiont. A host may provide nutrition to the parasite or symbiont, or it may simply provide a place in which to live.

VECTOR Any agent that carries and transmits parasites and diseases. Also, an organism or chemical used to transport a gene into a new host cell.

Disease History, Characteristics, and Transmission

EEE was first recognized in humans in 1938, although it had been diagnosed in horses since 1831. Transmission occurs via mosquitoes, and infection can cause a range of symptoms.

Generally, passerine birds act as hosts of the virus, and the mosquito *Culiseta melanura* acts as the vector. However, other mosquitoes, including the *Aedes* and *Coquillettidia* species, which more commonly feed on mammals such as horses and humans, can also transmit the disease. Horses and humans have a low level of the virus in their blood, making them ineffective as hosts for transmission. However, birds retain a high level of the virus and act as reservoirs for continued mosquito infection. Therefore, infection is more likely to occur from a mosquito that has fed on an infected bird than a mosquito that has fed on an infected mammal. Furthermore, infection in humans by blood transfusions is unlikely to occur. EEE tends to disappear during the winter months because low temperatures kill the vector populations. However, the infection tends to break out again when the weather becomes warm.

In some cases EEE infection does not result in illness. In other cases it causes mild to severe symptoms. Mild symptoms include fever, headache, and sore throat. Severe symptoms arise when the infection enters the central nervous system and causes sudden fever and headache, followed by seizures and coma. The outcome of a severe infection of EEE is mild to severe permanent neurological

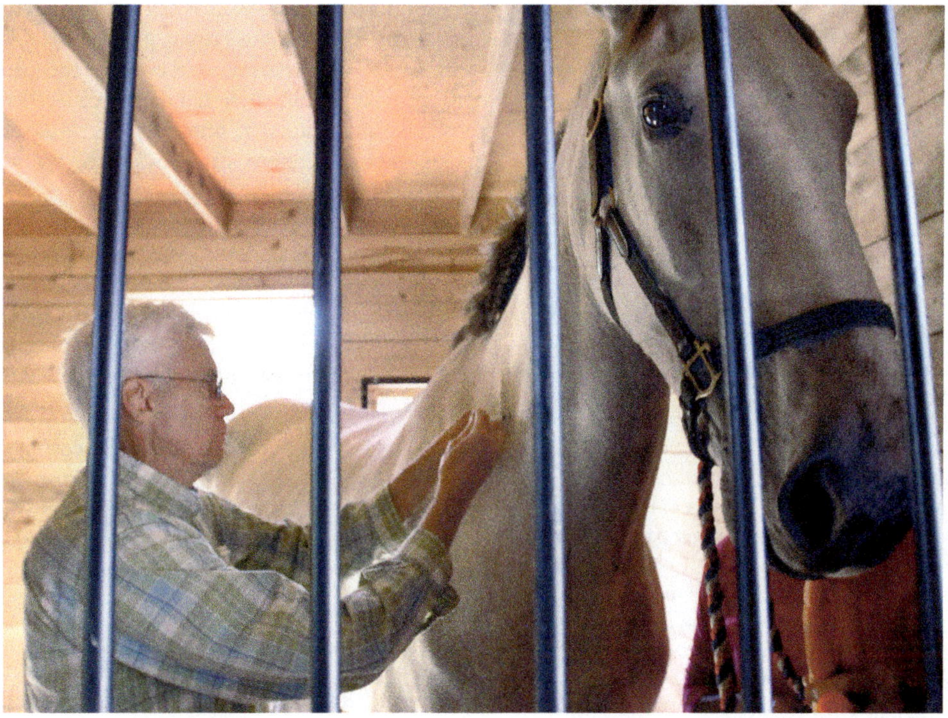

At the Woodlawn Farm in Gray, Maine, veterinarian David Jefferson administers the Eastern equine encephalitis (EEE) vaccine to a horse. EEE can also infect humans, though no human vaccine for the virus exists. © *John Patriquin/Portland Press Herald/Getty Images*

damage or death. The CDC has estimated that a third of severe cases of EEE are fatal, while half of those who survive a severe EEE infection will have mild to severe permanent neurological damage. Symptoms generally appear 3 to 10 days after the bite from an infected mosquito, and in severe cases rapid deterioration or death occurs soon after symptoms arise.

Scope and Distribution

The primary transmission cycle of the EEE virus, which involves the mosquito *Culiseta melanura* and passerine birds, occurs in freshwater, hardwood swamp environments. Therefore, EEE infections generally occur in these regions. EEE is found in North America, Central and South America, and the Caribbean. Within the United States the disease is most prevalent in the Atlantic and Gulf Coast states and the Great Lakes region.

The risk of infection in the United States has risen due to increased migration of people into previously undeveloped areas, especially previously uninhabited swampland. This has made EEE an emerging infectious disease. In 2010 the number of reported neuroinvasive cases of EEE virus in the United States rose to 10 after five consecutive years of 4 or fewer cases. In 2012 incidence of human EEE infection jumped to 15 cases, declining to 8 cases in 2013 and in 2014. The number dropped to 6 in 2015 and 7 in 2016. Of the 68 neuroinvasive cases of EEE virus reported between 2007 and 2016, 28 were fatal.

Outbreaks of EEE are more common among horses than humans. In 2006 an epidemic of 26 equine cases was reported in North Carolina. The scope of equine cases is argued to be underreported because owners may not consult a veterinarian when horses exhibit signs of EEE and thus no record is made of the infection.

Treatment and Prevention

As of 2017 there was no antiviral treatment for EEE infections in humans and no human vaccine, though there was a vaccine available for horses. Infection with the EEE virus is thought to confer lifelong immunity against reinfection with this virus. However, this immunity is limited to the EEE virus and does not confer protection against other viruses.

When EEE is symptomatic, treatment is given for the symptoms of the infection. This involves hospitalization, supportive care, prevention of secondary infections, and physical therapy. There are no antiviral drugs against EEE, and antibiotic drugs do not fight viral infections.

EEE infections can be prevented by avoiding mosquitoes. Most local health departments in EEE-endemic areas of the United States monitor mosquito populations by trapping them and continuously screening for EEE. If EEE viruses are detected, a health advisory

UNDERSTANDING EEE-CARRYING MOSQUITOES

Because mosquitoes transmit Eastern equine encephalitis (EEE), understanding how people can avoid contracting the virus largely depends on understanding which mosquitoes carry it and where those mosquitoes live. According to the US Department of Agriculture (USDA), scientists have narrowed the species of mosquito that carry EEE from the 3,000 total mosquito species to about 27. The most EEE-prone species of these 27 species is *Culiseta melanura*.

Understanding which mosquito species is most likely to carry EEE has helped scientists better identify where the disease is likely to spread: in swamps with lots of hardwood trees and muck. In the United States such swamps are most prevalent in New York, New Jersey, Maryland, Florida, and Michigan. Scientists have also come to understand that EEE outbreaks tend to occur in the summer months during hot and wet weather, when "weather conditions are ideal for expansion" of *Culiseta melanura* and other EEE-carrying mosquitos, according to the USDA report.

goes out to warn citizens about the risk and possible risk mitigation. Large-scale actions may be taken, such as the spraying of insecticides across regions known to be infected, to reduce the likelihood that humans will come into contact with infected mosquitoes. Smaller-scale methods to avoid mosquitoes include wearing protective clothing, using insect repellent, avoiding outdoor activities while mosquitoes are active, and removing standing bodies of water that may be used as breeding sites by mosquitoes.

■ Impacts and Issues

Because EEE infection has a high fatality rate (41 percent between 2007 and 2016) and survivors of severe infection may suffer permanent neurological damage, EEE is considered a major health concern in the United States despite its low incidence. However, there are some challenges associated with control of the disease, namely the lack of a vaccine. As a result, prevention of infection relies on avoidance of mosquitoes, and recovery depends on the extent of infection. Prevention and control methods of EEE infection are expensive and controversial, as the most common control method is large-scale use of insecticides to reduce mosquito populations. A conflict of interest arises between laws mandating wetland protection and the need to apply toxic insecticides for mosquito control.

Another emerging issue is associated with the increased migration of humans into previously uninhabited swamplands. The transmission cycle of the EEE virus occurs naturally within these habitats because *Culiseta melanura*, the mosquito that transmits this virus among birds, breeds there. Therefore, exposure to the virus increases as humans move into these areas.

The extent to which the disease is present among bird and horse populations is also uncertain. The prevalence of infection in horses is likely to be understated as owners fail to report cases of EEE. This may affect the extent to which a region prepares itself for the possibility of transmission of the EEE virus into the human population.

SEE ALSO *Arthropod-Borne Disease; Emerging Infectious Diseases; Encephalitis; Host and Vector; Japanese Encephalitis; Mosquito-Borne Diseases; St. Louis Encephalitis; Vaccines and Vaccine Development; Vector-Borne Disease; Viral Disease*

BIBLIOGRAPHY

Books

Bauerfeind, Rolf, and Alexander von Graevenitz. *Zoonoses: Infectious Diseases Transmissible from Animals to Humans.* Washington, DC: ASM, 2015.

Periodicals

Berlin, Daniel, et al. "A Difficult Case: Eastern Equine Encephalitis." *Practical Neurology* 17 (2017).

Deresiewicz, Robert L., et al. "Clinical and Neuroradiographic Manifestations of Eastern Equine Encephalitis." *New England Journal of Medicine* 336 (June 26, 1997): 1867–1874. This article can also be found online at http://www.nejm.org/doi/full/10.1056/NEJM199706263362604#t=abstract (accessed December 17, 2017).

Websites

"Disease Outbreak Alerts." Equine Disease Communication Center. http://www.equinediseasecc.org/alerts/outbreaks (accessed December 17, 2017).

"Eastern Equine Encephalitis." Centers for Disease Control and Prevention, April 5, 2016. https://www.cdc.gov/easternequineencephalitis/index.html (accessed December 17, 2017).

"Epidemiology and Ecology of Eastern Equine Encephalomyelitis." US Department of Agriculture, April 2004. https://www.aphis.usda.gov/animal_health/emergingissues/downloads/EEE042004.pdf (accessed December 17, 2017).

MacKay, Robert. "Eastern Equine Encephalitis (EEE)." University of Florida Large Animal Hospital. http://largeanimal.vethospitals.ufl.edu/eastern-equine-encephalitis-eee/ (accessed December 17, 2017).

"Mosquitoes Found with Eastern Equine Encephalitis Virus." Associated Press, July 14, 2017. https://www.usnews.com/news/best-states/rhode-island/articles/2017–07-14/mosquitoes-found-with-eastern-equine-encephalitis-virus (accessed December 17, 2017).

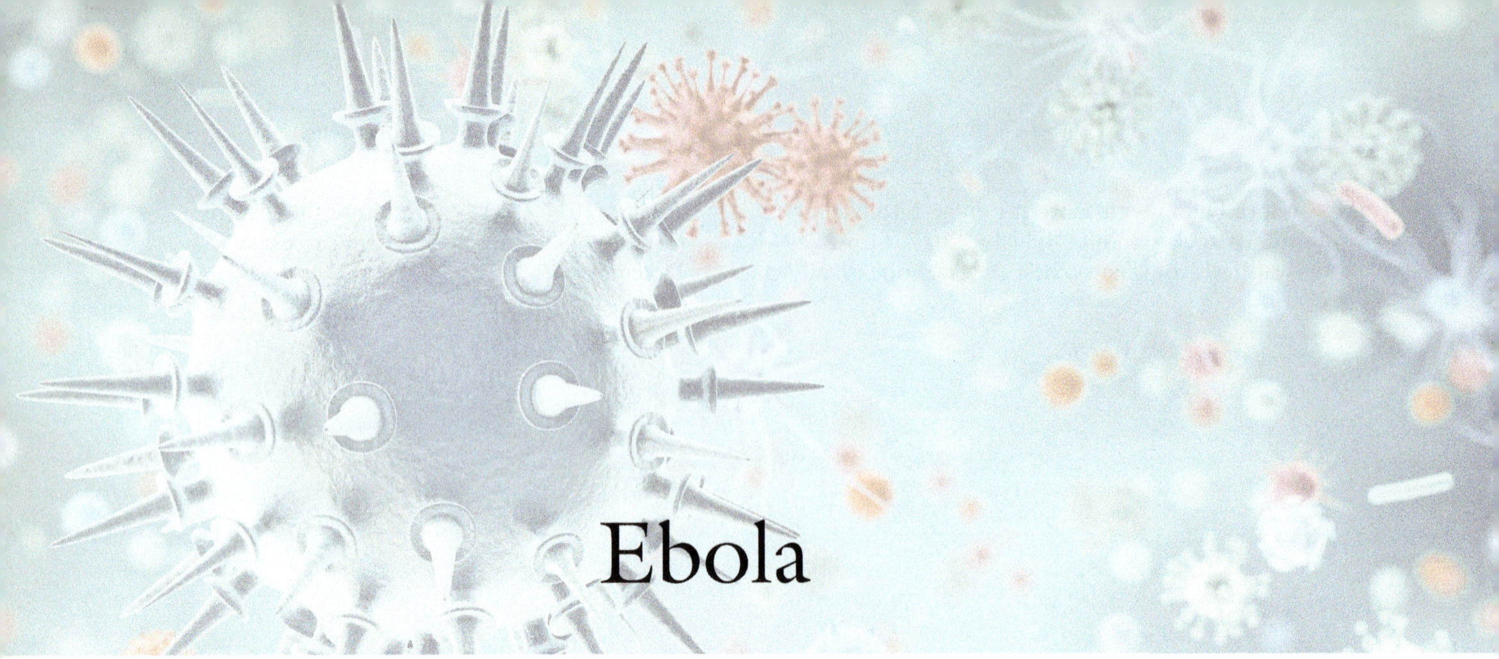

Ebola

Introduction

Ebola is a type of hemorrhagic fever caused by four subtypes of a virus called Ebola virus. The virus is one of two members of Filoviridae, a family of ribonucleic acid (RNA) viruses. The name of the virus comes from a river located in the Democratic Republic of the Congo, formerly called Zaire, where the virus was first discovered during an outbreak of the disease.

Ebola is a terrifying disease that can progress steadily toward death. The destruction of internal organs caused by the infecting virus produces a great deal of internal bleeding and can cause bleeding from various parts of the body, such as the eyes, gums, and nose. The disease caused by Ebola-Zaire, the first of the four types of the virus yet discovered, is fatal more than 90 percent of the time.

The progression from health to death within a few weeks for those unlucky enough to contract the infection is

WORDS TO KNOW

AMPLIFICATION A process by which something is made larger or the quantity of something is increased.

ANTIBODIES Antibodies, or Y-shaped immunoglobulins, are proteins found in the blood that help to fight against foreign substances called antigens. Antigens, which are usually proteins or polysaccharides, stimulate the immune system to produce antibodies. The antibodies inactivate the antigen and help to remove it from the body. While antigens can be the source of infections from pathogenic bacteria and viruses, organic molecules detrimental to the body from internal or environmental sources also act as antigens. Genetic engineering and the use of various mutational mechanisms allow the construction of a vast array of antibodies (each with a unique genetic sequence).

ANTIGEN A substance, usually a protein or polysaccharide, that stimulates the immune system to produce antibodies. While antigens can be the source of infections from pathogenic bacteria and viruses, organic molecules detrimental to the body from internal or environmental sources also act as antigens.

ANTISENSE DRUG A drug that binds to messenger RNA (mRNA), thereby blocking gene activity. Some viruses have mRNA as their genetic material, so an antisense drug can inhibit their replication.

BUSHMEAT The meat of terrestrial wild and exotic animals, typically those that live in parts of Africa, Asia, and the Americas. Also known as wild meat.

HEMORRHAGIC FEVER A high fever caused by viral infection that features a high volume of bleeding. The bleeding is caused by the formation of tiny blood clots throughout the bloodstream. These blood clots, also called microthrombi, deplete platelets and fibrinogen in the bloodstream. When bleeding begins, the factors needed for the clotting of the blood are scarce. Thus, uncontrolled bleeding (hemorrhage) ensues.

HOST An organism that serves as the habitat for a parasite or possibly for a symbiont. A host may provide nutrition to the parasite or symbiont, or it may simply provide a place in which to live.

RESERVOIR The animal or organism in which a virus or parasite normally resides.

VECTOR Any agent that carries and transmits parasites and diseases. Also, an organism or chemical used to transport a gene into a new host cell.

one terrifying aspect of Ebola. Another is that much about the virus remains unknown. Although the disease was discovered in 1976, the virus's origin, its reservoir, and how it can be prevented are still largely mysterious. The main reason for this is the infrequency of outbreaks and the speed of their appearance and disappearance. The infection quickly spreads from person to person through a local population and, because of the high death rate, soon disappears after running out of new hosts to infect. This pattern has made the study of Ebola difficult.

It is thought that the virus is transmitted to humans from a natural host by a vector. This route of transmission occurs in some other diseases. One example is malaria, which is transferred to a susceptible person from an infected animal or person via mosquitoes. Ebola may be naturally present in chimpanzees. At least two outbreaks of Ebola-Zaire were determined to be due to contact between humans and infected chimpanzees. However, it may be that chimpanzees are not the natural host but are themselves infected by the virus, which is transmitted to them from another host.

Evidence is growing that fruit bats of the Pteropodidae family are the natural host, although as of 2017 this had not been proven. Likewise, studies by the World Health Organization (WHO) and the US Centers for Disease Control and Prevention (CDC) had not yet identified the vector that carries the virus from that host to humans. What is clear from the ferocity of past outbreaks is that, once someone has been infected with Ebola, the virus is easily transferred from person to person.

Disease History, Characteristics, and Transmission

As of 2017 five species had been identified within the genus *Ebolavirus*: Zaire, Bundibugyo, Sudan, Reston, and Taï Forest. Only the first three had caused outbreaks. The outbreak in 2014–2016 was caused by Ebola-Zaire. The species are slightly different in the sequence of their genetic material and in the composition of the proteins present on their surface. This is consistent with the slightly different antibody patterns in the blood obtained from people during the various outbreaks that have occurred.

The first Ebola virus discovered was Ebola-Zaire. It was isolated near the Ebola River in the Democratic Republic of the Congo during an outbreak in 1976. There were 318 reported cases. Of these, 280 people died (a mortality rate of 88 percent). Other known occurrences of Ebola due to Ebola-Zaire include:

- Democratic Republic of the Congo, 1977 (1 case, 1 death)
- Gabon, 1994 (52 cases, 31 deaths)
- Democratic Republic of the Congo, 1995 (315 cases, 250 deaths)
- Gabon, January–April 1996 (37 cases, 21 deaths)
- Gabon, July 1996–January 1997 (60 cases, 45 deaths)

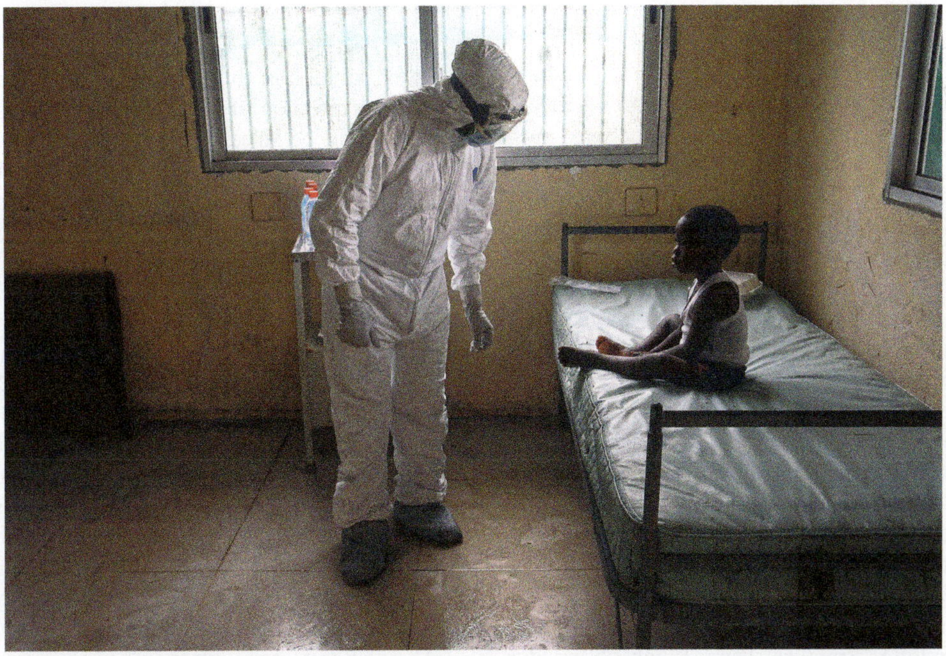

Wearing an anti-contamination suit at Redemption Hospital in Monrovia, Liberia, a worker for the nation's Ministry of Health talks to a four-year-old child suspected of having contracted the Ebola virus. According to the Centers for Disease Control and Prevention, more than 11,000 people died of the virus during an outbreak in West Africa between 2014 and 2016. © John Moore/Getty Images

- South Africa, 1996 (2 cases, 1 death; the disease was contracted in the Democratic Republic of the Congo)
- Gabon and the Democratic Republic of the Congo, October 2001–March 2002 (53 cases, 53 deaths in the Gabon outbreak; 57 cases, 43 deaths in the Congo outbreak)
- Democratic Republic of the Congo, December 2002–April 2003 (143 cases, 128 deaths)
- Democratic Republic of the Congo, 2003 (35 cases, 29 deaths)
- Guinea, Sierra Leone, Liberia, 2014–2016 (15,227 laboratory-confirmed cases, 11,310 deaths)

The 2014–2016 outbreak was the largest as of 2017 and had a mortality rate of 74.3 percent.

The second type of Ebola virus discovered was Ebola-Sudan. It was discovered in 1976 during an outbreak that occurred in Sudan (284 cases, 151 deaths). Other outbreaks involving Ebola-Sudan include:

- England, 1976 (1 case; a lab technician studying the virus accidentally contracted the virus from a needle puncture)
- Sudan, 1979 (34 cases, 22 deaths)
- Uganda, 2000–2001 (425 cases, 224 deaths)
- Sudan, 2004 (17 cases, 7 deaths)

The third type of Ebola virus discovered was Ebola-Reston. Outbreaks of Ebola occurred simultaneously in 1989 in three animal facilities in the United States that had received monkeys imported from the Philippines. One of the facilities was in Reston, Virginia. The virus took its name from the outbreak among the primates at this facility. No humans died in the outbreak, although four were infected, as shown by the antibodies they developed to the virus. This outbreak formed the basis for the best-selling book *The Hot Zone* (1994) by Richard Preston and the motion picture *Outbreak* (1995). Other outbreaks of Ebola-Reston in 1990, 1992, and 1996 involved deaths of primates but no human fatalities (although some people had produced antibodies to the virus). As of 2017 Ebola-Reston had not caused human illness.

Ebola-Taï Forest (formerly termed Ivory Coast) was discovered in 1994 in Côte d'Ivoire. As of 2017 the virus was still almost completely restricted to chimpanzees, in which it causes a severe infection. Only one human infection had been attributed to the virus, a nonlethal infection involving a scientist who had conducted an autopsy of an infected chimpanzee.

Ebola viruses are all filoviruses. One characteristic of filoviruses is their long, stringlike shape. When observed with the high magnification power of an electron microscope, the virus may appear coiled, circular, U-shaped, or even shaped like a cane (or a shepherd's crook). The different shapes may not be natural but rather may be formed artificially during purification of the virus.

The molecular details of the Ebola infection have been clarified. This work can only be done in a few laboratories in the world that are designed for research involving highly dangerous and infectious microorganisms. The infection begins when a protein on the surface of the virus recognizes a host molecule. It is not known whether the host molecule is another protein, lipid, or carbohydrate. Following the linkage between the viral protein and the host receptor, the viral genetic material enters the host cell. It is not known how this occurs. Increased understanding of these early steps is vital because subsequent infection may be stopped by blocking the viral attachment to the host cell or the transfer of the genetic material into the host cell. Efforts to develop a vaccine have focused on these steps. For example, blocking the adherence of a microbe to a host cell has proven successful in the development of a preliminary vaccine for cattle against a bacterium called *Escherichia coli* O157:H7, which can cause a lethal infection in humans, popularly known as hamburger disease.

Ebola viruses contain RNA. For the manufacture of a new virus, the infecting virus must use the host cell's genetic machinery to read the viral payload of RNA and to manufacture one of the viral proteins. Once this so-called nonstructural protein is made, it can decode the remaining viral genetic material to manufacture seven other proteins. These proteins are described as structural because they are used to form the new virus. The new virus particles are eventually released from the host cell when the cell bursts, and another cycle of infection begins as new cells are infected. How the virus, with just eight proteins, manages to make new copies of itself and evade the attempts by the host's immune system to stop the infection is unclear.

In its natural host the Ebola virus presumably does not cause serious infection. If it did, it would not persist because the host would be killed. However, in humans the resulting infection can be devastating. Within days Ebola-Zaire and Ebola-Sudan produce high fever, headache, generalized muscle aches (myalgia), abdominal pain, tiredness, and diarrhea. Cells lining the intestinal tract and stomach may be damaged, causing bloody diarrhea and vomiting of blood. At this stage some people recover. But for many the infection worsens. Massive internal bleeding sends a person into shock and can cause heart damage. Death soon follows.

One of the challenges to combating an Ebola outbreak is the fact that early symptoms of the infection are similar to those of the flu, malaria, typhoid fever, and several bacterial infections, which occur more often and are not as serious. By the time the true nature of the infection becomes known, many people in a community may have been infected.

The swiftness of the infection has been noted by some authors. Others feel, however, that the two-week course of the infection is not unusually quick. The latter view is true when a patient is near medical care in a developed country.

However, in rural regions of Africa where Ebola is most common, medical care may be days in coming and even then may not be capable of dealing with a severe infection. In that situation even a disease that develops within a week is swift and serious.

In some Ebola outbreaks the initial infection has been traced to contact between humans and an animal (usually a primate) that harbors the virus. The contagious person-to-person transmission of the virus subsequently occurs via infected blood or body fluids. This transfer can occur directly, with someone coming into contract with blood or body fluids during handling and care of a patient. Accidental infection during study of the virus also has occurred.

The rapid spread of Ebola is also aided by the location of most of the outbreaks. The areas in Africa where Ebola appears are poor and rural and do not have medical facilities close by. The health care facilities that are available are not likely to have space available to isolate the infected patient from other patients, which can contribute to the spread of the infection.

The pattern of the Ebola-Reston outbreak that occurred in Virginia in 1989 indicates that the virus may be capable of airborne spread. In that outbreak at least one of the primates who became ill was never in contact or even in the same room as the other sick primates. Lab studies have demonstrated that aerosols of the virus can infect test animals. Whether this route plays a major role in Ebola is unclear, but the general feeling is that airborne transmission is not as important as transmission by body fluids.

CULTURAL CONNECTIONS

Because the Ebola virus is transmitted by direct contact with the body fluids (blood, secretions, etc.) of infected persons, living or dead, various cultural practices can facilitate Ebola transmission. In 2017 the World Health Organization (WHO) stated, "Burial ceremonies that involve direct contact with the body of the deceased can also contribute in the transmission of Ebola. People remain infectious as long as their blood contains the virus."

WHO also reported, "Ebola virus is known to persist in immune-privileged sites in some people who have recovered from Ebola virus disease. These sites include the testicles, the inside of the eye, and the central nervous system. In women who have been infected while pregnant, the virus persists in the placenta, amniotic fluid, and fetus. In women who have been infected while breastfeeding, the virus may persist in breast milk."

WHO recommended, "Ebola survivors and their sexual partners should either: abstain from all types of sex, or observe safe sex through correct and consistent condom use until their semen has twice tested negative."

Scope and Distribution

Almost all confirmed cases of Ebola through 2017 have been in Africa. However, the infection may also occur in the western Pacific because the Reston outbreaks were caused by monkeys imported from the Philippines.

The rapid deterioration of a person following the appearance of symptoms and the fact that the affected villages can be difficult to reach has meant that response to infections by disease control officials from organizations such as WHO and the CDC occurs long after the disease has begun. This has made the discovery of Ebola's origin difficult. As of 2017 the source of the Ebola viruses remained unknown. The general agreement among scientists who study Ebola is that, because other filoviruses can infect African monkeys, macaques, and chimpanzees without causing harm to these hosts, the host for Ebola viruses may be similar. However, Ebola does harm some primates. Furthermore, an intensive 12-year-long sampling of tens of thousands of amphibians, mammals, birds, reptiles, and insects failed to detect the viruses.

Bats have also been considered as Ebola's natural host. The people who first became ill in two of the outbreaks worked in buildings where bats lived and may have come into contact with the bats. Furthermore, in a study that deliberately introduced Ebola virus into a number of vertebrates, the virus persisted only in bats. More evidence supporting the involvement of bats was published in *Nature* in 2006. The study reported on a survey of more than 1,000 animals from Gabon and Republic of the Congo, including more than 650 bats. Of these, Ebola virus RNA was found in 13 fruit bats. Bats also can harbor several other viruses that are related to Ebola. This evidence for the involvement of bats as the natural host of Ebola is still circumstantial. As of 2017 there was no evidence that infected bats were capable of infecting other animals, such as primates.

Treatment and Prevention

As of 2017 there was no known cure for Ebola. Treatment consists of keeping the patient as comfortable and free of pain as possible and minimizing the spread of infection. Additional treatment measures include restoring lost fluids, minimizing bleeding, and dealing with any secondary infections that may occur.

The outbreak that began in 2014 was the largest to date. Initially, the outbreak spread rapidly. But with time and with the mobilization of relief and medical aid from nations including the United States, the outbreak was contained. The outbreak also featured a clinical trial of a human vaccine designated recombinant vesicular stomatitis virus–Zaire Ebola virus (rVSV-ZEBOV). The trial involved 11,841 people in Guinea who were not yet infected but who had likely been in contact with someone who developed the infection. Of these, 5,837 received the vaccine, while the others did not. Of those who were vaccinated, none subsequently developed the infection, compared to 23 cases that occurred in the nonvaccinated group. The trial was important not only for its outcome but for demonstrating that a scientifically sound clinical trial could be performed during an epidemic.

The vaccine was created at the National Microbiology Laboratory in Winnipeg, Manitoba, Canada. The vaccine was based on vesicular stomatitis viruses that had been genetically engineered to express a glycoprotein component of Ebola-Zaire. The rationale was that, when the recombinant virus was injected into someone, the immune system would produce an antibody to the glycoprotein, which would protect the person from infection. As of late 2017, however, the vaccine was not yet commercially available.

■ Impacts and Issues

Ebola affects people in the most basic way. It strikes with little warning and can sweep through a village in a short time. In rural settings where the disease usually occurs, medical care is minimal and health care providers are stretched to their limits to contain the infection and provide basic comforts to those who are ill.

Although the book *The Hot Zone* and the movie *Outbreak* were somewhat sensational, they address the lethality of Ebola. These popular depictions of Ebola helped make the average person more aware of infectious diseases in general and Ebola specifically.

Ebola is a striking example of how human encroachment on regions that were previously uninhabited can bring people into contact with microorganisms to which they had not been previously exposed. Another example of this phenomenon is the emergence of avian influenza in humans. Long a disease transferred between certain species of poultry, closer human contact with poultry enabled the avian flu virus to adapt so that it became capable of, initially, bird-to-human transmission and later human-to-human transmission.

In the case of Ebola, human encroachment on previously uninhabited areas has increased contact with the natural host of the disease. The blurring of boundaries between the human and natural worlds has brought people into closer contact with primates, which are either the natural reservoir of the virus or which acquire the infection from the natural reservoir, possibly the fruit bat. The virus can spread to humans who kill and eat apes or chimpanzees. Rural Africans have long eaten bushmeat, including the meat of primates, and its sale is still an important part of the rural economy. In addition, bushmeat has become increasingly popular as a delicacy in the Western world.

The link between the consumption of bushmeat and the spread of Ebola has spurred efforts to restrict poaching. A 2005 meeting involving 23 African nations and representatives of the United Nations addressed the problem of the declining great ape population and urged stricter controls on poaching and deforestation (which increases people's access to ape territory). However, the effectiveness of the campaign was debatable. Ape meat is still available for sale in many local markets in regions of Africa and is sought by buyers in Western countries.

Whereas some species may naturally harbor the Ebola virus without harm, other species have been decimated by the disease. Beginning in 2002 conservationists in some regions of Africa noted a die-off of Western gorillas and common chimpanzees. Between 1983 and 2000 the great ape population in the African nation of Gabon declined by half, with Ebola and poaching cited as the most likely causes. Without a concerted effort, these near-human creatures may become extinct within decades. Efforts to eliminate poaching by organizations such as the World Wildlife Fund have had some benefit, but poaching of gorillas and chimpanzees has nevertheless continued.

Part of the reason for the ferocity of an Ebola outbreak is a lack of understanding of the disease among those most affected by it. More education targeting those who are at risk of acquiring the infection is still needed. For example, burial customs in many African cultures include an open viewing of the deceased, which potentially exposes the mourners to the virus. This practice can amplify the spread of the virus. Amplification is an important means by which a variety of viral and bacterial diseases can spread. In the case of Ebola and mourning customs, learning to pay respect to the deceased person without touching or even seeing the body would help reduce the spread of Ebola.

The infection of health care workers is a common aspect of Ebola outbreaks. During some initial outbreaks, medical personnel have inadvertently spread the virus. The use of protective measures, such as masks and gloves, lessens the risk of passing the infection to caregivers. In some rural clinics, however, such measures are a luxury, though they are commonplace in medical clinics in developed countries. This problem was highlighted in the early phase of the response to the 2014 outbreak.

Another issue concerning serious infections, including Ebola, is the potential of the microbe to be used as a weapon. Indeed, Ebola was considered for development as a biological weapon by both the United States and the Soviet Union. Members of the Japanese cult Aum Shinrikyo, who released sarin gas in the Tokyo subway system in 1995, killing 12 people and injuring almost 1,000, visited Zaire in 1992. Under the guise of offering medical aid to victims of an Ebola outbreak, they instead tried to acquire some virus to use as a terrorist weapon.

SEE ALSO *Antiviral Drugs; Emerging Infectious Diseases; Hemorrhagic Fevers; Vector-Borne Disease*

BIBLIOGRAPHY

Books

Preston, Richard. *The Hot Zone.* New York: Anchor, 1994.

Quammen, David. *Ebola: The Natural and Human History of a Deadly Virus.* New York: Norton, 2014.

Richards, Paul. *Ebola: How a People's Science Helped End an Epidemic.* London: Zed, 2016.

Shah, Sonia. *Pandemic: Tracking Contagions, from Cholera to Ebola and Beyond.* New York: Sarah Crichton Books/Farrar, Straus and Giroux, 2016.

Periodicals

Collier, Beth-Ann, et al. "Clinical Development of a Recombinant Ebola Vaccine in the Midst of an Unprecedented Epidemic." *Vaccine* (August 16, 2017): 4465–4469.

Leroy, E. M., et al. "Fruit Bats as Reservoirs of Ebola Virus." *Nature* (December 1, 2005): 575–576.

Regules, Jason A., et al. "A Recombinant Vesicular Stomatitis Virus Ebola Vaccine." *New England Journal of Medicine* 376 (2017): 330–341.

Websites

"Ebola Virus Disease." World Health Organization, June 2017. http://www.who.int/mediacentre/factsheets/fs103/en/ (accessed November 15, 2017).

"Final Results Confirm Ebola Vaccine Provides High Protection against Disease." World Health Organization, December 23, 2016. http://www.who.int/mediacentre/news/releases/2016/ebola-vaccine-results/en/ (accessed November 15, 2017).

Brian Hoyle

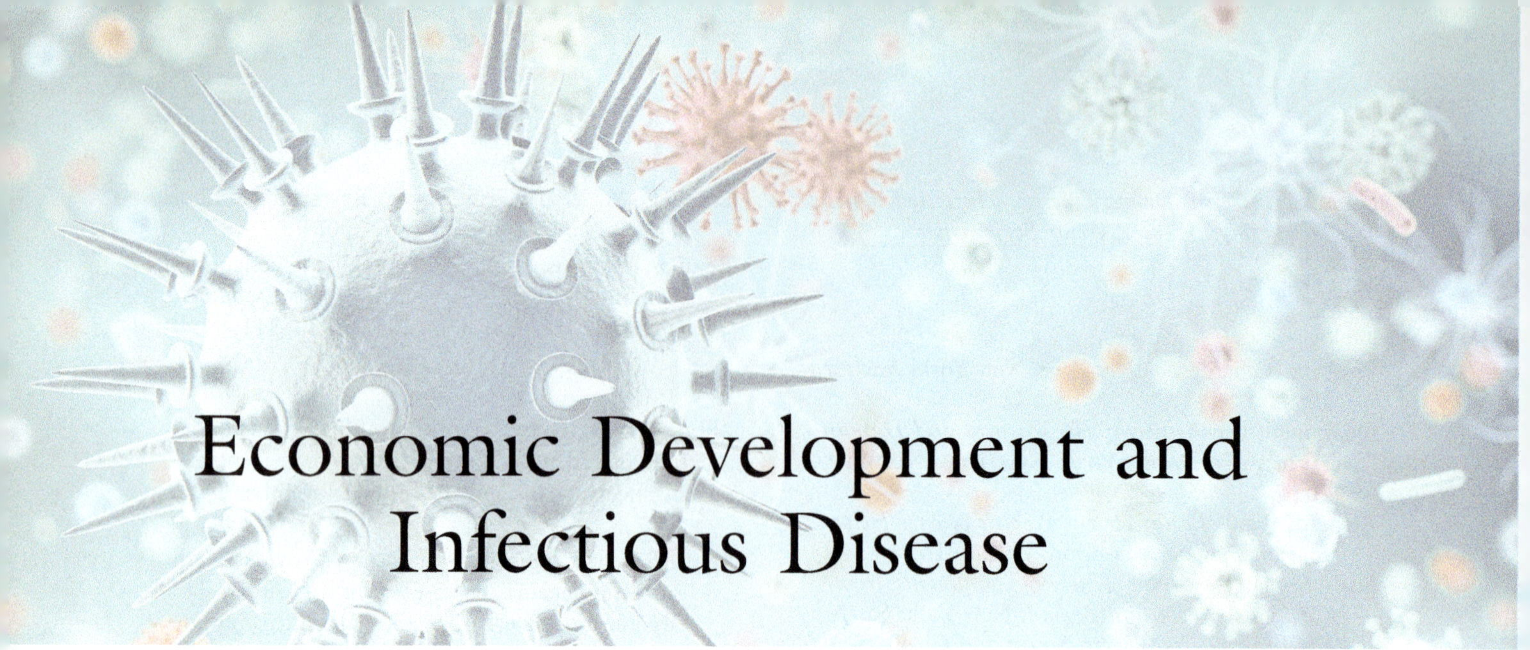

Economic Development and Infectious Disease

Introduction

There is a global relationship between national and personal income and health. Developed nations often have lower average morbidity (illness) and mortality (death) rates than developing nations. Mortality rates drop over time as countries increase in wealth. Within countries, wealthier people typically live longer than poorer people.

In the case of infectious disease, the causal relationship between poverty and public health can cut both ways. In some instances, endemic infections and catastrophic epidemics can stymie economic development. In others, lack of economic development can undermine the development of infrastructure that could promote healthful conditions and prevent mortality and morbidity from infectious disease.

WORDS TO KNOW

ENDEMIC Present in a particular area or among a particular group of people.

EPIDEMIC From the Greek *epidemic*, meaning "prevalent among the people," it is most commonly used to describe an outbreak of an illness or a disease in which the number of individual cases significantly exceeds the usual or expected number of cases in any given population.

MORBIDITY From the Latin *morbus*, "sick," it refers to both the state of being ill and the severity of the illness. A serious disease is said to have high morbidity.

MORTALITY The condition of being susceptible to death. The term *mortality* comes from the Latin word *mors*, which means death. Mortality can also refer to the rate of deaths caused by an illness or injury (e.g., "Rabies has a high mortality rate").

PATHOGEN A disease-causing agent, such as a bacterium, a virus, a fungus, or another microorganism.

SOCIOECONOMIC Concerning both social and economic factors.

History and Scientific Foundations

Economists have approached the relationship between disease and income using econometric analysis, an important methodology for guiding policy and foreign aid decisions. Econometric studies have consistently supported the correlation between income and health and have attempted to disentangle the complex processes that have produced this statistical relationship that exists both within and between nations.

The impact of economic conditions on health status has long been recognized, based on studies of the effects of food scarcity, shelter, and living space. Although economic conditions have been deemphasized as factors in mortality and morbidity because of the dissemination of medical technologies, there is increasing evidence that this diffusion of health knowledge and technology has had differential effects in developed and underdeveloped nations. Studies of this topic typically focus on national income (the value of all goods and services produced in a given period). Secondly, per capita income (income per person) is the leading indicator of economic development and motivates many health policy decisions. Therefore, many observers are calling for greater global economic development. Critics assail the emphasis on economic development over public health, but others assert that public health initiatives are too often thwarted by political and economic instability and food scarcity.

Studies have found a significant positive correlation between income and health status in both developed and developing economies. In more developed countries, the causal path typically goes from health status to income, with feedback from income to health. Healthier people are wealthy, but wealthy people may have increased access to health care and wellness resources. However, whether income "buys" better health and just how this may occur has proven difficult for economists to quantify, especially for adults in the workforce. In developed countries the most documented connection between income and health is based on studies of infant mortality rates, the scope of which cannot support a robust analysis of the feedback from health to income.

The mechanisms producing a relationship between money and health are complex. Variables such as race, education, and urban or rural status may also influence income or health for many individuals. The causes of poor health status in developing countries may be different from the factors that undermine health in industrialized countries. In developing countries infectious disease, lack of clean drinking water, and inadequate diet may present the greatest public health risks. In developed nations lifestyle-related chronic diseases and reduced physical activity may present the greatest public health threats.

The connecting mechanisms underlying the relationship between health and income are sometimes not specific to the level of industrialization. This relationship in "middle income" or transition economies may be particularly hard to analyze because people in the same communities, and even in the same households, can be disproportionately affected by problems common to both developed and developing regions. For example, obese women may be neighbors or even housemates of malnourished children. Thus, the scientific underpinnings of the relationship among development, income, and health are best served by focusing on universal mechanisms, or mechanisms likely to be found in every society and community, such as psychosocial stress (stress caused by social, psychological, and environmental factors).

A study of data sponsored by the World Health Organization (WHO) confirms a link between income and health, casting light on the interplay between wealth and health. In particular, the study focused on how income improves health apart from the availability of medical services. The study results indicate that increased earnings capacity, along with policies that provide for income transfers to those less wealthy, may be as important for health outcomes as additional funds for service provision. Within countries income is strongly correlated with health outcomes, especially in settings where the health services delivery is weak. This correlation exists apart from the presence of vital public health campaigns to provide clean water, eradicate malaria, vaccinate children, or deliver medicine to treat acquired immunodeficiency syndrome (AIDS) in developing countries.

In view of the possible independence of income as a factor in improving health, a question arises regarding the efficiency of public and private funds aimed at health promotion. For example, investment in economic development, employment opportunities, and income support for the poor might have equal or greater impact on health than would public expenditures on health services availability. People with more income may spend income on goods and services associated with better health, such as more nutritious food, better housing, exercise, or leisure activities.

■ Applications and Research

An experiment reported by Princeton University that illuminates the relationship between income and health dealt with the institution of larger pension payments to all elderly South Africans. To determine whether income has a causal effect on health, WHO-sponsored investigators identified state old-age pension payments as a source of income that is not determined by a respondent's health status. According to the report, in South Africa women aged 60 or older and men aged 65 or older are eligible for a monthly cash transfer if they do not have an employer-based pension, and over 80 percent of eligible people take up this source of income. In communities where unemployment reaches up to 40 percent, this is the only stable and considerable source of income.

The health survey showed that pension income had a protective effect on the self-reported health of all adults in which the pension income was pooled with that of other household members. For pensioners living in households in which income was not pooled, the beneficial health effects of the pension accrued only to the pensioners after they started receiving the pension. These effects persisted regardless of geographic location, race, educational level, and income level.

The researchers investigated whether higher income tended to have an impact on four major areas of daily life: medical care, water and sanitation, nutrition, and psychosocial stress. They found no evidence from the survey data suggesting that higher incomes enabled respondents to spend more time and money seeking out better health services such as private physicians and better-equipped clinics. Also, access to cleaner water was apparently not improved, although higher and pooled income families were more likely to have a flush toilet. However, higher and pooled income families were more likely to report improved nutrition and fewer skipped meals, which were correlated with better health status. Finally, income was correlated with reduced self-reported depression symptoms connected to psychosocial stress. Depression has been associated with increased all-cause medical symptoms in many studies. Thus, the researchers concluded that income has a causal effect on health status, which is mediated by a combination of improved sanitation, nutrition, and the reduction of psychosocial stress.

Examination of how specific infections have materially affected the economic well-being and income of societies shows that, despite the success of vaccination programs for polio, diphtheria, and other childhood diseases, diseases such as AIDS, malaria, tuberculosis, acute respiratory infections, and diarrheal disease continue to cause high mortality rates in Africa. But mortality figures do not provide a complete measure of the burden of infectious diseases such as lymphatic filariasis, leishmaniasis, schistosomiasis, and sleeping sickness. The global toll of these diseases includes health impacts such as disabilities and deformities, productivity loss, and the cost of care and treatment. The prevalence of these infectious diseases is directly correlated with the economic performance of African countries: the nations with the highest prevalence of these diseases have the lowest per capita income. The burden of these diseases is devastating because it affects all facets of human development, including income, health, and education. Therefore, it seems counterproductive and circuitous to focus on either health care assistance or economic development to the exclusion of one another. Striking the right balance between the two can be key to improving the standard of living and quality of life in developing countries.

■ Impacts and Issues

Social Inequality and Infectious Disease

Evidence is mounting that social inequalities contribute significantly to disease emergence. These inequalities have affected not only the distribution of infectious diseases but also the severity and outcome of disease in affected people. Analyses of outbreaks of Ebola, AIDS, and tuberculosis indicate that disease emergence is influenced by specific events and processes, subject to local variation. Close examination of mutations in microorganisms often shows that human actions have been key factors in increasing the spread of disease and resistance to antibiotics. For example, tropical diseases such as malaria generally affect people in lower socioeconomic brackets, whereas people with higher incomes may purchase mosquito nets and insect repellants or live in areas with better drainage and fewer mosquitoes.

The distribution of Ebola outbreaks affects people living in poverty and health care workers who serve the poor but often not others in close physical proximity. For example, the 1976 outbreak in Zaire affected 318 people. The cases could be traced to failure to follow contact precautions and improper sterilization of syringes and other equipment and supplies. Once these measures were taken, the outbreak was terminated. This explanation suggests that Ebola does not always emerge randomly. Rather, the likelihood of coming into contact with unsterile syringes (for example, in health clinics) is inversely proportional to social status. Population groups with access to high-quality medical services are unlikely to contract Ebola even in Ebola-affected regions.

After an outbreak of Ebola in West Africa began in 2014, researchers were again able to observe a strong connection between poverty and infection. In their 2015 article in *PLOS Neglected Tropical Disease*, Mosoka P. Fallah et al. found that "infected individuals residing in these most impoverished settings are associated with three times more Ebola transmission, as well as greater dissemination of disease between communities of different socioeconomic levels."

The reemergence of tuberculosis is another powerful example of the impact of social inequality on the epidemiology of infections. For decades the disease was largely absent in Western Europe and North America but remained endemic in many developing nations worldwide. World trade, increased migration, and international travel have reintroduced tuberculosis to regions where the disease had once been eliminated. As of 2016 tuberculosis had surpassed HIV to become the world's deadliest infectious disease.

Therefore, socioeconomic inequality within nations may have helped foster the virulence of old and new infectious diseases. Economic inequality between nations may also accentuate differences in the distribution of infectious diseases. National borders cannot keep out all pathogens but can be substantial boundaries to infectious disease response and the provision of health care.

Economic Development's Impact on Tuberculosis in India

In 2016 there were 2.7 million new tuberculosis cases in India and nearly half a million deaths from the disease. While this represented a 12 percent annual decline in mortality from tuberculosis in India, the country remained ranked number one among the world's nations in deaths from the disease. India has increased its investment in fighting tuberculosis, but observers have connected the country's outsize tuberculosis problem to a lack of sufficient funds to support both treatment and prevention.

Until the 21st century, fewer than 50 percent of people with tuberculosis received an accurate diagnosis. Less than half of these people received effective treatment. A study by the Ministry of Health and Family Welfare analyzed the impact of health policies promulgated in 1993 that devoted increased resources such as improved diagnosis, case management of treatment, and the use of uniform anti-tuberculosis treatments, as well as improved case reporting methods. The program trained more than 200,000 health workers and improved access to services for 436 million people, more than 40 percent of India's population. Under the program's auspices, about 3.4 million patients were evaluated for tuberculosis.

By late 2001 nearly 800,000 had received treatment, with a success rate greater than 80 percent. Thus, India's tuberculosis control program has succeeded in improving access to care, the quality of diagnosis, and the probability of successful treatment. This has translated into the prevention of 200,000 deaths and the alleviation of indirect medical costs, such as productivity and caregiving costs, of more than $400 million, an order of magnitude greater than the cost of program implementation.

In spite of the program's success, ministry officials observe that it will be challenging to sustain and expand the program due to the country's current limited primary health care system and large, but mainly unregulated, private health care system. Furthermore, India continued to struggle with an increase in incidence of HIV and multidrug-resistant tuberculosis.

The advance of public health systems and spread of advanced medical knowledge and technology has resulted in improvements in health status worldwide. However, lack of economic development and vast income inequalities across and within national boundaries continue to present major obstacles to public health. Poverty has prevented equality in health care among nations. Infectious diseases continue to be the major cause of death worldwide, with 25 percent of all deaths and 30 percent of the global disease burden attributed to communicable diseases. More than 95 percent of these deaths, the majority of which are preventable, occur in the poorest areas of developing nations. HIV/AIDS, tuberculosis, and malaria are the three most lethal infectious diseases in these regions.

Health assistance to developing countries, especially for these three diseases, has been based on advocacy for the principles of social justice and the human right to health in the developing world. Given the increasing integration of the global economy, economic development in lower-income countries will increase profitable investment opportunities for wealthier countries in the developing world. Improved public health in developing countries also has political and international security benefits for developed nations.

A 2017 study published in *Nature Ecology & Evolution* titled "General Ecological Models for Human Subsistence, Health and Poverty" considered the relationship between population, health, and economic growth, modeling how infectious disease affects the world's poor. According to the authors, "The models show that feedbacks between the biological and economic systems can lead to a state of persistent poverty." Their analysis described the ways in which disease undermines the economic aspirations of the rural poor, not only directly by making them sick and unable to work but also indirectly by affecting the livestock and crops that they rely on for sustenance and possible economic gain. As a result, the authors noted, improving access to health care has important potential for promoting economic growth among the world's poorest people.

In 2009 WHO produced the "WHO Guide to Identifying the Economic Consequences of Disease and Injury," which aimed to "help to identify possible strategies for reducing the cost of disease or injury via appropriate preventive action or treatment strategies." The organization planned to unveil a "new, improved tool" for analyzing the relationship between disease and economic development in 2018.

SEE ALSO *Developing Nations and Drug Delivery; Public Health and Infectious Disease; World Trade and Infectious Disease*

BIBLIOGRAPHY

Books

Boutayeb, A. "The Impact of Infectious Diseases on the Development of Africa." In *Handbook of Disease Burdens and Quality of Life Measures*, edited by Victor R. Preedy and Ronald Ross Watson, 1171–1188. New York: Springer-Verlag, 2010.

Lopez, Alan D., Colin Mathers, and Majid Ezzati, eds. *Global Burden of Disease and Risk Factors.* New York: World Bank Group, 2006.

Periodicals

Adler, Nancy E., and Joan M. Ostrove. "Socioeconomic Status and Health: What We Know and What We Don't." *Annals of the New York Academy of Sciences* 896 (1999): 3–15.

Fallah, Mosoka P., et al. "Quantifying Poverty as a Driver of Ebola Transmission." *PLOS Neglected Tropical Disease* 9, no. 12 (2015): e0004260. This article can also be found online at https://doi.org/10.1371/journal.pntd.0004260 (accessed March 5, 2018).

Farmer, P. "Social Inequalities and Emerging Infectious Diseases." *Emerging Infectious Diseases* 2, no. 4 (October–December 1996): 259–269. This article can also be found online at https://wwwnc.cdc.gov/eid/article/2/4/pdfs/96-0402.pdf (accessed February 26, 2018).

Ngonghala, Calistus N., et al. "General Ecological Models for Human Subsistence, Health and Poverty." *Nature Ecology & Evolution* 1 (2017): 1153–1159.

Smith, J. P. "Healthy Bodies and Thick Wallets: The Dual Relationship between Health and Economic Status." *Journal of Economic Perspectives* 13, no. 2 (1999): 145–166.

Websites

Sachdev, Chhavi. "Why Does India Lead the World in Deaths from TB?" NPR, November 9, 2017. https://www.npr.org/sections/goatsandsoda/2017/11/09/561834263/why-does-india-lead-the-world-in-deaths-from-tb (accessed March 5, 2018).

"TB Statistics India—National, Treatment Outcome & State Statistics." TBFacts.org. https://www.tbfacts.org/tb-statistics-india/ (accessed March 5, 2018).

"UN Millennium Development Goals." United Nations. http://www.un.org/millenniumgoals/ (accessed June 8, 2007).

"WHO Guide to Identifying the Economic Consequences of Disease and Injury." World Health Organization, 2009. http://www.who.int/choice/publications/d_economic_impact_guide.pdf?ua=1 (accessed February 8, 2018).

Kenneth T. LaPensee

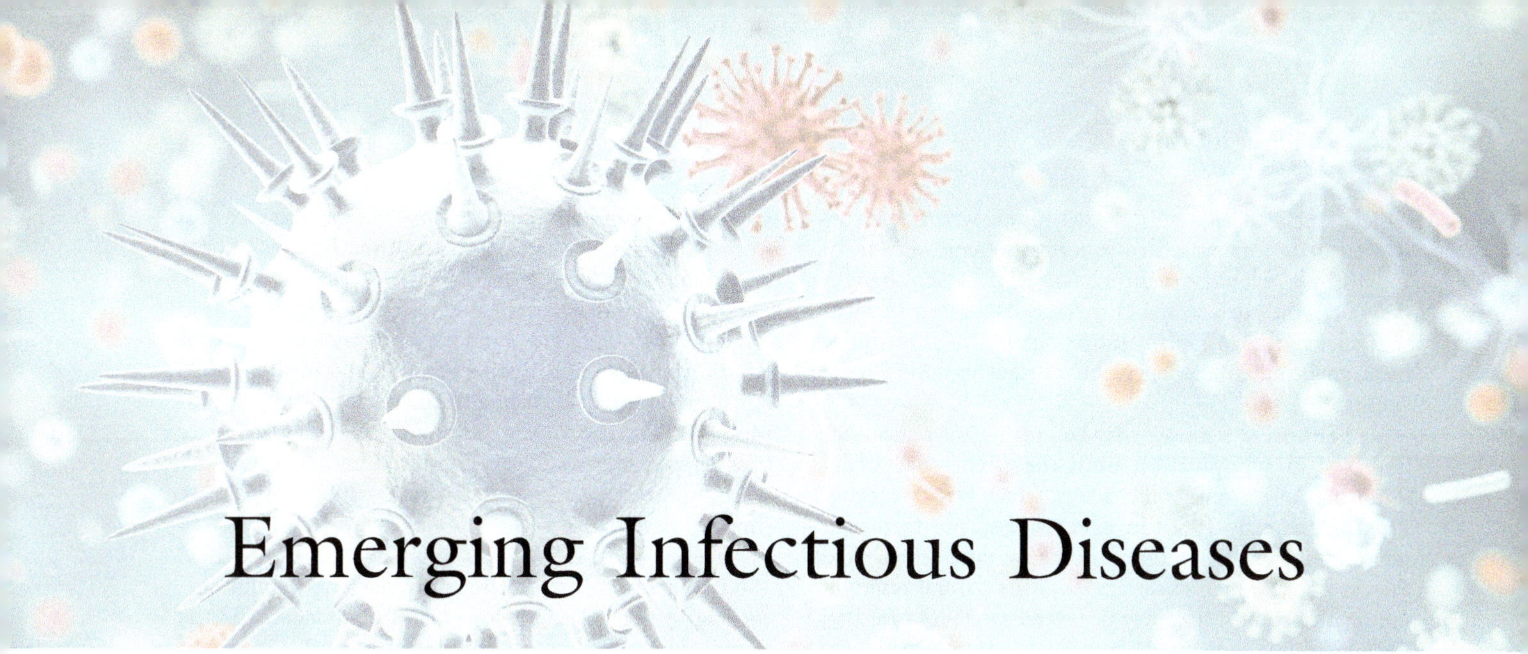

Emerging Infectious Diseases

Introduction

Emerging infectious diseases are human diseases caused by pathogens (disease-causing organisms) that have increased in prevalence in the preceding two decades or microbial diseases that are either becoming more widespread or threatening to become widespread. These diseases can be new, previously unrecognized, or reemergent (diseases that were once under control but have reappeared and have become a concern).

Infectious diseases that have emerged since 1990 include avian influenza, a viral disease that was originally a problem in poultry and has evolved to be capable of infecting humans. Tuberculosis (TB) is an example of a reemergent disease. Incidence of TB has increased in many regions, and several strains that are highly drug resistant have developed. Other emerging diseases include Ebola virus disease, Middle East respiratory syndrome (MERS), chikungunya virus, and H1N1 influenza virus (also known as swine flu).

History and Scientific Foundations

Microbial diseases appear and spread throughout a population for several reasons. Emergence may be genuine, meaning that the microbe changes in some way that makes it capable of causing disease or being transmitted. An example is *Escherichia coli* O157:H7,

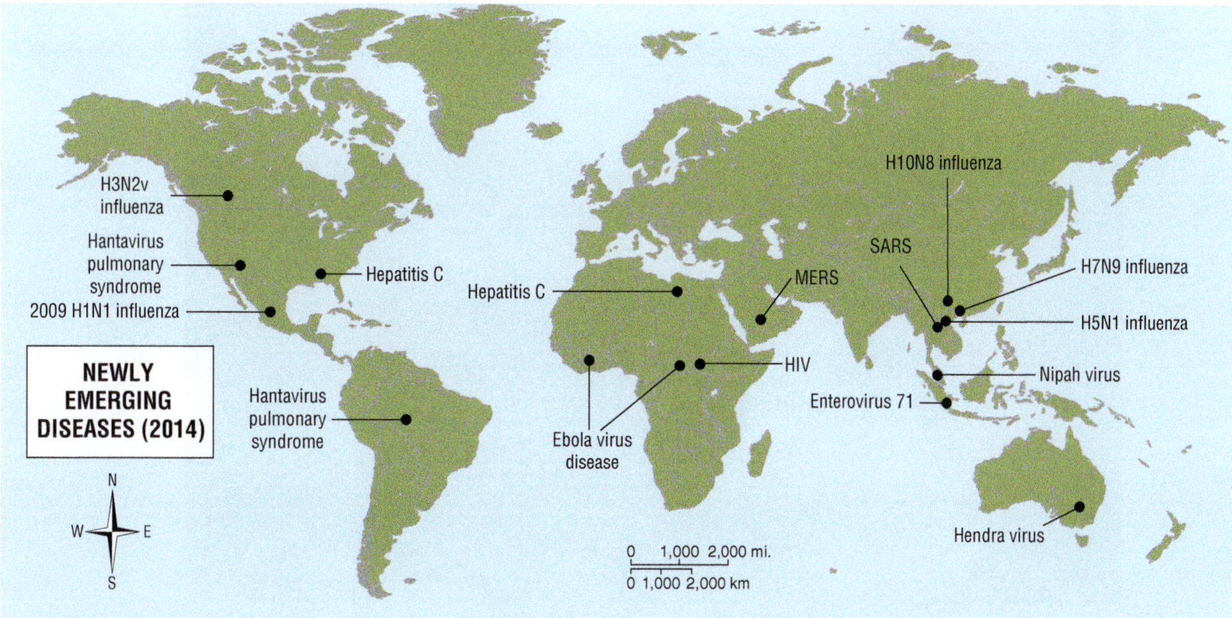

SOURCE: Adapted from Marston, Hilary D., et al. "Emerging Viral Diseases: Confronting Threats with New Technologies." *Science Translational Medicine,* September 10, 2014. Available from: http://stm.sciencemag.org/content/6/253/253ps10.full

which emerged as a serious pathogen when a toxin-coding gene was passed to a nonpathogenic version of *E. coli* by a related organism, *Shigella*. Other changes may alter the surface structure of a bacterium or virus that makes the organism more capable of infecting a host, environmentally hardy, or resistant to antibacterial agents.

Alternatively, a disease may be present but remain undetected in a population until the occurrence of an outbreak. An example is hantavirus, which was first recognized in the early 1950s in Korea and sprang to prominence during a 1993 outbreak in the southwestern United States. Ebola, which likely existed in its natural reservoir (an unaffected host that may be several species of fruit bat) for a long time, was not recognized as a human pathogen until a large human outbreak occurred in Uganda in 2000–2001. Another outbreak that began in 2014 claimed more than 11,000 lives.

Emerging infectious disease can also involve once-problematic diseases that were controlled but have re-emerged as a problem. In addition to TB, other examples of reemerging infectious diseases include malaria, influenza, and gonorrhea.

Approximately 75 percent of all emerging infectious diseases are zoonotic in nature, meaning they are transmitted from animals to people. As humans increasingly encroach on wild habitats, the opportunity to contract such infectious organisms increases. This is the main reason for the increased prevalence in the United States of the infections caused by the water-borne protozoa of the genera *Cryptosporidium* and *Giardia* and of the appearance and spread of Lyme disease, which is caused by a tick-borne bacterium.

All infectious diseases have been emerging diseases at some point in time. Polio and smallpox are two examples. By 1980 smallpox had been eradicated, and by 2011 polio remained endemic (occurring naturally) in only three countries: Afghanistan, Nigeria, and Pakistan. Other examples of emerging diseases include acquired immunodeficiency syndrome (AIDS) and variant Creutzfeldt-Jakob disease (nv-CJD or v-CJD).

The first report of AIDS in science literature was in 1981. Even then the disease was already spreading. According to the Bill & Melinda Gates Foundation and the World Health Organization (WHO), as of 2017 an estimated 37 million people globally were living with the human immunodeficiency virus (HIV), the virus linked to AIDS. Efforts to combat HIV/AIDS include more than $3 billion contributed by the Bill & Melinda Gates Foundation to various global agencies and the foundation's contribution of more than $1.6 billion to the Global Fund to Fight AIDS, Tuberculosis and Malaria. By mid-2017 efforts by WHO had helped 21 million people living in the most affected regions of the world, including Africa and India, achieve treatment for HIV/AIDS.

Malaria is considered a reemerging disease because of its increasing prevalence. It disproportionately affects pregnant women and young children in underdeveloped and developing countries. According to WHO, there were an estimated 216 million cases of malaria in 91 countries in

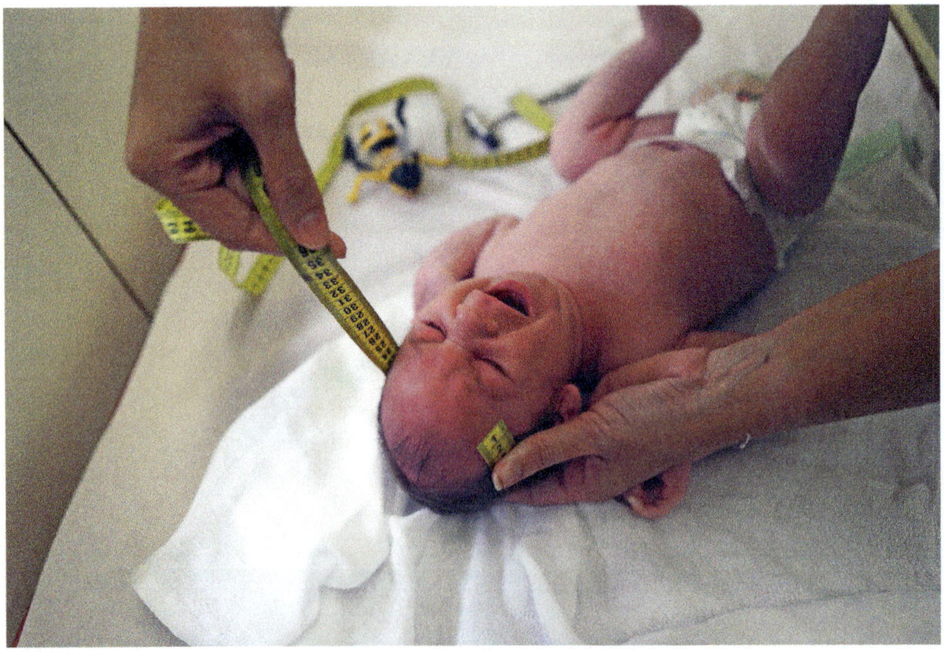

In January 2016, in Recife, Brazil, Dr. Vanessa Van Der Linden measures the head of a two-month-old baby with microcephaly, a condition in which a child is born with an abnormally small head. An outbreak of microcephaly beginning in late 2016 has been attributed to the Zika virus, an emerging infectious disease spread by mosquitoes. © Mario Tama/Getty Images

2016, representing an increase of about 5 million cases from 2015. There were approximately 445,000 deaths due to malaria in 2015 and 2016. Also according to WHO, an estimated 10.4 million people acquired TB and 1.7 million people died of the disease in 2016. That year the disease was ranked in the top 10 causes of death globally, with 95 percent of deaths occurring in poorer nations. The appearance of *M. tuberculosis* that is resistant to multiple antibiotics is of great concern to agencies such as WHO. In May 2007 two cases of TB that were resistant to every drug available to treat the disease were reported. By 2016 WHO estimated that there were 600,000 new cases of multidrug-resistant TB infections. An even more resistant version designated extensively drug resistant (XDR-TB) was still rare as of 2017, though researchers have predicted that the number of cases will increase.

In 2009 an H1N1 influenza virus outbreak began in Mexico and spread north into the United States. Before being contained near the end of that year, more than 18,000 people had died. The virus was first transferred from infected swine to humans, but human-to-human transmission did not occur. However, by around 2005 the virus had acquired the ability for contagious transmission between people, which laid the foundation for an outbreak.

WORDS TO KNOW

ENDEMIC Present in a particular area or among a particular group of people.

PATHOGEN A disease-causing agent, such as a bacterium, virus, fungus, or other microorganism.

RESERVOIR The animal or organism in which a virus or parasite normally resides.

RESISTANT ORGANISM An organism that has developed the ability to counter something trying to harm it. Within infectious diseases, the organism, such as a bacterium, has developed a resistance to drugs, such as antibiotics.

SELECTIVE PRESSURE The tendency of an organism that has certain characteristics to be eliminated from an environment or to increase in number. An example is the increased prevalence of bacteria resistant to multiple kinds of antibiotics.

SENTINEL An epidemiological method in which a subset of the population is surveyed for the presence of communicable diseases. Also, an animal used to indicate the presence of disease within an area.

STRAIN A subclass or a specific genetic variation of an organism.

ZOONOSES Diseases of microbiological origin that can be transmitted from animals to people. The causes of the diseases can be bacteria, viruses, parasites, or fungi.

■ Applications and Research

Scientists have been able to isolate the genetic material from a variety of infectious microorganisms and determine the genetic sequence of the material, a process that can now be completed in just a few days. This development allows researchers to identify the sequences that are important in emerging infectious diseases. The discipline of proteomics, in which the structure and function of proteins are determined, is helping to identify targets for antimicrobial drugs and to design vaccines and other antimicrobial agents that prevent or treat infections.

Disease surveillance is important in monitoring the appearance and spread of emerging infectious diseases. Organizations such as WHO and the US Centers for Disease Control and Prevention (CDC) receive data from global agencies to track the development and spread of infections. This scrutiny is necessary in the era of global travel. Someone infected in one region of the globe can spread the disease within a few days to distant locales via international air travel. Changing climatic conditions also affect the transmission of diseases by mosquitoes and other insects. The movement of Zika virus and avian influenza from more tropical regions of Central and South America to North America is one example.

■ Impacts and Issues

The emergence or reemergence of infectious diseases is influenced by several factors. A nation's economy affects the type and availability of health care. Inadequate vaccination programs and lack of general health care can make it easier for a disease to become established. In addition, the overall heath and nutritional status of citizens in developing nations may be compromised, making them more susceptible to infectious disease.

Of the estimated 37 million people infected with HIV at the end of 2016, two-thirds lived in sub-Saharan Africa. Widespread poverty exacerbates the HIV/AIDS crisis in Africa as drug treatments are typically expensive. Efforts by organizations such as WHO, the United Nations Children's Fund (UNICEF), the CDC, and some pharmaceutical companies are helping make HIV/AIDS drugs less expensive and more widely available in Africa.

One well-known agent of emerging infectious diseases is the increased resistance of a variety of bacteria to antibiotics. The resistance has been driven by the overuse and misuse of antibiotics, such as when combating a viral infection or when antibiotic therapy is stopped too soon. This selective pressure encourages the development of changes in bacteria that confer resistance and aid the proliferation of newly resistant bacteria.

Political change or conflict can favor the proliferation of an existing disease or the spread of an emerging one. Military conflict disables access to food, water, and adequate health care and results in the mass movement of people. Malnutrition and densely populated refugee or displaced persons camps, many of which lack proper sanitation, may exacerbate disease outbreaks. An example is the influenza epidemic that occurred in the aftermath of World War I (1914–1918). Troops returning from the battlefield spread influenza across Europe and to Russia, the United States, Australia, and New Zealand. The pandemic eventually spread worldwide. From 1918 to 1919 influenza claimed at least 20 million people, more than had been killed in the war.

The delivery of health services can be interrupted by changes other than war. For example, the global effort to eradicate polio suffered a setback in 2003 when the government halted vaccination of people in rural regions of Nigeria as a rumor circulated that the vaccine could cause sterility or AIDS. By the time these fears had been quelled and vaccination had resumed in 2004, nearly 700 children had become infected with polio, representing almost 75 percent of the total number of cases reported that year worldwide. In 2005 WHO had reinitiated the polio vaccination campaign in Nigeria. On National Immunization Day in May 2005, approximately 140,000 WHO-sanctioned volunteers went door to door to inoculate every Nigerian child under five years of age.

WHO's Epidemic and Pandemic Alert and Response initiative is responsible for the global coordination of efforts to eradicate emerging infectious diseases such as avian influenza. Its global scope is necessary in the era of rapid travel, as diseases can quickly spread around the globe.

See Also *AIDS (Acquired Immunodeficiency Syndrome); Avian Influenza; Bioterrorism; Climate Change and Infectious Disease; Globalization and Infectious Disease; Pandemic Preparedness; Reemerging Infectious Diseases; Virus Hunters*

BIBLIOGRAPHY

Books

Bayry, Jagadeesh. *Emerging and Re-emerging Infectious Diseases of Livestock.* Cham, Switzerland: Springer, 2017.

Pulcini, Céline, et al, eds. *Antimicrobial Stewardship.* Vol. 2 of *Developments in Emerging and Existing Infectious Diseases.* London: Elsevier/AP, 2017.

Periodicals

Chan, Emily H., et al. "Global Capacity for Emerging Infectious Disease Detection." *Proceedings of the National Academy of Sciences of the United States of America* 107, no. 50 (2010): 21701–21706.

Staples, J. Erin, Robert F. Breiman, and Ann M. Powers. "Chikungunya Fever: An Epidemiological Review of a Re-emerging Infectious Disease." *Clinical Infectious Diseases* 49, no. 6 (2009): 942–948.

Websites

"NIAID Emerging Infectious Diseases/Pathogens." National Institute of Allergy and Infectious Diseases. https://www.niaid.nih.gov/research/emerging-infectious-diseases-pathogens (accessed November 15, 2017).

Brian Hoyle

Encephalitis

Introduction

Encephalitis is a type of acute brain inflammation that is most often the result of an infection caused by a virus. Inflammation occurring in the spinal cord is myelitis, inflammation in both the spinal cord and the brain is encephalomyelitis, and an infection in both areas is encephalitis. The swelling in the brain that occurs in encephalitis can be serious and even life-threatening: brain damage, strokes, seizures, coma, and death can result. Encephalitis often accompanies bacterial meningitis (an infection of the meninges, or lining of the brain).

Disease History, Characteristics, and Transmission

There are two types of encephalitis: a primary form and a secondary form. Primary (or acute) encephalitis is directly due to a new viral infection. This form of encephalitis can be localized in just one region of the brain or spinal cord (focal infection) or can be more widely distributed (diffuse infection).

Secondary encephalitis, or post-infective encephalitis, arises as a consequence of an ongoing viral infection or from an immunization procedure that utilizes a virus. The

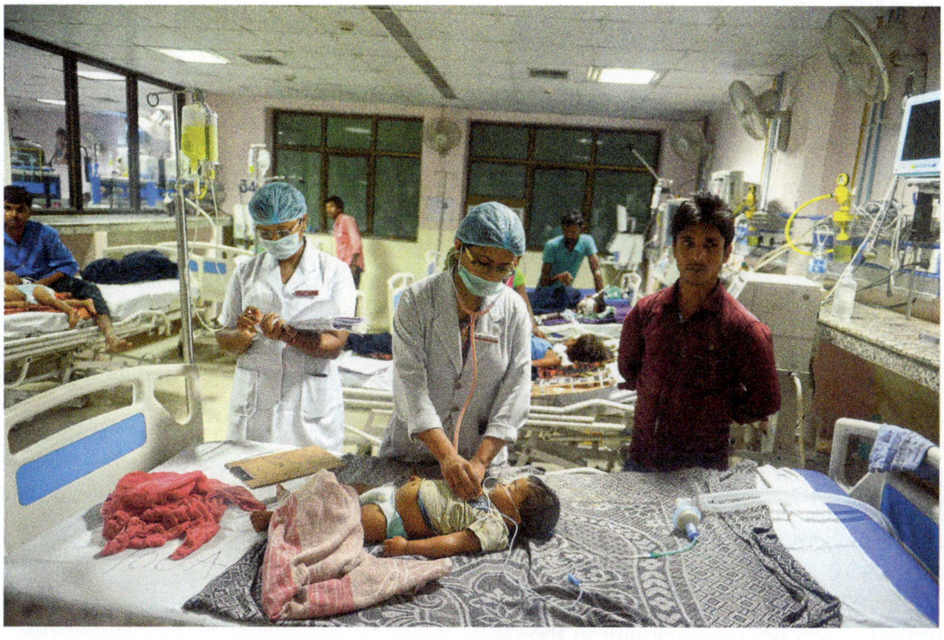

At the Baba Raghav Das Hospital in the northern Indian city of Gorakhpur, staff attend to a child admitted in the hospital's encephalitis ward. *© SANJAY KANOJIA/AFP/Getty Images*

WORDS TO KNOW

ACUTE INFECTION An infection of rapid onset and of short duration that either resolves or becomes chronic.

ARTHROPOD-BORNE DISEASE A disease caused by one of a phylum of organisms characterized by exoskeletons and segmented bodies.

ENTEROVIRUS A group of viruses that contain ribonucleic acid as their genetic material. They are members of the picornavirus family. The various types of enteroviruses that infect humans are referred to as serotypes, in recognition of their different antigenic patterns. The different immune response is important, as infection with one type of enterovirus does not necessarily confer protection to infection by a different type of enterovirus. There are 64 different enterovirus serotypes. The serotypes include polio viruses, coxsackie A and B viruses, echoviruses, and a large number of what are referred to as non-polio enteroviruses.

LATENT Potential or dormant, as in a condition that is not yet manifest or active.

MENINGITIS An inflammation of the meninges, the three layers of protective membranes that line the spinal cord and the brain. Meningitis can occur when there is an infection near the brain or spinal cord, such as a respiratory infection in the sinuses, the mastoids, or the cavities around the ear. Disease organisms can also travel to the meninges through the bloodstream. The first signs may be a severe headache and neck stiffness followed by fever, vomiting, a rash, and then convulsions leading to loss of consciousness. Meningitis generally involves two types: nonbacterial meningitis, or aseptic meningitis, and bacterial meningitis, or purulent meningitis.

VECTOR Any agent that carries and transmits parasites and diseases. Also, an organism or a chemical used to transport a gene into a new host cell.

latter uses a virus that has been altered to be incapable of causing harm. However, in rare cases the vaccine itself becomes harmful. Secondary encephalitis, or acute disseminated encephalitis, typically appears two to three weeks following the first infection or the immunization injection.

Encephalitis caused by herpes simplex virus (HSV) is the most common form of primary encephalitis in the United States, with about 2,000 cases each year. This represents about 10 percent of all cases of encephalitis in the United States. Worldwide, herpes simplex encephalitis also causes about 10 percent of all cases of the disease, although more than half of these cases result in death. Children can develop encephalitis after a bout of measles, mumps, or rubella. These occurrences are rare—approximately 1 in every 1,000 cases, according to the US Centers for Disease Control and Prevention (CDC).

Many cases of encephalitis involve the reactivation of an earlier infection by an HSV that became latent (this occurs when the viral genetic material is incorporated into the host's genetic material). Upon reactivation, production of new copies of the virus resumes, and symptoms associated with the infection appear.

The original infection may occur with herpes simplex type 1 (HSV-1), which commonly causes cold sores and facial blistering. Encephalitis related to this virus can occur in anyone but is most prevalent in people under 20 years of age and older than 40. The disease is contagious, being spread most often by inhalation of water droplets expelled by a cough or sneeze. The person who contracts the infection develops a headache and fever that can last almost a week. Subsequently, changes in personality and behavior, seizures, and delusions may appear, and severe brain damage may result. Encephalitis due to herpes simplex type 2 (HSV-2) is typically spread through sexual contact. Less commonly, a newborn can contract the virus from his or her infected mother during birth.

In the United States and Canada, Powassan encephalitis is transmitted to humans by ticks, which have previously acquired the virus from infected deer. The symptoms of Powassan encephalitis—headache, fever, nausea, and disorientation—begin within two weeks following the tick bite. Paralysis and coma also can occur. About 50 percent of those who contract Powassan encephalitis will have permanent brain damage, and more than 15 percent of those who become infected die of the infection. The illness is rare. According to the CDC, only 100 cases were reported between 2007 and 2017, mostly in the northeastern United States and around the Great Lakes.

In the United States there are four types of mosquito-borne viral encephalitis: equine encephalitis, La Crosse encephalitis, St. Louis encephalitis (SLEV), and West Nile encephalitis (WNE).

Rarely (less than 1 case per 1 million people), a viral form of the disease, infectious limbic system encephalitis, occurs. Areas of the brain that become inflamed include the hippocampus and amygdala. Brain functions that are affected include memory and learning. The primary symptom of this form of encephalitis is memory impairment similar to what is seen in individuals suffering from Alzheimer's disease or Creutzfeldt-Jacob disease. A variation of limbic encephalitis, paraneoplastic limbic encephalitis, is linked to the development of cancer.

■ Scope and Distribution

In the United States there are several thousand reported cases of encephalitis every year. However, according to the US National Institute of Neurological Disorders and Stroke (NINDS), the actual tally is likely much higher because many people do not seek medical help for cases that produce mild symptoms or no symptoms at all.

Encephalitis occurs in many regions of the world. Mosquito-borne forms of encephalitis are present in North and South America, Europe, Russia, Asia, India, Northern Africa, and Australia.

In the United States encephalitis is usually caused by an enterovirus, by HSV-1 and HSV-2, by an arbovirus that is transmitted from an infected animal to humans via a vector such as a mosquito (as occurs in West Nile disease) or tick, or by the bite of a rabid animal such as a raccoon that is infected with the rabies virus. Lyme disease, which is caused by the bacterium *Borrelia burgdorferi*, can also cause encephalitis.

One factor that has contributed to the global distribution of encephalitis is the fact that it is contagious and can be passed from person to person by coughing or sneezing, which release contaminated droplets into the air. In addition, the microorganisms that cause encephalitis can contaminate food and water.

Viral encephalitis that is transmitted to humans via a vector (such as a mosquito or tick) is more common in the United States. One such vector-borne encephalitis is equine encephalitis. As its name implies, equine encephalitis can affect horses. In horses this disease can be serious and often comes before the detection of the disease in humans. A form called Eastern equine encephalitis (EEE) is prevalent along the eastern coastal region of the United States and the coast of the Gulf of Mexico. Fever, muscle aches, and headache develop 3 to 10 days after a person is bitten by a virus-carrying mosquito. The headache becomes progressively worse, and in severe cases a person can lapse into a coma and die. The disease is still rare, despite having been known to occur in the United States since the 1930s. The CDC reported 15 cases in 2012, 8 in both 2013 and 2014, 6 in 2015, and 7 in 2016. Nearly half of those infected died.

The natural host of the EEE virus is still not precisely known, but the virus tends to infect birds that live near freshwater swamps. Whether the virus can survive the winter in northern climates is also unknown. Surveys of birds that live year-round in the northern climates have not detected the virus, and scientists suspect that returning migratory birds in the spring bring the virus back to these areas.

Western equine encephalitis is distributed in the western and central states of the United States. The virus was isolated in the United States in 1930 from an infected horse. Both horses and humans can be affected by this disease. The virus normally resides in a number of species of animals and birds and is transmitted by mosquitoes. Symptoms begin about a week following infection. Children are particularly at risk of developing a severe form of the disease that can produce permanent brain damage.

The prevalence of Western equine encephalitis has been influenced by agricultural practices. For example, the increasing irrigation of land has created more regions of stagnant water, which become breeding grounds for mosquitoes. In addition, the land becomes populated by bird species that naturally carry the virus.

Another form of equine encephalitis, Venezuelan equine encephalitis, has sickened thousands of people in epidemics in Central and South America that have occurred over the past half century. An outbreak in 1962 in Columbia and Venezuela sickened over 23,000 people and resulted in about 160 deaths. In 1992 the same countries experienced another outbreak that affected an estimated 100,000 people; 3,000 experienced brain damage, and approximately 300 died. Smaller outbreaks have continued to occur in Central and South America, Mexico, and Peru. Survivors can have permanent brain damage.

La Crosse encephalitis is another form of vector-borne encephalitis found in the United States. It is named for La Crosse, Wisconsin, where the disease was first detected in 1963. It is typically distributed in midwestern states including Illinois, Indiana, Ohio, Iowa, and Wisconsin but has also occurred in eastern states. The virus is passed to mosquitoes from infected chipmunks and squirrels. Children and adolescents under 16 years of age are most at risk. Headache, fever, vomiting, and fatigue develop about one week following the mosquito bite. In more severe cases a person can experience seizures. About 60 to 100 cases are reported in the United States each year, according to the CDC.

St. Louis encephalitis (SLEV) is another mosquito-borne viral infection. The CDC reported 8 cases in 2010, 4 in 2011, 1 in both 2012 and 2013, 6 in 2014, 19 in 2015, and 7 in 2016. Outbreaks can occur. A 1975 epidemic caused nearly 2,000 reported illnesses in Ohio and central states along the Mississippi River. The disease is transferred to mosquitoes from infected birds. In contrast to other forms of encephalitis, adults are affected more severely than are children. Symptoms include headache, fever, and, in more serious cases, mental disorientation, muscle tremors, convulsions, and unconsciousness.

The final mosquito-borne encephalitis is West Nile disease. Its geographical distribution in the United States has expanded since it was first detected in 1999 with 62 cases in New York state. In 2016 only the state of Alaska had no reported cases, according to the CDC. From 1999 to 2016, 46,086 cases were reported. California reported 6,031 cases, followed by Colorado with 5,362, Texas with 5,277, Nebraska with 3,653, and the remainder spread across all other US states. The disease is also found in Canada, Africa, the Middle East, Russia, India, and Indonesia. People whose immune systems are impaired are most at risk. In addition to transmission by mosquito, the virus can be present in transplanted organs or transfused blood and blood products.

INFLAMMATION AS A NONSPECIFIC DEFENSE

Inflammation is a localized, defensive response of the body to injury, usually characterized by pain, redness, heat, swelling, and, depending on the extent of trauma, loss of function. The process of inflammation, the inflammatory response, is a series of events, or stages, that the body performs to attain homeostasis (the body's effort to maintain stability). The body's inflammatory response mechanism serves to confine, weaken, destroy, and remove bacteria, toxins, and foreign material at the site of trauma or injury. As a result, the spread of invading substances is halted, and the injured area is prepared for regeneration or repair. Inflammation is a nonspecific defense mechanism; the body's physiological response to a superficial cut is much the same as with a burn or a bacterial infection. The inflammatory response protects the body against a variety of invading pathogens and foreign matter and should not be confused with an immune response.

Japanese encephalitis is the most common cause of encephalitis worldwide. Approximately 68,000 cases occur each year with a death rate of up to 30 percent, according to the World Health Organization (WHO). This form of encephalitis is common in certain regions of Asia, including China, Korea, Japan, Taiwan, Sri Lanka, and southern India. It also occurs on some Pacific Islands. The disease is especially prevalent where rice production and pig rearing occur. This is because the mosquitoes that spread the disease can breed in the rice paddies, and pigs are a host of the virus. The mosquitoes acquire the virus when taking a blood meal from a pig and then can spread the virus to humans. Vaccines are available. In the United States the IXIARO vaccine has been approved for people 17 years of age and older since March 2009 and for those 2 months to 16 years of age since May 2013.

■ Treatment and Prevention

The diagnosis of encephalitis involves an assessment of nerve function, hearing, speech, vision, balance and coordination, mental capability, and changes in behavior. The examination of bodily fluids, such as urine and blood, and a swab from the throat can be useful in revealing a bacterial or viral infection.

Tests that rely on the growth of bacteria or the appearance of clear zones in a layer of bacterial growth (clear zones being places where virus production has destroyed the bacteria) take two to three days. Antibody-based tests to detect protein components of the target bacteria or viruses and the use of polymerase chain reaction to amplify and detect specific regions of the viral or bacterial genetic material can produce results in as little as a day.

Other diagnostic procedures rely on imaging the brain or spinal cord. The two most widely used imaging procedures are computed tomography (CT) and magnetic resonance imaging (MRI). These techniques can be sensitive enough to detect inflammation of the meninges. These examinations need to be done promptly, as the inflammation associated with encephalitis can cause damage rapidly.

If viral encephalitis is suspected, treatment usually involves the antiviral drugs acyclovir, ganciclovir, or foscarnet. These drugs are similar in their three-dimensional structure to certain building blocks of the viral genetic material. Incorporation of the drug into the replicating genetic material instead of the normal building block inhibits the activity of an enzyme that is vital for the continued replication of the virus.

Milder cases of encephalitis are treated with bedrest and over-the-counter medications to relieve headache and to make the person feel as comfortable as possible. In more severe cases, hospitalization may be necessary, and drugs may be given to control or prevent seizures. The swelling of the meninges can be reduced using corticosteroids, which are usually administered intravenously to get the drug to the site of swelling quickly and to maintain an effective concentration of the drug.

The best way to prevent encephalitis is to minimize contact with vectors of the disease. Examples of preventive measures include using mosquito repellent, wearing protective clothing when outdoors, and eliminating sources of stagnant water (which can become breeding grounds for mosquitoes). While crucial in helping to avoid contact with vectors, these and other preventive measures are difficult to maintain.

As of 2017 several vaccine formulations were available. In the United States one formulation (IXIARO) was available.

■ Impacts and Issues

Encephalitis can be a devastating disease when it causes lasting effects such as brain damage. A person can be incapable of resuming work or study and can require assistance to perform routine daily tasks. This can place a burden on caregivers and can affect the person's capabilities as a family member and worker.

Sizable outbreaks of encephalitis can occur. In 1995 an outbreak of Venezuelan equine encephalitis in Venezuela and Colombia sickened an estimated 90,000 people. The size of such an outbreak imposes yet another burden on developing countries, particularly those where acquired immunodeficiency syndrome (AIDS) is prevalent. The impaired immune system function that is characteristic of AIDS makes individuals with the disease more susceptible to a wide range of other maladies, including encephalitis.

West Nile encephalitis is an emerging health hazard in the United States. The disease has spread geographically and in the number of reported cases. It has replaced St. Louis encephalitis as the most prevalent form of the disease in the United States. The number of cases reported by the CDC jumped from 66 in 2001 to 4,156 in 2002, which may reflect heightened awareness and more dedicated surveillance of the disease. Since then the annual tally has fluctuated from a high of 9,862 cases in 2003 to 712 in 2011. The tally in 2016 was 2,149 cases.

SEE ALSO *Arthropod-Borne Disease; Climate Change and Infectious Disease; Eastern Equine Encephalitis; Emerging Infectious Diseases; Encephalitis; Japanese Encephalitis; Meningitis, Viral; Mosquito-Borne Diseases; Vector-Borne Disease; West Nile*

BIBLIOGRAPHY

Books

Crosby, Molly Caldwell. *Asleep: The Forgotten Epidemic that Remains One of Medicine's Greatest Mysteries.* Berkley, CA: Berkley Books, 2011.

Periodicals

Aguilar, Patricia V., et al. "Endemic Venezuelan Equine Encephalitis in the Americas: Hidden under the Dengue Umbrella." *Future Virology* 6 (2011): 721–740.

Kennedy, Peter G. E., Phenix-Lan Quan, and W. Ian Lipkin. "Viral Encephalitis of Unknown Cause: Current Perspective and Recent Advances." *Viruses* 9, no. 6 (2017): 138.

Rice, Philip. "Viral Meningitis and Encephalitis." *Medicine* 45, no. 11 (November 2017): 664–669.

Shives, Katherine D., Kenneth L. Tyler, and J. David Beckham. "Molecular Mechanisms of Neuroinflammation and Injury during Acute Viral Encephalitis." *Journal of Neuroimmunology* 308 (July 2017): 102–111.

Websites

"Japanese Encephalitis." World Health Organization. 2015. http://www.who.int/mediacentre/factsheets/fs386/en/ (accessed November 16, 2017).

"West Nile Virus." Centers for Disease Control and Prevention. https://www.cdc.gov/westnile/index.html (accessed November 16, 2017).

Brian Hoyle

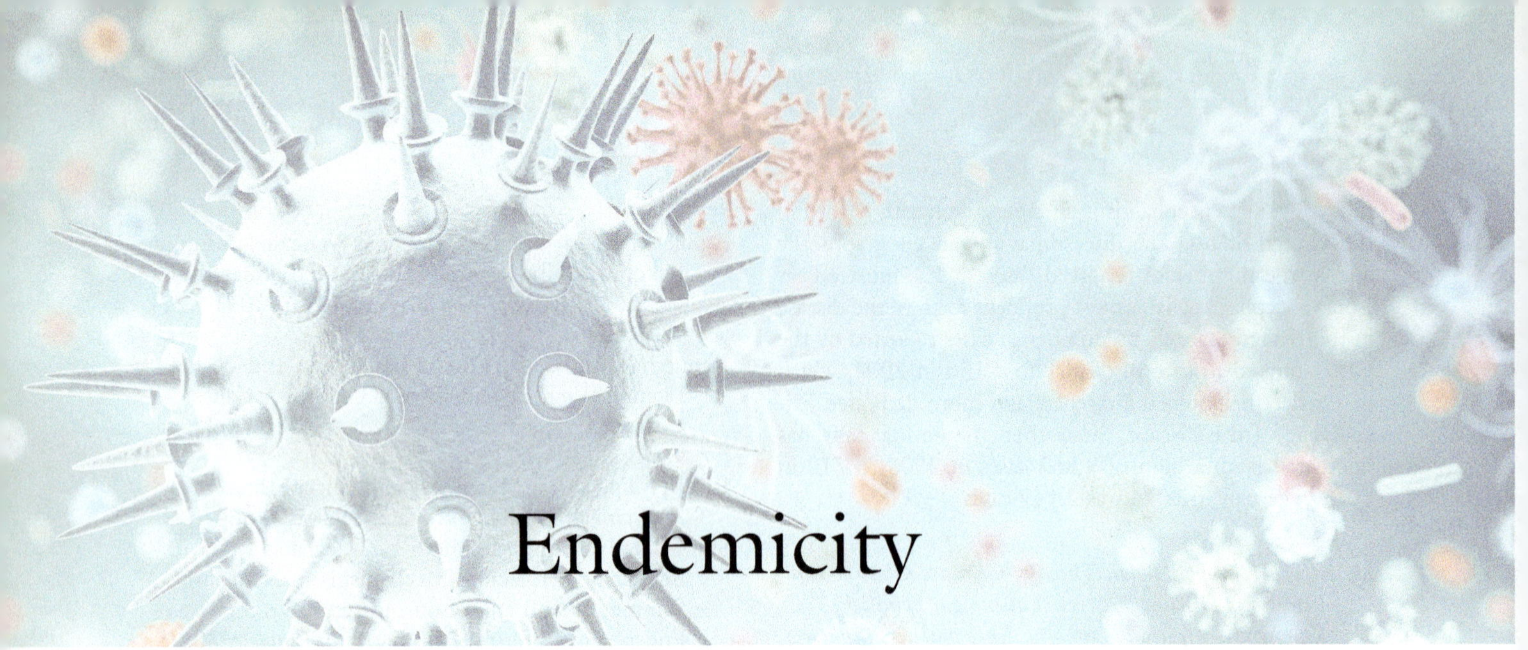

Endemicity

■ Introduction

An endemic disease is one that occurs naturally in a community. This is opposed to an epidemic disease, in which the rate of infection suddenly increases in a community. Endemicity can be measured by determining how common an infection is or by determining the change in rates of infection over time.

The endemicity of a disease may be altered by a number of factors. Human intervention has led to many previously endemic diseases being eradicated from specific regions. This has been achieved by vaccination, as well as by the elimination of the cause of the disease, such as a vector (the organism that aids in the transmission of the disease).

However, endemic diseases can also develop in previously non-endemic regions or can develop into epidemics. This often occurs when infections are introduced or undergo mutation or when conditions within a community change due to events such as wars or natural disasters. The extent to which the change persists influences whether the change in endemicity will be long term.

■ History and Scientific Foundations

An endemic disease is one with a constant rate of infection in a community. When new individuals are born into that community, they become infected, cured, and eventually recover and retain the infection for life or obtain immunity. Conversely, an epidemic occurs when a disease is introduced to a community and multiplies or when the rate of infection of an existing disease increases and causes an excess of cases in a community.

Endemicity can be measured by examining the prevalence rate or incident rate of a disease. Some communities may have higher levels of endemicity, which indicates a higher prevalence of infection. The incident rate refers to the change in the level of infection over time. Many infections tend to show seasonal incident rates, in which the level of infection increases during certain periods. When the incident rate increases above a certain threshold, the disease becomes an epidemic.

Within a community there can be foci, or areas of increased prevalence. Host focality refers to areas in which hosts have more severe infections than other hosts. For example, the infection schistosomiasis is characterized by infection with parasite eggs. Some hosts suffer heavier parasite loads due to more severe infections. When these heavier infections occur in specific areas, they form host foci. Geographic focality refers to a higher prevalence rate of the disease in certain regions. For example, malaria tends to show varying prevalence rates in urban versus rural regions.

The foci of a disease affect the treatment and eventual containment of the disease. If treatment methods aim to treat the entire community to the same extent, foci will maintain the infection. On the other hand, targeting foci will ensure that the infection is contained.

■ Applications and Research

Endemic diseases may not always remain endemic. In some cases, transmission of the disease may increase, causing the disease to become an epidemic. On the other hand, transmission of the disease may decrease, causing the number of cases in the community to go below an endemicity threshold. Many factors can influence the endemicity of a disease. Eradication techniques have played a major role in decreasing the endemicity of certain diseases in the world. Within the United States, measles, which was endemic prior to 1997, is no longer considered an endemic disease due to vaccination efforts. Similarly, malaria, which is still endemic in some regions of the world, has been eradicated from the United States and some Western European countries following large-scale eradication efforts.

The viral disease measles is highly communicable among humans. As a result, it is endemic in many regions of the world. In the United States, measles was once a common childhood disease, with over 90 percent of children under the age of 12 infected. However, following the introduction of a measles vaccine in 1963, measles outbreaks have decreased. Vaccination is an effective way of increasing the immunity of a population and causing a decrease in the transmissibility of an infection. As a result, when most or all of a population is vaccinated against a certain disease, that disease does not retain its endemic state. However, in 2008, 2011, and 2013 through 2015, there were more cases of measles in the United States than normal. This uptick was caused in part by a small number of people choosing not to vaccinate their children and by international travelers bringing the disease home with them from countries where there were measles outbreaks.

Vaccinations have not been developed for all infectious diseases. As a result, other methods must be used to control some endemic diseases. Malaria is an example of an endemic infectious disease that cannot be controlled by vaccination. This disease is transmitted via mosquitoes, which infect new hosts when they feed on them. Eradication efforts involved spraying human living spaces with dichlorodiphenyltrichloroethane (DDT), a toxic insecticide that kills mosquitoes (DDT was banned from use in most developing countries in the 1980s). This technique was designed to remove the mode of transmission for the disease (in this case, the mosquito vector), with the expectation that this would prevent the spread of the disease.

Worldwide efforts to completely eradicate malaria have not been as successful. A variety of problems, such as mosquito tolerance to DDT, banning of DDT use, outbreaks of war, lack of funding, and population movements, have hindered efforts to eradicate malaria worldwide. Health authorities now attempt to control outbreaks of malaria rather than to eradicate it completely.

Ren Minghui, the assistant director-general for HIV/AIDS, Tuberculosis, Malaria and Neglected Tropical Diseases at the World Health Organization (WHO), noted in a 2016 article for WHO that eliminating endemic diseases has numerous barriers, but it is possible to eliminate many diseases that still negatively affect humankind, such as malaria. He wrote, "From the outset, the fight against infectious diseases has been dogged by social, legal and economic barriers, and funding gaps have been significant. These are a major reason why HIV, TB [tuberculosis], malaria, viral hepatitis and neglected tropical diseases (NTDs) still kill more than 4 million people every year."

In the 21st century, developing nations often are more affected by endemic infectious diseases than developed countries. In addition, because many developing countries are located in or adjacent to the tropics, they are especially affected by neglected tropical diseases, which receive less study than diseases that affect the developed world.

WORDS TO KNOW

ENDEMIC Present in a particular area or among a particular group of people.

EPIDEMIC From the Greek *epidemic*, meaning "prevalent among the people," is most commonly used to describe an outbreak of an illness or a disease in which the number of individual cases significantly exceeds the usual or expected number of cases in any given population.

FOCI In medicine, a focus is a primary center of some disease process (for example, a cluster of abnormal cells). Foci is pleural for focus (more than one focus).

GEOGRAPHIC FOCALITY The physical location of a disease pattern, epidemic, or outbreak; the characteristics of a location created by interconnections with other places.

HOST FOCALITY The tendency of some animal hosts, such as rodents carrying hantavirus and other viruses, to exist in groups in specific geographical locations, acting as a local reservoir of infection.

INCIDENCE The number of new cases of a disease or an injury that occur in a population during a specified period of time.

PREVALENCE The actual number of cases of disease (or injury) that exist in a population.

VECTOR Any agent that carries and transmits parasites and diseases. Also, an organism or a chemical used to transport a gene into a new host cell.

■ Impacts and Issues

Endemicity can develop in countries in which the disease did not previously exist or only existed in low numbers. A disease may be introduced to countries with no history of the disease and thus no immunity against it. Endemicity may develop as the disease spreads unchecked throughout the community. If transmission continues to infect an increasing number of people, the endemic disease may develop into an epidemic. This happened with the Zika virus in 2015, a disease spread by certain mosquitoes.

ENDEMIC DISEASE AND THE PANAMA CANAL

Endemic diseases such as yellow fever, plague, and malaria had frustrated earlier French attempts to build a canal through the Isthmus of Panama by disabling and killing thousands of project workers and managers. William Crawford Gorgas (1854–1920), chief of sanitary affairs for the American project, made the canal possible by organizing public health and sanitation efforts. It was not ignorance of public health principles that had doomed earlier efforts to build the canal but a lack of effective public health organization and the thorough implementation of disease control measures.

Endemicity may also develop when a disease that is usually only transmitted from animal to human begins to be transmitted between humans, causing an increased rate of human infection. For example, avian influenza, or bird flu, tends to be predominantly spread between birds and occasionally from bird to human. However, the virus that causes this disease may mutate, allowing it to be transmitted more easily between birds and humans and, perhaps, between human hosts. Therefore, avian influenza is being closely monitored to keep it from becoming endemic—and possibly—an epidemic.

Not only can certain conditions cause a disease to become endemic, but some conditions may prompt an endemic disease to develop into an epidemic. Climate change and disasters, such as floods or wars, may cause changes that favor disease transmission. Some diseases, such as malaria, are dependent on an arthropod vector to spread among hosts. A change in the climate, such as increased temperature or moisture, may be favorable to the vector, causing an increased number of vectors in a region. This increases the chance that a human will become infected. If a disease is already endemic in the region, an increase in the number of cases may result in an epidemic.

Disasters, such as war or floods, may also cause other, more favorable conditions for a disease. For example, during war or following a flood or earthquake, a large number of people are often required to live together in close quarters, often with only basic sanitation. As a result, diseases are more easily transmitted. Airborne diseases benefit from the close proximity of people, orally transmitted diseases benefit from the poor sanitation conditions, and vector-borne diseases benefit from conditions that promote vector breeding. Therefore, diseases may erupt during these times. However, when people are allowed to return to their homes, conditions change again and may no longer favor the transmission of infectious diseases. This can cause the transmission rate to decrease and thus a disease may no longer be endemic or an epidemic.

SEE ALSO *Arthropod-Borne Disease; Avian Influenza; Bilharzia (Schistosomiasis); Climate Change and Infectious Disease; Epidemiology; Host and Vector; Immigration and Infectious Disease; Influenza; Influenza Pandemic of 1918; Influenza, Tracking Seasonal Influences and Virus Mutation; Malaria; Measles (Rubeola); Mosquito-Borne Diseases; Pandemic Preparedness; Sanitation; Travel and Infectious Disease; United Nations Millennium Goals and Infectious Disease; Vector-Borne Disease; War and Infectious Disease*

BIBLIOGRAPHY

Books

Bennett, John E., Raphael Dolin, and Martin J. Blaser. *Mandell, Douglas, and Bennett's Principles and Practice of Infectious Diseases.* 8th ed. Philadelphia: Elsevier/Saunders, 2015.

Harrison, Mark. *Contagion: How Commerce Has Spread Disease.* New Haven, CT: Yale University Press, 2012.

Nelson, Kenrad E., and Carolyn F. Masters Williams, eds. *Infectious Disease Epidemiology: Theory and Practice.* 3rd ed. Sudbury, MA: Jones and Bartlett, 2014.

Periodicals

Cohen, Jon. "Zika Has All but Disappeared in the Americas. Why?" *Science* (August 16, 2017). This article can also be found online at http://www.sciencemag.org/news/2017/08/zika-has-all-disappeared-americas-why (accessed February 9, 2018).

Leventhal, Gabriel E., et al. "Evolution and Emergence of Infectious Diseases in Theoretical and Real-World Networks." *Nature Communications* 6, no. 6101 (2015). This article can also be found online at https://www.nature.com/articles/ncomms7101 (accessed February 9, 2018).

Paules, Catharine I., and Anthony S. Fauci. "Emerging and Reemerging Infectious Diseases: The Dichotomy between Acute Outbreaks and Chronic Endemicity." *Journal of the American Medical Association* 317, no. 7 (February 2017): 691–692. This article can also be found online at https://jamanetwork.com/journals/jama/article-abstract/2598516?redirect=true (accessed February 9, 2018).

Websites

"Avian Influenza." Centers for Disease Control and Prevention, April 13, 2017.http://www.cdc.gov/flu/avian/gen-info/pdf/avian_facts.pdf (accessed February 9, 2018).

"Malaria." Centers for Disease Control and Prevention, January 26, 2018. https://www.cdc.gov/malaria/ (accessed February 9, 2018).

Minghui, Ren. "Endemic Infectious Diseases: The Next 15 Years." World Health Organization, August 17, 2016. http://www.who.int/mediacentre/commentaries/2016/Endemic-infectious-diseases-next-15-years/en/ (accessed February 9, 2018).

Tony Hawas
Claire Skinner

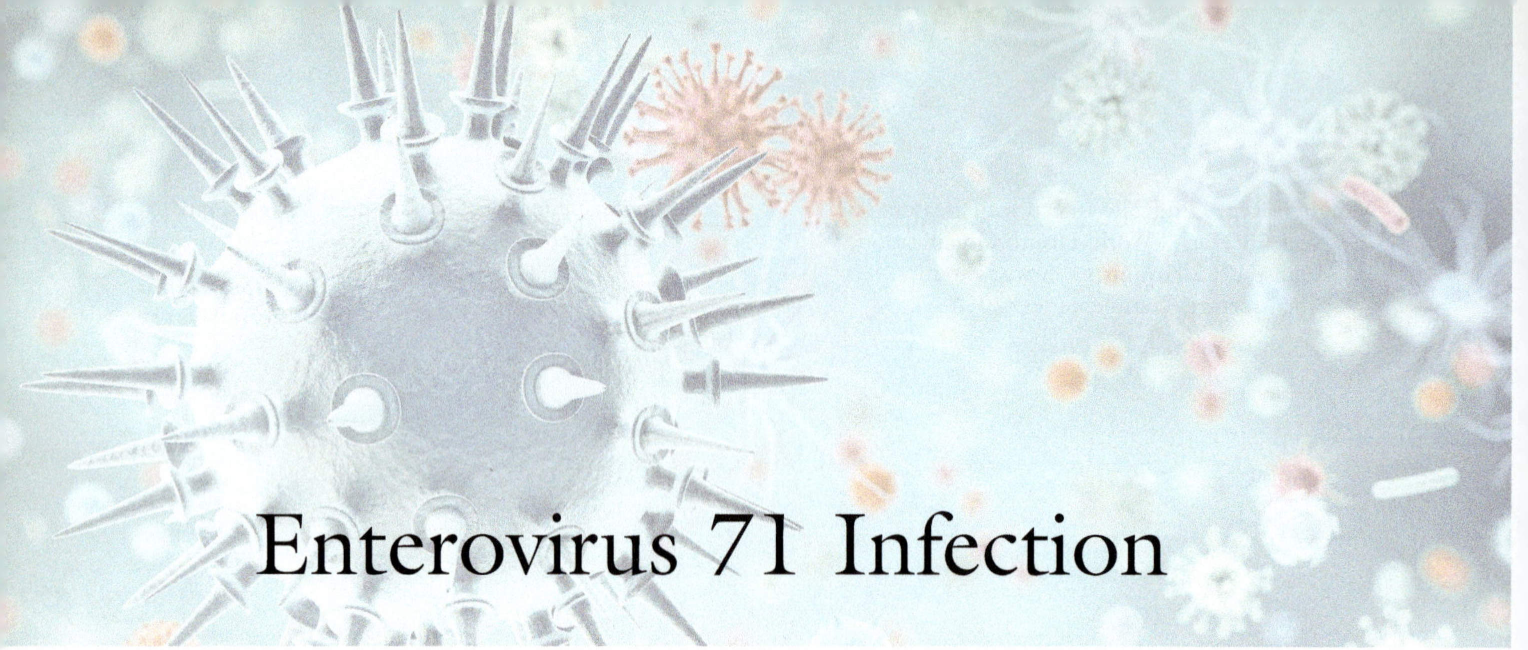

Enterovirus 71 Infection

■ Introduction

Enterovirus 71 infection is an infection caused by the enterovirus 71 (EV71) virus. The virus is part of a large family of viruses called Picornaviridae, within the genus *Enterovirus*. The virus is classified as human enterovirus species A, which is abbreviated HEV-A. EV71 inhabits the gastrointestinal tract (gut) of humans.

EV71 is a small, non-enveloped virus made of a single strand of ribonucleic acid (RNA). EV71 infection, considered a neurological disease, is common in infants and young children. EV71 is one of many pathogens that cause hand, foot, and mouth disease (HFMD), which creates sores in the mouth and a rash on the hands and feet. Although cases and outbreaks of EV71 infection are rare, the virus can produce illnesses ranging from the very mild to

WORDS TO KNOW

EPIDEMIC From the Greek meaning "prevalent among the people," an outbreak of an illness or a disease in which the number of individual cases significantly exceeds the usual or expected number of cases in any given population.

FECAL-ORAL TRANSMISSION The spread of disease through the transmission of minute particles of fecal material from one organism to the mouth of another organism. This can occur by drinking contaminated water, eating food that was exposed to animal or human feces (perhaps by watering plants with unclean water), or by the poor hygiene practices of those preparing food.

PATHOGEN A disease-causing agent, such as a bacterium, a virus, a fungus, or another microorganism.

RIBONUCLEIC ACID (RNA) Any of a group of nucleic acids (complex molecules that contain a cell's genetic information and the instructions for carrying out cellular processes) that carry out important tasks in the synthesis of proteins. Unlike deoxyribonucleic acid (DNA), RNA has a single strand. In eukaryotic cells RNA and DNA work together to direct protein synthesis. Although DNA contains the instructions for directing the synthesis of specific structural and enzymatic proteins, several types of RNA carry out the processes required to produce these proteins. These include messenger RNA (mRNA), ribosomal RNA (rRNA), and transfer RNA (tRNA). Further processing of the various RNAs is carried out by another type of RNA called small nuclear RNA (snRNA). The structure of RNA is very similar to that of DNA; however, instead of the base thymine, RNA contains the base uracil.

VIRUS Nonliving repositories of nucleic acid that require the presence of a living prokaryotic or eukaryotic cell for the replication of the nucleic acid. A number of different viruses challenge the human immune system and may produce disease in humans. A virus is a small, infectious agent that consists of a core of genetic material—either deoxyribonucleic acid (DNA) or ribonucleic acid (RNA)—surrounded by a shell of protein. Very simple microorganisms, viruses are much smaller than bacteria that enter and multiply within cells. Viruses often exchange or transfer their genetic material (DNA or RNA) to cells and can cause diseases such as chickenpox, hepatitis, measles, and mumps.

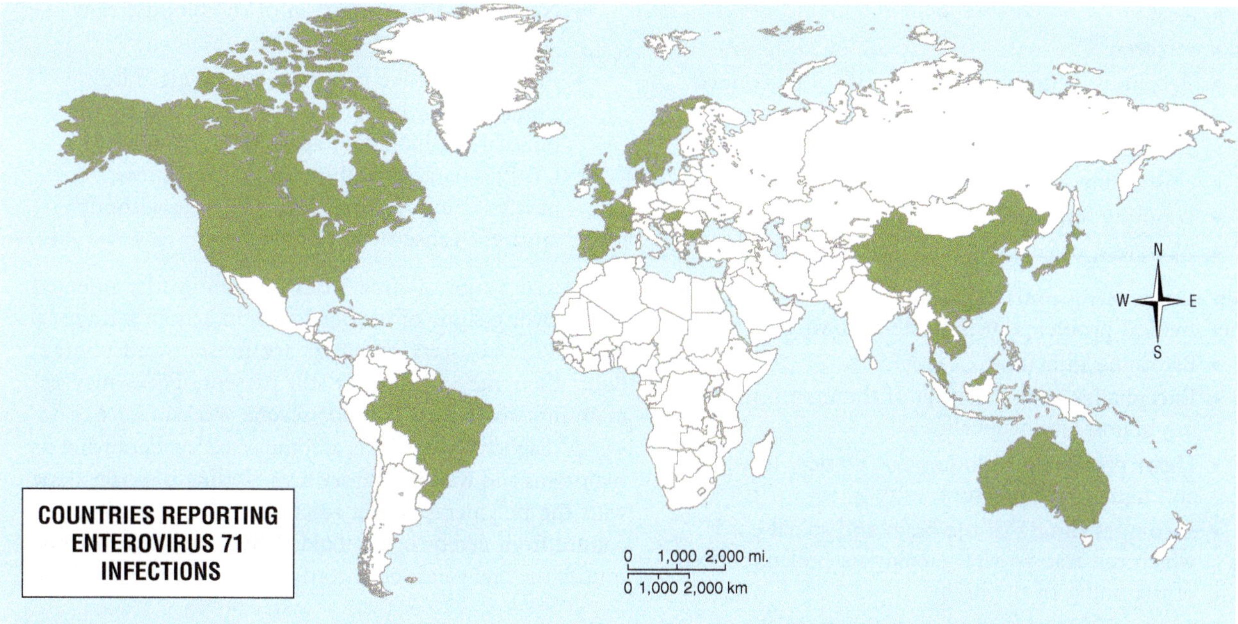

SOURCE: Adapted from Pen-Nien Huang and Shin-Ru Shih. "Update on Enterovirus 71 Infection." *Current Opinion in Virology* 5 (April 2014): 98–104.

the very serious, including life-threatening situations, permanent brain damage, or even death.

Disease History, Characteristics, and Transmission

EV71 was first isolated in the United States in 1969. Since then it has been reported around the world as a major cause of HFMD in infants and young children. It is frequently found in Asia, Australia, Europe, and the United States.

According to a 2010 article in the *Journal of Virology*, fatalities from the newly isolated EV71 virus, which had evolved into HFMD, were reported in Bulgaria in 1975, Hungary in 1978, Malaysia in 1997, and Taiwan in 1998. Forty-one deaths of children were reported in Malaysia.

In the early 21st century, higher fatality rates were reported in the Asia-Pacific region after a series of EV71-associated HFMD epidemics. From 2008 to 2009, China disclosed about 1.5 million infections and 2,457 deaths from EV71-associated HFMD. Since that time EV71 epidemics have been described outside of the Asia-Pacific region, specifically in France, Hungary, the Netherlands, Norway, the United Kingdom, and the United States.

EV71 is transmitted from person to person primarily through contaminated hands or objects that contain infected feces. Once a person touches the virus, he or she may take it in through the mouth or throat, or it may be spread through nasal liquids such as mucus (produced by the nose and sinuses), phlegm (produced by the lower airways), or saliva (produced by the glands). EV71 infection is most frequently found in young children. The infection process is called fecal-oral transmission.

Symptoms of mild cases of EV71 infection, which are similar to symptoms found in HFMD, include the following:

- Fever, usually slight in nature
- Loss of appetite
- Rash, usually located on the palms of the hands and the soles of the feet but sometimes also on the buttocks and genitals
- Sores within the mouth, usually before the appearance of blisters or ulcers
- Tiredness or sleepiness
- Ulcers or blisters, especially on the hands and feet and inside the mouth (mostly inside the cheeks, on the gums, and on the tongue), usually appearing as small, red spots with blisters followed by the formation of ulcers

Normally, the EV71 infection causes a mild illness in healthy adults and older children. However, younger children, those under the age of five years and especially those under two years, are at exceptionally higher risk for developing severe cases of the infection.

Symptoms of severe cases of EV71 infection include the following:

- Cough
- Fever, especially if persistent or with extremely high temperatures
- Irritability
- Paralysis

- Rash
- Seizures
- Sleepiness or drowsiness, especially if prolonged and persistent
- Stiff neck
- Unsteadiness
- Vomiting, especially if repeating
- Weakness, usually within the extremities

Such serious symptoms can lead to neurological and other medical problems such as the following:

- Breathing difficulties
- Encephalitis (inflammation of the brain), including brainstem encephalitis
- Heart problems, including fast or slow heart rate and high blood pressure
- Meninges (lining of the brain and spinal cord), which can lead to viral meningitis (inflammation of the lining of the brain)
- Myocarditis (inflammation of the middle layer of the heart muscle)
- Neonatal sepsis (infection of the bloodstream within a newborn baby)
- Poliomyelitis-like paralysis (a paralytic state similarly found in polio but not caused by the poliovirus), including acute flaccid paralysis (AFP), characterized by sudden weakness, paralysis, and decreased muscle tone without apparent cause

The usual range of time from becoming first infected and showing signs of having EV71 infection is three to five days. If blisters or ulcers are present and contain fluid, then the infection is still present. Feces may remain infected with EV71 for several weeks.

A diagnosis of EV71 is accomplished by identifying its symptoms and with laboratory tests. Testing is usually done with the polymerase chain reaction (PCR) test or with a culture from cerebrospinal fluid (CSF), the fluid that surrounds the brain and spinal cord; feces; or throat secretions.

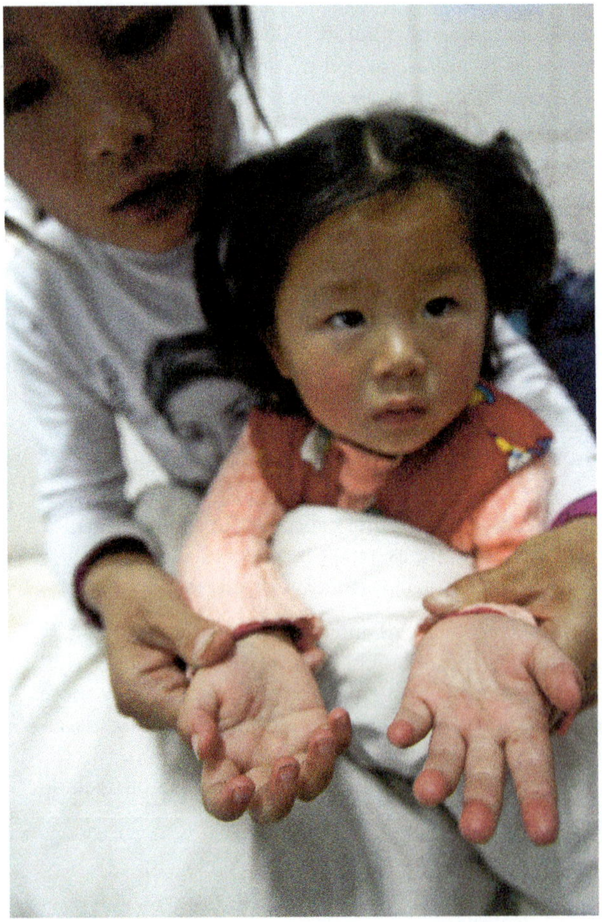

A two-year-old Chinese girl who has contracted enterovirus 71 shows her blistered hands, which are one symptom of the sometimes lethal intestinal virus. © *China Photos/Getty Images*

■ Scope and Distribution

EV71 infection is commonly found in the Asia-Pacific region and especially in Southeast Asia. It is prevalent during the late spring, summer, and early fall months. However, in tropical climates, it may be present throughout the year.

Outbreaks of EV71 infection are frequently reported in, but not limited to, Australia, China, Malaysia, Singapore, and Taiwan. As of February 2018, the most recent outbreak of EV71 neurological disease in Australia was in Perth in 1999. At that time 14 cases were reported.

■ Treatment and Prevention

Treatment for EV71 infection is the same as for any viral infection. As of 2018 a special treatment for EV71 infection was not available. If the symptoms become severe, then hospitalization is necessary to ensure that complications to the brain and spinal cord do not occur.

As of 2018 clinical trials for a vaccine for EV71 infection were ongoing. Phase 3 clinical trials (those that test drugs on patients to evaluate effectiveness, efficacy, and safety) for three potential vaccines had been completed in China, but approval of any of these vaccines had yet to be reached.

People with EV71 should remain home and avoid public or social situations until their blisters have dried up. To prevent the spread of EV71, people should take the following precautions:

- Avoid close contact with other people.

- Cover coughs and sneezes with disposable tissues, or cover them with an arm (not a hand). Dispose of used tissues immediately, followed with thorough washing of the hands.
- Maintain personal hygiene, such as thorough washing of hands with soap and water for at least 20 seconds, especially after using the toilet, before eating or handling food, after coughing or sneezing, and after touching blisters or ulcers.
- Regularly clean surfaces, such as toys, furniture, kitchen counters, and other common household items, with detergent and warm water, especially after contamination has occurred, such as from coughing or sneezing.
- Use separate towels and other personal items instead of sharing. Dispose of or clean them immediately.

■ Impacts and Issues

Children with EV71 neurological disease should stay away from all school and other outside-the-home activities until a doctor or public health official has approved them returning to such normal activities. That clearance means that the virus is no longer present in the child's excrement.

Because the EV71 virus is one of the main causes of HFMD in infants and young children, it is considered a major emerging threat to global public health. In fact, in a study published in *Scientific Reports*, Kang Li Lu Han and colleagues declared, "In the absence of efficacious therapy for severe infections and preventive vaccines, outbreaks and recurrent EV71 epidemics are major threats to public health and cause widespread panic during epidemics."

SEE ALSO *Immune Response to Infection; Public Health and Infectious Disease; Viral Disease*

BIBLIOGRAPHY

Books

David, Michael, and Jean-Luc Benoit, eds. *The Infectious Disease Diagnosis: A Case Approach*. Cham, Switzerland: Springer, 2018.

MacLachlan, N. James, and Edward J. Dubovi. *Fenner's Veterinary Virology*. 5th ed. Amsterdam: Academic Press, 2016.

Tselis, Alex C., and John Booss, eds. *Neurovirology*. Amsterdam: Elsevier, 2014.

Periodicals

Lee, Kyung Yeon. "Enterovirus 71 Infection and Neurological Complications." *Korean Journal of Pediatrics* 59, no. 10 (October 2016): 395–401. This article can also be found online at https://www.ncbi.nlm.nih.gov/pmc/articles/PMC5099286/ (accessed February 5, 2018).

Lu Han, Kang Li, et al. "Human Enterovirus 71 Protein Interaction Network Prompts Antiviral Drug Repositioning." *Scientific Reports* 7, no. 43143 (2017). This article can also be found online at https://www.nature.com/articles/srep43143 (accessed February 5, 2018).

Tee, Kok Keng, et al. "Evolutionary Genetics of Human Enterovirus 71: Origin, Population Dynamics, Natural Selection, and Seasonal Periodicity of the VP1 Gene." *Journal of Virology* 84, no. 7 (2010): 3339–3350. This article can also be found online at http://jvi.asm.org/content/84/7/3339.full (accessed February 5, 2018).

Websites

"Enterovirus 71 (EV71) Infection—Including Symptoms, Treatment and Prevention." SA Health, Government of South Australia. http://www.sahealth.sa.gov.au/wps/wcm/connect/public+content/sa+health+internet/health+topics/health+conditions+prevention+and+treatment/infectious+diseases/enterovirus+71+ev71+infection/enterovirus+71+%28ev71%29+infection+-+inlcuding+symptoms+treatment+and+prevention (accessed February 5, 2018).

"Enterovirus 71 (EV71) Neurological Disease." Queensland Government, December 10, 2017. http://conditions.health.qld.gov.au/HealthCondition/condition/14/217/45/Enterovirus-71-EV71-Neurological-Disease (accessed February 5, 2018).

"Hand, Foot & Mouth Disease." Centers for Disease Control and Prevention, June 26, 2017. https://www.cdc.gov/features/handfootmouthdisease/index.html (accessed February 5, 2018).

William Arthur Atkins

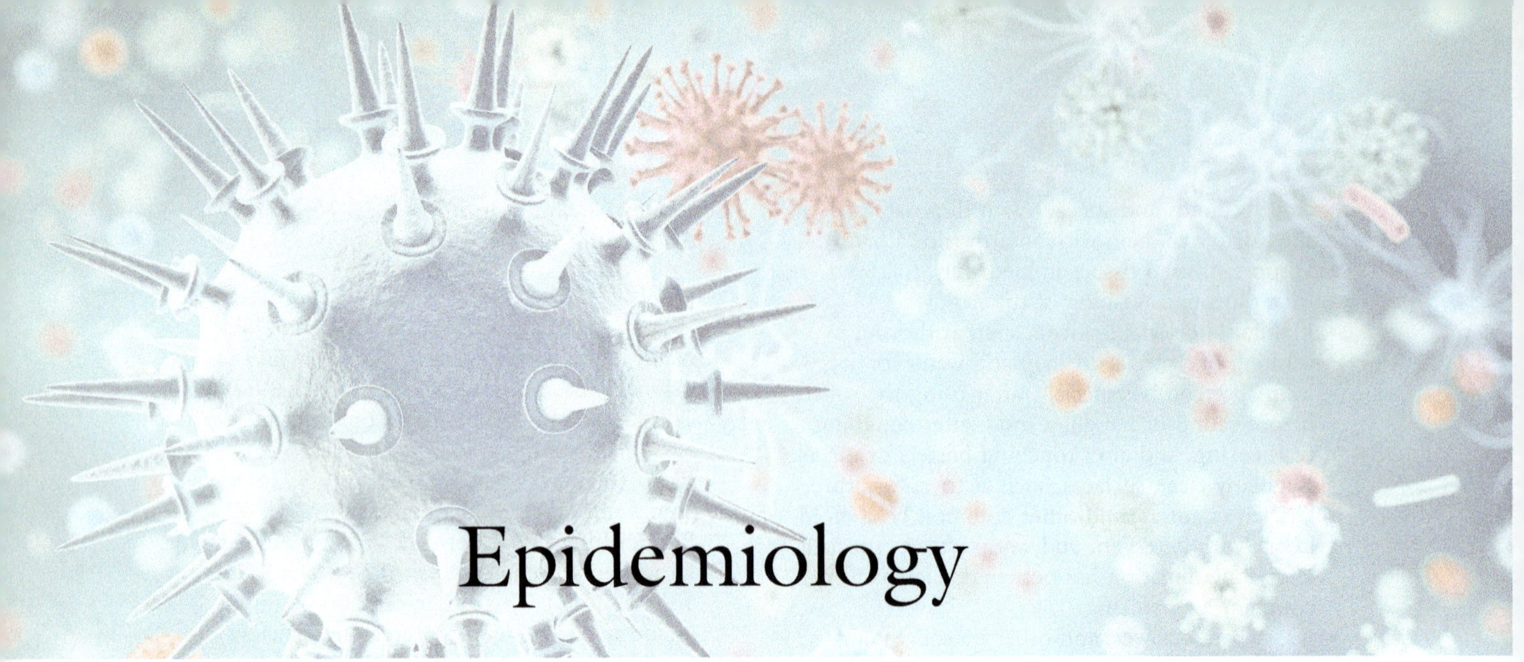

Epidemiology

Introduction

Epidemiology is the study of the causes and distribution of illness and injury. It constitutes the scientific underpinning of public health practice. According to noted British epidemiologist Sir Richard Doll (1912–2005), "Epidemiology is the simplest and most direct method of studying the causes of disease in humans, and many major contributions have been made by studies that have demanded nothing more than an ability to count, to think logically and to have an imaginative idea." In practice, epidemiology is applied in the three main areas of public health: safety and injuries, chronic disease, and infectious disease.

WORDS TO KNOW

INCIDENCE The number of new cases of a disease or an injury that occur in a population during a specified period.

MORBIDITY From the Latin word *morbus*, meaning "sick," the state of being ill and the severity of the illness. A serious disease is said to have a high morbidity.

MORTALITY The condition of being susceptible to death. The term comes from the Latin word *mors*, which means "death." Mortality can also refer to the rate of deaths caused by an illness or injury.

NOTIFIABLE DISEASES Diseases that the law requires must be reported to health officials when diagnosed, including active tuberculosis and several sexually transmitted diseases; also called reportable diseases.

PREVALENCE The number of cases of disease or injury that exist in a population.

SURVEILLANCE The systematic analysis, collection, evaluation, interpretation, and dissemination of data. In public health, surveillance assists in the identification of health threats and the planning, implementation, and evaluation of responses to those threats.

History and Scientific Foundations

The first physician known to consider the fundamental concepts of disease causation was the ancient Greek Hippocrates (c. 460 BCE–c. 377 BCE), when he wrote that medical thinkers should consider the climate and seasons, the air, the water that people use, the soil, and people's eating, drinking, and exercise habits in a region. Subsequently, these causes of diseases were often considered but, until the 20th century, not quantitatively measured. In 1662 John Graunt (1620–1674), a London haberdasher, published an analysis of the weekly reports of births and deaths in London, the first statistical description of population disease patterns. Among his findings, he noted a higher death rate for men than women, a high infant mortality rate, and seasonal variations in mortality. His study, with its meticulous counting and disease pattern description, set the foundation for modern public health practice.

Graunt's data collection and analytical methodology was furthered by physician William Farr (1807–1883), who assumed responsibility for medical statistics for England and Wales in 1839 and set up a system for the routine collection of the numbers and causes of deaths. In analyzing statistical relationships between disease and such circumstances as marital status, such occupations as mining and working with earthenware, and such physical characteristics as elevation above sea level and imprisonment, he addressed many of the basic methodological issues that contemporary epidemiologists deal with. These issues include defining populations at risk for disease and the relative disease risk between population groups, as well as considering whether associations between disease and the factors mentioned above might be caused by other factors, such as age, length of exposure to a condition, or overall health.

A generation later public health research came into its own as a practical tool when another British physician, John Snow (1813–1858), tested the hypothesis that a cholera epidemic in London was being transmitted by contaminated water. By examining death rates from cholera, he realized that they were significantly higher in areas supplied with water by the Lambeth and the Southwark and Vauxhall companies, which drew their water from a part of the Thames River that was grossly polluted with sewage. When the Lambeth Company changed the location of its water source to another part of the river that was relatively less polluted, rates of cholera in the areas served by that company declined, while no change occurred among the areas served by Southwark and Vauxhall. Areas of London served by both companies experienced a cholera death rate that was intermediate between the death rates in the areas supplied by just one of the companies. The geographic pattern of infections was carefully recorded and plotted on a map of London. In recognizing the grand but simple natural experiment posed by the change in the Lambeth Company water source, Snow was able to make a uniquely valuable contribution to epidemiology and public health practice.

After Snow's seminal work, investigations by epidemiologists have come to include many chronic diseases with complex and often still unknown causal agents, and the methods of epidemiology have become similarly complex. In the 21st century, researchers use genetics, molecular biology, and microbiology as investigative tools, and the methods used to establish relative disease risk make use of the most advanced statistical techniques available. Yet, reliance on meticulous counting and categorizing of cases and the imperative to think logically and avoid the pitfalls in mathematical relationships in medical data remain at the heart of all of the research used to show elevated disease risk in population subgroups and to prove that medical treatments are safe and effective.

Basic Epidemiological Concepts and Terms

The most basic concepts in epidemiology are the measures used to discover whether a statistical association exists between various factors and disease. These measures include various kinds of rates, proportions, and ratios. Mortality (death) and morbidity (disease) rates are the raw material that researchers use in establishing disease causation. Morbidity rates are most usefully expressed in terms of disease incidence (the rate with which members of a population or research sample contract a disease) and prevalence (the proportion of the group that has a disease over a given period).

The most important task in epidemiology is the assessment or measurement of disease risk. The population at risk is the group of people that could potentially contract a disease, which can range from the entire world population (as in the case of the flu) to a small group of people within a remote and isolated community (as in the case of an ecologically restricted parasite). The most basic measure of

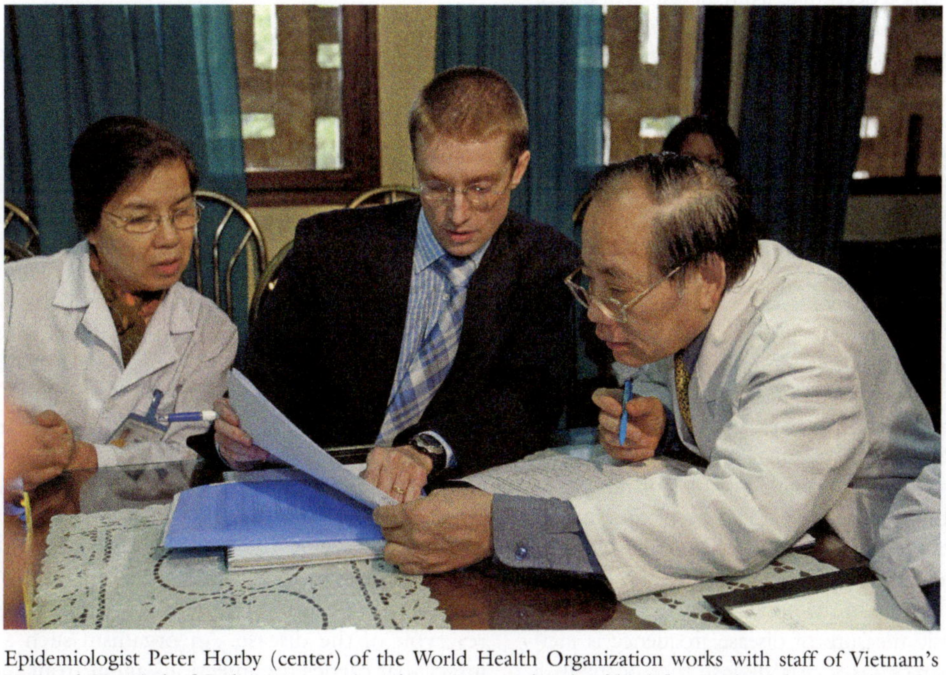

Epidemiologist Peter Horby (center) of the World Health Organization works with staff of Vietnam's National Hospital of Pediatrics to review data on an outbreak of bird flu. Epidemiology involves the study of how and why diseases spread within populations. *© Paula Bronstein/Getty Images*

a population group's risk for a disease is relative risk, or the ratio of the prevalence of a disease in one group with particular biological, demographic, or behavioral characteristics to the prevalence in another group with different characteristics.

The simplest measure of relative risk is the odds ratio, which is the ratio of the odds that a person in one group has a disease to the odds that a person in a second, comparator group has the disease. The odds for contracting a disease are the ratio between the proportion of people in a population group that share particular characteristics that put them at risk for a disease to the proportion of people in a reference or control population (often the general population in a certain region or jurisdiction). For example, patients with chronic obstructive pulmonary disease (COPD), an inflammatory condition of the lungs associated with smoking and long exposure to air pollution, are at significantly greater risk of contracting community-acquired pneumonia (CAP) compared to a general population group matched on age and gender. Thus, for a sample of subjects that includes both COPD patients and subjects who do not have COPD, epidemiologists expect that the odds ratio for the COPD patients contracting CAP would be significantly greater than 1.0 (the numeric value denoting equal risk).

The mortality rate is the ratio of the number of deaths in a population, either in total or disease-specific, to the total number of members of that population. It is usually given in terms of a large population denominator, so that the numerator may be expressed as a whole number. In 1982 the number of deaths from all causes was 1,973,000, and the number of people in the United States was 231,534,000, yielding a death rate from all causes of 852.1 per 100,000 per year. That same year there were 1,807 deaths from tuberculosis, yielding a disease-specific mortality rate of 7.8 per million per year.

Assessing disease frequency is more complex because of the factors of time and disease duration. For example, disease prevalence can be assessed at a point in time (point prevalence) or over a period, usually a year (period prevalence, annual prevalence). This is the prevalence that is usually measured in illness surveys that are reported to the public in the news. Researchers can also measure prevalence over an indefinite period, as in the case of lifetime prevalence, which is the prevalence of a disease over the course of the entire life of the people in the population under study up to the point in time when the researchers make the assessment. Researchers calculate this by determining for each person in the study sample whether or not he or she has ever had the disease or by checking lifetime health records for everybody in the population for occurrence of the disease and then counting the occurrences and dividing by the number of people in the population.

The other basic measure of disease frequency is incidence, the number of cases of a disease that occur in a given period. Incidence is a critical statistic in describing the course of a fast-moving epidemic, in which medical decision makers must know how quickly a disease is spreading. The incidence rate is the key to public health planning because it enables officials to understand what the prevalence of a disease is likely to be in the future. Prevalence is mathematically related to the cumulative incidence of a disease over a period, as well as the expected duration of a disease, which can be a week in the case of the flu or a lifetime in the case of juvenile-onset diabetes. Therefore, incidence not only indicates the rate of new disease cases but also is the basis of the rate of change of disease prevalence.

Epidemiologists use statistical analysis to discover associations between death and disease in populations and various factors—including environmental (e.g., pollution), demographic (e.g., age and gender), biological (e.g., body mass index [BMI] and genetics), social (e.g., educational level), and behavioral (e.g., tobacco smoking, diet, or type of medical treatment)—that could be implicated in causing disease.

Familiarity with basic concepts of probability and statistics is essential in understanding health care and epidemiological research. Statistical associations take into account the role of chance in contracting disease. Researchers compare disease rates for two or more population groups that vary in their environmental, genetic, pathogen exposure, or behavioral characteristics and observe whether a particular group characteristic is associated with a difference in rates that is unlikely to have occurred by chance alone.

■ Applications and Research

Applications in Public Health Practice

Certain concepts are basic to infectious disease epidemiology. These include the infectious agent, which is the organism that can develop within a human host and be passed along to other people via a particular mode of transmission—for example, by air, food, or sexual intercourse. Infectious diseases have geographic scope, or occurrence, and take a certain length of time to result in disease symptoms, called the incubation period. After this incubation period, there is a period during which the individual can pass the infection to others, called the period of communicability. The infectivity of a disease is the probability that an infected individual will pass the infection to an uninfected person, and the virulence of an infectious agent is the relative power and pathogenicity possessed by the organism, or the specific traits of the organism that contribute to making the host ill. Populations of animals or human groups that harbor the infectious agent constitute the reservoir of the disease. An organism such as a tick or insect that carries the infectious agent from such a reservoir to vulnerable individuals is called a vector.

Once an epidemic is underway, public health officials attempt to control it even as they continue to gather epidemiological information about its cause and distribution. These control efforts consist of preventive measures for individuals and groups, which are measures designed to prevent further spread of the disease, and treatment to minimize the period of communicability of the infection and reduce morbidity and mortality. Control of patient contacts and the immediate environment are foremost among such preventive measures, which can extend to patient isolation and observance of universal precautions, including handwashing, wearing of gloves and masks, and sterilization in dangerous instances. Epidemic measures, including the necessary abrogation of civil rights as in quarantines, are sometimes necessary to contain a communicable disease that has spread within an area, a state, or a nation. The epidemic may become a disaster if effective preventive actions are not initiated, and the scope of actions can be international, requiring the coordination of disparate public health capabilities across national boundaries.

Screening Programs

Screening a community using relatively simple diagnostic tests is one of the most powerful tools that health care professionals and public health authorities have in preventing or combating disease. Familiar examples of screening include HIV testing to help prevent AIDS, tuberculin testing to screen for tuberculosis, and hepatitis C testing by insurers to detect subclinical infection that could result in liver cirrhosis over the long term. In undertaking a screening program, authorities must always judge whether the benefits of preventing the illness in question outweigh the costs and the number of cases that have been mistakenly identified (false positives).

The ability of the test to identify true positives (sensitivity) and true negatives (specificity) makes screening a valuable prevention tool. However, the usefulness of the screening test is proportional to the disease prevalence in the population at risk. If the disease prevalence is low, there will likely be more false positives than true positives, which would cast doubt on the usefulness and the cost-effectiveness of the test. For example, if the prevalence of a disease in the population is only 2 percent and a test with a false positive rate of 4 percent is given to everyone (normally a good rate for a screening test), then individuals falsely identified as having the disease would be twice as frequent as individuals accurately identified with the disease. This would render the test results virtually useless. Public health officials deal with this situation by screening only population subgroups that have a high risk of contracting the disease. In infectious disease, screening tests are valuable for infections with a long latency period (the period during which an infected individual does not show disease symptoms) or with a lengthy and ambiguous symptomatic period.

Clinical Trials

Clinical trials are the experimental branch of epidemiology in which scientific sampling with randomized selection of research subjects is combined with prospective study design and experimental controls involving a placebo or comparator active treatment control group. The statistical analysis used in clinical trials is similar to that used in other types of epidemiological studies and usually involves simply counting cases that improve or deteriorate and comparing morbidity and mortality rates between the trial treatment groups.

Clinical trials in infectious disease are most common when a significant follow-up period is available. One such trial was a rigorous test of the effectiveness of condoms in the prevention of human immunodeficiency virus (HIV) and acquired immunodeficiency syndrome (AIDS). This experiment was reported in 1994 in the *New England Journal of Medicine.* Although in the United States and Western Europe, the transmission of AIDS has been largely within certain high-risk groups, including drug users and homosexual males, worldwide the predominant mode of HIV transmission is heterosexual intercourse. The effectiveness of condoms to prevent HIV transmission is generally acknowledged. But even decades after the epidemic began, many people remained ignorant of the scientific support for the preventive value of condoms.

A group of European scientists conducted a prospective study of HIV-negative subjects who had no risk factor for AIDS other than having a stable heterosexual relationship with an HIV-infected partner. A sample of 304 HIV-negative subjects (196 women and 108 men) was followed for an average of 20 months. During the trial 130 couples (42.8 percent) ended sexual relations, usually due to the illness or death of the HIV-infected partner. Of the remaining 256 couples who continued having exclusive sexual relationships, 124 (48.4 percent) consistently used condoms. None of the seronegative partners among these couples became infected with HIV. By contrast, among the 121 couples who inconsistently used condoms, the seroconversion rate was 4.8 per 100 person-years.

Because none of the seronegative partners among the couples who used condoms consistently became infected, this trial presents extremely powerful evidence of the effectiveness of condom use in preventing AIDS. However, there appear to be several major reasons why some of the couples did not use condoms consistently, highlighting the question of why so many couples do not use condoms in view of the obvious risks. Couples with infected partners who got their infection through drug use were much less likely to use condoms than when the seropositive partner got infected through sexual relations. Couples with more seriously ill partners at the beginning of the study were significantly more likely to use condoms consistently. Finally, the longer the couple had been together before the start of the trial was positively associated with condom use.

■ Impacts and Issues

The control of infectious disease is an urgent mission for epidemiologists employed in various state and federal public health agencies and their partners in private industry and research foundations. The American Public Health Association (APHA) provides guidance for the epidemiology and control of more than 100 communicable diseases that confront public health practitioners.

Infectious disease epidemiology requires accurate and timely incidence and prevalence data such as those provided with comprehensive disease surveillance of usual and emerging diseases. Although the development of an organized surveillance system is critical to the provision of these data, the system's effectiveness depends on the willingness and ability of health care providers to detect, diagnose, and report the incidence of cases that the system is supposed to track. A reporting system functions at four levels: (1) the basic data is collected in the local community where the disease occurs; (2) the data are assembled at the district, state, or provincial levels; (3) information is aggregated under national auspices (e.g., the US Centers for Disease Control and Prevention); and (4) for certain prescribed diseases, the national health authority reports the disease information to the World Health Organization.

The reporting of cases at the local level is mandated for notifiable illnesses that come to the attention of health care providers. Case reports provide patient information, suspect organisms, and dates of onset with basis for diagnosis, consistent with patient privacy rights. Collective case reports are compiled at the district level by diagnosis stipulating the number of cases occurring within a prescribed time. Any unusual or group expression of illness that may be of public concern should be reported as an epidemic, whether the illness is included in the list of notifiable diseases and whether it is a well-known identified disease or an unknown clinical entity.

Because of the emergence or reemergence of HIV/AIDS and resistant strains of tuberculosis, malaria, gonorrhea, and *E. coli*, among others, infectious disease epidemiology, once thought to be waning in importance due to significant advances in public sanitation and immunization programs, has reemerged as an urgent challenge. Infectious diseases currently threaten to destroy social order in some developing nations and pose extremely difficult public health problems even in the wealthiest societies. Hantavirus infections, thought to be a serious problem primarily in Asia, have emerged as an epidemic in the southwestern United States. Lyme disease has continued to afflict ever larger populations in the northeastern United States. Ebola virus has jumped from monkeys to humans in Africa, and pneumococci have continued to become resistant to the antibiotics used to treat infections.

Air travel has enabled travelers to return home from areas where particular pathogens are endemic within the incubation period of every infectious disease, which can potentially precipitate an epidemic.

Despite impressive improvements in global surveillance and response logistics, disease outbreaks may be unexpectedly difficult to respond to and control, as demonstrated by the international response to the 2014 Ebola epidemic in western Africa. The response to this outbreak illustrates many of the issues affecting the epidemiology, surveillance, and response to infectious disease outbreaks. It demonstrates the relationships between disease tracking and both effective and ineffective public health action to combat the spread of an extremely dangerous epidemic.

The Ebola outbreak occurred in numerous densely populated areas of Liberia, Guinea, and Sierra Leone, causing thousands of deaths. A British parliamentary report illustrated the difficulty and pitfalls in the global response to serious disease outbreaks in developing countries that might not have occurred had the outbreaks taken place in developed nations with advanced health care and disease surveillance organization.

Although the 2014–2015 British-led Ebola response effort ultimately achieved success, a parliamentary committee termed it "totally inadequate," saying that the UK Department for International Development's (DFID) response was "far too slow" and may have contributed to the loss of lives. The committee charged that the British government failed to release funds quickly enough to deal with the crisis and that its decision to suspend flights to areas affected by the outbreak had been "political."

The British government defended its actions, saying that the program in Sierra Leone had saved, rather than cost, lives and had reduced weekly reported cases from 537 in November 2014 to 70 by mid-February 2015. Still, the DFID, which oversaw the United Kingdom's involvement in the Ebola outbreak, was described in the committee's report as having inadequate "experience and capability" to contend with the epidemic. Further, the committee said that there had been an "unfortunate time lag between the department's recognition that it had to act and its allocation of funding to deal with the outbreak." The committee concluded, "Had the department acted sooner, both lives and money would have been saved."

While the report praised the bravery of British volunteers and armed forces members working in Sierra Leone, it said the government had not forged strong partnerships with nongovernmental organizations on the scene, such as Médecins Sans Frontières (Doctors Without Borders), which warned of the seriousness of the outbreak and described the suspension of flights to areas affected by Ebola as having "no scientific justification."

The parliamentary committee advocated that the DFID lead the international community's efforts to learn from and improve on the outcomes of the Ebola outbreak response by developing procedures and protocols to quickly respond to developing public health emergencies in countries that receive assistance from the United Kingdom. The government was advised to create and maintain a detailed contingency plan for sudden-onset medical emergencies and make investment in local health infrastructure for developing countries in receipt of UK aid a priority. In general, the committee recommended that developing countries should be supported to prevent future public health disasters and that a comprehensive evaluation of the UK's response to the crisis should be published after the outbreak subsided.

PRIMARY SOURCE

Instances of the Communication of Cholera through the Medium of Polluted Water at Newburn on the Tyne

SOURCE: *Snow, John.* On the Mode of Communication of Cholera. *2nd ed. London: John Churchill, 1855.*

INTRODUCTION: *John Snow (1813–1858) was an English physician who advanced understanding of the spread of disease, especially cholera. When the first cholera pandemic reached Great Britain in 1831, there was widespread public fear, and little was known about how the disease was transmitted. Snow's research led to the understanding that polluted water was a major source of cholera. The following excerpt from his 1849 essay "On the Mode of Communication of Cholera" outlines one case that he observed.*

John Snow

There is no spot in this country in which the cholera was more fatal during the epidemic of 1832 than the village of Newburn, near Newcastle-upon-Tyne. We are informed, in an excellent paper on the subject by Dr. David Craigie, that exactly one-tenth of the population died. The number of the inhabitants was five hundred and fifty; of these, three hundred and twenty suffered from the epidemic, either in the form of diarrhea or the more confirmed disease, and the deaths amounted to fifty-five. Being aware of this mortality, I wrote, about the beginning of the year 1849, to a friend in Newcastle—Dr. Embleton—to make inquiries respecting the water used at Newburn, and he kindly procured me some information from the Rev. John Reed, of Newburn Vicarage, which I received in February, as well as an answer from Mr. Davison, surgeon, of Newburn, to whom I had written in the meantime. I learnt from these communications that the people were supplied with water in 1832, as they still were, from three wells, two of which were very little used, and that the water in the third well was derived from the workings of an old coal mine near the village. The water of this well, as I was informed, although generally good when first drawn, became putrid after being kept two days. It was considered that the evacuations of the people could not get into any of the wells; but the vicar thought that the water of a little brook which runs past the village, and falls into the Tyne immediately afterwards, might find its way into that well which is chiefly resorted to. Putrefaction, on being kept a day or two, is so much the character of water containing animal matter, that, after receiving confirmation of my views respecting the communication of cholera by water from many other places, I wrote to Mr. Davison again on the subject, and he kindly took a great deal of trouble to investigate the matter further. He informed me that the brook was principally formed by water which was constantly pumped from coal pits in the neighborhood. About half a mile before reaching Newburn it received the refuse of a small village, and between that village and Newburn it ran through a privy used by the workmen of a steel factory. In Newburn this brook received the contents of the open drains or gutters from the houses. The drain which conveyed water from a coal mine or drift had not worked for a great number of years, to the well mentioned above, passed underneath the brook at one part of its course, and from that point ran alongside of the brook to the well—a distance of about three hundred yards. Mr. Davison said that it was disputed whether there was any communication between the drain and the brook, but that it was highly probable that there might be; and that an occurrence which took place a few months previously seemed to prove that there was. Some gas-water from the steel manufactory mentioned above got by accident into the brook, and some of the people affirmed that the water in the well was strongly impregnated with it.

The first case of cholera in Newburn was that of a young man living close to the brook, about a hundred yards above the place at which it passes the well. He was taken ill on the 29th December, 1831, and died, in the stage of consecutive fever, on January 4th, 1832. There were some cases of diarrhea in the village, but no new cases of cholera till the night of January the 9th, during which night and the following morning thirteen persons were taken ill. During the night of the 12th four persons were attacked; by the 15th there were fourteen new cases, and on this day the late vicar died—the Rev. John Edmonston. By the next day at noon there were at least fifty new cases. A few days after this the disease began to subside, and by the 2nd of February had almost disappeared. As several days elapsed between the first case of cholera and the great outbreak, it is probable that the water in which the soiled linen must have been washed, and which would necessarily run into the brook, was the means of communicating the disease to the thirteen persons taken ill on the night between the 9th and 10th of January; unless, indeed, the intermediate cases of diarrhea could transmit the disease.

SEE ALSO *Demographics and Infectious Disease; Public Health and Infectious Disease; Notifiable Diseases*

BIBLIOGRAPHY

Books

Bennenson, A. S., ed. *Control of Communicable Diseases Manual.* 20th ed. Washington, DC: American Public Health Association, 2014.

Graunt, J. *Natural and Political Observations Made upon the Bills of Mortality.* 1662. Reprint, Baltimore: Johns Hopkins Press, 1939.

Hennekens, C. H., and J. E. Buring. *Epidemiology in Medicine.* Boston: Little, Brown, 1987.

Shephard, David A. E. *John Snow: Anaesthetist to a Queen and Epidemiologist to a Nation.* Cornwall, Canada: York Point, 1995.

Tuberculosis Statistics: States and Cities, 1984. Atlanta: Centers for Disease Control, 1985.

Periodicals

De Vincenzi, I. "A Longitudinal Study of Human Immunodeficiency Virus Transmission by Heterosexual Partners." *New England Journal of Medicine* 331 (August 11, 1994): 341–346.

Websites

"Health Systems Dangerously Inadequate for Dealing with Emergencies Like Ebola." UK Parliament, Commons Select Committee, December 18, 2014. http://www.parliament.uk/business/committees/committees-a-z/commons-select/international-development-committee/news/report-responses-to-ebola-crisis/ (accessed February 10, 2018).

"John Snow." UCLA Department of Epidemiology, Fielding School of Public Health. http://www.ph.ucla.edu/epi/snow.html (accessed March 30, 2007).

Kenneth T. LaPensee

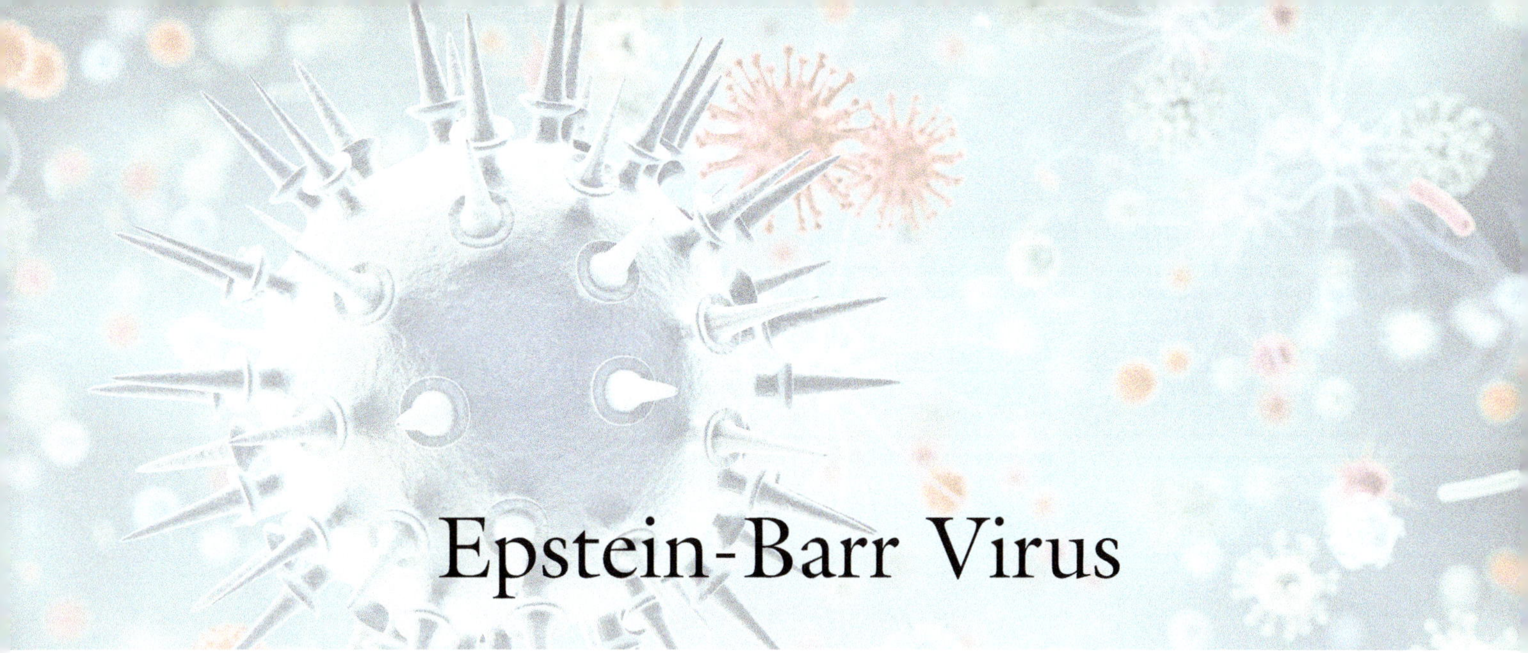

Epstein-Barr Virus

Introduction

Epstein-Barr virus (EBV), also known as human herpesvirus 4 (HHV-4), is one of the most common viruses present in humans. The US Centers for Disease Control and Prevention (CDC) estimates that about 50 percent of children five years of age or younger and about 90 percent of all adults in the United States will be infected by EBV. Most people infected with EBV during childhood either show no symptoms or suffer a brief illness with symptoms indistinguishable from other mild, common illnesses.

In teenagers and young adults, EBV can result in mononucleosis, commonly called mono, with prolonged and more severe symptoms. Teenagers and young adults typically acquire EBV from infected cells in the mouth. Because EBV is often transmitted through contact with saliva, mononucleosis is often called "the kissing disease."

Disease History, Characteristics, and Transmission

EBV was first discovered in 1964 by Michael Epstein and Yvonne Barr while they were studying Burkitt's lymphoma, a form of cancer that is relatively common in Africa. The virus's role as the cause of infectious mononucleosis was later identified.

The virus is extremely prevalent in humans. The infection can persist because EBV may remain latent for years. In response to triggers that are still not fully known, EBV can reinitiate an active infection. Latency and recurrence occur most often in individuals with compromised immune systems.

An EBV infection begins when the virus infects the thin layer of epithelial cells that line the mouth, throat, and cervix and then makes new copies of the virus. The infection then expands to include B cells, a type of cell that participates in the body's immune response. The virus becomes latent by integrating its DNA into the DNA of the B cells. As the host (B cell) DNA duplicates by cell division, so does the viral DNA. The virus particles made in the B cells escape to other cells in the body. Virus production in these other cells affects the functioning of the tissue, producing some of the symptoms of infection.

EBV can be spread from person to person. Transmission typically occurs through contact with saliva. Contact with infected cervical cells through sexual activity may also transmit EBV. Transmission via blood transfusions is rare.

WORDS TO KNOW

ANTIBODIES Also called Y-shaped immunoglobulins, proteins found in the blood that help to fight against foreign substances called antigens. Antigens, which are usually proteins or polysaccharides, stimulate the immune system to produce antibodies. The antibodies inactivate the antigen and help to remove it from the body. While antigens can be the source of infections from pathogenic bacteria and viruses, organic molecules detrimental to the body from internal or environmental sources also act as antigens. Genetic engineering and the use of various mutational mechanisms allow the construction of a vast array of antibodies (each with a unique genetic sequence).

HETEROPHILE ANTIBODY An antibody found in the blood of someone with infectious mononucleosis, also known as glandular fever.

LATENT Potential or dormant, as in a condition that is not yet manifest or active.

Diseases Linked to Epstein-Barr Virus Infection

The Epstein-Barr virus (EBV) has been linked to many diseases in addition to infectious mononucleosis. The list below shows diseases for which a link to EBV has been proposed. Studies of the relationship between these diseases and the virus are ongoing.

Malignant Diseases	Autoimmune Diseases	Neurological Disorders	Hematologic Disorders
Burkitt's lymphoma	Dermatomyositis	Encephalitis	Hemophagocytic lymphohistiocytosis
Gastric carcinoma	Multiple sclerosis	Guillain-Barré syndrome	Lymphomatoid granulomatosis
Hodgkin lymphoma	Sjögren's syndrome	Optic neuritis	
Leukemia	Systemic lupus erythematosus	Transverse myelitis	
Pyothorax-associated lymphoma	Rheumatoid arthritis		
T-cell lymphoproliferative disorder (LPD)			
Undifferentiated nasopharyngeal carcinoma			

Scope and Distribution

EBV can be present almost anywhere in the world. Most people are exposed to EBV early in life, when infection is most likely to cause only mild illness. In developing countries infection occurs earlier in life than in developed countries. Around 90 percent of children in developing countries develop antibodies to EBV within the first few years of life. By contrast, in the United States only 50 percent of the population is positive for antibodies to the virus by the age of five.

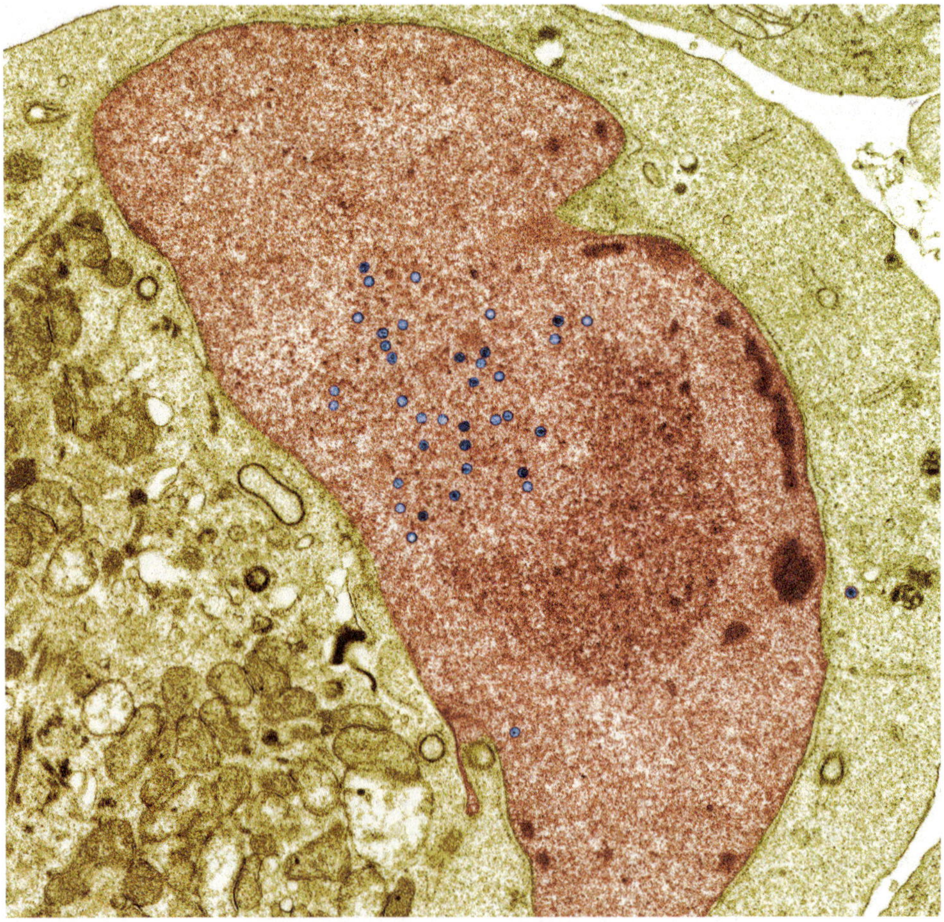

A colored transmission electron micrograph shows, in blue, Epstein-Barr virus particles within the nucleus (orange) of a cancerous white blood cell. Though Epstein-Barr virus is often latent, it can lead to lymphomas, nasopharyngeal carcinomas, and glandular fevers under certain conditions. *© Steve Gschmeissner/Science Source*

Treatment and Prevention

Infection is determined by detecting the presence of the antibodies produced by the immune system in response to the virus. The level of a particular antibody in the blood known as the heterophile antibody is a reliable indicator of the intensity of an infection. Even though the virus is common in the cells of the mouth and throat, samples of cells taken from these areas are not a reliable means of detecting the virus.

Treatment of EBV infection is difficult, as the virus can become latent for months or years. As of 2017 there were no available vaccines or antiviral drugs to prevent or treat EBV. Teenagers and young adults suffering from infectious mononucleosis are typically given medications to ease symptoms such as fever, aches, and fatigue, which can persist for up to four weeks.

Impacts and Issues

EBV affects just about everyone at some time. In most people the infection is brief and may produce either no symptoms or a brief, mild illness. The most severe symptoms associated with EBV occur in people aged 10 to 21 who were not exposed to EBV in early childhood and who develop mononucleosis. Infectious mononucleosis can have a more serious impact on people living in developing regions by making them more susceptible to other dangerous infectious diseases in their environment.

The virus has been linked to several cancers, including Burkitt's lymphoma, Hodgkin's lymphoma, stomach cancer, and nasopharyngeal carcinoma; ear infections in children; Guillain-Barré syndrome; and multiple sclerosis. Whether the virus is the cause of these illnesses was still unknown as of 2017.

SEE ALSO *Mononucleosis; Viral Disease*

BIBLIOGRAPHY

Books

Crawford, Dorothy H., Alan B. Rickinson, and Ingolfur Johannessen. *Cancer Virus: The Discovery of the Epstein-Barr Virus.* Oxford, UK: Oxford University Press, 2014.

Esterson, Joseph. *Epstein-Barr Virus (Mononucleosis): A Reference Guide.* Washington DC: Capitol Hill Press, 2015.

Periodicals

Balandraud, Nathalie, and Jean Roudier. "Epstein-Barr Virus and Rheumatoid Arthritis." *Joint Bone Spine* (May 9, 2017). This article can also be found online at https://www.sciencedirect.com/science/article/pii/S1297319X17300933 (accessed December 26, 2017).

Chan, K. C. Allen, et al. "Analysis of Plasma Epstein-Barr Virus DNA to Screen for Nasopharyngeal Cancer." *New England Journal of Medicine*, 377 (August 10, 2017): 513–522. This article can also be found online at http://www.nejm.org/doi/full/10.1056/NEJMoa1701717 (accessed December 26, 2017).

Young, Lawrence S., Lee Fah Yap, and Paul G Murray. "Epstein-Barr Virus: More Than 50 Years Old and Still Providing Surprises." *Nature Reviews Cancer* 16, no. 12 (2016): 789–802.

Websites

"Epstein-Barr Virus and Infectious Mononucleosis." Centers for Disease Control and Prevention, January 7, 2014. http://www.cdc.gov/epstein-barr/index.html (accessed November 16, 2017).

Brian Hoyle

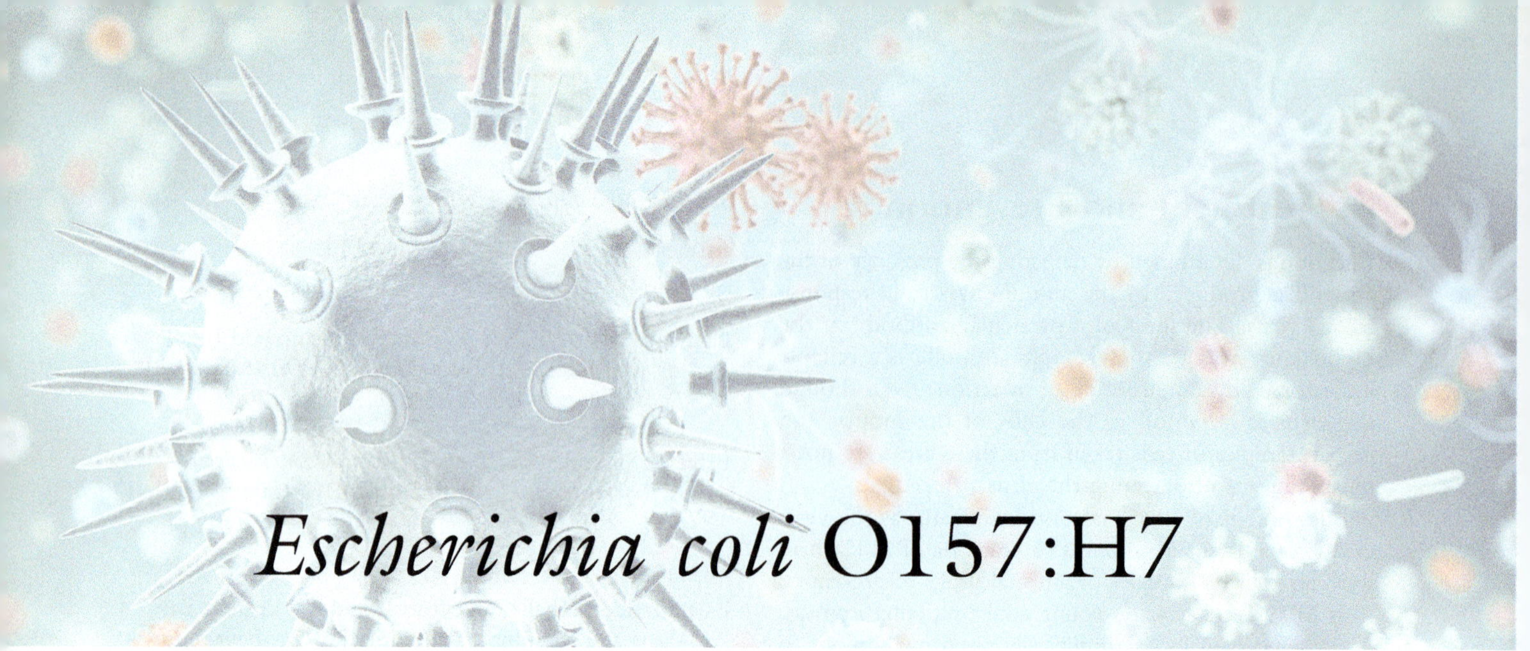

Escherichia coli O157:H7

Introduction

Escherichia coli is a gram-negative bacterium that normally inhabits the intestinal tracts of humans and other warm-blooded animals. There are hundreds of different types (strains) of *E. coli* that differ from one another only slightly in their composition. Most of these strains are harmless, and many are beneficial because they can manufacture some vitamins that are needed for proper functioning of the body. Strain O157:H7 is an exception. In contrast to many of the other strains, *E. coli* O157:H7 does not normally reside in the intestinal tract of humans. It is generally found in the intestinal tract of cattle. While harmless in cattle, *E. coli* O157:H7 can be dangerous to people. Ingesting food or water that is contaminated with O157:H7 can produce a severe, even life-threatening infection.

The descriptor O157 is a code that refers to lipopolysaccharide, a structure that is located on the outer surface of the bacterium. Different configurations of lipopolysaccharide are possible, which can affect the disease-causing ability of the bacterium. The other descriptor, H7, refers to a form of the bacteria's flagellum.

Since it was first described in the early 1980s, the illness caused by *E. coli* O157:H7 has sickened thousands, and more than a thousand people have died as a result of the infection, which can destroy intestinal and kidney cells. *E. coli* O157:H7 can be found around the world. In the United States, the Centers for Disease Control and Prevention (CDC) estimates that there are about 73,000 illnesses each year, with around 50 deaths. In the United Kingdom, a June 2016 outbreak of *E. coli* O157 PT34, which is closely related to O157:H7, sickened 158 people and caused two deaths.

WORDS TO KNOW

FLAGELLUM A hairlike structure in a cell that serves as an organ of locomotion.

GRAM-NEGATIVE BACTERIA Bacteria whose cell walls are composed of an inner and outer membrane that are separated from one another by a region called the periplasm. The periplasm also contains a thin but rigid layer called the peptidoglycan.

STRAIN A subclass or a specific genetic variation of an organism.

TOXIN A poison produced by a living organism.

Disease History, Characteristics, and Transmission

E. coli O157:H7 is one of four types of the bacterium that can infect the gastrointestinal tract, causing a disease called gastroenteritis. Additionally, O157:H7 is enterohemorrhagic, or able to destroy the cells lining the intestinal tract, which causes copious bleeding.

The severe intestinal damage that occurs during an infection by *E. coli* O157:H7 is the result of the production of powerful toxins. These toxins, verotoxin and shiga-like toxin, are similar to the destructive toxin produced by another disease-causing bacterium, *Shigella dysenteriae.*

The similarity of the toxins in the two different bacteria reflects how strain O157:H7 came into existence. The strain was discovered in Argentina in 1977. Studies of the sequences of the genetic material in O157:H7 and *S. dysenteriae* support the idea that, likely in the intestinal tract of a cow, a typical *E. coli* acquired genetic material from a neighboring *S. dysenteriae.* The acquired genetic material included the gene that coded for the destructive *Shigella* toxins. The genetically altered *E. coli*, O157:H7, was capable of producing the toxins.

In 1982 strain O157:H7 was first identified as a cause of illness when an outbreak of severe diarrhea in several states in the United States was traced to undercooked hamburgers. The disease became known as "hamburger disease." It later became clear that other foods, including various kinds of produce, fruits, unpasteurized juices and milk, and cheese products, can be contaminated with strain O157:H7. Produce and fruits can become contaminated when sprayed with sewage-containing water during their growth. If the food is not washed prior to being eaten, the bacteria can be ingested. In 2006, for example, a multistate illness outbreak caused by O157:H7 was traced to organically grown lettuce. Some consumers had eaten the lettuce without first washing it. The CDC estimates that up to 85 percent of all O157:H7 infections are food-borne infections.

When cattle are slaughtered, intestinal contents can splatter on the carcass. In whole cuts of meat, such as T-bone steaks, the bacteria-contaminated surface can be made safe to eat by properly cooking the meat. However, when surface-contaminated meat is ground, bacteria, including O157:H7, can be distributed throughout the meat. The only way to kill all these bacteria is to adequately cook the meat. Any undercooked meat can still contain living O157:H7 that are capable of causing infection.

O157:H7 can also contaminate drinking water. This occurs when O157:H7-containing feces mixes with the drinking water. If the water is not properly treated to remove or kill the bacteria, drinking the water can sicken a person. In the summer of 2000, one of the wells in the community of Walkerton, Ontario, Canada, was contaminated by storm runoff from a cattle field. Improper treatment of the water caused thousands of people to become ill, and seven people died. Some of the survivors had permanent kidney damage caused by the O157:H7 toxins.

In a few instances in the United States and Canada, O157:H7 infection has been traced to children's petting zoos. Stroking fur that is soiled by feces can be dangerous if children put their unwashed hands in their mouths.

The toxins are so destructive because they not only damage the host cells they contact, but they also prevent repair of the damage by shutting down the manufacture of host cell proteins. The toxins can damage the cells because the bacteria bind tightly to the cells. This strong association enables the bacteria to remain in position and establish the infection.

Another aspect of the disease-causing ability of *E. coli* is the presence of fimbriae, hairlike structures that stick out from the surface of each bacterium. The fimbriae are made up in part of proteins termed adhesions, which bind to other proteins on the surface of the cells that line the intestinal tract. This binding is another way the bacteria can be locked into position along the intestinal tract. Once this occurs the bacterium can inject proteins into the host cell, which forces the host cell to cooperate in the ensuing infection. The host cell produces extensions of the cell wall. These are called pedestals. An *E. coli* bacterium will perch at the top of the pedestal, which allows the bacterium free access to nutrients in the intestinal tract while remaining firmly attached to the lining of the intestinal tract.

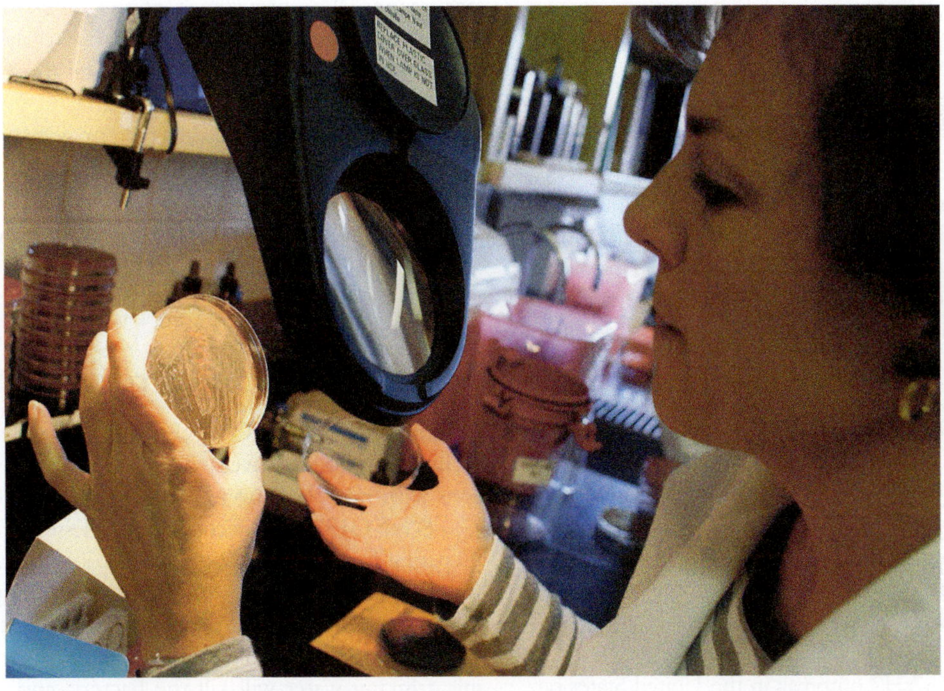

Michelle Males, a medical laboratory technologist in North Bay, Ontario, examines a petri dish while testing for *Escherichia coli* O157:H7, a strain of *E. coli* that can cause severe and even fatal illness. *© Pawel Dwulit/Toronto Star/Getty Images*

REAL-WORLD FACTORS IN REPORTING DISEASE

Public health inspectors and scientists use variations of DNA fingerprinting on bacteria to determine the source of an *E. coli* infection. By comparing samples from exposed patients and potential sources, investigators can often identify a common source of an outbreak.

There is always a delay, typically two to three weeks, between infection and source identification. The Centers for Disease Control and Prevention (CDC) publishes the following timeline of identification procedures so that, in part, the number of cases possible during an outbreak may be more accurately estimated:

1. Incubation time: The time from eating the contaminated food to the beginning of symptoms. For *E. coli* O157:H7, this is typically three to four days.
2. Time to treatment: The time from the first symptom until the person seeks medical care, when a diarrhea sample is collected for laboratory testing. This time lag may be one to five days.
3. Time to diagnosis: The time from when a person gives a sample to when *E. coli* O157:H7 is obtained from it in a laboratory. This may be one to three days from the time the sample is received in the laboratory.
4. Sample shipping time: The time required to ship the *E. coli* O157:H7 bacteria from the laboratory to the state public health authorities that will perform DNA fingerprinting. This may take up to seven days depending on transportation arrangements within a state and the distance between the clinical laboratory and public health department.
5. Time to complete DNA fingerprinting: The time required for the state public health authorities to perform DNA fingerprinting on the *E. coli* O157:H7 and compare it with the outbreak pattern. Ideally this can be accomplished in one day. However, many public health laboratories have limited staff and space and experience multiple emergencies at the same time. Thus, the process may take one to four days.

An early symptom of the infection, which occurs as the intestinal cells become damaged, is watery diarrhea. Destruction of intestinal cells causes the diarrhea to become bloody. An infected person can also experience nausea and vomiting. The fluid loss and pain can be debilitating, and intake of fluids is important to prevent more serious problems. In most people these symptoms fade within several weeks, as the body's immune system is able to successfully deal with the infection. People whose immune systems are immature or malfunctioning can develop a more widespread infection. The kidney damage that can occur can be so extensive that the kidney stops functioning. This occurs in 10 to 15 percent of those who contract the infection. The infection can also affect the pancreas, brain, and other organs; this assault can be overwhelming and can cause death.

Approximately 10 to 15 percent of those infected with strain O157:H7 develop hemolytic uremic syndrome. The syndrome is the leading cause of sudden-onset kidney failure in children worldwide. Elderly people can develop thrombocytopenic purpura, a condition that results in fever and nerve damage. In the elderly this complication of *E. coli* O157:H7 infection can kill almost half of those who become infected.

An *E. coli* O157:H7 outbreak in the United States occurred in January and February 2017, when contaminated peanut butter caused illness in 16 people in nine states. Of the 16 people, 8 needed hospital care.

■ Scope and Distribution

E. coli O157:H7 is worldwide in distribution and occurrence. The prevalence of the illness is higher in countries where agriculture is more prominent and where standards of infection control in food sources are not as stringent.

There is no evidence that race or gender makes any difference in susceptibility to infection. However, those with immune systems that are relatively inefficient can be at increased risk. This includes children, the elderly, and those whose immune systems have been impaired by surgery or during the course of caring for another illness.

■ Treatment and Prevention

Treatment of *E. coli* O157:H7 infection is supportive, including blood replacement and kidney dialysis in persons with hemolytic uremic syndrome.

E. coli O157:H7 infections can be lessened by properly preparing food (such as by adequate cooking until the center of a hamburger is no longer red), washing preparation surfaces that have been in contact with raw ground meat, and handwashing. O157:H7 is readily killed by heat; boiling drinking water will kill the bacteria and destroy the toxins.

Vaccines that have been developed to prevent *E. coli* infection in cattle may have benefits in preventing the attachment of *E. coli* to the wall of the intestinal tract in humans. By occupying the site on the intestinal wall to which *E. coli* binds, the vaccine can outcompete the bacterium for attachment, which is necessary to establish an infection. As of 2018 the strategy remained in the research phase.

Impacts and Issues

The CDC has estimated that the illness caused by strain O157:H7 afflicts more than 70,000 Americans each year. Of these, over 2,000 require hospitalization, and approximately 60 die. For those who become infected, the best that can be expected is a bout of severe diarrhea. Fortunately, for many people recovery is complete and the misery of the infection becomes a memory. For others the infection can damage the kidney or completely destroy kidney function. If that happens, dialysis or a kidney transplant is needed.

E. coli O157:H7 highlights the necessity of proper hygiene, particularly proper handwashing after using the bathroom. Many food-borne cases of the illness could be prevented if food preparation was accomplished with clean hands. Furthermore, the infection can be easily prevented by cooking ground meat thoroughly. Since the initial outbreak in 1982, many restaurants no longer serve hamburgers that are not cooked to an internal temperature of 160°F (71.1°C) or are not considered "well done."

In 2007 a Canadian biopharmaceutical company announced the successful development and testing of a vaccine for cattle. The vaccine operates by blocking the binding of the bacteria to the intestinal epithelial cells. The stranded bacteria are washed out of the intestinal tract. Through vaccination of cattle herds, the reservoir of O157:H7 could gradually be eliminated, and outbreaks from beef would be a thing of the past. As of 2017 the vaccine was available, although it was not in widespread use because there has been no indication that vaccinated cattle fare any better in terms of sales than cattle that are not vaccinated. Food safety scientists are also studying other methods to decrease contamination of meat on the farm and in the slaughterhouse and to encourage the use of irradiation to keep the ground beef supply safe.

A human vaccine for O157:H7 was being tested as of 2014. No results had been reported as of 2017.

See Also *Food-Borne Disease and Food Safety; Vaccines and Vaccine Development; Water-Borne Disease*

BIBLIOGRAPHY

Books

Benedict, Jeff. *Poisoned: The True Story of the Deadly* E. coli *Outbreak That Changed the Way Americans Eat.* New York: Inspire, 2011.

Periodicals

Gally, David L., and Mark P. Stevens. "Microbe Profile: *Escherichia coli* O157:H7—Notorious Relative of the Microbiologist's Workhorse." *Microbiology Society* 163 (2017): 1–3.

Min, Sea C., et al. "In-Package Inhibition of *E. coli* O157:H7 on Bulk Romaine Lettuce Using Cold Plasma." *Food Microbiology* 65 (2017): 1–6.

Sharapov, Umid M., et al. "Multistate Outbreak of *Escherichia coli* O157:H7 Infections Associated with Consumption of Fresh Spinach: United States, 2006." *Journal of Food Protection* 79 (2016): 2024–2030.

Websites

"*E. coli (Escherichia coli).*" Centers for Disease Control and Prevention. http://www.cdc.gov/ecoli/index.html (accessed January 12, 2018).

Brian Hoyle

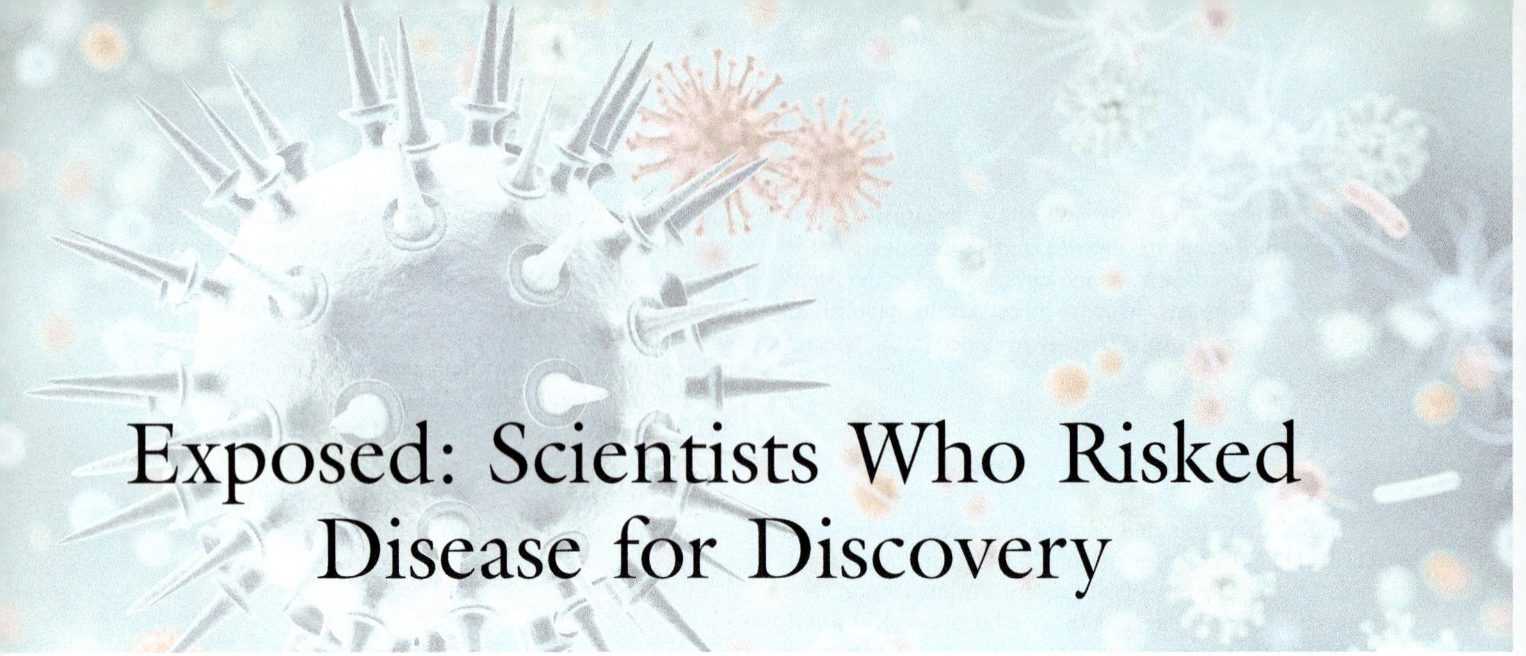

Exposed: Scientists Who Risked Disease for Discovery

Introduction

Most physicians would not find much commonality between yellow fever and stomach ulcers. Yellow fever is a viral illness spread by the bite of an infected mosquito, and spiral-shaped bacteria living in the extremely acidic environment of the stomach cause the majority of stomach ulcers. The common thread lies in the stories of the medical researchers who solved the mysteries presented by these otherwise distinct ailments by purposefully infecting themselves with the disease to prove what causes it.

Modern medical researchers still study diseases that spring from deadly bacteria and viruses. In the early 21st century, experimental designs minimize the risks of exposure to these pathogens. Special containment facilities (biosafety laboratories) ensure that accidental exposures do not occur easily. Special animal models are built by genetic techniques, negating the need for human experimentation. However, a need may always exist for scientists to take risks to solve serious medical problems.

WORDS TO KNOW

BIOSAFETY LABORATORY A place for scientific study of infectious agents. A biosafety laboratory is specially equipped to contain infectious agents, prevent their dissemination, and protect researchers from exposure.

COLONIZATION The process of occupation and increase in number of microorganisms at a specific site.

HELSINKI DECLARATION A set of ethical principles governing medical and scientific experimentation on human subjects. It was drafted by the World Medical Association and was originally adopted in 1964.

INFORMED CONSENT An ethical and informational process in which a person learns about a procedure or clinical trial, including potential risks or benefits, before deciding to voluntarily participate in a study or undergo a particular procedure.

History and Scientific Foundations

Yellow Fever

Yellow fever is a viral disease now preventable by vaccination, but, until the early 20th century, this virus caused epidemics of severe disease and death. Called "yellow jack," yellow fever caused yearly summer epidemics in American coastal cities. The disease struck year-round in the tropics. The US Army lost more troops to yellow fever during the 1898 Spanish American War than to any other single cause. Some regiments lost over 50 percent of their men to yellow fever. The initial attempt by French engineers to build the Panama Canal in the 1880s failed in large part due to yellow fever and malaria that put a majority of canal workers in either the hospital or the grave. When the United States began to plan resuming construction of the canal in the 1890s, medical officials realized the need to find a cure for yellow fever.

In 1900 US Army Surgeon General George Sternberg (1838–1915) appointed four army physicians to serve on the fourth Yellow Fever Commission. The physicians—Walter Reed (1851–1902), James Carroll (1854–1907), Aristides Agramonte (1868–1931), and Jesse Lazear (1866–1900)—received orders to travel to Cuba and initiate experiments to discover the cause of yellow fever. The prevailing medical wisdom asserted that yellow fever infected people when they came in contact with clothing or bedding contaminated by those afflicted with yellow fever. A competing theory taught that the bite of infected mosquitoes spread the disease. In 1897 physicians Ronald Ross (1857–1932) and Patrick Manson (1844–1922) showed that the *Anopheles* mosquito carried malaria. This was in line with the beliefs of Carlos Finley (1833–1915), a Cuban physician, who thought that yellow fever was also carried by a mosquito.

The four physicians of the Yellow Fever Commission quickly found evidence refuting the contaminated bedding theory, but they soon discovered that providing evidence for the mosquito transmission theory would require dramatic actions. Yellow fever affected only humans; this meant animals could not be used to prove their theory that mosquitos spread the disease. To show that the bite of infected mosquitoes caused yellow fever, human volunteers needed to allow themselves to be bitten. The physicians agreed to experiment on themselves before requesting human volunteers. Agramonte was immune to yellow fever because he had acquired the disease years earlier, and Reed had traveled back to Washington, D.C., to complete a report to Surgeon General Sternberg. As the only physicians available, Lazear and Carroll began the experiments with humans.

The doctors obtained mosquitoes that had fed on those suffering from yellow fever, and in late August 1900

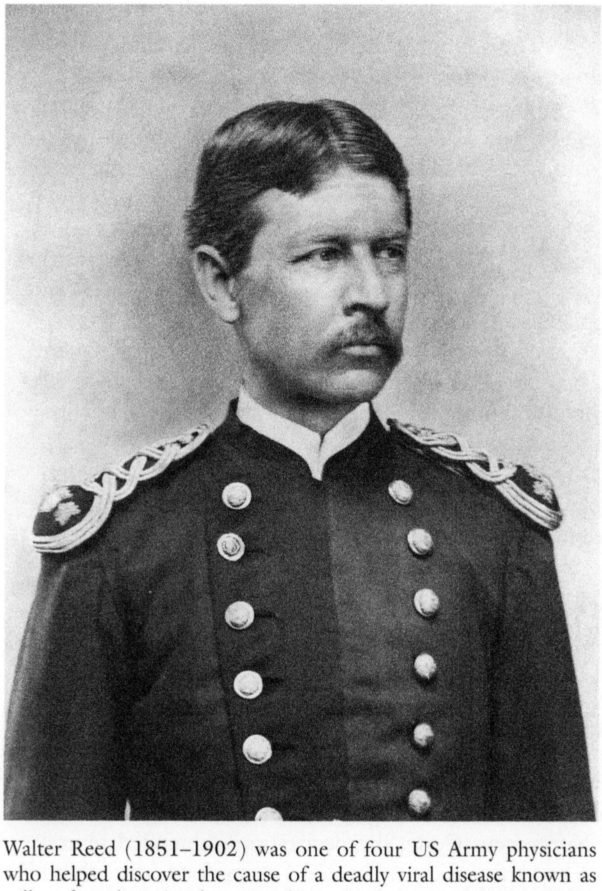

Walter Reed (1851–1902) was one of four US Army physicians who helped discover the cause of a deadly viral disease known as yellow fever by using human subjects in their experiments. *© Bettmann/Getty Images*

Carroll allowed these mosquitoes to bite him. He fell sick a few days later. Two days later a second human volunteer, Private William Dean, also contracted yellow fever after a deliberate exposure to infected mosquitoes. Both Carroll and Dean recovered; however, Carroll's coworker, the physician Lazear, developed a fatal case of the disease. Lazear's exposure was officially ruled accidental, but many historians argue that the doctor allowed himself to be a human test subject (the determination of accidental exposure would have allowed life insurance payments to his family). Reed, Carroll, and Agramonte went on to carry out a series of experiments that conclusively showed that the *Aedes aegypti* mosquito transmitted yellow fever.

The research did not provide the cause of yellow fever, however. Many years would pass before research determined yellow fever to be due to a virus, but showing that mosquitoes spread the disease provided a means to control the disease. Public health physicians rapidly declared war on the mosquito populations in American cities. The summer epidemics of yellow fever along the southern and gulf coasts soon became a thing of the past. The building of the Panama Canal in the early 20th century proceeded without the large death toll of malaria and yellow fever due to aggressive control of the mosquito population there.

Stomach Ulcers

In the 1980s another physician—pathologist J. Robin Warren (1937–)—used his own body to test if a bacteria caused stomach ulcers, a painful condition that can cause problems such as internal bleeding. His theory—that ulcers were caused by bacteria—was radical for the time. Most physicians assumed that stress, together with poor diet, resulted in stomach ulcers. The theory was that excessive acid in the stomach due to stress, diet, or smoking corroded the stomach lining and produced an ulcer. Treating patients with acid-lowering drugs seemed to confirm this thinking: ulcers responded to this treatment. But, when patients stopped the drugs, the ulcers recurred.

Despite the commonly-held belief that ulcers were caused by diet and lifestyle, Warren continued to research the connection between bacteria and ulcers. He found odd bacteria present in the stomachs of many patients with stomach ulcers and gastritis (inflammation of the stomach lining). These bacteria proved difficult to explain because conventional medical wisdom said bacteria could not survive in the highly acidic environment of the stomach. Another Australian physician, Barry Marshall (1951–), became interested in these novel bacteria, which eventually were given the name *Helicobacter pylori.* Marshall and Warren began to collect evidence that the spiral-shaped bacteria caused stomach ulcers.

Because the medical establishment already "knew" the cause of ulcers, Marshall's ideas were viewed with considerable skepticism. The medical community derided Marshall's ideas and provided him little funding for research. Despite the obstacles, from 1981 to 1984, Marshall gathered evidence implicating *H. pylori* as a cause of stomach ulcers and gastritis. The bacteria were present in biopsy specimens taken from ulcer patients and grown in pure culture from these specimens. However, like the case with yellow fever, no animal model existed to study stomach ulcers. Marshall could not inoculate an ulcer-free animal with the *H. pylori* bacteria and show that ulcers or gastritis developed. This experiment was essential to show that *H. pylori* did indeed cause stomach ulcers and that the bacteria were not just colonizing the human stomach.

By 1984 Marshall and Warren had a good circumstantial case implicating *H. pylori* as the causative agent of most stomach ulcers. They also developed a treatment strategy, which clearly both destroyed the bacteria in the stomach and healed the ulcers and gastritis. What they still lacked was definitive proof that, when *H. pylori* infected someone, ulcers or gastritis developed. Marshall knew he would not likely be able to get permission to experiment on humans, so he decided to swallow a pure culture of *H. pylori.* He would be the animal model to see if ulcers developed (he had already determined that his stomach did not harbor *H. pylori*). Within a week of ingesting the bacteria, Marshall had classic symptoms of gastritis. Biopsies from his stomach showed bacteria and infection where previously there had been a healthy stomach lining.

Soon after Marshall published the result of his self-experimentation, he was able to obtain funding for a more detailed experiment to determine the role of *H. pylori* in stomach disease. Marshall and Warren later discovered the way the bacteria cause infections and disease. They also determined why many people harbor the bacteria in their stomachs but never develop disease. Other researchers confirmed their findings, and, by the early 1990s, the role *H. pylori* played in stomach ulcers and chronic gastritis was well established. For their research Marshall and Warren shared the Nobel Prize in Physiology or Medicine in 2005.

■ Issues and Impact

These stories dramatically illustrate medical research using human volunteers. At the time Carroll and Lazear contracted yellow fever, medical research using the scientific method was scarcely a few decades old. No guidelines on using human volunteers existed when Carroll exposed himself to a deadly disease in the name of science. Many decades would elapse before guidelines established what truly constitutes informed consent.

The physicians of the Yellow Fever Commission obtained consent of the volunteers. This was unusual at the time. The consent documents established a contract between individual volunteers and the Yellow Fever Commission, represented by Reed. Each volunteer was at least 25 years old, and each explicitly volunteered to participate in the research. The documents discussed the near certainty of contracting yellow fever while being in Cuba versus the risks of developing the disease as part of the experiment. The volunteers received promises of expert and timely medical care, and the volunteers had to remain at Camp Lazear, the site of the experiments, for the duration of the studies. The volunteers received $100 "in American gold," with an additional $100 if they developed yellow fever. This money represented a near fortune for many at the time. A family member could receive the money in case of death, but, if the volunteer deserted prior to completion of the experiment, they forfeited all payments.

This consent is quite coercive by modern-day standards. Essentially, the volunteers heard that they would likely get yellow fever anyway, so if they volunteered they would receive both money and better medical care than the average soldier or immigrant would likely obtain. No organization overseeing human research would allow such a means of obtaining volunteers for research in the 21st century. This "informed consent" has elements of coercion, forceful persuasion, and manipulation, particularly among the military, with officers asking enlisted personnel to participate. However, the involved physicians truly put themselves first in line, and at that time obtaining any consent was remarkable.

The modern practice of informed consent in human research did not come into being until after the revelations of the abuse of human subjects in the middle of the 20th century. The well-documented atrocities committed by German and Japanese physicians during World War II (1939–1945) made the names Josef Mengele (1911–1979) and Shiro Ishii (1892–1959) synonymous with torture in the name of medical science. Perhaps less well documented are the experiments during World War II by American physician Stafford Warren (1896–1981). In attempts to learn of radiation effects, researchers injected plutonium into humans without their consent. Experiments on American troops using mustard gas were conducted with the "volunteers" not knowing what they were volunteering for. Unlike the example of Carroll, none of the physicians involved in these experiments stepped forward to experiment first on themselves.

Knowledge of the abuse of human subjects in the Nazi concentration camps resulted in the drafting of the 1947 Nuremberg Code. Perhaps one of the most important of the 10 principles in the code is the assertion that consent to participate in medical research must be given free of coercive influence. Also directed in the code is the assertion that the benefits of the research should exceed the risk to the human volunteers.

In 1964 medical leaders drafted another, somewhat more thorough set of guidelines, the Declaration of Helsinki. This document set forth ethical principles for medical research involving human subjects. Together with the Nuremberg Code, the declaration—amended several times and most recently in 2013—sets forth the ethical principles to which medical research using human beings must adhere.

Marshall discussed the ethics of his decision to experiment on himself in his Nobel Lecture. He stated, "I had to be my own guinea pig." He felt that he was the only one who could make truly informed consent to his own experiment, and this thinking confirmed his approach to the problem of using human subjects to prove the role of *H. pylori* in stomach disease.

PRIMARY SOURCE

The Prevention of Yellow Fever

SOURCE: *Reed, Walter, and James Carroll. "The Prevention of Yellow Fever."* Public Health Papers and Reports *27 (1901): 113–130. This article can also be found online at https://www.ncbi.nlm.nih.gov/pmc/articles/PMC2329408/pdf/pubhealthpap00030-0119.pdf (accessed February 13, 2018).*

INTRODUCTION: *The following is an excerpt from Walter Reed and James Carroll's 1901 article in* Public Health Papers and Reports. *In the excerpt, Reed and Carroll describe how they proved their hypothesis that mosquitoes were responsible for transmitting yellow fever. They also strongly recommend that measures be taken to reduce certain mosquito populations that spread the disease in the United States.*

Continuing our studies, especially as regards the means by which yellow fever is spread from individual to individual, and as to the manner in which houses become infected, we were able, under strict rules of isolation and quarantine, to bring about an attack of yellow fever in ten non-immune individuals (and always within the period of incubation of this disease) out of a total of thirteen (76.84%) whom we attempted to infect by means of the bites of mosquitoes—Stegomyia Fasciata—that had previously been fed with the blood of yellow fever patients during the first, second and third days of their attacks. These results were reported in part to the Pan-American Congress held in Havana during February of this year and in part to the Association of American Physicians at its last meeting held in the city of Washington.

It will be seen that we were able to establish in the most conclusive manner that the mosquito serves as the intermediate host for the parasite of yellow fever. At this same Experimental Sanitary Station we were also able to demonstrate that an attack of yellow fever cannot be induced by the most intimate and prolonged contact with the clothing and bedding of yellow fever patients, even though these articles had been previously thoroughly soiled with the excreta of such patients.

In other words, we were able to prove that the garments worn, and the bedding used, by yellow fever patients were no more concerned in propagating this disease, than the clothing and bedding of patients suffering from malarial fever are concerned in the spread of the latter malady. The doctrine of the spread of yellow fever by fomites having, at the first touch of actual experiment on human beings, burst like a bubble, we may hereafter cast it aside, with other exploded beliefs, to the very great simplification of the problem how to prevent yellow fever. Indeed, in our opinion, the time has now arrived when the latter problem may be reduced to measures which shall prevent the propagation of this disease by mosquitoes. Although the specific agent of yellow fever has not, as yet, been discovered, this must remain largely a matter of scientific interest, and does not, in the least, lessen the efforts which we, as sanitarians, are now able for the first time, to bring into action for the prevention of the spread of this disease; since in dealing with the mosquito, we are dealing with the intermediate host which carries the specific agent from the sick to the well.

In considering, then, in a broad way, the prevention of yellow fever, the natural order would be to give our attention, first, to measures which will prevent the importation of this disease from infected places into the seaports of the United States; and secondly, to measures which will most effectually prevent the spread of this disease, provided it should gain a lodgment in one of the cities of this country.

With your permission, however, we will reverse the order of consideration above suggested, and will later refer in the briefest manner to the prevention of the importation of yellow fever into the United States from foreign ports, since this part of the subject will be presented by the health officer of the port of New York, who, from long experience, will be able to deal more intelligently than we with this part of the problem.

Since the mosquito, especially that species of Stegomyia which has recently been designated by Theobald as Stegomyia Fasciata (formerly known to entomologists as Culex Fasciatus), has become so prominent a factor in the spread of yellow fever, it becomes necessary to consider this insect from the point of view of his identification; its habitat; its breeding places; the length of its generation; its hours of feeding; the influence of temperature upon both its propagation and stinging; the interval after contamination before the insect becomes capable of propagating the disease; the length of time during which it remains dangerous; the measures that should be used not only to protect the sick against the bites of these insects, but also to prevent the latter from infecting the healthy individual; and finally, a consideration of the several agents which may be successfully employed both to prevent the breeding of mosquitoes as well as directed towards their destruction in the adult stage.

Aside from the standpoint of scientific interest, it is certainly a matter of hygienic importance, in taking up the question of how to prevent the spread of yellow fever, when imported into the United States, that the health authorities of our several coast cities, and, indeed, of some of our inland towns, should be able to determine whether the only species of mosquito, which, up to the present time, has been shown capable of conveying yellow fever, is or is not present in these cities. If it should hereafter be proven that only species of the genus Stegomyia are capable of acting as intermediate hosts for the specific agent of yellow fever, as appears to have been demonstrated for the genus Anopheles in the spread of malaria, the presence or absence of the former genus will definitely determine whether yellow fever will or will not spread in a given locality. The presence or absence of mosquitoes that can propagate the disease is the only intelligible explanation of what has heretofore been considered an inexplicable problem, viz., the capability of this disease to propagate itself in certain localities, while in other places it could be introduced with perfect impunity to the public health. In other words, our present knowledge of this question solves, at last, the problem of the portability or non-portability of yellow fever.

SEE ALSO *Helicobacter pylori*; Malaria; Public Health and Infectious Disease; Yellow Fever

BIBLIOGRAPHY

Books

Emanuel, Ezekiel J. *The Oxford Textbook of Clinical Research Ethics.* New York: Oxford University Press, 2011.

Periodicals

Ghooi, Ravindra B. "The Nuremberg Code—A Critique." *Perspectives in Clinical Research* 2, no. 2 (April–June 2011): 72–76. This article can also be found online at https://www.ncbi.nlm.nih.gov/pmc/articles/PMC3121268/ (accessed February 12, 2018).

Shuster, Evelyn. "Fifty Years Later: The Significance of the Nuremberg Code." *New England Journal of Medicine* 337 (November 13, 1997): 1436–1440. This article can also be found online at http://www.nejm.org/doi/full/10.1056/NEJM199711133372006 (accessed February 12, 2018).

Websites

"45 CFR 46." US Department of Health & Human Services, January 15, 2009. https://www.hhs.gov/ohrp/regulations-and-policy/regulations/45-cfr-46/index.html (accessed February 12, 2018).

"The Nuremberg Code." National Institutes of Health, 1949. https://history.nih.gov/research/downloads/nuremberg.pdf (accessed February 12, 2018).

"WMA Declaration of Helsinki—Ethical Principles for Medical Research Involving Human Subjects." World Medical Association, March 29, 2017. https://www.wma.net/policies-post/wma-declaration-of-helsinki-ethical-principles-for-medical-research-involving-human-subjects/ (accessed February 12, 2018)

Lloyd Scott Clements
Claire Skinner

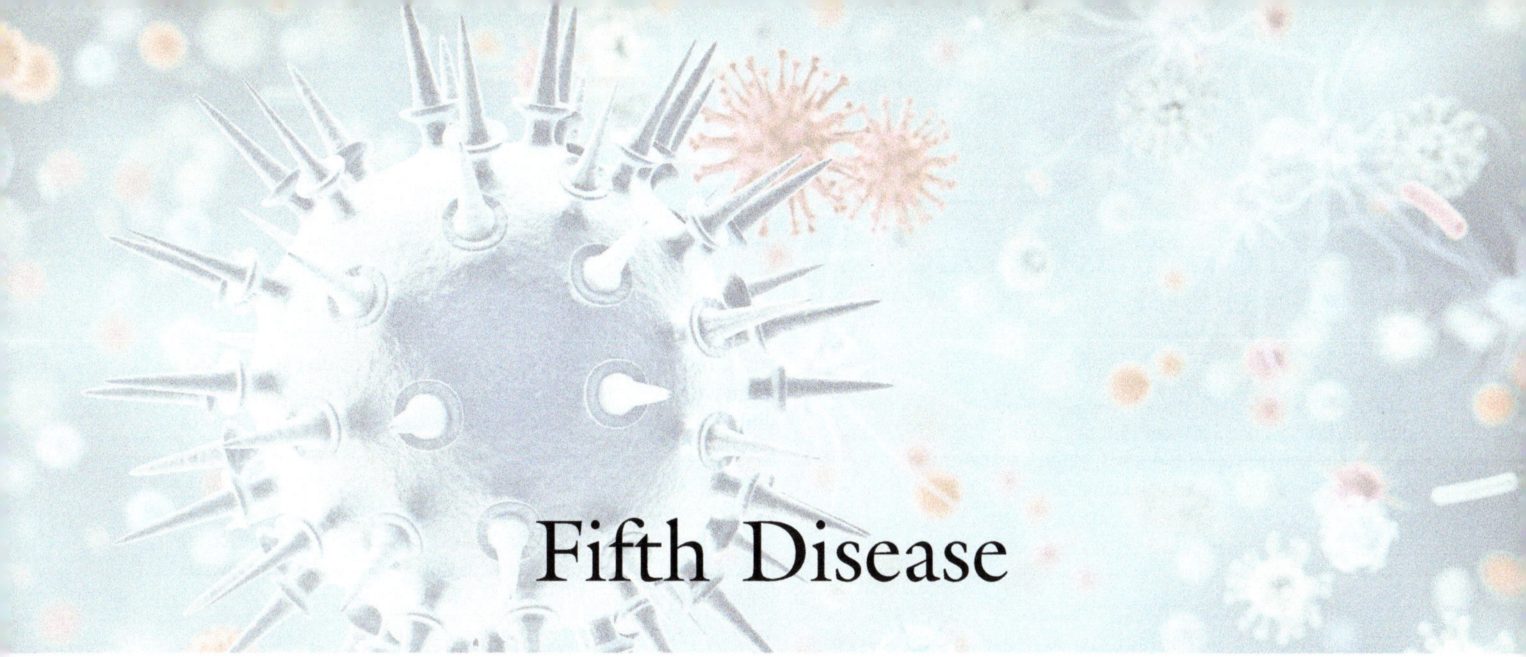

Fifth Disease

Introduction

Fifth disease, or erythema infectiosum (infectious redness), is a common childhood viral infection that is characterized by a mild rash. The infection lasts less than two weeks. Fifth disease is also known as slapped cheek syndrome because of the characteristic redness of the face that develops.

The illness can also occur in adults, where it can involve the joints. In people with some forms of anemia or immune system malfunction, fifth disease can become a more serious condition.

Disease History, Characteristics, and Transmission

While fifth disease is likely ancient in origin, its cause has been known only since 1975. Fifth disease is caused by human Parvovirus B19. Only humans can be infected by this virus, although other types of parvovirus infect dogs and cats. Parvovirus B19 cannot be spread from humans to dogs and cats, nor can the parvoviruses that infect dogs and cats be passed to humans.

The designation *fifth disease* arose because, when the prevalence of childhood rash-producing illnesses were determined, it was fifth in occurrence behind scarlet fever and three forms of measles.

A hallmark feature of fifth disease is the presence of a bright red rash on the cheeks. A duller rash can also be present on the arms, legs, stomach, and back. The rash sometimes fades, only to be reactivated by stresses such as sunlight, exercise, and heat.

A child with fifth disease may also develop a mild fever and coldlike symptoms and become tired in the days before the appearance of the rash. Other symptoms can include swollen glands, red eyes, sore throat, and diarrhea.

Some adults who are infected with Parvovirus B19 do not develop symptoms. Others develop the characteristic rash. In others, joints become swollen and painful in a way that is similar to arthritis. Still other adults develop both the rash and the joint discomfort.

WORDS TO KNOW

ANTIBODIES Also called Y-shaped immunoglobulins, proteins found in the blood that help to fight against foreign substances called *antigens*. Antigens, which are usually proteins or polysaccharides, stimulate the immune system to produce antibodies. The antibodies inactivate the antigen and help to remove it from the body. While antigens can be the source of infections from pathogenic bacteria and viruses, organic molecules detrimental to the body from internal or environmental sources also act as antigens. Genetic engineering and the use of various mutational mechanisms allow the construction of a vast array of antibodies (each with a unique genetic sequence).

DROPLET A drop of water or other fluid that is fewer than 5 microns (a millionth of a meter) in diameter.

IMMUNOSUPPRESSION A reduction of the ability of the immune system to recognize and respond to the presence of foreign material.

INCUBATION PERIOD The time between exposure to a disease-causing virus or bacteria and the appearance of symptoms of the infection. Depending on the microorganism, the incubation time can range from a few hours (for example, food poisoning due to *Salmonella*) to a decade or more (for example, acquired immunodeficiency syndrome, or AIDS).

EFFECTIVE RULES AND REGULATIONS

The National Center for Infectious Diseases, Respiratory and Enteric Viruses Branch states, "Excluding persons with fifth disease from work, child care centers, or schools is not likely to prevent the spread of the virus, since people are contagious before they develop the rash."

Fifth disease is contagious, at least until the rash appears. This can occur as early as four days after infection with the parvovirus, but some people can be symptom-free for almost three weeks. Person-to-person transmission is likely during this time, especially among children who may be in close contact with each other in a day care or other facility, because both the child and the caregiver are usually unaware that an infection is present, so no special precautions are yet being taken. By the time the rash has appeared, a child or an adult is no longer contagious.

The incubation period for the disease is 4 to 20 days from the time of exposure. Transmission of the virus occurs via contaminated droplets, by the passage of saliva, sputum, or mucous from the nose from one person to another. Likely routes also include sharing eating utensils or drink containers.

Scope and Distribution

Fifth disease occurs worldwide and is a common childhood illness. It tends to be seasonal, occurring more frequently in late winter and early spring. However, cases can occur any time of the year. During outbreaks in schools, 10 to 60 percent of students acquire the disease.

Fifth disease occurs more commonly among children ages 5 to 14 but also occurs in preschool-age children and their parents. About 50 percent of tested adults show antibodies in their blood to the disease, meaning they have already contracted it and are immune.

Treatment and Prevention

Treatment is usually not necessary, as the infection passes within a week or two. In some adults with fifth disease, joint swelling and pain can last for several months. Over-the-counter medications can be helpful in easing joint discomfort. In those with more serious symptoms, treatment with Parvovirus B19 antibodies can be useful. As of 2017 there was no vaccine for fifth disease.

Options for infected pregnant women and their unborn children should be discussed with a personal physician. As of 2017 the US Centers for Disease Control and Prevention (CDC) stated that the disease is usually not a problem for pregnant women and their babies. About half of pregnant women are immune to Parvovirus B19, so they and their babies are usually protected from getting the virus and fifth disease. The CDC further noted that pregnant women who are not immune usually have only mild illness if they are exposed to fifth disease, and their babies usually do not have any problems. In rare cases (less than 5 percent of all pregnancies involving women with Parvovirus B19 infection), severe anemia can occur.

A bout of fifth disease protects a person from a further illness, as the immunity that is built up to the parvovirus lasts for a person's lifetime.

Impacts and Issues

Fifth disease is an almost-universal aspect of childhood. Fortunately for the millions of children around the world who contract the infection every year, the illness is not severe and resolves on its own.

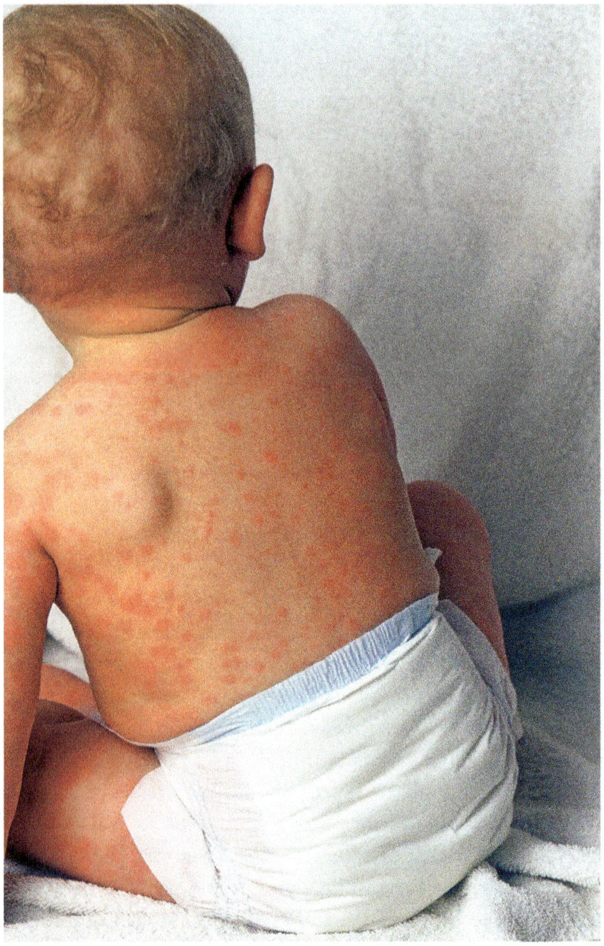

A baby suffering from fifth disease, a mild rash common in children, caused by a type of virus called Parvovirus B19. © *Loisjoy Thurstun/Alamy Stock Photo*

Children with fifth disease are sometimes excluded from school when the characteristic rash appears on the face, in an effort to reduce the chance of spreading the disease. In fact, the contagious period is earlier, when cold or flulike symptoms are present. Once the rash appears, the children are no longer able to spread the disease.

For people with anemia (a condition where the transport of oxygen by the blood is impaired), fifth disease can cause the anemia to become more severe. People whose immune system is not functioning efficiently due to illness, such as acquired immunodeficiency syndrome (AIDS), or deliberate immunosuppression, which is used, for example, to lessen the chance of rejection of a transplanted organ, can develop anemia with fifth disease that is more long-lasting.

SEE ALSO *Childhood-Associated Infectious Diseases, Immunization Impacts; Viral Disease*

BIBLIOGRAPHY

Books

Aronson, Susan, and Timothy R. Shope. *Managing Infectious Disease in Child Care and School: A Quick Reference Guide.* Elk Grove Village, IL: American Academy of Pediatrics, 2016.

Cherry, James, and Gail J. Demmler-Harrison. *Feigen and Cherry's Textbook of Pediatric Infectious Disease.* Philadelphia: Elsevier Saunders, 2014.

Long, Sarah S., and Charles G. Prober. *Principles and Practice of Pediatric Infectious Disease.* Philadelphia: Elsevier, 2017.

Periodicals

Khorsandi, Danial, and Ghasemi Mahtab. "Childhood Skin Disorders: Genetic Study of the Erythema Infectiosum (Fifth Disease)." *Journal of Pregnancy and Child Health* 4 (2017): 1–4.

Websites

"Parvovirus B19 and Fifth Disease." Centers for Disease Control and Prevention. http://www.cdc.gov/parvovirusb19/fifth-disease.html (accessed November 16, 2017).

Brian Hoyle

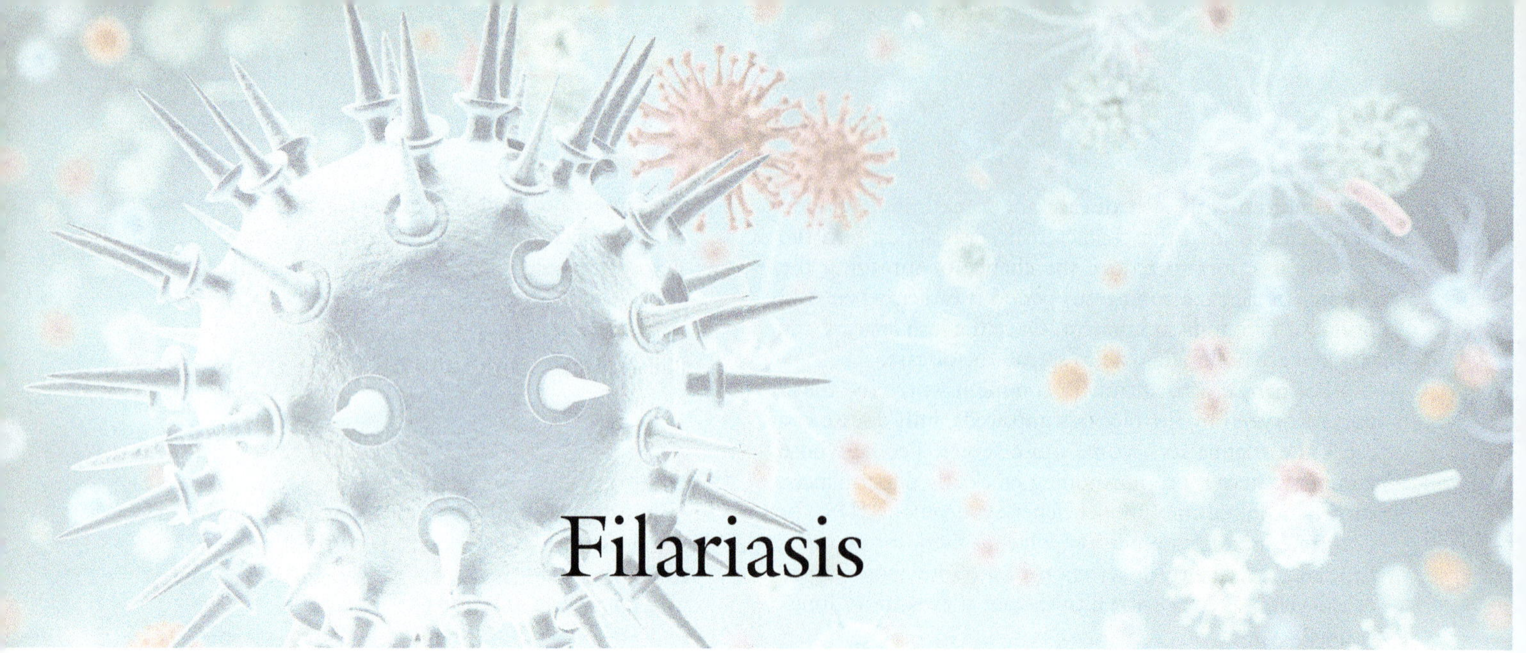

Filariasis

Introduction

Filariasis, or lymphatic filariasis, is a preventable parasitic disease caused by the nematodes (roundworms) *Wuchereria bancrofti*, *Brugia malayi*, and *Brugia timori*. It is considered to be among the most significant causes of permanent disability in the developing world. While filariasis has historically been endemic in more than 70 countries, a global effort to eliminate the disease has helped dramatically reduce its prevalence, and some countries, including China and South Korea, have successfully achieved targets for its elimination.

When symptomatic, patients may present with severe lymphatic swelling (lymphedema) and severe limb swelling (elephantiasis). The disfigurations resulting from elephantiasis and lymphedema raise issues among some communities and add to the socioeconomic impacts of this debilitating disease. It is one of the leading causes of global disability.

Infection is transmitted through mosquito bites, where both the vector (disease carrier) and the human host are necessary in the successful completion of the parasitic life cycle. Antiparasitic treatment is available but expensive. It can take about a year to eliminate the parasites.

WORDS TO KNOW

LYMPHATIC SYSTEM The body's network of organs, ducts, and tissues that filter harmful substances out of the fluid that surrounds body tissues. Lymphatic organs include the bone marrow, thymus, spleen, appendix, tonsils, adenoids, lymph nodes, and Peyer's patches (in the small intestine). The thymus and bone marrow are called primary lymphatic organs because lymphocytes are produced in them. The other lymphatic organs are called secondary lymphatic organs. The lymphatic system is a complex network of thin vessels, capillaries, valves, ducts, nodes, and organs that runs throughout the body, helping protect and maintain the internal fluids system of the entire body by both producing and filtering lymph and by producing various blood cells. The three main purposes of the lymphatic system are to drain fluid back into the bloodstream from the tissues, to filter lymph, and to fight infections.

SOCIOECONOMIC Concerning both social and economic factors.

VECTOR Any agent that carries and transmits parasites and diseases. Also, an organism or a chemical used to transport a gene into a new host cell.

Disease History, Characteristics, and Transmission

Filariasis was first recognized in its infectious form in 1866 when filarial larvae were detected in urine and identified as the causative agent.

The infection is usually acquired in childhood but takes years to manifest. It typically remains asymptomatic until adulthood. Once developed, symptoms may include chronic swelling of the lymph nodes and swelling of the arms, legs, and genitals. Elephantiasis refers to the thickening of skin and underlying tissue and often accompanies symptoms. Without presentation of symptoms, internal damage to the kidneys and the lymphatic system may also develop.

Transmission of filariasis occurs through mosquito bites, whereby the larval form is drawn out of blood by mosquitos, develops to the infective stage, and is injected into a new host. Here the larvae develop into the adult form, migrate to the lymph nodes, mate, and release millions of larvae into the host's bloodstream. Adult worms may live up to six years, during which time the host will remain a source of infection for others.

Scope and Distribution

Filariasis is a disease largely associated with poverty. Though the disease was commonly found in some 73 countries, incidence in these countries has declined in the early 21st century because of initiatives such as the Global Programme to Eliminate Lymphatic Filariasis (GPELF), which the World Health Organization (WHO) launched in 2000. As of 2017 18 of these 73 countries were "conducting surveillance to validate elimination," according to WHO.

Infection caused by *W. bancrofti* is endemic in tropical regions of Southeast Asia, Africa, India, and Central and South America, while *B. malayi* and *B. timori* are generally limited to areas of Southeast Asia. This disease state is rare in Western countries. According to the US Centers for Disease Control and Prevention (CDC), the infection disappeared in the United States in the early 20th century.

Filariasis has been recognized as the leading cause of permanent disability worldwide, with up to 54 million people affected as of 2017. That year, according to WHO, 25 million men worldwide remained affected by swelling in the scrotum (hydrocele) caused by filariasis, and more than 15 million people by lymphedema.

Disease distribution is also affected by habitat suitability for the various forms of mosquitoes responsible for transmission of the parasite and by the extent of mass drug administration in areas where infection is endemic.

RELATED DISEASE GROUPS

Filariasis is a group of tropical diseases caused by thread-like parasitic roundworms (nematodes of the superfamily Filarioidea, commonly called filariae) and their larvae. The group affects humans and animals. The larvae transmit the disease to humans through a mosquito bite. Filariasis is characterized by fever, chills, headache, and skin lesions in the early stages and, if untreated, can progress to include gross enlargement of the limbs and genitalia in a condition called elephantiasis. There are hundreds of described filarial parasites but only eight that cause infections in humans: *Brugia malayi, Wucheria bancrofti, Brugia timori, Onchocerca volvulus, Loa loa, Mansonella streptocerca, Mansonella ozzardi*, and *Mansonella perstans.*

Treatment and Prevention

Treatment of filariasis consists of a multifaceted approach. Treatment of the infection itself may be achieved with a concurrent dosage of strong antiparasitic drugs such as diethylcarbamazine citrate (DEC), DEC-fortified salt, and albendazole. This combination

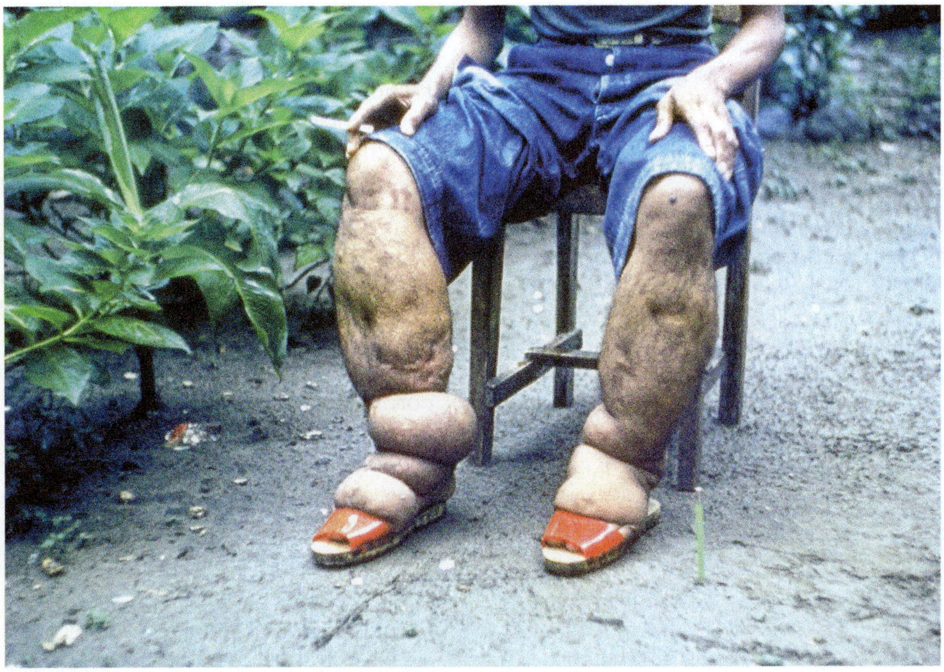

In Luzon, Philippines, a person who has contracted filariasis displays this painful and disfiguring disease's most prominent symptom: elephantiasis of the leg. © Smith Collection/Gado/Getty Images

of drugs proves to be 99 percent effective in removing microfilaria from the blood after one year of treatment.

Lymphodema and elephantiasis are often exacerbated due to bacterial and fungal infections taking advantage of the patient's compromised lymphatic condition. Following rigorous hygiene routines as prevention against infection from opportunistic pathogens and completing exercises to improve lymph flow often helps to reduce these causes of swelling. Surgery may be necessary for treatment of severe genital swelling in men.

Prevention of filariasis is achievable by reducing exposure to mosquito bites and treating endemic communities, in total, to remove the pool of infection. Some means of prevention are relatively simple and inexpensive. Using mosquito netting in sleeping areas, wearing clothing that covers the arms and legs, applying mosquito repellant on exposed skin, and remaining indoors during peak times of mosquito activity all reduce the risk of exposure to filariasis. These measures are the basis of a global campaign to eradicate filariasis.

■ Impacts and Issues

Filariasis causes permanent—and often painful—disability in more than 40 million people worldwide. Most cases occur in developing or underdeveloped regions. Many people disabled by filariasis cannot regularly farm, work, or attend school. Malnourishment rates are often higher among those affected by filariasis than in the surrounding noninfected population.

The social impacts of filariasis present not only in the loss of work labor due to incapacitation but also in community relations. People disfigured by the disease are frequently shunned by society, and chronic complications are often deemed shameful. Marriage is considered a near impossibility among those suffering genital manifestations, which then puts growth and development of the community at risk.

Filariasis is a disease with potential for eradication, and the international community has made eliminating the disease a priority. In 1997 WHO identified filariasis as one of six "eradicable or potentially eradicable" infectious diseases. The World Health Assembly followed suit the same year with a call for countries to eradicate the disease. The result was the creation of the GPELF in 2000. The program aimed to implement mass drug administration, reduce infection "below a threshold at which transmission is not sustainable," and provide care for those who are infected. Also in 2000 a public-private initiative known as the Global Alliance to Eliminate Lymphatic Filariasis was formed to help provide technical assistance to the GPELF. The United Nations has also targeted eliminating filariasis as part of its 2000–2015 Millennium Development Goals and its 2015–2030 Sustainable Development Goals.

Such efforts have begun to pay off. In 2007 China reported filariasis had been eliminated. A year later South Korea did the same. According to WHO, as of 2017 18 other countries were seeking to verify that the disease had been eradicated, and 22 countries had completed mass drug administration and were "on track to achieve elimination." Despite such progress, filariasis remains endemic in poor communities in countries that have not completed mass drug administration initiatives.

In 2017 researchers made an important breakthrough in the understanding of the relationship between *B. malayi*, one of the worms that causes filariasis, and *Wolbachia*, the bacteria these worms carry. Alexandra Grote and her coauthors examined the "molecular interplay" between the worms and the bacteria. The results of their study "highlighted specific pathways to which both *Wolbachia* and *B. malayi* contribute concurrently over the life cycle of the parasite, paving the way for the development of novel intervention strategies."

See Also *Demographics and Infectious Disease; Economic Development and Disease; Helminth Disease; Host and Vector; Opportunistic Infection; Parasitic Diseases*

BIBLIOGRAPHY

Books

Mandell, G. L., J. E. Bennett, and R. Dolin, eds. *Principles and Practice of Infectious Diseases.* 7th ed. Philadelphia: Elsevier, 2010.

Periodicals

Babu, Subash, and Thomas B. Nutman. "Immunology of Lymphatic Filariasis." *Parasite Immunology* 36, no. 8 (2014): 338–346. This article can also be found online at https://www.ncbi.nlm.nih.gov/pmc/articles/PMC3990654/ (accessed January 22, 2018).

Grote, Alexandra, et al. "Defining *Brugia Malayi* and *Wolbachia* Symbiosis by Stage-Specific Dual RNA-Seq." *PLOS Neglected Tropical Diseases* 11, no. 3 (2017). This article can also be found online at https://doi.org/10.1371/journal.pntd.0005357 (accessed January 22, 2018).

Hoerauf, Achim. "Filariasis: New Drugs and New Opportunities for Lymphatic Filariasis and Onchocerciasis." *Current Opinion in Infectious Disease* 21, no. 6 (2008): 673–681. This article can also be found online at https://insights.ovid.com/pubmed?pmid=18978537 (accessed January 22, 2018).

Websites

"Filariasis." National Organization for Rare Disorders. https://rarediseases.org/rare-diseases/filariasis/ (accessed January 22, 2018).

Hotez, Peter, and Serap Aksoy. "Eliminating Lymphatic Filariasis in Cameroon." Speaking of Medicine Community Blog, June 29, 2017. http://blogs.plos.org/speakingofmedicine/2017/06/29/eliminating-lymphatic-filariasis-in-cameroon/ (accessed January 22, 2018).

"Lymphatic Filariasis." Centers for Disease Control and Prevention, June 14, 2013. https://www.cdc.gov/parasites/lymphaticfilariasis/ (accessed January 22, 2018).

"Lymphatic Filariasis." World Health Organization. http://www.who.int/lymphatic_filariasis/en/ (January 22, 2018).

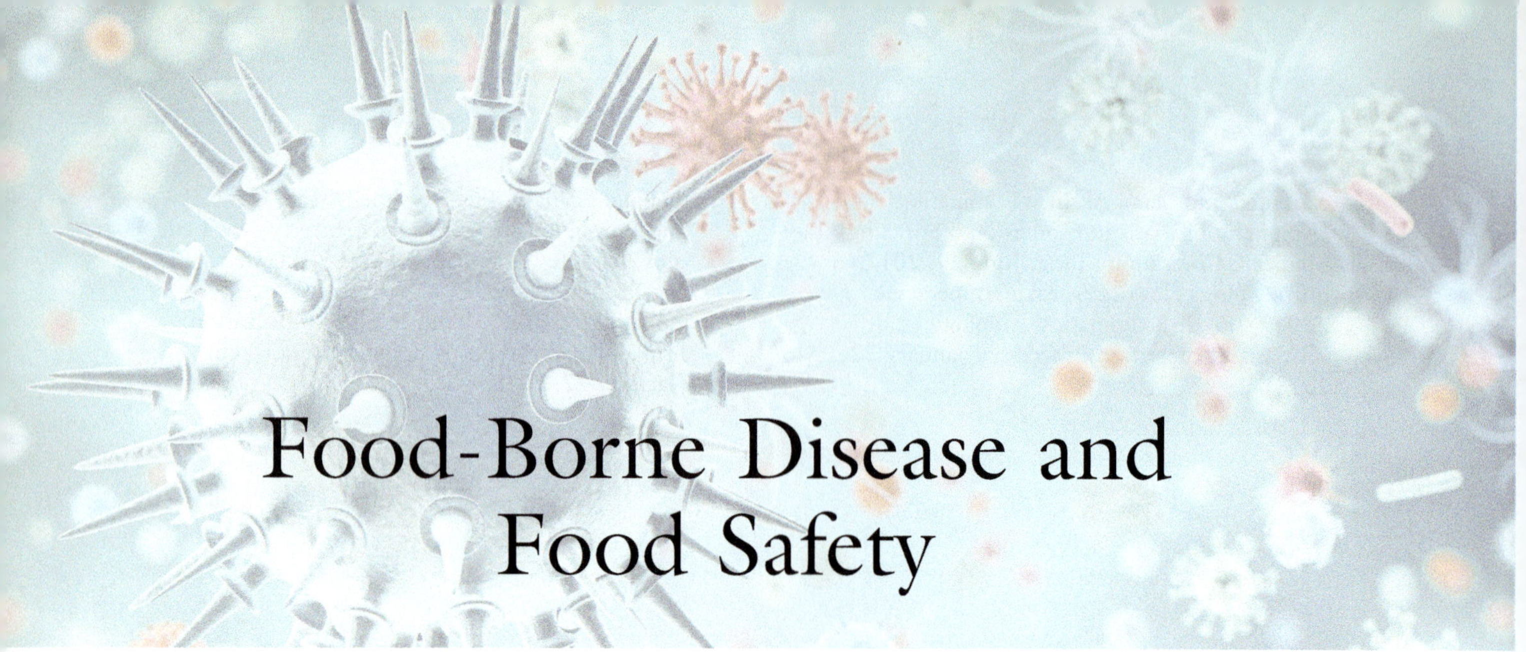

Food-Borne Disease and Food Safety

■ Introduction

Food is necessary for human growth and survival. The nutrients in many foods that are vital to humans, however, also provide a meal for microorganisms. The organic (carbon-containing) compounds and moisture content of many foods permit the growth of microbes. Sometimes this coexistence is beneficial. For example, bacteria in the genus *Lactobacillus* help produce yogurt. However, the presence of some microorganisms in foods threatens the food supply and the health of those who eat it.

Some bacteria that can form spores can survive for extended periods of time in foods that are too acidic to permit growth of the bacteria. If the food is eaten, the spores can germinate, and growth can resume in the more hospitable environment of the intestinal tract.

Bacteria, viruses, parasites, and poisons (toxins) produced by some microbes cause more than 200 different food-borne diseases. This is a serious health threat worldwide. For example, in the United States, 2017 statistics from the Centers for Disease Control and Prevention (CDC) indicate that there are an estimated 48 million food-borne diseases every year. These diseases affect about one of every six Americans, with about 128,000 requiring hospital care and 3,000 dying.

WORDS TO KNOW

ANAEROBIC BACTERIA Bacteria that grow without oxygen, also called anaerobic bacteria or anaerobes. Anaerobic bacteria can infect deep wounds, deep tissues, and internal organs where there is little oxygen. These infections are characterized by abscess formation, foul-smelling pus, and tissue destruction.

FOOD PRESERVATION Any one of a number of techniques used to prevent food from spoiling, such as canning, pickling, drying or freeze-drying, irradiation, pasteurization, smoking, and the addition of chemical additives. Food preservation has become an increasingly important component of the food industry as fewer people eat foods produced on their own lands and as consumers expect to purchase and consume foods that are out of season.

IONIZING RADIATION Any electromagnetic or particulate radiation capable of direct or indirect ion production in its passage through matter. In general use: Radiation that can cause tissue damage or death.

IRRADIATION A method of preservation that treats food with low doses of radiation to deactivate enzymes and to kill microorganisms and insects.

SPORE A dormant form assumed by some bacteria, such as anthrax, that enables the bacterium to survive high temperatures, dryness, and lack of nourishment for long periods of time. Under proper conditions, the spore may revert to the actively multiplying form of the bacteria.

■ Disease History, Characteristics, and Transmission

Food-borne diseases tend to be from microorganisms that usually live in the intestinal tract. Generally, the illnesses produce intestinal upset, often with nausea and vomiting. Food-borne illnesses are commonly called food poisoning. However, the term *food poisoning* obscures the fact that there are several types of food-borne diseases that vary in cause and severity. While mild to moderate illnesses tend to pass after a few days, more serious illnesses can cause kidney damage or failure, muscle paralysis, and death.

Death most often results from the excessive loss of fluid that occurs with diarrhea. A person can lose fluid at a rate that is difficult to replace by drinking water. If the person cannot get medical attention (such as the continual provision of fluids intravenously), he or she can go into shock and suffer organ failure.

In many countries, including the United States and Canada, the majority of food-borne diseases are caused by the Norwalk-like virus (norovirus) and by bacteria including *Campylobacter* (mainly *C. jejuni*), *Salmonella* species, *Escherichia coli*, species of *Listeria*, and *Clostridium* species.

The most common cause of food-borne disease in the United States is norovirus. The virus normally lives in the human intestinal tract and is usually spread to food when the food is handled by people who have not washed their hands properly after a bowel movement. More than 9 million infections are estimated to occur each year in the United States alone. Most of these could be eliminated by proper handwashing. Globally, the World Health Organization (WHO) estimates that there are 35,000 deaths each year resulting from food contaminated by norovirus.

Another major source of food-borne disease is poultry that is contaminated with *C. jejuni*. The bacterium is a normal resident in the intestinal tract of poultry. During the slaughtering process, the intestinal contents of the poultry can be spread onto the skin. Even with washing of the carcasses, bacteria can remain stuck in crevasses and other areas on the surface. Indeed, monitoring studies have reported that about half to 90 percent of the poultry that reaches supermarket shelves is contaminated with *Campylobacter* strains.

Even with the hundreds of millions of poultry meals eaten in the United States each year, the number of illnesses produced by *C. jejuni* is relatively low. Because the bacteria are susceptible to heat, thorough cooking will kill the bacteria long before the meal is eaten. However, improper cooking and the recontamination of cooked meat by, for example, laying the meat on a cutting board that has not been washed after use, sickens millions of Americans annually.

Salmonella species cause about 1 million cases of food-borne disease each year in the United States, and contamination with *Salmonella* is a major cause of food-borne disease globally. There are hundreds of species of *Salmonella*, and dozens of them are capable of causing illness. For example, *S. enteritidis* is commonly associated with egg-containing prepared salad dressings or custards that have been left for several hours at room temperature. This allows the contaminating bacteria to grow to numbers that cause disease when eaten.

From May to early October 2017, an outbreak of food-borne illness caused by *Salmonella*-contaminated papayas shipped from Mexico sickened 220 people in 23 US states. Sixty-eight people were hospitalized, and one died. Globally, WHO estimates that about 52,000 deaths occur each year due to *Salmonella* food poisoning.

Escherichia coli O157:H7 and related *E. coli* strains can cause severe intestinal illnesses (they are collectively known as enterohemorrhagic *E. coli*, or EHEC). Still other varieties of *E. coli* are normally found in the intestinal tract of humans and animals but are usually harmless. However, strain O157:H7 arose in the 1970s when genetic material from another bacterium, *Shigella*, was transferred to *E. coli*. The genetic material coded for the production of a potent toxin and made the new *E. coli* extremely dangerous. The toxin damages intestinal cells, which causes bleeding, and

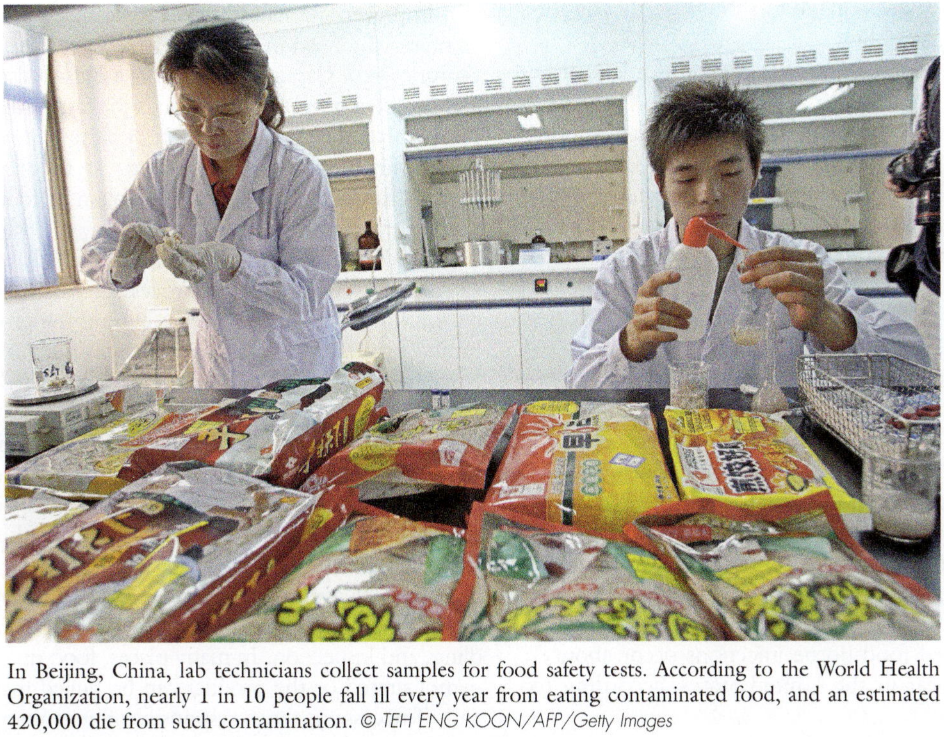

In Beijing, China, lab technicians collect samples for food safety tests. According to the World Health Organization, nearly 1 in 10 people fall ill every year from eating contaminated food, and an estimated 420,000 die from such contamination. *© TEH ENG KOON/AFP/Getty Images*

SCIENTIFIC, POLITICAL, AND ETHICAL ISSUES

Although food irradiation is opposed by some advocacy groups, the practice has become widespread. According to the Food and Drug Administration (FDA), "Irradiation does not make foods radioactive, compromise nutritional quality, or noticeably change the taste, texture, or appearance of food. In fact, any changes made by irradiation are so minimal that it is not easy to tell if a food has been irradiated."

Food is irradiated by applying ionizing radiation that destroys potentially harmful microorganisms. The FDA has procedures in place for the initial determination that irradiation is safe for a particular food, as well as for regulating the sources of radiation used in the process.

can spread via the bloodstream to the kidneys, potentially causing permanent organ damage or failure.

O157:H7 can be a normal part of the bacterial community found in the intestinal tract of cattle. The illness is usually produced when cattle feces contaminate drinking water. The bacterium can also contaminate ground beef during slaughter and packaging. As with *Campylobacter*, inadequate cooking allows the bacteria to remain alive. Vegetables can also become contaminated by manure supplied as fertilizer. Raw vegetables should be thoroughly washed before consumption.

Globally, WHO estimates that 37,000 deaths can be attributed to *E. coli* annually.

Some bacteria in the genus *Listeria* also cause food-borne illnesses. *Listeria monocytogenes* causes listeriosis, a rare but serious illness. *Listeria* especially threatens people with compromised immune systems, the elderly, and pregnant women. In addition to the usual symptoms associated with food poisoning, listeriosis can cause a severe form of meningitis. *Listeria* bacteria flourish in temperatures between 39°F (4°C) and 98.6°F (37°C).

Clostridium species such as *C. perfringens* and *C. botulinum* are anaerobic. These bacteria can contaminate canned food that has been inadequately prepared. The bacterium can form an environmentally hardy form called a spore. Spores are dormant and can survive for years in conditions that would kill the growing form of the bacterium. When conditions become more favorable, the spore can revive, and growth and division resume. The resuscitated bacteria are capable of causing disease. *Clostridium*-related food-borne infections occur about 1 million times a year in the United States, according to CDC data.

■ Scope and Distribution

Food-borne infections can affect anyone, anywhere. WHO estimates that more than 2 million people around the world die each year from diarrhea caused by food-borne infections. Most deaths from food-borne illnesses occur in developing nations.

Because food-borne illnesses are mainly caused by microorganisms that are residents of the intestinal tract, most outbreaks are related to fecal contamination of food and water rather than to the time of year or particular aspect of a culture. Worldwide, poor hygiene is the culprit.

■ Treatment and Prevention

Prevention of food-borne illness depends on several factors. The type of disease-causing organism can be important. For example, *Campylobacter* can be effectively treated by the proper cooking of foods, whereas spore-forming *Clostridium* may still be capable of causing an infection even after the food is heated. The environment is another factor; temperature and the amount of moisture in the food can influence the type of organisms that can thrive. Environment also includes the various places that the food passes through on its way to the dinner table. A food entering a processing plant may be safe, then become contaminated during processing. These factors are interrelated. For example, protecting a food from questionable environments but failing to decontaminate the food does little to lessen the chance of a food-borne illness.

Treatment of foods prior to eating is absolutely important in preventing illness. Some treatments, such as drying or preserving food in salt prior to a sea voyage, were done centuries ago. Canning of foods as a means of preservation and protection from spoilage began in the 18th century. In the 19th century the association of an unhygienic environment and disease was recognized. As food began to be shipped further to market, the problem of food deterioration during transit became apparent.

Food safety owes a great deal to Louis Pasteur (1822–1895), who developed the process of pasteurization. Pasteurization began in the 1890s. During the process milk is heated for a short time at temperatures high enough to be lethal to those microbes that would be expected to be contaminants without altering the taste or appearance of the milk. Milk is now routinely pasteurized before sale. Innovations in the pasteurization technique have increased the shelf-life of refrigerated milk and developed means of transporting and storing milk without the need for refrigeration.

Another prevention strategy is the development and legal enforcement of standards of food preparation, handling, and inspection. In many places, food quality must be demonstrated or the product can be pulled from the shelf and, if necessary, those responsible for its manufacture or distribution can be prosecuted. In the United States, the Food and Drug Administration (FDA) regulates processing and labeling of most foods. The US Department of Agriculture (USDA) regulates and oversees the safety of all meat, poultry, and egg products. The two agencies work together to ensure the safety of food produced within and imported into the United States. Both agencies also provide assistance to international organizations and developing nations that wish to implement or strengthen food safety programs.

While government agencies monitor the safety of food as it is produced and sold, monitoring food preparation and hygienic practices in the home must be done by individuals. Improper storage of foods prepared with raw or undercooked eggs can cause growth of microorganisms in the food. Improper cleaning of cutting boards and other preparation surfaces can cross-contaminate one food by another. Many cases of food poisoning with *Clostridium botulinum* are related to improper home canning of foods; the spores of the bacterium can survive the food preparation steps and remain capable of causing illness when the food is eaten, even years later.

■ Impacts and Issues

The impact of food-borne illnesses on the individual is substantial. The estimated 48 million food-borne illnesses that are thought to occur each year in the United States (likely an underestimate, as many people who suffer from an illness do so without seeking medical attention) result in the hospitalization of 128,000 people and the death of about 3,000, according to the CDC. Globally, WHO data from 2015 indicated that the annual global rate of food-borne diseases is 10 percent. An estimated 125,000 deaths occur in children less than five years of age.

In underdeveloped countries, where medical care is not as available or advanced as it is in developed countries, food-borne illnesses can be even more devastating. Diarrheal illnesses afflict millions of people every year, and many of them are children. The illnesses are a major cause of the malnutrition that is a part of everyday life in many underdeveloped regions.

A food safety issue that has become more urgent since the 2001 terrorist attacks in the United States is the monitoring of foods to ensure their safety from deliberate tampering. The supply chain from the field to the supermarket leaves food vulnerable to the deliberate addition of microbiological agents that cause illness or death. While storage conditions, monitoring programs, and even the design of packing that can detect contamination are useful in protecting foods from accidental contamination, it is difficult to protect food from deliberate harm.

See Also Campylobacter *Infection;* Clostridium difficile *Infection;* Escherichia coli *O157:H7; Listeriosis;* Salmonella *Infection (Salmonellosis)*

BIBLIOGRAPHY

Books

Dodd, Christine E. R., et al. *Foodborne Diseases.* 3rd ed. New York: Academic Press, 2017.

Redman, Nina E., and Michele Morrone. *Food Safety: A Reference Handbook.* 3rd ed. Santa Barbara, CA: ABC-CLIO, 2017.

Periodicals

Min, Sea C., et al. "In-Package Inhibition of *E. coli* O157:H7 on Bulk Romaine Lettuce Using Cold Plasma." *Food Microbiology* 65 (2017): 1–6.

Sharapov, Umid M., et al. "Multistate Outbreak of *Escherichia coli* O157:H7 Infections Associated with Consumption of Fresh Spinach: United States, 2006." *Journal of Food Protection* 79 (2016): 2024–2030.

Skarp, C. P. Astrid, et al. "Campylobacteriosis: The Role of Poultry Meat." *Clinical Microbiology and Infection* 22 (2016): 103–109.

Websites

"Estimates of Foodborne Illness in the United States." Centers for Disease Control and Prevention. http://www.cdc.gov/foodborneburden/burden/index.html (accessed November 16, 2017).

U.S. Food and Drug Administration. https://www.fda.gov/ (accessed March 15, 2018).

Brian Hoyle

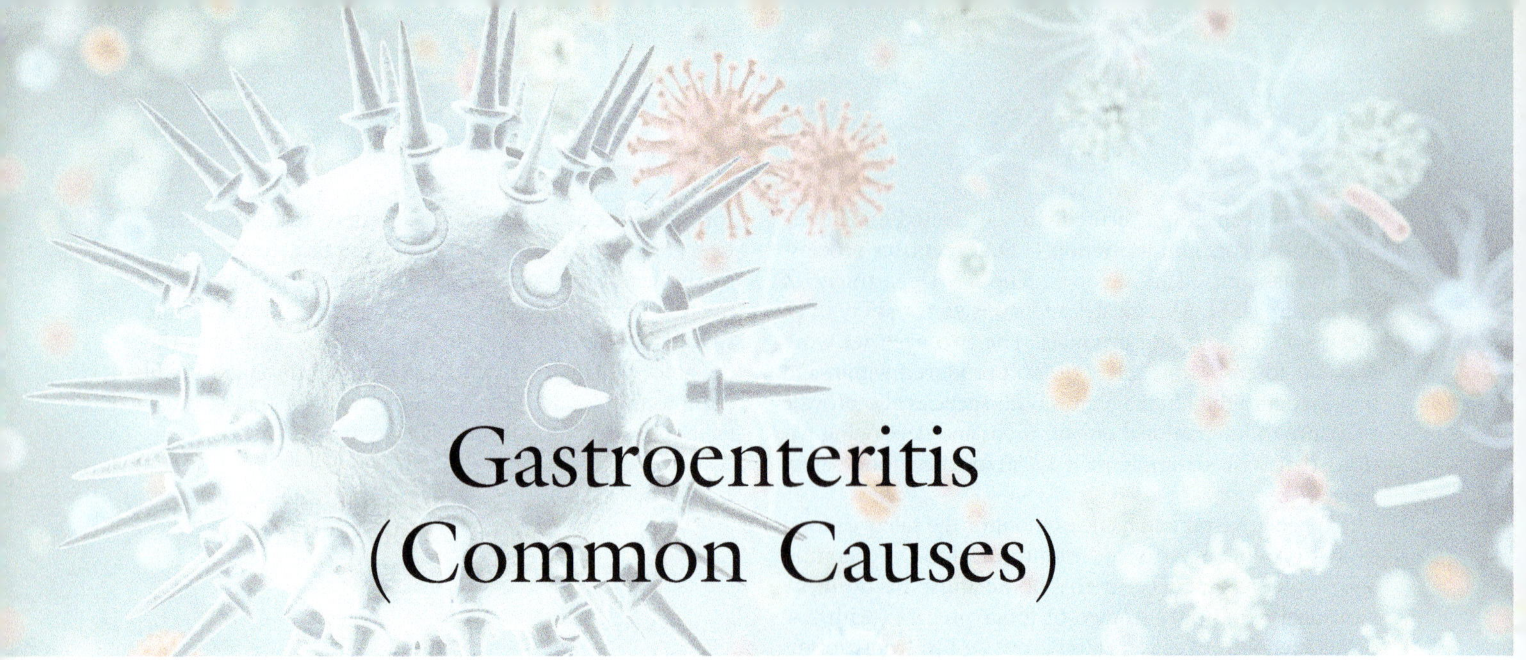

Gastroenteritis (Common Causes)

Introduction

Gastroenteritis is an inflammation of the stomach and the intestines that is produced by the immune system's response to an infection caused by a number of bacteria or viruses. Gastroenteritis is sometimes referred to as the stomach flu, but it is not caused by influenza viruses.

The symptoms of gastroenteritis include stomach or intestinal upset, vomiting, and often diarrhea, or watery feces. In developing regions of the world, and especially among children, gastroenteritis-induced diarrhea can be fatal. Millions of deaths of newborns and children resulting from gastroenteritis occur each year in Asia, Africa, parts of the Indian subcontinent, and Latin America.

Disease History, Characteristics, and Transmission

Gastroenteritis is a part of everyday life, but outbreaks of illness do occur. A well-known example that occurs periodically is gastroenteritis caused by norovirus, which spreads through the consumption of virus-contaminated food or water. Outbreaks that occur on cruise ships are particularly newsworthy, as the afflicted are at sea and are unable to escape the outbreak. Outbreaks that occur in nursing homes are also serious because the elderly residents can be in poor health, less robust, and therefore in greater danger of developing a serious, even life-ending, infection. According to the US Centers for Disease Control and Prevention (CDC), as of the end of 2015, norovirus was causing about 20 million cases of gastroenteritis in the United States each year, with an estimated 56,000 to 71,000 people hospitalized for treatment and about 600 to 800 of the cases resulting in death. Death typically occurs among the very young and the elderly.

Gastroenteritis is caused mainly by viruses, but it can also be caused by infection with bacteria and protozoa. The viruses that cause gastroenteritis include rotaviruses, enteroviruses, adenoviruses, caliciviruses, astroviruses, Norwalk virus, and a group of Norwalk-like viruses. Of these, rotavirus infections are the most common.

The symptoms of viral gastroenteritis usually appear quickly, within a few days of ingesting the virus in contaminated water or food. The illness tends to pass quickly, usually within a week. However, people whose immune system function is inefficient (such as the young and the elderly), people who are ill with another ailment such as acquired immunodeficiency syndrome (AIDS), or someone whose immune system has been deliberately subdued (such as someone who has received an organ transplant, to reduce the chances of organ rejection) can be ill for a longer time.

Rotavirus is a member of the Reoviridae family of viruses, all of which contain ribonucleic acid (RNA) as the genetic material. When the virus infects a host cell, the host's genetic machinery is used to make deoxyribonucleic acid (DNA) from the viral RNA; the viral DNA can then be transcribed and translated with host DNA to produce the components that will make new virus particles. There are three main groups of rotavirus that differ from each other slightly in the composition of the protein shell that surrounds the genetic material. These differences mean that a host's immune system will produce different antibodies to the different viruses. Group A rotavirus causes more than 3 million cases of gastroenteritis in the United States annually. Group B rotavirus causes diarrhea that is more prevalent in adults. It has caused several large outbreaks in China. Group C causes diarrhea in children and adults but is less common than the other two types of rotaviral gastroenteritis.

Prior to the introduction of a vaccine for rotavirus, 55,000 to 70,000 children were hospitalized for gastroenteritis caused by the virus every year in the United States. The main reason that rotaviral gastroenteritis is so common is the contagious nature of the virus. Rotavirus is easily spread from person to person, usually when fecal material gets into the mouth. This is known as the fecal-oral route of transmission. Not surprisingly, this type of gastroenteritis occurs frequently in day care facilities, where touching of soiled diapers and hand-to-mouth contact are common.

In older children and adults, improper hygiene, particularly handwashing, is the main reason for the spread of the virus. People who are infected can excrete (or shed) high numbers of virus particles in diarrhea and spread the infection. Also, handling of utensils and preparation of food with hands that are soiled spreads the virus to the diner.

Another route of transmission that is not related to hygiene is the consumption of shellfish. Shellfish are filter feeders—they filter water through an apparatus that traps small food particles. The filter can also trap rotavirus that is present in contaminated water. As the shellfish feeds, more and more virus can accumulate, until the shellfish becomes toxic to anyone eating it. The danger is especially pronounced in shellfish such as oysters, which some people prefer to eat raw.

Following the introduction of the rotavirus vaccine in 2006 and the widespread vaccination of infants, the number of cases of gastroenteritis dropped in the United States. The CDC estimates that 40,000 to 50,000 hospitalizations are prevented every year through vaccination.

Globally, rotavirus is still a killer, causing over 450,000 deaths each year in children younger than five years of age.

Another virus that causes gastroenteritis is the Norwalk virus. This form of the illness tends to be more common in adults, although surveys of children using sophisticated molecular techniques of viral detection have revealed the presence of Norwalk antibodies, meaning the children had been exposed to the virus or to a protein that is similar to the Norwalk viral protein.

Bacteria also cause gastroenteritis. Common examples include certain strains of *Escherichia coli*, *Salmonella*, *Shigella*, and *Vibrio cholerae*. Bacterial gastroenteritis occurs less in developed countries, in part because the treatment of drinking water and the treatment and disposal of sewage water tend to be much better than in underdeveloped regions. In developing nations bacterial gastroenteritis caused by contaminated water remains a significant concern. Bacterial gastroenteritis can also be caused by eating contaminated food. Examples include foods such as potato salad that has been left at room temperature for some time prior to the meal and contaminated with *Salmonella* and the presence of a type of *E. coli* designated O157:H7 in undercooked meat (a toxin produced by O157:H7 damages the cells lining the intestinal tract, causing bloody diarrhea).

Cryptosporidium parvum, a protozoan that resides in the intestinal tract of some animals, also causes gastroenteritis when it contaminates drinking water. This type of gastroenteritis is becoming more prevalent in the United States. One reason is the continuing expansion of urban

WORDS TO KNOW

ANTIBODIES Proteins found in the blood that help fight against foreign substances called antigens. Antigens, which are usually proteins or polysaccharides, stimulate the immune system to produce antibodies, or Y-shaped immunoglobulins. The antibodies inactivate the antigen and help remove it from the body. While antigens can be the source of infections from pathogenic bacteria and viruses, organic molecules detrimental to the body from internal or environmental sources also act as antigens. Genetic engineering and the use of various mutational mechanisms allow the construction of a vast array of antibodies (each with a unique genetic sequence).

CYST Refers to either a closed cavity or sac or the stage of life during which some parasites live inside an enclosed area. In a protozoan's life, it is a stage when it is covered by a tough outer shell and has become dormant.

FECAL-ORAL ROUTE The spread of disease through the transmission of minute particles of fecal material from one organism to the mouth of another. This can occur by drinking contaminated water; eating food exposed to animal or human feces, such as food from plants watered with unclean water; or preparing food without practicing proper hygiene.

ORAL REHYDRATION THERAPY Patients who have lost excessive water from their tissues are said to be dehydrated. Restoring body water levels by giving the patient fluids through the mouth (orally) is oral rehydration therapy. Often, a special mixture of water, glucose, and electrolytes called oral rehydration solution is given.

VIRAL SHEDDING The movement of the herpes virus from the nerves to the surface of the skin. During shedding the virus can be passed on through skin-to-skin contact.

Causes of Gastroenteritis

Type	Hosts	Type	Hosts
Bacterial	*Campylobacter* *Escherichia coli* *Salmonella* *Shigella* *Vibrio cholerae*	Parasitic	*Cryptosporidium parvum* *Giardia*
		Viral	Adenovirus Astrovirus Calicivirus Herpesvirus Rotavirus
Fungal	*Candida* *Histoplasma* *Microsporidium*		

areas into regions that were previously wild, which brings humans into closer contact with wildlife and the *C. parvum* they carry. Another reason is that the protozoans can form an environmentally hardy form called a cyst that allows the protozoan to persist through water treatments such as chlorination and, because of the small diameter of the cysts, to pass through filters used in water filtration. Once inside a person, the cyst can rejuvenate into the growing form that is the cause of the illness.

The symptoms of gastroenteritis always include diarrhea. Fever and vomiting are also common. Typically these symptoms last several days, then progressively lessen over the next few days as the infection abates. The diarrhea in gastroenteritis is very loose and watery. Bowel movements occur frequently, even several times an hour, as fluid pours out of the cells lining the intestine as a consequence of the infection and as an attempt to flush out the infecting bacteria or virus. Dehydration is not usually a problem in an adult, who will instinctively drink water. If dehydration occurs quickly or if infected individuals are so sick that they are unable to take care of themselves, they can become very ill. Hospitalization of a child for diarrhea is usually because of complications of the excessive fluid loss rather than any direct effect of the stomach and intestinal infection.

Scope and Distribution

Gastroenteritis is global in distribution. However, it primarily affects people living in the developing world, most of whom are children. Estimates put the death toll of children from gastroenteritis-related diarrhea at 1 million to 2 million each year, and the majority of these deaths occur in developing countries. Still, this is much less than the nearly 5 million deaths that occurred annually until the 1980s, when oral hydration therapy, drinking a solution containing salts and sugars that helps replenish the body's essential electrolytes and fluids that are lost due to diarrhea, was introduced.

The differences in the severity of the infection and the death rates in developed versus developing countries highlight the influence of living conditions, hygiene, and cultural practices on the consequences of gastroenteritis. Age is another factor. The very young and the elderly are particularly susceptible because they may be physically unable to seek prompt relief from the dehydration caused by diarrhea.

Treatment and Prevention

In the treatment of gastroenteritis, it is important to distinguish whether the infection is caused by a bacterium, a virus, a protozoan, or some other nonbiological factor. An example of the latter is lactose intolerance. Antibiotics are effective against bacteria but are not useful against viruses and can actually make the disease worse, as antibiotics can remove normal intestinal bacteria that can help clear a viral infection.

Antibiotics such as fluoroquinolone are useful in treating bacterial forms of gastroenteritis, and over-the-counter compounds that lessen diarrhea can also be beneficial. Making sure a person is receiving plenty of fluids is a crucial part of the treatment.

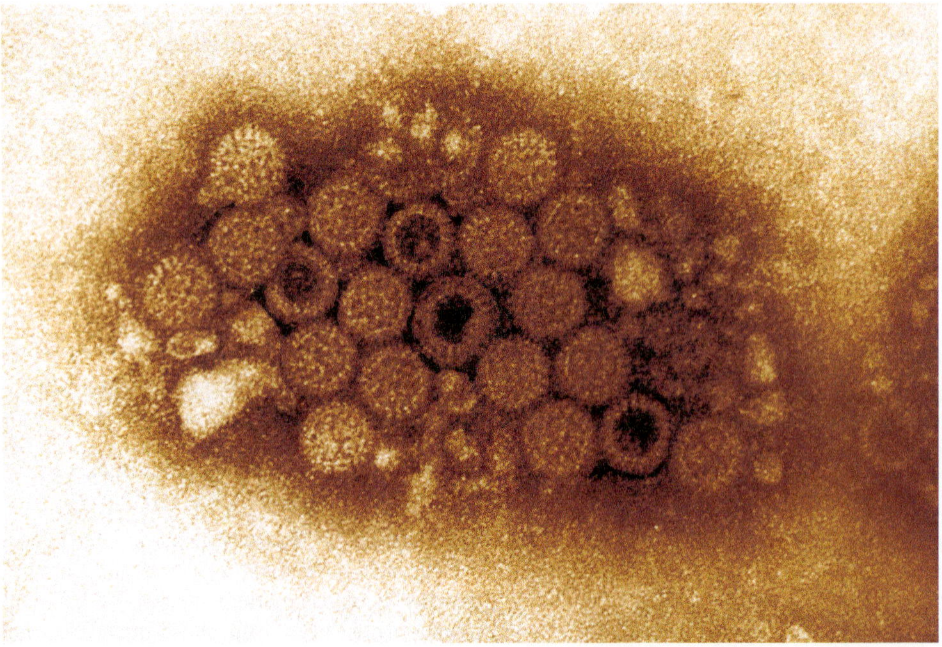

An RNA virus responsible for benign infectious gastroenteritis in children. *© BSIP/UIG/Getty Images*

A vaccine for rotaviral gastroenteritis was approved for use in 1998, but complications in some children who received the vaccine resulted in its withdrawal from the market a few years later. In 2006 two rotavirus vaccines were licensed for use by the European Medicines Agency and the US Food and Drug Administration (FDA). Both are taken orally and consist of a weakened version of the virus. The vaccines are incapable of causing an infection but stimulate the immune system to develop protective antibodies against rotavirus.

Impacts and Issues

The overwhelming impacts of gastroenteritis are its prevalence and the high death toll among children in underdeveloped and developing countries due to the debilitating effects of diarrhea. Diarrheal diseases are the second most common cause of death each year in children age five years and under, according to the World Health Organization (WHO), resulting in more than 2 million child deaths. Earlier and larger death tolls have been reduced by the use of oral rehydration therapy, which is spearheaded by organizations such as the United Nations Children's Fund.

Despite the availability of vaccines against rotavirus, the diarrheal gastroenteritis that is caused by this virus still kills over 450,000 children each year, and more than 2 million children require hospitalization because of the severity of the infection. Overwhelmingly the deaths occur in developing countries, where the vaccines and treatment are not as readily available as in developed countries.

Beginning in 2003 a number of agencies, including the CDC and WHO, initiated the Rotavirus Vaccination Program, which sought to make rotavirus vaccines more widely available. The program ran until 2008. Beginning in 2005 the Pan American Health Organization commenced an annual campaign of immunization that includes the FDA-licensed rotavirus vaccine.

Another vaccine initiative began in 2011 through the Global Alliance for Vaccines and Immunization (GAVI), which has received over $1.5 billion in funding from the Bill & Melinda Gates Foundation. The goal was to support the introduction of rotavirus vaccine to 33 underdeveloped/developing countries in Africa, as well as Bangladesh and Pakistan, by the end of 2015. This goal was met in 2014, and by the end of 2016, the vaccine had been introduced in 40 countries.

SEE ALSO *Bacterial Disease; Cholera; Escherichia coli O157:H7; Food-Borne Disease and Food Safety; Norovirus Infection; Salmonella Infection (Salmonellosis); Sanitation; Shigellosis; Water-Borne Disease*

BIBLIOGRAPHY

Books

Kaslow, Richard A., Lawrence R. Stanberry, and James W. LeDuc. *Viral Infections of Humans: Epidemiology and Control.* New York: Springer, 2014.

Payne, Susan. *Viruses: From Understanding to Investigation.* New York: Academic Press, 2017.

Periodicals

Leshem, Eyal, et al. "National Estimates of Reductions in Acute Gastroenteritis–Related Hospitalizations and Associated Costs in US Children After Implementation of Rotavirus Vaccines." Journal of the American Pediatric Infectious Diseases Society 91 (2017): 6.

Websites

"Diarrhoea." World Health Organization. http://www.who.int/topics/diarrhoea/en (accessed November 16, 2017).

"Rotavirus." Centers for Disease Control and Prevention. https://www.cdc.gov/rotavirus/index.html (accessed November 16, 2017).

"Rotavirus Vaccine Support." Global Alliance for Vaccines and Immunization. http://www.gavi.org/support/nvs/rotavirus (accessed November 16, 2017).

Brian Hoyle

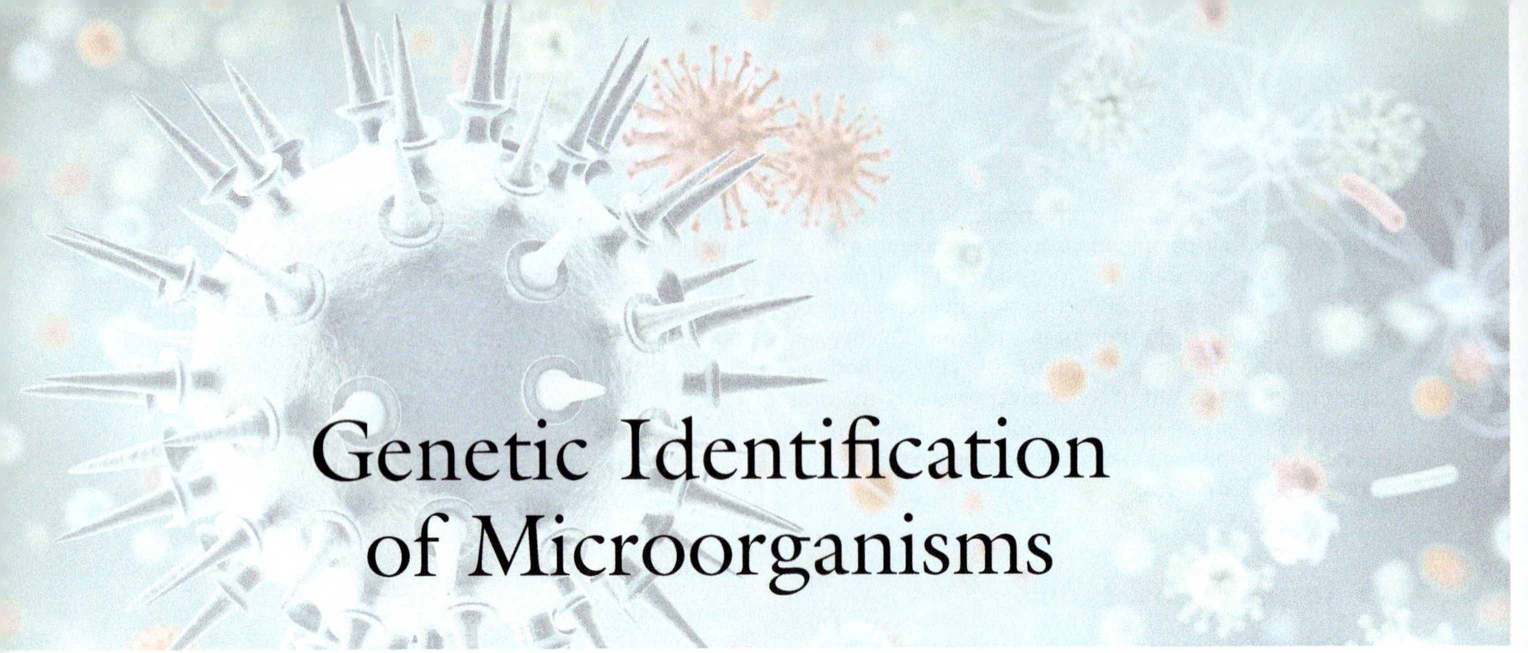

Genetic Identification of Microorganisms

Introduction

Genetic identification of microorganisms uses molecular technologies to evaluate specific regions of a microbial genome and determine to which genus, species, or strain a microorganism belongs. The techniques used are adapted from deoxyribonucleic acid (DNA) fingerprinting technology, which is also used for genetic identification of humans and other living organisms such as microbes. These technologies have enhanced the ability to diagnose diseases quickly and accurately compared to the traditional laboratory culture methods.

WORDS TO KNOW

ASSAY A determination of an amount of a particular compound in a sample (e.g., to make chemical tests to determine the relative amount of a particular substance in a sample). A method used to quantify a biological compound.

CHEMILUMINESCENT SIGNAL The production of light from a chemical reaction. A variety of tests to detect infectious organisms or the target components of such organisms relies on the binding of a chemical-containing probe to the target and the development of light following the addition of a reactive compound.

DNA FINGERPRINTING A range of techniques used to show similarities and dissimilarities between the deoxyribonucleic acid (DNA) present in different individuals or organisms.

DNA PROBES Substances or agents that bind directly to a predefined specific sequence of nucleic acids in deoxyribonucleic acid (DNA).

GENOME All of the genetic information contained in a cell or organism. The complete sequence of genes within a cell or virus.

HYBRIDIZATION The process of combining two or more different molecules or organisms to create a new molecule or organism. Often called a hybrid organism.

POLYMERASE CHAIN REACTION (PCR) A widely used technique in molecular biology involving the amplification of specific sequences of genomic deoxyribonucleic acid (DNA).

QUANTITATED An act of determining the quantity of something, such as the number or concentration of bacteria in an infectious disease.

REVERSE TRANSCRIPTASE An enzyme that makes it possible for a retrovirus to produce deoxyribonucleic acid (DNA) from ribonucleic acid (RNA).

SOUTHERN BLOT ANALYSIS An electrophoresis technique in which pieces of deoxyribonucleic acid (DNA) created by enzyme digestion are separated from one another on the basis of size, followed by the transfer of the DNA fragments to a flexible membrane. The membrane can then be exposed to various probes to identify target regions of the genetic material.

History and Scientific Foundations

The process of microbial identification has largely depended on culture methods followed by microscopy. This method remains common at small clinical laboratories for identifying microbes in stool or blood samples. However, a major disadvantage of this method is the human error that may result in misidentification, especially when managing a large sample number.

The process of genetic identification of microorganisms is a comparison study. The key deoxyribonucleic acid (DNA) sequences of an unknown organism are compared to DNA sequences from known organisms, and the percentage of similarity is calculated. An exact match occurs when the DNA sequences from the two organisms are the same. Related individuals have genetic material that is identical for some regions and dissimilar for others. Unrelated individuals will have significant differences in the DNA regions being evaluated.

Databases of DNA and protein sequences of disease-causing pathogens have been developed by researchers across the globe and shared in public domains. One such shared DNA repository is the GenBank, which is a collection of DNA sequences maintained by the National Center for Biotechnology Information (NCBI) at the National Institutes of Health (NIH). GenBank also has shared information from the DNA Data Bank of Japan (DDBJ) and the European Nucleotide Archive (ENA).

In the 21st century there are many bioinformatic tools available to search and retrieve genetic information, including DNA and protein sequences. Such searches are commonly referred to as basic local alignment search tool (BLAST) searches, which allow the sequences obtained in laboratory testing to be compared to already available sequences across the data banks. This has made identification and diagnosis easy, accurate, and less time consuming for many microbes.

TERRORISM AND BIOLOGICAL WARFARE

The capability for detecting and identifying microorganisms quickly and accurately is required to protect both troops on the battlefield and civilians confronted with terrorist attacks using biological agents. Because the systems available for sensing biological molecules rely on technologies that require several steps to identify biological weapons, the procedures are both labor and time intensive. The Defense Advanced Research Projects Agency (DARPA) initiated the Biosensor Technologies Program in 2002 to develop fast, sensitive, automatic technologies for the detection and identification of biological warfare agents. The program focuses on a variety of technologies including surface receptor properties, nucleic acid sequences, identification of molecules found in the breat,h and mass spectrometry.

Applications and Research

Depending on the level of specificity required, molecular assays can provide information on the genus, species, or strain of a microorganism. The most basic type of identification is classification to a genus, which can be useful in a variety of situations. For example, if a person is thought to have tuberculosis, a test to determine if *Mycobacterium* cells (the genus that includes the tuberculosis-causing organism) are present in a sputum sample can be used to confirm the diagnosis. However, if there are several species within a genus that cause similar diseases but require different drug therapies, a more specific test is needed.

In some instances it is important to take the analysis one step further to detect genetically distinct subspecies or strains. Variant strains usually arise out of physical separation and evolution of the genome. If one homogeneous sample of cells is split and sent to two different locations, changes (mutations) may occur over time, distinguishing the two populations as unique entities. The importance of this issue can be appreciated when considering tuberculosis (TB). Since the late 1980s, there has been a resurgence of this disease accompanied by the appearance of several new strains that are resistant to the standard antibiotic treatments, known as MDR-TB or multidrug-resistant TB. The use of genetic identification for rapid determination of which strain is present has been essential to protect health care workers and provide appropriate therapy for affected individuals.

The tools used for genetic studies include standard molecular technologies. Total sequencing of an organism's genome is one approach, but this method is time consuming and expensive. Southern blot analysis, or specific sequencing of DNA using gel separation and hybridization, was used originally, but in most laboratories this has been replaced by newer technologies such as polymerase chain reaction (PCR). PCR is a technique that uses an enzyme called a taq polymerase to amplify a single copy of a segment of DNA to several thousands or millions. This technique has revolutionized the world of diagnostics and research in molecular biology.

Solution-phase hybridization using DNA probes has proven effective for many organisms. In this procedure, probes labeled with a reporter molecule are combined with cells in solution, and, upon hybridization with target cells, a chemiluminescent signal that can be quantitated by a luminometer is emitted. A variation of this scheme is to capture the target cells by hybridization to a probe followed by a second hybridization that results in precipitation of the cells for quantitation. These assays are rapid, relatively inexpensive, and highly sensitive. However, they require the presence of a relatively large number of organisms to be effective.

Amplification technologies such as PCR, ligase change reaction (LCR), and, for viruses with a ribonucleic acid (RNA) genome, reverse transcriptase PCR (RT-PCR) allow detection of very low concentrations of organisms from cultures or patient specimens such as blood or body tissues. Primers, or small, specific sequences matching a small part of the microbial sequence to be detected, are designed to selectively amplify genomic sequences unique to each species. By screening unknown organisms for the presence or absence of these regions, the unknown organism may be identified. To speed up the process, multiplex PCR can be used to differentiate between several different species in a single amplification reaction. Going a step further, microarray technology will allow comparisons among much larger numbers of microorganisms and may be more successful at identifying specimens that contain more than one species.

■ Impacts and Issues

Microorganism identification technologies were important during the investigation of the anthrax outbreak in the United States in the fall of 2001. Because an anthrax infection can mimic cold or flu symptoms, the earliest victims did not realize they were harboring a deadly bacterium. After confirmation that anthrax was the causative agent in the first death, genetic technologies were used to confirm the presence of anthrax in other locations and for other potential victims. Results were available more rapidly than would have been possible using standard microbiological methodology, and appropriate treatment regimens could be established immediately. Furthermore, unaffected individuals were quickly informed of their status, alleviating unnecessary anxiety.

Sequencing technologies have offered advantages when identifying microorganisms of pathogenic importance. It is often unclear whether these are new or whether they were misclassified previously due to lack of proper tools. While genetic identification through gene amplification, such as with PCR, and gene sequencing is an important tool, these techniques may be challenging when the genus or the family (taxonomy) is large and complex. It is also becoming clear that databases such as GenBank, MicroSEQ, and SmartGene have many advantages as well as limitations. For example, GenBank is a large, enormously popular public database but at times offers poor-quality reference sequences, which may lead to misidentification.

BIBLIOGRAPHY

Books

Dale, Jeremy W., and Simon F. Park. *Molecular Genetics.* 5th ed. Chichester, UK: Wiley-Blackwell, 2010.

James, Jenny Lynd. *Microbial Hazard Identification in Fresh Fruits and Vegetables.* New York: Wiley-Interscience, 2006.

Persing, David H., et al., eds. *Molecular Microbiology: Diagnostic Principles and Practice.* 3rd ed. Washington, DC: ASM, 2016.

Periodicals

Barth Reller, L., et al. "Detection and Identification of Microorganisms by Gene Amplification and Sequencing." *Clinical Infectious Diseases* 44 (2007): 1108–1114.

Frederick, Adzitey, Nurul Huda, and Gulam Rusul Rahmat Ali. "Molecular Techniques for Detecting and Typing of Bacteria, Advantages and Application to Foodborne Pathogens Isolated from Ducks." *3 Biotech* 3, no. 2 (2013): 97–107.

Jernigan, D. B., et al. "Investigation of Bioterrorism-Related Anthrax, United States, 2001: Epidemiologic Findings." *Emerging Infectious Diseases* 8, no. 10 (October 2002): 1019–1028.

Peplies, Jorg, Frank Oliver Glockner, and Rudolf Amann. "Optimization Strategies for DNA Microarray-Based Detection of Bacteria with 16S rRNA-Targeting Oligonucleotide Probes." *Applied and Environmental Microbiology* 69 (2003): 1397–1407.

Read, Timothy D., et al. "Comparative Genome Sequencing for Discovery of Novel Polymorphisms in *Bacillus anthracis.*" *Science* 296 (June 14, 2002): 2028–2033.

Websites

"GenBank Overview." National Center for Biotechnology Information (NCBI). https://www.ncbi.nlm.nih.gov/genbank/ (accessed February 28, 2018).

Constance Stein
Kausalya Santhanam

Genital Herpes

Introduction

Genital herpes is a common sexually transmitted infection (STI). According to the US Centers for Disease Control and Prevention (CDC), more than one in six people between the ages of 15 and 49 had genital herpes in 2017. Genital herpes is caused most often by infection with the herpes simplex 2 virus (HSV-2), but occasionally the herpes simplex 1 (HSV-1) virus is also responsible. Often, people infected with these herpes viruses have no symptoms. When symptoms of genital herpes do appear, they usually involve blisters in the area of the genitals or rectum. The blisters are normally fluid-filled at first and then break to form tender, itchy ulcers that can take up to a month to heal. Although infection with HSV-1 or HSV-2 can last a lifetime in the body, future outbreaks of genital herpes blisters usually decline in frequency and severity. Genital herpes is spread among sexual partners when the virus is released from a blister (or occasionally from intact skin) during sexual contact. It is not possible to contract genital herpes from toilet seats, swimming pools, or shared clothing or towels.

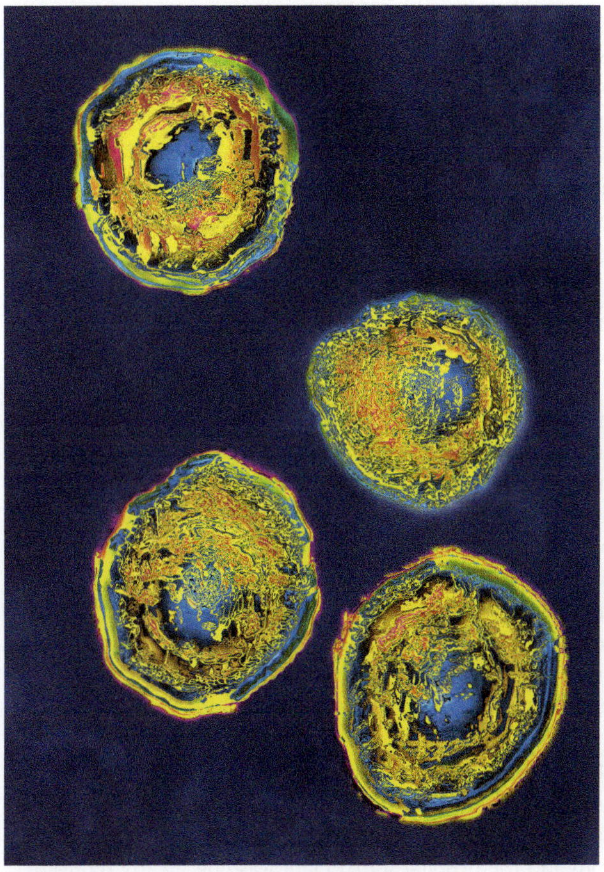

This image made under a transmission electron microscope shows the herpes simplex virus type 2, which is responsible for approximately 70 percent of cases of genital herpes. *© BSIP/UIG/Getty Images*

Genital herpes infection can lead to miscarriage, and mothers infected with genital herpes can pass the virus to their newborns during vaginal birth (vertical transmission). Individuals who are infected with HSV-2 are more vulnerable to the human immunodeficiency virus (HIV). According to the CDC, persons with genital herpes who are genitally exposed to HIV have an estimated twofold to fourfold increased risk of acquiring HIV.

Although daily antiviral drugs such as acyclovir, famciclovir, and valacyclovir can prevent or shorten outbreaks, there is no cure or vaccine for genital herpes. As of 2018 several promising potential vaccines were undergoing animal or human studies.

Editor's note: Further information about genital herpes can be found in the articles about the specific causative agents, Herpes Simplex 2 Virus and Herpes Simplex 1 Virus.

SEE ALSO *Herpes Simplex 1 Virus; Herpes Simplex 2 Virus*

BIBLIOGRAPHY

Websites

"Genital Herpes." Centers for Disease Control and Prevention, September 1, 2017. https://www.cdc.gov/std/herpes/stdfact-herpes.htm (accessed January 29, 2018).

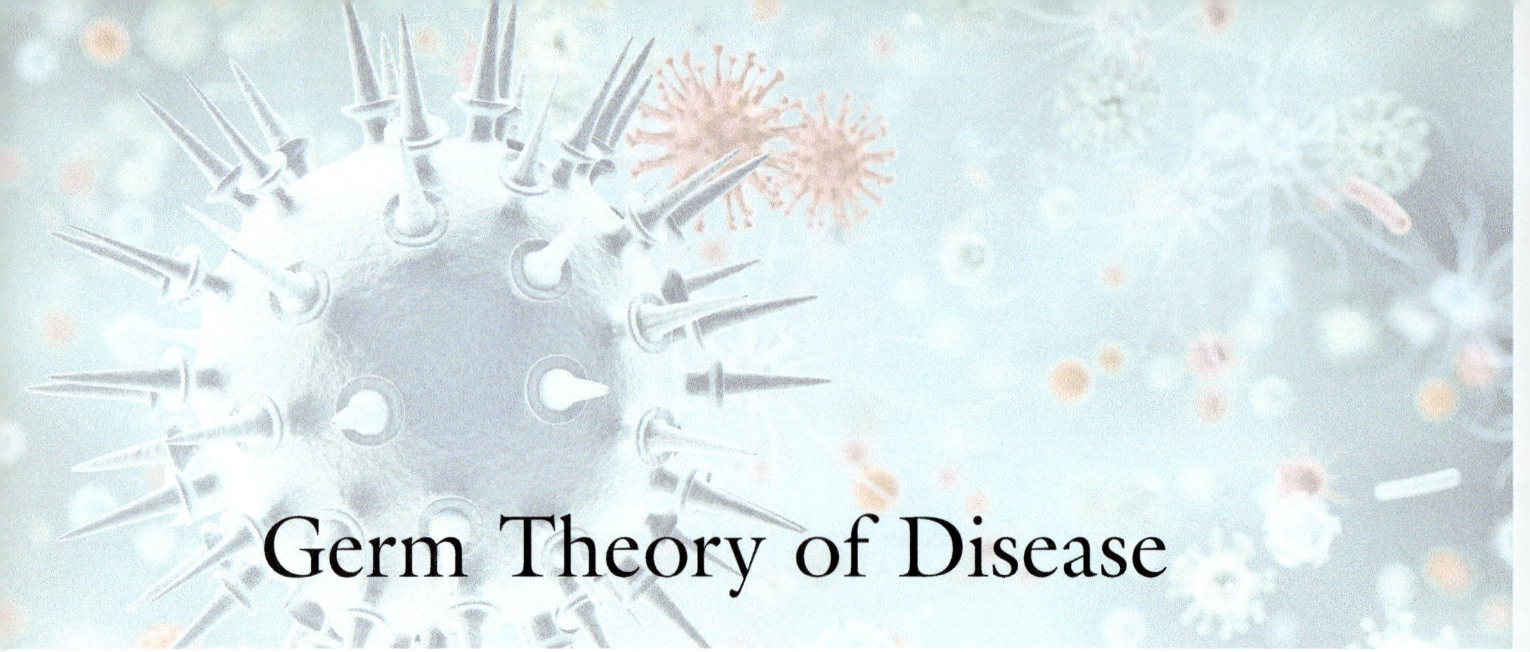

Germ Theory of Disease

Introduction

The germ theory of disease states that microorganisms —organisms that, with only one known exception, are too small to be seen without the aid of a microscope —are the cause of many diseases. Microorganisms include bacteria, viruses, fungi, algae, and protozoa. The germ theory of disease also states that the microbes that cause disease are capable of being recovered and will cause the same disease when introduced into another creature. This theory has withstood scientific scrutiny for centuries. Indeed, it is known with certainty that many diseases are caused by microorganisms. Two examples are anthrax, which is caused by the bacterium *Bacillus anthracis*, and bacterial meningitis, which is caused by *Neisseria meningitidis*.

While an accepted part of infectious disease microbiology and the foundation of a variety of disciplines, such as hygiene and epidemiology (the study of the origin and spread of infections), the exact reasons why some microbes cause disease remain poorly understood and are still being investigated.

History and Scientific Foundations

Millenia ago, when microorganisms were unknown, some diseases were thought to be a consequence of divine punishment for a person's bad behavior. Illnesses that affected groups of people were sometimes attributed to the foul-smelling gases from a nearby swamp or the vapors from a sewage lagoon. While some microbes can become airborne and cause disease when inhaled (anthrax is one example), this was not recognized for many years. Other purported causes of disease included vapors created by the rotation of Earth or disturbances within the planet, which was thought to be hollow.

A publication dating back to 36 BCE proposed that some illness was the result of the inhalation of tiny creatures present in the air. However, this farsighted view was the exception for centuries. With the development of the microscope in the 17th century by Robert Hooke (1635–1703) and Antoni van Leeuwenhoek (1632–1723), it became possible to examine specimens, such as water, and to visually detect living organisms.

At that time the prevailing view was that life and disease arose spontaneously from nonliving material. Then, in 1668, Italian scientist Francisco Redi (1627–1697) showed that maggots did not appear if decaying meat was kept in a sealed container but that the maggots appeared if the meat was placed in the open air. This implied that the maggots were present in the air that contacted the meat rather than spontaneously appearing on the meat.

Early in the 18th century, it was observed that people could be protected from developing smallpox by exposing them to pus from the lesions of other people with the illness. While this is now understood as the basis of vaccination, at the time the idea—that something in the illness could protect others from the malady—was revolutionary. English physician Edward Jenner (1749–1823) is recognized as the founder of the practice of vaccination. Jenner noticed that dairy workers who had been exposed to cowpox, a milder disease similar to smallpox, seldom contracted smallpox. He showed that injecting people with fluid from the cowpox blisters (which was subsequently shown to contain the cowpox virus, which is related to the smallpox virus) conferred protection against smallpox.

In 1848 Hungarian physician Ignaz Semmelweis (1818–1865) discovered that the disease puerperal fever could be spread from corpses to living patients by attendants who did not wash their hands between the autopsy room and the hospital ward. Handwashing greatly reduced the number of these infections. In 1854 English physician John Snow (1813–1858) demonstrated that an ongoing cholera epidemic in London was caused by water coming

WORDS TO KNOW

ASEPSIS Without germs, more specifically without microorganisms.

CARBOLIC ACID An acidic compound that, when diluted with water, is used as an antiseptic and a disinfectant.

COWPOX A disease that is caused by the cowpox or catpox virus. The virus is a member of the orthopoxvirus family. Other viruses in this family include the smallpox and vaccinia viruses. Cowpox is a rare disease and is mostly noteworthy as the basis of the formulation, over 200 years ago, of an injection by Edward Jenner that proved successful in curing smallpox.

EPIDEMIOLOGY The study of various factors that influence the occurrence, distribution, prevention, and control of disease, injury, and other health-related events in a defined human population. By the application of various analytical techniques, including mathematical analysis of the data, the probable cause of an infectious outbreak can be pinpointed.

INFECTION CONTROL Policies and procedures used to minimize the risk of spreading infections, especially in hospitals and health care facilities.

MICROORGANISM With only a single currently known exception (i.e., *Epulopiscium fishelsonia*, a bacterium that is billions of times larger than the bacteria in the human intestine and is large enough to view without a microscope), microorganisms are minute organisms that require microscopic magnification to view. To be seen, they must be magnified by an optical or electron microscope. The most common types of microorganisms are viruses, bacteria, blue-green bacteria, some algae, some fungi, yeasts, and protozoans.

PUERPERAL FEVER A bacterial infection present in the blood (septicemia) that follows childbirth. The Latin word *puer*, meaning "boy" or "child," is the root of this term. Puerperal fever was much more common before the advent of modern aseptic practices, but infections still occur. Louis Pasteur showed that puerperal fever is most often caused by *Streptococcus* bacteria, which is now treated with antibiotics.

SPONTANEOUS GENERATION Also known as abiogenesis; the incorrect discarded assumption that living things can be generated from nonliving things.

VACCINATION The inoculation, or use of vaccines, to prevent specific diseases within humans and animals by producing immunity to such diseases. It is the introduction of weakened or dead viruses or microorganisms into the body to create immunity by the production of specific antibodies.

from a particular pump. When the water flow from the pump was shut off, the outbreak ended.

However, even with the accumulating weight of evidence that some agent was responsible for various diseases, many physicians continued to maintain that these agents did not exist because they could not be seen with the unaided eye. If they did not exist, then they could not be the cause of disease. It remained for Agostino Bassi (1773–1856), Louis Pasteur (1822–1895), and Robert Koch (1843–1910) to perform the research necessary to finally convince the scientific community that germs did, indeed, cause disease.

In 1835 Bassi proposed the germ theory for the first time, when he hypothesized that a lethal disease of silkworms was due to a microscopic living organism. The agent was subsequently shown to be the fungus *Beauveria bassiana*. Then, in a series of experiments in the middle of the 19th century, Pasteur convincingly demonstrated that the spoilage of wine, beer, and foods were caused by something in the air and not by the air itself.

In 1875 concrete evidence for the germ theory was provided by Koch, who showed that *Bacillus anthracis* was the cause of anthrax in cattle and sheep. Koch's step-by-step approach to his experiments laid the foundation for a series of conditions that must be met to demonstrate that a particular microorganism is the cause of a particular disease. The following conditions came to be known as Koch's postulates.

Koch's postulates drove the nail into the coffin of the theory of spontaneous generation. Once scientists accepted that the germ theory of disease was valid and began to search for more examples of microbial-caused diseases, the floodgates opened. By the end of the 19th century, it had been established that microbes were responsible for cholera, typhoid fever, diphtheria, pneumonia, tetanus, meningitis, and gonorrhea, as a few examples.

Also in the 19th century, English physician Joseph Lister (1827–1912) demonstrated that the development of infections in patients following surgery could be drastically reduced if a spray of carbolic acid was applied over the wound during surgery and surgical dressing put on the wound was soaked in the chemical. Because carbolic acid was known to kill microbes present in sewage, Lister helped convince people that microorganisms were important in postoperative infections.

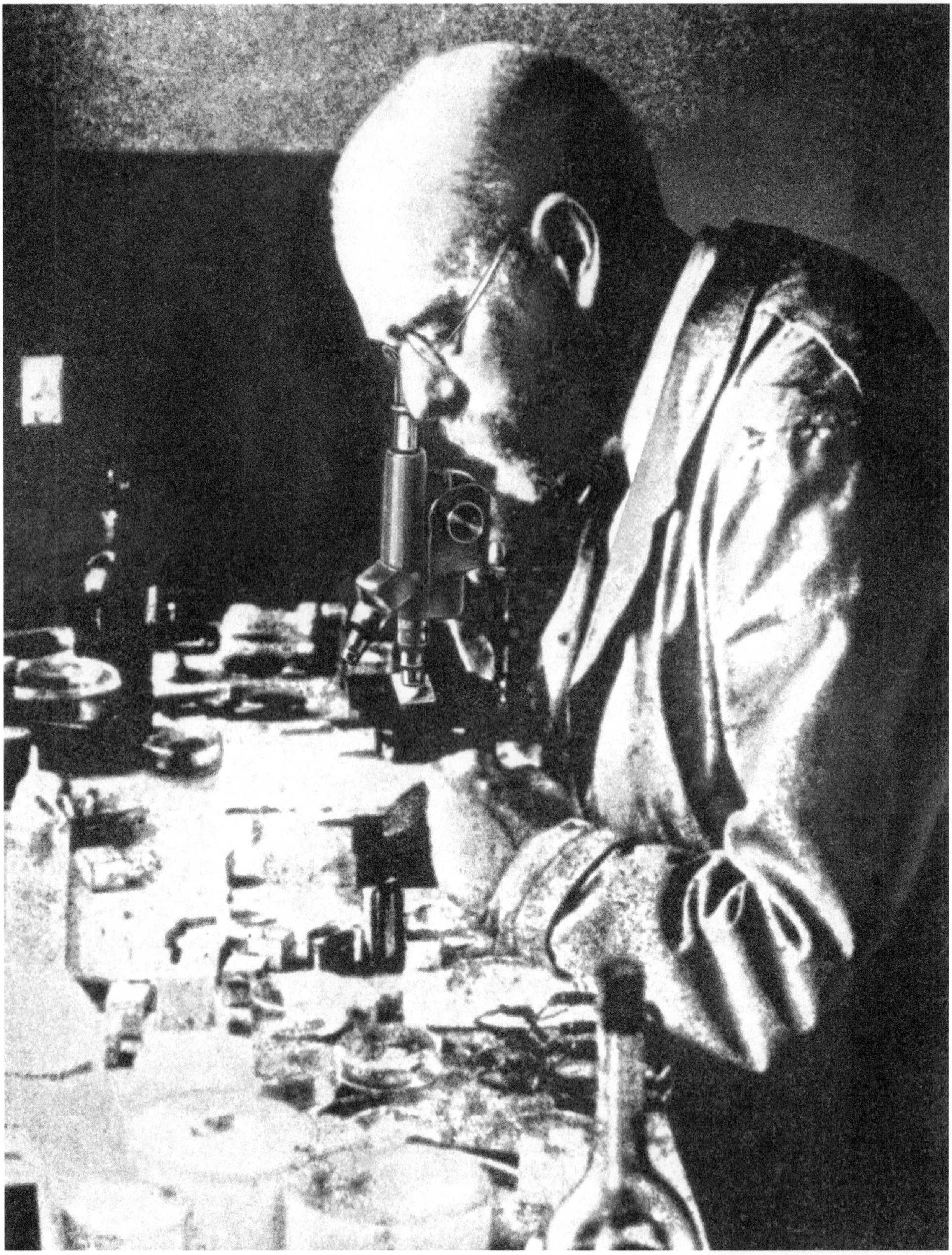

Dr. Robert Koch, whose research on the anthrax bacteria *Bacillus anthracis* helped popularize the germ theory of disease in the late 19th century. © *Sueddeutsche Zeitung Photo/Alamy Stock Photo*

■ Applications and Research

The germ theory is applied to infection control in hospitals, the treatment of food and water, and efforts to control the spread of infection in natural settings. Examples of the latter are the various vaccination and disease prevention programs that are spearheaded by agencies such as the World Health Organization (WHO) and the US Centers for Disease Control and Prevention (CDC). Even in the 21st century, research continues to identify the microbes responsible for diseases, to rapidly and accurately detect their presence, and to devise strategies that will minimize or completely prevent the particular diseases.

■ Impacts and Issues

The germ theory is profoundly important in understanding and preventing a variety of diseases. Knowledge that microorganisms can cause disease spawned efforts to prevent the microbes from coming into contact with people, food, water, and other materials. The practices of disinfection, sterilization, personal hygiene, and proper food preparation have their basis in germ theory.

Knowledge that many diseases are caused by microorganisms and that the microbes can be spread from person to person and from an inanimate surface to a person spurred the development of techniques to minimize or prevent microbial spread. One example is asepsis—the treatment of living and nonliving surfaces to kill or prevent the growth of associated microorganisms. Aseptic technique is one of the cornerstones of research microbiology and is crucially important in medicine. Up until the middle of the 19th century, the absence of aseptic techniques during operations made surgery a risky procedure. However, after the adoption of techniques to minimize microbial contamination of wounds and the airborne spread of microorganisms, the mortality rate following surgery plummeted. The infection control practices that are routine in hospitals in the 21st century are a result of the germ theory.

Similarly, knowledge that some disease-causing bacteria, viruses, and protozoa—particularly those that normally reside in their intestinal tract—can be spread via the contamination of water by feces prompted the implementation of techniques of water treatment. Filtration, chlorination, and exposure of water to ozone or ultraviolet light are techniques used to kill potentially harmful microbes in the water.

The techniques of modern-day molecular biology have an important place in germ theory. Detection and identification of microorganisms based on the presence of target sequences of genetic material is making infection control more rapid and efficient. Furthermore, the use of antibodies and other compounds to block the adherence of microbes to living and nonliving surfaces is useful in minimizing the spread of infections.

The discipline of epidemiology is rooted in the germ theory. Epidemiology is essentially the germ theory in reverse. Rather than tracing the path from the source of a microbe to the disease, an epidemiologist begins with a disease and then, by various means, determines the source and geographical dissemination of that particular disease. Epidemiology is also important in designing strategies to combat an ongoing disease outbreak and in minimizing the chances of future illnesses.

Strategies to minimize the spread of disease-causing microorganisms are often wise. However, concern with the potential for microbial safety in the home and workplace has fostered a sense of urgency that is out of proportion to the risk posed by the microbes. Supermarket shelves are lined with antibacterial products designed to keep a home almost free of microbes. While this may seem sensible, it has, in fact, spawned the development of increased resis-

GERMAN PHYSICIAN ROBERT KOCH (1843–1910)

Robert Koch is considered one of the founders of the field of bacteriology. He pioneered principles and techniques in studying bacteria and discovered the specific agents that cause tuberculosis, cholera, and anthrax. For this he is also regarded as a pioneer of public health, aiding legislation and changing prevailing attitudes about hygiene to prevent the spread of various infectious diseases. For his work on tuberculosis, he was awarded the Nobel Prize in 1905.

Koch's postulates

1. The particular microorganism must be present in every case of the disease.
2. That microorganism must be able to be isolated from a person or other creature host with the particular disease and must be capable of being grown in a pure form free from other organisms. (This condition has since been modified because not all organisms can be grown in the laboratory. However, with molecular techniques of organism identification that are based on the detection of certain unique sequences of genetic material, the microbe does not always need to be grown to fulfill this condition.)
3. The microorganism that is recovered from the pure culture is capable of causing the disease when introduced into a previously healthy test creature.
4. The microorganism can be recovered from the infected creature and can be shown to be the same as the originally recovered or detected microbe.

tance of some microbes to the chemicals being used to control or kill them. In addition, evidence is accumulating that the human immune system requires exposure to microorganisms to keep the system primed and capable of a rapid and efficient response. The strategy of disinfecting a house may be contributing to an increase in allergic diseases because the immune system may overreact when confronted by a foreign substance, such as a microorganism.

SEE ALSO *Bloodborne Pathogens; Disinfection; Koch's Postulates*

BIBLIOGRAPHY

Books

Allman, Toney. *The Importance of Germ Theory.* San Diego, CA: ReferencePoint, 2016.

Fitzharris, Lindsey. *The Butchering Art.* New York: Scientific American, 2017.

Gaynes, Robert P. *Germ Theory: Medical Pioneers in Infectious Diseases.* Washington, DC: ASM, 2011.

Periodicals

Santer, Melvin. "Joseph Lister: First Use of a Bacterium as a 'Model Organism' to Illustrate the Cause of Infectious Disease of Humans." *Notes and Records of the Royal Society of London* 64, no. 1 (March 2010): 59–65.

Websites

"Germ Theory." *Contagion: Historical Views of Diseases and Epidemics.* Harvard University Library. http://ocp.hul.harvard.edu/contagion/germtheory.html (accessed December 1, 2017).

Brian Hoyle

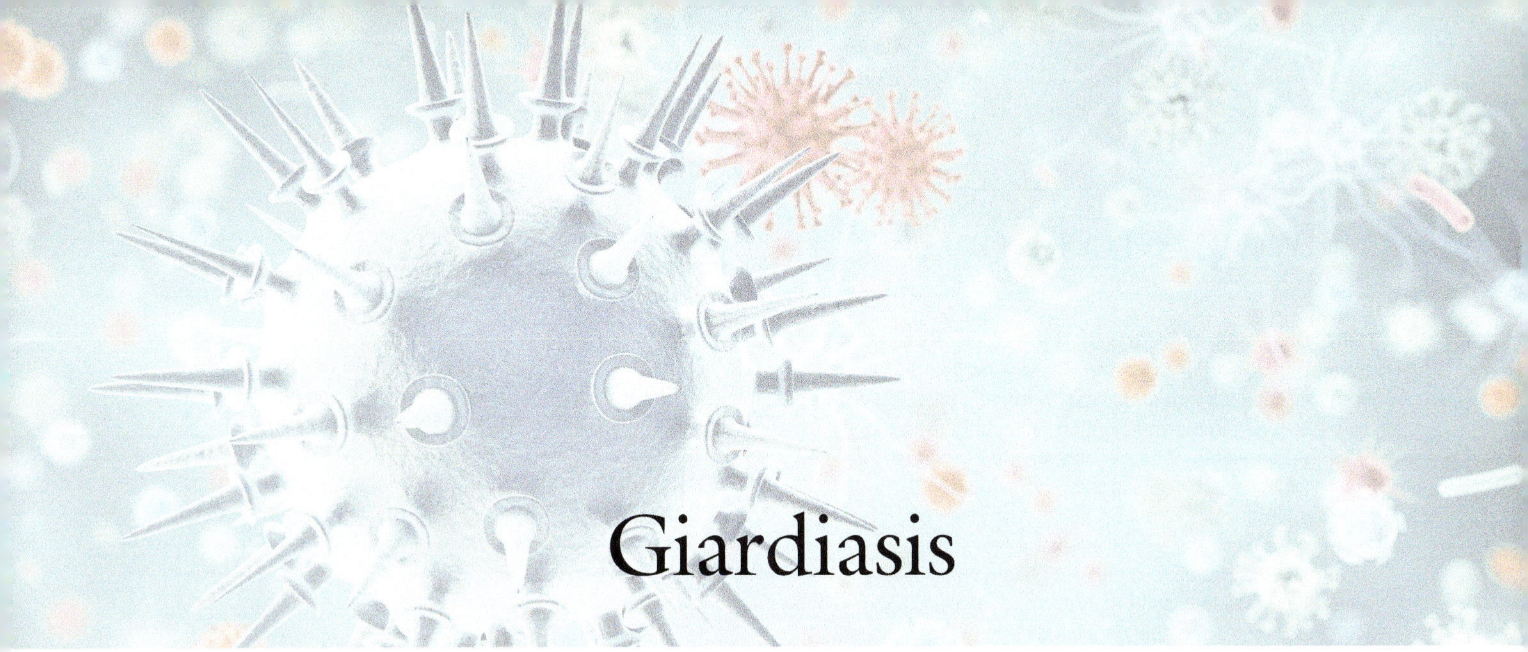

Giardiasis

■ Introduction

Giardiasis (GEE-are-DYE-uh-sis) is an intestinal infection with the protozoan parasite *Giardia lamblia* (also called *Giardia intestinalis* or *Giardia duodenalis*). Sometimes the parasite is simply referred to as *Giardia* (gee-ARE-dee-uh). Protozoa are single-celled animals with more complex features and behavior than bacteria, which are also single-celled organisms. Giardiasis is a waterborne disease found almost everywhere in the world. Its symptoms include diarrhea, gas, stomach cramps, fatigue, weight loss, and nausea.

Giardiasis is transmitted by ingestion of cysts (extremely small, dormant, seedlike objects) that have been shed in the feces of an infected person or animal. Several drugs can be used to treat giardiasis, but healthy individuals can usually overcome the disease without treatment. The symptoms of untreated giardiasis usually last from two to six weeks. Postinfection issues, such as the development of irritable bowel syndrome (IBS), can occur.

Giardia is a protozoan flagellate—that is, a one-celled animal that propels itself using tiny, rapidly waving hairs called flagella. It exists in two forms: the trophozoite and the cyst. A *Giardia* cyst is a microscopic, oval object about 1 to 12 μm (millionths of a meter) long and 7 to 10 μm wide. A *Giardia* infection occurs when a sufficiently large number of these cysts are ingested by an animal or a human.

In the duodenum, the part of the small intestine just below the stomach, each cyst hatches and divides into two trophic individuals, or trophozoites. A *Giardia* trophozoite is shaped somewhat like a limpet with a short, pointed tail. It attaches its flat surface to the cells of the intestinal wall and feeds on them. After a few days the trophozoites detach from the intestinal wall and divide into two identical individuals. Some are carried downstream through the digestive tract to the large intestine, where feces are formed. The harsh chemical conditions in the large intestine signal the trophozoites to become cysts. Cysts can survive for months in surface waters such as lakes and streams.

■ Disease History, Characteristics, and Transmission

Giardiasis has probably been endemic since before modern humans evolved. *Giardia* were first described by Dutch scientist Antoni van Leeuwenhoek (1632–1723), who significantly improved the microscope and was the first person to observe single-celled organisms. He found *Giardia* living in his own feces. The organism was originally named *Cercomonas intestinalis* by Czech physician Wilhelm Lambl (1824–1895) in 1859. It was renamed *Giardia lamblia* in 1915 to honor both Lambl and French physician Alfred Giard (1846–1908), another early researcher of *Giardia*. The term *Giardia intestinalis* is usually preferred by 21st-century scientists.

In the 20th century five species of *Giardia* were identified. *Giardia intestinalis*, the species that afflicts humans, can be hosted by mammals, reptiles, and possibly birds.

REAL-WORLD RISKS

The US Centers for Disease Control and Prevention states that "anyone may become infected with *Giardia*. However, those at greatest risk are:

1. Travelers to countries where giardiasis is common
2. People in childcare settings
3. Those who are in close contact with someone who has the disease
4. People who swallow contaminated drinking water
5. Backpackers or campers who drink untreated water from lakes or rivers
6. People who have contact with animals who have the disease
7. Men who have sex with men."

WORDS TO KNOW

BACTERIA Single-celled microorganisms that live in soil, water, plants, and animals and whose activities range from the development of disease to fermentation. They play a key role in the decay of organic matter and the cycling of nutrients. Bacteria exist in various shapes, including spherical, rod-shaped, and spiral. Some bacteria are agents of disease. Different types of bacteria cause many sexually transmitted diseases, including syphilis, gonorrhea, and chlamydia. Bacteria also cause diseases such as typhoid, dysentery, and tetanus. Bacterium is the singular form of bacteria.

CYST A closed cavity or sac or the dormant stage of life of some parasites when they live inside an enclosed area, covered by a tough outer shell

FLAGELLUM A hairlike structure in a cell that serves as an organ of locomotion.

PROTOZOA Single-celled, animal-like microscopic organisms that live by taking in food rather than making it by photosynthesis and must live in the presence of water. (Singular: protozoan.) Protozoa are a diverse group of single-celled organisms, with more than 50,000 different types represented. The vast majority are microscopic, many measuring less than 5 one-thousandth of an inch (0.005 millimeters), but some, such as the freshwater Spirostomun, may reach 0.17 inches (3 millimeters) in length, large enough to enable it to be seen with the naked eye.

TROPHOZOITE The amoeboid, vegetative stage of the malaria protozoa.

Giardia infection usually lasts two to six weeks. In some cases, however, the infection can become chronic or ongoing. Exactly how *Giardia* cause the symptoms of giardiasis is not known. Many people infected with *Giardia* have no symptoms.

During bouts of diarrhea caused by giardiasis, both trophozoites and cysts exit the body in the feces. The trophozoites die outside the body, but the cysts may be ingested by another animal and continue the life cycle. Many stool samples of infected persons do not contain detectable levels of *Giardia* at all. However, authors of a 2016 article for the *BMJ* stated that "the number of patients detected with *Giardia* will increase as routine testing of stool samples using highly sensitive diagnostic tests becomes more widespread."

Cysts are almost always transmitted by the fecal-oral route (the ingestion of fecal material, generally in a very small or diluted amount, through the mouth). This may occur through feces-hand-oral contact (common among children or those caring for children) or in drinking water. The drinking water route is common worldwide but less so in developed countries. *Giardia* cysts may also be foodborne.

Giardia is common in pets, wild mammals, and farm animals, but there is little evidence that these are important sources of human infection, despite the association in the United States of *Giardia* with drinking open waters containing fecal matter from beavers. (The disease is sometimes called "beaver fever" in the United States.) Whether pets such as cats and dogs are significant in spreading *Giardia* is debated.

■ Scope and Distribution

Giardia is present in most surface waters of the world at varying rates.

Infection with *Giardia intestinalis* is one of the most commonly reported protozoan parasite infections worldwide. Each year *Giardia* infects about 280 million people across the globe (or about 3.5 percent of the world's population of 7.6 billion). Around 33 percent of people who live in developing countries are infected.

In industrialized countries giardiasis is most common among people in childcare environments (including both caregivers and children), in people who live with or who are in close contact with people with the disease, and in those who have recently traveled to countries with high rates of the disease. It can also be contracted by people who drink untreated lake or stream water while visiting wilderness areas. However, drinking such water does not usually result in infection. The body can usually fend off infection if it has ingested only a small to moderate number of cysts.

■ Treatment and Prevention

The primary public health approach to preventing giardiasis is to keep *Giardia* cysts out of drinking water supplies. This is accomplished by keeping water sources used for drinking water from *Giardia* contamination by sewage or livestock waste and by treating drinking water before distributing it. Because *Giardia* and other protozoan cysts are resistant to chemicals such as chlorine at the levels ordinarily used to treat water, the primary means of treating water is filtering. Portable, hand-operated filters can be used by people in wilderness areas to filter out not only *Giardia* cysts but also other parasites and bacteria. The US Centers for Disease Control and Prevention recommends not drinking recreational water, untreated surface water, or untreated ice or drinking water while traveling in developing countries.

For healthy individuals treatment for giardiasis is usually not necessary, as the body is capable of freeing itself

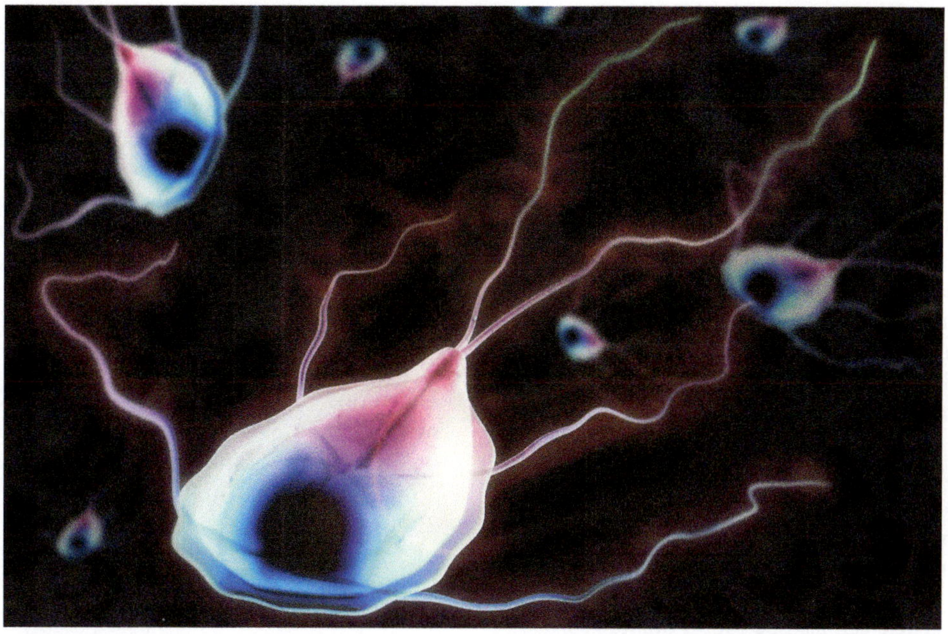

This image shows the structure of the giardiasis parasite, which causes gastroenteritis. © *3D4Medical/Science Source*

from the infection. Where treatment is needed or desired, a number of drugs are available, including tinidazole, metronidazole, and nitazoxanide. Of these, tinidazole is the most effective and has the fewest side effects, according to Karlyn D. Beer and colleagues in a 2017 study published in *Clinical Infectious Diseases.*

A 2016 study in the journal *Nature* demonstrated that dogs, cats, and gerbils could successfully be vaccinated against giardiasis. The authors suggested the success of the animal vaccinations indicated a human vaccination could successfully be developed. In addition, the authors found that vaccinating dogs in locations where *Giardia* was common reduced the transmission of the disease to human children.

Impacts and Issues

In the 2010s members of the medical community expressed increasing concern that *Giardia* was becoming resistant to drugs. Studies showed that people who had been infected with giardiasis could experience postinfection issues, such as IBS, chronic fatigue syndrome, and food allergies. At the same time, evidence suggested that experiencing giardiasis could protect people from contracting other diseases that cause diarrhea.

Beer and her coauthors also noted that "giardiasis care infrequently follows all aspects of clinical recommendations. Multiple differences between pediatric and adult care, despite age-agnostic recommendations, suggest opportunities for provider education or tailored guidance."

In 2018 health enthusiasts and those worried about chemical contaminants in public drinking water in industrialized countries promoted the benefits of drinking "raw water," or water that had not been chemically treated or filtered. However, doctors warned that ingesting raw water could cause drinkers to contract giardiasis and other waterborne infections.

See Also *CDC (Centers for Disease Control and Prevention); Cryptosporidiosis; Parasitic Diseases; Protozoan Diseases; Waterborne Disease*

BIBLIOGRAPHY

Books

Erlandsen, Stanley L., and Ernest A. Meyer. *Giardia and Giardiasis: Biology, Pathogenesis, and Epidemiology.* New York: Springer-Verlag, 2013.

Luján, Hugo D., and Staffan Svärd, eds. *Giardia: A Model Organism.* New York: Springer, 2011.

Periodicals

Ansell, Brendan R. E., et al. "Drug Resistance in *Giardia duodenalis.*" *Biotechnology Advances* 33, no. 6 (2015): 888–901.

Beer, Karlyn D., et al. "Giardiasis Diagnosis and Treatment Practices among Commercially Insured Persons in the United States." *Clinical Infectious Diseases* 64, no. 9 (May 1, 2017): 1244–1250. This article can also be found online at https://academic.oup.com/cid/article-abstract/64/9/1244/3000619 (accessed January 17, 2018).

Corrado, Minetti, et al. "Giardiasis." *BMJ* 355 (2016): i5369. This article can also be found online at http://www.bmj.com/content/355/bmj.i5369 (accessed January 16, 2018).

Einarsson, Elin, Showgy Ma'ayeh, and Staffan G. Svärd. "An Update on *Giardia* and Giardiasis." *Current Opinion in Microbiology* 34 (December 2016): 47–52.

Ordóñez-Mena, José M., Noel D. McCarthy, and Thomas R. Fanshawe. "Comparative Efficacy of Drugs for Treating Giardiasis: A Systematic Update of the Literature and Network Meta-Analysis of Randomized Clinical Trials." *Journal of Antimicrobial Chemotherapy* (November 27, 2017). This article can also be found online at https://academic.oup.com/jac/advance-article-abstract/doi/10.1093/jac/dkx430/4662983?redirectedFrom=fulltext (accessed January 17, 2018).

"Raw Water: The Unsterilised Health Craze That Could Give You Diarrhea." *Guardian* (January 3, 2018). This article can also be found online at https://www.theguardian.com/lifeandstyle/shortcuts/2018/jan/03/raw-water-the-unsterilised-health-craze-that-could-give-you-diarrhoea (accessed January 16, 2018).

Serradell, Marianela C., et al. "Vaccination of Domestic Animals with a Novel Oral Vaccine Prevents *Giardia* Infections, Alleviates Signs of Giardiasis and Reduces Transmission to Humans." *Nature* (September 15, 2016). This article can also be found online at https://www.nature.com/articles/npjvaccines201618?utm_source=feedburner&utm_medium=feed&utm_campaign=Feed%3A+npjvaccines%2Frss%2Fcurrent+(npj+Vaccines) (accessed January 17, 2018).

Watkins, Richard R., and Lars Eckmann. "Treatment of Giardiasis: Current Status and Future Directions." *Current Infectious Disease Report* 16, no. 2 (2014): 396. This article can also be found online at https://link.springer.com/article/10.1007/s11908-014-0396-y (accessed January 17, 2018).

Websites

"Parasites: Giardia." US Centers for Disease Control and Prevention, July 22, 2015. https://www.cdc.gov/parasites/giardia/index.html (accessed January 16, 2018).

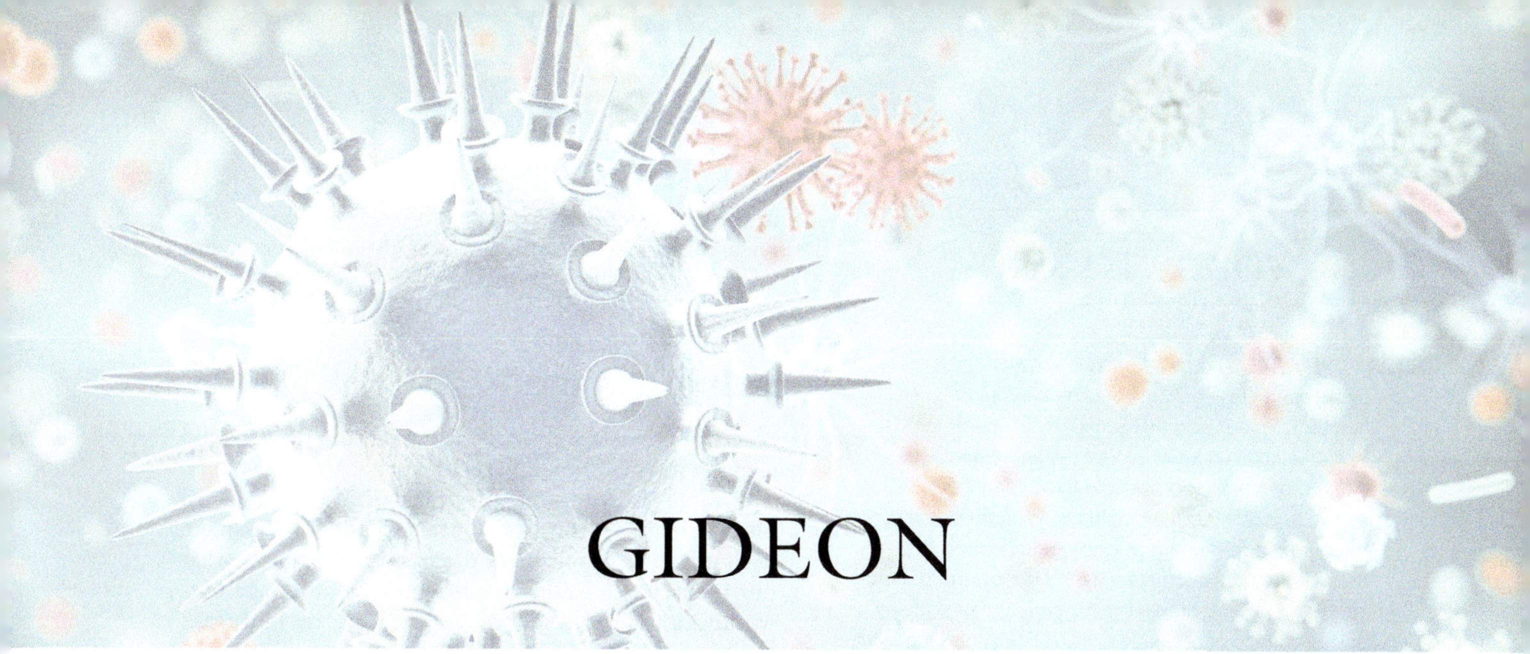

GIDEON

Introduction

The Global Infectious Diseases and Epidemiology Online Network (GIDEON) is a web-based software system designed for use in geographic medicine, a branch of medicine that deals with international public health issues including infectious and tropical diseases. GIDEON, located at www.gideononline.com, helps physicians diagnose any recognized infectious disease occurring in the world.

The first module of GIDEON generates a ranked list of potential diagnoses based on signs, symptoms, laboratory tests, country of acquisition, incubation period, exposure (foods, animals, insects), and other relevant details. This list is not intended to replace the expertise of health care workers but rather to present a comprehensive group of diseases that can focus further analysis of the case, suggest additional diagnostic tests, and offer in-depth analysis of each individual disease. At this point the user can query GIDEON about why additional diseases are not listed, search for information on the country-specific status of each disease listed, or access links to specific therapy and diagnostic options.

Additional options allow the user to generate a list of diseases compatible with bioterrorism and to simulate disease scenarios not associated with a specific patient. For example, the user might access a list of all infectious diseases associated with diarrhea or diseases associated with diarrhea in the United States and then limit the listing to agents of diarrhea associated with water or diarrhea that might develop in the United States within 24 hours of ingesting water.

The second GIDEON module presents the epidemiology of individual diseases, including descriptive text (infective agent, route of infection, incubation period, diagnostic tests, therapy, and vaccines), a global and historical overview of the disease, and the disease's status in every country and region. Country notes include specific regions of activity within each country; local foods, insects, etc., involved in transmission; reported incidence and rates (cases per 100,000 population per year); and a chronology of regional outbreaks. The vaccination standards for every relevant disease in every country are also listed. As of December 2017 the epidemiology module contained about 3 million words of text concerning 357 diseases, 316 drugs, and 71 vaccines. The microorganisms included 1,607 bacteria, 139 mycobacteria, and 128 yeasts. Reference numbers are electronically linked to available abstracts and titles in the medical literature. Thirty-two thousand graphs and about 350 maps are automatically generated to follow the status of all diseases, both worldwide and in each specific country. More than 4,200 images include life-cycle charts, photomicrographs, X-rays, skin lesions, and the like. More than 22,000 outbreaks and 58,000 surveys are listed—for example, all outbreaks of measles reported in scientific literature, prevalence studies of hookworm, acquired immunodeficiency syndrome (AIDS) and liver fluke in African countries, and studies concerning food contamination in all European countries.

The third module follows the pharmacology and usage of all anti-infective drugs and vaccines. Drugs of choice, contraindications, doses for special patient groups, and interaction with other drugs are presented in great detail. An index of all drug trade names (more than 10,000) reflects the international nature of the program. The user may access a list of drugs for a specific indication, such as AIDS or tuberculosis, or antibiotics associated with a specified form or toxicity or drug interaction.

The vaccines module presents similar information regarding all vaccines, including lesser-known preparations used to prevent diseases such as Kyasanur Forest disease (KFD), a viral hemorrhagic fever transmitted by ticks, and Argentine hemorrhagic fever (AHF), a zoonotic infectious disease spread by the corn mouse. Dosage schedules, boosters, side effects, and trade names are accessed through interactive menus.

WORDS TO KNOW

BIOINFORMATICS The development of new database methods to store genomic information (information related to genes and the genetic sequence), computational software programs, and methods to extract, process, and evaluate this information. Also known as computational biology, bioinformatics also refers to the refinement of existing techniques to acquire the genomic data. Finding genes and determining their function, predicting the structure of proteins and sequence of ribonucleic acid (RNA) from the available sequence of deoxyribonucleic acid (DNA), and determining the evolutionary relationship of proteins and DNA sequences are aspects of bioinformatics.

GEOGRAPHIC MEDICINE Also called geomedicine, the study of how human health is affected by climate and environment.

INCIDENCE The number of new cases of a disease or injury that occur in a population during a specified period of time.

INCUBATION PERIOD The time between exposure to a disease-causing virus or bacteria and the appearance of symptoms of the infection. Depending on the microorganism, the incubation time can range from a few hours, such as with food poisoning due to *Salmonella*, to a decade or more, such as with acquired immunodeficiency syndrome (AIDS).

OUTBREAK The appearance of new cases of a disease in numbers greater than the established incidence rate or the appearance of even one case of an emergent or rare disease in an area.

PATHOGEN A disease-causing agent, such as a bacterium, a virus, a fungus, or another microorganism.

The fourth module is designed to identify, compare, and characterize all species of bacteria, mycobacteria (tuberculosis-like organisms), and yeasts. Technical material used in evaluating susceptibility standards of bacteria to anti-infective agents is also available.

All text, maps, images, and graphs are designed for transfer to PowerPoint, word processors, or email for preparation of publications, syllabi, student handouts, and other formats. A built-in network option allows for installation on any computer network. Network managers can add custom notes in their own languages to the program regarding any disease, drug, or pathogen relevant to their institutions. A text box allows users to append custom notes in their own fonts and languages to the GIDEON text, including contact information, submission of specimens, pricing, or ongoing outbreaks.

Impacts and Issues

As GIDEON is a web-based program, the server could easily be adopted to follow all diseases analyzed by users. This form of "syndromic surveillance" is an example of bioinformatics (using computers as tools to manage data and solve problems in the biological sciences) that can be useful to health departments or other agencies worldwide for rapid identification of disease outbreaks or unusual disease patterns in the community.

GIDEON is a rich source of information that has proven popular for clinicians in hospitals, researchers in academic and commercial research labs, teachers, and health care professionals. It has been used to investigate the global spread of infectious diseases, to refine the treatment of drinking water by surveying illness outbreaks related to contaminated drinking water, and to clarify knowledge concerning the spread of disease-causing microorganisms from domesticated animals to people. GIDEON is also crucial in helping researchers find the potential sources of future diseases.

PRIMARY SOURCE

Global Infectious Diseases and Epidemiology Network (GIDEON): A World Wide Web–Based Program for Diagnosis and Informatics in Infectious Diseases.

SOURCE: *Edberg, Stephen C. "Global Infectious Diseases and Epidemiology Network (GIDEON): A World Wide Web–Based Program for Diagnosis and Informatics in Infectious Diseases."* Clinical Infectious Diseases *40, no. 1 (January 2005): 123–126.*

INTRODUCTION: *How does GIDEON work? In the following excerpt from an article published in the medical journal* Clinical Infectious Diseases*, Stephen C. Edberg of the Yale University School of Medicine discusses how GIDEON makes a diagnosis.*

The Diagnosis module is designed to generate a ranked differential diagnosis on the basis of signs, symptoms, laboratory tests, incubation period, and country of disease origin. Options in the data entry screen are organized by body system, country of disease acquisition, and details of exposure. The lower "personal notes" box is used to record additional case data, and notes can be written in the user's own language. The resulting differential diagnosis list allows the reader options that include a hard-copy or e-mail report generation of a table comparing the clinical features of the diseases listed, and queries concerning the omission or ranking of specific diseases. If the user clicks on a disease name, additional screens describe the disease itself and its clinical epidemiology.

The differential diagnosis list in GIDEON is based on a Bayesian formula that compares the mathematical product of disease incidence times the rate of symptom occurrence for all relevant infectious diseases within a given country. Additional options allow for analysis of a worldwide scenario (e.g., a list of the complete differential diagnoses of eosinophilia and splenomegaly or of arthralgia with rash). A "bioterrorism" option produces the differential diagnosis of signs and symptoms associated with suspected bioterrorism scenarios. Interestingly, the latter option is not based on a Bayesian formula, because the concept of "incidence" is not relevant.

As the manufacturers point out, the module should not substitute for clinical acumen, and should be considered an "expert" or "decision support" system. In many cases, the correct diagnosis does, in fact, appear as the first item on GIDEON's list. In a blinded study of 500 cases conducted by the developer of GIDEON, the correct diagnosis appeared in the differential diagnosis in 94.7% of cases and was ranked first in 75%. A later study, which examined 86 hospitalized patients, found that the correct diagnosis appeared in only 69% of cases and was ranked first in only 60%. For this reason, a "why not" option was added to GIDEON to analyze why certain diagnoses are not listed.

SEE ALSO *Globalization and Infectious Disease; Notifiable Diseases; ProMED; Public Health and Infectious Disease; Travel and Infectious Disease*

BIBLIOGRAPHY

Books

Kudva, Indira T., et al., eds. *Virulence Mechanisms of Bacterial Pathogens.* 5th ed. Washington, DC: ASM, 2016.

Shah, Sonia. *Pandemic: Tracking Contagions, from Cholera to Ebola and Beyond.* New York: Sarah Crichton Books/Farrar, Straus and Giroux, 2016.

Periodicals

Felitti, Vincent J. "GIDEON: Global Infectious Diseases and Epidemiology Online Network." *JAMA* 293 (2005): 1674–1675.

Ross, John J., and Daniel S. Shapiro. "Evaluation of the Computer Program GIDEON for the Diagnosis of Fever in Patients Admitted to a Medical Service." *Clinical Infectious Diseases* 26, no. 3: (March 1998): 766–767.

Websites

"GIDEON Content-Outbreaks." GIDEON, 2018. https://www.gideononline.com (accessed December 11, 2017).

Stephen A. Berger
Brian Hoyle

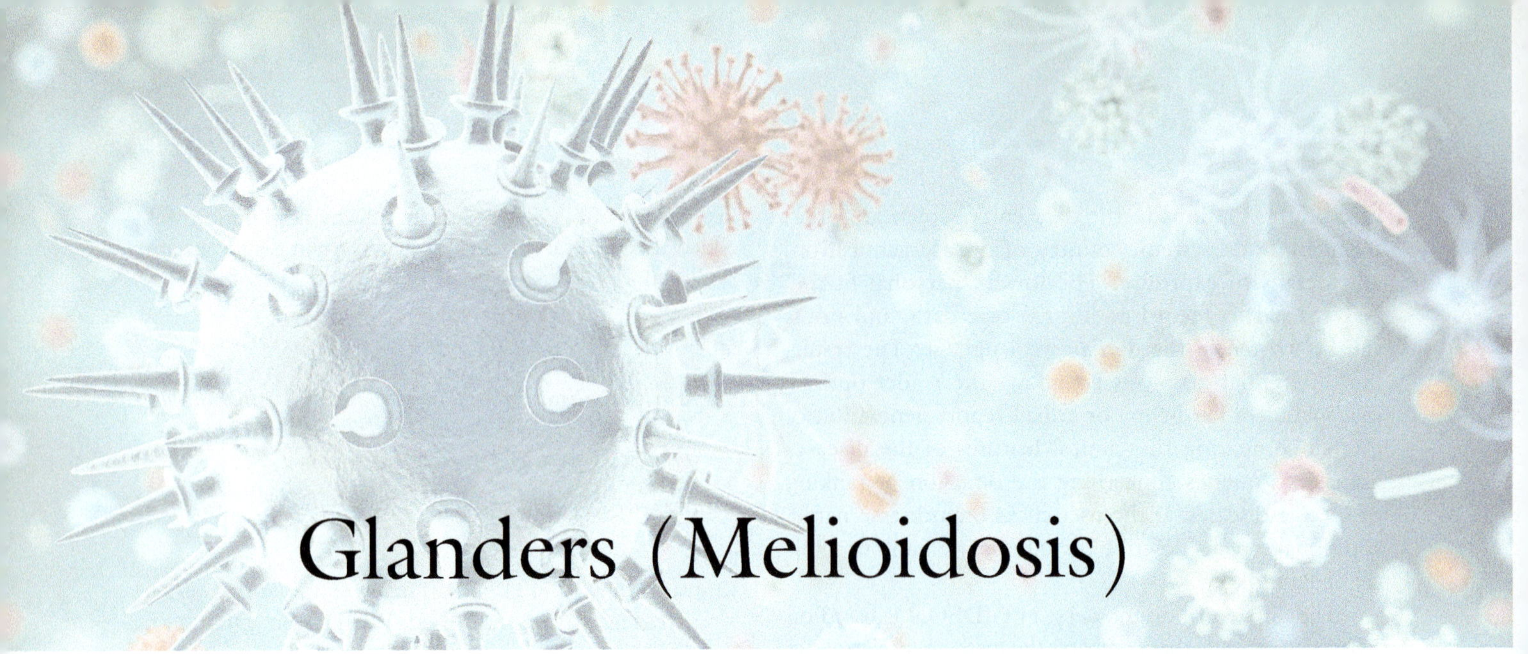

Glanders (Melioidosis)

Introduction

Glanders and melioidosis are related infectious diseases caused by bacterial species in the *Burkholderia* genus. Both diseases produce similar symptoms and are diagnosed, treated, and prevented similarly. However, glanders and melioidosis differ with respect to where they originate and how they spread.

WORDS TO KNOW

ABSCESS A pus-filled sore, usually caused by a bacterial infection, that results from the body's defensive reaction to foreign material. Abscesses are often found in the soft tissue under the skin, such as in the armpit or the groin. However, they may develop in any organ, and they are commonly found in the breast and gums. Abscesses are far more serious and call for more specific treatment if they are located in deep organs such as the lung, liver, or brain.

ACUTE Of rapid onset and short duration, which either resolves or becomes chronic.

CHRONIC Chronic infections persist for prolonged periods of time—months or even years—in the host. This lengthy persistence is due to a number of factors, which can include masking of the disease-causing agent (e.g., bacteria) from the immune system, invasion of host cells, and the establishment of an infection that is resistant to antibacterial agents.

MORTALITY The condition of being susceptible to death. The term *mortality* comes from the Latin word *mors*, which means death. Mortality can also refer to the rate of deaths caused by an illness or injury (e.g., "Rabies has a high mortality rate").

NODULE A small, roundish lump on the surface of the skin or of an internal organ.

Glanders is caused by the bacterium *Burkholderia mallei*. The bacterium is found only in infected host animals and is not found in plants, soil, or water. Glanders primarily infects horses but can also infect donkeys, mules, cats, dogs, sheep, and goats. Humans contract glanders when they make contact with the body fluids or tissue of animals carrying the disease. While cases of glanders in humans are rarely reported, occasional cases occur in Africa, Asia, South and Central America, and the Middle East.

Melioidosis, which is also sometimes known as Whitmore's disease, is caused by the bacterium *Burkholderia pseudomallei*. Most animals that contract melioidosis do so by ingestion of contaminated food, soil, or water. Humans become infected with both glanders and melioidosis through openings in the skin, the mucosal surfaces, or inhalation. Melioidosis is most commonly found in northern Australia and Southeast Asia, where it is considered an infectious disease of major public health importance, but it is also found in other parts of the world. Epidemiologists believe melioidosis is a chronically underreported disease.

Numerous nations, including the United States, have studied the potential for weaponizing both glanders and melioidosis. Their potential as agents of biological warfare derives from their resistance to most antibiotic treatments and the ease with which they can be converted into aerosolized form. The US National Institute of Allergy and Infectious Diseases has classified *B. mallei* and *B. pseudomallei* as category B pathogens because they "are moderately easy to disseminate," "result in moderate morbidity rates and low mortality rates," and "require specific enhancements for diagnostic capacity and enhanced disease surveillance."

Disease History, Characteristics, and Transmission

The earliest-known descriptions of glanders can be found in Greek texts from the 5th century BCE, when it was known only as a disease that affected horses. In

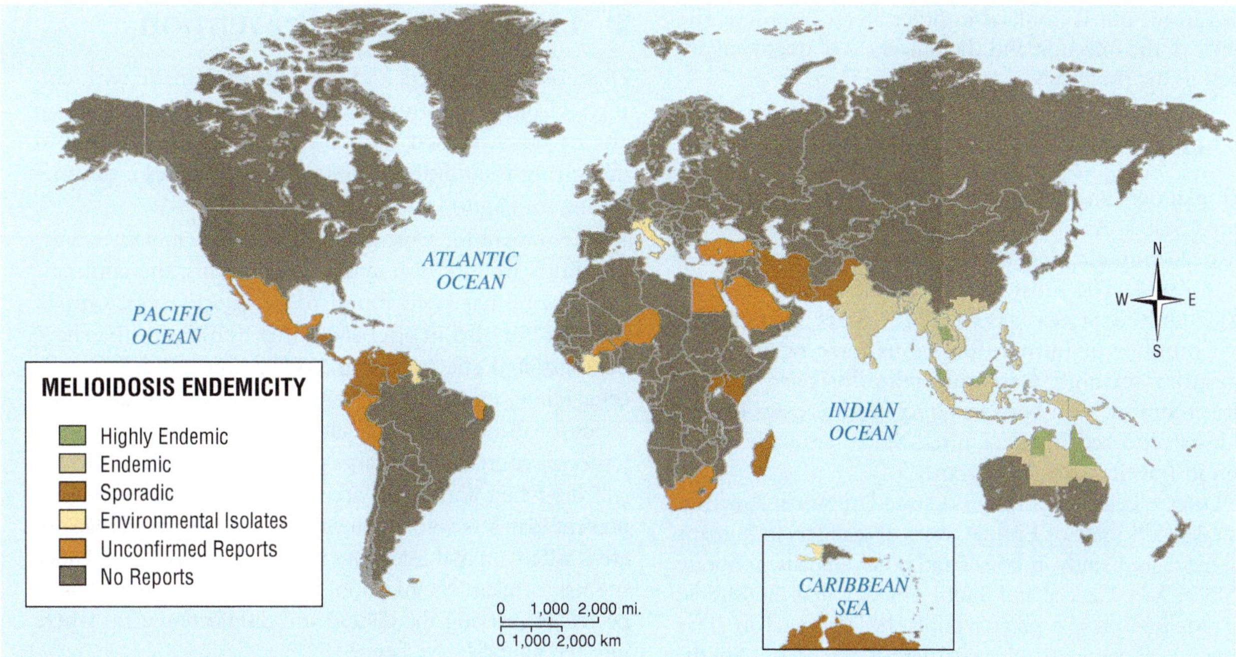

SOURCE: Adapted from "Endemicity of Melioidosis Infection." US Centers for Disease Control and Prevention. Available from: https://www.cdc.gov/melioidosis/prevention/index.html

the centuries since, glanders has been known by many names, to many different civilizations and societies. However, it was not until 1882 that scientists were able to identify *B. mallei* as the disease's cause. Several decades later, in 1911, while working in what was then Rangoon, Burma (present-day Yangon, Myanmar), Alfred Whitmore (1876–1946) and C. S. Krishnaswami described a similar disease caused by a similar, but different, bacteria. That disease has since come to be known as melioidosis. The bacteria that causes it was given the name *B. pseudomallei* in 1992.

Historically, glanders was known largely as a disease that affected horses. However, transmission to other animals, including humans, can occur via direct contact with infected animals. *B. mallei* bacteria enter the human body through breaks in the skin or through the mucosal surfaces of the eyes and nose. Melioidosis is transmitted by direct contact with contaminated soil and surface waters, and the bacteria are thought to enter the body through breaks in the skin, inhalation of contaminated soil, and ingestion of contaminated water. Person-to-person transmission of glanders and melioidosis, though rare, also have been documented. Symptoms depend on the amount of bacteria in the human system. A few bacteria inside the body rarely cause any symptoms. When more organisms are present, more symptoms appear.

In glanders infection, symptoms appear in about one to five days, whereas melioidosis symptoms may not develop for years. When symptoms occur their characteristics depend on the mode of transmission (skin or mucosal surfaces) into the body and the form of the infection (acute or chronic).

An acute localized infection with glanders results in swollen lymph glands, fever, sweats, muscle pains, and coughing. Other symptoms include eye tearing, light sensitivity, and diarrhea. Entrance into the body through the eyes, nose, and respiratory tract causes excessive and sometimes infectious mucus. The infection may also enter the bloodstream. This more serious bacterial infection in the bloodstream is called septicemia. Septicemia caused by *B. mallei* will usually cause death within 7 to 10 days.

An acute localized infection with melioidosis causes respiratory problems, headache, diarrhea, fever, pus-filled skin lesions, muscle soreness, and confusion. Usually the infection is resolved in a short time. However, people with unrelated serious illnesses such as renal failure, diabetes, and human immunodeficiency virus (HIV) infection can go into septic shock, resulting in multiple organ collapse and death.

Acute pulmonary infections in both glanders and melioidosis can cause symptoms ranging from mild bronchitis to severe pneumonia. Symptoms include fever, headache, anorexia, pulmonary abscesses, and muscle soreness.

Chronic infections of both diseases cause multiple abscesses within the arm and leg muscles or in the spleen or liver. For glanders, nasal and subcutaneous nodules form, followed by ulceration. Death can follow within a few months. Symptoms of chronic melioidosis are often similar to tuberculosis. Lung or spleen abscesses often cause abdominal pain and fever, while brain abscesses often cause neurological problems. When bacteria enter the bloodstream, glanders is usually fatal within a week to 10 days. Melioidosis infection also may travel into the bones, brain, lungs, and joints. It usually causes death when it infects the bloodstream but is nonfatal in other areas. However, the severity of the infection and the timeliness of treatment are critical in the prognosis.

Scope and Distribution

Both glanders and melioidosis are extremely rare in the United States. As of 2018 the most recent case of naturally occurring glanders in a human in the United States was in 1934. The most recent case of equine glanders in the United States was in 1942. Since that time a small number of human infections have occurred in laboratory settings. Cases of melioidosis are slightly more common, with between zero and five cases of melioidosis reported in the United States annually, most often in travelers and immigrants.

Despite being essentially eradicated in North America, Australia, and most of Europe, cases of glanders in humans and, more frequently in horses and other animals, continue in Africa, Asia, Central and South America, and the Middle East. Melioidosis is a greater public health threat in areas where it is endemic, such as northern Australia and Southeast Asia. While reports of melioidosis are most common in Thailand, Australia, Singapore, and Malaysia, public health officials believe infections are also common but underreported in a number of other areas, including India, southern China, Laos, and Cambodia. It is also occasionally found in Central and South America, the Caribbean, Africa, the Middle East, and the South Pacific. Evidence suggests that melioidosis infections increase during the rainy season in the areas of Southeast Asia and Australia, where it is most prevalent.

Treatment and Prevention

Diagnosis of glanders and melioidosis is made with cultures of blood, sputum, or urine. A pus culture from an abscess also is used with melioidosis. Detecting and measuring the number of bacterial antibodies is another means to diagnosis.

Treatment for acute glanders is limited, in part because infections are rare in humans. Despite this, the antibiotic sulfadiazine has been found to be effective not only in humans but also in animals. Other antibiotics that have demonstrated effectiveness in combatting glanders include ceftazidime, imipenem, novobiocin, and tetracyclines. Statistics for glanders are difficult to obtain, but medical professionals contend that a large percentage of people infected still die when antibiotics are not given. The best way to prevent glanders is to eliminate the infection in animals. In areas where animal infections do occur, people can reduce the risk of glanders infection by quarantining animals suspected of carrying the disease and disinfecting areas where infected animals have been.

Treatment of acute melioidosis often begins with intravenous antibiotics, often ceftazidime or meropenem. Antibiotics are typically administered intravenously for 10 to 14 days. After the initial course of antibiotics is completed, patients are usually prescribed oral antimicrobial medication such as doxycycline or trimethoprim-sulfamethoxazole. Antimicrobial therapy typically lasts 12 to 24 weeks.

Before the use of antibiotics, acute melioidosis had a death rate of about 90 percent. By the 21st century, antibiotics had reduced the likelihood of dying from melioidosis.

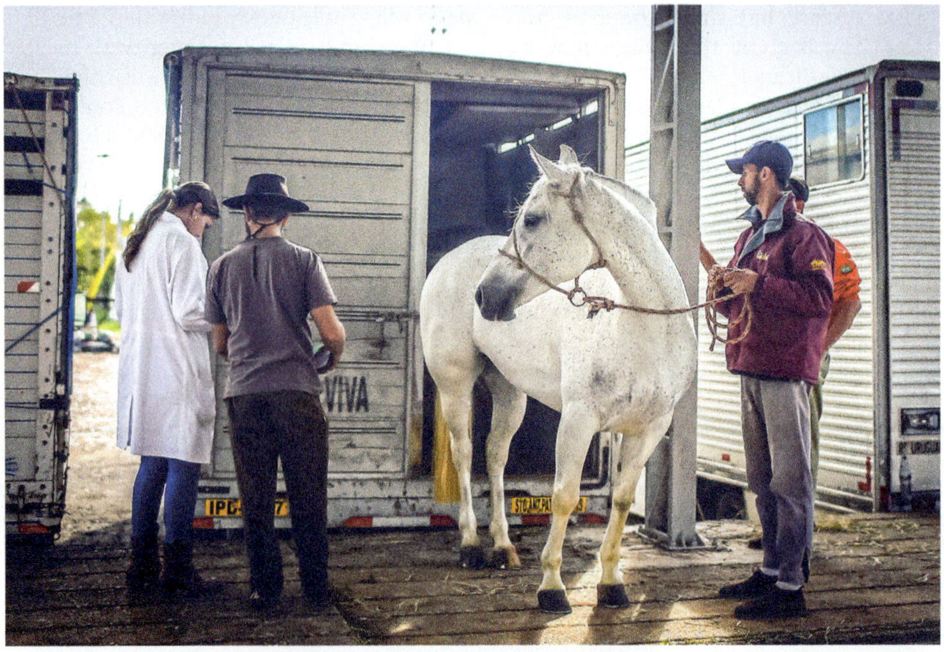

In Esteio, Brazil, a sanitary inspection team checks a horse for glanders (melioidosis), a highly contagious disease that can infect not only horses but also humans. © *JEFFERSON BERNARDES/AFP/Getty Images*

However, death rates vary by country and even within countries due to differences in patient access to health care. For example, the mortality rate in Australia was 16 percent between 1990 and 2002, whereas in Thailand the mortality rate was 43 percent between 1997 and 2006, according to a 2016 article in the *British Medical Bulletin* by Direk Limmathurotsakul and Sharon J. Peacock. In northeastern Thailand, melioidosis is the third-most frequent cause of death. In countries where melioidosis is prevalent, contact with soil, mud, floodwaters, and surface waters should be avoided to prevent infection.

As of 2017 medical researchers had not developed vaccines for either glanders or melioidosis.

■ Impacts and Issues

Both glanders and melioidosis are considered potential biological weapons in warfare and terrorism due to the high incidence of death in infected humans and the ease with which *Burkholderia* bacteria can be aerosolized. During the 20th century, the United States, the Soviet Union, Japan, and other countries intensively studied how *B. mallei* might be weaponized. While it is not definitively known whether *Burkholderia* was ever used in warfare, evidence suggests the German military deliberately infected horses and mules of the Russian army with *B. mallei*. Evidence also indicates Japan used *B. mallei* as a weapon of biological warfare in China during World War II (1939–1945), infecting prisoners of war, civilians, and animals. The Soviet Union was also accused of deploying glanders in weaponized form in Afghanistan during the Soviet-Afghan War. International treaties ban the use of biological weapons. The US National Institute of Allergy and Infectious Diseases classifies glanders and melioidosis as category B pathogens, the second-most dangerous class of biological organisms.

In the 21st century glanders was classified as a reemerging zoonotic disease, becoming increasingly common in horses and a growing threat to humans. To control infections in horses, some observers have advocated for improved testing and culling strategies and for improved safety measures for those who regularly work around experimental or domestic animals, such as animal caretakers, laboratory personnel, and veterinarians.

Melioidosis may remain dormant for many years before producing symptoms. Thus, it can be contracted without any visible signs of infection. As a result, travel to countries where melioidosis frequently occurs is considered risky. People with a higher-than-normal incidence of melioidosis infection include those engaging in frequent sexual activity with multiple partners and intravenous drug users. Numerous observers have pointed to disparities in mortality rates from melioidosis as evidence of the importance of improving access to treatment in areas where it is lacking.

See Also *Bacterial Disease; Emerging Infectious Diseases; Tropical Infectious Diseases; World Health Organization (WHO)*

BIBLIOGRAPHY

Books

Bannister, Barbara A. *Infection: Microbiology and Management.* Malden, MA: Blackwell, 2006.

Lindler, Luther E., Frank J. Lebeda, and George W. Korch, eds. *Biological Weapons Defense: Infectious Diseases and Counterbioterrorism.* Totowa, NJ: Humana, 2005.

Periodicals

Cheng, Allen C., and Bart J. Currie. "Melioidosis: Epidemiology, Pathophysiology, and Management." *Clinical Microbiology Reviews* 18 (April 2005): 383–416. This article can also be found online at http://cmr.asm.org/cgi/content/full/18/2/383 (accessed February 7, 2018).

Elschner, Mandy C., Heinrich Neubauer, and Lisa D. Sprague. "The Resurrection of Glanders in a New Epidemiological Scenario: A Beneficiary of 'Global Change.'" *Current Clinical Microbiology Reports* 4, no. 1 (2017): 54–60.

Limmathurotsakul, Direk, and Sharon J. Peacock. "Melioidosis: A Clinical Overview." *British Medical Bulletin* 99, no. 1 (2011): 125–139. This article can also be found online at https://doi.org/10.1093/bmb/ldr007 (accessed February 7, 2018).

Raja, N. S., M. Z. Ahmed, and N. N. Singh. "Melioidosis: An Emerging Infectious Disease." *Journal of Postgraduate Medicine* 51, no. 2 (2005): 140–145. This article can also be found online at http://www.jpgmonline.com/article.asp?issn=0022-3859;year=2005;volume=51;issue=2;spage=140;epage=145;aulast=Raja (accessed February 7, 2018).

Van Zandt, Kristopher E., Marek T. Greer, and H. Carl Gelhaus. "Glanders: An Overview of Infection in Humans." *Orphanet Journal of Rare Diseases* 8 (2013): 131. This article can also be found online at https://doi.org/10.1186/1750-1172-8-131 (accessed February 7, 2018).

Wilkinson, Lise. "Glanders: Medicine and Veterinary Medicine in Common Pursuit of a Contagious Disease." *Medical History* 25 (1981): 363–384. This article can also be found online at https://www.ncbi.nlm.nih.gov/pmc/articles/PMC1139069/pdf/medhist00089-0026.pdf (accessed February 18, 2018).

Websites

"Burkholderia Mallei and Pseudomallei (Glanders and Melioidosis)." Center for Health Security, December 1, 2013. http://www.centerforhealthsecurity.org/our-work/publications/glanders-and-melioidosis-fact-sheet (accessed February 7, 2018).

"Glanders." Centers for Disease Control and Prevention, October 31, 2017. https://www.cdc.gov/glanders/index.html (accessed February 7, 2018).

"Melioidosis." Centers for Disease Control and Prevention, January 26, 2012. https://www.cdc.gov/melioidosis/index.html (accessed February 7, 2018).

"NIAID Emerging Infectious Diseases/Pathogens." National Institute of Allergy and Infectious Diseases, October 28, 2016. https://www.niaid.nih.gov/research/emerging-infectious-diseases-pathogens (accessed February 7, 2018).

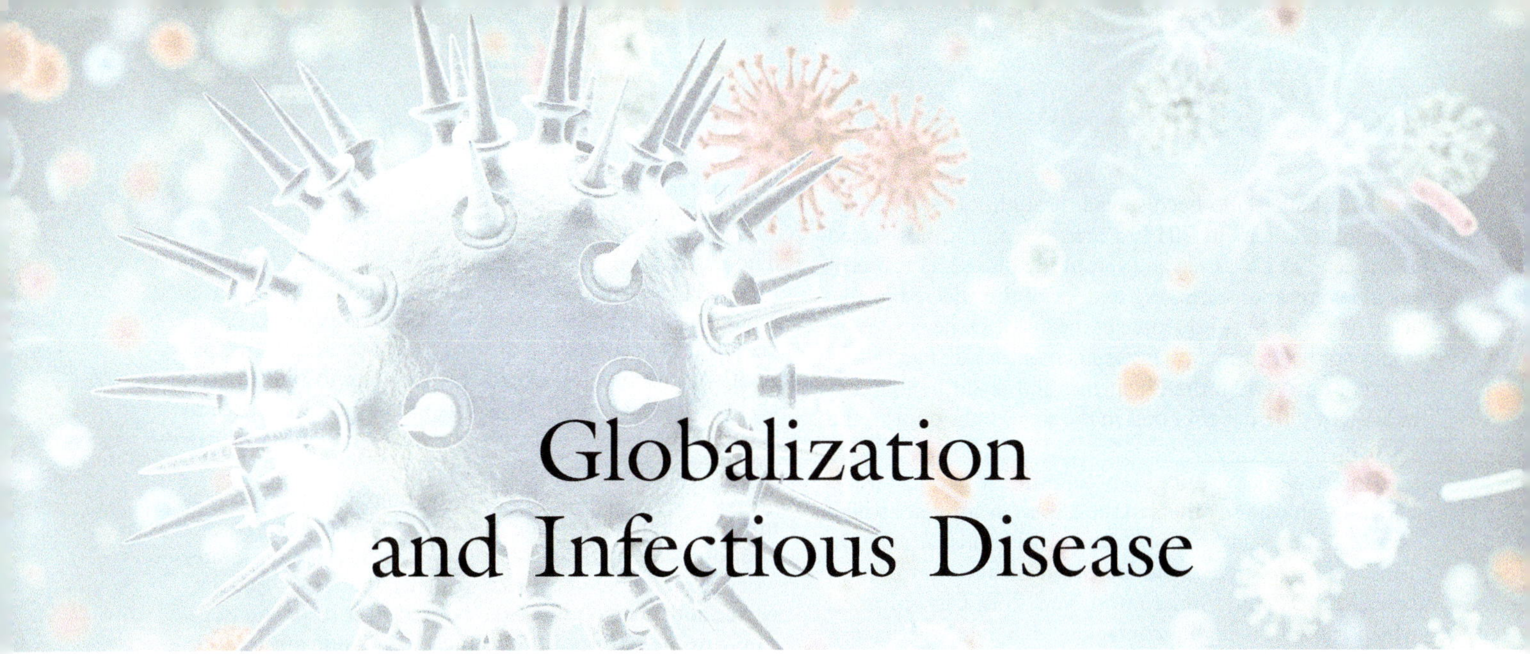

Globalization and Infectious Disease

Introduction

The rise of globalization has contributed significantly to the spread of infectious disease. As the acquired immunodeficiency syndrome (AIDS) epidemic has illustrated, a disease that emerges or reemerges anywhere in the world can move rapidly around the globe. With the increased ease of air travel and the growth of international trade, infectious diseases have more opportunities to spread than in previous eras. Dangerous microbes (pathogens) can arrive in people, insects, exotic animals, or shipments of fruits, meats, or vegetables.

With globalization, diseases no longer have borders. Nations and international health organizations must work together to prevent and control the spread of infectious diseases.

Disease History, Characteristics, and Transmission

Trade and travel can transmit infectious diseases. Travel is a bigger business than oil exports, food products, or automobiles, according to the World Tourism Organization (WTO). It takes less than 36 hours to travel to almost any destination on the globe, far shorter than the usual incubation period for most infectious diseases. A person can become infected in Sierra Leone, travel through Europe, and die in the United States within the space of a few days, as American traveler Joseph Ghoson demonstrated in 2004.

Lassa fever killed Ghoson. A zoonotic, or animal-borne, disease, Lassa fever can also be spread through person-to-person contact. Transmission occurs when a person comes into contact with the blood, tissue, secretions, or excretions of an infected individual. In epidemics of Lassa fever, as many as 50 percent of infected individuals may die. When Lassa fever was confirmed as Ghoson's cause of death, the US Centers for Disease Control and Prevention (CDC) rushed to compile a list of 188 people known to have had contact with him while he was infectious. They included five family members; 139 health care workers at the hospital where he died; 16 employees of commercial laboratories in Virginia and California, where Ghoson's blood samples were tested; and 19 people on the flight he took home from London to Newark, New Jersey. If infected, these individuals could spread Lassa fever.

The CDC could not locate every person who had contact with Ghoson in part because of reporting problems. It does not have electronic access to airline records or flight manifests without special arrangement. Accordingly, investigators from the CDC's Division of Global Migration and Quarantine had to fly to Newark to sift through documents to identify Ghoson's fellow travelers. There was no way to identify other people who might have come into contact with Ghoson on his trek back from Africa.

WORDS TO KNOW

EMERGING INFECTIOUS DISEASE A new infectious disease such as severe acute respiratory syndrome (SARS) or West Nile virus, as well as a previously known disease such as malaria, tuberculosis, or bacterial pneumonia that is appearing in a new form that is resistant to drug treatments.

PATHOGEN A disease-causing agent, such as a bacterium, a virus, a fungus, or another microorganism.

VECTOR Any agent that carries and transmits parasites and diseases. Also, an organism or a chemical used to transport a gene into a new host cell.

ZOONOTIC A disease that can be transmitted between animals and humans. Examples of zoonotic diseases are anthrax, plague, and Q fever.

Measles has also been spread through travel. Over the Christmas holiday in 2014, a person with measles visited Disneyland in California and spread the disease to 125 others in seven other states. Eighty-four of the affected people were hospitalized. The source of the initial Disney exposure could not be identified, but the strain of measles had caused a recent outbreak in the Philippines and could be found in at least 14 different countries in the six months prior to the incident.

International visitors from countries where measles is endemic can expose others to the disease in any place where people gather, such as airports and other tourist attractions. In 2018 an Australian tourist spread measles throughout several hotels and a museum in New York City. Measles, which can kill, is highly contagious, but high vaccination rates usually protect Americans from the disease. In 2013 an outbreak in New York City affected an Orthodox Jewish community that did not support vaccination. The 57 people who became ill were linked to an unvaccinated person who had caught measles while traveling in London. Both Australia and England have high vaccination rates, so the initial sources for both episodes may be other travelers who remain unidentified.

■ Scope and Distribution

The exact scope of infectious diseases spread through globalization is unknown. Many cases probably go unreported each year because surveillance is passive. Physicians must recognize a disease, inquire about the patient's travel history, obtain proper diagnostic samples, and report the case. A physician who does not expect to see an illness that is rare or unknown in his country could misidentify the disease.

Additionally, inspections of cargo are declining even as imports, legal and illegal, increase. Monkeypox is a zoonotic disease that first appeared in the United States when contaminated African rodents that had been imported into the country were housed next to prairie dogs. The virus passed from the prairie dogs to humans in 2003 after the animals were sold as pets. Tens of thousands of exotic animals are smuggled into the United States each year as part of a global black market. Meanwhile, the globalization of food production has created a boom in food import and export without an accompanying rise in inspectors. However, an infected insect or small animal in a corner of a large crate might elude even the most eagle-eyed official.

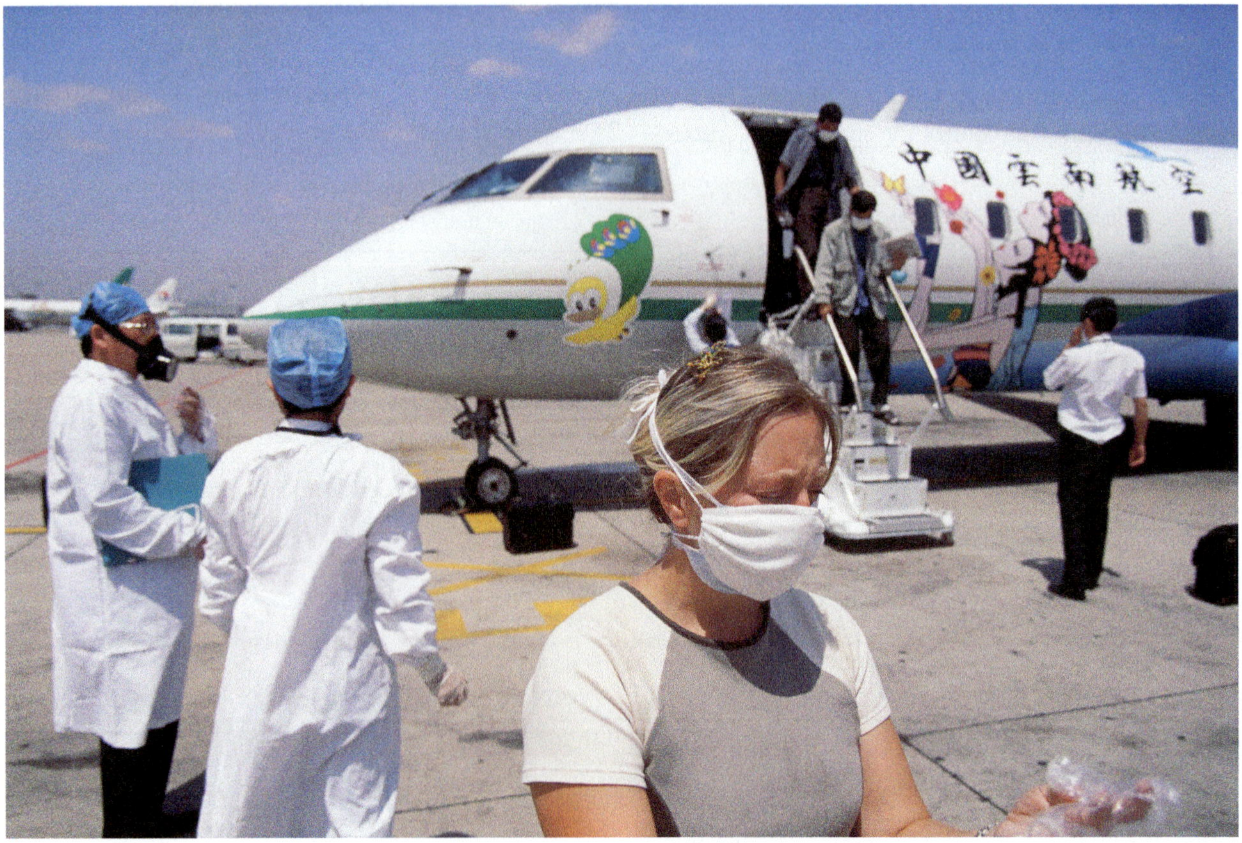

At an airport in Kunming, China, officials take part in measures designed to control the spread of SARS, an infectious disease that spread around the world in 2003. *© Travel Ink/Getty Images*

Treatment and Prevention

The CDC has revised its infectious disease priorities in response to globalization. International outbreak assistance is now a top priority. The CDC has strengthened its diagnostic facilities and enhanced its capacity for epidemiological investigations overseas. The CDC offers follow-up assistance after infectious disease outbreaks as part of an effort to control new pathogens. It has also increased research on diseases that are uncommon in the United States. For example, the CDC has worked in West Africa to fight the Ebola epidemic that began in 2014. Transmission of the virus apparently stopped in 2016, but the CDC established a surveillance system to monitor the region in the event that Ebola reappears. Ebola killed about 40 percent of the people who were infected, making it particularly terrifying.

The CDC also launched the International Emerging Infections Program, targeting disease sources in developing countries and working with international health organizations to prevent the spread of disease through travel, migration, and trade. It is also coordinating disease control and eradication efforts to stop the spread of malaria and tuberculosis.

The CDC is also attempting to strengthen preventive procedures at home. Prompted in part by the SARS epidemic of 2003 and the Ghoson incident, the CDC has asked the US Congress to toughen laws on disease reporting, increase the number of inspectors and quarantine stations, and require common carriers such as airlines and ships to maintain lists of passengers for longer periods. However, legislative success has been limited.

The CDC also expanded regional disease surveillance networks into a global network that could provide early warning of infectious diseases. With this strategy the CDC works closely as a technical consultant with WHO. Like the CDC, WHO is charged with addressing health threats in the changing global landscape, and it has focused on creating new strategies to coordinate response efforts.

Impacts and Issues

Coordination is the major issue that faces government agencies as they attempt to protect public health. The CDC's Geographic Medicine and Health Promotion Branch has warned that there is inadequate national surveillance for zoonotic diseases. Human diseases are handled by the CDC, whereas animal diseases are addressed by the US Department of Agriculture.

Monkeypox is just one example of a zoonotic disease that has infected humans. Avian influenza, also known as H5N1, or bird flu, is a zoonotic disease that has the potential to cause enormous disruptions around the world. CDC preparations for a pandemic include avian influenza because the risk is so high.

Vaccines offer a promising means of stopping infectious disease. Under the long-established WHO system, countries send influenza specimens to the agency, which then makes these samples available to the global community for public health purposes, including vaccine development. However, some developing countries have been reluctant to share viral samples for vaccine research because they want to ensure that their citizens have access to vaccines at affordable prices. A long-term WHO goal is that developing countries obtain enough technology and scientific training to produce vaccines.

Globalization also has positive effects for combating disease. Pharmaceutical companies have reached agreements with several nations and international health organizations to provide drugs and vaccines for some epidemic diseases at reduced cost. Increasing international attention on neglected diseases has garnered support for research and development of drugs and vaccines to fight illnesses rare in industrialized nations but endemic in underdeveloped nations. International agencies are better able to communicate vaccine and drug needs. Finally, an increasing amount of companies are producing vaccines and manufacturing therapeutic drugs in a growing number of nations. India is poised to become one of the world's major suppliers of pharmaceuticals in the next several decades.

Increase in worldwide trade has posed unique challenges for disease prevention. In 1986 CDC investigators began an investigation of rising numbers of certain Asian mosquitoes in the United States. The invasive species served as vectors (transmitters) of disease, causing illnesses such as West Nile and dengue fever. Both illnesses were extremely rare in the United States, typically occurring only in people who traveled abroad. CDC researchers discovered that ports of entry in California, Florida, New York, and Texas all had sizable populations of daytime-biting mosquitoes native to Asia. Cargo ships were identified as the means of transport, especially those ships carrying large box containers or old tires.

To combat invasive species and vectors of disease, there are now more stringent laws governing inspection, decontamination, and quarantine of imported cargo. However, several invasive species have managed to establish substantial populations across the United States. The *Aedes albopictus* mosquito, associated with dengue virus, is found in varying numbers in Hawaii and throughout the southeastern United States. Researchers tracked a sharp increase in the presence of daytime biting mosquitoes to shipments of bamboo plants to California plant nurseries. Immediate control measures such as insecticide application and quarantine and decontamination of other shipments prevented the mosquitoes from establishing large local populations.

Health officials warned nursery workers to use insect repellant and wear covering clothing to minimize the risk of bites. No cases of illness were linked to the event.

PRIMARY SOURCE

CDC Travel Notice: MERS in the Arabian Peninsula

SOURCE: *"MERS in the Arabian Peninsula." Centers for Disease Control and Prevention, June 28, 2017. https://wwwnc.cdc.gov/travel/notices/alert/coronavirus-saudi-arabia-qatar (accessed February 28, 2018).*

INTRODUCTION: *The US Centers for Disease Control and Prevention (CDC) is responsible for issuing travel notices to warn international travelers about health issues they may face in the countries to which they are traveling. The CDC has three levels of notice: Warning Level 3 (Avoid Nonessential Travel), Alert Level 2 (Practice Enhanced Precautions), and Watch Level 1 (Practice Usual Precautions). The following is an Alert Level 2 notice regarding an outbreak of Middle East respiratory syndrome (MERS) in the Arabian Peninsula. The notice describes the outbreak and outlines precautions that travelers should take when visiting the region.*

June 2017

As of June 2017, nearly 2,000 cases of MERS (Middle East Respiratory Syndrome) have been identified in multiple countries in the Arabian Peninsula, including in travelers to the region. In about one-third of the cases, the patients have died. For more information, see CDC's MERS website.

It is not clear how people are exposed to MERS coronavirus, which causes MERS. However, evidence of transmission to humans from direct contact with camels has been steadily increasing. Most instances of person-to-person spread have occurred in healthcare workers and other close contacts (such as family members and caregivers) of people sick with MERS.

CDC does not recommend that travelers change their plans because of MERS. If you are concerned about MERS, you should discuss your travel plans with your doctor.

What is MERS?

MERS is a viral respiratory illness first reported in Saudi Arabia in 2012. The virus that causes MERS is different from any other virus that has been previously found in people. Symptoms of MERS include fever, cough, and shortness of breath. CDC is working with the World Health Organization (WHO) and other partners to understand the public health risks from this virus.

What can travelers do to prevent MERS?

All travelers can take these everyday actions to help prevent the spread of germs and protect against colds, flu, and other illnesses:

- Wash your hands often with soap and water. If soap and water are not available, use an alcohol-based hand sanitizer.
- Avoid touching your eyes, nose, and mouth. Germs spread this way.
- Avoid close contact with sick people.
- Be sure you are up-to-date with all of your shots and, if possible, see your healthcare provider at least 4–6 weeks before travel to get any additional shots.
- Visit CDC's Travelers' Health website for more information on healthy travel.

SEE ALSO *Developing Nations and Drug Delivery; Emerging Infectious Diseases; Reemerging Infectious Diseases; World Trade and Infectious Disease*

BIBLIOGRAPHY

Books

Davies, Sara E., Adam Kamradt-Scott, and Simon Rushton. *Disease Diplomacy: International Norms and Global Health Security.* Baltimore, MD: Johns Hopkins University Press, 2015.

Price-Smith, Andrew T. *Contagion and Chaos: Disease, Ecology, and National Security in the Era of Globalization.* Boston: MIT Press, 2008.

Websites

"Lassa Fever." Centers for Disease Control and Prevention. https://www.cdc.gov/vhf/lassa/pdf/factsheet.pdf (accessed February 27, 2018).

Caryn E. Neumann

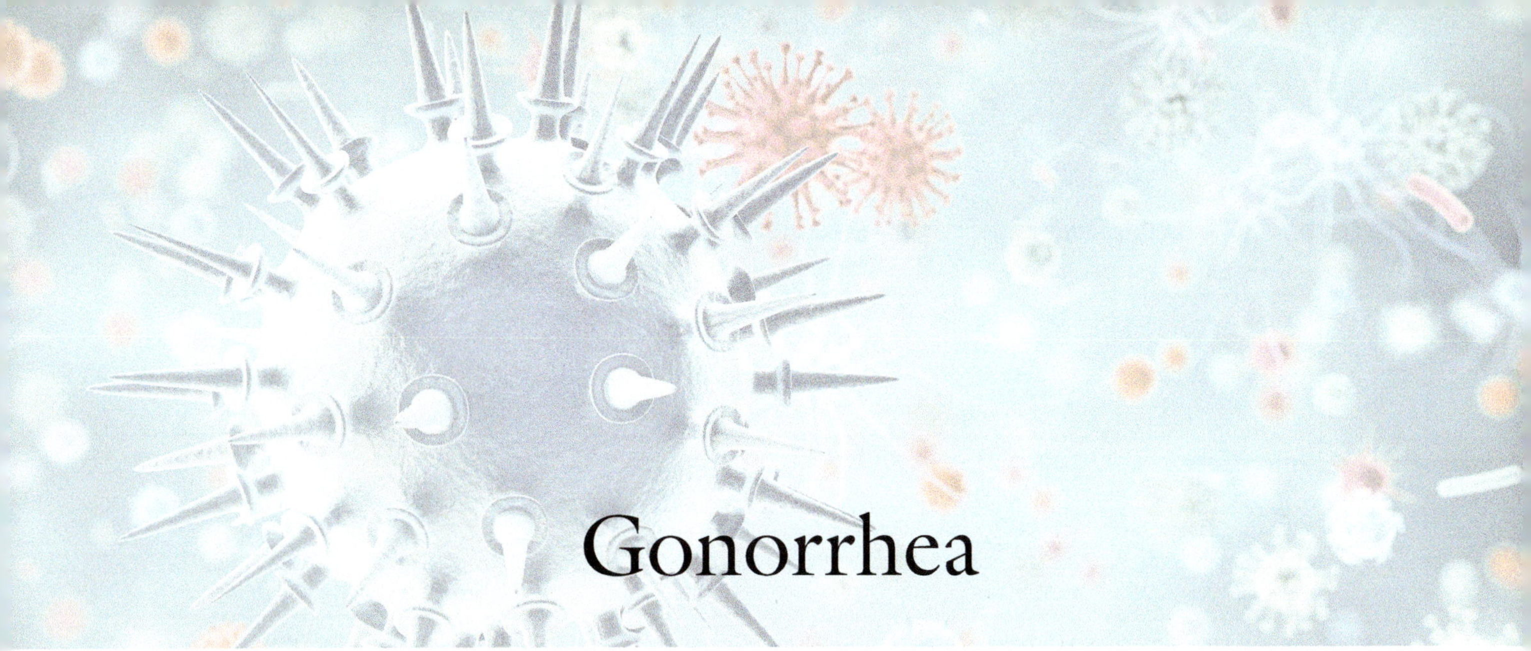

Gonorrhea

Introduction

Gonorrhea is one of the most common sexually transmitted infections (STIs). It is caused by the bacterium *Neisseria gonorrhoeae*, which infects the mucous membranes of the cervix, uterus, and fallopian tubes in women and the urethra in both men and women. *N. gonorrhoeae* is spread by sexual contact or from mother to infant during childbirth. It results in substantial morbidity and economic loss worldwide.

N. gonorrhoeae, sometimes known as gonococcus, is one of two pathogenic species in the *Neisseria* genus. The other, *N. meningitides*, is a leading cause of acute bacterial meningitis, an inflammation of the membranes covering the brain and spinal cord. Gonorrhea is curable, and treatment is important, as the disease can cause serious complications, leading to both female and male infertility. Treatment must extend to the sexual partners of those who are diagnosed with the disease to help control its spread. Certain strains of gonorrhea have become resistant to antibiotics, which is a major emerging threat in combating the disease.

Disease History, Characteristics, and Transmission

The word *gonorrhea* comes from the Greek words *gono* for "seed" and *rhoea*, meaning "flow." The disease was first described in 170 CE by Greek physician and philosopher Galen (c. 129–216). It was thought that the characteristic discharge of gonorrhea in men consisted of semen. The causative agent, *N. gonorrhoeae*, was discovered in 1879 by Albert Neisser (1855–1916), who gave the bacterium its name. This was just one of many important advances during the late 19th and early 20th centuries in the understanding of the causes of venereal diseases (now known as sexually transmitted infections, or STIs). *N. gonorrhoeae* is a round-shaped bacterium that is Gram-negative (a term that describes the way it is stained for microscopic examination).

Infection with *N. gonorrhoeae* causes urethritis (inflammation of the lining of the urethra) among men and cervicitis (inflammation of the cervix) in women. The time of onset of symptoms following infection varies from 1 to 30 days. The first symptom of gonorrhea in both men and women is usually painful urination, followed by a thick, purulent (pus-containing) discharge from the urethra. The

WORDS TO KNOW

ECTOPIC PREGNANCY A complication of pregnancy in which the embryo attaches outside the uterus. Classic signs and symptoms include abdominal pain and vaginal bleeding. Also known as a tubal pregnancy.

GRAM-NEGATIVE BACTERIA Bacteria whose cell walls are composed of an inner and outer membrane that are separated from one another by a region called the periplasm. The periplasm also contains a thin but rigid layer called the peptidoglycan.

PURULENT Any part of the body that contains or releases pus. Pus is a fluid produced by inflamed, infected tissues and is made up of white blood cells, fragments of dead cells, and a liquid containing various proteins.

SEXUALLY TRANSMITTED INFECTION (STI) Infections that vary in their susceptibility to treatment, their signs and symptoms, and the consequences if they are left untreated. Some are caused by bacteria. These usually can be treated and cured. Others are caused by viruses and can typically be treated but not cured.

Percentage of US *Neisseria gonorrhoeae* Isolates with Reduced Ceftriaxone Susceptibility (2000–2014)

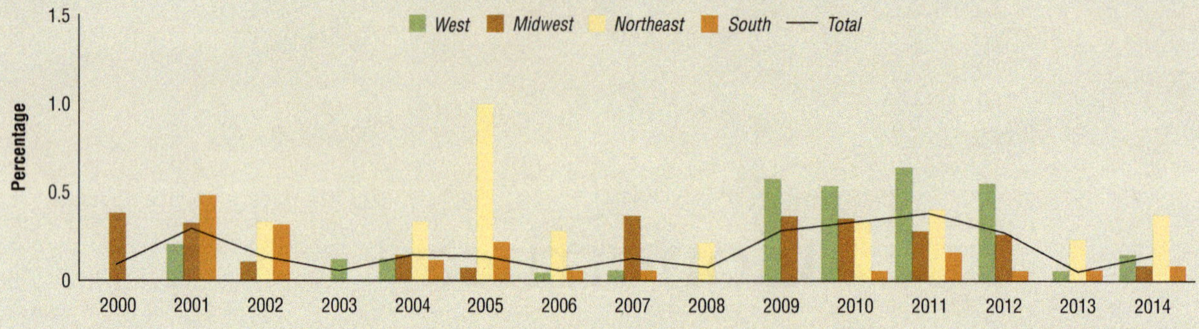

SOURCE: Adapted from "Neisseria Gonorrhoeae Antimicrobial Susceptibility Surveillance—The Gonococcal Isolate Surveillance Project, 27 Sites, United States, 2014." US Centers for Disease Control and Prevention. 2016. Available from: https://www.cdc.gov/mmwr/volumes/65/ss/ss6507a1.htm#F1_down

presence of pus makes the discharge yellow, white, or green, and it may be flecked with blood. In most cases both men and women have no symptoms. Affected men may experience swelling in the testicles. In women there may be vaginal discharge and possible bleeding. Sometimes the symptoms in women are so minor that they are mistaken for a vaginal or urinary infection.

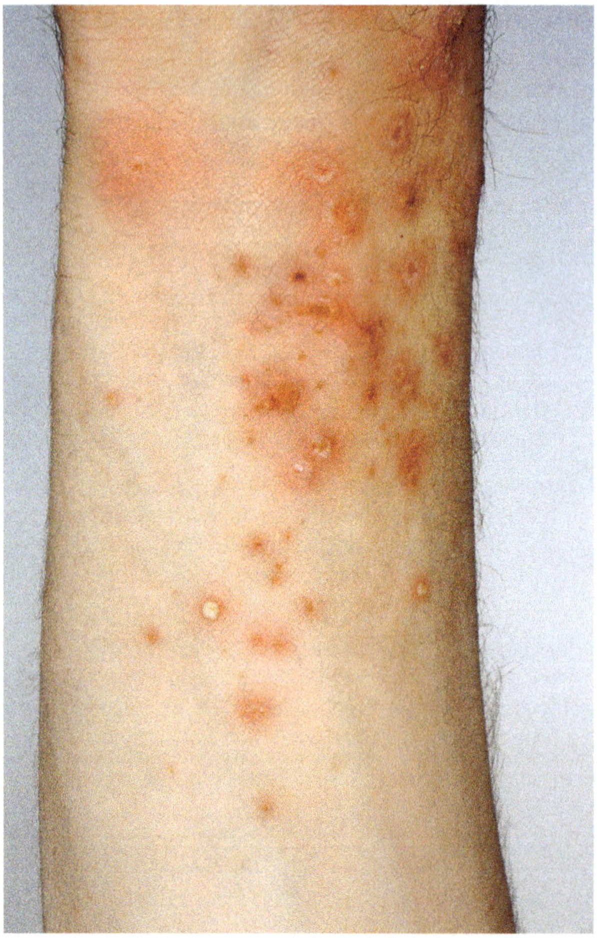

A patient infected with gonorrhea shows the skin abscesses a gonococcal infection can cause. *© Clinical Photography, Central Manchester University Hospitals NHS Foundation Trust, UK/Science Source*

With early intervention and appropriate therapy, such as treatment with the antibiotic cephalosporin, complete cure from the disease is possible. However, late, delayed, or inappropriate therapy may lead to significant morbidity and, on rare occasions, death. Untreated, gonorrhea tends to resolve after several weeks. However, during this time complications may set in, and the person remains infectious. In men the epididymis (coiled tube leading sperm from the testicles) may become inflamed, which can lead to infertility. In around 1 percent of cases, gonorrhea spreads throughout the body and causes severe arthritis and skin lesions. Neonatal gonorrhea contracted during childbirth causes severe conjunctivitis, an inflammation of the conjunctiva (the mucus membrane that lines the inner surface of the eyelid) covering the cornea and may lead to blindness.

Gonococcemia is the presence of *N. gonorrhoeae* bacterium in the bloodstream. It may lead to a condition known as disseminated gonococcal infection (DGI). Severe DGI occurs in approximately 1 percent of genital infections. Symptoms of DGI include rash, fever, arthralgia, migratory polyarthritis, septic arthritis, tendonitis, tenosynovitis, endocarditis, or meningitis and fatal septic shock. Patients who are pregnant or menstruating may be particularly prone to gonococcemia. *N. gonorrhoeae* disperse from a primary site, such as the endocervix, the urethra, the pharynx, or the rectum, and spread to the blood to infect other end organs. Usually multiple sites, such as the skin and the joints, are infected.

Untreated gonorrhea in women can lead to salpingitis, an inflammation of the fallopian tubes. It is also a leading cause of pelvic inflammatory disease (PID), which affects around 1 million women a year in the United States. Symptoms of PID can include severe abdominal pain and fever, and the condition may lead to the development of pus-filled abscesses, long-lasting pelvic pain, and infertility. PID can also scar the fallopian tubes, increasing the risk of ectopic pregnancy. In men *N. gonorrhoeae* commonly leads to uncomplicated infections such as urogenital, anogenital, or pharyngeal infection. Gonorrhea can also spread throughout the body to cause localized and disseminated disease.

Gonorrhea is spread through contact with the anus, mouth, penis, or vagina—typically from various forms of unprotected sexual intercourse. Ejaculation is not necessary for infection to occur. A few "core" transmitters may spread the disease by having unprotected sex with many different partners. Those without symptoms are more likely to spread the disease than those who do have symptoms. As the infection affects the cervix in women, an infected woman can transmit the disease to the fetus during childbirth. Other risk factors of disease include unsafe sex, multiple sex partners, male homosexuality, low socioeconomic status, history of concurrent or past STIs, drug abuse, and early age of onset of sexual activity.

MONITORING TREATMENT

Researchers are increasingly concerned about antimicrobial resistance shown by *Neisseria gonorrhoeae.* The problem presents an important global public health challenge in the struggle to control gonorrhea.

According to data collected between 2009 and 2014 by the World Health Organization's (WHO) Gonococcal Antimicrobial Surveillance Programme, disease-resistant strains were present in 97 percent of countries, with 81 percent reporting growing resistance to azithromycin, highlighting the grim situation in controlling the infection. Furthermore, 66 percent of infections were resistant to cefixime or injectable ceftriaxone. As of 2016 WHO has recommended a treatment regimen of two antibiotics: ceftriaxone and azithromycin.

■ Scope and Distribution

After chlamydia, gonorrhea is the most common sexually transmitted infection in the United States. In 2015 the Centers for Disease Control and Prevention (CDC) recorded 400,000 new cases. Due to underreporting, the true estimate is about 800,000 cases each year. Worldwide, there are around 98 million new cases of gonorrhea every year. Teenagers and young adults between the age of 15 and 24 appear to be most at risk of gonorrhea. It is also more common within lower socioeconomic groups. Gonorrheal infection may also increase the risk of contracting human immunodeficiency virus (HIV) infection.

■ Treatment and Prevention

Penicillin was the first treatment for gonorrhea. Many other antibiotics, including ceftriaxone and ciprofloxacin, are used, but they can only treat the primary infection, not the complications. World Health Organization (WHO) guidelines recommend the combination of a single oral dose of cefixime and azithromycin to minimize the development of drug resistance. It is important that any sexual partners of the infected person are traced and treated to stop the spread of infection. Strains of *N. gonorrhoeae* have become resistant to penicillin and the fluoroquinolone antibiotics in recent years, making the infection harder to treat.

Emergence of drug-resistant infections has been rising, thus limiting the treatment options for gonorrhea. In 2016 the Gonococcal Isolate Surveillance Project (GISP) noted the emergence of bacterium resistant to antibiotics, including azithromycin. The GISP reported that 0.3 percent of the tested isolates in Hawaii show resistance to ceftriaxone and a high level of resistance to azithromycin.

N. gonorrhoeae can be diagnosed by culturing bacterium from clinical samples taken from the patient, such as urine and vaginal swabs, under laboratory conditions. Samples can also be tested using nucleic acid amplification (NAA) tests, which identify gonorrhea-specific DNA. NAA tests are quick and highly sensitive and can be done using a variety of clinical samples. Pregnant women should be tested for gonorrhea and treated to prevent the infection from passing to the baby. Newborns are routinely treated with antibiotic drops such as erythromycin to prevent conjunctivitis, which can result from maternal infections including gonorrhea.

Sexual abstinence or a monogamous sexual relationship with an uninfected partner are the most effective means of preventing the spread of gonorrhea. Condoms, used correctly and consistently, can also help prevent infection. The CDC recommends annual gonorrhea screenings for sexually active men and women in high-risk groups to prevent the spread of the disease in the community. In 2012 WHO initiated a global action plan to reduce antibiotic resistance to *N. gonorrhoeae* infection that includes early detection, effective treatment, fostering patient compliance, and education along with increased surveillance. Vaccines and microbicides against *N. gonorrhoeae* are under development. A 12-year study involving more than 14,730 young people found that a meningitis B vaccine known as MeNZB provided 31 percent protection against contracting gonorrhea.

■ Impacts and Issues

Gonorrhea remains a serious health problem despite public health initiatives that began in the mid-1970s and resulted in declining incidence of the disease. It can inflict long-term complications on the female and, to a lesser extent, male reproductive systems without an individual being aware that he or she is infected. According to a 2016 WHO report, each year an estimated 78 million are reported to have gonorrheal infection globally. There may be no symptoms associated with either the primary infection or the complications, which further complicates early treatment options. According to the CDC, 468,514 cases of gonorrhea were reported in the United States in 2016, an 18.5 percent increase over the prior year. The increase in cases is attributed to a decrease in the use of condoms and inadequate or failed treatment (due to drug resistance). Early diagnosis techniques and newer antibiotics are needed alongside prevention practices to stop the spread of the disease.

Gonorrhea and HIV infection are closely related; those with both conditions are more likely to transmit HIV. People with gonorrhea who are HIV negative are also more likely to become infected with HIV than people without gonorrhea. Without a vaccine against *N. gonorrhoeae*, prevention efforts focused on safer sex practices, regular STI testing, and routine gynecological examination.

SEE ALSO *Antibiotic Resistance; Bacterial Disease; HIV; Meningitis, Bacterial; Sexually Transmitted Infections*

BIBLIOGRAPHY

Books

Wilson, Walter Ray, et al. *Current Diagnosis & Treatment in Infectious Diseases.* New York: McGraw-Hill Professional, 2011.

Periodicals

Dalke, Brian, et al. "Gonorrhea: Treatment and Management Considerations for the Male Patient." *U.S. Pharmacist* 41, no. 8 (2016): 41–44.

Petousis-Harris, Helen, et al. "Effectiveness of a Group B Outer Membrane Vesicle Meningococcal Vaccine against Gonorrhoea in New Zealand: A Retrospective Case-Control Study. *Lancet* 39, no. 10102 (September 20, 2017): 1603–1610. This article can also be found online at http://www.thelancet.com/journals/lancet/article/PIIS0140-6736(17)31449-6/fulltext?elsca1=tlpr (accessed January 31, 2018).

Workowski, K. A., and Bolan, G. A. "Sexually Transmitted Diseases Treatment Guidelines, 2015." *Morbidity and Mortality Weekly Report* 64, no 3 (June 5, 2015): 1–137. This article can also be found online at https://www.cdc.gov/std/tg2015/default.htm (accessed January 28, 2017).

Websites

"Diagnosis and Management of Gonococcemia: Differential Diagnoses." Medscape, 2010. https://www.medscape.org/viewarticle/724973 (accessed January 21, 2017).

"Fact Sheet: Gonorrhea." Centers for Disease Control and Prevention (CDC), June 2017. https://www.cdc.gov/std/gonorrhea/Gonorrhea-FS-June-2017.pdf (accessed January 21, 2017).

"Gonococcal Isolate Surveillance Project (GISP) Supplement & Profiles." Centers for Disease Control and Prevention (CDC), Division of STD Prevention, February 2016. https://www.cdc.gov/std/gisp2014/gisp-2014-text-fig-tables.pdf (accessed January 21, 2017).

Lo, Bruce M. "Emergent Management of Gonorrhea." Medscape, March 24, 2016. https://emedicine.medscape.com/article/782913-overview#a1 (accessed January 21, 2017).

"Sexually Transmitted Infections (STIs)." World Health Organization, August 2016. http://www.who.int/mediacentre/factsheets/fs110/en/ (accessed January 31, 2018).

"WHO: Antibiotic-Resistant Gonorrhoea on the Rise, New Drugs Needed." World Health Organization, July 7, 2017. http://www.who.int/mediacentre/news/releases/2017/Antibiotic-resistant-gonorrhoea/en/ (accessed February 5, 2018).

"WHO Guidelines for the Treatment of *Neisseria gonorrhoeae*, 2016." World Health Organization. http://apps.who.int/iris/bitstream/10665/246114/1/9789241549691-eng.pdf?ua=1 (accessed January 21, 2017).

Susan Aldridge
Kausalya Santhanam

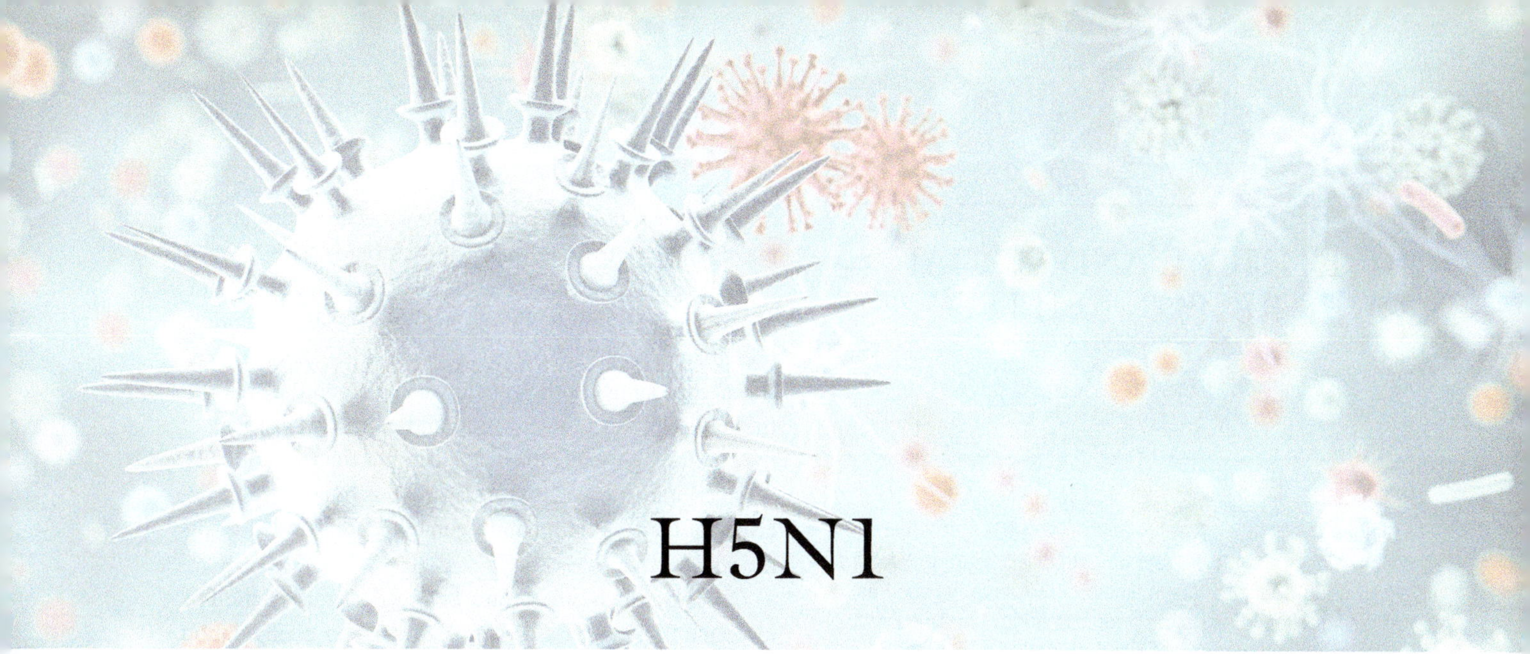

H5N1

■ Introduction

The H5N1 virus is classified as an influenza A virus. This type of virus is normally found in avian species (birds) and is both highly contagious and highly lethal to bird populations ranging from wild migrating birds to chickens on commercial poultry farms.

The disease has spread to some humans. According to the World Health Organization (WHO), the influenza in humans resulting from H5N1 infection is highly lethal, with a mortality rate of 60 percent, although some outbreaks have had higher rates. Between 2003 and 2018, there were 860 cases of H5N1 reported and 454 deaths.

As of 2017 H5N1 was not easily transmissible to humans. Most of the cases of human infection with H5N1 involved infections resulting from close contact with infected bird populations—for example, situations in which people lived in proximity to infected birds (mostly poultry), handled infected birds, or had contact with H5N1-contaminated surfaces. Globally, epidemiologists had documented only a few cases of human-to-human transmission of H5N1, and all of the documented cases involved close contact (e.g., a family member caring for an infected relative, etc.).

■ History and Scientific Foundations

Genetic testing of the H5N1 flu virus shows it to be a highly mutable virus. The virus has been documented to infect pigs, which serve as a host for flu viruses that historically mutate easily into a form that can infect humans. Accordingly, WHO has made the study and containment of H5N1 and other avian flu viruses originating in Asia a top priority. WHO officials fear a potentially devastating global pandemic if H5N1 is able to mutate into a form easier to transmit to humans or a form easier for humans to transmit to other humans.

WORDS TO KNOW

ANTIVIRAL DRUGS Compounds that are used to prevent or treat viral infections, via the disruption of an infectious mechanism used by the virus, or to treat the symptoms of an infection.

CELL MEMBRANE The cell is bound by an outer membrane that, as described by a membrane model termed the fluid mosaic model, is composed of a phospholipid lipid bilayer with proteins—molecules that also act as receptor sites—interspersed within the phospholipid bilayer. Varieties of channels exist within the membrane. In eukaryotes (cells with a true nucleus) there are a number of internal cellular membranes that can partition regions within the cells' interior. Some of these membranes ultimately become continuous with the nuclear membrane. Bacteria and viruses do not have inner membranes.

EPIDEMIOLOGIST One who studies the various factors that influence the occurrence, distribution, prevention, and control of disease, injury, and other health-related events in a defined human population. By the application of various analytical techniques, including mathematical analysis of the data, the probable cause of an infectious outbreak can be pinpointed.

GLYCOPROTEIN A protein that contains a short chain of sugar as part of its structure.

HEMAGGLUTININ Often abbreviated as HA, hemagglutinin is a glycoprotein.

MUTABLE VIRUS A virus whose DNA changes rapidly so that drugs and vaccines against it may not be effective.

NEURAMINIDASE Also abbreviated (NA), neuraminidase is a glycoprotein.

ETHICAL AND SOCIAL RESPONSIBILITY

As of 2017 the H5N1 virus was easy to avoid among most populations. However, people who work closely with poultry, especially poultry in countries where H5N1 is endemic, are at risk for developing the disease.

The World Health Organization (WHO) states that, "for avian influenza viruses, the primary risk factor for human infection appears to be direct or indirect exposure to infected live or dead poultry or contaminated environments, such as live bird markets. Slaughtering, defeathering, handling carcasses of infected poultry, and preparing poultry for consumption, especially in household settings, are also likely to be risk factors." WHO also states that contracting H5N1 from eating infected poultry products, such as eggs or meat, is low if they are properly cooked, as high temperatures kill the virus. For this reason, "rare" meat and eggs with "runny" yokes are to be avoided. Although freezing some meats will kill viruses, H5N1 will not be destroyed when frozen.

The avian flu viruses attack human cells by first attaching themselves to the outer cell membrane with pointed probe-like hemagglutin molecules that are capable of binding to specific sites on the cell membrane. Hemagglutinin (designated as HA) and neuraminidase (designated as NA) are glycoproteins. Both protrude from the outer surface of the influenza virus, and neuraminidase is a constituent of the enveloping membrane that surrounds the viral contents. A typical influenza virus particle contains hundreds of molecules of hemagglutinin and neuraminidase studded across the viral surface.

Because the binding must be specific—that is, the HA molecule must be of a certain structure and configuration to bind to the membrane receptor sites—the vast majority of viruses that infect birds are not capable of binding to human cell membranes. Small and subtle changes, driven by the process of mutation, in either the protein structure or protein configuration (the protein's shape in three-dimensional space) can, however, permit binding to human cell membranes. This allows the virus to infect the human cell and make the jump from birds to humans.

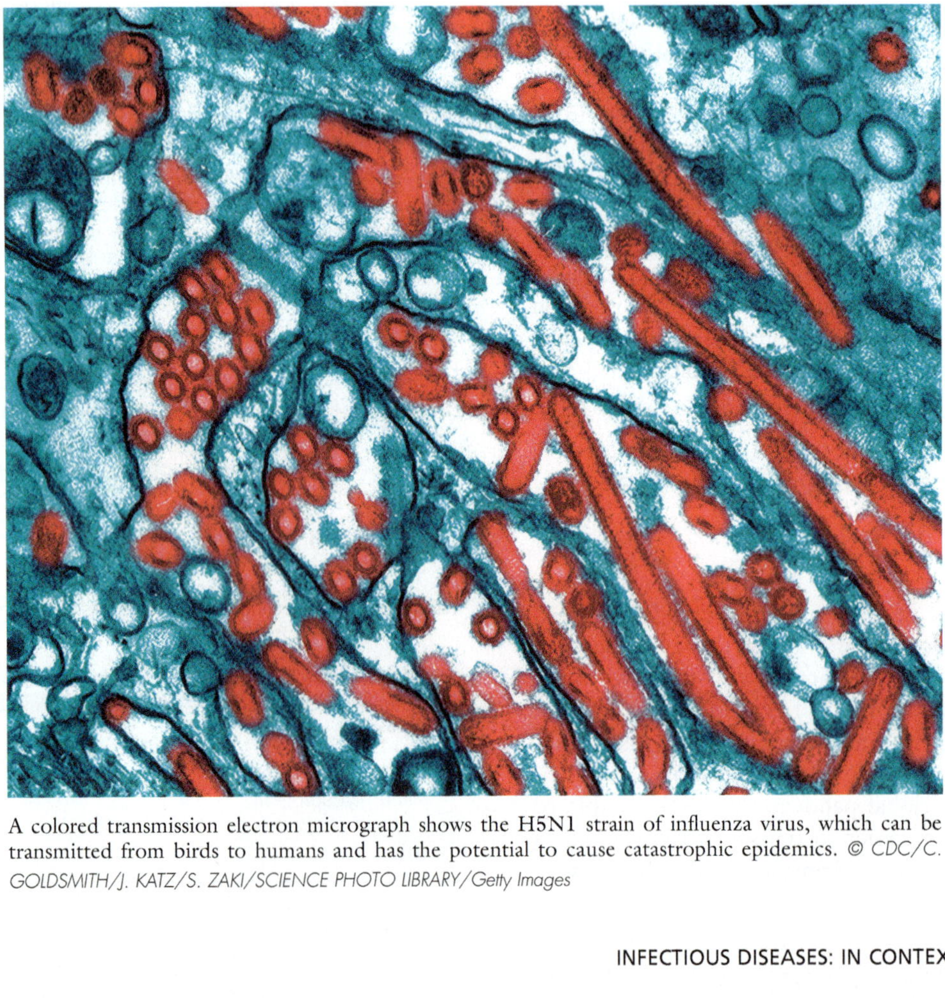

A colored transmission electron micrograph shows the H5N1 strain of influenza virus, which can be transmitted from birds to humans and has the potential to cause catastrophic epidemics. *© CDC/C. GOLDSMITH/J. KATZ/S. ZAKI/SCIENCE PHOTO LIBRARY/Getty Images*

■ Applications and Research

Researchers and health officials are optimistic about containing the current outbreaks of flu. However, scientists remain vigilant—and public health officials remain concerned—because the changes required to make the jump to humans also occurred in the viruses responsible for global outbreaks of influenza in 1957 and 1968. There is also concern that the transmission mode of the virus will change and become easier to transmit, thus increasing the likelihood of a global pandemic. Because of these concerns, WHO operates the Global Influenza Surveillance and Response System to monitor H5N1 and other avian influenzas.

In 2012 two groups of scientists working separately were able to mutate the virus so that it could be transmitted through the air between ferrets. The research showed that it would be simple for the virus to evolve on its own and become transmittable through the air among humans.

■ Impacts and Issues

Biologically, there is little that can be done to stop the virus from spreading and mutating, except to reduce its host environment. Governments of countries where the disease is endemic in bird populations (Bangladesh, China, Egypt, India, Indonesia, and Vietnam) have often ordered the wholesale slaughter of sick, potentially infected, and exposed birds as a response to avian flu outbreaks (the disease H5N1 causes in avian populations).

Millions of chickens, for example, have been culled to attempt to inhibit the spread to other flocks as governments imposed prompt and sometimes severe quarantine restrictions. In other countries chickens have been given vaccines (some with questionable effectiveness) against the disease in an attempt to minimize the potentially overwhelming negative economic impacts of H5N1 on commercial bird species.

The specific H5N1 virus linked to human deaths is especially dangerous because it is resistant to both amantadine and rimantadine, two commonly used antiviral drugs used to treat influenza. Other antiviral medications, oseltamavir (Tamiflu®) and zanamavir, have shown effectiveness in reducing mortality. As of 2017 no vaccine against H5N1 was yet formally approved for use in humans.

See Also *Avian Influenza; Developing Nations and Drug Delivery; Emerging Infectious Diseases; Influenza; Influenza, Tracking Seasonal Influences and Virus Mutation; Influenza Pandemic of 1918; Notifiable Diseases; Pandemic Preparedness; Vaccines and Vaccine Development*

BIBLIOGRAPHY

Books

Bennett, John E., Raphael Dolin, and Martin J. Blaser. *Mandell, Douglas, and Bennett's Principles and Practice of Infectious Diseases.* 8th ed. Philadelphia: Elsevier/Saunders, 2015.

Periodicals

Herfst, Sander, et al. "Airborne Transmission of Influenza A/H5N1 Virus between Ferrets." *Science* 336, no. 6088 (June 22, 2012): 1534–1541. This article can also be found online at http://science.sciencemag.org/content/336/6088/1534.full (accessed February 22, 2018).

Russell, Colin A., et al. "The Potential for Respiratory Droplet–Transmissible A/H5N1 Influenza Virus to Evolve in a Mammalian Host." *Science* 336, no. 6088 (June 22, 2012): 1541–1547. This article can also be found online at http://science.sciencemag.org/content/336/6088/1541 (accessed February 22, 2018).

Websites

"Cumulative Number of Confirmed Human Cases for Avian Influenza A(H5n1) Reported to WHO, 2003–2018." World Health Organization, January 25, 2018. http://www.who.int/influenza/human_animal_interface/2018_01_25_tableH5N1.pdf?ua=1 (accessed February 22, 2018).

"Highly Pathogenic Asian Avian Influenza A (H5N1) Virus." Centers for Disease Control and Prevention, October 14, 2015. https://www.cdc.gov/flu/avianflu/h5n1-virus.htm (accessed February 22, 2018).

"Influenza (Avian and Other Zoonotic)." World Health Organization, January 2018. http://www.who.int/mediacentre/factsheets/avian_influenza/en/ (accessed February 22, 2018).

Paul Davis
Claire Skinner

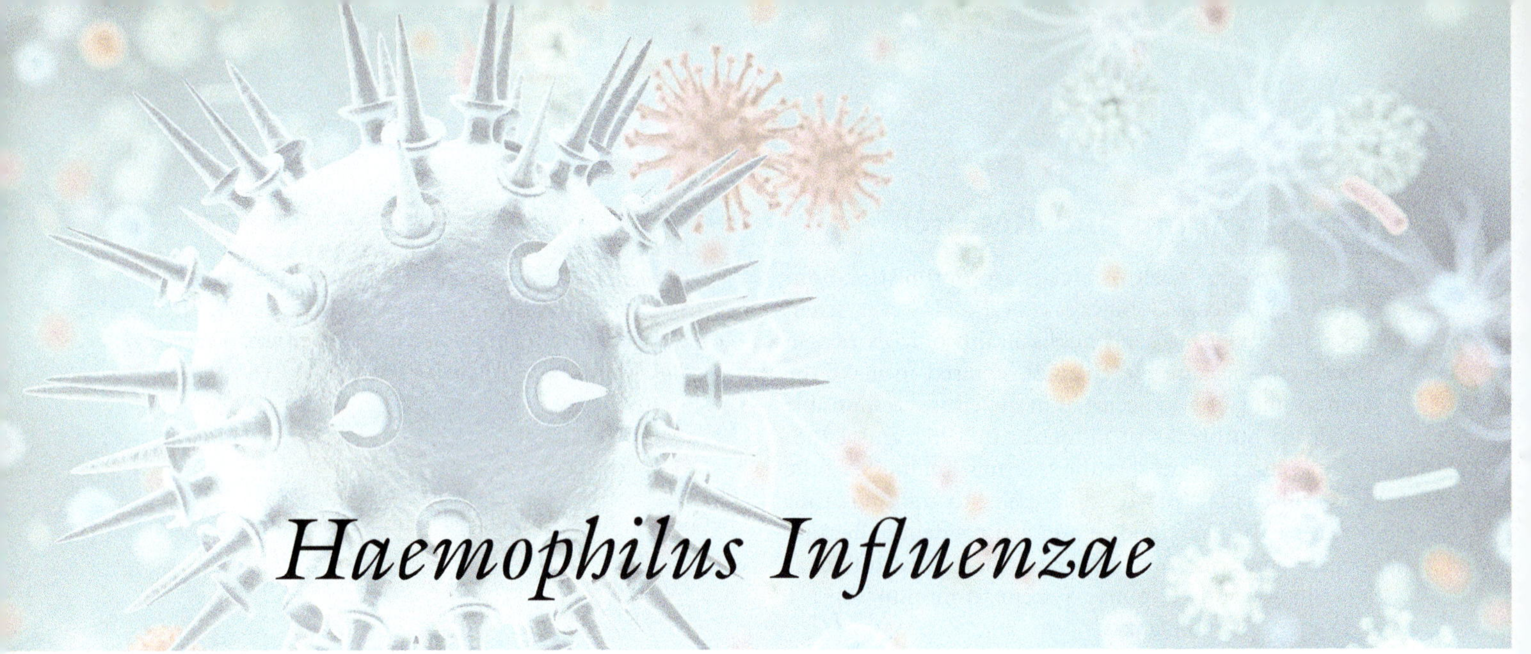

Haemophilus Influenzae

Introduction

Haemophilus influenzae is a bacterium that can cause upper respiratory disease mainly in young children. *H. influenzae* type b, or Hib, is one of the main causes for meningitis. Meningitis can also be caused by viral infections, injuries, cancer, and some drugs.

H. influenzae are gram-negative, which means their cell walls consist of two membranes on either side of a thin but strong layer, the peptidoglycan. The bacteria are pleomorphic, meaning they can be shaped like ovals or can adopt different shapes. When grown on a solid nutrient, clumps of bacteria tend to form in the vicinity of another bacterium called *Staphylococcus* when the latter are present. This behavior can be important in identifying *H. influenzae.*

While vaccination against Hib has reduced the occurrence of infections in developed countries, *H. influenzae* remains responsible for many lower respiratory infections in children in other regions of the world. According to statistics from the World Health Organization (WHO), in 2000, prior to the vaccine's introduction in developing nations, Hib was responsible for at least 8 million illnesses and 371,000 deaths of children under age four years. In 2008, in 136 countries using the vaccine, an estimated 203,000 children under age five died. In the United States the death rate in children under age five following introduction of the vaccine dropped from about 1,000 a year to fewer than 40 children in 2013, 49 in 2014, and 41 in 2015, according to the US Centers for Disease Control and Prevention (CDC).

WORDS TO KNOW

DROPLET A drop of water or other fluid that is fewer than 5 microns (a millionth of a meter) in diameter.

GRAM-NEGATIVE BACTERIA Bacteria whose cell wall is composed of an inner and outer membrane that are separated from one another by the periplasm region. The periplasm also contains a thin but rigid layer, the peptidoglycan.

PATHOGENIC Causing or capable of causing disease.

STRAIN A subclass or a specific genetic variation of an organism.

Disease History, Characteristics, and Transmission

H. influenzae was first described by Richard Friedrich Johannes Pfeiffer (1858–1945) in 1892 during an influenza epidemic. The name for the bacterium reflects an early misunderstanding that it was the cause of the flu. In 1933 scientists demonstrated that influenza was instead caused by a virus. *H. influenzae*, however, was subsequently shown to be the cause of several other diseases.

Some types (strains) of *H. influenzae* are surrounded by a sugary coat, or capsule, while other strains do not have a capsule. The strains with a capsule tend to be more of a health concern because the capsule helps protect a bacterium from attack by a host's immune system. Nonetheless, some strains without a capsule are also pathogenic and can cause bronchitis, ear infections, and epiglottitis, an inflammation in the esophagus. Complications of epiglottis can produce a blockage of the airway that can be fatal in children under the age of five.

H. influenzae is normally found in the throat and nose of many people. The bacteria residing there are usually harmless. However, if the bacteria spreads to other areas of the body, or if a person's immune system is compromised the bacteria can cause infection. Thus, *H. influenzae* is an opportunistic pathogen.

Only humans are known to be susceptible to *H. influenzae* infections. This has complicated research on the mechanisms of infection and vaccine development, as animal models of the disease cannot be established.

H. influenzae can be spread from person to person in the droplets that are expelled when someone coughs or sneezes. The infection is usually caused by types of the bacterium that have a capsule. The capsule makes *H. influenzae* harder to kill in the body. The resulting lung infection often affects young children because their immune system may not be fully developed yet. More seriously, the bacteria can infect the blood and spread. Joints can be affected, producing arthritis. The heart infection pericarditis can occur. *H. influenzae* infections may also attack the lining of nerves such as those in the brain. The resulting inflammation is a form of bacterial meningitis, an infection of the covering (membrane) around the spinal cord and brain. Bacterial meningitis is a potentially life-threatening complication. Stiffness in the neck accompanied by flu-like symptoms can be an early indication of bacterial meningitis.

Hib infections were previously a much more common and dangerous threat. The availability of infant- and childhood-based vaccines against Hib—and their widespread use beginning in the late 1990s, which are typically included in the series of vaccinations many children receive during their first decade of life—has reduced the prevalence of Hib meningitis dramatically. In the United States CDC data showed that the incidence of Hib infections in children under five years old has dropped from 40 to 100 children per 100,000 in the 1990s to about 2 of every 100,000 children from 2006 to 2015 (the last year statistics were kept). In 2015 only one death occurred in this age group. Globally, data are harder to come by. In 2008, according to the latest data from WHO, about 200,000 deaths of children under age five were due to *H. influenza*. The risk of infection is higher throughout Africa.

DISEASE IN DEVELOPING NATIONS

The World Health Organization (WHO) states that "*Haemophilus influenzae* type b (Hib) has been shown to be an important cause of childhood meningitis and a major cause of bacterial pneumonia in children. Although little population-based incidence data are available from most of Asia and the Newly Independent States, Hib is estimated to cause at least 3 million cases of serious disease and hundreds of thousands of deaths annually, worldwide. The most important manifestations of Hib disease, namely pneumonia and meningitis, are seen mainly in children under 5 years of age, particularly infants."

■ Scope and Distribution

H. influenzae is worldwide in distribution. Most affected are children who are in close contact with one

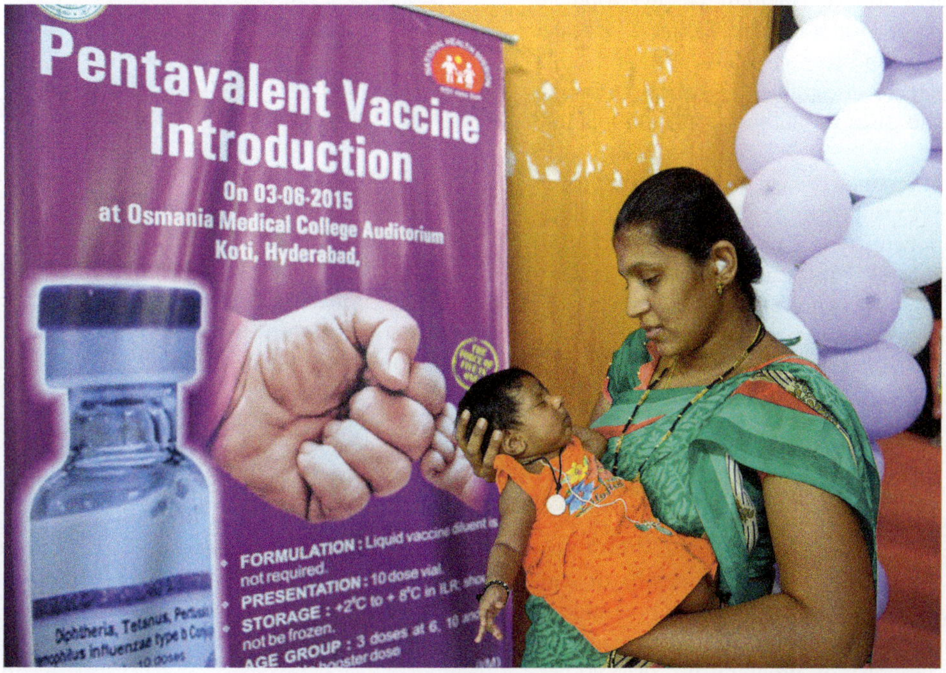

A mother and child in Hyderabad, India, await vaccination for a range of illnesses, including *Haemophilus influenzae* type B (Hib). Vaccinations against Hib have helped to dramatically reduce the prevalence of Hib-related deaths among children since the 1990s. © NOAH SEELAM/AFP/Getty Images

another. There is no indication that girls, boys, or members of any racial group are more susceptible to infection.

H. influenzae pneumonia and meningitis are greater problems in developing countries. Agencies including the CDC and WHO assist countries in determining the prevalence and geographical distribution of infections, which helps assist infection control programs. Infection control strategies include vaccination and avoiding close contact with someone who is coughing or sneezing due to illness (because the bacterium is spread through the air). Vaccination efforts involving WHO, the Global Alliance for Vaccines and Immunization (GAVI), and local agencies in more than 100 countries in Africa, Asia, and South America has resulted in the incorporation of *H. influenzae* vaccination in the routine vaccination schedule in these countries.

Treatment and Prevention

H. influenzae can be treated by a number of different antibiotics, although there have been reports of antibiotic resistance. In Canada antibiotic-resistant *H. influenzae* was present in about 45 percent of infections between 2007 and 2014. Studies conducted in the last 10 years from Poland, China, Thailand, and the United Kingdom have revealed similar rates, with about half of *H. influenzae* infections (including both pneumonia and meningitis) being antibiotic resistant.

Hib pneumonia and meningitis are preventable. Vaccination in a series of inoculations, which can begin as early as six months of age, protects children. The development and widespread use of Hib conjugate vaccines—vaccines that provide combined protection against Hib and other diseases that children are susceptible to—have been invaluable in reducing the cases of childhood pneumonia and meningitis.

Conjugate Hib vaccines contain a purified component of the outer layer (capsule) of the Hib bacterium along with purified components of one or more bacteria or virus that causes other diseases. Hib vaccination is done in combination with the diphtheria/tetanus/pertussis vaccine and with the vaccine for hepatitis C virus.

Impacts and Issues

Despite the overwhelming success of Hib vaccines in combating meningitis, *H. influenzae* continues to be a problem in developing countries. In 2012 WHO estimated that Hib caused about 200,000 deaths of children under five years of age, mainly due to pneumonia.

In 2007 the vaccination rate for the approximately 90 countries with Hib vaccination programs was over 90 percent, while the rate in developing regions such as sub-Saharan Africa was less than 10 percent. This situation is changing with the aid of organizations like GAVI. By 2009 GAVI support had helped begin vaccination programs in 62 developing nations. By 2014 all 73 nations that had been targeted had introduced Hib vaccination.

SEE ALSO *Bacterial Disease; Childhood Infectious Diseases, Immunization Impacts; Developing Nations and Drug Delivery; Meningitis, Bacterial*

BIBLIOGRAPHY

Books

Artenstein, Andrew W. *In the Blink of an Eye: The Deadly Story of Epidemic Meningitis.* New York: Springer, 2012.

Wadman, Meredith. *The Vaccine Race: Science, Politics, and the Human Costs of Defeating Disease.* New York: Viking, 2017.

Periodicals

Townsend-Payne, Kelly, et al. "Children with *Haemophilus Influenzae* Type B (Hib) Vaccine Failure Have Long-Term Bactericidal Antibodies against Virulent Hib Strains with Multiple Capsular Loci." *Vaccine* 34 (July 2016): 3931–3934

Whittaker, Robert, et al. "Epidemiology of Invasive *Haemophilus influenza* Disease, Europe, 2007–2014." *Emerging and Infectious Disease* 23 (March 2017): 396–404.

Websites

Buensalido, Joseph Adrian L. "Haemophilus Influenzae Infections Treatment & Management." Medscape. Last modified November 29, 2017. https://emedicine.medscape.com/article/218271-treatment (accessed November 17, 2017).

"*Haemophilus Influenzae* Disease (Including Hib)." Centers for Disease Control and Prevention (CDC). https://www.cdc.gov/hi-disease/index.html (accessed November 17, 2017).

"Haemophilus Influenza Type B (Hib)." World Health Organization. http://www.who.int/immunization/diseases/hib/en/ (accessed November 17, 2017).

"Hib Initiative: A GAVI Success Story." Global Alliance for Vaccines and Immunization. http://www.gavi.org/library/news/roi/2010/hib-initiative--a-gavi-success-story/ (accessed November 17, 2017).

Brian Hoyle

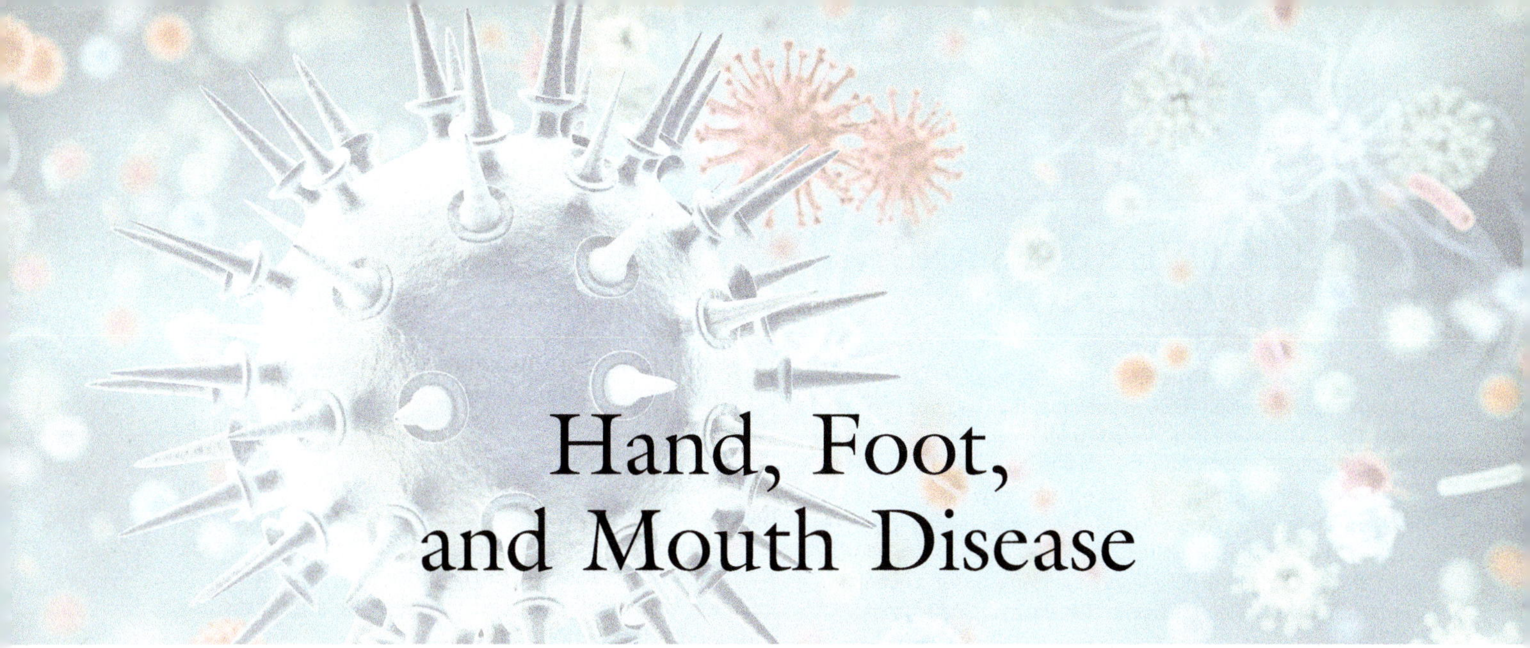

Hand, Foot, and Mouth Disease

■ Introduction

Hand, foot, and mouth disease (HFMD) is a mild, self-limiting disease caused by the enterovirus family of viruses. HFMD usually affects infants and children under the age of 10. It is endemic around the world with periodic outbreaks. Symptoms include fever, nausea, ulcers in the mouth, and sores on the hands and feet. Infected individuals generally recover within two weeks, and complications are rare. The disease is considered contagious and spreads through contact with fluids from infected persons.

Although there is no treatment for the disease and no formal preventive measures, most people with HFMD recover without any complications. However, more severe strains of enteroviruses have emerged, causing potentially fatal diseases and highlighting the need to monitor HFMD.

HFMD is not to be confused with foot-and-mouth disease, which is an unrelated disease that only affects cattle, sheep, and swine.

■ Disease History, Characteristics, and Transmission

HFMD was first diagnosed during an outbreak in Canada in 1957, but the name was not assigned until 1960 when Birmingham, England, suffered a similar outbreak. Individual cases of HFMD occur worldwide, with peak occurrence typically in late summer and early fall.

The disease, most common in children, results from infection by a group of enteroviruses, namely coxsackievirus A16. More severe forms of infection have appeared because of human enterovirus-71, which has caused epidemics with fatalities from HFMD-associated meningitis or encephalitis in countries such as Japan, Taiwan, Singapore, Malaysia, and Indonesia.

The onset of disease symptoms is usually three to seven days, after which children will suffer from a mild fever, loss of appetite, nausea, abdominal cramping, and a sore throat. After one to two days, the fever will heighten. In addition, painful sores will develop on the tongue, gums, and cheeks; these begin as small dots but quickly blister and ulcerate. At this point patients will usually also display a rash affecting the palms of hands, soles of feet, and often the buttocks.

WORDS TO KNOW

ANTIGEN A substance, usually a protein or polysaccharide, that stimulates the immune system to produce antibodies. While antigens can be the source of infections from pathogenic bacteria and viruses, organic molecules detrimental to the body from internal or environmental sources also act as antigens.

COHORT A group of people (or any species) sharing a common characteristic. Cohorts are identified and grouped in cohort studies to determine the frequency of diseases or the kinds of disease outcomes over time.

ENTEROVIRUS A group of viruses that contain ribonucleic acid as their genetic material. They are members of the picornavirus family. The various types of enteroviruses that infect humans are referred to as serotypes, in recognition of their different antigenic patterns. The different immune response is important, as infection with one type of enterovirus does not necessarily confer protection to infection by a different type of enterovirus. There are 64 different enterovirus serotypes. The serotypes include polio viruses, coxsackie A and B viruses, echoviruses and a large number of what are referred to as non-polio enteroviruses.

EFFECTIVE RULES AND REGULATIONS

Regarding public health concerns, the Centers for Disease Control and Prevention (CDC) states that the CDC has "no specific recommendations regarding the exclusion of children with HFMD from child care programs, schools, or other group settings. Children are often excluded from group settings during the first few days of the illness, which may reduce the spread of infection, but will not completely interrupt it. Exclusion of ill persons may not prevent additional cases since the virus may be excreted for weeks after the symptoms have disappeared. Also, some persons excreting the virus, including most adults, may have no symptoms. Some benefit may be gained, however, by excluding children who have blisters in their mouths and drool or who have weeping lesions on their hands."

HFMD is considered moderately to highly contagious during the first week of infection and can be transmitted through contact with nose and throat discharge, blister fluids, and stools of those affected. There is no evidence of transmission from mother to infant during pregnancy, but mothers infected just prior to delivery may pass the virus on to the newborn baby. The risk of severe infection among babies is highest during the first two weeks of life.

■ Scope and Distribution

The people most commonly infected with HFMD are infants and children under the age of 10, although some cases may occur in adults. Children are the most susceptible to the disease because of their lack of previous exposure to the antigens and their consequent lack of inbuilt immune defense.

The development of outbreaks and epidemics of this infection is rapid among cohorted children attending childcare facilities and schools because of the high degree of physical contact and child interaction aiding transmission. The ratio of boys affected to girls is 1:1, and there does not appear to be a higher susceptibility to infection among certain races or ethnic groups.

Both individual cases and outbreaks of HFMD occur worldwide, with no regions demonstrating a higher predisposition to the disease caused by infection with the coxsackievirus. However, HFMD presents two different disease states depending on the specific enterovirus-causing infection and demonstrates a varied distribution.

The more severe illness, which is caused by the human enterovirus-71, presented in the first outbreak in Singapore in 1970, then occurred in Malaysia in 1997, in Taiwan in 1998, again in Singapore and Malaysia in 2000, and in Malaysia in 2003. As an example of the scope of this disease, 1.5 million people were reportedly affected during the outbreak in Taiwan, which included 78 child fatalities. In nearly all the above-mentioned outbreaks, fatalities resulted from infections leading to viral meningitis or encephalitis. The mortality rates and chances of complication were higher in later epidemics than those previous, which raised much concern among health care facilities in these countries.

Despite the fatalities resulting from outbreaks associated with this disease, HFMD caused by coxsackievirus infection is generally still considered to be a mild disease with global distribution.

■ Treatment and Prevention

HFMD is caused by a viral infection, and there is no specific treatment for it. The infection is self-limiting, which means it has a known usual timeline of duration and is followed by resolution on its own accord. Patients usually recover once the virus has run its course, most often within 10 days. The most common complication of HFMD is dehydration due to the pain experienced when swallowing. As such, it is important for patients to maintain adequate fluid intake during the course of the illness. Medication may also be administered to manage symptoms, such as nonsteroidal anti-inflammatory medication for pain and fever.

There is no vaccination or formal prevention available for HFMD, but transmission may be minimized by hygiene practices such as cleaning contaminated surfaces and preventing the sharing of utensils. It is also important to limit the exposure of those infected, so infected children should avoid group environments until sores have healed and the fever has subsided.

In cases of disease with a strong potential for outbreak, prevention must be maintained at both the individual and societal levels. Health ministries in Singapore have been made aware of the possible severity of enterovirus infection and have made laws requiring childcare centers and general practitioners to report any suspected outbreaks of HFMD. This creates a heightened awareness among the community of the possibility of infection and increases the chances of preventing an epidemic.

■ Impacts and Issues

One important feature of HFMD is the speed and ease with which it can be transmitted. In addition to the weeklong incubation period, during which infected persons display no symptoms, the virus may remain present in the saliva for up to 10 days and in the stool for months. This combination means that children may be contagious for months, even if symptoms have been displayed only for a short time, making implementation of successful prevention strategies difficult.

Once a person has had HFMD, he or she will no longer be susceptible to infection from that particular strain of enterovirus. However, the person will remain susceptible to infection from other enteroviruses, which means a previous infection does not indicate complete immunity. Studies into outbreaks of HFMD involving human enterovirus-71 have suggested that previous infection by other enteroviruses, including coxsackievirus A16, may cause increased sensitivity to the disease, as well as increased severity.

Although generally HFMD enterovirus infection is mild and self-limiting, there has been an emergence of more critical forms of the disease. The high number of fatalities among later outbreaks suggests that certain strains of infection are gaining virulence, while populations remain defenseless against them. Discrepancies exist among symptoms and presentation of symptoms in people with HFMD in epidemics involving fatalities. Some patients display the usual symptoms of HFMD before experiencing further complications, while others display no signs at all. The onset of complicating viral meningitis, encephalitis, or endocarditis following enterovirus infection is rapid, which further limits the treatment opportunities for people affected with these strains of enterovirus.

See Also *Childhood-Associated Infectious Diseases, Immunization Impacts; Contact Precautions; Emerging Infectious Diseases; Handwashing; Microbial Evolution; Notifiable Diseases; Polio (Poliomyelitis); Viral Disease*

BIBLIOGRAPHY

Books

Bennett, John E., Raphael Dolin, and Martin J. Blaser. *Mandell, Douglas, and Bennett's Infectious Disease Essentials.* Philadelphia: Elsevier, 2016.

Bennett, John E., Raphael Dolin, and Martin J. Blaser. *Mandell, Douglas, and Bennett's Principles and Practice of Infectious Diseases.* 8th ed. Philadelphia: Elsevier, 2014.

Murray, Patrick R., Ken S. Rosenthal, and Michael A. Pfaller. *Medical Microbiology.* Philadelphia: Elsevier, 2015.

Wilson, Walter R., and Merle A. Sande. *Current Diagnosis and Treatment in Infectious Diseases.* New York: McGraw-Hill, 2014.

Periodicals

Phutthichayanon, Thanyada, and Surapol Naowarat. "Effects of Hand Washing Campaign on Dynamical Model of Hand Foot Mouth Disease." *International Journal of Modeling and Optimization* 5, no. 2 (2015): 104–108.

Slomski, Anita. "Vaccines for Enterovirus 71." *JAMA* 311, no. 16 (2014): 1602.

Wong, K. T. "Enterovirus Encephalitis Including Enterovirus 71 and D68." *International Journal of Infectious Diseases* 45 (2016): 25.

Websites

"Hand, Foot, and Mouth Disease." Centers for Disease Control and Prevention, January 6, 2017 https://www.cdc.gov/hand-foot-mouth/index.html (accessed December 8, 2017).

Laura J. Cataldo

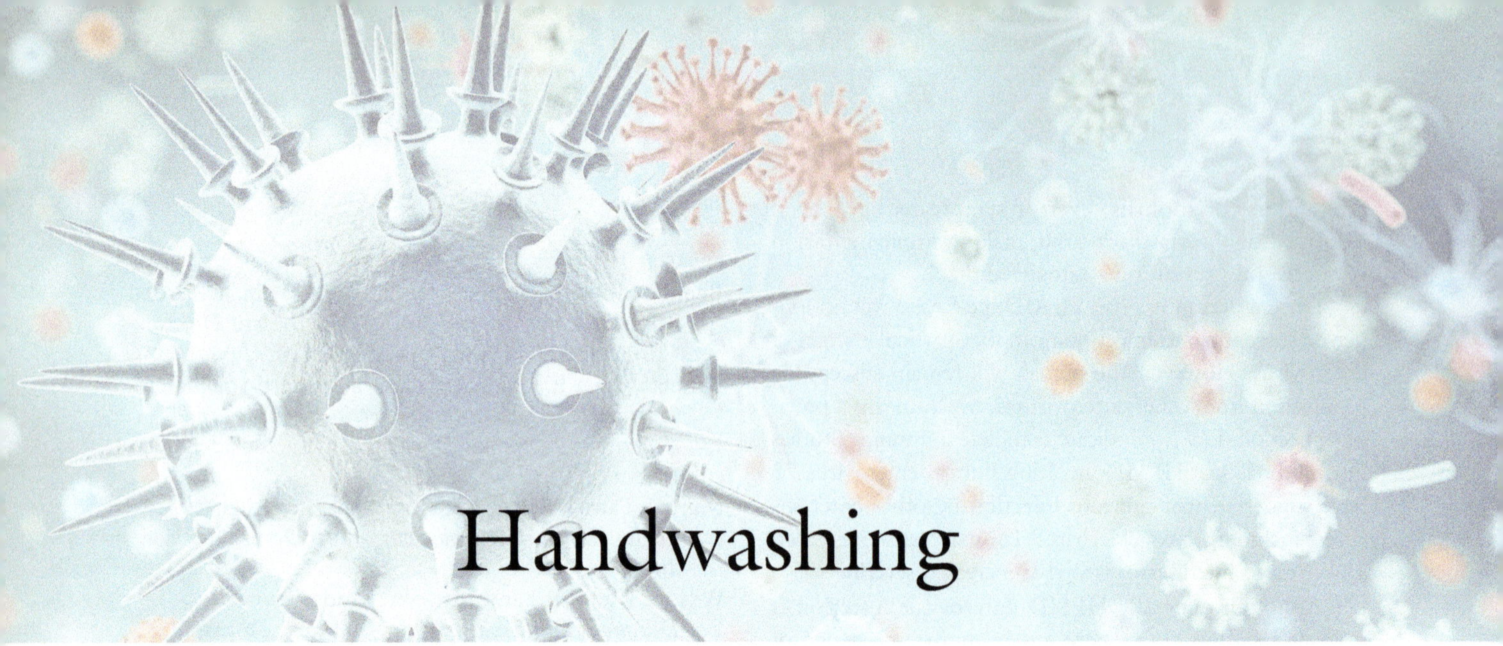

Handwashing

Introduction

Handwashing, or hand hygiene, is the most important method of preventing the spread of infection, whether in the hospital, at home, or in the community. Experts agree that regular and proper handwashing using soap and water is the simplest and most effective way to promote personal hygiene and reduce infections at school and in most workplaces. However, studies have shown that using alcohol-based hand sanitizers in a hospital setting is also effective in reducing the number of transient pathogens (infectious microorganisms) on the hands. Because hand sanitizers are quick and easy to use, busy hospital personnel use them more often.

WORDS TO KNOW

BROAD SPECTRUM A series of objects or ideas with great variety between them. In medicine the term is often applied to drugs that act on a large number of disease-causing agents.

ELBOW BUMP A personal greeting that involves two people touching elbows instead of shaking hands. It is recommended by the World Health Organization for use by researchers handling highly infectious organisms such as Ebola virus.

FOMITE An object or a surface to which infectious microorganisms such as bacteria or viruses can adhere and be transmitted. Papers, clothing, dishes, and other objects can all act as fomites. Transmission is often by touch.

PATHOGEN A disease-causing agent, such as a bacterium, a virus, a fungus, or another microorganism.

Handwashing minimizes the spread of pathogens between people, as well as between people and other living things. Fomites, or inanimate objects and surfaces such as contaminated computer keyboards, desktops, stair rails, and cutlery, often provide surfaces that harbor microorganisms that are easily transferred to membranes of the mouth, nose, and eyes via the hands.

History and Scientific Foundations

As early as the mid-19th century, doctors and nurses began to assert that handwashing could reduce illness. Florence Nightingale (1820–1910), an English pioneer of the nursing profession, wrote about the relationship between unsanitary conditions and disease she perceived during her nursing experiences in the Crimean War (1853–1856). At about the same time, Viennese physician Ignaz Philipp Semmelweis (1818–1865) noted a connection between deaths among hospital patients and contact with physicians who moved from patient to patient without washing their hands. After introducing handwashing with a solution containing chloride, Semmelweis found the incidence of mortality due to puerperal fever (infection after childbirth) diminished from 18 percent to less than 3 percent.

British surgeon and scientist Joseph Lister (1827–1912) also changed the role of surgery by demonstrating the value of infection control. When he applied a spray of disinfectant over a patient's wound during surgery, he showed that postoperative infections could be markedly reduced. Later this was shown to be due to the killing of bacteria present in the air of the operating room or on the clothing or gloves of health care providers. By killing the bacteria before or immediately after they contacted the wound, health care providers could minimize the infection. In the decades after Lister's method became popular, postoperative patient deaths dropped to less than 1 percent. This was the beginning of the modern concept of aseptic technique.

By the 21st century handwashing protocols had become a cornerstone of the infection control program of health care facilities. Because the most basic concept of infection control assumes that all body fluids are potential sources of infection, standard precautions state that handwashing should occur both before and after routine contact with body fluids, even though latex gloves are worn. For surgery and related procedures, handwashing is accomplished with a nonirritating antimicrobial preparation that has fast, long-lasting, broad-spectrum activity against pathogens.

Proper handwashing is the most effective way to prevent the spread of infection. In the home a combination of household soap and vigorous scrubbing of the hands for 30 to 60 seconds has been shown to eliminate most microorganisms of concern from the hands. This is especially important for those involved in food preparation because fecally acquired bacteria and viruses can contaminate food during handling. In a related step, the cleaning of cutting boards and utensils such as knives helps prevent transfer of microbes. For example, failure to properly wash cutting boards used to process raw poultry is one of the main reasons for the millions of cases of food-borne contamination with the bacterium *Campylobacter jejuni* that occur each year in the United States. Bacteria on the surface of the board may be transferred to other food, which if not cooked or if undercooked can cause illness when eaten.

Applications and Research

To maximize effectiveness, careful attention must be paid to proper handwashing technique. The act of handwashing is best accomplished by vigorous rubbing together of the hands and fingers. This is because the removal of microorganisms is accomplished not only by the presence of the soap or antiseptic but also by the friction of the opposing skin surfaces rubbing together. Warm water, soap, and friction loosen dirt and grime. The soap does not need to be specifically labeled antibacterial. Liquid soap lasts longer without hosting bacterial growth than bar soap.

Far more important than the type of soap is the effort put into washing. Friction is key, and it is important to work the soap into lather on both sides of the hands and wrists, between the fingers, and on the fingertips. Careful attention should also be given to areas around nail beds that may harbor bacteria in broken cuticles. Contact time is often critical in effectively killing germs. It is important to wash for about 15 seconds before rinsing well, without touching the faucet or sides of the washbasin, and drying with an air dryer or disposable towel (preferred) or a clean cloth towel. Equally important is avoiding recontamination by turning the water faucet off with the paper towel or

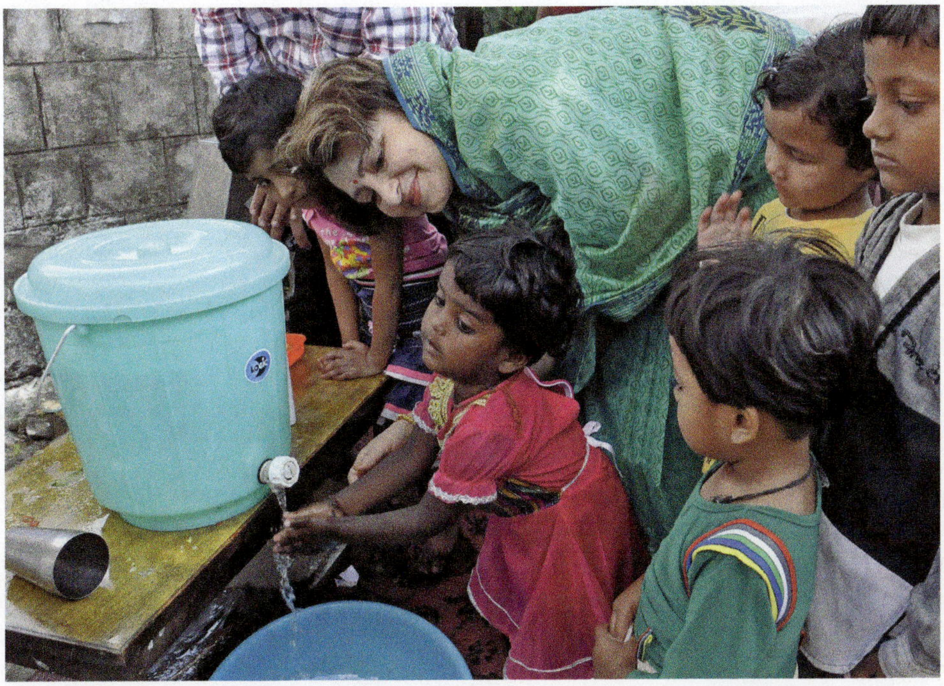

Maya Singh, India's Women and Child Development minister, helps a child wash her hands on Global Handwashing Day in 2014. The October 15 event helps educate children about the importance of handwashing. © Mujeeb Faruqui/Hindustan Times/Getty Images

Proper Handwashing Technique

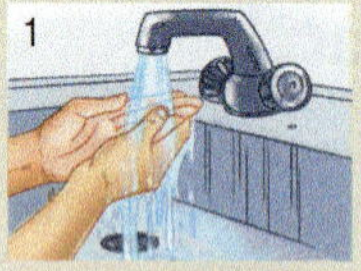

Wet hands.

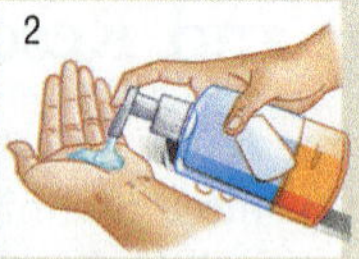

Apply soap. Be sure to cover the entire surface of your hand.

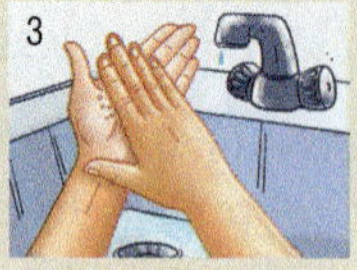

Rub your palms together.

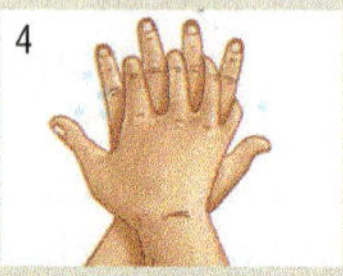

Put your right palm over your left hand and interlace your fingers. Rub. Repeat with your left palm on top.

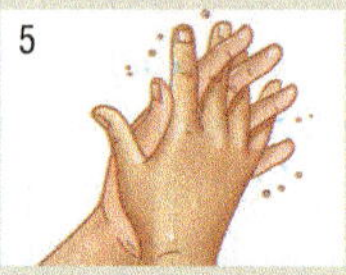

Put your palms together with your fingers interlaced. Rub.

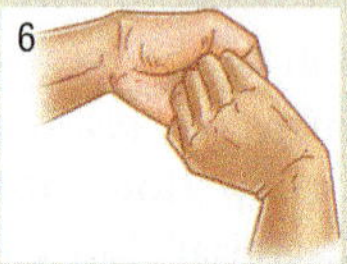

Put the backs of your fingers against the palm of the opposite hand. Interlock your fingers and rub your hands up and down.

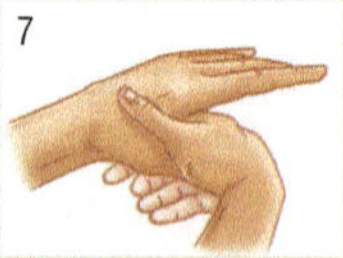

Clasp your left thumb in your right hand and rub. Repeat with your right thumb and left hand.

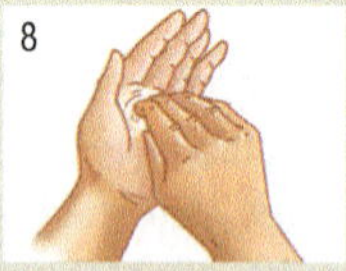

Use the fingers of your right hand to scrub your left palm. Repeat with the fingers of your left hand and your right palm.

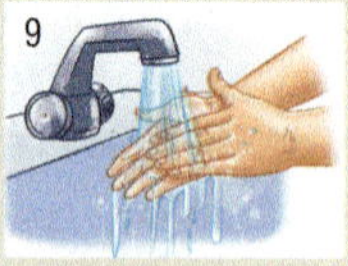

Rinse your hands thoroughly.

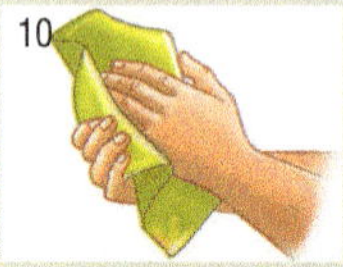

Dry your hands thoroughly with a paper towel.

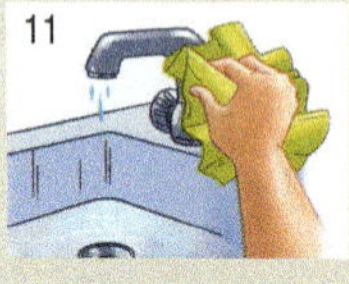

Use the paper towel to turn off the water.

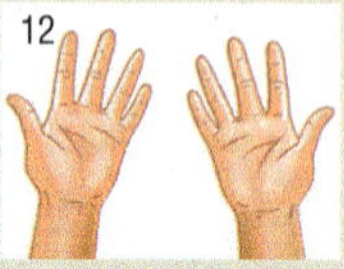

Your hands are clean and safe.

SOURCE: Adapted from "Clean Hands Protect against Infection." World Health Organization (WHO). Available from: http://www.who.int/gpsc/clean_hands_protection/en/

cloth. Children can be taught to count, repeat a simple rhyme, or softly sing a song to make sure they invest the needed time in washing.

Washing with an alcohol-based solution has become popular in hospitals because it can kill organisms on skin within about 10 seconds. This has proven popular with physicians and nurses, who often do not have much time for the traditional soap-and-water handwashing. Many hospitals are equipped with an alcohol-based washstand at the foot of each patient bed or in the room.

In the hospital setting, handwashing is done according to US Centers for Disease Control and Prevention (CDC) guidelines. The guidelines specify that health care providers wash their hands before and after seeing each patient and, if gloves have been worn, as the final step after removing gloves and disposing of them in the proper container.

■ Impacts and Issues

Although it is difficult to estimate the financial impact of proper hygienic practices, conservative estimates by the CDC place savings due to successful handwashing in clinical settings at over $1 billion per year. More than 30 million school days are lost due to flu in the United States each year, which means the savings generated by proper handwashing in schools and in the workplace could exceed this figure by a significant factor.

Especially during influenza season, both the CDC and World Health Organization (WHO) recommend the elbow bump greeting as a replacement for the handshake. Cold and influenza viruses that remain on the hands after a sneeze are often passed on through a handshake. The recipient is then infected after touching his or her eyes or mouth with the contaminated hand. Because it is difficult to contaminate the elbow with a sneeze, bumping elbows transfers fewer pathogens. WHO and CDC scientists responding to outbreaks of infectious disease in places where infrastructure is lacking commonly use the elbow bump greeting. In the event of an influenza pandemic, the US government recommends the elbow bump greeting as a measure of social distancing, in addition to regular handwashing, to prevent the spread of infection.

See Also *Antimicrobial Soaps; Infection Control and Asepsis*

BIBLIOGRAPHY

Books

Amer, Fatma. *Hospital Infection Control, Part 1*. 3rd ed. Saarbrücken, Germany: Noor, 2017.

Saint, Sanjay, and Sarah L. Krein. *Preventing Hospital Infections: Real-World Problems, Realistic Solutions.* New York: Oxford University Press, 2014.

Periodicals

Fox, Cherie, et al. "Use of a Patient Hand Hygiene Protocol to Reduce Hospital-Acquired Infections and Improve Nurses' Hand Washing." *American Journal of Critical Care* 24 (2015): 216–224.

Goldmann, Donald. "System Failure versus Personal Accountability—The Case for Clean Hands" *New England Journal of Medicine* 355 (July 13, 2006): 121–123.

Seibert, Grace, et al. "What Do Visitors Know and How Do They Feel about Contact Precautions?" *American Journal of Infection Control* 46, no. 1 (January 2018): 115–117.

Websites

"Hand Hygiene in Healthcare Settings." Centers for Disease Control and Prevention, March 24, 2017. https://www.cdc.gov/handhygiene/index.html (accessed January 16, 2017).

"Handwashing: Clean Hands Save Lives." Centers for Disease Control and Prevention, December 8, 2017. https://www.cdc.gov/handwashing/index.html (accessed December 4, 2017).

"Hand-washing: Do's and Don't's." Mayo Clinic. https://www.mayoclinic.org/healthy-lifestyle/adult-health/in-depth/hand-washing/art-20046253 (accessed December 11, 2017).

"Transmission-Based Precautions" Centers for Disease Control and Prevention, February 28, 2017. https://www.cdc.gov/infectioncontrol/basics/transmission-based-precautions.html (accessed December 4, 2017).

Brenda Wilmoth Lerner
Brian Hoyle

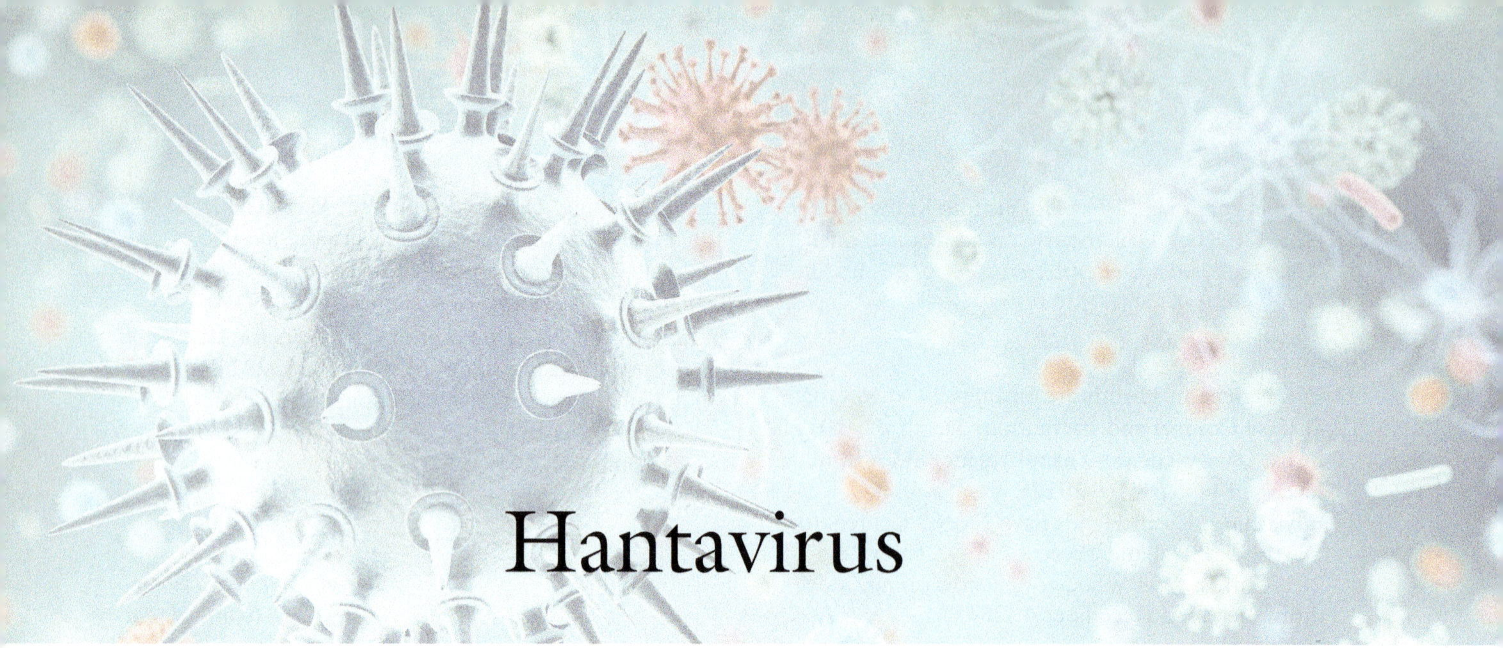

Hantavirus

■ Introduction

During the 1950s more than 6,000 United Nations (UN) military personnel serving in Korea were stricken by a mysterious illness characterized by high fever, kidney failure, and spontaneous bleeding. This disease continues to claim victims in the region, with around 400 cases reported each year between 2006 and 2017. A group of viruses has been identified as the cause of this so-called "Korean hemorrhagic fever." The group was named Hantaan virus, after the Hantaan River, which flows through Gangwon and Gyeonggi provinces.

Similar illnesses of varying severity in Asia and Europe were found to be caused by a number of distinct viruses, and the group came to be known as *hantaviruses.* In 1993 a new illness was reported in the southwestern United States. Unlike the Korean disease, prominent features of the new illness included rapidly progressive lung infection with high death rates. Despite the unique nature of the disease, a viral agent was discovered that had all the common biological features of the older hantavirus group. The new illness was therefore referred to as *hantavirus pulmonary syndrome* (HPS). As of January 2017, 728 cases of hantavirus infection (including both HPS and nonpulmonary hantavirus infection) have been reported in the United States. Thirty-six percent of these cases have resulted in death. As in the Asian variety, a large number of additional hantavirus species have since been identified in the United States, as well as in Central and South America, though the exact number is not known.

■ Disease History, Characteristics, and Transmission

Regardless of differences in clinical presentation and geographic occurrence, all hantaviruses are found in rodents. Humans acquire the disease through inhalation of dried rodent excreta or occasionally through ingestion of milk and other foods that have been contaminated by these animals. In fact, the ability of the virus to survive in dust and the contagious nature of infected material have suggested hantaviruses as potential agents of bioterrorism.

■ Scope and Distribution

The following is a summary of the clinical features, distribution, and epidemiology of hantaviruses that infect humans. Specific viruses are arranged alphabetically.

Old World Hantaviruses

Clinical features Infection by the European and Asian hantaviruses is characterized by sudden onset with intense headache, backache, fever, and chills. Hemorrhage is manifested during the febrile phase as a flushing of the face or an injection of the conjunctiva (membranes lining the eye) and mucous membranes. A petechial rash (tiny, red dots) may appear on the palate and axillary (underarm) skin folds. Extreme albuminuria (protein in the urine), typically appearing on the fourth day, is characteristic of severe hemorrhagic fever renal syndrome (HFRS).

As the febrile stage ends, low blood pressure may develop and last for hours to days, accompanied by nausea and vomiting. One-third of deaths occur during this phase, related to vascular bleeding and shock. Approximately 50 percent of deaths occur during the subsequent oliguric phase (when the kidneys produce very little urine). Patients who survive and progress to the diuretic phase show improved renal function but may still die of shock or pulmonary complications. The final phase can last weeks to months.

Case fatality rates range from less than 0.1 percent for HFRS caused by Puumala virus (a virus transmitted by the bank vole) to approximately 5 to 10 percent for HFRS caused by Hantaan virus.

Epidemiology Dobrava-Belgrade virus causes severe hemorrhagic fever with renal syndrome. The reservoirs, the yellow-necked mouse (*Apodemus flavicollis*) and the striped field mouse (*Apodemus agrarius*), are found from England and Wales through northwestern Spain, France, southern Scandinavia, European Russia to the Urals, southern Italy, the Balkans, Syria, Lebanon, and Israel.

Hantaan virus causes epidemic hemorrhagic fever (Korean hemorrhagic fever and hemorrhagic fever with renal syndrome). The striped field mouse is found in Central Europe south to Thrace, the Caucasus and Tien Shan Mountains, the Amur River to East Xijiang and East Hunnan, West Sichuan, and Fujian (China), and Taiwan.

Puumala virus causes nephropathia epidemica (a usually less severe form of hemorrhagic fever). The reservoir, the bank vole (*Clethrionomys glareolus*), is found in the West Palearctic from France and Scandinavia to Lake Baikal, southern to northern Spain, northern Italy, the Balkans, western Turkey, northern Kazakhstan, the Altai and Sayan Mountains, Great Britain, and southwestern Ireland. The house mouse (*Mus musculus*) is implicated in Serbia, and the northern red-backed vole (*Clethrionomys rutilus*) in western Russia. The muskrat (*Ondatra zibethicus*) has been implicated as a disease reservoir in Germany. The Puumala virus may remain infective in the environment for as long as 12 to 15 days.

Saaremaa virus has been associated with human disease in Estonia and is closely related to Dobrava virus.

Seoul virus causes less severe hemorrhagic fever with renal syndrome. The reservoir, the common rat (*Rattus norvegicus*), is found worldwide. Wounds inflicted by other rats appear to be a major source for transmission among rats.

Thailand virus has been identified in humans and bandicoot rats (*Bandicota indica* and *Bandicota savilei*) in Thailand.

WORDS TO KNOW

CASE FATALITY RATE The rate of patients suffering disease or injury that die as a result of that disease or injury during a specific period of time.

EPIDEMIOLOGY The study of the various factors that influence the occurrence, distribution, prevention, and control of disease, injury, and other health-related events in a defined human population. By the application of various analytical techniques, including mathematical analysis of the data, the probable cause of an infectious outbreak can be pinpointed.

FEBRILE Pertaining to a fever.

HEMORRHAGIC FEVER A high fever caused by viral infection that features a high volume of bleeding. The bleeding is caused by the formation of tiny blood clots throughout the bloodstream. These blood clots, or *microthrombi*, deplete platelets and fibrinogen in the bloodstream. When bleeding begins, the factors needed for the clotting of the blood are scarce. Thus uncontrolled bleeding (hemorrhage) ensues.

PRODROME A symptom indicating the disease's onset; it may also be called a prodroma. For example, painful swallowing is often a prodrome of infection with a cold virus.

RESERVOIR The animal or organism in which a virus or parasite normally resides.

STRAIN A subclass or a specific genetic variation of an organism.

Hantavirus Pulmonary Syndrome (HPS)

Clinical features The typical illness is characterized by fever, chills, headache, and occasionally gastrointestinal symptoms. Five days after onset, patients have difficulty breathing, with rapid progression to pulmonary edema/acute respiratory distress syndrome (ARDS) within as little as 24 hours. In the twenty-first century, cases of prodromic infection (having symptoms of oncoming disease) without severe pulmonary disease have been reported. According to the US Centers for Disease Control and Prevention (CDC), HPS is fatal in 38 percent of infections.

Epidemiology Andes virus is transmitted by the long-tailed pygmy rice rat (*Oligoryzomys longicaudatus*), found in Chile, Argentina, and possibly Uruguay.

Bermejo virus (reservoir *Oligoryzomys* species) has been associated with human infections in Bolivia.

Bayou virus is transmitted by the rice rat (*Oryzomys palustris*) in Louisiana and eastern Texas.

Black Creek Canal virus is transmitted by the cotton rat (*Sigmodon hispidus*), found in the eastern and southern United States from southern Nebraska to central Virginia, south to southeastern Arizona and peninsular Florida, and from central to eastern Mexico through Central America and central Panama to northern Colombia and northern Venezuela.

Caño Delgadito virus (clinical significance unknown) is found in rodents in central Venezuela.

Central Plata virus is associated with human infections in Uruguay and is transmitted by the yellow pygmy rice rat (*Oligoryzomys flavescens*).

Choclo virus (reservoir *Oligoryzomys fulvescens*) is implicated in human infections in Panama. Calabazo virus (clinical significance unknown) has been identified in *Zygodontomys brevicauda* (short-tailed cane mouse) in Panama.

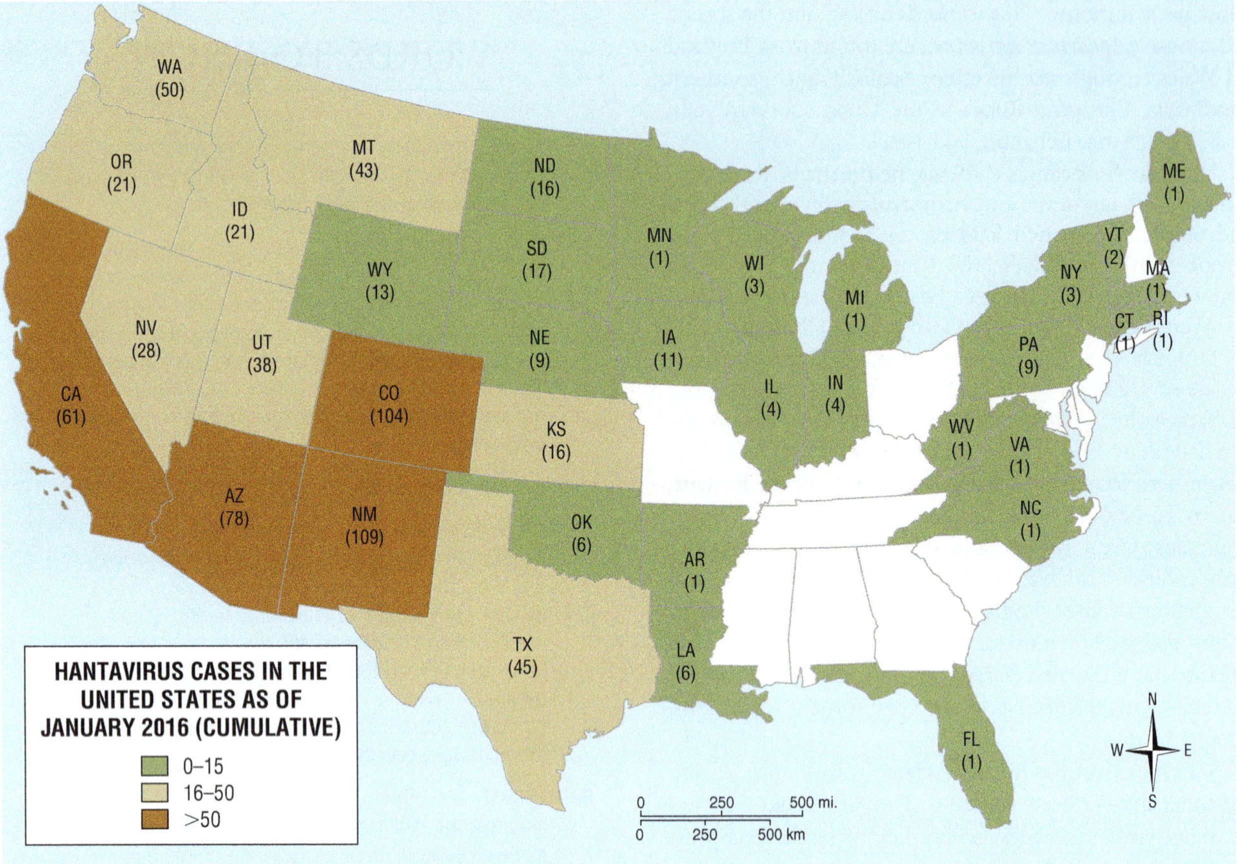

SOURCE: Adapted from "Hantavirus Disease, by State of Reporting." US Centers for Disease Control and Prevention. 2017. Available from: https://www.cdc.gov/hantavirus/surveillance/reporting-state.html

Convict Creek virus (similar and possibly identical to Sin Nombre virus, a previously unknown type of hantavirus [Spanish for "without name"]) has been identified in California and was implicated in a fatal case in Ontario, Canada.

Juquitiba virus, Araraquara virus, and Castelos dos Sonhos virus have been implicated in human infections in Brazil; HU39694 remains unnamed, and reservoirs are still unknown.

Laguna Negra virus has caused human disease in Argentina, Chile, and Paraguay and is transmitted by the vesper mouse (*Calomys laucha*). This rodent is found in northern Argentina and Uruguay, southeastern Bolivia, Chile, western Paraguay, and west-central Brazil.

Maporal virus (clinical significance unknown) has been identified in the fulvous pygmy rice rat (*Oligoryzomys fulvescens*) in western Venezuela.

Monongahela virus (similar and possibly identical to Sin Nombre virus) is found in the eastern United States and Canada and is carried by the white-footed mouse (*Peromyscus leucopus*) and possibly the deer mouse (*Peromyscus maniculatus nubiterrae*).

New York–1 virus is transmitted by the white-footed mouse (*Peromyscus leucopus*), found in the central and eastern United States to southern Ontario, southern Alberta, Quebec, and Nova Scotia, and in northern Durango and along the Caribbean coast of Mexico to the Isthmus of Tehuantepec and Yucatan Peninsula.

Oran virus (reservoir *Oligoryzomys longicaudatus*), Lechiguanas virus (reservoir *Oligoryzomys flavescens*), and Andes virus (reservoir *Oligoryzomys longicaudatus*) are found in Argentina.

Rio Mamore virus (reservoir *Neacomys spinosus*) has been associated with human infections in Peru.

Seoul virus is also a rodent-borne virus. As of 2017 it had sickened 17 people in seven states, according to the CDC.

Sin Nombre virus is transmitted by the deer mouse (*Peromyscus maniculatus*) in the southwestern United States. The reservoir is found from the Alaska panhandle across northern Mexico, Canada, and most of the continental United States to southernmost Baja California and north-central Oaxaca, Mexico. The mouse itself shows evidence of pneumonia. The virus has also been found in *Pseudallescheria boylii* (a species of fungus), *Peromyscus truei* (the pinyon mouse), *Reithrodontomys* spp. (harvest mice), *Mus musculus* (the house mouse), and *Tamias* spp. (chipmunks).

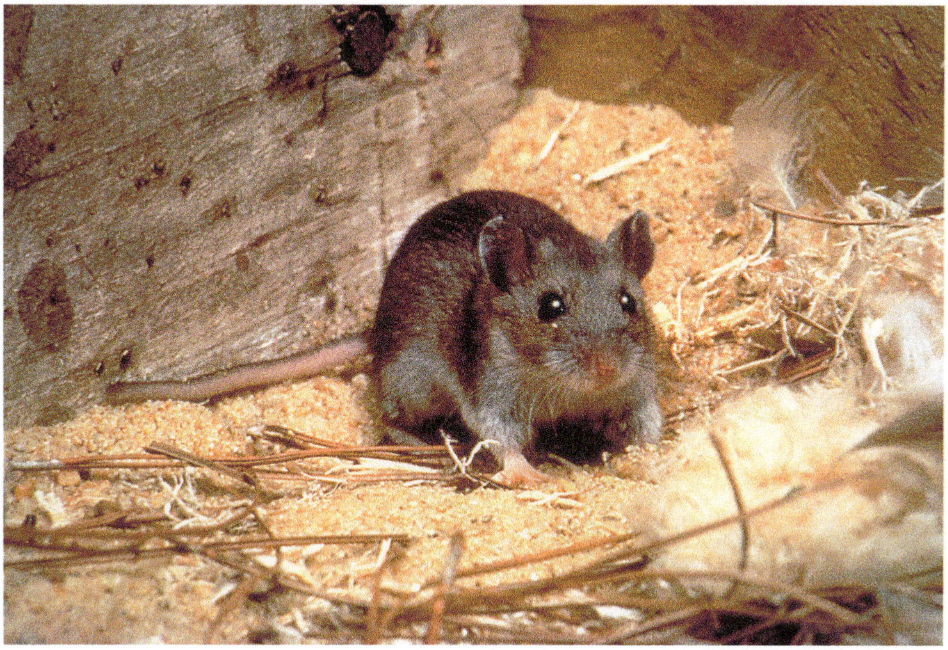

Sin Nombre virus, a strain of hantavirus common in the southwestern United States, is carried by the deer mouse. *© Smith Collection/Gado/Getty Images*

■ Treatment and Prevention

Although the viruses in this group can be cultivated using standard techniques, viral culture is limited to a small number of institutions that meet strict standards of biosafety. Diagnosis can also be established through testing for serum antibodies in specialized laboratories. Treatment is directed at support of renal, pulmonary, and other systems affected by the viruses. The value of specific antiviral agents is not proven, but some authorities have suggested ribavirin in the treatment of the Old World hantaviruses, including Seoul virus and Hantaan virus. As of 2017 there was not specific treatment, cure, or vaccine for hantavirus infection.

■ Impacts and Issues

HPS was first identified in May 1993 in the so-called "Four Corners" region of the United States, where the states of New Mexico, Utah, Arizona, and Colorado meet. Initially it was unclear what was so rapidly killing healthy adults in the region. Virologists from the CDC used techniques that analyze a virus at the molecular level to link the pulmonary illness to the previously unknown hantavirus Sin Nombre.

In addition to molecular and clinical studies, scientists are studying HPS through the study of rodent populations (which often requires trapping and collecting various mice species), weather patterns, and climate change. Research in the southwestern United States has linked the years having higher levels of precipitation with a larger population of rodents. The moisture leads to a greater supply of food for rodents, as well as higher vegetation growth, which provides ample habitat and protection for the rodents. Associated with the weather phenomenon El Niño in 1991 and 1993, rainfall levels increased in the southwestern United States. The population density of deer mice in New Mexico then increased from 1 deer mouse per 2.5 acres (1 hectare) to 20 to 30 per 2.5 acres during that time period. It is thought that this large population of mice led to the first identified outbreak of HPS in May 1993.

Although rare, HPS has since been found throughout the United States. As of May 2017 rodent control remains the primary defense against hantavirus.

See Also *Emerging Infectious Diseases; Hemorrhagic Fevers*

BIBLIOGRAPHY

Books

Hopkins, Donald R., and Alexandra M. Levitt. *Deadly Outbreaks: How Medical Detectives Save Lives Threatened by Killer Pandemics, Exotic Viruses, and Drug-Resistant Parasites.* New York: Skyhorse, 2015.

Periodicals

Anderson, Dustin, et al. "A Neuropathic Pain Syndrome Associated with Hantavirus Infection." *Journal of Neurovirology* 23 (December 2017): 919–921.

Websites

"Hantavirus." Centers for Disease Control and Prevention. http://www.cdc.gov/hantavirus/hps/index.html (accessed December 11, 2017).

"Hantavirus Pulmonary Syndrome." Mayo Clinic. https://www.mayoclinic.org/diseases-conditions/hantavirus-pulmonary-syndrome/symptoms-causes/syc-20351838 (accessed December 11, 2017).

Stephen A. Berger
Brian Hoyle

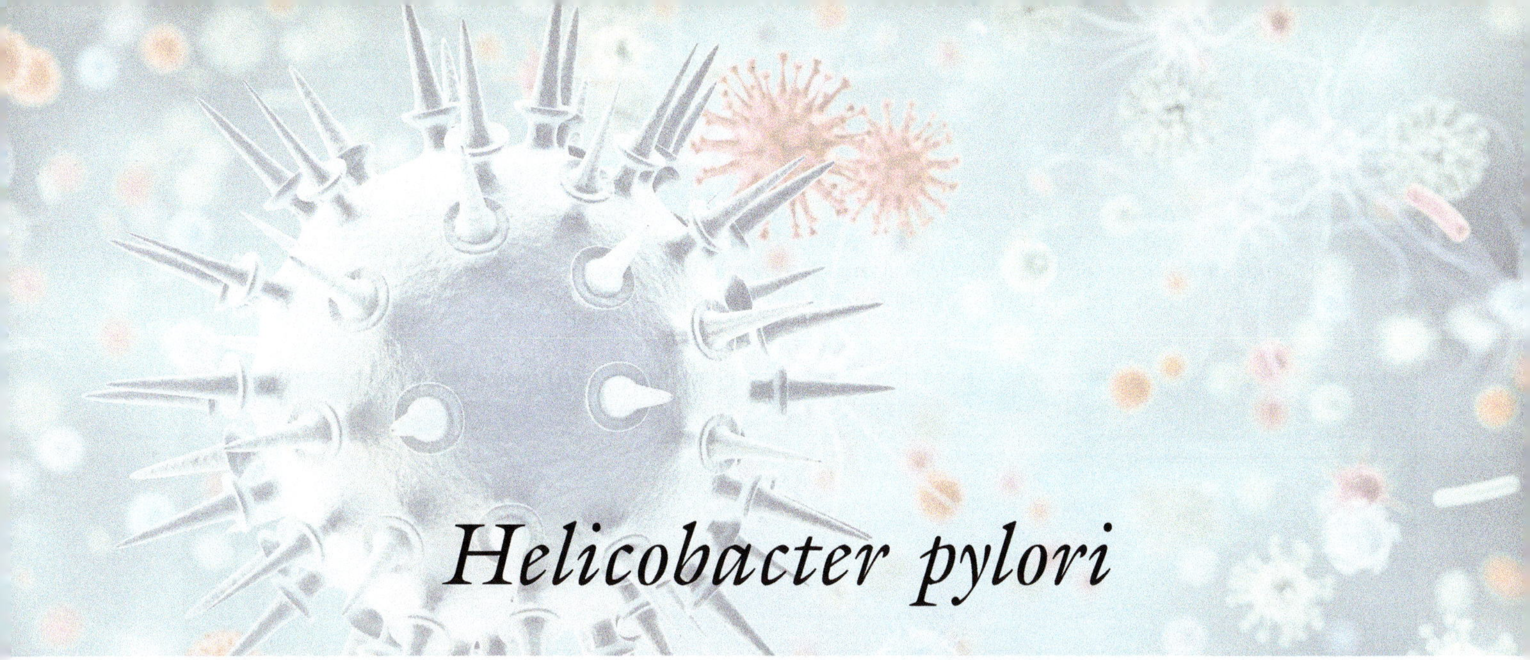

Helicobacter pylori

Introduction

Helicobacter pylori are bacteria that live in the lining of the stomach and sometimes cause stomach inflammation and ulcers. The discovery of *H. pylori* in 1982 changed scientists' thinking about the nature of stomach ulcers. The scientists who discovered the bacteria earned a Nobel Prize, not only because of the insight their discovery offered about the cause of peptic ulcers but also because it led to the broader study of bacteria and other pathogens (infectious agents) as possible contributors to other well-known diseases, including heart disease and some types of cancer.

H. pylori is present in more than half of the world's population, making it one of the most common pathogens in humans. However, the presence of the bacteria is far more common in underdeveloped countries than in developed parts of the world. In addition to acting as the principal cause of ulcers, *H. pylori* has been linked to gastritis, cancer, and other conditions.

History and Scientific Foundations

In 1975 J. Robin Warren (1937–) of Australia discovered the presence of helical (spiral-shaped) bacteria in the antrum, the section of the stomach that empties into the duodenum (the top part of the upper intestine) through the pyloric valve. At that time Warren observed that the bacteria were present in 50 percent of people who had stomach biopsies and that infected people invariably showed signs of stomach inflammation. Later, he named the bacterium *Helicobacter pylori* after working with fellow Australian Barry J. Marshall (1951–) to cultivate the species from biopsied patients.

The two scientists hypothesized that an *H. pylori* infection played a role in stomach disorders, including gastritis and peptic ulcers. In 1982 they presented evidence supporting this theory. However, many of their peers in the medical community considered this hypothesis to be preposterous because the existing scientific consensus held both that no bacteria could survive in the highly acidic environment of the stomach and that ulcers were caused by lifestyle and psychological stress. Perhaps the greatest barrier to acceptance of such a simple explanation as a bacterial infection was the simplicity of the potential cure, a course of antibiotics and acid secretion inhibitors, for a chronic and often disabling condition.

The belief that stress and lifestyle caused stomach ulcers was so pervasive and impervious to new evidence that Marshall took drastic action, putting himself at risk to demonstrate the role of *H. pylori* in disease. He allowed colleagues to obtain a sample of his stomach tissue in a biopsy to show that he was free of infection, then infected himself with the bacterium and, subsequently, contracted gastritis. This act of personal commitment and courage had a decisive impact on the medical community, which began to accept his work, although the *H. pylori* hypothesis as a major cause of peptic ulcers did not gain worldwide acceptance until 1991.

Applications and Research

Subsequent studies have shown that about half of all humans have chronic *H. pylori* infection, and clinical experience confirms that this infection and the consequent destruction of the stomach lining and predisposition for stomach cancer can be halted by antibiotic treatment. Thus, Warren and Marshall brought about a paradigm shift, or a fundamental change in thinking, regarding the relative importance of infectious agents as opposed to psychosocial factors in the cause and origin of gastric disease. This paradigm shift in turn led to a marked improvement in health and quality of life for the large number of stomach ulcer sufferers around the world. It also led to research about the possible role of infectious agents in other diseases. For example, scientists are studying the potential role of infectious agents in inflammation of the walls of blood vessels that could relate to heart disease and stroke.

A 2007 study in which gastric biopsies were evaluated showed that the presence of *H. pylori* is strongly associated with both acute and chronic inflammation. The presence of neutrophils (immune cells that release a bacteria-killing chemical) on biopsy is predictive of the presence of *H. pylori* as well as the extent of inflamed tissue. Long-term

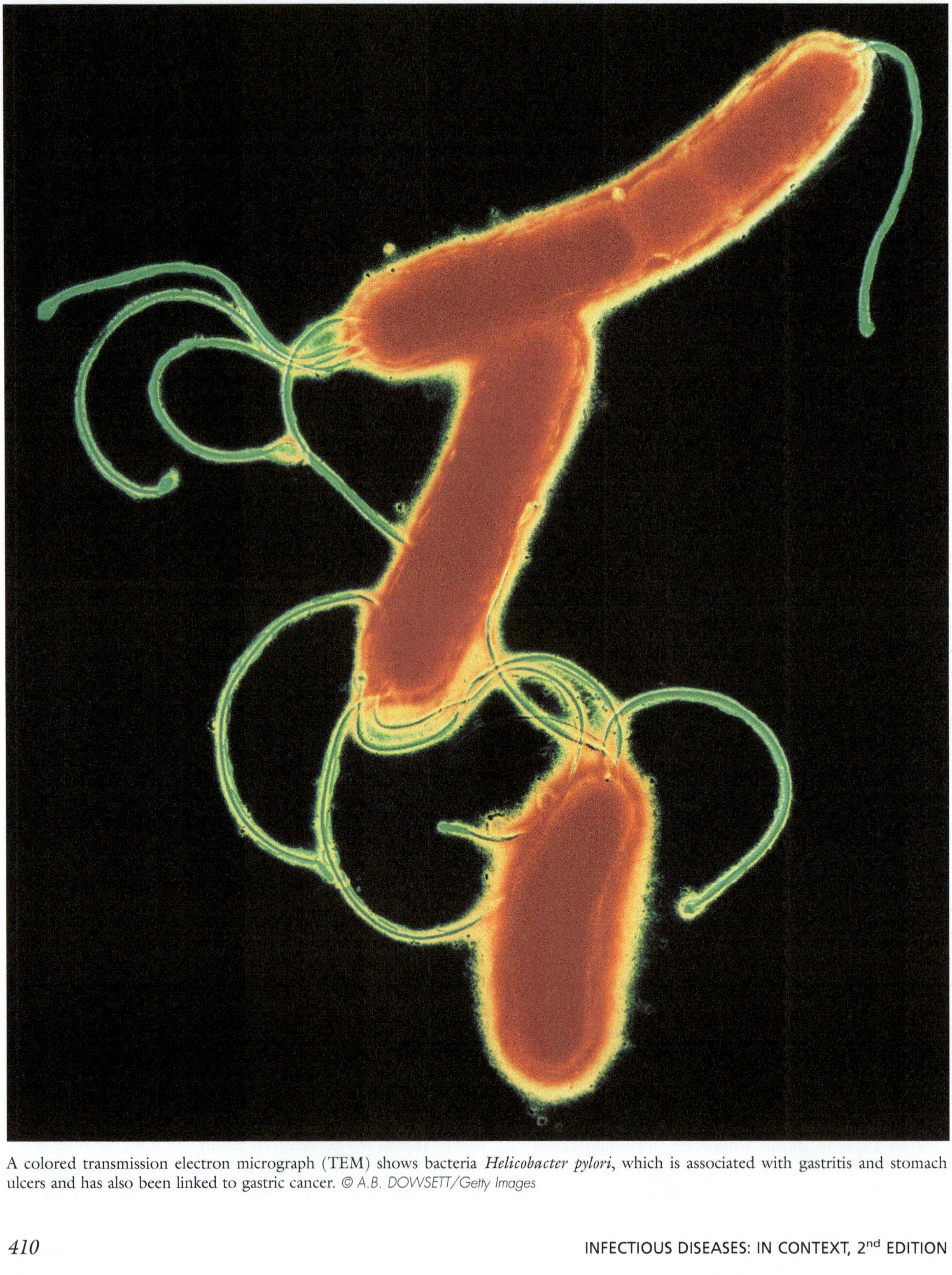

A colored transmission electron micrograph (TEM) shows bacteria *Helicobacter pylori*, which is associated with gastritis and stomach ulcers and has also been linked to gastric cancer. *© A.B. DOWSETT/Getty Images*

inflammation leads to atrophy (wasting, or decreasing size) of the stomach lining. This persistent inflammation appears to be due either to a weakness in the immune system, thus preventing the predisposed individual from eliminating the bacterium, or a physiological weakness in the structure of the stomach lining that fosters the growth of *H. pylori* colonies (populations).

Treatment

Available treatments for *H. pylori*–caused gastritis include antibiotics that destroy the bacteria, such as amoxicillin, clarithromycin, metronidazole, tetracycline, or tinidazole. Typically, physicians prescribe two drugs from this group. Doctors may also prescribe drugs that reduce stomach acid, called proton pump inhibitors (PPIs), such as dexlansoprazole (Dexilant), esomeprazole (Nexium), lansoprazole (Prevacid), omeprazole (Prilosec), pantoprazole (Protonix), and rabeprazole (Aciphex). Medication to block the chemical histamine, which prompts the stomach to make more acid, may also be used. Examples include cimetidine (Tagamet), famotidine (Fluxid, Pepcid), nizatidine (Axid), or ranitidine (Zantac). Over-the-counter medications known as bismuth subsalicylates, which are sold under the brand name Pepto-Bismol, may also help kill *H. pylori* when used with antibiotics.

According to the CDC, treatment usually consists of a combination of medications, including one to two antibiotics and a bismuth subsalicylate or a PPI for between 10 and 14 days. However, if patients do not take all of the prescribed antibiotics in the correct way, bacteria in their bodies can become resistant to them. This makes infections harder to treat.

WORDS TO KNOW

ATROPHY Decreasing in size or wasting-away of a body part or tissue.

CHRONIC Chronic infections persist for prolonged periods of time—months or even years—in the host. This lengthy persistence is due to a number of factors, which can include masking of the disease-causing agent (e.g., bacteria) from the immune system, invasion of host cells, and the establishment of an infection that is resistant to antibacterial agents.

COLONIZATION The process of occupation and increase in number of microorganisms at a specific site.

CYTOKINE One of a family of small proteins that mediate an organism's response to injury or infection. Cytokines operate by transmitting signals between cells in an organism. Minute quantities of cytokines are secreted, each by a single cell type, to regulate functions in other cells by binding with specific receptors. Their interactions with the receptors produce secondary signals that inhibit or enhance the action of certain genes within the cell. Unlike endocrine hormones, which can act throughout the body, most cytokines act locally near the cells that produced them.

NEUTROPHIL A type of white blood cell that phagocytizes foreign microorganisms, releasing a bacteria-killing chemical known as lysozyme. Neutrophils are prominent in the inflammatory response.

PATHOGEN A disease-causing agent, such as a bacterium, a virus, a fungus, or another microorganism.

Impacts and Issues

As a persistent colonizer of the human stomach, *H. pylori* also contributes to the development of gastric cancer as well as extra-intestinal diseases. Despite awareness that *H. pylori* is a risk factor for developing gastric cancer, which is highly lethal, researchers have had difficulty understanding why a small number of people develop this disease relative to the large number of people who harbor the bacteria. In 2010 Lydia E. Wroblewski, Richard M. Peek Jr., and Keith T. Wilson published "*Helicobacter pylori* and Gastric Cancer: Factors That Modulate Disease Risk," an article in which they sought to "identify high-risk subpopulations" that are most susceptible to developing gastric cancer. Among the factors identified as contributing to increasing risk of developing cancer from *H. pylori* infection were "host polymorphisms, alterations to the apical-junctional complex, and the effects of environmental factors." However, more work remains to fully understand why certain people develop cancer as a result of *H. pylori* and others do not. In a review article on the link between the bacteria and gastric cancer published in 2015, Sauid Ishaq and Lois Nunn noted the continued and "urgent need for future research to focus on the genetic changes that are occurring in parallel to the inflammatory process to improve the outcomes of this killer disease."

H. pylori is implicated not only in gastric cancer but also in childhood lymphomas. The latter type of cancer may arise due to the proliferation of lymphocytes in the stomach lining as a result of the inflammatory response to chronic infection. Such proliferation could raise the probability of a lymphocyte replication error that results in cancer.

Paradoxically, scientists have found an inverse association between *H. pylori* infection and esophageal cancer. This inverse relationship has been attributed to reduced

THE POSITIVE ROLE OF BACTERIA

The work of Barry J. Marshall (1951–) and J. Robin Warren (1937–) has been crucial to improved treatment of peptic ulcers and other stomach conditions. However, understanding of *Helicobacter pylori* has also played an important role in a new strain of scientific inquiry: identifying the *positive* role bacteria have played, and continue to play, in human biology over the course of history. In a 2012 article for the *New Yorker*, Michael Specter noted that *H. pylori* "has been intertwined with our species for at least two hundred thousand years." This long history of coexistence suggests that *H. pylori* may actually have benefited humanity by inhabiting so many stomachs. Discussing the work of the American microbiologist Martin J. Blaser (1948–), Specter proposed that greater understanding of *H. pylori* holds the promise to "focus attention on the critical, and usually positive, role that these organisms play in human evolution."

Though scientists do not yet fully understand the positive effects of the bacteria, Blaser and others have suggested that there may be a correlation between declining rates of *H. pylori* infections in developed countries and rising asthma and obesity rates in those parts of the world. The possibility that *H. pylori* aids some biological functions in humans has raised the possibility that there may be some downside to treating *H. pylori* too aggressively, especially in developed countries, where rates of infection have plummeted. In the United States, for example, only 5 percent of the population carries *H. pylori*. As researchers uncover new evidence about the negative effects of reducing the bacteria's presence in humans, Specter observed, "they have transformed the vanishing bacterium into a cautionary symbol of what can happen when we tinker with the ecological communities inside us."

stomach acidity, which is often seen after years of *H. pylori* infection. Stomach acid can damage the esophagus because of the atrophy of the gastric lining.

Chronic infection with *H. pylori* illustrates the damage that can occur when the genetic variability of individuals results in favorable conditions for a pathogen that is harmless to a large proportion of the human population. The inability of the immune system and even antibiotic treatment to conclusively end the infection in these individuals can result in severe tissue damage and possibly cancer. Perhaps the larger lesson to be taken from *H. pylori* infection is that humans and microbes are in a constant struggle to adapt to one another, and some of the resulting infections resemble a chronic and desultory war that eventually wears down the host. The work of Marshall and Warren is all the more important for having provided the basis for relieving a significant amount of the misery caused by this stubborn microbial foe. In 2005 Marshall and Warren were awarded the Nobel Prize for the discovery of the role of *H. pylori* infection in the development of stomach ulcers.

Current antibiotic therapies against *H. pylori* have been limited by antibiotic resistance and recurrence of infection, probably due to predisposing factors in susceptible individuals. Consequently, promising vaccine development programs have been mounted as an effective preventive measure. As of 2017, however, developmental vaccines had failed the transition from animal models to human trials.

SEE ALSO *Cancer and Infectious Disease; Exposed: Scientists Who Risked Disease for Discovery*

BIBLIOGRAPHY

Books

Sutton, Philip, and Hazel M. Mitchell, eds. Helicobacter pylori *in the 21st Century. Cambridge, MA: CABI, 2010.*

Yamaoka, Yoshio, ed. Helicobacter Pylori*: Molecular Genetics and Cellular Biology*. Norfolk, UK: Caister Academic Press, 2008.

Periodicals

Ishaq, Sauid, and Lois Nunn. "*Helicobacter pylori* and Gastric Cancer: A State of the Art Review." *Gastroenterology and Hepatology from Bed to Bench* 8, Suppl. 1 (2015): S6–S14. This article can also be found online at https://www.ncbi.nlm.nih.gov/pmc/articles/PMC4495426/ (accessed March 6, 2018).

Specter, Michael. "Germs Are Us." *New Yorker* (October 22, 2012). This article can also be found online at https://www.newyorker.com/magazine/2012/10/22/germs-are-us (accessed March 6, 2018).

Weintraub, Pamela. "The Dr. Who Drank Infectious Broth, Gave Himself an Ulcer, and Solved a Medical Mystery." *Discover* (April 8, 2010). This article can also be found online at http://discovermagazine.com/2010/mar/07-dr-drank-broth-gave-ulcer-solved-medical-mystery (accessed March 6, 2018).

Wroblewski, Lydia E., Richard M. Peek Jr., and Keith T. Wilson. "*Helicobacter pylori* and Gastric Cancer: Factors That Modulate Disease Risk." *Clinical Microbiology Reviews* 23, no 4 (2010): 713–739. This article can also be found online at https://www.ncbi.nlm.nih.gov/pmc/articles/PMC2952980/ (accessed March 6, 2018).

Zagari, Rocco Maurizio, Stefano Rabitti, Leonardo Henry Eusebi, and Franco Bazzoli. "Treatment of *Helicobacter pylori* infection: A Clinical Practice Update." *European Journal of Clinical Investigation* 48, no. 1 (2018). This article can also be found online at http://onlinelibrary.wiley.com/doi/10.1111/eci.12857/full (accessed March 6, 2018).

Websites

Helicobacter Foundation. http://www.helico.com/ (accessed March 6, 2018).

"*Helicobacter pylori* (*H. pylori*) infection." Mayo Clinic, May 17, 2017. https://www.mayoclinic.org/diseases-conditions/h-pylori/symptoms-causes/syc-20356171 (accessed March 6, 2018).

"The Nobel Prize in Physiology or Medicine 2005." Nobelprize.org, October 3, 2005. https://www.nobelprize.org/nobel_prizes/medicine/laureates/2005/press.html (accessed March 6, 2018).

Santacroce, Luigi. "*Helicobacter pylori* Infection." Medscape, October 12, 2017. https://emedicine.medscape.com/article/176938-overview (accessed March 6, 2018).

Kenneth T. LaPensee

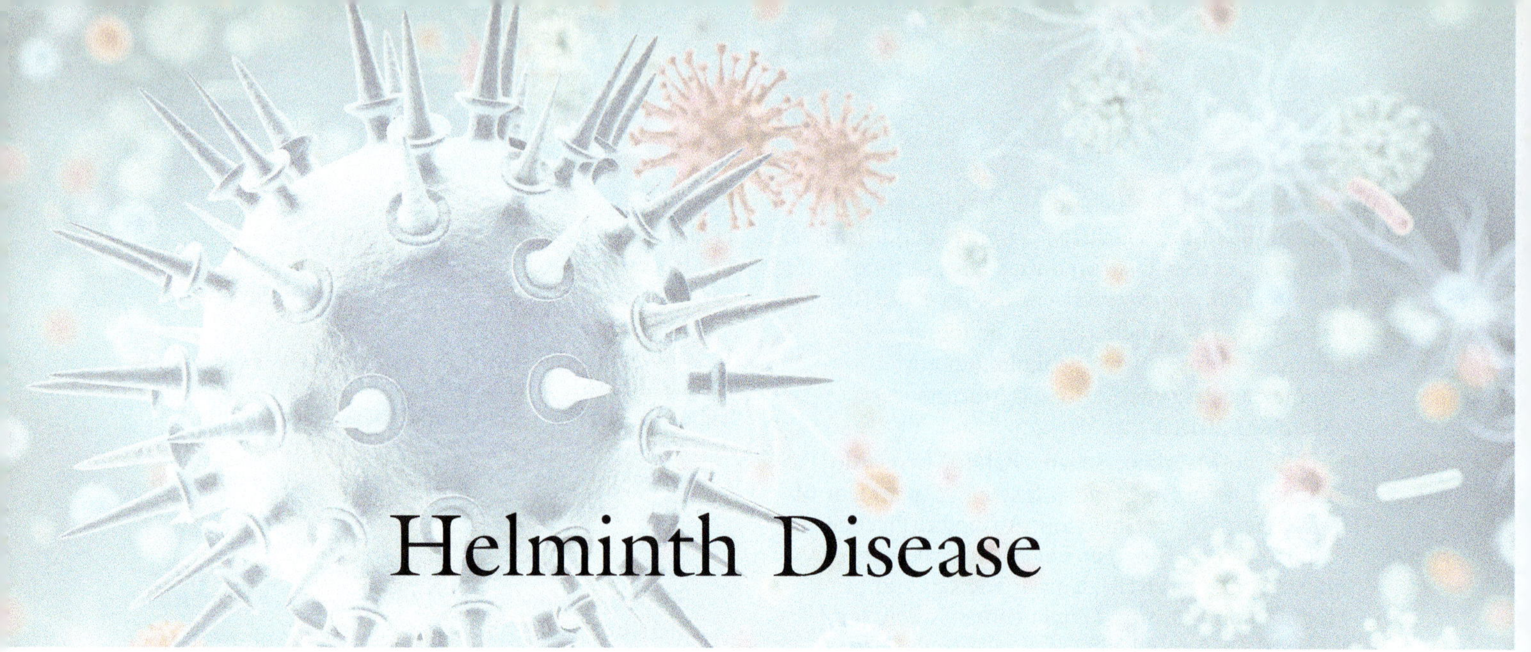

Helminth Disease

■ Introduction

Helminth diseases are caused by parasitic worms known as helminths. Helminths are the most common infectious agent in the developing world. Helminth infections of light intensity typically do not lead to any symptoms. Helminths are categorized into three main categories: roundworms (nematodes), tapeworms (cestodes), and flukes (trematodes). Transmission of helminths typically involves direct contact with the parasite or ingestion of the parasite via contaminated food or water. In some cases the parasites can pass through human skin from infected water or soil.

Symptoms and their severity depend on the type of helminth causing the infection and the overall health of the person infected. While full recovery is possible from some infections, death or debilitating disabilities occur with other infections. Treatment, when possible, usually involves administration of anti-inflammatory drugs alone or in combination with anthelmintic drugs that kill the existing parasites.

Helminths cause human disease worldwide, although climate conditions limit many species of helminths to tropical or semitropical areas. However, with changes in climate, certain infections are becoming widespread. Developing or poverty-stricken countries are heavily affected with helminth diseases. The burden of helminth diseases in these countries is often compounded by lack of education, funding, and additional challenges such as human immunodeficiency virus (HIV) infection, lagging infrastructure, political instability, and war.

WORDS TO KNOW

HELMINTH A representative of various phyla of wormlike animals.

HYGIENE Health practices that minimize the spread of infectious microorganisms between people or between other living things and people. Inanimate objects and surfaces such as contaminated cutlery or a cutting board may be a secondary part of this process.

MORPHOLOGY The study of form and structure of animals and plants. Also, the outward physical form possessed by an organism.

SANITATION The use of hygienic recycling and disposal measures that prevent disease and promote health through sewage disposal, solid waste disposal, waste material recycling, and food processing and preparation.

■ Disease History, Characteristics, and Transmission

Evidence from mummified remains suggests helminths have been present in humans since before recorded history. In addition, early human writings from Egypt, Greece, and the Middle East contain descriptions of what appear to be helminth disease. Helminth infections have since been identified around the world, with a variety of these parasitic worms causing a range of diseases. During the 20th century, study of helminths increased, leading to an increase in the number of recognized helminths, from 28 to more than 300. Study of helminths has also led to a greater understanding of how pervasive helminth infections are and to a fuller picture of how helminth infections are transmitted and how they can be treated.

Most roundworms hatch and live in the intestines. The eggs of roundworms enter the body of the host and travel toward the intestines, where they hatch. Depending on the subtype, the roundworms remain in the intestine or migrate to other regions of the body. Transmission of roundworms occurs when contaminated material enters the body. This could be via ingestion of contaminated food or water, entry of eggs via the anal or genital tracts, or ingestion of (or contact with) contaminated soil. Symptoms of roundworm infection vary depending on the type of worm, such as hookworm, trichinosis, ascariasis, or filariasis.

Some cause general symptoms such as abdominal pain, diarrhea, fatigue, itching, or fever, whereas others can be more specific and may cause damage to certain regions of the body.

The mode of roundworm transmission varies depending on the kind of nematode that infects a person. There are three kinds of roundworm transmission. One kind of roundworm begins life as an egg laid outside a host organism, typically in soil, and matures outside the host before infection. A second kind of roundworm begins life outside a host but completes the maturation process after infecting a host. A third kind of roundworm moves directly from one host to another. Typically, roundworms do not reproduce within a host. As a result, hosts usually only develop symptomatic nematode infections due to extended exposure to roundworms.

Tapeworms generally live in the intestines. Their eggs are normally ingested when meat containing the parasites is undercooked or raw or when water is contaminated with tapeworm larvae or eggs. While symptoms usually do not occur or are mild, some patients experience abdominal pain, fatigue, and diarrhea. The most severe outcomes of tapeworm infection occur when larvae leave the intestines and infect tissue elsewhere in the body, including the brain, forming cysts that can lead to neurological issues such as headaches and even seizures.

Flukes can affect organs including the skin, brain, spleen, liver, lungs, eyes, and intestines. Flukes are classified according to the part of the host they infect. There are blood flukes, liver flukes, lung flukes, eye flukes, intestinal flukes, and pancreatic flukes, among other classifications. Blood flukes, which belong to the *Schistosoma* species, are the most common cause of disease in humans, which is known as schistosomiasis.

The flukes that infect humans are known as digenetic trematodes. They feature two suckers, which they use to adhere to their host. The life cycle of these worms begins in water, where eggs are laid and hatch, releasing larval flukes known as miracidium. Miracidium swim in water and infect snails or aquatic vertebrates such as fish or amphibians, which are required to serve as intermediate hosts. In snails the miracidium develop into a more mature form known as cercariae, which the snails then release into fresh water. This mature fluke larvae can then enter humans via contact with the skin.

Most cases of fluke infection cause mild, acute symptoms, such as blood in urine, abdominal pain, and diarrhea. Typically, the parasites pass out of the body quickly. However, reinfection can occur. If reinfection occurs continuously over time, it can cause damage to body organs. In symptomatic cases infection usually results in a rash, itching, muscle aches, coughing, chills, and fever. Severe infections involve flukes entering the liver, lung, or brain and spinal cord.

■ Scope and Distribution

Helminth diseases occur worldwide. However, different types of infections are present in different regions, depending largely on climate. Some helminths survive only in tropical climates, whereas others require temperate conditions. Regions that are in the midst of conflict or have low sanitation standards have a high prevalence of infection. Poverty-stricken countries in the developing world, located in Africa, China, East Asia, and the Americas, account for most of the world's helminth infections.

However, some infections of helminths are common in developed countries. For example, infection by the pinworm, a nematode that causes itching, is common in temperate areas such as Western Europe and North America. High infection rates are recorded for these regions. The CDC reported in 2013 that infection rates of children under age 18, their caregivers, and people who live in institutions may be as high as 50 percent. Despite its large prevalence in the temperate zone, this infection is rare in the tropics.

According to Peter J. Hotez and his colleagues in a 2008 article in the *Journal of Clinical Investigation*, hel-

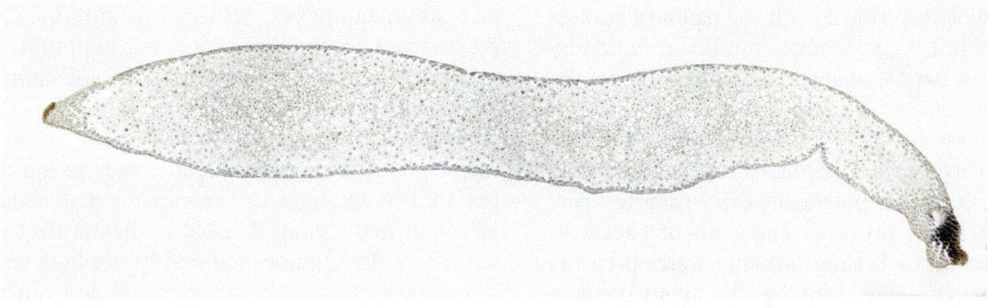

A light micrograph shows a roundworm, one of the three main kinds of helminth parasites that cause a range of diseases, most commonly in developing tropical and subtropical countries. *© Science Stock Photography/Science Source*

Helminth Life Cycles

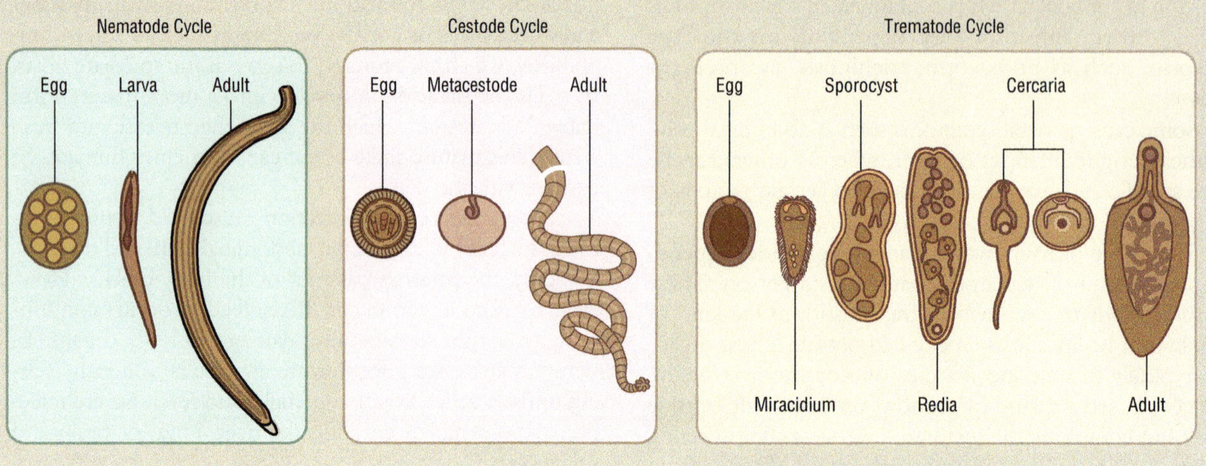

minths "are the most common infectious agents of humans in developing countries and produce a global burden of disease that exceeds better-known conditions, including malaria and tuberculosis." While it is impossible to know exactly how many people are infected with helminths, Christine Dubray noted in the *CDC Yellow Book 2018* that a "large part of the world's population is infected with 1 or more ... helminths." According to the World Health Organization (WHO), as of 2017 nearly a quarter of the world's population was infected with soil-transmitted helminths, which were the cause of most of the world's helminth disease burden.

Treatment and Prevention

Because a wide variety of helminths cause disease in humans, there is no universal treatment for helminth infection. However, most infections can be treated with vermifuges, which are antiworm drugs that effectively kill parasitic worms. In addition, while some helminth infections can be cured within a short period, others may take months or years to heal. In some cases patients are left with debilitating disabilities due to organ and limb damage.

There are several ways to prevent infection from helminths. First, avoiding contact with the parasites ensures that infection does not occur. Contact can be prevented by frequent washing of hands, maintaining a clean bathroom and kitchen, avoiding contact with infected animals, and wearing shoes when walking in areas where soil-transmitted helminths are known to be present. Furthermore, thorough cooking of foods that potentially carry parasites, particularly pork and beef, prevents ingestion of parasites. Chlorinating, filtering, or boiling drinking water prevents ingestion of parasites while drinking. To avoid parasite uptake while bathing or swimming in infected water, a problem particularly for fluke parasites, water can be boiled prior to bathing or avoided completely.

Another way to prevent infection is to lower the prevalence of helminths within a community. This is achieved through regular deworming, or mass administration of antiworm treatments to infected people. This can effectively reduce the long-term effects of the parasites on infected people, as well as reduce the prevalence of the parasite within a community.

To effectively implement prevention methods, communities affected by helminth infestations rely on education about hygiene, sanitation, and proper food preparation. Together with helminth treatments, these methods help reduce the prevalence of helminth infections.

Impacts and Issues

Parasitic infections are a worldwide issue. Millions of people become infected by helminths every year. Although knowledge about helminths is increasing, the prevalence of infections is also increasing.

One reason helminth infections are on the rise is the spread of HIV and acquired immunodeficiency syndrome (AIDS), which causes decreased immunity in infected people. This makes them more susceptible to infection by emerging parasites, which take advantage of weakened immune systems. Furthermore, existing helminth infections take advantage of people with low immunity and have increased as a result. This problem compounds when countries with a high prevalence of HIV infection also have a high prevalence of helminth infection.

Helminth invasion into new areas has also become a major contributor to global increases in infection. This is initiated by changes in the climate that make previously helminth-free regions suitable for helminths to survive and reproduce. In addition, war and its resulting social upheaval cause lower standards of sanitation and nutrition, which lead to reemergence of helminth infections in some populations. Helminth resistance to antiworm drugs has also caused issues in controlling and treating infections.

The US Centers for Disease Control and Prevention (CDC) estimated in 2016 that 780 million people worldwide lacked access to clean drinking water, and 2.5 billion people did not have access to improved sanitation. Water polluted by sewage, refuse, and agricultural by-products such as manure spreads some helminths. Several international organizations help communities build wells, water purification stations, and sewage collection systems.

Helminth diseases are most likely to strike children, especially in the developing world, causing malnutrition and illness. Malnutrition during childhood has lifelong effects on an estimated 155 million children worldwide, from increased rates of illness and stagnated development to disability and premature death. Thus, WHO, in partnership with the United Nations Children's Fund (UNICEF), focuses its antihelminth efforts on children and schools. In areas where helminths thrive in local water or soil, efforts to curb helminth diseases include food safety, hygiene, and sanitation education, as well as the widespread administration of anthelmintic drugs. Such comprehensive public health measures have reduced incidence of helminth diseases in parts of Indonesia by as much as 50 percent.

Several world leaders serve as advocates for international cooperative antihelminth efforts, including former US president Jimmy Carter (1924–), former Mali president Amadou Toumani Touré (1948–), and former Nigerian head of state Yakubu Gowon (1934–). The Carter Center's International Task Force for Disease Eradication, with support from the Bill & Melinda Gates Foundation, sponsors antihelminth programs with the aim of eradicating dracunculiasis (guinea worm disease) and lymphatic filariasis across the globe, eradicating onchocerciasis (river blindness) in the Americas, and controlling schistosomiasis.

While much of the research into helminths concerns stopping their transmission and treating people with infections, some scientists have begun to study the potential benefits of helminth infections. As Kate Baggelay noted in a 2017 article in *Popular Science*, various "researchers are investigating whether intestinal worms might be able to treat autoimmune and inflammatory conditions, from celiac disease to autism to allergies. The idea behind this experimental worm therapy is that squirmy creatures called helminths evolved alongside us and actually benefit our immune system." As of 2018, however, clinical trials were inconclusive about the effectiveness of using worms for therapeutic purposes.

See Also *AIDS (Acquired Immunodeficiency Syndrome); Bilharzia (Schistosomiasis); Climate Change and Infectious Disease; Dracunculiasis; Emerging Infectious Diseases; Handwashing; HIV; Hookworm (Ancylostoma) Infection; Liver Fluke Infections; Lung Fluke (Paragonimus) Infection; Opportunistic Infection; Pinworm (Enterobius vermicularis) Infection; River Blindness (Onchocerciasis); Roundworm (Ascariasis) Infection; Sanitation; Tapeworm Infections; War and Infectious Disease; Waterborne Disease*

BIBLIOGRAPHY

Books

Crompton, David William Thomasson, et al. *Controlling Disease Due to Helminth Infections.* Geneva: World Health Organization, 2003.

Dubray, Christine. "Helminths, Soil-Transmitted." In *CDC Yellow Book 2018: Health Information for International Travel.* Oxford, UK: Oxford University Press, 2017.

Macpherson, Calum N. L., and Philip S. Craig. *Parasitic Helminths and Zoonoses in Africa.* New York: Springer, 1991.

Periodicals

Baggelay, Kate. "Scientists Are Trying to Treat Autoimmune Disease with Intestinal Worms." *Popular Science* (July 28, 2017). This article can also be found online at https://www.popsci.com/can-intestinal-worms-treat-autoimmune-disease (accessed December 19, 2017).

Bartsch, Sarah M., et al. "The Global Economic and Health Burden of Hookworm Infection." *PLOS Neglected Tropical Diseases* 10, no. 9 (September 8, 2016). This article can also be found online at http://journals.plos.org/plosntds/article?id=10.1371/journal.pntd.0004922 (accessed December 19, 2017).

Hotez, Peter J. "Helminth Infections: The Great Neglected Tropical Diseases." *Journal of Clinical Investigation* 118, no. 4 (April 2008): 1311–1321. This article can also be found online at https://www.ncbi.nlm.nih.gov/pmc/articles/PMC2276811/ (accessed December 19, 2017).

Websites

"Enterobiasis (Also Known as Pinworm Infection): Epidemiology & Risk Factors." Centers for Disease Control and Prevention, January 10, 2013. https://www.cdc.gov/parasites/pinworm/epi.html (accessed March 10, 2018).

"Global WASH Fast Facts." Centers for Disease Control and Prevention, April 11, 2016. https://www.cdc.gov/healthywater/global/wash_statistics.html (accessed January 31, 2018).

"Helminth Parasites." Australian Society of Parasitology. http://parasite.org.au/para-site/contents/helminth-intoduction.html (accessed January 29, 2017).

"Soil-Transmitted Helminth Infections." World Health Organization, September 2017. http://www.who.int/mediacentre/factsheets/fs366/en/ (accessed January 29, 2018).

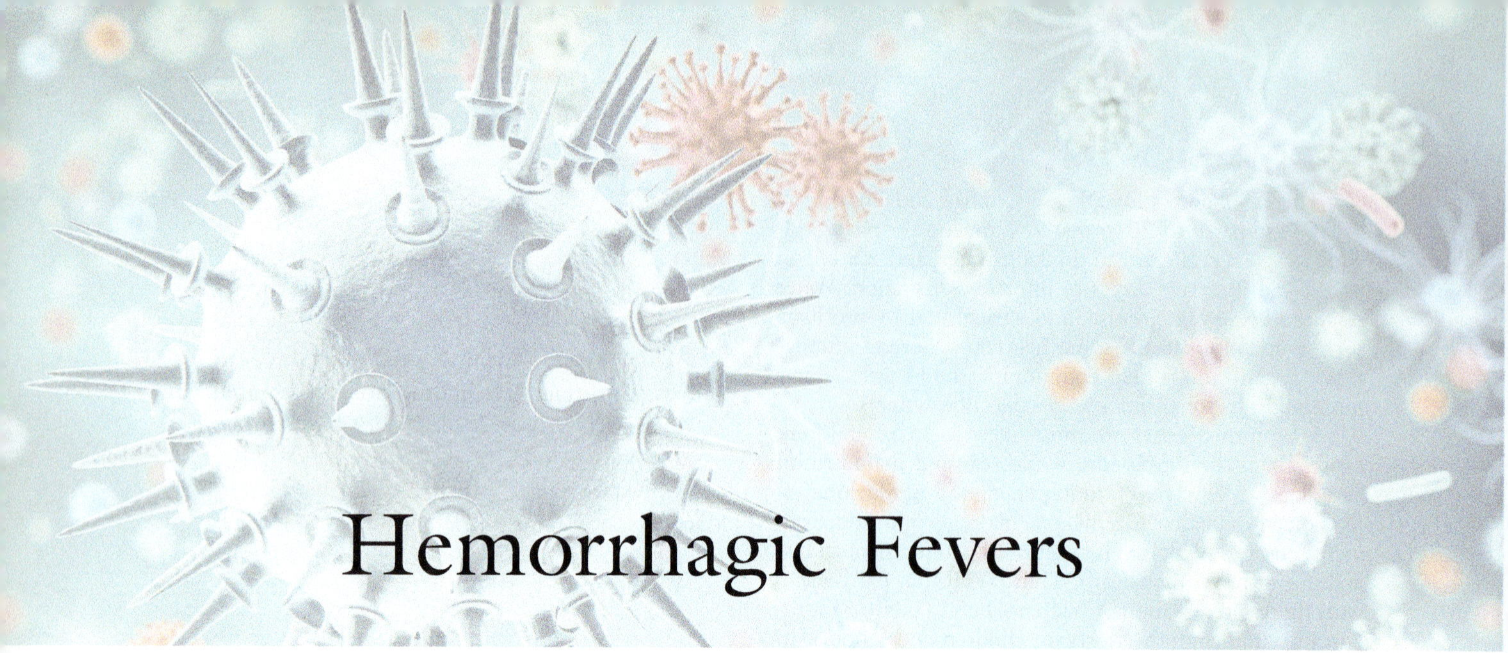

Hemorrhagic Fevers

Introduction

Hemorrhagic diseases are caused by infection with certain viruses and, rarely, bacteria. A central feature of hemorrhagic fevers, as implied by their name, is hemorrhage, or severe and uncontrolled bleeding. This uncontrolled bleeding is caused by the destruction of cells inside the body as the virus makes new copies of itself.

Hemorrhagic fevers are terrifying to those affected, those attempting to care for the sick, and those who read about or watch images of an outbreak. Hemorrhagic infections cause symptoms that appear and progress swiftly. Because outbreaks of hemorrhagic fever appear and sweep through a population very rapidly before disappearing, little is known of the details of the various viral infections.

WORDS TO KNOW

BIOSAFETY LEVEL 4 FACILITY A specialized biosafety laboratory that deals with dangerous or exotic infectious agents or biohazards that are considered high risks for spreading life-threatening diseases, either because the disease is spread through aerosols or because there is no therapy or vaccine to counter the disease.

HEMORRHAGE Very severe, massive bleeding that is difficult to control.

MYALGIA Muscular aches and pain.

ZOONOTIC A disease that can be transmitted between animals and humans. Examples of zoonotic diseases are anthrax, plague, and Q fever.

Disease History, Characteristics, and Transmission

Hemorrhagic diseases are mainly caused by viruses. They are also known collectively as viral hemorrhagic fevers (VHFs). Bacterial hemorrhagic infections are rare, but one example of such a disease is scrub typhus.

Viral hemorrhagic fevers are caused by viruses in four groups: arenaviruses, filoviruses, bunyaviruses, and flaviviruses. Arenaviruses are a family of RNA viruses (their genetic material is not composed of DNA, only RNA) that are associated with human diseases transmitted by rodents. They cause a number of hemorrhagic fevers, including Lassa fever (caused by the Lassa virus), Argentine hemorrhagic fever (caused by the Junin virus), Bolivian hemorrhagic fever (caused by the Machupo virus), Venezuelan hemorrhagic fever (caused by the Guananto virus), and Brazilian hemorrhagic fever (caused by the Sabia virus).

The first arenavirus was isolated in 1933 during an investigation into an outbreak of St. Louis encephalitis. The virus was found not to be the cause of the outbreak, but the severity of the health threat was revealed. The limited studies that have been done in the intervening decades (studies are limited because of the great danger in working with the viruses) have shown that arenaviruses are typically transmitted to humans via animals such as rodents. These viruses are characterized as zoonotic, which means they reside in another host (a wild or domesticated animal) but are capable of causing disease when transmitted to humans.

Bunyaviruses are a family of RNA viruses associated with rodent- or insect-borne diseases in humans. Viruses in this family are known to cause Crimean-Congo hemorrhagic fever, Rift Valley fever, and hantavirus pulmonary syndrome. Congo-Crimean fever, a disease known for many years in Eastern Europe and Central Asia, is caused by a virus that is transmitted to humans and a variety of domestic and wild animals by ticks. Humans can become infected when they come into close contact with infected

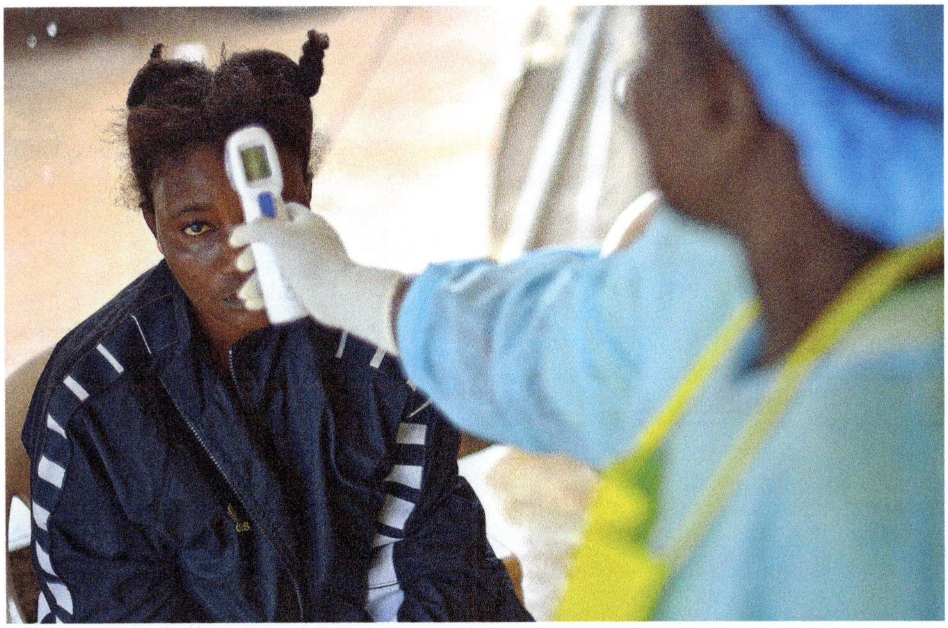

A government hospital worker in Sierra Leone checks the temperature of a girl suspected of having contracted the Ebola virus, which is one of various causes of deadly hemorrhagic fever. © CARL DE SOUZA/AFP/Getty Images

cattle, and slaughterhouses have been involved in disease outbreaks. Rift Valley fever is generally found in areas of eastern and southern Africa where cattle and sheep are raised. The virus responsible for the disease primarily affects livestock, but humans can also contract the disease when they are bitten by mosquitoes infected with the virus or when they come into contact with the blood or body parts of infected animals. Hantavirus disease is transmitted to humans mainly through the inhalation of aerosolized virus particles from dried mouse feces. Investigation of a disease outbreak that occurred in the United States in 1993 determined that a virus called the Sin Nombre virus (a type of hantavirus) was a cause. Another virus, Hantaan virus, causes hantavirus pulmonary syndrome. This virus was isolated during an investigation of a disease outbreak that occurred in the 1950s near the Hantan River in Korea.

Filoviruses cause severe hemorrhagic diseases in humans and other primates, including Ebola hemorrhagic fever and Marburg hemorrhagic fever. Flaviviruses cause a wide range of human diseases, including tick-borne encephalitis, yellow fever, dengue hemorrhagic fever, Kyasanur Forest disease, and Omsk hemorrhagic fever. Depending on the virus, the disease may be transmitted to humans via rodents, ticks, and mosquitoes. In some cases, such as Ebola, bats are the suspected natural reservoir of the virus. The Ebola outbreak that began in 2014 involved 15,227 laboratory-confirmed cases and 11,310 deaths. Initially, the outbreak spread rapidly. With time and with the mobilization of relief and medical aid from nations including the United States, the outbreak was contained. The 2014 outbreak was also noteworthy for the clinical trial of an Ebola vaccine that demonstrated effectiveness in protecting people from infection. As of 2017, however, the vaccine was not licensed for use.

The various viral hemorrhagic viruses differ in structure. For example, arenaviruses are spherical, while filoviruses, such as Marburg virus, may be U-shaped, O-shaped, or even shaped like the number 6. Although these hemorrhagic viruses differ, they share some common features. For example, they all contain ribonucleic acid (RNA) as their genetic material. In addition, humans are not their normal host. While the viruses can live without severely affecting natural hosts, such as cattle, the infection caused in humans is severe. This is the primary reason that human outbreaks of hemorrhagic fever disappear so rapidly. The high death rate makes it impossible for the virus to persist in a human population for very long once an outbreak has been recognized and treatment measures, such as isolation of those who are infected, are initiated.

Most hemorrhagic viruses share another feature in common. Once a human is infected, he or she can transfer the virus to other people, often via contaminated body fluids. Caregivers can become infected in this way. This transmission can occur in a hospital or clinic. Such hospital-acquired infections are called nosocomial infections.

While the various viral hemorrhagic fevers have their own distinct symptoms, they share some symptoms and a pattern of symptoms over time. The diseases typically begin with a sudden fever, a general feeling of fatigue, myalgia, dizziness, pain and stiffness in the neck and back, diarrhea, and severe headache (which can be so bad that a person becomes nauseated and vomits and becomes very sensitive to light). Some people recover, and recovery can be as

SCIENTIFIC QUESTIONS

Ebola virus and Marburg virus are the two known members of the filovirus family that cause hemorrhagic fevers. Ebola viruses were first isolated from humans during concurrent outbreaks of viral hemorrhagic fever (VHF) in northern Zaire and southern Sudan in 1976. An earlier outbreak of VHF caused by Marburg virus occurred in Marburg, Germany, in 1967 when laboratory workers were exposed to infected tissue from monkeys imported from Uganda. Two subtypes of Ebola virus (Ebola-Sudan and Ebola-Zaire) previously were associated with disease in humans. In 1994 a single case of infection from a newly described Ebola virus occurred in a person in Côte d'Ivoire. In 1989 an outbreak among monkeys imported into the United States from the Philippines was caused by another Ebola virus but was not associated with human disease.

Initial clinical manifestations of Ebola hemorrhagic fever include fever, headache, chills, myalgia (muscle aches throughout the body), and malaise. Subsequent manifestations include severe abdominal pain, vomiting, and diarrhea. In reported outbreaks between 50 percent and 90 percent of cases have been fatal.

The natural reservoir for these viruses is suspected to be the fruit bat. Transmission of the virus to secondary cases occurs through close personal contact with infectious blood or other body fluids or tissue. In previous outbreaks, secondary cases occurred among people who provided medical care for patients. Secondary cases also occurred among patients exposed to reused needles. Although aerosol spread has not been documented among humans, this mode of transmission has been demonstrated among nonhuman primates. Based on this information, the high fatality rate, and lack of a specific treatment or vaccine, laboratory work with this virus requires biosafety level 4 containment.

rapid as the onset of the disease. Others deteriorate further and begin to hemorrhage from the mouth, eyes, and ears. This bleeding is the external manifestation of the massive bleeding that is occurring inside the body as various organs become infected. In the final stages of hemorrhagic fever, organs fail and the nervous system breaks down, leading to coma, seizures, and death.

■ Scope and Distribution

The filoviruses that cause Marburg hemorrhagic fever and Ebola are found in various regions of Africa. Three of the four known species of Ebola are named for the regions in which they were first discovered: Ivory Coast, Sudan, and Zaire.

The occurrence of viral hemorrhagic fevers in areas as widespread as Korea, Arizona, and Africa highlight the global distribution of the virus that causes hemorrhagic fevers. However, particular viruses may be more localized. For example, the viruses that cause Ebola appear to be localized to a few regions in Africa. However, because so little is still known about viral hemorrhagic fevers in 2017, it is possible that the true distribution of the various viruses is not yet known.

■ Treatment and Prevention

Hemorrhagic diseases are difficult to treat because outbreaks occur quickly, often in remote regions of the world. The speed and ferocity of the infection often means that patients are near death by the time they are seen by a health care provider. Vaccines are available only for yellow fever and Argentine hemorrhagic fever. For the remaining hemorrhagic fevers, the best prevention is to avoid contact with animals that are known hosts of the particular virus. However, in many cases a population has little knowledge of the infections and their exposure risks, making prevention virtually impossible. One exception is hantavirus pulmonary syndrome in the United States. This disease has been well publicized, and many people are aware that it is spread by rodents. When insects are involved in the transmission of a virus, spraying programs that kill insect populations, especially during their breeding season, can be helpful.

When combating an outbreak, isolating infected patients from other patients can help reduce the spread of the disease. In addition, all protective clothing and soiled material used in patient treatment should be stored in a secure container until it can be destroyed (usually by incineration).

■ Impacts and Issues

As of 2017 little is known about hemorrhagic fevers. One reason for this lack of knowledge is that the infections are very difficult to study during an outbreak. Health care providers faced with an outbreak struggle to mount a quick and efficient response that can save lives. Sometimes cultural norms and taboos in remote regions hinder efforts to contain outbreaks and study their cause. For instance, during the 2005 Ebola outbreak, medical workers from United Nations (UN) aid agencies arrived at the scene wearing white protective biohazard suits and were met with skepticism and hostility, as the color white is associated with evil in the remote village where the outbreak first occurred. Also, the custom of handling the body of a deceased person before burial can be difficult to prevent and likely contributes to the spread of the virus from the body to the unprotected person handling the body.

Viral hemorrhagic fevers can only be studied in a few specialized laboratories known as biosafety level 4 (BSL-4) laboratories. These laboratories are designed with safety and containment features that make it safe for researchers to work with the viruses and prevent escape of the viruses from the lab. In BSL-4 laboratories hemorrhagic fevers are studied in a high-containment environment, where incoming and outgoing airflow is controlled and where researchers wear protective clothing that includes one-piece positive pressure suits with separate ventilation systems. Protocols for studying the viruses that cause hemorrhagic fevers include restricted access to the laboratory, working under Class III biological safety cabinets, and decontamination following work with the virus. As of 2017 there were 50 BSL-4 laboratories in the world, with the majority in the United Kingdom, Europe, and the United States.

See Also *Ebola; Marburg Hemorrhagic Fever*

BIBLIOGRAPHY

Books

Quammen, David. *Ebola: The Natural and Human History of a Deadly Virus.* New York: Norton, 2014.

Richards, Paul. *Ebola: How a People's Science Helped End an Epidemic.* London: Zed, 2016.

Shah, Sonia. *Pandemic: Tracking Contagions, from Cholera to Ebola and Beyond.* New York: Sarah Crichton Books/Farrar, Straus and Giroux, 2016.

Periodicals

Regules, Jason A., et al. "A Recombinant Vesicular Stomatitis Virus Ebola Vaccine." *New England Journal of Medicine* 376 (2017): 330–341.

Websites

"*Haemophilus influenzae* Disease (Including Hib)." Centers for Disease Control and Prevention. https://www.cdc.gov/hi-disease/index.html (accessed November 17, 2017).

"Haemorrhagic Fevers, Viral." World Health Organization. http://www.who.int/topics/haemorrhagic_fevers_viral/en (accessed November 17, 2017).

"Hib Initiative: A GAVI Success Story." Global Alliance for Vaccines and Immunization. http://www.gavi.org/library/news/roi/2010/hib-initiative--a-gavi-success-story/ (accessed November 17, 2017).

Brian Hoyle

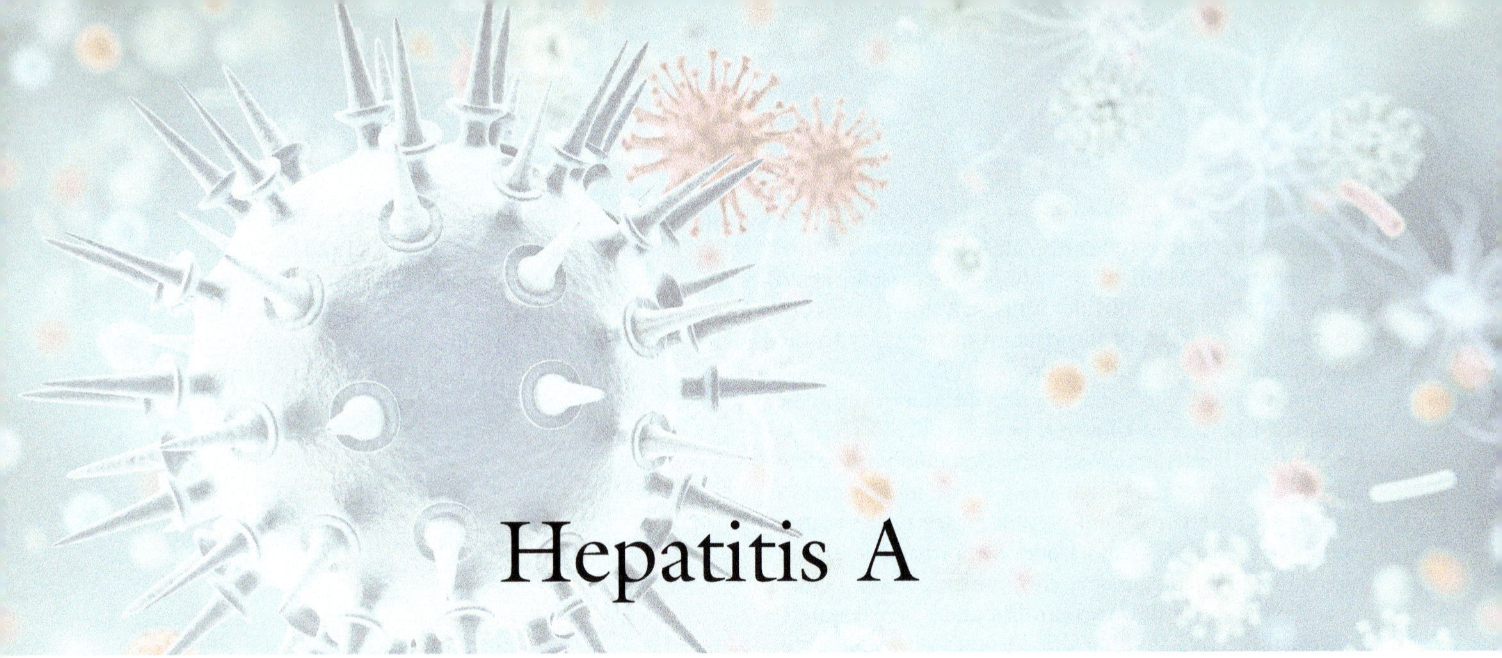

Hepatitis A

■ Introduction

Hepatitis is an inflammation of the liver that can be caused by exposure to chemicals (including alcohol) or by any one of six hepatitis viruses. Hepatitis A infection, which was formerly known as infectious hepatitis, is caused by the Hepatitis A virus (HAV). HAV was discovered in the early 1970s in the stool of a patient incubating the disease. Hepatitis A is primarily contracted through oral contact with the feces of a person carrying HAV. Such fecal-oral contact often occurs via food or water contaminated with HAV-positive fecal matter, via sexual activity, or via intravenous drug use.

Hepatitis A is an acute disease, with symptoms including nausea, malaise, diarrhea, and enlarged liver. Some infected people, particularly children, have no symptoms. Unlike other forms of hepatitis, it does not progress to chronic disease, which damages the liver. Typically, symptoms of hepatitis A pass within two months, without treatment, though some are affected for up to six months.

Hepatitis A has been on the decline in developed countries since the 1970s, although epidemics still occur, especially under conditions of overcrowding and poor hygiene. It is still a risk to travelers, as HAV can be spread through certain foods that have been in contact with contaminated water. Those at risk can be protected through vaccination against HAV.

WORDS TO KNOW

FECAL-ORAL ROUTE The transmission of minute particles of fecal material from one organism (human or animal) to the mouth of another organism.

IMMUNE GLOBULIN Globulins are a type of protein found in blood. Immune globulins (also called immunoglobulins) are Y-shaped globulins that act as antibodies, attaching themselves to invasive cells or materials in the body so that they can be identified and attacked by the immune system. There are five immune globulins, designated IgM, IgG, IgA, IgD, and IgE.

INACTIVATED VIRUS A virus that is incapable of causing disease but still stimulates the immune system to respond by forming antibodies.

JAUNDICE A condition in which a person's skin and the whites of the eyes are discolored a shade of yellow due to an increased level of bile pigments in the blood, resulting from liver disease. Sometimes called icterus, from a Greek word for the condition.

RNA VIRUS A virus whose genetic material consists of either single- or double-stranded ribonucleic acid (RNA) rather than deoxyribonucleic acid (DNA).

■ Disease History, Characteristics, and Transmission

Hepatitis A is a single-stranded RNA virus unrelated to the other hepatitis viruses. During its average incubation time of 28 days, it first infects the intestines and then passes through the blood into the liver. The onset of symptoms, such as nausea, loss of appetite, diarrhea, and fever, is acute. A person with hepatitis A may have an enlarged liver with pain and tenderness in the upper-right abdomen. Many people later develop jaundice, a yellowing of the skin and eyes resulting from liver inflammation. An individual's urine may be dark, and stools a pale clay color.

The vast majority of cases of hepatitis A clear up within a week or so, although 15 percent are prolonged and relapse over a period of months. The disease does not, however, become chronic like hepatitis B and hepatitis C. Between 0.3 and 1.5 percent of HAV infections prove fatal, usually due to liver failure. Factors that increase the likelihood of mortality include coinfection with hepatitis B or hepatitis C, advanced age, and being female. Hepatitis A is transmitted through the fecal-oral route, commonly through eating seafood or raw fruits, or vegetables that have come into contact with water contaminated with infected sewage.

Scope and Distribution

Adults are more likely than children to develop symptoms of hepatitis A. Household and sexual partners of those with hepatitis A are at elevated risk of contracting the disease, as are men who have sex with men and both injecting and non-injecting drug users. Epidemics of hepatitis A are fairly common in institutions such as prisons and nursing homes and among those of low socioeconomic status living in overcrowded conditions.

According to data from the Centers for Disease Control and Prevention (CDC), there were 1,390 reported US cases of hepatitis A in 2015. (The CDC estimated that, in fact, there were 2,800 new HAV infections that year due to unreported cases.) Although the reported cases represent a 12.2 percent increase from the previous year, hepatitis A cases have declined precipitously over the course of the early 21st century. However, the CDC and other health agencies continue to confront new outbreaks. In 2016 and 2017, for example, hepatitis A outbreaks in the United States were traced to raw scallops, frozen strawberries, homelessness, and drug use.

Despite such outbreaks, hepatitis A is on the decline throughout the developed world. For residents of such countries, hepatitis A most often represents a risk for those who are traveling into less developed countries where the disease remains common. In developing countries up to 90 percent of children under the age of 10 have been infected with HAV, according to the World Health Organization (WHO). Infection rates are highest in areas where sanitary conditions and hygienic practices are poor.

Treatment and Prevention

There is no definitive treatment for hepatitis A, and often the disease resolves with adequate nutrition and rest. Those at risk of infection can be given either immune serum globulin, prepared from pooled plasma, or a vaccine against hepatitis A (or both). There are two hepatitis A vaccines, both made of inactivated virus. One protects against hepatitis A only; the other is a combined hepatitis A and hepatitis B vaccine. As of 2016 16 countries routinely immunized children against HAV, according to WHO. In addition to vaccinating children, some governmental organizations recommend that at-risk populations (such as drug users, men who have sex with men, those with chronic liver disease, and travelers to countries with high rates of infection) receive vaccines. Studies of the efficacy of HAV vaccines have found them to be highly effective, with efficacy rates found to be as high as 100 percent.

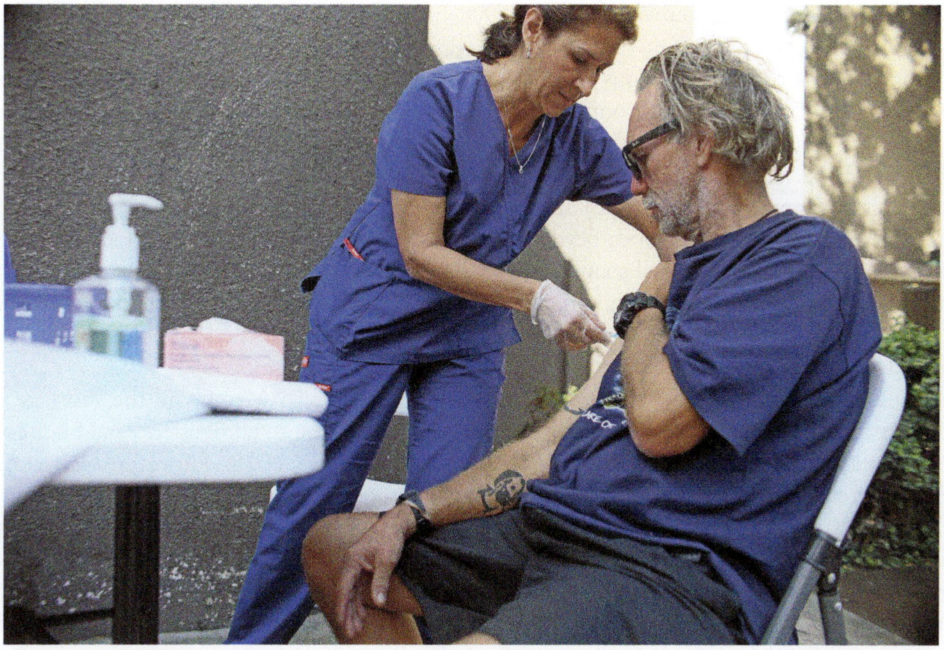

During a 2017 hepatitis A outbreak within the San Diego, California, homeless community, a nurse gives a man a vaccine against the liver disease. © *Sandy Huffaker/The Washington Post/Getty Images*

Impacts and Issues

People travel more widely in the 21st century than ever before, which means they may be exposed to diseases they otherwise would not be. For travelers, hepatitis A is the most common preventable infection. The extent of the risk depends on the length of stay, the living conditions in the place visited, and the level of hepatitis A in the country visited. In general, the risk of contracting hepatitis A is low in North America (except Mexico), New Zealand, Australia, and developed European countries. However, epidemics still occur even on standard tourist itineraries. Travelers to other places are advised to check out the latest information for the area from public health departments and the CDC.

In destinations where high standards of hygiene and sanitation may be lacking, it is recommended to stick to bottled water and avoid ice, seafood, raw fruits and vegetables, and foods sold by street vendors. Personal hygiene, such as thorough handwashing after using the bathroom and before eating or preparing food, can also prevent transmission of HAV.

Despite food safety measures, outbreaks of hepatitis A sometimes occur wherever food is prepared and served. In February 2007 an employee at a well-known catering company in Los Angeles, California, was diagnosed with hepatitis A, sparking an investigation into events the company had catered during the concurrent Hollywood entertainment industry awards season. Health authorities contacted several celebrities and movie industry executives, recommending immune globulin injections to prevent hepatitis A infection after they were possibly exposed to the disease by food served during the festivities.

In August 2016 an outbreak of HAV infections began in southeastern Michigan. As of early 2018, the outbreak had led to 677 cases, 81.5 percent of which resulted in hospitalization. In addition, 22 had died from infection. According to the Michigan Department of Health and Human Services, "No common sources of food, beverages, or drugs have been identified as a potential source of infection. Transmission appears to be through direct person-to-person spread and illicit drug use. Those with history of injection and non-injection drug use, homelessness or transient housing, and incarceration are thought to be at greater risk in this outbreak setting." Beginning in November 2016, Southern California also suffered an HAV outbreak, with 688 reported cases, 449 hospitalizations, and 21 deaths as of early 2018. According to the CDC, infections were being transmitted from person to person rather than via contaminated food or drug use. The outbreak in California also spread to Utah and other southwestern states.

These outbreaks led to an increased demand for the HAV vaccine, which created a shortage of the vaccine's supply. According to a 2018 CNN story, manufacturers of the HAV vaccine aimed to prioritize delivery of the vaccine to high-risk populations and to increase production.

PRIMARY SOURCE

Michigan hit hard by deadly hepatitis A outbreak

SOURCE: *LaMotte, Sandee. "Michigan Hit Hard by Deadly Hepatitis A Outbreak. CNN, January 16, 2018. http://www.cnn.com/2018/01/11/health/hepatitis-a-outbreak-michigan-bn/index.html (accessed February 2, 2018).*

INTRODUCTION: *This article from CNN describes the challenges recent outbreaks of hepatitis A in the United States have posed to health officials and HAV-vaccine manufacturers.*

Hepatitis A outbreaks have hit several states across the country, killing dozens of people and potentially sickening thousands. Michigan has been hardest-hit in terms of deaths, with 22.

The outbreak there began in August 2016 and, after a dropoff during the winter, continued to climb last year, according to the Michigan Department of Health and Human Services.

"We currently have 677 cases in Michigan and continue to see approximately 15–20 cases matching into the cluster every week," Lynn Sutfin, spokeswoman for the Michigan Department of Health and Human Services, wrote in an email. "The Michigan outbreak now includes 15 different county jurisdictions. We believe that person-to-person transmission is the primary route of infection."

Fighting the outbreak was challenging in some jurisdictions due to a national shortage of the vaccine for hepatitis A.

"Vaccine supply is still 'constrained,'" Sutfin wrote. "We continue to prioritize vaccine to the highest risk individuals that have been identified and focus our vaccination efforts in the parts of the state who are experiencing the largest number of cases."

Vaccine supplier Merck said the shortage of prefilled syringes, the easiest to administer, would not ease until the second quarter of 2018. However, vials containing 10 single doses are available.

"The company is taking steps to continue to increase our capacity to meet demand globally in 2018," Merck spokeswoman Pamela Eisele wrote in an email. "We apologize for any inconvenience this supply availability may be causing."

The only other vaccine maker, GlaxoSmithKline, said it has adult hepatitis A vaccine in prefilled syringes is in stock and is "working diligently to increase our supply." The company is also working closely with the US Centers for Disease Control and Prevention, spokeswoman Robin Gaitens wrote in an email, to ensure that its vaccines "are directed to areas of greatest need."

California epicenter: San Diego

In California, the outbreak can be traced to transient camps and illicit drug users in San Diego, officials say. Now, the state is in the middle of the biggest person-to-person outbreak of hepatitis A since the vaccine first became available in the mid-'90s, according to the California Department of Public Health. Though the virus has spread across the state, San Diego has seen the most deaths: 21, out of a reported 686 cases.

Officials say movement among the homeless population has also spread the virus to Utah, Arizona and Colorado. Cases of hepatitis A in Colorado doubled in 2017, specifically among "gay, bisexual and other men who have sex with unvaccinated men," said health officials. However, only one of those cases was linked to San Diego, according to Shannon Barbare of the Colorado Disease Control and Environmental Epidemiology Division, and the outbreak now appears to be over.

Over the weekend, officials in Utah announced a new outbreak at a convenience store in Salt Lake County that can be traced to San Diego.

"We have 97 outbreak-related cases in our county," Salt Lake County Health Department spokesman Nicholas Rupp said, adding that those cases were tied to a worker at a 7-Eleven who tested positive for the same strain of the virus as that in San Diego. "We are seeing similar hospitalization rates as San Diego, about 60%, but we have fortunately not seen any deaths."

Just south of Salt Lake, workers at two Utah County restaurants also tested positive for the virus in late December.

"In Utah, we don't require vaccinations for food workers against hepatitis A, but we are encouraging everyone who handles food to be vaccinated, and this is why," Rupp said. "And everyone should practice handwashing after being in public places to protect themselves from exposure."

Consumers who used the restroom at or ate at the two restaurants are at risk, health officials said, and those who visited the 7-Eleven and consumed any self-serve beverage, fresh fruit or items from the hot food case, such as pizza, hot dogs or chicken wings, may have been exposed. Packaged foods are not affected, according to the Health Department.

Rupp said the Salt Lake County Health Department has fielded hundreds of phone calls since it announced the 7-Eleven exposure Sunday and referred about 70% of those callers for vaccination.

"If they receive the vaccine within 14 days of exposure, the vaccine will act as a preventative to the virus," Rupp said, adding that exposure could only have occurred December 26 through January 3.

The state of Utah has confirmed 152 total cases as part of this outbreak; no deaths have been reported.

SEE ALSO *Food-Borne Disease and Food Safety; Hepatitis B; Hepatitis C; Travel and Infectious Disease*

BIBLIOGRAPHY

Books

Achord, James L. *Understanding Hepatitis.* Oxford: University of Mississippi Press, 2002.

Horn, Lyle W. *Deadly Diseases and Epidemics: Hepatitis.* Philadelphia: Chelsea House, 2005.

Periodicals

Delzo, Janissa. "Utah Hit by National Hepatitis Outbreak That Has Left 41 Dead in California and Michigan." *Newsweek* (November 30, 2017). This article can also be found online at http://www.newsweek.com/utah-hit-national-hepatitis-outbreak-which-has-left-41-dead-california-and-727616 (accessed January 22, 2018).

Ishak, Kamal, et al. "Histological Grading and Staging of Chronic Hepatitis." *Journal of Hepatology* 22, no. 6 (1995): 696–699.

Websites

"Hepatitis A." World Health Organization, July 2017. http://www.who.int/mediacentre/factsheets/fs328/en/ (accessed January 22, 2018).

LaMotte, Sandee. "During a Hepatitis A Emergency, There's a Nationwide Shortage of Vaccine." CNN, January 12, 2018. http://www.cnn.com/2017/11/15/health/hepatitis-a-outbreak-vaccine-shortage/index.html (accessed January 22, 2018).

"Michigan Hepatitis A Outbreak." Michigan Department of Health and Human Services, January 17, 2018. http://www.michigan.gov/mdhhs/0,5885,7-339-71550_2955_2976_82305_82310-447907--,00.html (accessed January 22, 2018).

"Viral Hepatitis." Centers for Disease Control and Prevention, September 29, 2017. https://www.cdc.gov/hepatitis/hav/index.htm (accessed January 22, 2018).

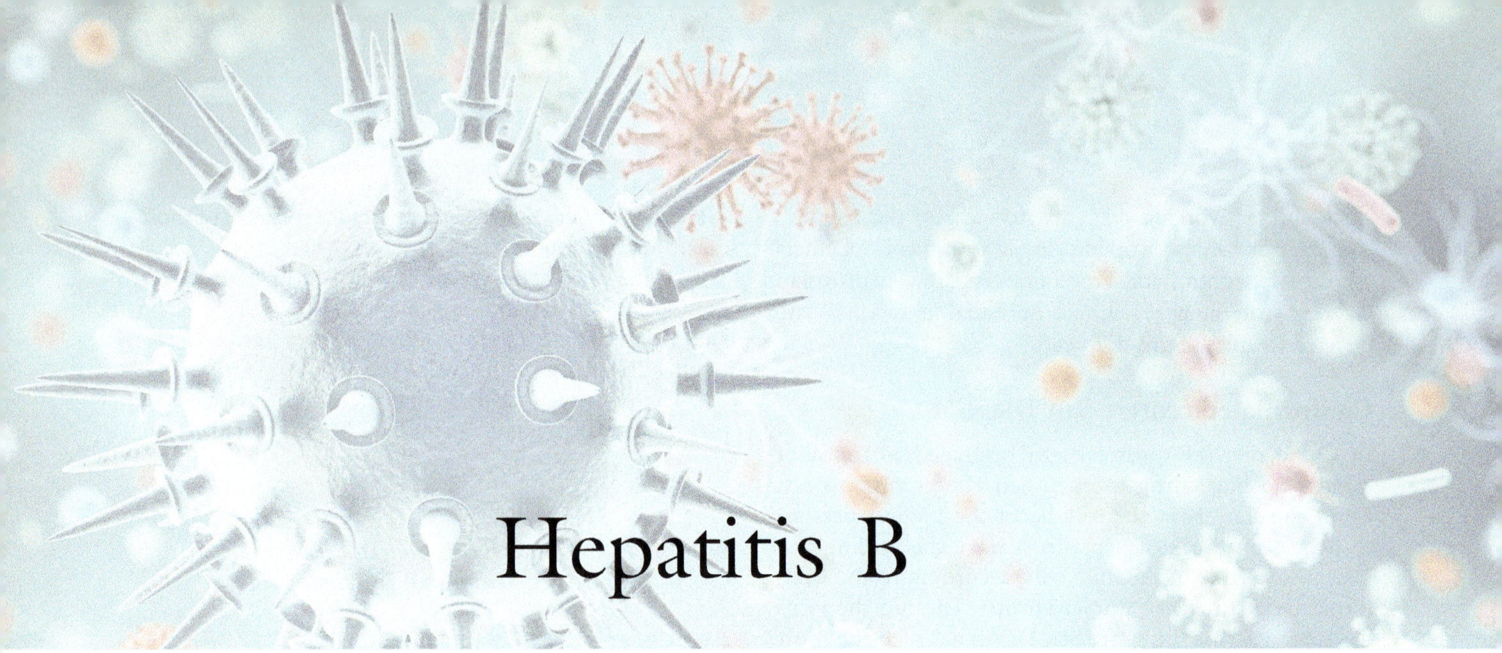

Hepatitis B

■ Introduction

Hepatitis B (HBV) is one of five viruses that cause hepatitis, an inflammation of the liver. Formerly known as posttransfusion or serum hepatitis, HBV is transmitted through infected blood and other body fluids rather than by food or casual contact. Infection can cause acute disease, with symptoms including nausea, malaise, diarrhea, joint pain, and abdominal pain. In some cases HBV infection progresses to chronic disease, damaging the liver and causing cirrhosis and liver cancer, which may be fatal. According to the US Centers for Disease Control and Prevention (CDC), chronic HBV infection causes premature death in 25 percent of those infected in childhood and in 15 percent of those who become infected during adulthood.

WORDS TO KNOW

CIRRHOSIS A chronic, degenerative, irreversible liver disease in which normal liver cells are damaged and are then replaced by scar tissue. Cirrhosis changes the structure of the liver and the blood vessels that nourish it. The disease reduces the liver's ability to manufacture proteins and process hormones, nutrients, medications, and poisons.

INTRAVENOUS In the vein. For example, the insertion of a hypodermic needle into a vein to instill a fluid, withdraw or transfuse blood, or start an intravenous feeding.

JAUNDICE A condition in which a person's skin and the whites of the eyes are discolored a shade of yellow due to an increased level of bile pigments in the blood as a result of liver disease. Jaundice is sometimes called icterus, from a Greek word for the condition.

Since the advent of screening of blood for HBV in developed countries, rates of infection have gone down. However, people may still come into contact with HBV through intravenous drug use and through sexual contact. An effective vaccine helps to protect high-risk groups, including babies at risk due to mother-to-child transmission, those who work with blood in laboratory environments, intravenous drug users, and people who live in areas where HBV is endemic.

■ Disease History, Characteristics, and Transmission

HBV is unrelated to any known human virus, although similar liver viruses are found in other animal species. It exists as spherical particles with double-stranded deoxyribonucleic acid (DNA) as the genetic material. Approximately 30 to 50 percent of those above the age of five infected with HBV will develop symptoms around 90 days after exposure. Children younger than age five and immunocompromised people are less likely to have symptoms. Symptoms include nausea, diarrhea, joint pain, abdominal discomfort, fatigue, and loss of appetite. Jaundice, a yellowing of the skin and whites of the eyes, may also develop, along with dark urine and clay-colored stools. The symptoms may continue for several months.

The HBV infection causes chronic viral hepatitis in around 90 percent of people infected with the disease as newborns, 25 to 50 percent of people infected from the ages of one to five years old, and 5 percent of people infected as adults. Around 15 to 25 percent of those who develop chronic HBV will die of the disease due to cirrhosis (scarring) of the liver or liver cancer.

Transmission of HBV occurs through infected blood and other body fluids. As such, the disease can be contracted through sexual contact with an infected person and by sharing needles or syringes with an infected person. It

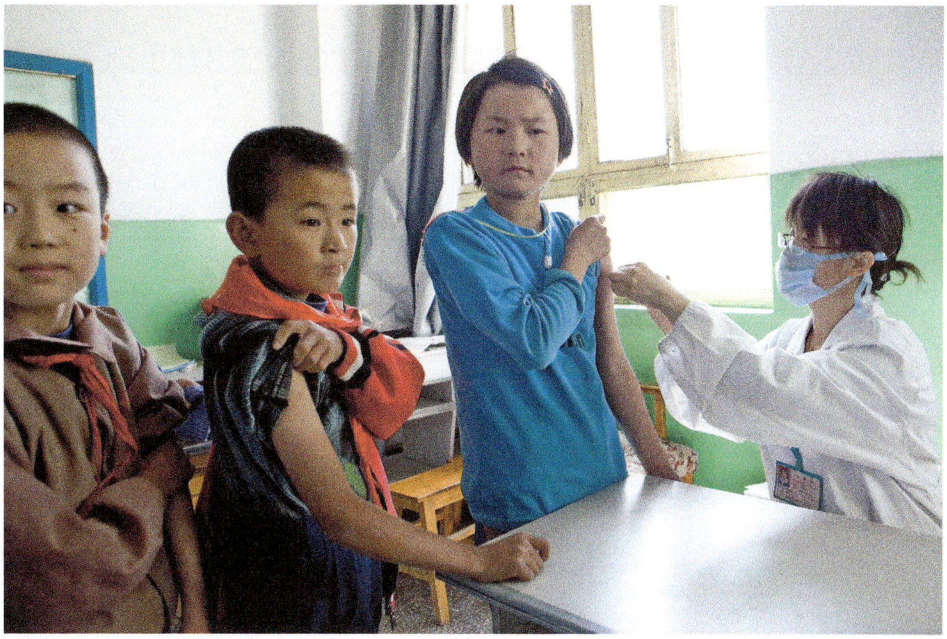

In Ledu, China, schoolchildren await epatitis B vaccinations as part of a large-scale campaign to reduce incidence of the potentially fatal liver disease in the country. © Aaron Deemer/Bloomberg/Getty Images

can also be transmitted from mother to child during childbirth or by sharing toothbrushes and razors with an infected person.

The virus is highly infectious. Experiments have shown that it can be spread through a mere 0.0001 milliliters of blood. For most people the HBV infection clears up within a few weeks. However, those with chronic disease remain infectious, even if they do not have symptoms.

Scope and Distribution

According to the CDC, an estimated 248 million people around the world had HBV in 2017, and 887,000 people die each year from the disease. It is especially common in sub-Saharan Africa, as well as in East Asia and the Western Pacific. Around 6 percent of the adults in those regions have HBV. In general, HBV causes 45 percent of all liver cancer and 30 percent of all liver cirrhosis.

In 2015 the CDC recorded 3,370 new cases of acute HBV infection in the United States. However, after adjusting for underreporting, the CDC estimated that there were actually around 21,900 total new acute HBV infections that year. Between 2011 and 2012, 847,000 noninstitutionalized people in the United States had acute HBV. The CDC estimates that 14,000 people in the United States die of complications of chronic HBV infection such as liver cirrhosis and liver cancer each year.

Infants are most at risk of developing chronic HBV infection, even though they are unlikely to have symptoms of acute disease. Others at high risk include sexual and household partners of those with chronic HBV, men who have sex with men (especially if they have more than one sexual partner), intravenous drug users, and people whose work brings them into contact with blood, such as health care workers. Around 7.4 percent of those with the human immunodeficiency virus (HIV) are also chronic carriers of HBV.

Treatment and Prevention

There is no specific treatment for acute HBV infection once acquired. Adequate nutrition and rest are most often recommended to ease symptoms.

Chronic HBV (sometimes referred to as CHB) is treated with antiviral medications. The purpose of the treatment is to prevent the hepatitis B virus from replicating itself and thereby prevent the disease from progressing and causing problems, such as liver cirrhosis. Although HBV cannot be cured, it can be managed so that there are no symptoms. Because chronic HBV does not progress linearly, the disease must be continually monitored by a qualified health care professional.

Treatment of chronic HBV is determined by the phase of the disease. To assess this, measurements are taken of the patient's HBV DNA levels, alanine aminotransferase (ALT) levels, anti-HBV antibodies, and the presence or absence of HBeAg (the HBV antigen, a type of protein that is present in the blood when someone is infectious). An assessment of the liver can determine whether it is inflamed and if there is scarring (called fibrosis). Because one measurement may not give a complete picture of the disease, multiple measurements should be taken over time so that an appropriate antiviral therapy can be used.

SOCIAL AND PERSONAL RESPONSIBILITY

The best way to avoid contracting hepatitis B is to get vaccinated. The vaccination is recommended for the following groups of people:

1. "All infants, starting with the first dose of hepatitis B vaccine at birth
2. All children and adolescents younger than 19 years of age who have not been vaccinated
3. People whose sex partners have hepatitis B
4. Sexually active persons who are not in a long-term, mutually monogamous relationship.
5. Persons seeking evaluation or treatment for a sexually transmitted disease
6. Men who have sex with men
7. People who share needles, syringes, or other drug-injection equipment
8. People who have close household contact with someone infected with the hepatitis B virus
9. Health care and public safety workers at risk for exposure to blood or blood-contaminated body fluids on the job
10. People with end-stage renal disease, including predialysis, hemodialysis, peritoneal dialysis, and home dialysis patients
11. Residents and staff of facilities for developmentally disabled persons
12. Travelers to regions with moderate or high rates of hepatitis B
13. People with chronic liver disease
14. People with HIV infection
15. Anyone who wishes to be protected from hepatitis B virus infection"

There are four phases of chronic HBV: (1) the immune-tolerant phase, characterized by high HBV DNA levels, normal ALT levels, and mild liver scarring and liver inflammation; (2) the HBeAg-positive immune-active phase, characterized by high HBV DNA levels, high ALT levels, and medium to acute liver fibrosis and liver inflammation; (3) the inactive CHB phase, characterized by low HBV DNA levels, normal ALT levels, and the presence of anti-HBV antibodies; and (4) the HBeAg-negative reactivation phase, characterized by high HBV DNA levels, high ALT levels, and medium to acute liver fibrosis and liver inflammation.

There are two types of antiviral medications: interferon (IFN) and nucleoside/nucleotide analogues (NAs), which are newer. NAs, particularly entecavir and tenofovir, are recommended in most cases. They can be taken orally and have fewer side effects than IFN. Not all people with chronic HCB should receive antiviral therapy, however. For example, it is not recommended for people with immune-tolerant CHB or for those who have no evidence of cirrhosis, normal ALT levels, and low levels of HBV DNA replication. People with immune-tolerant CHB should be tested every six months to see if the disease has progressed to the HBeAg-positive immune-active phase or the inactive CHB phase.

Prevention of hepatitis B is possible. The hepatitis B vaccine is manufactured through genetic engineering, a process that involves inserting the HBV gene into yeast cells. It was introduced in 1982 and is highly effective against infection. In most cases the vaccine is given in three doses. According to the World Health Organization (WHO), "the complete vaccine series induces protective antibody levels in more than 95% of infants, children and young adults. Protection lasts at least 20 years and is probably lifelong."

Impacts and Issues

HBV is a bloodborne infection. Those who are infected with HCV should not donate blood, organs, or tissue.

In the United States, some regions heavily affected by the opioid epidemic have seen dramatic increases in HBV infections. For example, the CDC reported that, between 2009 and 2013, incidents of HBV in Kentucky, Tennessee, and West Virginia increased by 114 percent, in correlation with the opioid epidemic in those states. Needle exchange programs in some countries have demonstrated limited success in reducing incidence of HBV among intravenous drug users.

HBV can never be cured, only managed. As such, the disease requires constant monitoring, and people without access to antiviral medications can face lifelong effects. Care of patients with chronic HBV is costly, and populations with a high rate of infection experience significant social and economic effects. HBV is one of the few viruses that can lead to cancer. HBV-related liver cancer (due to the virus damaging cells in the liver) and cirrhosis increase demand for liver transplants in an environment already strained by a lack of suitable donor organs.

SEE ALSO *Blood Supply and Infectious Disease; Bloodborne Pathogens; Hepatitis A; Hepatitis C; Hepatitis E*

BIBLIOGRAPHY

Books

Liaw, Yun-Fan, and Fabien Zoulim, eds. *Hepatitis B Virus in Human Diseases.* New York: Humana, 2015.

Shetty, Kirti, and George Y. Wu. *Chronic Viral Hepatitis.* 2nd ed. New York: Humana, 2012.

Periodicals

Brouwer, Willem Pieter, et al. "Adding Pegylated Interferon to Entecavir for Hepatitis B e Antigen-Positive Chronic Hepatitis B: A Multicenter Randomized Trial (ARES Study)." *Hepatology* 61, no. 5 (May 2015): 1512–1522. This article can also be found online at http://onlinelibrary.wiley.com/doi/10.1002/hep.27586/full (accessed February 2, 2018).

Buti, Maria, et al. "Seven-Year Efficacy and Safety of Treatment with Tenofovir Disoproxil Fumarate for Chronic Hepatitis B Virus Infection." *Digestive Diseases and Sciences* 60, no. 5 (May 2015): 1457–1464. This article can also be found online at https://link.springer.com/article/10.1007/s10620-014-3486-7 (accessed February 2, 2018).

Harris, Aaron, M., et al. "Increases in Acute Hepatitis B Virus Infections—Kentucky, Tennessee, and West Virginia, 2006–2013." *Morbidity and Mortality Weekly Report* 65, no. 3 (2016): 47–50. This article can also be found online at https://www.cdc.gov/mmwr/volumes/65/wr/mm6503a2.htm (accessed February 2, 2018).

Terrault, Norah A., et al. "AASLD Guidelines for Treatment of Chronic Hepatitis B." *Hepatology* 63, no. 1 (2016): 261–283. This article can also be found online at https://www.aasld.org/sites/default/files/Terrault_et_al-2016-Hepatology.pdf (accessed February 2, 2018).

Websites

"Guidelines for the Prevention, Care and Treatment of Persons with Chronic Hepatitis B Infection." World Health Organization (WHO), March 2015. http://apps.who.int/iris/bitstream/10665/154590/1/9789241549059_eng.pdf?ua=1&ua=1 (accessed February 2, 2018)

"Hepatitis B." World Health Organization (WHO), July 2017. http://www.who.int/mediacentre/factsheets/fs204/en/ (accessed February 2, 2018).

"Viral Hepatitis: Hepatitis B Information." Centers for Disease Control and Prevention (CDC), May 31, 2015. https://www.cdc.gov/hepatitis/hbv/index.htm (accessed February 2, 2018).

"Viral Hepatitis and Young Persons Who Inject Drugs." Centers for Disease Control and Prevention (CDC), April 17, 2017. https://www.cdc.gov/hepatitis/featuredtopics/youngpwid.htm (accessed February 2, 2018).

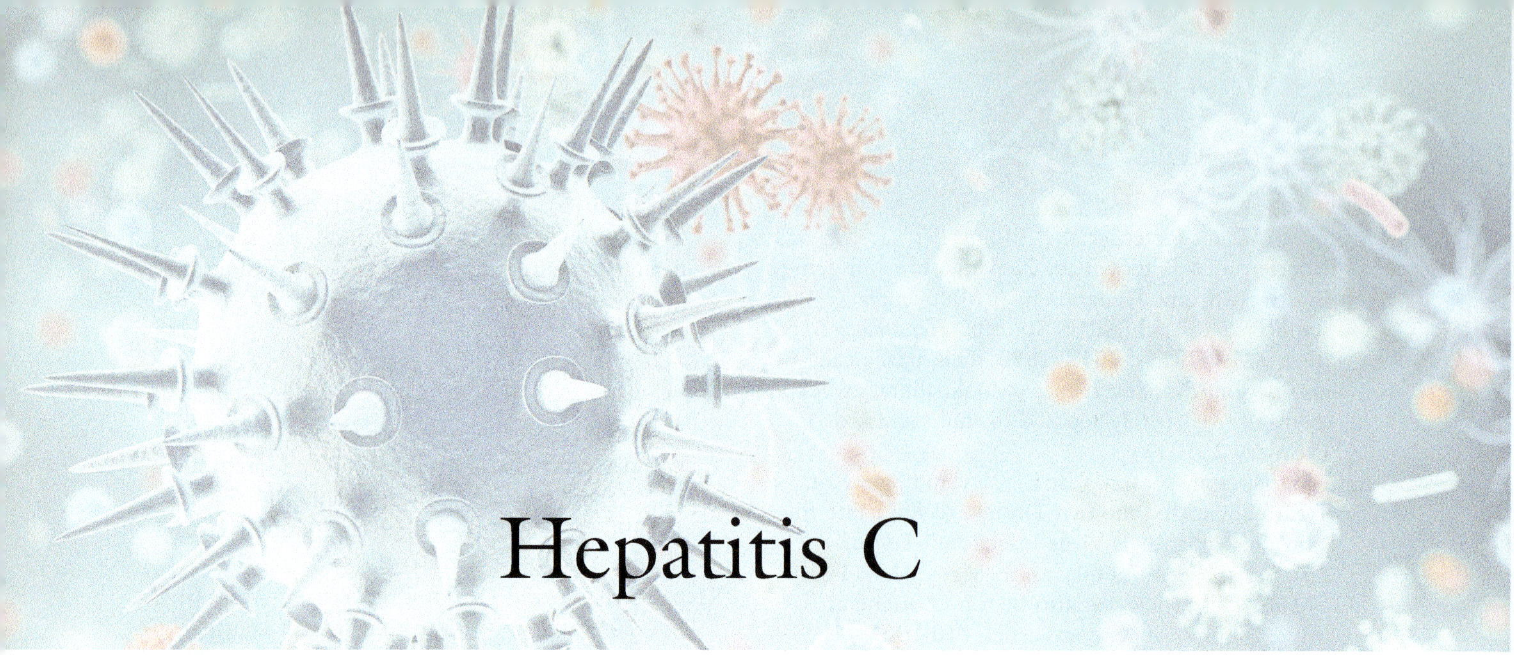

Hepatitis C

Introduction

The hepatitis C virus (HCV) is one of five viruses that cause hepatitis, an inflammation of the liver. HCV is transmitted through blood. For that reason, people who inject drugs are particularly at risk of contracting HCV, which is very infectious.

Unlike hepatitis A and hepatitis B, hepatitis C rarely causes an acute infection. A majority of HCV cases progress without any symptoms to become chronic hepatitis, which can cause liver damage and eventually lead to liver problems, including scarring and cancer. Direct-acting antiviral treatment is available for HCV, but there is no vaccine to protect against the disease.

For many people around the world, hepatitis C is a silent killer because even those with chronic infection may have no symptoms until liver disease is well advanced.

WORDS TO KNOW

BLOODBORNE PATHOGENS Disease-causing agents carried or transported in the blood. Bloodborne infections are those in which the infectious agent is transmitted from one person to another via contaminated blood.

INCUBATION PERIOD The time between exposure to a disease-causing virus or bacterium and the appearance of symptoms of the infection. Depending on the microorganism, the incubation time can range from a few hours, such as with food poisoning due to *Salmonella*, to a decade or more, such as with acquired immunodeficiency syndrome (AIDS).

STRAIN A subclass or a specific genetic variation of an organism.

Disease History, Characteristics, and Transmission

Formerly known as non-A non-B hepatitis (HCV was not discovered until 1989), HCV is an RNA virus, meaning that its genetic material consists of ribonucleic acid (RNA) rather than deoxyribonucleic acid (DNA). It is also a flavivirus, a type of virus related to the viruses that cause yellow fever and dengue. HCV exists in six different genotypes, which have varying distributions around the world and which respond differently to treatment. Genotype 1a is the most common in the United States.

The incubation period for HCV is an average of 4 to 12 weeks, and most acute infections do not cause any symptoms. If symptoms do occur, they may be mild enough to be ignored or mistaken for another illness. Symptoms include fever, nausea and abdominal pain, changes in the color of urine and stool, and jaundice, among others. In 75 to 85 percent of cases, HCV becomes chronic over a period of several years, during which time the liver becomes progressively inflamed and damaged. Around 60 to 70 percent of those who are chronically infected with HCV will develop significant liver disease, including cirrhosis (scarring) or liver cancer.

HCV is a bloodborne pathogen, a disease-causing organism transmitted through infected blood and body fluids that may contain blood. With the screening and treatment of blood and blood products, transmission of HCV by blood transfusion or receipt of blood clotting factors has become rare. However, because around 5 percent of all medical injections given around the world by health care workers are unsafe, HCV is sometimes spread accidentally in medical settings.

Intravenous drug use is a risk factor for contracting HCV. The sharing of needles and drug preparation supplies such as syringes, tourniquets, and drug cookers (including spoons) facilitates the transmission of infected blood from one person to another.

Occupational exposure, through needlestick injuries by health care workers, may be a transmission method for HCV. Hepatitis C can also pass from an infected mother to her baby during childbirth, although the risk is relatively low.

To a much lesser extent, hepatitis C is transmitted through body fluids during sexual contact and through sharing items such as toothbrushes on which miniscule amounts of blood may be present. Hepatitis C is not spread through coughing, sneezing, kissing, or casual contact between people.

■ Scope and Distribution

HCV is a global disease. The World Health Organization (WHO) estimated that around 71 million people had chronic HCV in October 2017. There are around 1.75 million new HCV infections each year. WHO also stated that an estimated 399,000 people die each year from end-stage HCV infection. Of the people who die, approximately 31 percent have a history of intravenous drug use. Europe and the eastern Mediterranean have the highest prevalence of the disease.

The majority of people with HCV do not know they have the disease, according to WHO. Of the people who have been diagnosed with HCV, about 8 percent receive treatment.

The US Centers for Disease Control and Prevention (CDC) estimated that there were 33,900 new HCV infections in 2015 in the United States. Between 2.7 million and 3.9 million people in the United States have chronic hepatitis C. Between 2010 and 2015, the rate of new cases of HCV almost tripled. The CDC reports that people born between 1945 and 1965 are six times more likely to have HCV than the general population (many of these baby boomers contracted the disease through blood transfusions and other injections prior to discovery of the disease). The disease is also spreading rapidly in people ages 20 to 29, largely caused by use of intravenous drugs.

Some groups of people are at a higher risk for contracting HCV than others. At-risk populations include intravenous drug users, incarcerated people, some indigenous communities, and immigrants who move from a country where HCV is common to a country where it is not. Men who have sex with men are also at a higher risk for contracting HCV than the general population.

■ Treatment and Prevention

In many cases HCV can be cured with appropriate treatment. Treatment of HCV is tailored to the genotype. Treatment regimens also take into account whether there is liver damage, including cirrhosis.

Prior to the creation of direct-acting antivirals (DAAs), treatment for hepatitis C consisted of injections of interferon, an immune system protein, which may have been combined with the oral antiviral drug ribavirin over a period of months. The treatment regimen was long and marked by side effects, some of which were severe enough to cause patients to discontinue taking their medicine. Cure rates were only 40 to 65 percent.

DAAs, which are administered orally, target specific receptors in the HCV genome. The first generation of

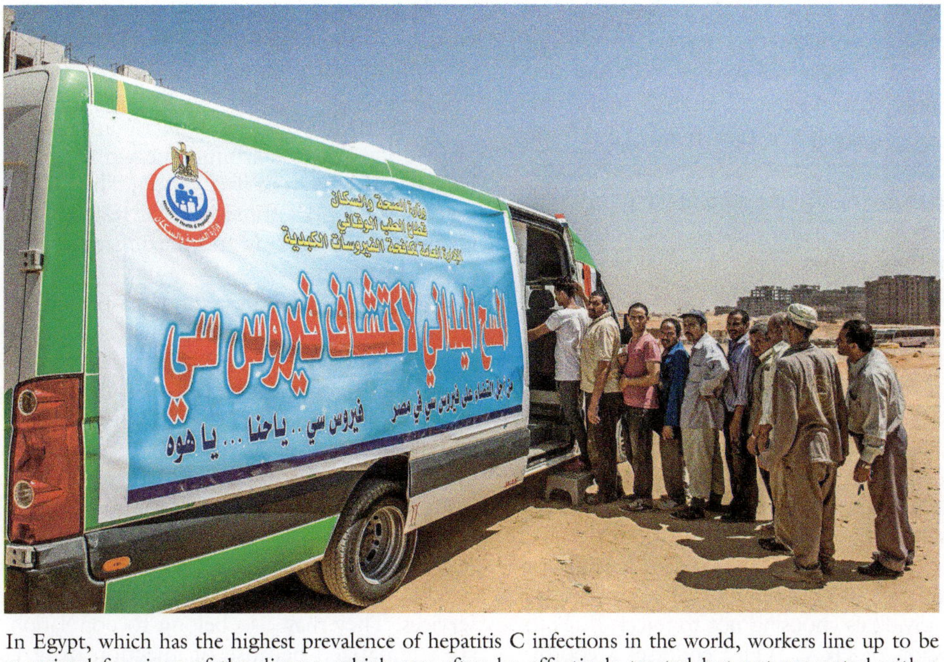

In Egypt, which has the highest prevalence of hepatitis C infections in the world, workers line up to be examined for signs of the disease, which can often be effectively treated but not prevented with a vaccine. *© KHALED DESOUKI/AFP/Getty Images*

PERSONAL RESPONSIBILITY AND PREVENTION

According to the US Centers for Disease Control and Prevention (CDC), the following groups are at an elevated risk for contracting HCV:

1. Current or past injection drug users (injection drug use is the most common way that HCV is spread)
2. People who have received donated blood, blood products, or organs (this form of transmission decreased dramatically after the advent of blood screening in 1992)
3. People who were given a blood product made before 1987 to treat clotting issues
4. People who are currently undergoing or have previously undergone hemodialysis
5. People who have body piercings or tattoos that were performed with improperly sterilized equipment
6. People who have been exposed to HCV, including health care workers and recipients of HCV-positive blood, blood products, or organs
7. People with HIV
8. Children of HCV-infected mothers

DAAs (namely, boceprevir and telaprevir) were only able to treat HCV genotype 1. They were administered orally in conjunction with interferon and ribavirin and caused serious side effects. Second-generation DAAs, which were the recommended treatments for HCV as of 2018, can be used without the addition of interferon and ribavirin (although interferon and ribavirin may also be recommended in a few cases). Some second-generation DAAs only treat one genotype, while others are effective on multiple genotypes. In general, treatment of HCV involves a cocktail of second-generation DAAs that are administered for up to about three months. Drugs include daclatasvir, sofosbuvir, and dasabuvir, among others. Cure rates with second-generation DAAs are around 95 percent.

Not all HCV must be treated to be cured. Some people are naturally able to clear the virus from their system after infection. The majority of people with HCV, however, require treatment.

To reduce the risk of spreading HCV, all donated blood should be screened for it. In addition, health care workers should follow best practices when giving injections to avoid accidentally spreading the disease.

People who inject drugs should not share needles or other drug-related items. WHO, however, notes that it will take more than individuals choosing not to inject drugs to slow the transmission of HCV. WHO endorses a coordinated public health response from governments that supports "prevention of initiation of injection drug use, prevention of stigma and discrimination, and the provision of a full spectrum of harm reduction interventions." Harm reduction interventions include offering free clean needles to injection drug users.

Toothbrushes, razors, and other personal items that could contain invisible traces of blood should not be shared. A person with hepatitis C should not donate blood, organs, or tissue. Condoms provide some protection to those having sex with an infected person. Occupational exposures for health care workers can be avoided by following the appropriate guidance on cleaning up blood spills, using needles with protective shields, and following other infection control procedures. Because there is no vaccine against HCV, these practical precautions against infection offer the most efficient protection strategies.

■ Impacts and Issues

Although second-generation DAAs are effective at treating and curing HCV in most cases, many people in developed countries cannot afford them. Not all insurance programs cover the costs. For example, *Pharmacy Times* reported that one pill of sofosbuvir cost US$1,000 in February 2017. A full treatment of sofosbuvir would accordingly cost US$84,000. In developing countries, however, there are sometimes generic, less expensive versions of the DAAs available. In India, for example, a single dose of sofosbuvir costs only US$4. A promising drug called Mavyret is relatively less expensive than other treatments. It was approved by the US Food and Drug Administration (FDA) in 2017 for treatment of people with HCV genotypes 1 through 6 who do not have cirrhosis.

Hepatitis C is known as a silent killer because many people do not realize they are infected and can pass the virus on to others. Moreover, the infection causes progressive damage to the liver but may not produce any symptoms for many years. HCV is a common cause of unexplained liver disease around the world and is responsible for many deaths from liver cancer. The CDC recommends that those at risk of infection be tested for HCV to help identify infections early and maximize the chances for successful treatment.

In the United States, about 25 percent of people who are infected with the human immunodeficiency virus (HIV) are also infected with HCV. In addition, about 50 to 90 percent of people with HIV who inject drugs also have HCV. Coinfection (i.e., being infected with both HCV and HIV at the same time) increases the risk of HCV-caused liver problems and accelerates their development. WHO stated in a 2017 report about viral hepatitis that "persons with HIV–[Hepatitis B] or HIV–HCV coinfection are at risk for accelerated disease progression, stigma and, in some instances, compromised access to health services. They may also belong to population groups that are stigmatized because of injection drug use or sexual behaviours."

SEE ALSO *Blood Supply and Infectious Disease; Bloodborne Pathogens; Hepatitis B*

BIBLIOGRAPHY

Books

Thomas, Howard C., et al., eds. *Viral Hepatitis.* 4th ed. Chichester, UK: John Wiley Blackwell, 2014.

Periodicals

Gupta, Neil, and Paul Farmer. "We Can Cure Hepatitis C. But We're Now Making the Same Mistake We Did with AIDS." *Washington Post* (July 28, 2017). This article can also be found online at https://www.washingtonpost.com/opinions/we-can-cure-hepatitis-c-but-were-now-making-the-same-mistake-we-did-with-aids/2017/07/28/503a4b02-72f9-11e7-9eac-d56bd5568db8_story.html (accessed February 20, 2018).

Toich, Laurie. "Will Hepatitis C Virus Medication Costs Drop in the Years Ahead?" *Pharmacy Times* (February 8, 2017). This article can also be found online at http://www.pharmacytimes.com/resource-centers/hepatitisc/will-hepatitis-c-virus-medicaton-costs-drop-in-the-years-ahead (accessed February 20, 2018).

Zezima, Katie. "Another Outbreak Related to the Nation's Opioid Crisis: Hepatitis C." *Washington Post* (October 17, 2017). This article can also be found online at https://www.washingtonpost.com/national/another-outbreak-related-to-the-nations-opioid-crisis-hepatitis-c/2017/10/17/eb24e7b6-a063-11e7-9083-fbfddf6804c2_story.html (accessed February 20, 2018).

Websites

Andrews, Michelle. "FDA's Approval of a Cheaper Drug for Hepatitis C Will Likely Expand Treatment." NPR. https://www.npr.org/sections/health-shots/2017/10/04/555156577/fdas-approval-of-a-cheaper-drug-for-hepatitis-c-will-likely-expand-treatment (accessed February 20, 2018).

"Genotypes of Hepatitis C." Hepatitis C Trust. http://www.hepctrust.org.uk/information/about-hepatitis-c-virus/genotypes-hepatitis-c (accessed February 19, 2018).

"Global Hepatitis Report, 2017." World Health Organization. http://apps.who.int/iris/bitstream/10665/255016/1/9789241565455-eng.pdf?ua=1 (accessed February 19, 2018).

"Guidelines for the Screening, Care and Treatment of Persons with Chronic Hepatitis C Infection." World Health Organization. http://apps.who.int/iris/bitstream/10665/205035/1/9789241549615_eng.pdf?ua=1 (accessed February 19, 2018).

"Hepatitis C." World Health Organization. http://www.who.int/mediacentre/factsheets/fs164/en/ (accessed February 19, 2018).

"HIV and Viral Hepatitis." Centers for Disease Control and Prevention. https://www.cdc.gov/hiv/pdf/library/factsheets/hiv-viral-hepatitis.pdf (accessed February 20, 2018).

Kodjak, Alison. "Hepatitis Drug among the Most Costly for Medicaid." NPR. https://www.npr.org/sections/health-shots/2015/12/15/459873815/hepatitis-drug-among-the-most-costly-for-medicaid (accessed February 20, 2018).

"New Hepatitis C Infections Nearly Tripled over Five Years." Centers for Disease Control and Prevention. https://www.cdc.gov/nchhstp/newsroom/2017/Hepatitis-Surveillance-Press-Release.html (accessed February 20, 2018).

"Viral Hepatitis: Hepatitis C Information." Centers for Disease Control and Prevention. https://www.cdc.gov/hepatitis/hcv/index.htm (accessed February 19, 2018).

Susan Aldridge
Claire Skinner

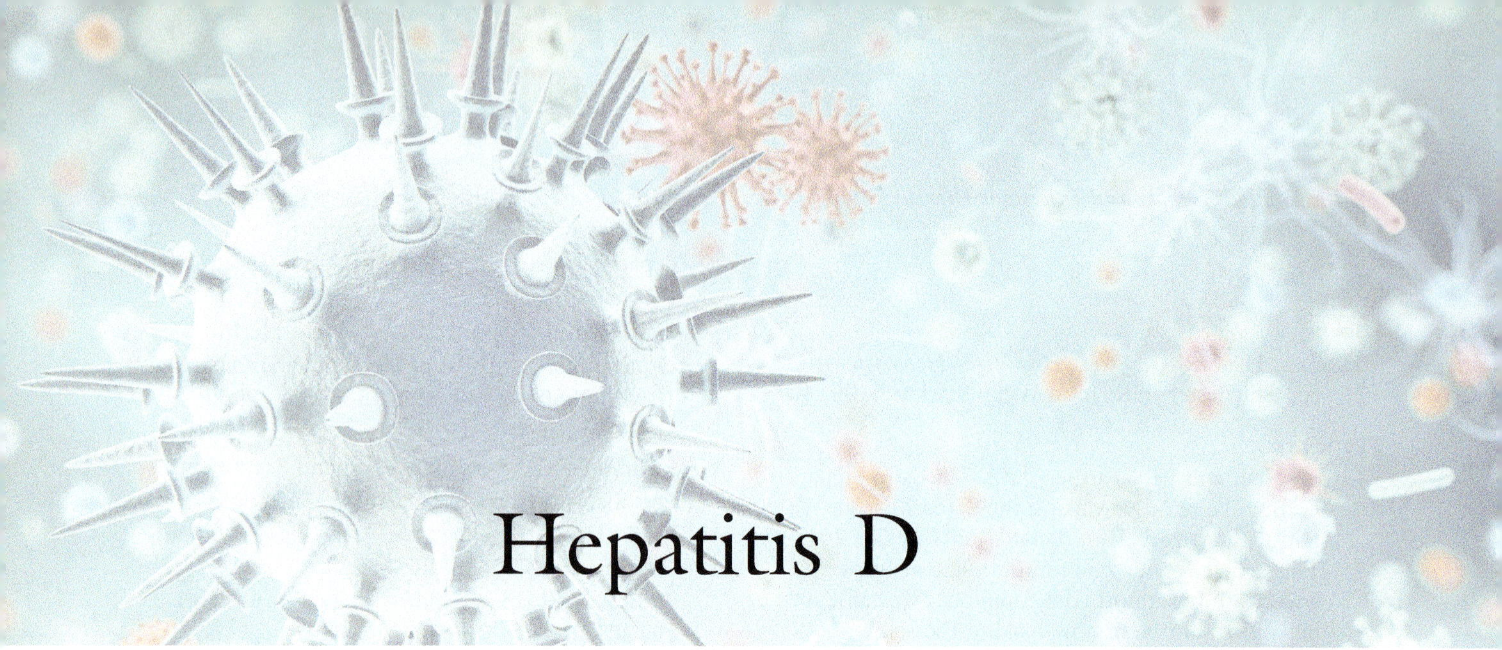

Hepatitis D

■ Introduction

The hepatitis D virus (HDV), also known as hepatitis delta virus, is one of six viruses that cause hepatitis, an inflammation of the liver. It is unusual in that it is found only with hepatitis B virus (HBV) infection. HDV is transmitted in a similar way to HBV, through infected blood and other body fluids, rather than by food or casual contact. HDV infection can cause acute disease with symptoms similar to that of HBV, including nausea, malaise, diarrhea, joint pain, and abdominal pain. People with HBV and HDV tend to be at higher risk of serious liver damage and death than those with HBV alone. HDV is uncommon in the United States, though its prevalence is likely underreported because of a lack of routine screenings. Most cases occur in injecting drug users.

WORDS TO KNOW

BLOOD-BORNE PATHOGENS Disease-causing agents carried or transported in the blood. Blood-borne infections are those in which the infectious agent is transmitted from one person to another via contaminated blood.

FULMINANT An infection that appears suddenly and whose symptoms are immediately severe.

RNA VIRUS A virus whose genetic material consists of either single or double-stranded ribonucleic acid (RNA) rather than deoxyribonucleic acid (DNA).

SUPERINFECTION When a new infection occurs in a patient who already has some other infection. For example, a bacterial infection appearing in a person who already had viral pneumonia would be a superinfection.

■ Disease History, Characteristics, and Transmission

HDV is a single-stranded RNA virus that exists as one of seven genotypes (genetic identities). It was first identified by Italian virologist Mario Rizzetto (1945–) in 1977. There are two types of HDV infection. HDV may occur as a coinfection (occurring simultaneously with HBV) or as a superinfection (occurring in someone who already has chronic HBV infection). The symptoms of acute HDV infection are difficult to distinguish from those of hepatitis A virus (HAV) and HBV and include jaundice (a yellowing of the skin and whites of the eyes), fatigue, abdominal pain, loss of appetite, nausea, vomiting, joint pain, and dark urine. Fulminant hepatitis, a sudden, severe form of the disease with rapid onset, is more likely to develop from acute HDV infection than with HAV or HBV. Superinfection causes a worsening in the severity and progression of HBV; those affected are likely to develop chronic cirrhosis of the liver or liver cancer.

Because the virus is transmitted via infected blood and other body fluids, having sexual contact with an infected person or injecting drugs with shared needles is strongly associated with HDV transmission. Rarely, HDV infection can pass from mother to child through contact with infected blood during childbirth (vertical transmission).

■ Scope and Distribution

The World Health Organization (WHO) estimated that there were approximately 15 million people chronically coinfected with HDV and HBV worldwide in 2017. That year the Hepatitis B Foundation (HBF) reported an estimated 20,000 people coinfected with the viruses in the United States, where there is no routine HDV surveillance data. HDV is also rare in northern Europe and Japan. It is found mainly in southern Europe, Africa, and South America. Those at risk include injecting

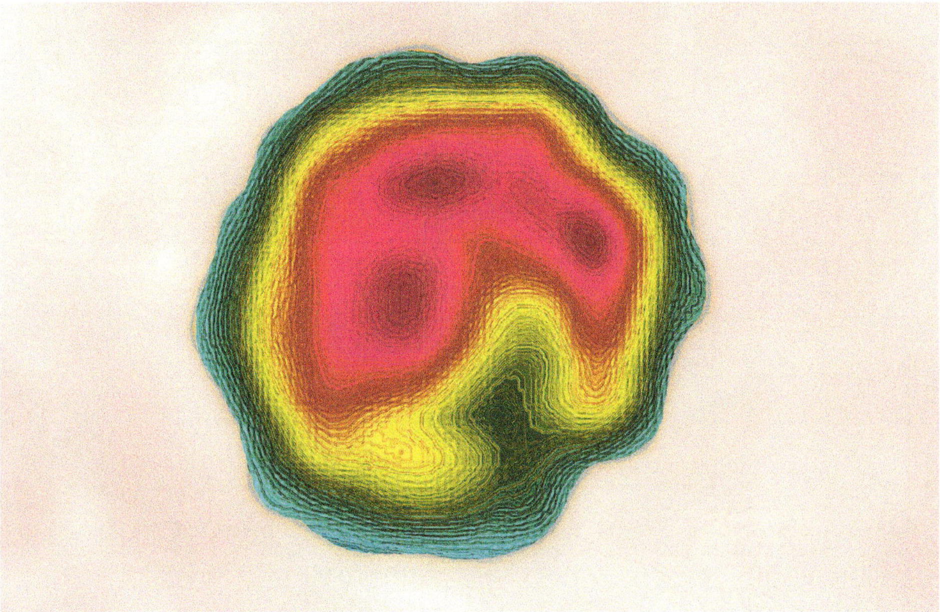

The hepatitis D virus is unlike the other viruses that cause hepatitis, in that it is found only with hepatitis B virus infection. People with both hepatitis D and B tend to be at higher risk of serious liver damage and death than those with hepatitis B alone. *© BSIP/UIG/Getty Images*

drug users, those on hemodialysis (the purifying of blood by a machine), those who have had sexual contact with infected people, men who have sex with men, and those who may be exposed to HDV through their occupations.

Treatment and Prevention

As of 2017 there was no treatment for HDV infection other than rest and adequate nutrition, although researchers were working to develop therapies specific to the virus. Chronic infection can be treated with the drug interferon, although response is less effective than if the person is infected only with HBV. Higher doses of interferon may be necessary with coinfection. Liver failure can be treated with a liver transplant. Transmission of HDV is prevented in the same way as is HBV, by preventing contact with infected blood.

Blood is not screened specifically for HBV and HDV in all countries, so this is a possible route of infection for someone who already has HBV, particularly when traveling abroad. If someone is protected against HBV, then that individual is automatically protected from HDV as well. Therefore, the HBV vaccine is an effective method of preventing HDV transmission. As of 2018 researchers were working on a vaccine specific for HDV.

Impacts and Issues

HDV is an unusual virus in that it cannot infect people on its own. It requires the presence of HBV. Those who are at risk of HBV infection may also be at risk of HDV if they live in an area where the virus is common. Being infected with both viruses leads to a poorer prognosis than being infected with HBV alone. According to WHO in 2017, the superinfection of HDV with chronic HBV leads to the progression of more severe hepatitis in 70 to 90 percent of patients. Some studies have indicated that HDV infection may make HBV infection more difficult to control.

In those parts of the world where HDV is common, such as southern Europe, Africa, and South America, more widespread access to HBV vaccine and screening and treatment of the blood supply could considerably cut the death toll from liver disease. Research has suggested a decrease in HDV among drug users and prostitutes in Taipei, Taiwan (Republic of China). However, the virus has a new potential reservoir (the animal or organism in which the virus normally resides) among the populations of male and immigrant prostitutes moving into the area. Increased surveillance of the health of these groups could help stop the spread of HDV in the area.

In 2016 the World Health Assembly adopted a new strategy to combat hepatitis around the world. The Global Health Sector Strategy on Viral Hepatitis, 2016–2021 outlines a vision for reducing new infections by 90 percent and reducing the death rate from viral hepatitis by 65 percent by 2030. To meet these goals, WHO has promoted increased awareness of viral hepatitis, creation of evidence-based health policy, and increased screenings and access to treatment.

HDV screenings are not widely performed in the United States. There is growing awareness, however, that

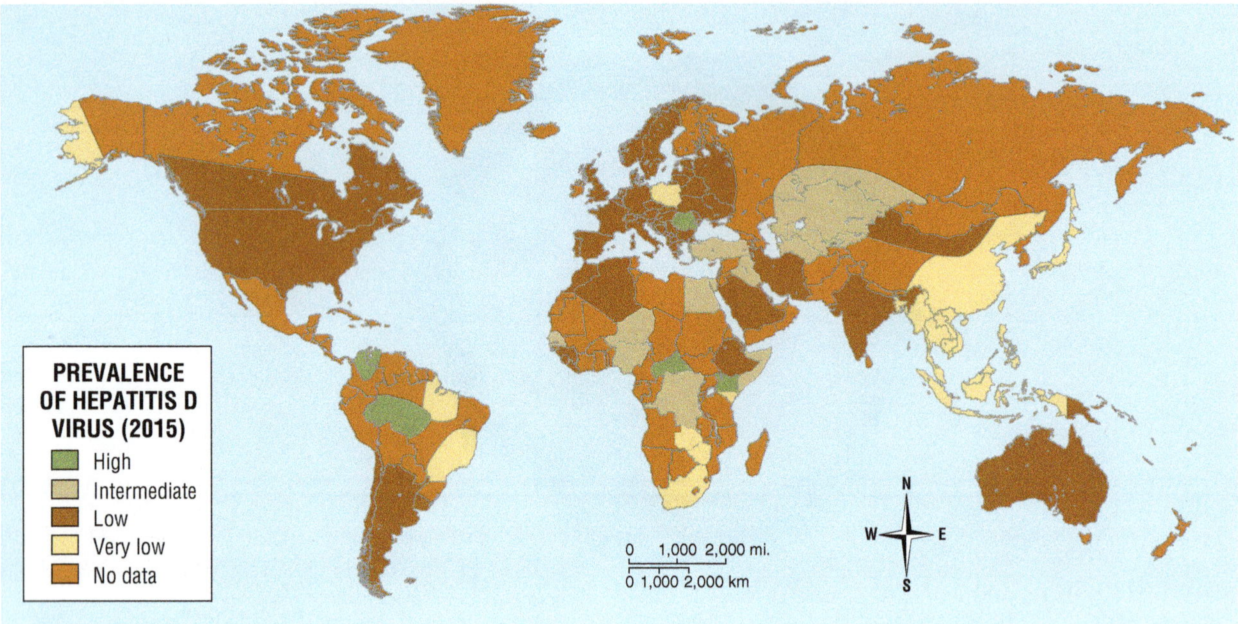

SOURCE: Hepatitis B Foundation

the virus is not as rare as once believed, with some doctors and researchers calling for routine testing in all patients with chronic HBV infection, as well as patients from countries where HDV is prevalent.

See Also *Blood Supply and Infectious Disease; Bloodborne Pathogens; Hepatitis B*

BIBLIOGRAPHY

Books

Horn, Lyle W., and Alan Hecht. *Hepatitis.* New York: Chelsea House, 2011.

Thomas, Howard C., et al., eds. *Viral Hepatitis.* 4th ed. Chichester, UK: Wiley, 2014.

Periodicals

Ahn, Joseph, and Robert G. Gish. "Hepatitis D Virus: A Call to Screening." *Journal of Gastroenterology and Hepatology* 10, no. 10 (October 2014): 647–686.

Bahcecioglu, I. H., and A. Sahin. "Treatment of Delta Hepatitis: Today and in the Future." *Infectious Diseases* 49, no. 4 (April 2017): 241–250.

Websites

"Hepatitis D." Centers for Disease Control and Prevention, December 8, 2015. https://www.cdc.gov/hepatitis/hdv/index.htm (accessed January 9, 2018).

"Hepatitis D." World Health Organization, July 2017. http://www.who.int/mediacentre/factsheets/hepatitis-d/en/ (accessed January 9, 2017).

Hepatitis Delta. http://hepatitis-delta.org/ (accessed January 10, 2017).

"What Is Hepatitis D?" Hepatitis B Foundation. http://www.hepb.org/research-and-programs/hepdeltaconnect/whatishepatitisd/ (accessed January 9, 2017).

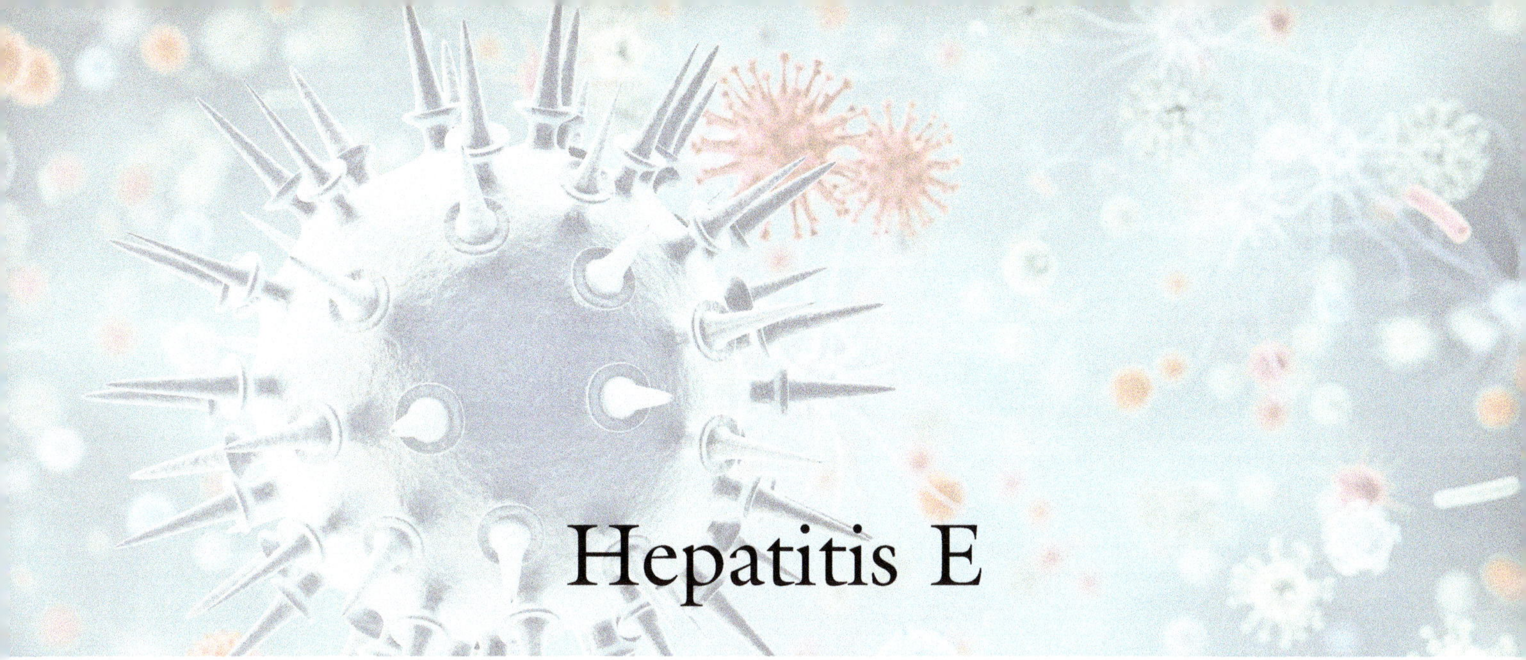

Hepatitis E

Introduction

hepatitis is an inflammation of the liver that can be caused by exposure to chemicals, including alcohol, or by any one of five hepatitis viruses. Hepatitis E infection is caused by the hepatitis E virus (HEV). It was shown to be a separate form of hepatitis in 1980.

Like hepatitis A, HEV is primarily spread through water and occasionally through food. It is the greatest risk to people who live in or who travel to areas where sanitation standards are poor. Hepatitis E infection is always acute. Symptoms include nausea, malaise, diarrhea, and an enlarged liver. Occasionally HEV infection can be severe, especially among pregnant women, as well as immunocompromised people and those with a history of liver problems.

HEV occurs worldwide and is most prevalent in East Asia and South Asia. Outbreaks of the disease may occur. There is a commercially available vaccine against HEV in China, but it is not licensed for use elsewhere. For most people prevention requires avoiding potential sources of exposure.

Disease History, Characteristics, and Transmission

The hepatitis E virus is a single-stranded ribonucleic acid (RNA) virus, with no outer envelope, but is distinguished by the appearance of spike-like structures on its surface. The virus has four known genotypes: genotype 1, genotype 2, genotype 3, and genotype 4.

The incubation time of HEV following exposure is 2 to 10 weeks. Infection may or may not cause symptoms. Symptoms of HEV infection can include jaundice, nausea, vomiting, diarrhea, fatigue, fever, dark urine, pale stools, and a slightly enlarged, tender liver. Symptomatic infection with HEV is most common in the 15 to 40 age group. Children get infected also but are more likely to be asymptomatic. In a small minority of cases, HEV infection is fulminant—that is, resulting in acute liver failure. Fulminant hepatitis E is fatal to mother and fetus in about 20 to 25 percent of cases if it occurs during late pregnancy. It can also result in miscarriage and stillbirth. In rare cases it can progress to chronic disease, primarily in immunocompromised people.

In general, hepatitis E is transmitted by the fecal-oral route, usually via contaminated water. It can also be transmitted through certain uncooked or undercooked meat, from mother to child, and from receiving transfusions of blood that has the virus. Unlike hepatitis B and hepatitis C, hepatitis E is not transmitted sexually.

Scope and Distribution

According to the World Health Organization (WHO), there are about 20 million cases of HEV each year. Only about 3.3 million of these cases cause symptoms.

WORDS TO KNOW

FECAL-ORAL ROUTE The transmission of minute particles of fecal material from one organism (human or animal) to the mouth of another organism.

FULMINANT INFECTION An infection that appears suddenly and whose symptoms are immediately severe.

JAUNDICE A condition in which a person's skin and the whites of the eyes are discolored a shade of yellow due to an increased level of bile pigments in the blood resulting from liver disease. Jaundice is sometimes called icterus, from a Greek word for the condition.

Hepatitis E Genotypes

Characteristics	Genotype 1	Genotype 2	Genotype 3	Genotype 4
Geographic Location	Africa, Asia	Mexico, West Africa	Developed Countries	China, Taiwan, Japan
Transmission Route	Waterborne, Fecal-oral, Person to person	Waterborne, Fecal-oral	Food-borne	Food-borne
Groups at High Risk for Infection	Young adults	Young adults	Older adults (>40 years), Males, Immunocompromised people	Young adults
Zoonotic Transmission	No	No	Yes	Yes
Chronic Infection	No	No	Yes	No
Occurrence of Outbreaks	Common	Smaller-scale outbreaks	Uncommon	Uncommon

SOURCE: Adapted from "Viral Hepatitis: Hepatitis E." US Centers for Disease Control and Prevention. April 28, 2015. Available from: https://www.cdc.gov/hepatitis/hev/index.htm

HEV occurs around the world, and each genotype of the disease has a geographical range. According to the US Centers for Disease Control and Prevention (CDC), genotype 1 is more common in Africa and Asia; genotype 2, Mexico and West Africa; genotype 3, developed countries; and genotype 4, China, Japan, and Taiwan.

The risk of contracting the disease is highest where access to clean water is restricted and where sanitation is poor. Therefore, HEV is a greater problem in some developing countries. In addition, isolated cases of HEV can occur in developed countries when people eat certain uncooked or undercooked meat, especially organ meat (HEV tends to be genotypes 3 or 4 in these cases).

When water sources have been contaminated by fecal matter, outbreaks of the disease can occur. Outbreaks are the most common in Asia and Africa. A 1986–1988 outbreak in China infected 119,000 people, 707 of whom died. There have been a few small outbreaks in Latin America. Outbreaks are generally caused by genotype 1 and, to a much lesser extent, genotype 2. In 2017 WHO stated that "some of these outbreaks have occurred in areas of conflict and humanitarian emergencies, such as war zones, and in camps for refugees or internally displaced populations (IDP), situations where sanitation and safe water supply pose special challenges."

■ Treatment and Prevention

Hepatitis E infection is usually self-limiting, and there is no specific treatment for it for most people, other than rest and adequate nutrition. For immunocompromised people who have chronic HEV, antiviral drugs are recommended. A vaccine against HEV is available only in China.

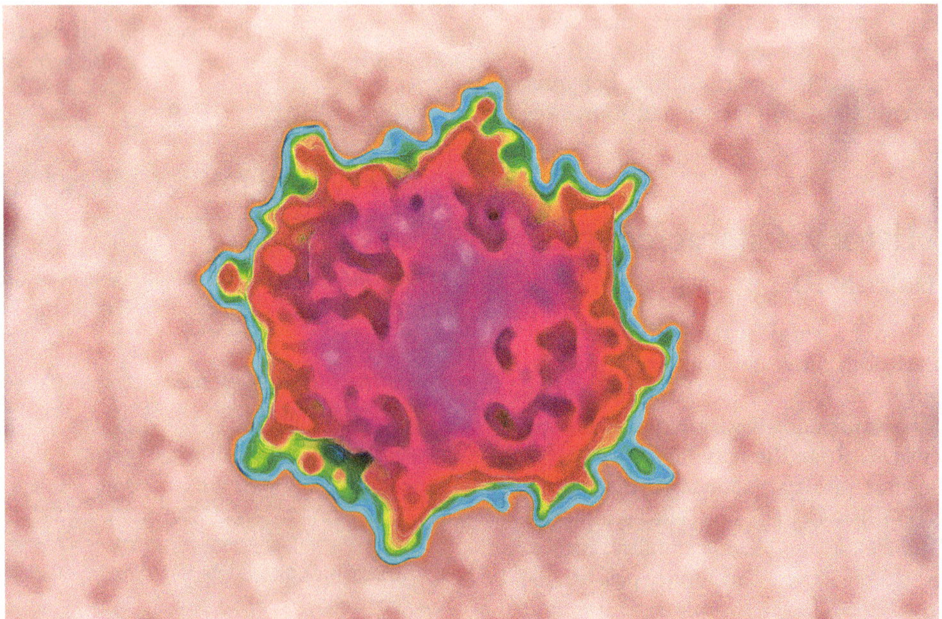

The hepatitis E virus is spread through contaminated water. The symptoms are typically not severe and include nausea and diarrhea. *© BSIP/UIG/Getty Images*

In the absence of a widely available vaccine, prevention of HEV infection requires adequate sanitation systems. To a lesser extent, prevention depends on maintaining a good standard of personal hygiene. Handwashing after using the bathroom and before eating or preparing food is recommended. Avoiding uncooked or undercooked meat is also advised.

Impacts and Issues

Hepatitis E is rare in developed countries, but those who live in or travel to developing countries may be at risk of exposure. In destinations where high standards of hygiene and sanitation may be lacking, it is best to drink bottled water and avoid ice, seafood, and raw fruit and vegetables. For those who live in developing countries, improvement of the infrastructure with respect to access to clean drinking water and adequate sanitation is the most effective method of preventing outbreaks with viruses such as HEV.

See Also *Hepatitis A; Hepatitis B; Hepatitis C; Travel and Infectious Disease*

BIBLIOGRAPHY

Books

Ruggeri, Franco Maria, et al. *Hepatitis E Virus: An Emerging Zoonotic and Foodborne Pathogen*. New York: Springer, 2013.

Wang, Youchun. *Hepatitis E Virus*. New York: Springer, 2016.

Periodicals

Cossaboom, Caitlin M., et al. "Risk Factors and Sources of Foodborne Hepatitis E Virus Infection in the United States." *Journal of Medical Virology* 88, no.9 (September 2016): 1641–1645.

Krain, Lisa J., Kenrad E. Nelson, and Alain B. Labrique. "Host Immune Status and Response to Hepatitis E Virus Infection." *Clinical Microbiology Reviews* 27, no. 1 (January 2014): 139–165. This article can also be found online at http://cmr.asm.org/content/27/1/139.full (accessed February 7, 2018).

Zhang, Jun, et al. "Long-Term Efficacy of a Hepatitis E Vaccine." *New England Journal of Medicine* 372 (2015): 914–922. This article can also be found online at http://www.nejm.org/doi/full/10.1056/nejmoa1406011 (accessed February 7, 2018).

Websites

"Hepatitis E." World Health Organization, July 2017. http://www.who.int/mediacentre/factsheets/fs280/en/ (accessed February 7, 2018).

"Viral Hepatitis: Hepatitis E." Centers for Disease Control and Prevention, April 28, 2015. https://www.cdc.gov/hepatitis/hev/index.htm (accessed February 7, 2018).

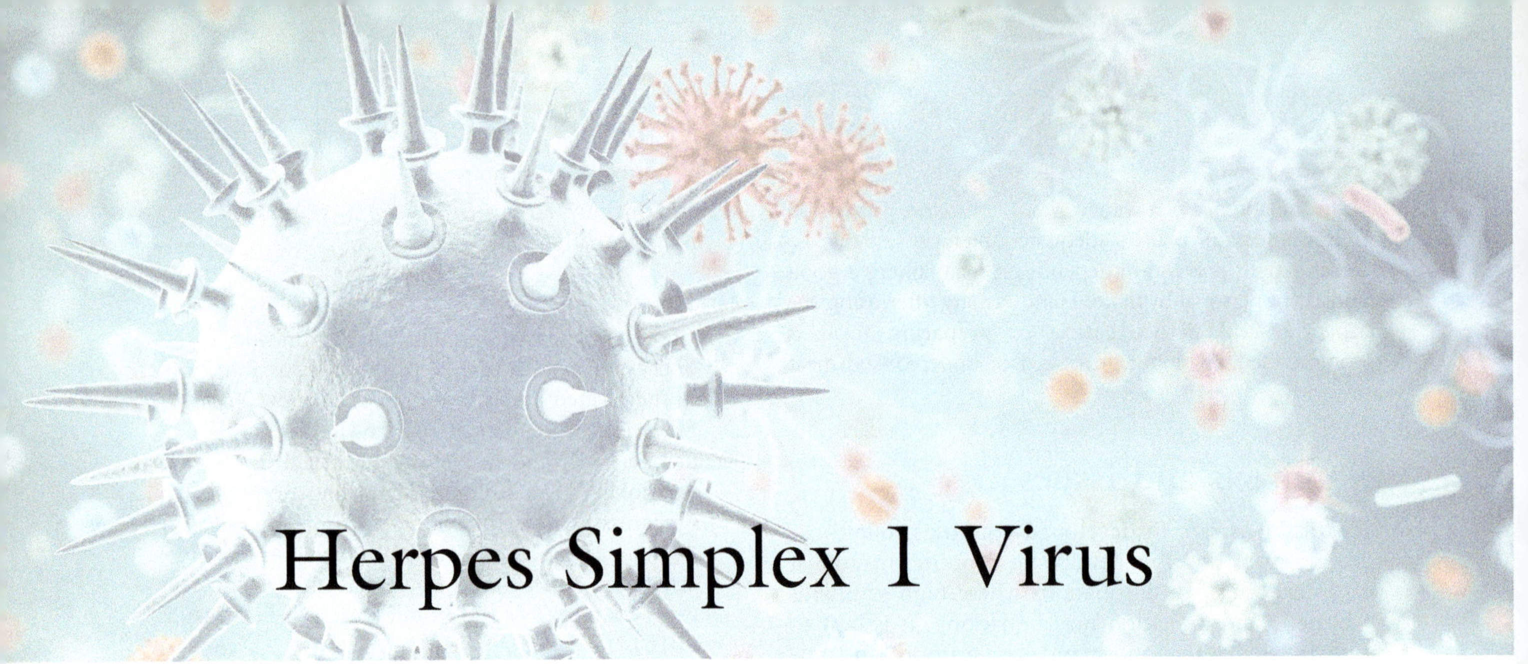

Herpes Simplex 1 Virus

■ Introduction

The herpes simplex virus, HSV-1 and HSV-2, belong to the herpes family of viruses, all of which exist as viral particles of a diameter around 200 nanometers, consisting of a protein exterior enclosing a molecule of double-stranded deoxyribonucleic acid (DNA). The herpes simplex 1 virus (HSV-1) causes painful sores, known as cold sores, on the skin or in the eyes. Less frequently, HSV-1 can cause genital ulcers. HSV-2 is the virus generally associated with similar lesions in the genital area (known sometimes just as herpes). Other significant herpes viruses include the varicella-zoster virus, which causes chickenpox; Epstein-Barr virus; and cytomegalovirus (CMV). The herpes virus invades cells, such as neurons, and may lie dormant for many years, causing no obvious symptoms. However, a herpes infection can be activated at any time and may often recur during life. Although the virus itself cannot be eliminated, symptoms of active infection, such as cold sores, can be treated with antiviral drugs.

■ Disease History, Characteristics, and Transmission

HSV-1 infection is transmitted through respiratory droplets or direct exposure to infected saliva or herpes

WORDS TO KNOW

ANTIBODIES Proteins found in the blood that help fight against foreign substances called antigens. Antigens, which are usually proteins or polysaccharides, stimulate the immune system to produce antibodies, or Y-shaped immunoglobulins. The antibodies inactivate the antigen and help remove it from the body. While antigens can be the source of infections from pathogenic bacteria and viruses, organic molecules detrimental to the body from internal or environmental sources also act as antigens. Genetic engineering and the use of various mutational mechanisms allow the construction of a vast array of antibodies (each with a unique genetic sequence).

DORMANT Inactive but still alive. A resting, nonactive state.

ENCEPHALITIS A type of acute brain inflammation, most often due to infection by a virus.

IMMUNOCOMPROMISED Having an immune system with reduced ability to recognize and respond to the presence of foreign material.

LATENT INFECTION An infection already established in the body but not yet causing symptoms or having ceased to cause symptoms after an active period.

OPPORTUNISTIC INFECTION An infection that occurs in people whose immune systems are diminished or are not functioning normally. Such infections are opportunistic insofar as the infectious agents take advantage of their hosts' compromised immune systems and invade to cause disease.

VIRAL SHEDDING The movement of the herpes virus from the nerves to the surface of the skin. During shedding, the virus can be passed on through skin-to-skin contact.

lesions. Contact with infected secretions from items such as cups, glasses, towels, and food is also a significant mode of transmission. In addition, HSV-1 can be transmitted from mother to infant during childbirth, resulting in potentially life-threatening infection of the newborn.

SV1 primarily causes oral lesions, including gingivostomatitis (infection of the mouth and gums), in approximately 80 percent of the population. Around 20 percent of cases also experience genital lesions mostly caused through oro-genital contact. Other diseases caused by HSV1 include encephalitis, chickenpox, and shingles. Severe HSV-1 infections such as encephalitis may occur in patients with a compromised immune system, wherein the mortality rate is estimated at 60 to 80 percent.

Primary infections are usually mild and asymptomatic. However, patients with a weakened immune system may develop a severe infection, resulting in painful blisters and sores. In both cases the virus may remain latent after primary infection and reside in cranial nerve cells. For 10 to 40 percent of patients, the virus may reactivate later in life under certain stress conditions. In a person with an intact immune system, symptoms of reactivation may not be apparent, but they still make new copies of the HSV-1 virus. This phenomenon is known as viral shedding and leads to people without symptoms spreading HSV-1 unknowingly through the usual modes of transmission.

Herpes virus induces breakdown of infected cells, leading to cell necrosis (death), and inflammatory response, resulting in fluid accumulation between the epidermal and dermal layers of the skin. This forms a blister, usually referred to as a fever blister or cold sore. Each blister contains millions of new virus particles and is highly infectious. A single blister or a cluster of them may occur, and they often recur around the same location on the upper or lower lip, nose, chin, cheeks, or inside of the mouth. The time between the warning signs and the appearance of the cold sore is typically a few hours to a day or so. Once the blister

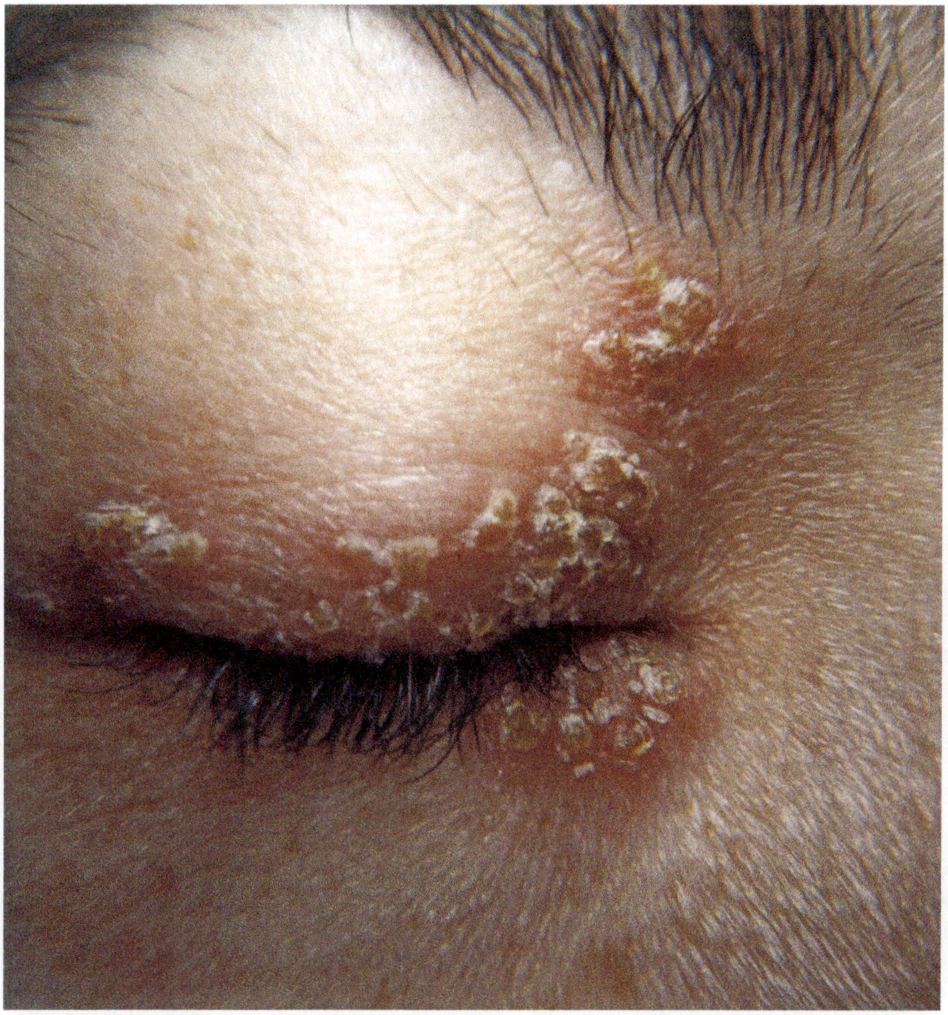

The herpes simplex 1 virus causes painful sores, known as cold sores, on the skin or in the eyes. *© John F. Wilson, MD/Science Source*

REAL-WORLD RISKS

The herpes simplex 1 virus is also the cause of a condition known as herpes gladiatorum, a skin infection common in wrestlers, rugby players, and other athletes playing sports with extensive skin contact between competitors. In this condition, lesions occur most often on the head and neck. Primary infection may cause symptoms such as fever, malaise, weight loss, and regional lymphadenopathy (a swelling of the lymph nodes). Ocular (eye) involvement includes keratitis (a swelling or inflammation of the transparent covering at the front of the eye that protects the iris and pupil), conjunctivitis (a swelling or inflammation of the conjunctiva often termed pink eye), and blepharitis (a swelling or inflammation of the eyelids). Transmission occurs primarily through skin-to-skin contact.

As recent as 2014, an outbreak of skin lesions caused by HSV-1 (leading to herpes gladiatorum) and bacteria (*Staphylococcus*) was reported in high school wrestlers in Arizona. The Centers for Disease Control and Prevention thus emphasizes infection control guidelines for athletes and coaches, including keeping infected skin lesions covered, using a dry dressing for lesions, and excluding athletes from competition when lesions cannot be covered.

has formed, it breaks and produces a yellow crust. This falls off within a few days, leaving behind pinkish skin that heals without forming a scar. The whole process normally takes 8 to 10 days, after which the skin is completely healed with no scar remaining. Patients may experience short-term local pain and irritation during primary infection. The virus reaches to nerve fibers from the primary site of infection. It may remain latent, waiting to reactivate later under various types of stress conditions.

The area around the fingernails (where the virus may enter through torn cuticles) is another common site of HSV-1 infection, which results in a painful condition known as herpetic whitlow. This area is especially vulnerable because it contains many nerve endings through which HSV-1 can be transmitted.

Scope and Distribution

Herpes simplex 1 infection is a highly contagious infection found all around the world, but prevalence is influenced by age and socioeconomic status. A 2017 estimate by the World Health Organization (WHO) indicates that about 3.7 billion people (accounting for 67 percent of global population) are infected with HSV-1. Prevalence of infection is highest in Africa (87 percent) and lowest in the Americas (40 to 50 percent).

People with weakened immunity, such as transplant recipients and human immunodeficiency virus (HIV)/acquired immunodeficiency syndrome (AIDS) patients, are more susceptible to serious HSV-1 infections. Thus, HSV-1 is often also listed as an opportunistic infection. Those with eczema—whose skin is frequently broken or damaged—are often affected with widespread HSV-1 infection, a condition known as eczema herpeticum, which requires prompt treatment with antiviral drugs.

Health care workers, such as anesthesiologists and dentists, are at risk of herpetic whitlow (lesions) if their fingers come into contact with patients who have cold sores or through viral shedding from patients who are infected but do not have symptoms.

Treatment and Prevention

There is no cure for HSV-1 infection. Once the virus is present in cells, it is there for life, even though it may not cause any symptoms. However, there are a number of antiviral drugs that can treat the symptoms of cold sores. The main ones are acyclovir, valacyclovir, and famciclovir; the former can be used as a cream, a tablet, or an intravenous injection, but the latter two are only available in tablet form. These drugs are most effective in treating the first episode of cold sores. An outbreak of cold sores can be prevented by using lip balm—to avoid broken skin—and minimizing stress and sun exposure.

Severe disease (e.g., HSV meningoencephalitis, disseminated infection, or pneumonitis) is treated with intravenous acyclovir for two to seven days or until clinical improvement is observed, followed by oral antiviral therapy to complete at least 10 total days of therapy. HSV encephalitis requires 21 days of intravenous therapy; impaired renal function due to treatment warrants adjustment in acyclovir dosage.

The TORCH test is a diagnostic test used to check for a panel of infectious diseases, including HSV, especially in infants. This blood test measures the presence of antibodies and their level of concentration in the blood. The TORCH test measures the levels of an infant's antibodies against five groups of chronic infections and is routinely used in hospitals to test newborns for HSV (and other) infections.

Patients with infection should be counseled to prevent HSV transmission to others. People who have cold sores should not kiss others and should keep any items such as cups, washcloths, and towels separate. Infected people should also abstain from oral sex to avoid transmitting the virus to the genitals of a sexual partner.

■ Impacts and Issues

HSV-1 is a common infection that usually lies dormant in the body within the nervous system. It causes health problems mainly in immunocompromised people, although the infection may be triggered in anyone carrying the virus through stress or sunlight exposure. People without symptoms may easily pass on the infection to those who are more vulnerable, so anyone who has ever had an outbreak of cold sores should consider themselves infected with HIV-1 and should take extra care with hygiene. HSV infection is a huge medical burden to society, with HSV genital infection in the United States alone resulting in more than $2.7 billion in health care costs in the year 2015. Neonatal HSV develops in 1 per 2,000 to 10,000 live births per year.

HSV-1 infection is occasionally life-threatening. Untreated, HSV-1 encephalitis has a mortality rate of 70 percent and requires intravenous acyclovir to bring the infection under control. Neonatal HSV-1 infection, although rare, can have a mortality rate of 60 percent, as the infant immune system is incapable of fighting it. Babies who survive often have severe neurological problems. Approximately 70 percent of cases of neonatal HSV occur when the mother is asymptomatically experiencing viral shedding near the time of delivery. The risk of neonatal transmission is increased if vaginal delivery occurs during acute maternal infection.

Although for many people HSV-1 infection is of little consequence, for those who are already vulnerable, it may be extremely serious.

See Also *Chickenpox (Varicella); CMV (Cytomegalovirus) Infection; Herpes Simplex 2 Virus; Shingles (Herpes Zoster) Infection*

BIBLIOGRAPHY

Books

Corey, Lawrence, and Anna Wald. "Genital Herpes." In *Sexually Transmitted Diseases*, edited by King K. Holmes, et al., 399–437. New York: McGraw-Hill, 2008.

Diefenbach, Russell J., and Cornel Fraefel. *Herpes Simplex Virus: Methods and Protocols.* New York: Humana, 2014.

Periodicals

Ahmad, F. A., G. A. Storch, and A. S. Miller. "Impact of an Institutional Guideline on the Care of Neonates at Risk for Herpes Simplex Virus in the Emergency Department." *Pediatric Emergency Care* 33, no. 6 (August 21, 2015): 396–401.

Mell, H. K. "Management of Oral and Genital Herpes in the Emergency Department." *Emergency Medicine Clinics of North America* 26, no. 2 (May 26, 2008): 457–473.

Jouan, Y., et al. "Long-Term Outcome of Severe Herpes Simplex Encephalitis: A Population-Based Observational Study." *Critical Care* 19 (September 21, 2015): 345.

Tronstein, Elizabeth, et al. "Genital Shedding of Herpes Simplex Virus among Symptomatic and Asymptomatic Persons with HSV-2 Infection." *Journal of the American Medical Association* 14 (April 13, 2011): 1441–1449.

Williams C., et al. "Notes from the Field: Outbreak of Skin Lesions among High School Wrestlers —Arizona, 2014." *Morbidity and Mortality Weekly Report* 64, no. 20 (May 29, 2015): 559–560. This article can also be found online at https://www.cdc.gov/mmwr/preview/mmwrhtml/mm6420a6.htm (accessed January 28, 2018).

Workowski, Kimberly A., and Gail A. Bolan. "Sexually Transmitted Diseases Treatment Guidelines, 2015." *Morbidity and Mortality Weekly Report* 64, no. 3 (June 15, 2015): 1–137. This article can also be found online at https://www.cdc.gov/mmwr/preview/mmwrhtml/rr6403a1.htm (accessed March 15, 2018).

Websites

"Herpes Simplex Virus." World Health Organization, January 2017. http://www.who.int/mediacentre/factsheets/fs400/en/ (accessed March 15, 2018).

Kohn, Melissa. "Herpes Simplex in Emergency Medicine." Medscape, June 26, 2017. https://emedicine.medscape.com/article/783113-overview (accessed January 27, 2018).

"What Is Herpes Keratitis?" American Academy of Ophthalmology, March 1, 2017. https://www.aao.org/eye-health/diseases/herpes-keratitis (accessed January 27, 2018).

Susan Aldridge
Kausalya Santhanam

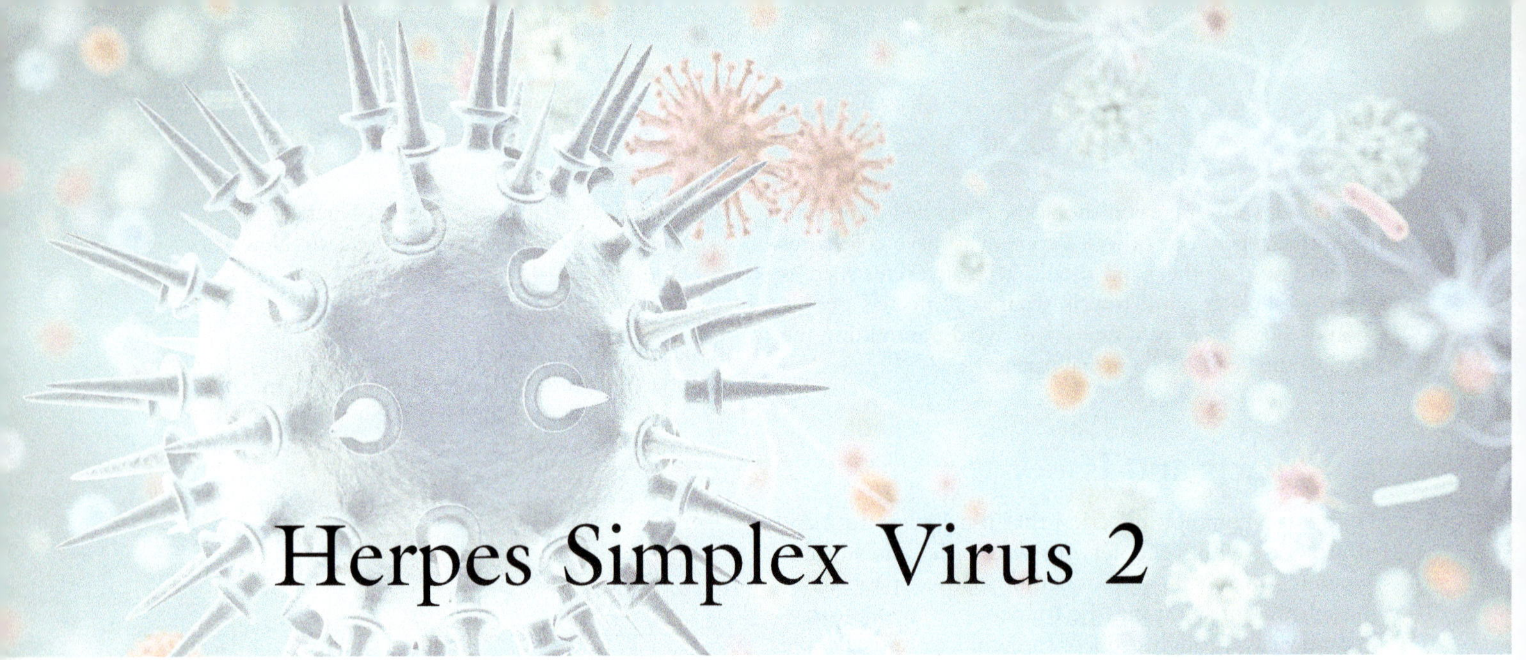

Herpes Simplex Virus 2

Introduction

Genital herpes (often known just as herpes) is an infection by the herpes simplex virus (HSV), which leads to the formation of painful sores in the genital area. Most cases of genital herpes are caused by herpes simplex virus 2 (HSV-2), but the closely related herpes simplex virus 1 (HSV-1), which normally causes cold sores, is occasionally involved. Both HSVs belong to the herpes family of viruses, all of which exist as viral particles of a diameter around 200 nanometers.

The herpes virus invades cells and may lie dormant for many years, causing no obvious symptoms. However, a herpes infection can be activated at any time and often recurs throughout life. Symptoms typically are present only when the herpes virus is active. Although the virus itself cannot be eliminated, symptoms of active infection, such as genital sores, can be treated with antiviral drugs.

WORDS TO KNOW

ASYMPTOMATIC A state in which an individual does not exhibit or experience symptoms of a disease.

DORMANT Inactive but still alive. A resting, nonactive state.

LATENT INFECTION An infection already established in the body but not yet causing symptoms or having ceased to cause symptoms after an active period.

LESION The tissue disruption or the loss of function caused by a particular disease process.

MUCOCUTANEOUS A region of the body in which mucosa (mucous membrane) transitions to skin. Mucocutaneous zones occur in animals, at the body orifices. In humans mucocutaneous zones are found at the lips, nostrils, conjunctivae, urethra, vagina (in females), foreskin (in males), and anus.

PRODROMAL SYMPTOMS The earliest symptoms of a disease.

Disease History, Characteristics, and Transmission

Like HSV-1, HSV-2 infection is a chronic and lifelong condition. The defense system of the body fails to eradicate the virus, resulting in latent infection. Most people infected with HSV-2 remain asymptomatic or experience only mild symptoms. Many people who have antibodies in their blood, indicating a past infection, have never been diagnosed with genital herpes.

HSV-2 infection is initiated in mucocutaneous zones such as the vagina, foreskin, mouth, and anus. From there it moves to nerve cells, where it remains latent before resulting in recurrent infection brought on by stress conditions. According to the US Centers for Disease Control and Prevention (CDC), about 20 percent of infected patients may experience flulike symptoms with fever, swollen lymph nodes, headache, and body aches. This is followed by development of one or more painless lesions around the mouth, genitals, and rectum. Other symptoms include intense pain, dysuria (difficulty in urination), itching, and vaginal discharge. Symptoms appear after an average incubation period of 2 to 12 days. Meningitis, an illness involving inflammation of the membranes covering the brain and spinal cord, is an occasional complication of genital herpes.

HSV-2 is a deoxyribonucleic acid (DNA) virus. It is primarily associated with genital disease, and humans are the only known reservoirs. Transmission of the infection also can occur through individuals who are asymptomatic but continue to shed viral particles. HSV-2 infection predisposes an individual to HIV infection by promoting replication of HIV in genital epithelial tissue, increasing the risk of transmission. HSV-2 infection is transmitted through vaginal, anal, or oral sex with an infected person. According to the CDC, women are more likely to contract infection than males. Other risk factors, such as duration of sexual activity, minority ethnicity, previous genital infection, socioeconomic status, and multiple sexual partners, are also determining factors of infection.

Scope and Distribution

HSV-2 infection is found around the world. According to the World Health Organization (WHO), approximately 417 million people were affected as of 2012. Estimates of HSV-2 infection may not be accurate because most cases of genital herpes remain unreported. According to a 2014 study, approximately 50 million Americans aged 12 years or older experience an episode of genital herpes, with 1.5 million new cases every year in the United States. According to WHO, Africa has the highest rate of prevalence, with about 31.5 percent of individuals infected with HSV-2. The percentage of infected individuals in the Americas is about 14.4 percent.

WHO estimates suggest that infection rates are increasing among adolescents. Symptoms of HSV-2 infection are usually most severe during the initial infection. Shorter duration flares with milder symptoms are generally reported in subsequent recurring infections. Because sexual transmission of HSV-2 infection from men to women is more common, the number of women affected (267 million) is almost double that of infected men (150 million). Herpes infection at birth, known as neonatal herpes, affects about 10 of every 10,000 births worldwide. The risk of transmitting the virus to a newborn is higher in mothers who contract the HSV-2 infection during pregnancy.

Treatment and Prevention

As of 2018 there was no cure or vaccine available for HSV-2 infection. However, trials were underway at the University of Pennsylvania for a new vaccine. A number of antiviral drugs can be used to treat outbreaks of genital herpes, such as acyclovir, valacyclovir, and famciclovir. Those who know they are infected because of past outbreaks can help protect their sexual partners by using condoms. People with active genital sores should not have sexual contact with others even if using a condom, because sores and lesions can appear outside of the area covered by the condom.

The Division of Sexually Transmitted Disease (STD) at the CDC recommends that "all pregnant women should be asked whether they have a history of genital herpes. At the onset of labor, all women should be questioned carefully about symptoms of genital herpes, including prodromal symptoms (early signs), and all women should be examined carefully for herpetic lesions."

Detection of the virus through a tissue culture is the definitive diagnostic approach, but such testing is feasible only during initial infection and not recurrent episodes of genital herpes.

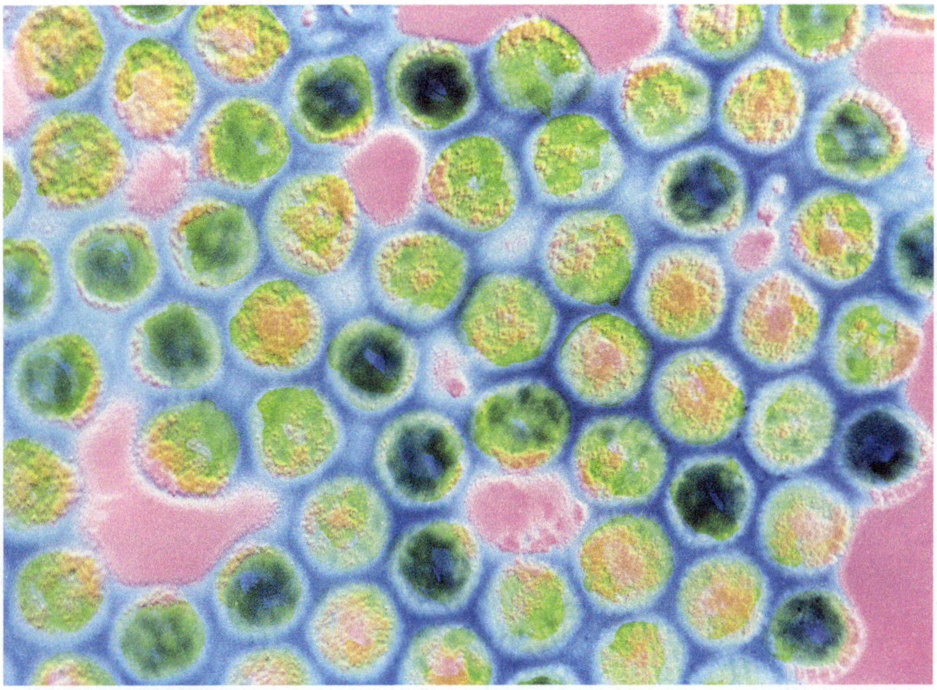

A false-color transmission electron micrograph (TEM) of numerous virions (virus particles) of the herpes simplex virus, a member of the herpes virus group. *© CNRI/Science Source*

REAL-WORLD RISKS

The US Centers for Disease Control and Prevention's 2015 Sexually Transmitted Diseases Treatment Guidelines states that the following recommendations apply to counseling of people with herpes simplex virus (HSV) infection:

- Persons who have genital herpes should be educated concerning the natural history of the disease, with emphasis on the potential for recurrent episodes, asymptomatic viral shedding, and the attendant risks of sexual transmission.
- Persons experiencing a first episode of genital herpes should be advised that suppressive therapy is available and is effective in preventing symptomatic recurrent episodes and that episodic therapy sometimes is useful in shortening the duration of recurrent episodes.
- All persons with genital HSV infection should be encouraged to inform their current sex partners that they have genital herpes and to inform future partners before initiating a sexual relationship.
- Sexual transmission of HSV can occur during asymptomatic periods. Asymptomatic viral shedding is more frequent in genital HSV-2 infection than in genital HSV-1 infection and is most frequent during the first 12 months after acquiring HSV-2.
- All persons with genital herpes should remain abstinent from sexual activity with uninfected partners when lesions or prodromal symptoms are present.
- The risk of HSV-2 sexual transmission can be decreased by the daily use of valacyclovir by the infected person.
- Recent studies indicate that latex condoms, when used consistently and correctly, might reduce the risk for genital herpes transmission.
- Sex partners of infected persons should be advised that they might be infected even if they have no symptoms. Type-specific serologic testing of asymptomatic partners of persons with genital herpes is recommended to determine whether risk for HSV acquisition exists.
- The risk for neonatal HSV infection should be explained to all persons, including men. Pregnant women and women of childbearing age who have genital herpes should inform their providers who care for them during pregnancy and those who will care for their newborn infant. Pregnant women who are not infected with HSV-2 should be advised to avoid intercourse during the third trimester with men who have genital herpes. Similarly, pregnant women who are not infected with HSV-1 should be counseled to avoid genital exposure to HSV-1 during the third trimester (e.g., oral sex with a partner with oral herpes and vaginal intercourse with a partner with genital HSV-1 infection).
- Asymptomatic persons diagnosed with HSV-2 infection by type-specific serologic testing should receive the same counseling messages as persons with symptomatic infection. In addition, such persons should be taught about the clinical manifestations of genital herpes.

Impacts and Issues

HSV-2 usually lies dormant within the body, leaving people unaware that they can infect others through sexual contact. As herpes infections can be life threatening in newborns and people with impaired immunity, the risk of infection is a serious concern. HSV-2 infection has also been found to promote HIV transmission. The link between genital ulcers and HIV has been known for more than 20 years. According to WHO, HSV-2 infected individuals have a threefold increased likelihood of contracting a new HIV infection. It is estimated that 60 to 90 percent of HIV patients have HSV-2 infections. Treatment with acyclovir, a relatively inexpensive drug, could help prevent reactivation of HSV-2, thereby potentially reducing the risk of HIV transmission.

Research also highlights the psychosocial impact of HSV-2 infection. Recurring symptoms of genital herpes may be painful and cause distress in sexual relationships. This often may lead to social stigma affecting the quality of life of infected individuals.

SEE ALSO *Herpes Simplex 1 Virus; Shingles (Herpes Zoster) Infection*

BIBLIOGRAPHY

Books

Gillespie, Stephen H., and Kathleen B. Bamford. *Medical Microbiology and Infection at a Glance.* 4th ed. Hoboken, NJ: Wiley Blackwell, 2012.

Knodel, Leroy C. "Sexually Transmitted Diseases." In *Pharmacotherapy: A Pathophysiologic Approach*, edited by Joseph T. DiPiro. New York: McGraw-Hill, 2014.

Periodicals

Bernstein, D., et al. "Epidemiology, Clinical Presentation, and Antibody Response to Primary Infection with Herpes Simplex Virus Type 1 and Type 2 in Young Women." *Clinical Infectious Diseases* 56 (2013): 344–351.

Li, De-Kun, et al. "Genital Herpes and Its Treatment in Relation to Preterm Delivery." *American Journal of Epidemiology* 180, no. 11 (2014): 1109–1117. This article can also be found online at https://academic.oup.com/aje/article/180/11/1109/147904 (accessed February 28, 2018).

Roett, M. A., M. T. Mayor, and K. A. Uduhiri. "Diagnosis and Management of Genital Ulcers." *American Family Physician* 85 (2012): 254–262.

Shin, H., and A. Iwasaki. "Generating Protective Immunity against Genital Herpes." *Trends in Immunology* 34 (2013): 487–494.

Workowski, Kimberly A., and Gail A. Bolan. "Sexually Transmitted Diseases Treatment Guidelines, 2015." *Morbidity and Mortality Weekly Report* 64, no. RR3 (June 5, 2015): 1–137.

Websites

"Genital Herpes: CDC Fact Sheet." Centers for Disease Control and Prevention, September 1, 2017. https://www.cdc.gov/std/herpes/stdfact-herpes.htm (accessed February 27, 2018).

"Genital HSV Infections." Centers for Disease Control and Prevention, June 8, 2015. http://www.cdc.gov/std/tg2015/herpes.htm (accessed February 17, 2018).

"Herpes Simplex Virus." World Health Organization, January 2017. http://www.who.int/mediacentre/factsheets/fs400/en/ (accessed February 27, 2018).

Susan Aldridge
Kausalya Santhanam

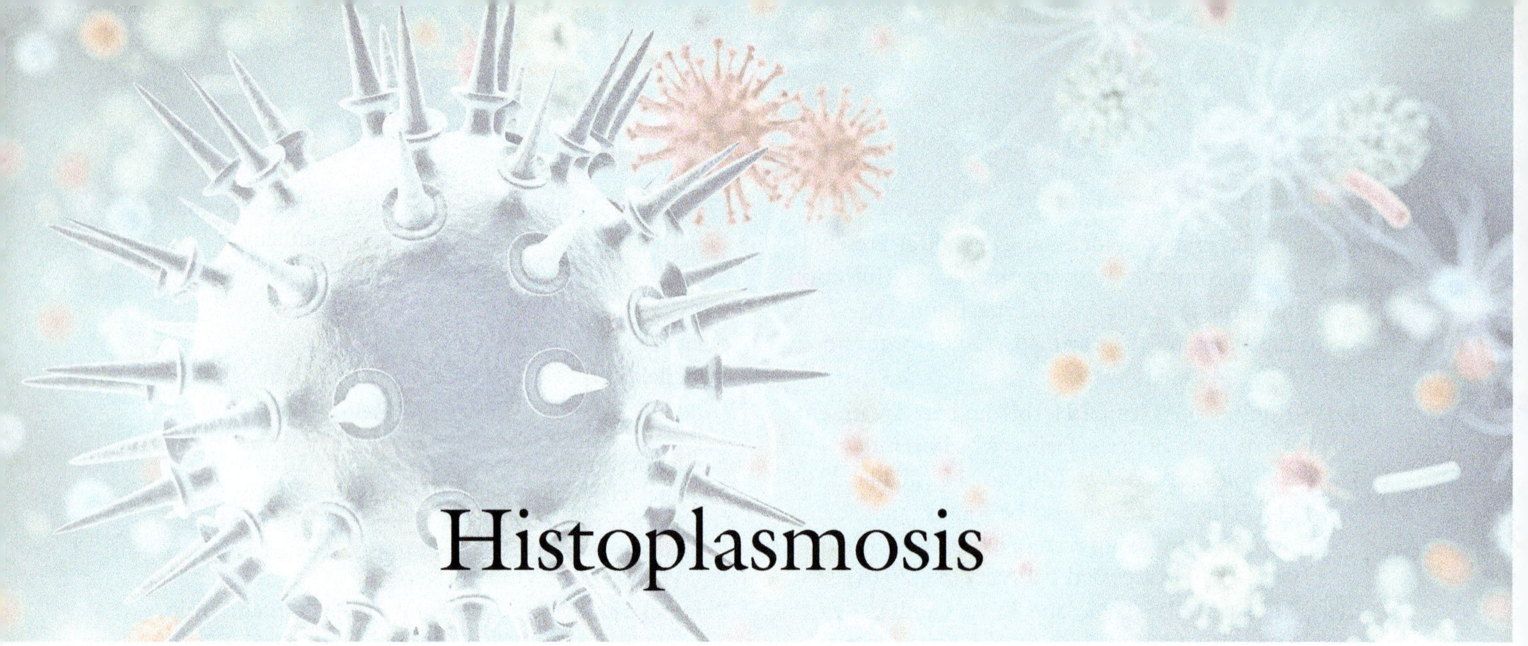

Histoplasmosis

Introduction

Histoplasmosis is a disease caused by a mycotic (fungal) infection of *Histoplasma capsulatum* fungal spores. The infection develops when fungal spores are inhaled, and the resulting disease affects the lungs. The fungus is found globally and is endemic in some areas. The key factor about these spores is their resilience in the environment and their ability to become airborne when the ground is disturbed. Typically, *Histoplasma* spores are concentrated in soil that contains the droppings of birds or bats. Such soil can often be found in caves, lending histoplasmosis the nickname "cave disease." The disease is not transmissible between humans.

In the majority of cases, infection will not result in disease, but in severe cases, which occur in fewer than 1 percent of patients, people with histoplasmosis may present with chronic flu- or tuberculosis-like symptoms. People with existing immune system problems are at an increased risk of the disease spreading to other organs of the body, which can be potentially fatal if untreated. Treatment commonly includes antifungal medication.

WORDS TO KNOW

ENDEMIC Present in a particular area or among a particular group of people.

IMMUNOSUPPRESSION A reduction of the ability of the immune system to recognize and respond to the presence of foreign material.

MYCOTIC Having to do with or caused by a fungus. Any medical condition caused by a fungus is a mycotic condition, also called a mycosis.

SPORE A dormant form assumed by some bacteria, such as anthrax, that enable the bacterium to survive high temperatures, dryness, and lack of nourishment for long periods of time. Under proper conditions, the spore may revert to the actively multiplying form of the bacteria.

Disease History, Characteristics, and Transmission

Histoplasmosis was first identified in 1905 and 1906, when the American physician Samuel Darling (1872–1925) identified *Histoplasma capsulatum* infections while performing autopsies on workers in the Panama Canal Zone. Histoplasmosis infections were first reported in the United States in 1926. The disease is believed to have originated in Latin America, but it occurs worldwide and is endemic in some parts of the United States. Risk of infection in North America is highest in the Ohio, Mississippi, and St. Lawrence river valleys, where *Histoplasma* is most prevalent. Histoplasmosis primarily affects the lungs but in some cases spreads to other organs in the body. Histoplasmosis is also known as cave disease, spelunkers' disease, Darling's disease, Ohio River Valley fever, Mississippi River Valley disease, and Appalachian Mountain disease.

Most people infected have no symptoms or have symptoms that heal spontaneously; in most cases these people will develop partial immunity against reinfection. If symptoms do occur, they will usually develop within 3 to 17 days. Acute symptomatic pulmonary histoplasmosis has a short duration, with possible symptoms including fever, chills, chest pain, and a nonproductive cough.

Chronic pulmonary histoplasmosis presents with longer-lasting symptoms that are similar to tuberculosis: chest pain, loss of breath, coughing, sweating, and fever. Disseminated histoplasmosis is the most serious form of the disease; it is only common among immunosuppressed people and can be fatal if left untreated. In these cases, the disease spreads from the lungs to other organs, and symptoms include neck stiffness, skin lesions, and mouth sores. When not treated, disseminated histoplasmosis is often fatal.

Histoplasmosis is contracted by inhalation of the *Histoplasma* fungal spores, which thrive in damp, organically rich soil, and some animal droppings, most commonly those of birds and bats. *Histoplasma* has also been found in the feces of both wild animals, such as baboons and raccoons, and domesticated animals, such as horses, dogs, and cats. Once these microscopic spores enter the lungs, they imbed in the small air sacs and trigger an immune reaction that, in serious cases, leads to inflammation, scarring, and calcium deposits on the lungs. The extent of histoplasmosis infection is dependent both on the number of spores inhaled and the immunity of the host.

■ Scope and Distribution

Histoplasmosis is primarily located in the temperate regions of the world and is endemic in areas of the United States, including the southeastern, mid-Atlantic, and central states of Arkansas, Kentucky, Missouri, Tennessee, West Virginia, Ohio, and Texas, as well as Central and South America. Most cases of the disease are sporadic, but point-source outbreaks have been previously described.

The fungal spores are commonly found in fertile soils, caves, poultry houses, bird roosts, and areas harboring bats. The spores frequently become airborne when disturbed, are extremely resilient, and remain viable in the environment for long periods of time. In fact, plants fertilized with droppings may contain spores and produce infectious smoke when burned. This gives the spores the ability to transfer large distances from the initial source and still retain viability in causing disease.

Due to the high prevalence of histoplasmosis fungi, infection is common, and 80 percent of people living in fungal-rich areas of the United States could exhibit a positive skin test for the presence of histoplasmosis fungi. However, development of disease is rare and is only considered a risk to people with weakened immune systems, such as very young children, elderly people, organ transplant patients, chemotherapy patients, patients with human immunodeficiency virus (HIV), and people with autoimmune

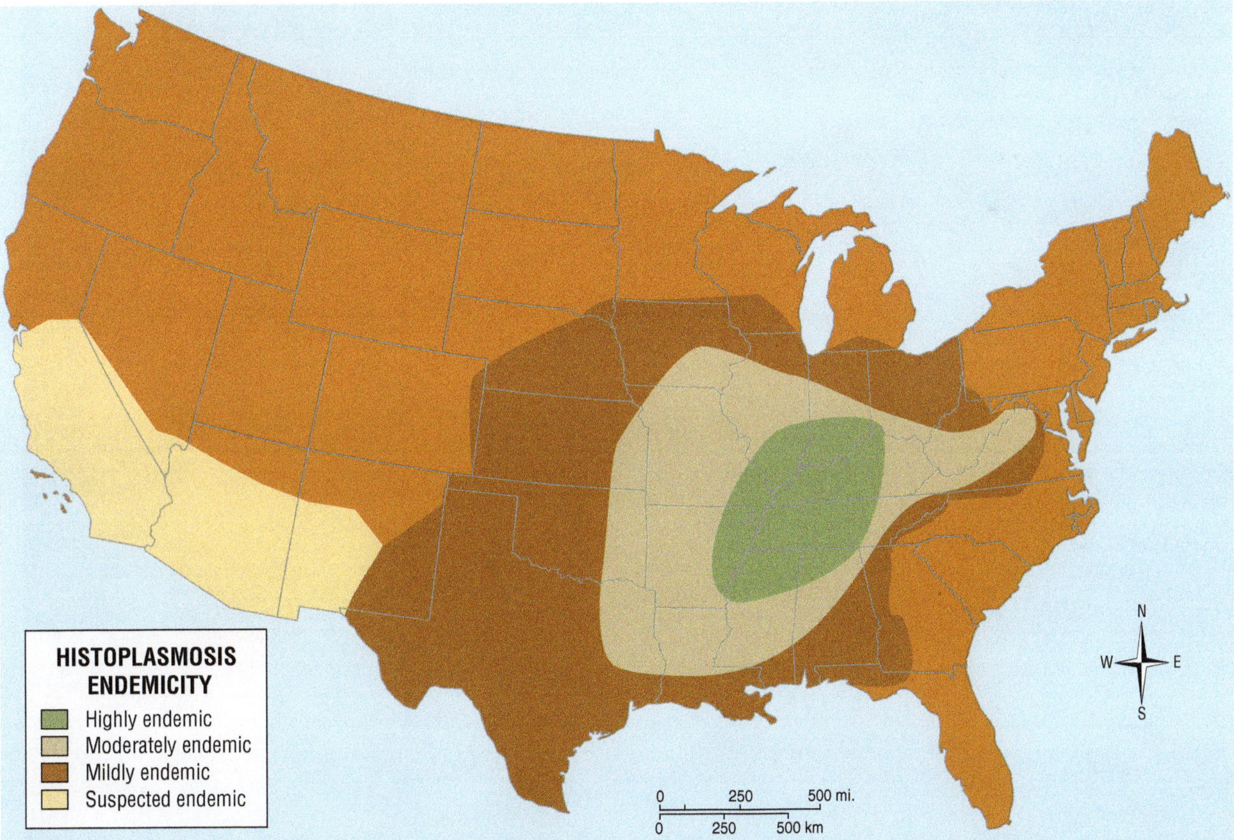

SOURCE: Adapted from "Areas Endemic for Histoplasmosis." US Centers for Diseases Control and Prevention. Available from: https://www.cdc.gov/fungal/diseases/histoplasmosis/images/histoplasmosis-lifecycle-maps-300px.jpg

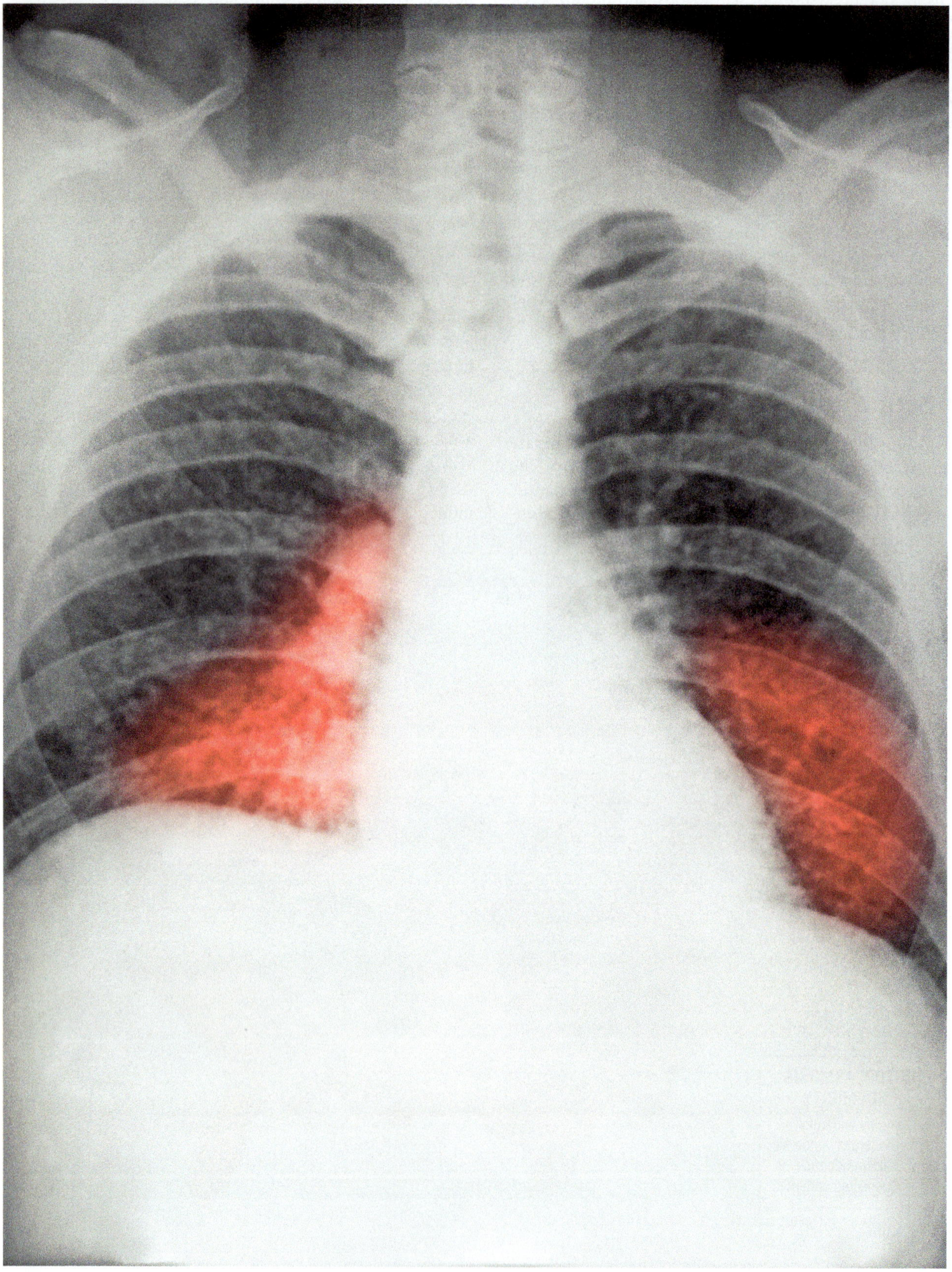

A chest X-ray shows a histoplasmosis fungal infection, which, in severe cases, can cause chronic tuberculosis-like symptoms. *© Scott Camazine/Science Source*

disease. The ages of people affected range from children to adults, and there is no increased incidence among either sex, although chronic lung infections are more common in men than women.

Although quite infrequent, outbreaks of histoplasmosis have been previously described and generally result from a single event, such as construction, clearing, cleaning, and cave exploration, that causes disruption of a large area housing the fungus. One such outbreak occurred in 2001 in Indiana and infected 523 school students. The cause of the outbreak was rototilling of a courtyard containing the fungus.

■ Treatment and Prevention

Histoplasmosis may present symptoms similar to other diseases, and, as such, diagnosis is achieved through blood tests or laboratory cultures. Generally, histoplasmosis fungal infections do not lead to the development of disease, and, even with mild cases that do develop, the disease usually resolves without treatment. When required, the most common treatment for histoplasmosis is antifungal medication such as itraconazole, which is administered for various lengths of time depending on the severity of infection. In most cases previous infection will result in partial protection against reinfection.

Awareness is a key factor in disease prevention, so the public is advised to investigate potential risk factors before beginning a job or an activity with a potential exposure to the histoplasmosis fungi. When working in areas carrying a high risk of making contact with the fungal spores, it is also important to wear appropriate protective clothing, such as disposable coveralls (to prevent transfer of the spores from the worksite) and a dust mask that covers both the nose and mouth (to filter out all particles larger than two microns in size).

Due to the natural widespread occurrence of *Histoplasma capsulatum*, it would be virtually impossible to decontaminate all infected sites. Prevention is commonly achieved by minimizing the disruption of soils in affected areas in addition to limiting the exposure of persons to dust in contaminated environments. In areas where soil disruption is unavoidable, spraying infected areas thoroughly with water mist prior to beginning excavation reduces the number of aerosols produced.

■ Impacts and Issues

Cases of chronic disease caused by histoplasmosis are on the rise and are attributed mainly to the increasing number of persons living with weakened immune systems due to HIV, chemotherapy, organ transplant, or autoimmune disease. Immunosuppression later in life may also result in reactivation of quiescent infection born from earlier exposure. As the number of people living with immune disorders increases, scientists expect there will be a proportional increase in the prevalence of chronic histoplasmosis.

Land use might also play a part in the resurgence of histoplasmosis. Development of lands traditionally used for farming in the nitrogen-rich belt of the central and southern United States could also be a factor in the increased number of reported cases.

Scientists have learned that histoplasmosis infection can also lead to ocular histoplasmosis syndrome (OHS). OHS is a condition that damages blood vessels in the eyes and leads to impaired vision. It is thought that the fungal spores travel from the lungs to the eye and lodge in the blood vessels leading to the retina. This causes no initial damage to eyesight, although it does leave recognizable histo spots on the blood vessels. Vision loss can occur years after the initial infection. Detecting the histo spots can indicate future vision loss, and photocoagulation laser eye surgery can reduce the likelihood of vision loss by more than 50 percent.

Awareness of this disease acts to minimize unnecessary exposure to contaminated areas and promote the use of protective equipment when required. In the United States the National Institute for Occupational Safety and Health, along with the Centers for Disease Control and Prevention (CDC), engages in promotions geared to educate employers and workers about the risks and prevention strategies for histoplasmosis.

SEE ALSO *AIDS (Acquired Immunodeficiency Syndrome); Emerging Infectious Diseases; HIV; Land Utilization and Disease; Opportunistic Infection; Tuberculosis*

BIBLIOGRAPHY

Books

Bennett, John E., Raphael Dolin, and Martin J. Blaser. *Mandell, Douglas, and Bennett's Principles and Practice of Infectious Diseases.* Vol. 2. Philadelphia: Elsevier, 2014.

Morris, Timothy A., Andrew L. Ries, and Richard A. Bordow, eds. *Manual of Clinical Problems in Pulmonary Medicine.* Philadelphia: Wolters Kluwer, 2014.

Periodicals

Chamany, S., et al. "A Large Histoplasmosis Outbreak among High School Students in Indiana, 2001." *Pediatric Infectious Disease Journal* 23, no. 10 (2004): 909–914.

Kandi, Venkataramana, et al. "Chronic Pulmonary Histoplasmosis and Its Clinical Significance: An Under-Reported Systemic Fungal Disease." *Cureus* 8, no. 8 (2016): e751. This article can also be found online at https://www.ncbi.nlm.nih.gov/pmc/articles/PMC5037059/ (accessed January 23, 2018).

Kauffman, Carol A. "Histoplasmosis: A Clinical and Laboratory Update." *Clinical Microbiology Reviews* 20, no. 1 (2007): 115–132. This article can also be found online at https://www.ncbi.nlm.nih.gov/pmc/articles/PMC1797635/ (accessed January 23, 2018).

Siegel-Itzkovich, Judy. "First-Ever Case of 'Cave Disease' Diagnosed in the Middle East." *Jerusalem Post* (December 11, 2017). This article can also be found online at http://www.jpost.com/HEALTH-SCIENCE/First-ever-case-of-cave-disease-diagnosed-in-the-Middle-East-517728 (accessed January 23, 2018).

Websites

"Histoplasmosis." Centers for Disease Control and Prevention, November 21, 2015. https://www.cdc.gov/fungal/diseases/histoplasmosis/index.html (accessed January 23, 2018).

"Histoplasmosis." Mayo Clinic. https://www.mayoclinic.org/diseases-conditions/histoplasmosis/symptoms-causes/syc-20373495 (accessed January 23, 2018).

Turbert, David. "Histoplasmosis." American Academy of Ophthalmology, September 1, 2017. https://www.aao.org/eye-health/diseases/what-is-histoplasmosis (accessed January 23, 2018).

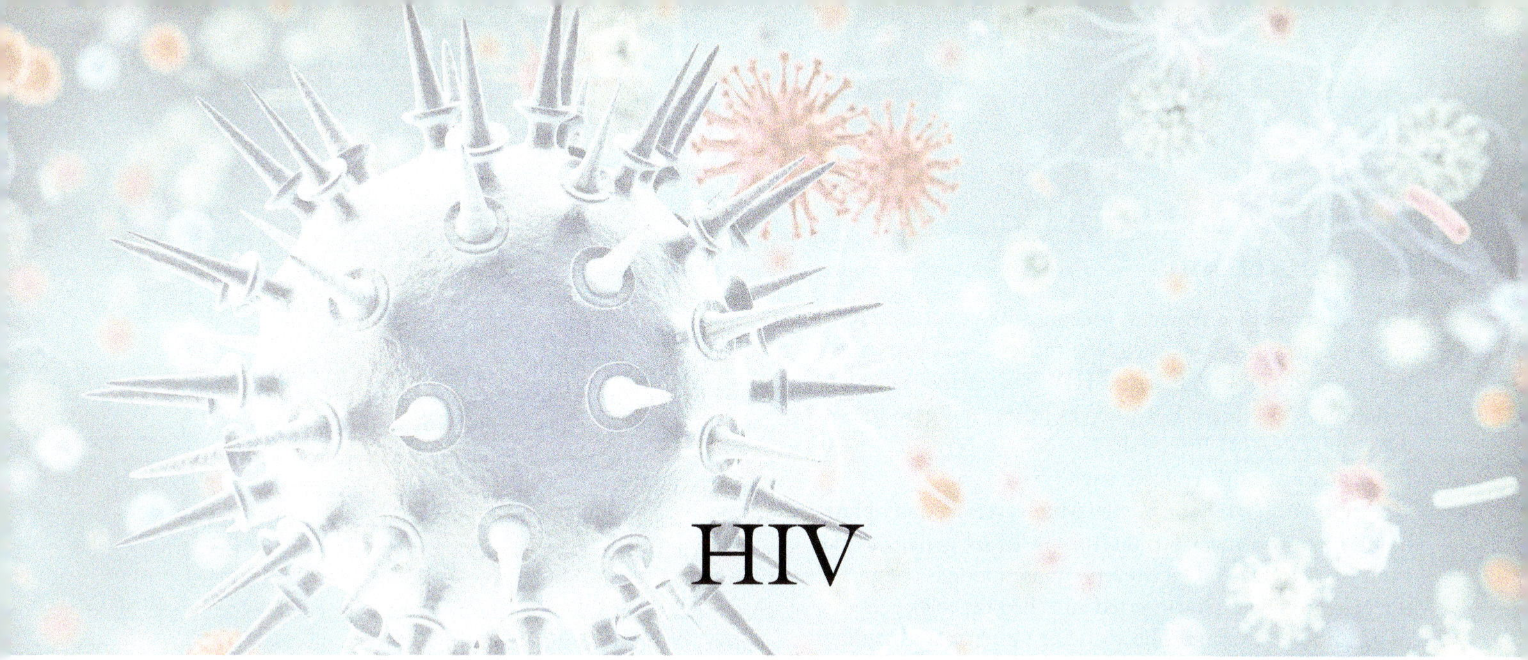

HIV

Introduction

Human immunodeficiency virus (HIV) is the microorganism responsible for acquired immunodeficiency syndrome (AIDS). HIV attacks the immune system and eventually leaves the body vulnerable to potentially fatal opportunistic infections. There are two major forms of HIV, known as HIV-1 and HIV-2. In 2017 the Joint United Nations Programme on HIV/AIDS (UNAIDS) estimated that 78 million people had been infected with HIV since the beginning of the epidemic in 1981. Of these people, 35 million had died of illnesses associated with AIDS.

WORDS TO KNOW

AUTOIMMUNITY A condition in which the immune system attacks the body's cells, causing tissue destruction. Autoimmune diseases are classified as either general, in which the autoimmune reaction takes place simultaneously in a number of tissues, or organ specific, in which the autoimmune reaction targets a single organ. Autoimmunity is accepted as the cause of a wide range of disorders and is suspected to be responsible for many more. Among the most common diseases attributed to autoimmune disorders are rheumatoid arthritis, systemic lupus erythematosus (lupus), multiple sclerosis, myasthenia gravis, pernicious anemia, and scleroderma.

CD4+ T CELLS A type of T cell found in the immune system that are characterized by the presence of a CD4 antigen protein on their surface. These are the cells most often destroyed as a result of HIV infection.

CYTOTOXIC Able to kill cells. Cytotoxic drugs kill cancer cells but may also have applications in killing bacteria.

GENOME All of the genetic information for a cell or organism. The complete sequence of genes within a cell or virus.

OPPORTUNISTIC INFECTION An infection that occurs in people whose immune systems are diminished or not functioning normally. Such infections are opportunistic insofar as the infectious agents take advantage of their host's compromised immune system and invade to cause disease.

PATHOGEN A disease-causing agent such as a bacterium, a virus, a fungus, or another microorganism.

RECOMBINATION A process during which genetic material is shuffled during reproduction to form new combinations. This mixing is important from an evolutionary standpoint because it allows the expression of different traits between generations. The process involves a physical exchange of nucleotides between duplicate strands of deoxyribonucleic acid (DNA).

RETROVIRUS Viruses in which the genetic material consists of ribonucleic acid (RNA) instead of the usual deoxyribonucleic acid (DNA). Retroviruses produce an enzyme known as reverse transcriptase that can transform RNA into DNA, which can then be permanently integrated into the DNA of the infected host cells.

History and Scientific Foundations

HIV is a type of retrovirus, meaning its genetic code is made of ribonucleic acid (RNA) rather than deoxyribonucleic acid (DNA). Because HIV has no DNA, which is necessary to create RNA copies of its viral genome, it uses the DNA of infected host cells to create a new RNA genome and replicate itself.

Retroviruses rely on the enzyme reverse transcriptase to perform the reverse transcription of its genetic code from RNA to DNA. Once reverse transcription is complete, the genetic code can be inserted into the host cell's genome using another enzyme. The virus then replicates as part of the cell's DNA. One of the major classes of HIV drugs targets reverse transcriptase, inhibiting the virus's ability to create the DNA segment for insertion into the infected cell's DNA.

One of the most important features of HIV replication is its ability to generate large numbers of new genetic combinations through a process known as recombination. This, together with a high rate of genetic mutation of individual genes, enables HIV to rapidly create new drug-resistant strains.

After HIV was identified as the cause of AIDS, researchers suspected that genetic recombination could also play a key role in the evolution of the virus. Studies of HIV infection worldwide have revealed that recombination frequencies are much higher than expected. Recombination is regarded as a central aspect of the HIV infectious cycle and the evolution of the virus. The recombination frequency of the HIV-1 genome has been observed to vary between 3 and 30 recombinations for each round of replication, depending on the infected cell type and the viral genome.

HIV has a globular structure with a spiked envelope. The spikes control the process by which the virus fuses with the targeted CD4+ cells, a type of white blood cell known as a T cell, which plays an important role in the immune system. These spikes contain a glycoprotein called gp120, which attaches to CD4, a protein found on the surface of T cells. It is also thought that the virus enters a host cell with the aid of a coreceptor on the T cell surface, either CCR5 or CXCR4 (fusin), which are chemokine receptors, or proteins that direct cell movement.

The HIV coat is formed by budding from the plasma membrane of an infected host cell. As HIV tries to enter a cell, interactions between cell surface molecules and viral envelope proteins enable the HIV envelope to fuse with the cell membrane. The HIV envelope protein gp41 plays a key role in this interaction.

Treatment and Prevention

Whereas many current therapies interrupt viral replication, new treatments target the ability of HIV to fuse with target cells. Laboratory researchers have begun testing two in vitro approaches that may help to block the CCR5 and CXCR4 receptors. One is to infuse more chemokines to people whose CD8+ cells (another type of T cell that aids in the immune response) are not

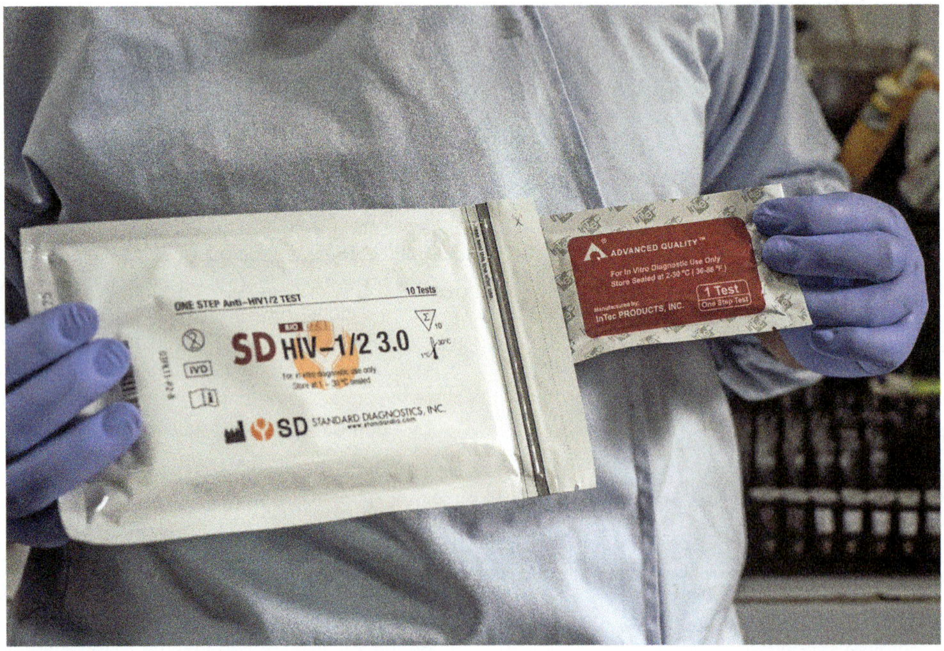

In Jakarta, Indonesia, in 2017, a laboratory technician shows a kit that tests for human immunodeficiency virus (HIV), the microorganism responsible for acquired immunodeficiency syndrome, or AIDS. While HIV can be fatal if left untreated, new medicines and vaccines have shown promise in combating the virus. *© Anton Raharjo/Anadolu Agency/Getty Images*

producing enough of these chemicals. The other is to directly block the receptors. Therapies employing these approaches should help prevent HIV from entering host cells.

An exciting new approach to prevent HIV from infecting cells employs chimeric antigen receptor T cell (CAR-T) gene therapy, also a highly promising immunological approach to cancer treatment. Researchers have begun bioengineering blood-forming stem cells that can transport CAR molecules to cells to eliminate the interaction between HIV and CD4. This means that the T cells derived from bone marrow stem cells will target the HIV-infected cells. When the CAR molecule attaches to HIV, other parts of the molecule activate the T cell to kill the HIV-infected cell.

The immune system has a so-called innate component (innate immunity) composed of white blood cells called phagocytes, which migrate to affected areas and engulf disease-causing organisms. Special cells of innate immunity called dendritic cells are particularly important for regulating immune response. When dendritic cells encounter foreign material, they have unique receptors that allow them to distinguish harmless and pathogenic organisms. These cells carry fragments of pathogen to the lymph nodes, where they stimulate a response by the adaptive immune system (called adaptive immunity), depending on the ability of the foreign material to cause disease.

If dendritic cells decide that the material is pathogenic (part of a virus or bacteria), they activate CD4+ helper T cells. Helper T cells can then stimulate another group of white blood cells, B cells, to produce antibodies, which bind to the specific antigen and immobilize it, preventing it from causing infection. Antibodies are specific for only one antigen. Memory cells are also produced to ensure faster and stronger immune response when the body is reexposed to the same pathogen.

Pathogens that escape antibody detection can enter and infect body tissue cells. The cell membranes of infected cells change in a way that is recognized by T cells. Cytotoxic T cells kill infected cells, preventing them from producing more pathogens. Cytotoxic T cells must interact with helper T cells to regulate the destruction of infected cells.

HIV specifically attacks helper T cells. Without an adequate number of helper T cells, the immune system cannot signal B cells to produce antibodies to kill infected cells. When HIV has critically depleted the helper T cell population, the body can no longer launch an adaptive immune response and becomes susceptible to many opportunistic infections, thus resulting in the immunodeficiency that characterizes AIDS.

Research shows that CD4+ membrane proteins are targets for HIV infection. Therefore, memory helper T cells are quickly infected and destroyed in the mucus membranes of tissues. Researchers have recognized that memory cell destruction occurs in the first several days after HIV infection, suggesting that therapies should begin as soon as the infection is detected.

Mysteries remain about how HIV causes disease, particularly the reason why there is uncontrolled viral replication in most infected patients. Investigation into HIV has focused on T regulatory (Treg) cells, a subset of CD4+ T cells, whose main function is to avoid autoimmunity. Data point to two main roles for Treg cells in HIV. One is that Treg cells have a detrimental effect in which HIV-specific immune responses are muted. The other is that Treg cells limit immune activation and therefore limit the helper T cell targets of HIV. Several promising in vitro trials developed since 2012 at the University of Texas could assist research in this area. It is possible that HIV takes advantage of a feature of the immune system that naturally limits immune response.

CDC RISK REDUCTION TOOL

The Centers for Disease Control and Prevention (CDC) offers an online tool to help users learn about human immunodeficiency virus (HIV) and HIV prevention, assess their lifestyle choices and risk factors, and gather information and resources, including those available in their local communities. The HIV Risk Reduction Tool (https://www.cdc.gov/hivrisk/) provides an overview of what it means to be infected with HIV and includes answers to frequently asked questions about how HIV is transmitted. The tool also details behaviors that can increase or decrease the risk of contracting the virus. The site offers practical advice for communicating with sexual partners, choosing less risky sexual practices, and correctly using condoms. Information on the site can be customized based on factors such as gender identity, HIV status, and sexual partners. Users can also enter a zip code to locate local services such as confidential HIV testing.

Impact and Issues

The level of specificity of the science required to provide breakthroughs in the battle against HIV is unprecedented. Most disease cures and treatments that have been discovered since the early 20th century have been based on limited knowledge of microbes' ability to cause disease. As with the fight against cancer, the effort to find a cure for AIDS is leading scientists into ever more minute aspects of the pathogen, all the way down to the atomic structure of viral envelope spikes and the molecular mechanisms of genetic replication.

HIV is an amazingly versatile and adaptive enemy, probably owing to millennia of evolution in nonhuman primates and its now relatively open ecological niche within humanity. While HIV transmission is preventable, a variety of social and behavioral factors have led to its becoming the worst epidemic in the history of the human species in terms of lives lost. Also, as with the struggle against cancer, contending with the perplexing mysteries of HIV will leave a mark not only on the history and future development of medicine but also on human behavior and social evolution for the foreseeable future.

SEE ALSO *AIDS (Acquired Immunodeficiency Syndrome); AIDS: Origin of the Modern Pandemic; Viral Disease*

BIBLIOGRAPHY

Books

Palladino, Michael A., and David Wesner. *HIV and AIDS*. Special Topics in Biology Series. San Francisco: Benjamin Cummings, 2005.

Periodicals

Collison, Lauren W., and Dario A. A. Vignali. "In Vitro Treg Suppression Assays." *Methods in Molecular Biology* 707 (2011): 21–37.

Sempere, J. M., V. Soriano, and J. M. Benito. "T Regulatory Cells and HIV Infection." *AIDS Reviews* 9, no. 1 (January–March 2007): 54–60.

Tran, D. Q. "In vitro Suppression Assay for Functional Assessment of Human Regulatory T Cells." *Methods in Molecular Biology* 979 (2013): 199–212.

Websites

"AIDS 2000, a Laboratory Simulation." University of Arizona. http://www.biology.arizona.edu/immunology/tutorials/AIDS (accessed March 6, 2018).

"Co-Receptors: CCR5—Understanding HIV." The Body Pro, January 2003. http://www.thebodypro.com/content/art4978.html (accessed March 6, 2018).

Padmanabha, Disha. "Gene Therapy Using CAR-T Could Interfere with the Ability of HIV to Infect Cells." BioTecNika, December 30, 2017. https://www.biotecnika.org/2017/12/gene-therapy-using-car-t-interfere-ability-hiv-infect-cells/ (accessed March 6, 2018).

Kenneth T. LaPensee

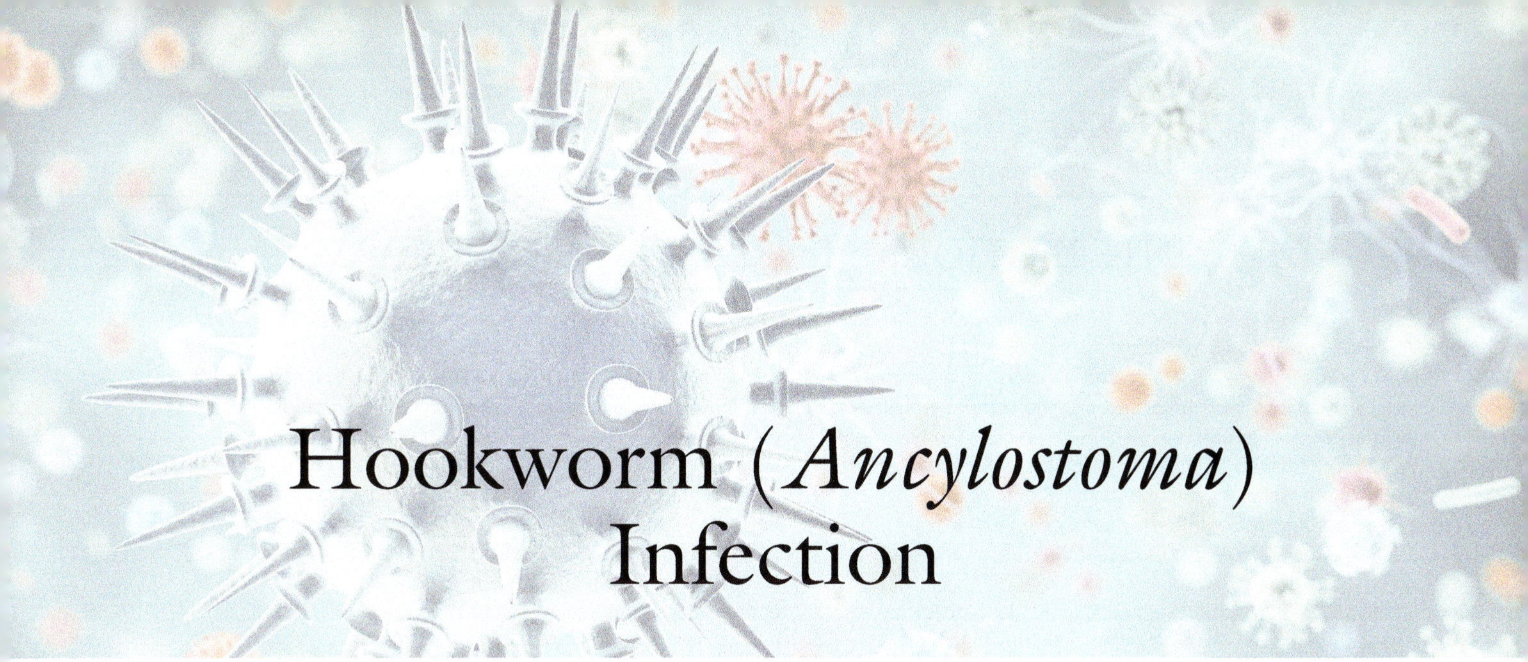

Hookworm (*Ancylostoma*) Infection

■ Introduction

Ancylostoma (an-cy-LO-sto-ma) infection, also called hookworm infection, is an infection of one of two roundworms: *Ancylostoma duodenale* or *Necator americanus.* Depending on maturity, the roundworms range from 0.3 to 0.5 inches (0.7 to 1.3 centimeters) in length.

Hookworms are parasitic roundworms that infest the intestines of their host. They have hooklike appendages, from which they take their name. Hookworms belong to the class Nematoda. Moderate infestation of hookworms in humans is considered by the World Health Organization (WHO) to be between 2,000 and 3,999 eggs per gram of feces. Heavy infestation is counted at 4,000 or more eggs per gram of feces.

Hookworm infection is most common in areas with rural poverty and low socioeconomic status, especially southern China, the Indian subcontinent, and parts of the Americas. As of 2016 approximately 500 million people worldwide were infected with hookworm, and another 5.1 billion were at risk of acquiring the infection.

■ Disease History, Characteristics, and Transmission

Hookworms deposit eggs in warm, moist, shaded soil. Such conditions allow the eggs to develop into larvae. The larvae are barely visible but can easily penetrate human skin. They frequently enter the body through the soles of the feet or when humans handle feces. Children often are infected because they play in the dirt and go barefoot. Humans cannot infect other humans with hookworm.

Once inside the body, the larvae travel through the bloodstream to the lungs and respiratory tract, then move on to the trachea. From there the larvae are coughed up and swallowed into the digestive tract and stomach, ending up in the small intestine. The trip from the skin to the intestines takes about one week. In the small intestine the larvae develop into adult worms about 0.5 inches (1.3 centimeters) in length. They attach themselves to the intestinal walls and feast on blood. One adult worm can produce thousands of eggs and live up to 10 years. The eggs are expelled in feces. Under the proper conditions, the eggs hatch, molt, and develop into infective larvae after 5 to 10 days.

WORDS TO KNOW

ANTHELMINTIC Medicines that rid the body of parasitic worms.

HELMINTH A representative of various phyla of wormlike animals.

MORBIDITY From the Latin *morbus*, "sick," it refers to both the state of being ill and the severity of the illness. A serious disease is said to have high morbidity.

PARASITE An organism that lives in or on a host organism and gets its nourishment from that host. The parasite usually gains all the benefits of this relationship, whereas the host may suffer from various diseases and discomforts or show no signs of infection. The life cycle of a typical parasite usually includes several developmental stages and morphological changes as the parasite lives and moves through the environment and one or more hosts. Parasites that remain on the surface of a host's body to feed are called ectoparasites, whereas those that live inside a host's body are called endoparasites. Parasitism is a highly successful biological adaptation. There are more known parasitic species than nonparasitic ones, and parasites affect just about every form of life, including most all animals, plants, and even bacteria.

THE INTERNATIONAL BURDEN OF HOOKWORM

While WHO and other organizations have sought to combat hookworm, especially in infants and children, many observers have argued that the international effort to combat the infection has lagged. In part, the insufficient response to hookworm has been attributed to uncertainty about the economic effects hookworm infection has on the global economy.

According to Sarah Bartsch and coauthors of a 2016 study for *PLOS Neglected Tropical Diseases*, "Without a better understanding of hookworm's economic burden worldwide, it is difficult for decision makers such as funders, policymakers, disease control officials, and intervention manufacturers to determine how much time, energy, and resources to invest in hookworm control." To create such an improved understanding, the authors analyzed hookworm infection data and found the economic impact of the infection to be in the billions of dollars. Although it is difficult to quantify exactly how much hookworm costs the global economy, the study authors estimated that total productivity losses from hookworm ranged from $7.5 billion to $138.9 billion. Because hookworm is most common in developing countries, the magnitude of these economic loses underscores the importance of combatting hookworm infections.

Most of the time there are no symptoms. However, symptoms may occur at any point within the worm's life cycle. Initial symptoms include itching and a rash at the larvae's entrance site to the host. Asthma- or pneumonia-like symptoms may occur when the worms are in the lungs. Symptoms from intestinal infection include anemia, loss of appetite, weight loss, excessive intestinal gases, cramps and abdominal pain, and diarrhea. In chronic infections symptoms may include malnutrition, breathing difficulties, dizziness, pale complexion, tiredness and weakness, swelling and bloating, impotence, enlargement of the heart, and irregular heartbeat.

The most serious health problems associated with hookworm are anemia and protein deficiency. Infection can be especially problematic for newborn and infant children, pregnant women, and people who are malnourished. Death is uncommon but may occur, especially in newborn and infant children. In addition, children's physical and mental development may be impeded by the lack of nutrients caused by hookworm.

■ Scope and Distribution

Hookworm infection occurs mostly in tropical and subtropical regions of the world. *Ancylostoma duodenale* is found in China, India, Japan, and Mediterranean countries. *Ancylostoma americanus* is located in the tropical areas of Africa, Asia, and the Americas. As of 2016 approximately half a billion people around the world carried hookworm infection.

■ Treatment and Prevention

Diagnosis is often accomplished by identifying hookworm eggs in a stool sample with the use of a microscope. A blood sample is also used because positive results show iron or protein deficiency.

Treatment consists of anthelmintic drugs. The drugs mebendazole and albendazole are the most common anthelmintic drugs used because they cause the immobilization and eventual death of the worms by restricting the ingestion of nutrients. These drugs are sold under the brand names Antiox®, Ovex®, Pripsen®, Vermox®, Benzole®, and Combantrin-A®. They are effective, able to cure the infection about 99 percent of the time when given twice a day for one to three days. For patients suffering from anemia, iron supplements and a high-protein diet are also typically recommended.

Hookworm infection is prevented by promoting safe, sanitary practices. Feces should be disposed of properly, and contaminated areas should be cleansed thoroughly. Wearing shoes, avoiding swimming in contaminated pools, and treating or boiling contaminated water before drinking also help prevent hookworm infection.

■ Impacts and Issues

Hookworm infection is the leading cause of iron deficiency anemia in developing countries. In countries where food is scarce, people with heavy hookworm infections are sometimes unable to eat enough calories to compensate for those lost due to intestinal iron and protein depletion brought on by hookworms. In the past hookworm infection was neglected due to its concentration among the world's poorest peoples. Generally, international coordination involving the infection was not accomplished. Since the 1990s, however, there has been increasing concern over the global incidence of hookworm infection. International efforts are increasing to control the occurrence of hookworm, flatworm, and related helminth infections. In 2017 WHO estimated that some 1.5 billion people worldwide suffered from illnesses associated with hookworms and other soil-transmitted helminths.

Children are especially susceptible to hookworm infection because of the amount of time they spend outdoors. WHO estimated that as of 2017 about 267 million preschool-age children and 580 million school-age children lived in "areas where these parasites are intensively transmitted, and are in need of treatment and preventive interventions." If infected, children often suffer morbidity that includes physical and mental problems such as anemia, attention deficits, learning disabilities, and school absenteeism. Children who are not properly treated are permanently affected.

In 2001 WHO adopted a resolution to target all countries where helminth infections occur most frequently. The project called Partners for Parasite Control (PPC) aimed to regularly treat at least 75 percent of all schoolchildren at risk by the year 2010 and to support local health facilities so that they have adequate supplies of anthelmintic drugs and perform regular treatment of high-risk groups. While WHO did not meet the PPC goal by 2010, the organization reported that some 30 percent of at-risk children (more than 300 million people) were treated with anthel-

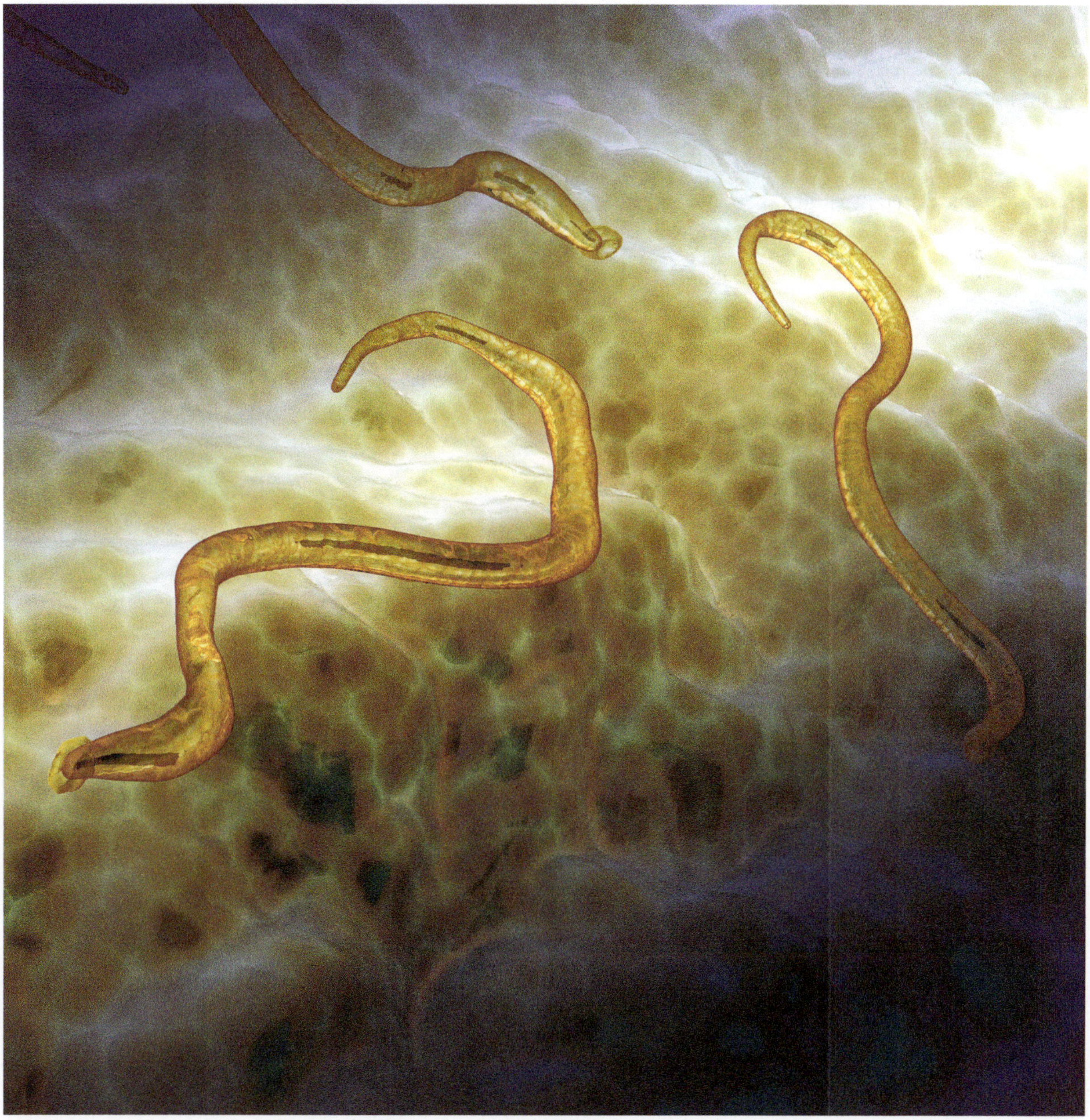

Hookworms are parasitic roundworms that range from 0.3 to 0.5 inches (0.7 to 1.3 centimeters) in length and infest the intestines of their host. *© Science Picture Co/Science Source*

mintic drugs in 2011. As of 2017 WHO was still pursuing the PPC's goal of treating 75 percent of children in an effort to eliminate morbidity resulting from hookworm and other helminthiases.

SEE ALSO *Bilharzia (Schistosomiasis); Helminth Disease; Roundworm (Ascariasis) Infection*

BIBLIOGRAPHY

Books

Freedman, David O., ed. *Immunopathogenetic Aspects of Disease Induced by Helminth Parasites.* New York: Karger, 1997.

Holland, Celia V., and Malcolm W. Kennedy, eds. *The Geohelminths: Ascaris, Trichuris, and Hookworm.* Boston: Kluwer Academic, 2002.

Periodicals

Bartsch, Sarah M., et al. "The Global Economic and Health Burden of Hookworm Infection." *PLOS Neglected Tropical Diseases* 10, no. 9 (September 8, 2016). This article can also be found online at http://journals.plos.org/plosntds/article?id=10.1371/journal.pntd.0004922 (accessed December 19, 2017).

Hotez, Peter J., et al. "Hookworm Infection." *New England Journal of Medicine* 351, no. 8 (August 19, 2004): 799–807.

Websites

"Hookworm." Centers for Disease Control and Prevention. https://www.cdc.gov/parasites/hookworm/ (accessed December 19, 2017).

"Intestinal Worms." World Health Organization. http://www.who.int/intestinal_worms/en/ (accessed December 19, 2017).

"Soil-Transmitted Helminth Infections Fact Sheet." World Health Organization, September 2017. http://www.who.int/mediacentre/factsheets/fs366/en/ (accessed December 19, 2017).

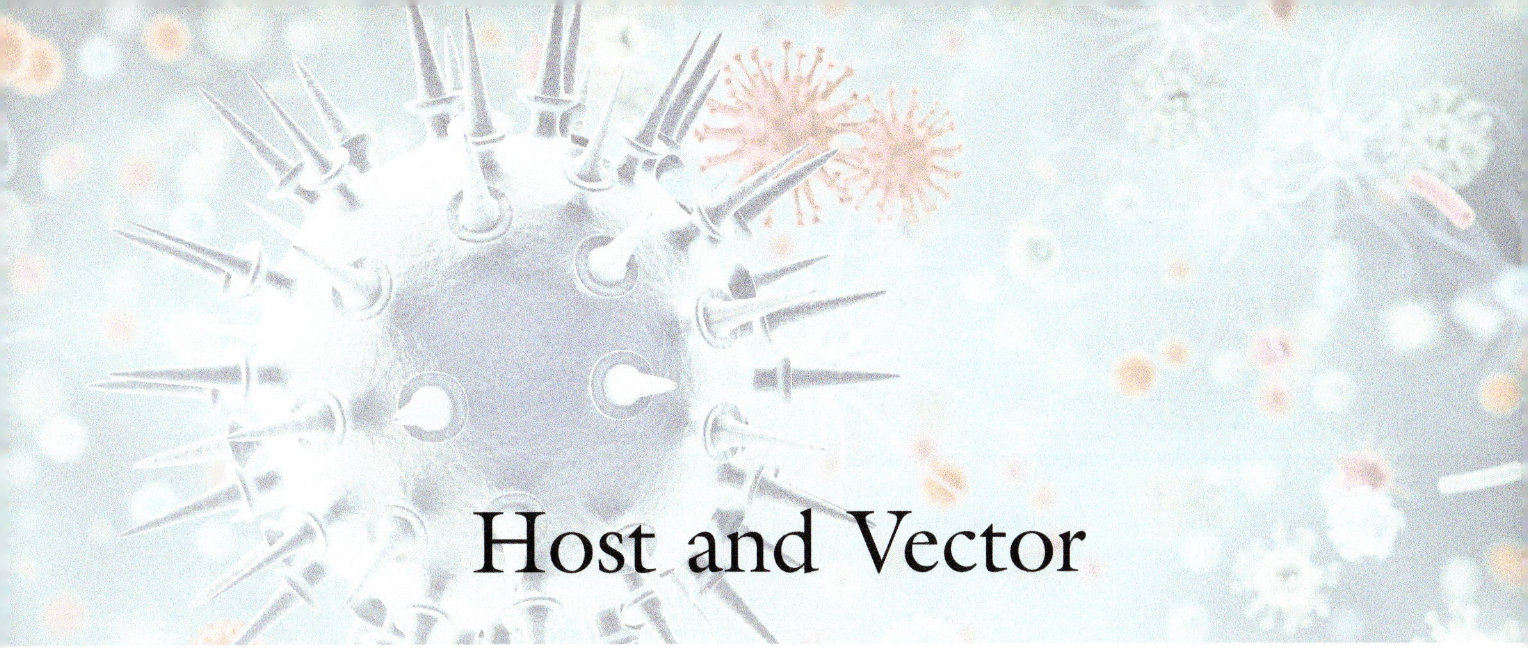

Host and Vector

Introduction

The terms *host* and *vector* refer to the route of transmission of some infectious diseases to humans and animals.

The host is the living being that the bacterium, virus, protozoan, or other disease-causing microorganism normally resides in. Some bird species, for example, are normal hosts to arboviruses such as West Nile virus. Typically, the microorganism does little or no harm to the host, which is important if the disease-causing organism is to successfully persist in that host over time. Occasionally, the host population maintains the organism even though some members suffer from infection caused by it. Several species of birds in North America have experienced West Nile infection although they are considered the natural host.

A reservoir host, or simply a reservoir, refers to a living (e.g., human, animal, insect, plant) or nonliving (e.g., soil, water) entity where a disease-causing organism normally lives and multiplies. A host in which a parasite resides to sexual maturity is called a primary host, and a host in which a parasite spends only part of its life cycle or does not reach sexual maturity is called an intermediate host. Certain species of snails, for example, are the intermediate host of the *Schistosoma* larvae that are responsible for causing the disease bilharzia in humans.

A vector is an organism that helps transmit infection from one host to another. For example, the mosquito serves as the vector to infect humans with the West Nile virus. The mosquito acquires the virus from birds when it takes a blood meal. If the same mosquito subsequently feeds on a human, the virus can be transferred, and the result can be West Nile disease in humans.

Disease History, Characteristics, and Transmission

The host-vector route of transmission is responsible for a number of diseases, including several types of encephalitis that sicken humans and horses (Western equine encephalitis, Eastern equine encephalitis, and St. Louis encephalitis). Malaria, which is caused by several protozoans of the genus *Plasmodium* (the most common and serious forms of malaria are caused by *P. falciparum* and *P. vivax*), is also a vector-borne disease. The vector for transmission of the malaria protozoa is also the mosquito. Typically, the host is another human whose blood harbors the protozoan. As with encephalitis, the mosquito acquires the microbe when it feeds on the infected host, and it transfers the microbe to a susceptible human host when it seeks another blood meal.

Mosquitoes also function as the vectors in the transmission of arbovirus species that cause yellow fever and dengue fever in humans. Other examples of potential disease vectors include flies, mites, fleas, ticks, rats, skunks, and even dogs.

WORDS TO KNOW

INTERMEDIATE HOST An organism infected by a parasite while the parasite is in a developmental form and not sexually mature.

PRIMARY HOST An organism that provides food and shelter for a parasite while allowing it to become sexually mature. By contrast, a secondary host is one occupied by a parasite during the larval or asexual stages of its life cycle.

RESERVOIR The animal or organism in which a virus or parasite normally resides.

VECTOR Any agent that carries and transmits parasites and diseases. Also, an organism or a chemical used to transport a gene into a new host cell.

A more recently emerging vector-borne disease is encephalitis caused by Zika virus, though Zika virus infection has been known for decades. If a pregnant woman is bitten by a mosquito that carries the virus, the fetus is at risk of a variety of birth defects, including brain malformation. The threat of Zika virus was highlighted by the refusal of some athletes to attend the 2016 Summer Olympics held in Rio de Janeiro because of fears of contracting the virus. At the time some regions of South America were experiencing a spike in the number of cases of birth defects attributed to the infection. The number of cases subsequently declined. The cause of the upsurge and decline in cases was not known as of 2017.

■ Scope and Distribution

The host-vector route of disease transmission occurs globally. Some diseases are confined to certain regions of the world. One example is malaria, which is associated with equatorial regions. Malaria has a significant impact. In 2016 the World Health Organization (WHO) reported 212 million new cases of malaria in 2015, with over 90 percent being in Africa. In 2015 there were an estimated 429,000 deaths due to malaria, with 92 percent occurring in Africa.

■ Treatment and Prevention

The best way to eliminate host-vector diseases is to break the vector-mediated chain of transmission between the infected host and the susceptible person or animal that will become a new host. In the case of malaria, for example, spraying areas that are breeding grounds for mosquitoes can help curb their population and thereby reduce the likelihood of disease transmission. In mid-2013 several African countries began spraying with dichlorodiphenyltrichloroethane (DDT) as a means of mosquito control. Despite the infamous history of DDT due to its overuse and resulting environmental harm, its controlled application was judged a relatively safe means of host-vector control.

Another means of malaria host-vector control that has become more widely practiced is the use of mosquito netting to protect people while they sleep. This inexpensive and easy-to-use method prevents the mosquito from feeding on a sleeping person and interrupts the transmission path of the *Plasmodium* protozoan. Similarly, protective clothing can minimize the chance that a vector will have access to unexposed skin.

More exotic vector control approaches are being explored by scientists. An example is an ongoing program to breed and release male mosquitoes that harbor a bacterium called *Wolbachia*, which makes them incapable of breeding. The rationale is that, because malaria is transmitted only by female mosquitoes, the lack of availability of a male breeding partner will drive down the female population over time. As of 2017 active releases of sterile mosquitoes have been done in regions of Africa and the United States to combat vector-borne diseases.

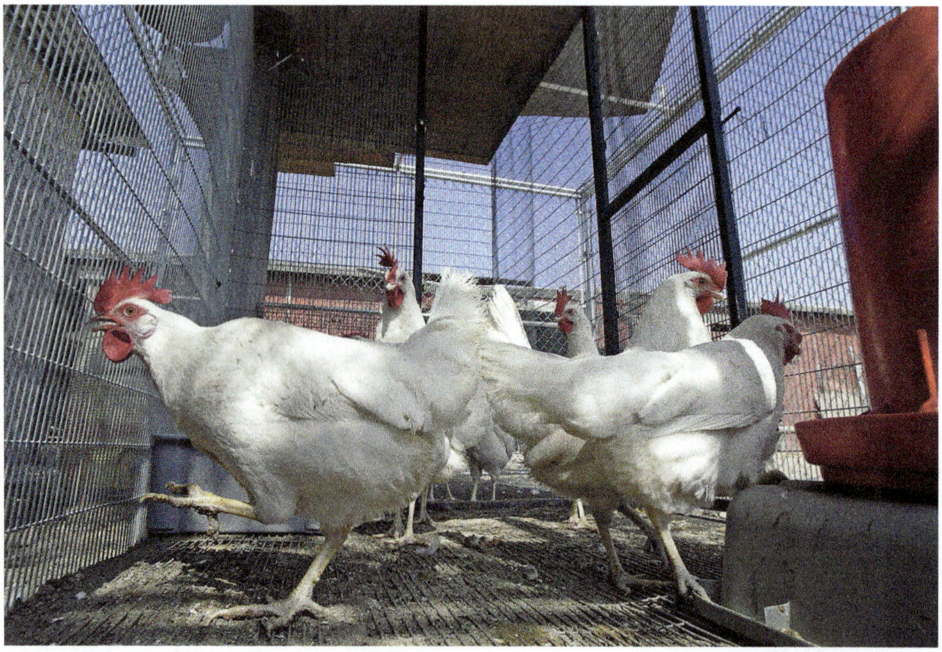

In San Bernardino County, California, a local vector control program holds and tests chickens for West Nile virus. Chickens serve as hosts for the virus, which can be transmitted to humans via mosquitoes. Mosquitoes serve as vectors for the virus. *© David McNew/Getty Images*

REDUCING COSTS AND RISKS OF VECTOR CONTROL

Integrated vector management (IVM) strategies are emerging as part of an effort to achieve effective disease control at costs countries can afford and at the same time minimize potential negative impacts on biodiversity, ecosystems, and public health (e.g., reduce risks related to pesticides or bioaccumulation of toxic or potentially toxic chemicals).

The World Health Organization (WHO) Global Strategic Framework for Integrated Vector Management defines IVM as a strategy to "improve the efficacy, cost-effectiveness, ecological soundness and sustainability of disease vector control. IVM encourages a multi-disease control approach, integration with other disease control measures and the considered and systematic application of a range of interventions, often in combination and synergistically."

The IVM approach is also designed to reduce the development of vector resistance to vector control measures (e.g., increasing resistance to pesticides).

Cost effectiveness is an important aspect of IVM strategy. For example, officials in Sri Lanka indicated that "costs of periodic river flushing to eliminate mosquito breeding habitats compared favourably with the use of insecticide-impregnated bednets as a mosquito-control measure."

■ Impacts and Issues

Changing the behavior of vectors influences the transmission of a disease. Knowledge of a vector's habitat, life cycle, behavior, and migratory patterns, for example, is vital to efforts to curb the spread of disease. Vector-borne diseases with simple transmission cycles can be difficult to treat and prevent. This is because the vectors are living things that are often capable of moving from one location to another, sometimes over thousands of miles.

Threats from vector-borne diseases with complicated transmission cycles that involve one or more intermediate hosts are sometimes easier to eliminate. This is because breaking only one link in the disease transmission chain will result in fewer infections. Guinea worm disease, for example, infected 3 to 5 million people in Asia and Africa in the mid-1980s. Through an international effort, ponds in endemic areas were treated with a simple insecticide that eliminated the intermediate host, a copepod or water flea, but left the water drinkable. By 2006 cases of guinea worm infection numbered fewer than 12,000 in Africa, and the disease was eliminated from Asia. An ongoing campaign that began in 2011 seeks to completely eliminate the disease in Africa.

A looming issue for host-vector diseases involves climate change. As vector-borne diseases such as malaria are associated with warmer climates, some researchers have warned that the increasing warming of Earth's atmosphere could expand the habitat of mosquito species and thereby increase the prevalence of mosquito-borne diseases such as malaria and Zika encephalitis.

Due to climate change, vector-borne diseases have increasingly spread from tropical regions to more northerly regions where the vector is now able to survive. One example is the mosquito-borne West Nile disease. The West Nile virus that causes this disease has spread as far north as Canada, where it can be transmitted by mosquitoes during the warmer months of the year and even during the cooler days of spring by mosquitoes that have survived the winter. In the United States West Nile virus was unheard of in the early 1990s. Between 1999 and 2017, more than 42,000 cases have been reported in the United States, according to the CDC.

Climate change also lengthens the breeding season of disease-carrying insects and increases the areas in which they can breed. In some regions of the globe, climate change has increased rainfall. The moistened ground helps facilitate the breeding of insect vectors such as mosquitoes.

SEE ALSO *Arthropod-Borne Disease; Bloodborne Pathogens; Climate Change and Infectious Disease; Dengue and Dengue Hemorrhagic Fever; Encephalitis; Malaria; Vector-Borne Disease; Zoonoses*

BIBLIOGRAPHY

Books

Diniz, Debora. *Zika: From the Brazilian Backlands to Global Threat.* London: Zed, 2017.

McNeil, Donald G., Jr. *Zika: The Emerging Epidemic.* New York: Norton, 2017.

Rocco, Fiammetta. *The Miraculous Fever-Tree: Malaria and the Quest for a Cure That Changed the World.* New York: HarperCollins, 2003.

Periodicals

Jiggins, Francis M. "The Spread of *Wolbachia* through Mosquito Populations." *PLOS Biology* 15 (June 2017): e2002780.

Metsky, Harold C., et al. "Zika Virus Evolution and Spread in the Americas." *Nature* 546 (June 2017): 411–415.

Websites

"Division of Vector-Borne Diseases." Centers for Disease Control and Prevention. https://www.cdc.gov/ncezid/dvbd/index.html (accessed December 6, 2017).

"Fact Sheet: World Malaria Report 2016." World Health Organization, December 13, 2016. http://www.who.int/malaria/media/world-malaria-report-2016/en/ (accessed December 6, 2017).

"Malaria Control: The Power of Integrated Action." World Health Organization. http://www.who.int/heli/risks/vectors/malariacontrol/en/ (accessed December 6, 2017).

"Zika Virus." Centers for Disease Control and Prevention. https://www.cdc.gov/zika/index.html (accessed November 17, 2017).

Brian Hoyle

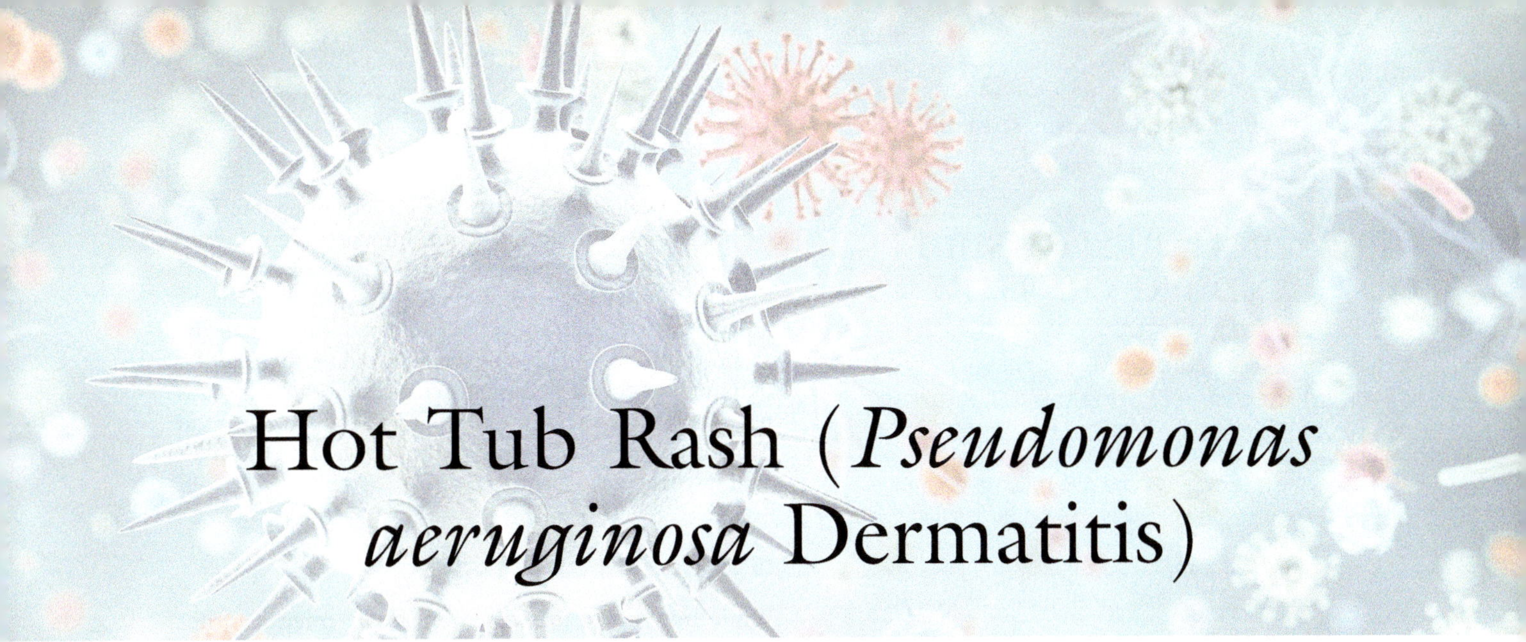

Hot Tub Rash (*Pseudomonas aeruginosa* Dermatitis)

■ Introduction

Hot tub rash is a form of skin irritation that results from an infection caused by the bacterium *Pseudomonas aeruginosa*. This bacterium is commonly found in environments such as water and soil.

■ Disease History, Characteristics, and Transmission

Hot tub rash is a skin infection known as dermatitis. The infected skin becomes itchy and a red rash develops 48 hours to several weeks after contact with contaminated water. The depressions in the skin that surround hair follicles can also become contaminated, which can lead to the development of pus-filled blisters, a condition known as folliculitis. Less commonly, hot tub rash can lead to other and more serious infections in the eye, breast, lung, and urinary tract.

The term *hot tub rash* reflects the prevalence of the infection in hot tubs, where warm water can provide ideal conditions for the growth of *P. aeruginosa*. However, hot tub rash is not exclusive to hot tubs and can result from swimming in a contaminated lake or pool. *P. aeruginosa* skin infections have also been documented in waterslides and bathtubs, as well as following the use of diving suits that have not been properly washed between uses, particularly when someone has a cut or scratch. Any opening on the skin surface increases the likelihood that *P. aeruginosa* can establish an infection. Skin that is covered by a bathing suit can develop a more severe infection, as the contaminated water is held in closer and has more prolonged contact with the skin.

Chemicals such as chlorine, which are added to keep the water free from microorganisms, lose their potency more quickly at the elevated water temperatures in hot tubs. Backyard or commercial hot tubs are sometimes inadequately disinfected, which also creates opportunity for the growth of *P. aeruginosa*.

The construction of a hot tub can contribute to *P. aeruginosa* growth. Even if the tub's inner wood or plastic surface looks smooth, the surface contains tiny cracks in which the bacteria can grow. When growing on surfaces, *P. aeruginosa* often produces a sugary coating called an exopolysaccharide. The resulting exopolysaccharide-enclosed population of bacteria (biofilm) can become resistant to chlorine and other disinfectants. Bacteria can slough off from the biofilm into the water; if someone is in the hot tub, the skin infection has an opportunity to develop. Even plastic hot tubs can have surface-adhering *P. aeruginosa* biofilms.

■ Scope and Distribution

Because *P. aeruginosa* is widespread in the environment, hot tub rash is common. The infection is of special concern in hospitals, especially for patients with malfunctioning immune systems. In these patients *P. aeruginosa* often causes infection in the moist tissues of the lung.

There is no age, race, gender, or geographical influence on the occurrence of hot tub rash.

WORDS TO KNOW

BIOFILM A population of microorganisms that forms following the adhesion of bacteria, algae, yeast, or fungi to a surface. These surface growths can be found in natural settings, such as on rocks in streams, and in infections, such as those that occur on catheters. Microorganisms can colonize living and inert natural and synthetic surfaces.

PERSONAL RESPONSIBILITY AND PREVENTION

To ensure safe and healthy use, the US Centers for Disease Control and Prevention (CDC) recommends that spa users observe the following rules to protect against recreational water illnesses:

- Refrain from entering a spa when you have diarrhea.
- Avoid swallowing spa water or even getting it into your mouth.
- Shower or bathe with soap before entering the spa.
- Observe limits, if posted, on the maximum allowable number of bathers.
- Exclude children less than five years of age from using spas.
- If pregnant, consult a physician before spa use, particularly in the first trimester.

■ Treatment and Prevention

Hot tub rash tends to clear without treatment in several weeks. However, some people can benefit from the use of an antibiotic-containing ointment that is rubbed onto the affected areas of the skin. This treatment may be ineffective, however, as some strains of *P. aeruginosa* are resistant to a variety of antibiotics.

For people at higher risk of more serious infection (such as those with an inefficient immune system), treatment with the antibiotic ciprofloxacin can be useful.

Hot tub rash can be prevented by avoiding environments where *P. aeruginosa*–contaminated water might be found. Most commonly this means avoiding the use of a domestic hot tub or not using a crowded hot tub. If this is not possible, then regular disinfection of the tub water and cleaning of the inside surface of the tub should be considered essential maintenance.

■ Impacts and Issues

While hot tub rash is often an inconvenience rather than a health concern, the infection can be serious for someone whose immune system is less able to fight off infection. In such people *P. aeruginosa* becomes an opportunistic pathogen, an organism that does not normally cause disease but is capable of causing disease under the appropriate circumstances.

In public environments such as hospitals or spas, whirlpools and hot tubs should be regularly maintained and the water tested for the presence of microorganisms. The CDC recommends maintaining the free-chlorine or bromine level of the hot tub or pool between 2 and 5 parts per million and maintaining the pH level of the water at 7.5 to 7.8. In addition, the whirlpool or tub should be located in a well-ventilated room, as the agitation of the hot water could create aerosolized bacteria, which are bacteria that have become suspended in the air. If the bacteria become aerosolized, they can be inhaled, which can result in a lung

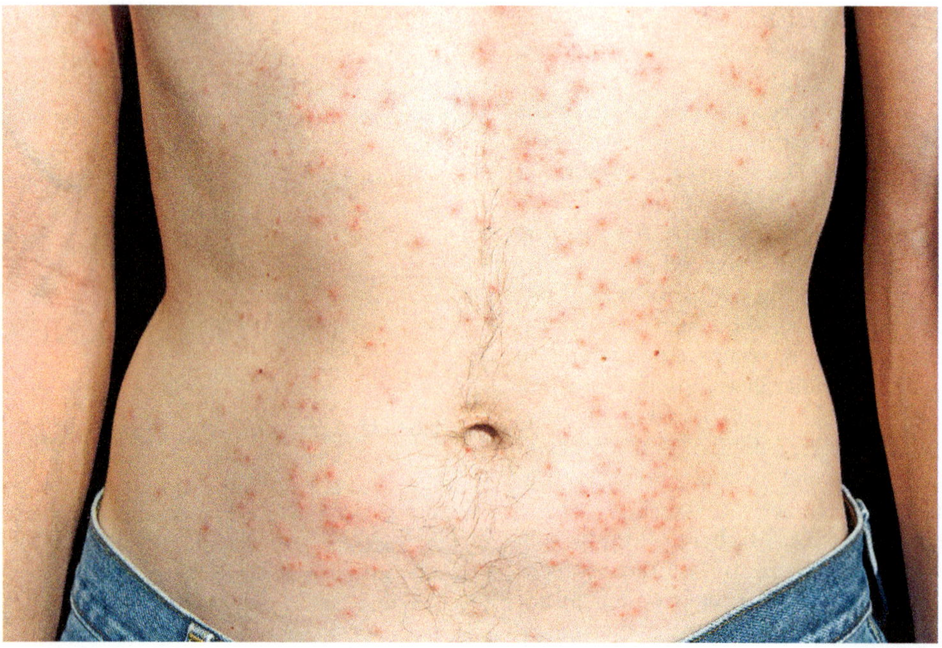

Folliculitis, an infection of the hair follicles, is a common side effect of hot tub rash, a skin infection caused by the bacterium *Pseudomonas aeruginosa*. © JCarillet/Getty Images

infection. The possibility of a lung infection is especially serious for persons who have cystic fibrosis, because *P. aeruginosa* can establish a persistent infection that can progressively damage the lung tissue.

SEE ALSO *Swimmer's Ear and Swimmer's Itch (Cercarial Dermatitis)*

BIBLIOGRAPHY

Books

Kahlon, Rachhpal. *Pseudomonas: Molecular and Applied Biology.* New York: Springer, 2016.

Tortora, Gerard, and Berdell R. Funke. *Microbiology: An Introduction.* New York: Pearson, 2016.

Periodicals

Gupta, P., et al. "Potentiation of Antibiotic against *Pseudomonas aeruginosa* Biofilm: A Study with Plumbagin and Gentamicin." *Journal of Applied Microbiology* 123 (July 2017): 246–261.

Metsky, Hayden C., et al. "Zika Virus Evolution and Spread into the Americas." *Nature* 546 (June 2017): 411–415.

Websites

"Healthy Swimming." Centers for Disease Control and Prevention. https://www.cdc.gov/healthywater/swimming/swimmers/rwi/rashes.html (accessed November 17, 2017).

Brian Hoyle

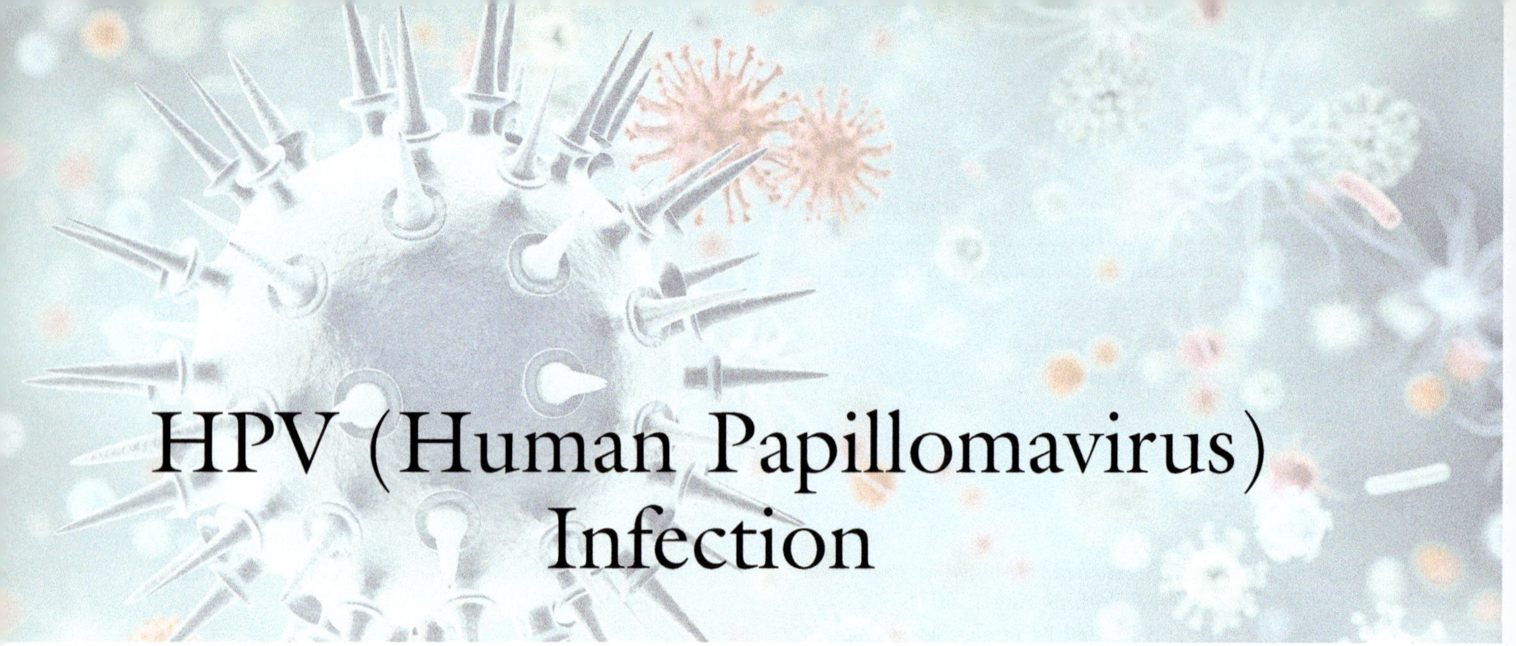

HPV (Human Papillomavirus) Infection

Introduction

The human papillomavirus (HPV) is one of the most common infectious diseases. Almost all people who are sexually active will acquire the disease at some point. It grows exclusively in the epithelial cells making up the surface of the skin, including the cervix, vagina, and anus. Although HPV infection often causes no symptoms, it sometimes triggers benign tumors known as papillomas or warts on the hands and feet or in the genital area.

Most HPV infections clear up on their own, but they are also capable of causing cancers in the cervix and, more rarely, in the vagina, vulva, penis, and anus. The link between HPV and cancer is not well understood, but the virus could trigger abnormal growth and multiplication in the cells it infects. The genetic material (DNA) of HPV has been found in the majority of cervical cancers studied, and the disease is a major killer of women in low- to middle-income countries. However, there is a vaccine that can protect children and young adults against the main types of HPV that cause both genital warts and cancer.

WORDS TO KNOW

DYSPLASIA Abnormal changes in tissue or cell development.

IMMUNOCOMPROMISED Having an immune system with reduced ability to recognize and respond to the presence of foreign material.

MORTALITY The condition of being susceptible to death. The term *mortality* comes from the Latin word *mors*, which means death. Mortality can also refer to the rate of deaths caused by an illness or injury (e.g., "Rabies has a high mortality rate").

PREVALENCE The actual number of cases of disease or injury that exists in a population.

SEXUALLY TRANSMITTED INFECTION (STI) Infections that vary in their susceptibility to treatment, their signs and symptoms, and the consequences if they are left untreated. Some are caused by bacteria. These usually can be treated and cured. Others are caused by viruses and can typically be treated but not cured.

Disease History, Characteristics, and Transmission

More than 200 types of HPV have been identified. Around 40 of these are spread through sexual contact. Some types of HPV cause skin warts and some genital warts, while others cause cancer. Most people with HPV infection will not have symptoms, although they can still transmit the infection to others. In addition, most people with HPV will clear the virus within two years.

HPV can cause skin warts. They are either flat (shallow) or plantar (deep), occurring mainly on the hands and feet in children and young adults. Sometimes papillomas grow in the mouth or on the larynx (voice box). Genital warts can occur anywhere in the external genitalia, in the vagina, on the cervix, or around the anus. They consist of soft, moist, pink or flesh-colored swellings. In an otherwise healthy person, these warts are benign. Ninety percent of anogenital warts are caused by HPV type 6 or HPV type 11.

HPV can also cause cancer: most commonly, cervical cancer in women, with HPV type 16 or HPV type 18 involved in around 66 percent of cases. Less commonly it can cause cancer of the anus, penis, vagina, vulva, and throat.

It takes about 15 to 20 years after infection with HPV for cervical cancer to develop in women that are not immunocompromised. Microscopic evaluation of cells from the cervix taken in a Pap test (a routine screen for cervical cancer) can reveal a series of changes that may lead to cervical cancer. The first stage is known as dysplasia, an abnormality that often reverts to normal by the time a second test is taken. However, these changes may progress to a condition known as cervical intraepithelial dysplasia (CIN), which is generally regarded as being precancerous and likely to develop into cervical cancer within 10 years if left untreated. Most genital HPV infections do not develop into cervical cancer, however.

HPV is usually transmitted through vaginal or anal sex. It can also be spread through oral sex. It can be transmitted even if the infected person has no signs or symptoms of the disease. Occasionally, the disease can be transmitted through genital-to-genital skin contact.

Scope and Distribution

Infection with HPV is common around the world. It is present in both men and women. Sexually active people are likely to encounter the disease at some point in their lifetime.

Globally HPV infection exacts a significant toll in the form of cervical cancer. Cervical cancer is the fourth-most-common cancer in women around the world. The World Health Organization states that there were an estimated 530,000 new cases of cervical cancer in 2012. Cervical cancer is responsible for 7.5 percent of all cancer deaths in women. Some 270,000 women die each year from the disease. The mortality rate for cervical cancer around the world is 52 percent; most deaths occur in developing countries.

Treatment and Prevention

There is a vaccine for HPV. There are three types of HPV vaccines available in the United States: Gardasil, Cervarix, and Gardasil 9. Gardasil is given to both sexes and is effective against HPV types 6, 11, 16, and 18. Cervarix is given only to women and is effective against HPV types 16 and 18. Gardasil 9 is given to both sexes and is effective against HPV types 6, 11, 16, 18, 31, 33, 45, 52, and 58. Gardasil and Gardasil 9 prevent HPV-caused cancer and genital warts. Cervarix prevents cervical cancer. Vaccines afford the highest level of protection against genital warts and cancer to those who have not become sexually active.

The CDC recommends that boys and girls between the ages of 11 and 12 receive two doses of the vaccine between six months and one year apart. (The vaccine is most effective at a younger age and prior to any sexual activity.) Three doses of the vaccine are recommended for people who begin vaccination after age 15 and who are immunocompromised. The HPV vaccine can be given to children as young as nine years old if they have been sexually abused.

There is no treatment for HPV, and often no treatment is needed for the symptoms of HPV infection because both skin and genital warts tend to disappear over time. Ninety percent are gone within two years. If warts are large

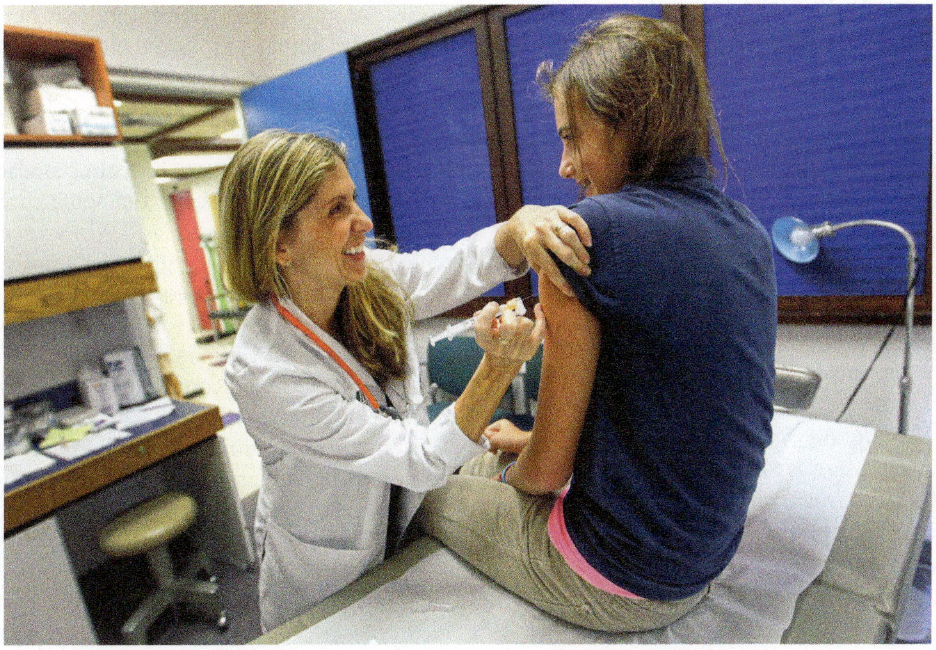

A young woman receives an HPV vaccination in Florida in 2011. The vaccine is designed to prevent infection with the human papillomavirus, which can cause cancer. *© Joe Raedle/Getty Images*

or painful, they can be destroyed by burning (electrocautery), freezing (cryotherapy), and chemical treatment. Laryngeal papillomas can be surgically removed.

Limiting the number of sexual contacts and using condoms will provide some protection. Women who are sexually active should have regular Pap smears to check for the early signs of cervical cancer. In countries that have a national screening program, cervical cancer has become far less common than it was previously, and cases tend to occur among women who have never had a Pap test.

It is important for those who have been vaccinated to still receive regular Pap tests because the current vaccine does not protect against all the HPV types that can cause cervical cancer.

■ Impacts and Issues

Vaccination against HPV has been shown to be effective in preventing genital warts and cancers in men and women and lowering the prevalence of HPV. A vaccine for girls was first introduced in 2006 in the United States and extended to boys in 2010. The CDC reported that in 2016 60 percent of adolescents ages 13 to 17 had received at least one dose of the vaccine. This was up from 56 percent in 2015. In general, adolescent girls are receiving the vaccine at a higher rate than adolescent boys, but the gap between the vaccination rates is narrowing over time. Adolescents in rural areas are less likely than their urban peers to have been vaccinated against HPV.

There is concern among public health professionals that not enough people are completing all doses of the vaccine. The CDC reports that only 43 percent of adolescents have received the complete HPV vaccination.

PRIMARY SOURCE

This Vaccine Can Prevent Cancer, but Many Teenagers Still Don't Get It

SOURCE: *Aubrey, Allison. "This Vaccine Can Prevent Cancer, But Many Teenagers Still Don't Get It." NPR, February 19, 2018. https://www.npr.org/sections/health-shots/2018/02/19/586494027/this-vaccine-can-prevent-cancer-but-many-teenagers-still-dont-get-it (accessed February 20, 2018).*

INTRODUCTION: *In the following article, the author reports that fewer than 50 percent of American teenagers in 2018 were receiving the full dosage of the HPV vaccine, despite its efficacy at preventing certain cancers. This is a major public health concern because the vaccine is most effective when it is given at a young age and when it is given before people have begun any sexual activity. The author emphasizes the fact that men, not just women, are at risk of developing HPV-related cancers as well.*

Each year, about 31,000 men and women in the U.S. are diagnosed with a cancer caused by an infection from the human papillomavirus, or HPV. It's the most common sexually transmitted virus and infection in the U.S.

In women, HPV infection can lead to cervical cancer, which leads to about 4,000 deaths per year. In men, it can cause penile cancer. HPV also causes some cases of oral cancer, cancer of the anus and genital warts.

The CDC says HPV vaccination can prevent many of these cancers, and urges pediatricians to recommend HPV vaccination for all their patients, beginning at age 11.

But a new analysis from the Blue Cross Blue Shield Association finds only 29 percent of the teens its members insure receive a first dose of the HPV vaccine by their 13th birthday. And the CDC finds, nationally, only 43 percent of teens are up-to-date on all the recommended doses of the vaccine.

"It's important for 12 and 13-year-olds to get the HPV vaccine to provide immunity so that when they may be exposed to HPV later in life, typically through sexual activity, they have protection," says Dr. Margaret Stager, of the Metro Health Medical Center in Cleveland. She's a pediatrician and spokesperson for the American Academy of Pediatrics.

The CDC summarizes the transmission of the virus bluntly: "People get HPV from another person during intimate sexual contact. Most of the time, people get HPV from having vaginal or anal sex. Men and women can also get HPV from having oral sex or other sex play."

HPV immunization rates have been rising in the decade or so since the first vaccine became available, but pediatricians still hear pushback from some parents. Stager says she's heard questions such as: "Why are we giving this vaccine to my [11-year-old] girl? She's not going to be having sex—so why are we doing this now?"

There are two reasons to vaccinate at this age. First, there's a more effective immune response if it is given in early adolescence. And second: "It works best if given before any sexual exposure."

Though gender differences in vaccine rates have narrowed, more girls than boys get the HPV vaccine. This may be because the recommendation to vaccinate boys began in 2011, years after it was first recommended for girls.

Meanwhile, it's clear that males are getting HPV-related cancers. "We're seeing a trend in adult men with oral cancers related to HPV," says Stager. These oropharyngeal cancers occur in the back of the throat, including the base of the tongue and tonsils. Oral HPV cancer is much more common in men than women.

"This is the [age] group of men that did not have the opportunity to get the HPV vaccine," she says.

So what's the connection between HPV and oral cancer? "It's related to oral sex," Stager explains.

The CDC has documented an increase in the cases of HPV-related cancers in men in recent years, with a significant increase in oropharyngeal cancer.

"The fastest growing segment of the oral and oropharyngeal cancer population are otherwise healthy, nonsmokers in the 25–50 age range," according to the Oral Cancer Foundation.

For young men and women, it may not be too late to get the vaccine.

The CDC says those who missed being vaccinated as teenagers, can still benefit from getting the HPV vaccine through their early and mid-20s.

SEE ALSO *Cancer and Infectious Disease; Sexually Transmitted Diseases*

BIBLIOGRAPHY

Books

Boruto, Franco, and Marc de Ridder, eds. *HPV and Cervical Cancer: Achievements in Prevention and Future Prospects.* New York: Springer, 2012.

World Health Organization. *Comprehensive Cervical Cancer Control: A Guide to Essential Practice.* Geneva: WHO Press, 2014. This book can also be found online at http://apps.who.int/iris/bitstream/10665/144785/1/9789241548953_eng.pdf?ua=1 (accessed February 20, 2018).

Periodicals

Dunne, Eileen F., et al. "CDC Grand Rounds: Reducing the Burden of HPV-Associated Cancer and Disease." *Morbidity and Mortality Weekly Report* 63, no. 4 (January 31, 2014): 68–72. This article can also be found online at https://www.cdc.gov/mmwr/preview/mmwrhtml/mm6304a1.htm?s_cid=mm6304a1_e (accessed February 20, 2018).

Giuliano, Anna R., et al. "Efficacy of Quadrivalent HPV Vaccine against HPV Infection and Disease in Males." *New England Journal of Medicine* 364 (2011): 401–411. This article can also be found online at http://www.nejm.org/doi/full/10.1056/nejmoa0909537 (accessed February 20, 2018).

Gray, Penelope, et al. "Evaluation of HPV Type-Replacement in Unvaccinated and Vaccinated Adolescent Females—Post-Hoc Analysis of A Community-Randomized Clinical Trial (II)." *International Journal of Cancer* (February 12, 2018). This article can also be found online at https://www.ncbi.nlm.nih.gov/pubmed/29377141 (accessed February 20, 2018).

Markowitz, Lauri E., et al. "Reduction in Human Papillomavirus (HPV) Prevalence among Young Women Following HPV Vaccine Introduction in the United States, National Health and Nutrition Examination Surveys, 2003–2010." *Journal of Infectious Diseases* 208, 3 (August 1, 2013): 385–393. This article can also be found online at https://academic.oup.com/jid/article/208/3/385/2192839 (accessed February 20, 2018).

Websites

Haelle, Tara. "CDC Endorses a More Effective HPV Vaccine to Prevent Cancer." NPR, February 1, 2016. https://www.npr.org/sections/health-shots/2016/02/01/465160937/cdc-endorses-a-more-effective-hpv-vaccine-to-prevent-cancer (accessed February 20, 2018).

"Human Papillomavirus (HPV)." Centers for Disease Control and Prevention, January 4, 2017. https://www.cdc.gov/std/hpv/default.htm (accessed February 20, 2018).

"Human Papillomavirus (HPV) and Cervical Cancer." World Health Organization, June 2016. http://www.who.int/mediacentre/factsheets/fs380/en/ (accessed February 20, 2018).

Susan Aldridge
Claire Skinner

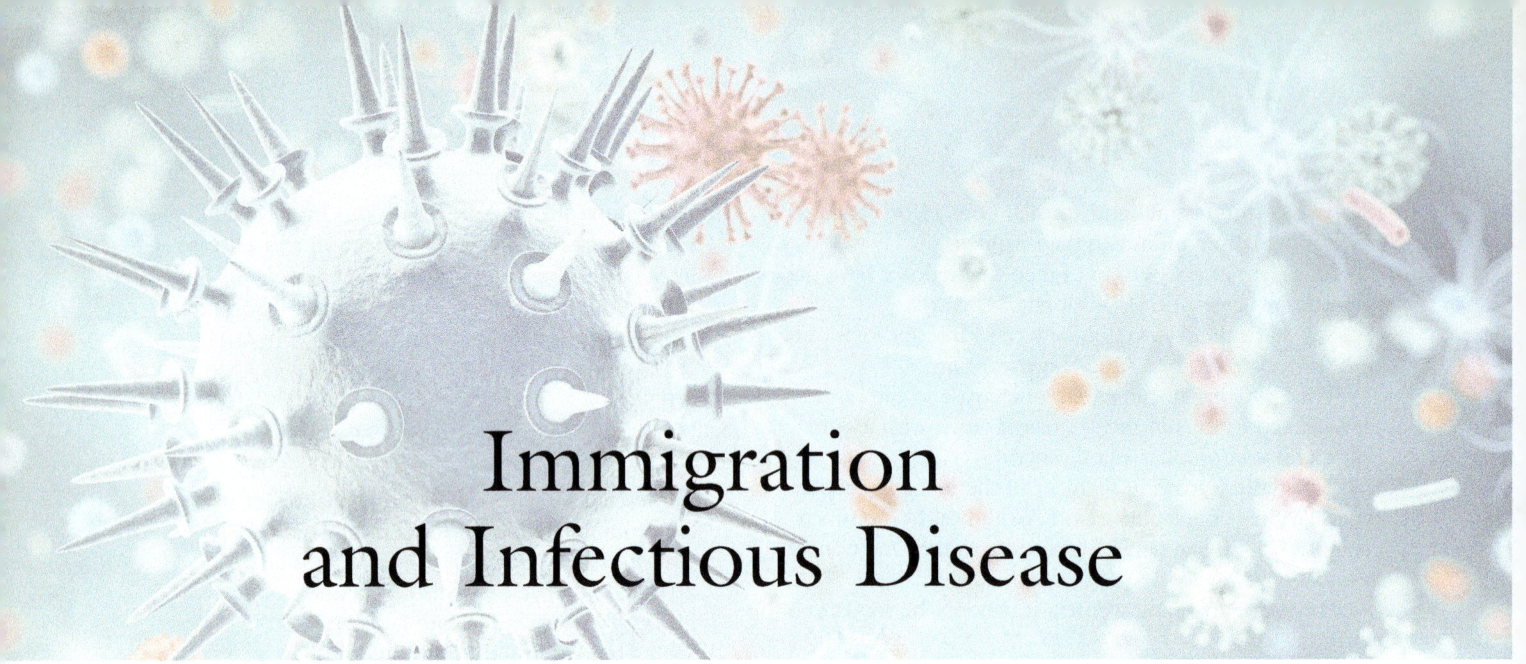

Immigration and Infectious Disease

Introduction

Every day an estimated 2 million people cross an international boundary. Many of these people are travelers on short visits. Others are immigrants, either refugees or voluntary migrants. Some migrants never cross national borders but are displaced within their own nations. As of 2016 there were at least 64 million internally displaced persons (IDPs) worldwide, the highest number since the United Nations (UN) began counting in 1950. IDPs typically migrate or are forced to move because of war, ecological disaster, disease, or economic collapse. The UN estimates that 20 people are driven from their home by violence or persecution every minute.

The increasing movement of people across the globe plays a significant role in the spread of disease. Since antiquity health hazards have moved across long distances through movement of people. Travel, trade, exploration, and war forged nations but also spread disease. Travel by horse or on foot was slow, serving as a limited barrier to the transport of infectious disease. Those who fell ill often died or were no longer ill by the time they reached other population centers. Ships spread diseases faster, as a disease could linger on a ship for months, infecting whole crews. In addition, the large cargo load of ships posed a unique disease risk. In the case of the Black Death (plague), rats aboard cargo ships likely hosted fleas responsible for spreading plague throughout Asia, the Middle East, and Europe. In the modern era, the spread of air travel and its reduced costs have greatly increased the number of travelers and have heightened the risk of disease. Air travel permits infected people and diseases to reach new populations, often in distant locations, within hours.

Immigration raises many of the same disease issues as voluntary travel. However, immigrants also have unique health needs. Some immigrant populations come from areas with parasites or other infectious diseases that are endemic to their homeland but have been eliminated in the industrialized world. Immigrants may not have had access to routine health care in their home countries. Providing effective health care to immigrant groups requires training health care professionals to recognize the health needs of diverse immigrant groups.

WORDS TO KNOW

IMMIGRATION The relocation of people to a different region or country from their native lands. Also, the movement of organisms into an area where they were previously absent.

IMPORTED CASE OF DISEASE An instance of disease in which an infected person who is not yet showing symptoms travels from his or her home country to another country and develops symptoms of the disease there.

INTERNATIONAL HEALTH REGULATIONS Regulations introduced by the World Health Organization (WHO) that aim to control, monitor, prevent, protect against, and respond to the spread of disease across national borders while avoiding unnecessary interference with international movement and trade.

ISOLATION Within the health community, precautions taken in the hospital to prevent the spread of an infectious agent from an infected or colonized patient to susceptible people. Isolation practices are designed to minimize the transmission of infection.

MIGRATION In medicine, the movement of a disease symptom from one part of the body to another, apparently without cause.

PREVALENCE The actual number of cases of disease or injury that exists in a population.

STRAIN A subclass or a specific genetic variation of an organism.

Disease History, Characteristics, and Transmission

Cholera, dysentery, typhoid, tuberculosis, human immunodeficiency virus (HIV)/acquired immunodeficiency syndrome (AIDS), and malaria are only a few of the infectious diseases that migration and immigration have helped to spread. Illnesses that have been largely eliminated from some areas, such as malaria or tuberculosis, can be reintroduced by migrants. Such cases of disease are labeled imported cases. For example, in the 2010s the World Health Organization (WHO) became concerned that refugees from the Boko Haram insurgency in Nigeria may spread polio to other Lake Chad basin countries and the rest of sub-Saharan Africa. The instability that creates refugees also hampers vaccination and other public health efforts.

Cholera, dysentery, and typhoid are major killers that are spread by poor sanitation. Densely packed refugee camps with improper sanitation and poor hygienic conditions foster outbreaks of infectious disease. Carelessness can also be deadly. In 2016 the UN accepted responsibility for spreading cholera in Haiti via peacekeepers from Nepal who were providing aid after a 2010 earthquake. Nepal had a cholera epidemic at the time, and human waste from the UN base leaked into the Meille River. The Haitian epidemic killed at least 10,000 people and sickened hundreds of thousands more.

The construction of latrines and treatment of wastewater has helped reduce some incidences of infectious disease. Such measures are not always possible at severely underresourced, overcrowded, and hastily constructed refugee camps. Food shortages and malnutrition in refugee and IDP camps also contribute to the spread of disease.

Scope and Distribution

It is difficult to measure the scope and distribution of infectious disease spread by immigrants because of reporting difficulties. Health care systems in some countries, including developing nations that have received large numbers of refugees from neighboring nations, are too inadequate to correctly identify diseases and complete the necessary procedures for effective reporting. However, the US Centers for Disease Control (CDC) and WHO have helped identify areas of concern.

Haiti has sent large numbers of economic and political refugees to the United States and to other Caribbean nations. In 2006 the Jamaican Health Ministry reported that there was a link between Haitian immigrants and a recent outbreak of malaria in Jamaica. Deoxyribonucleic acid (DNA) testing by the CDC tied an outbreak in Kingston to a single source consistent with the *Falciparum* malaria parasite found in Haiti. At least 302 Jamaicans were infected. The government conducted an island-wide surveillance of breeding sites for the *Anopheles* (malaria-spreading) mosquito and destroyed about 450 *Anopheles* breeding sites in 256 communities.

Tuberculosis, an infectious disease that in some forms is resistant to treatment, is spread through air droplets expelled when infected people cough, sneeze, speak, or sing. It had largely been eliminated from some nations, notably the United States and the United Kingdom, until

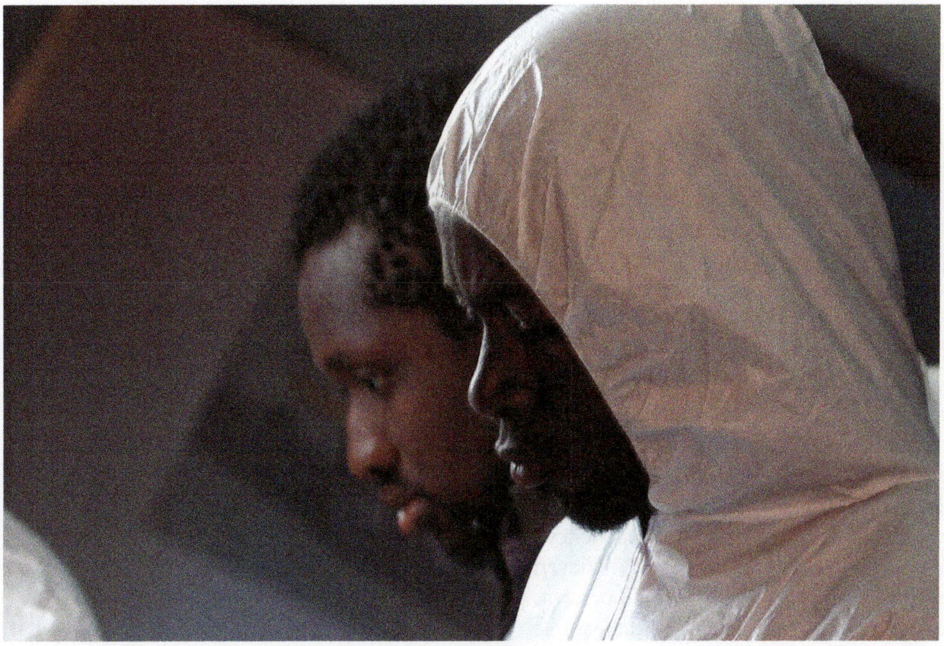

In Salerno, Italy, immigrants rescued from the Mediterranean Sea are place in quarantine to try to prevent the spread of disease. © *Carlo Hermann/KONTROLAB/LightRocket/Getty Images*

immigration brought it back. In 2001 61.4 percent of all tuberculosis cases in the Netherlands occurred among foreign citizens. Tuberculosis transmission during air travel has been documented by WHO.

Varicella, the chickenpox virus, is yet another disease that can be spread by immigrants. In tropical countries varicella does not generally infect in early childhood as it does in temperate zones. In the tropics infections typically occur in the late teens and 20s, meaning immigrants from those countries do not have the same high level of immunity to chickenpox as do young adults who grew up in temperate countries.

■ Treatment and Prevention

The International Health Regulations (IHR), a WHO-designed legal instrument, aims to provide maximum security against the international spread of diseases with a minimum interference with world traffic. The first IHR, approved in 1969, only targeted cholera, yellow fever, and plague. The rise of globalization prompted a revised IHR, which took effect in 2007 and is binding to 196 countries. Among its many measures, the IHR establishes a single code of procedures and practices for routine public health measures at international airports and ports and some ground crossings. The regulations focus on ensuring early detection, confirmation, investigation, and rapid response for any emergencies of international concern.

■ Impacts and Issues

Infectious diseases do not recognize borders. Accordingly, nations need to improve their medical surveillance to safeguard the health of their citizens. The IHR is one step in this direction. Screening and immunization programs would protect the health of immigrants and established residents. Canadian medical researchers have recommended that family doctors should ask young adult immigrants and refugees whether they have ever had chickenpox, test those who answer in the negative, and offer to vaccinate those who are susceptible to the disease.

For many years Somalia had an HIV prevalence rate of about 1 percent, which was lower than that of many African countries. After much cross-border movement of HIV-infected refugees from Ethiopia, however, the HIV infection rates in Somalia subsequently increased. Condoms are generally unavailable in Somalia, and there is a lack of adequate health care. Other African nations have experienced similar patterns of disease progression with HIV. Eleven African nations have HIV prevalence rates over 13 percent.

Political issues are also affecting international public health. Taiwan lacks full membership in WHO because of a historically strained relationship with mainland China. The island state has had more success than any other East Asian country in fighting H5N1, or avian influenza. Nevertheless, WHO has refused Taiwan's applications to attend avian flu–related international conferences, thus preventing Taiwan from effectively sharing its valuable experience in disease prevention. According to Taiwan's National Immigration Agency, an average of 1,200 people travel between Taiwan and China each day, and the number of Taiwanese traveling to the United States averages more than 1,600 per day.

In 2007 Andrew Speaker, an Atlanta man with a strain of tuberculosis that is highly resistant to current drug therapies, flew to France for his honeymoon against the advice of his physicians. While in Italy medical personnel determined that his tuberculosis was the extremely resistant type (XDR-TB). Fearing isolation in an Italian hospital, Speaker flew to Prague, Czech Republic, and Montreal, Quebec, before renting a car, driving to New York City, and checking into a hospital. The CDC tracked people who were in close contact with him, including his fellow aircraft passengers and the flight attendants. Speaker subsequently became the subject of the first federal order for isolation issued in the United States since 1963, raising questions about compulsory quarantines.

While immigration has the potential to spread disease, it also has brought attention to many health issues. Industrialized nations with large immigrant populations, including the United States, have renewed interest in combating neglected diseases (diseases that are rare or eliminated in developed nations) across the globe. For example, international cooperative projects have sought to reduce incidence of tuberculosis and endemic parasitic diseases in Central and South America, as well as encourage screening and treatment for immigrants from those regions.

PRIMARY SOURCE

Internationally Adopted Children—Immigration Status

SOURCE: *Miller, Laurie C. "Internationally Adopted Children—Immigration Status."* Pediatrics *103, no. 5 (May 1999): P1078(1).*

INTRODUCTION: *This letter to the editor of the journal* Pediatrics *highlights the special vaccination needs of children immigrating to the United States. Laurie C. Miller, a Boston-based physician specializing in internationally adopted children, wrote this letter in 1999 to raise awareness about a concern that remains in 2018. Miller is an associate professor of pediatrics and director of the International Adoption Clinic at Tufts University School of Medicine. She is the author of* The Handbook of International Adoption Medicine: A Guide for Physicians, Parents, and Providers *(2005).*

To the Editor,—

The number of internationally adopted children arriving in the United States has increased dramatically (13,620 in 1997, compared with 9,945 in 1986). Many children have received vaccines in their birth countries; however, the efficacy [effectiveness] of the vaccines and the accuracy of the records are sometimes questionable. Hostetter, et al. have reported protective diphtheria and tetanus titers in only 38 percent of Chinese, Russian, or Eastern European children with written evidence of age-appropriate vaccines.

We have observed that polio titers also may not be protective. Four children in our clinic with written evidence of 3 to 6 polio vaccines were found to have incompletely protective titers. The children were from Lithuania (1), Russia (2), and China (1). They ranged in age from 12 months to 8 years. In 3 children, protective titers to Type 1 and Type 2 polio were found, but no titers to Type 3 polio were measured. In one child, protective titers to Type 1 were absent, but were present for Types 2 and 3.

Although the *Red Book* recommends that "written documentation should be accepted as evidence of prior immunization," clinicians caring for internationally adopted children should be aware of the possibility of incomplete immunity to polio, and should either revaccinate or verify immunity to all 3 types of polio. Revaccination or verification of protective titers should be considered for all immunizations in this population.

LAURIE C. MILLER, MD
International Adoption Clinic
New England Medical Center
Boston, MA 02111

SEE ALSO *Airborne Precautions; Avian Influenza; Cholera; Contact Precautions; Dysentery; Isolation and Quarantine; Polio (Poliomyelitis); Reemerging Infectious Diseases; Tuberculosis; Typhoid Fever; War and Infectious Disease*

BIBLIOGRAPHY

Books

Bashford, Alison, ed. *Medicine at the Border: Disease, Globalization, and Security, 1850 to the Present.* New York: Palgrave Macmillan, 2006.

Markel, Howard. *When Germs Travel: Six Major Epidemics That Have Invaded America since 1900 and the Fears They Have Unleashed.* New York: Pantheon, 2004.

Periodicals

Waterman, Stephen H., et al. "A New Paradigm for Quarantine and Public Health Activities at Land Borders: Opportunities and Challenges." *Public Health Reports* 124, no. 2 (2009): 203–211.

Websites

"International Health Regulations (IHR)." World Health Organization. http://www.who.int/topics/international_health_regulations/en/ (accessed February 25, 2018).

"Tuberculosis and Air Travel: Guidelines for Prevention and Control." World Health Organization, 2006. http://www.who.int/tb/publications/2006/who_htm_tb_2006_363.pdf (accessed May 17, 2007).

Caryn E. Neumann

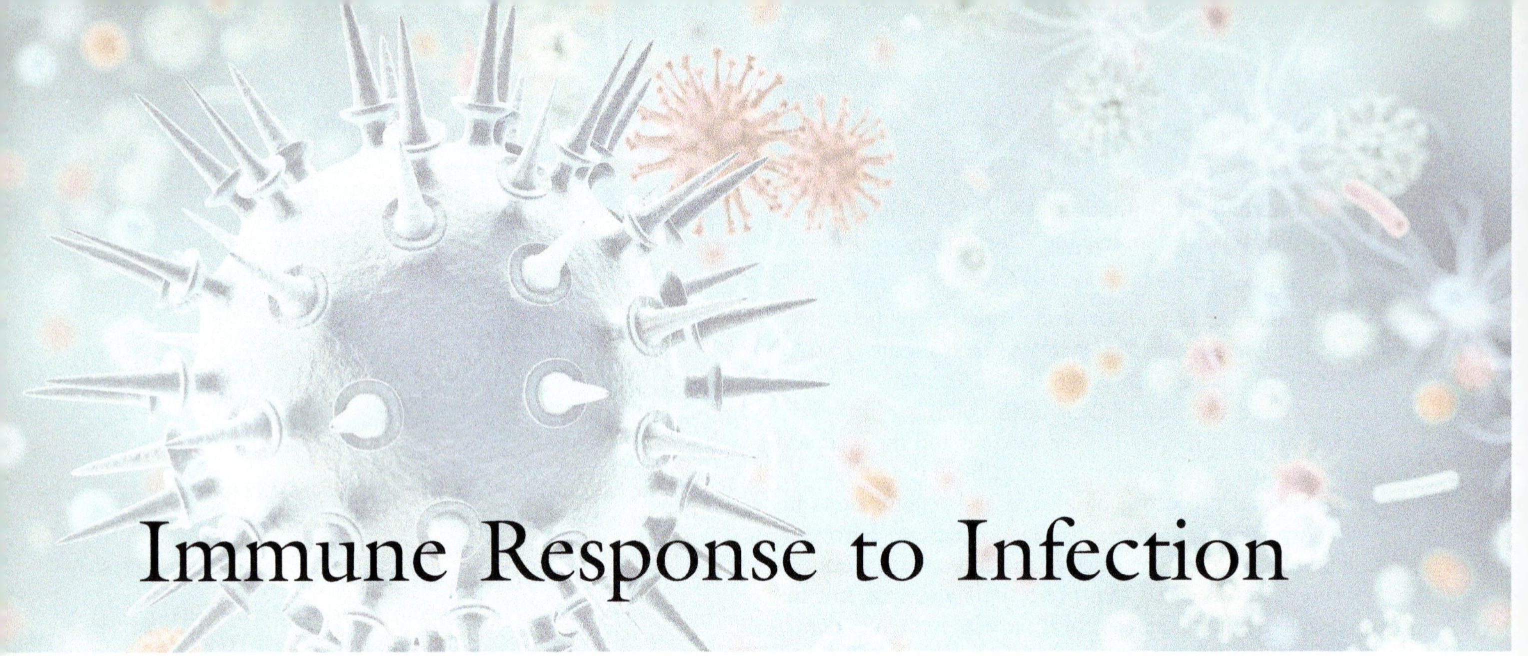

Immune Response to Infection

Introduction

The immune system is a series of cells, tissues, organs, and processes in the body that differentiates the self from foreign bodies, fights infections, and develops immunity against future attack. The function of the immune system is to identify pathogens of all types and to destroy them through immune processes. Bacteria, viruses, fungi, parasites, cancerous cells, and single-celled organisms such as amoebas can all attack the body and cause disease. The immune system must recognize and act on these pathogens without attacking its own healthy tissues, thereby causing illness. The immune system also works to keep dangerous pathogens out of the body, resisting, trapping, and killing microorganisms to prevent them from causing disease. This is an important function of the skin and mucous membranes, which have high concentrations of immune system cells.

Scientific Foundations

One of the most important jobs of the immune system is to differentiate the self from the nonself. Almost all the cells of the body have specific proteins on their surfaces that identify them as part of the self. These proteins are part of the major histocompatibility complex (MHC). Foreign bodies such as bacteria, viruses, or cells belonging to another organism lack the appropriate MHC protein and are thus identified as

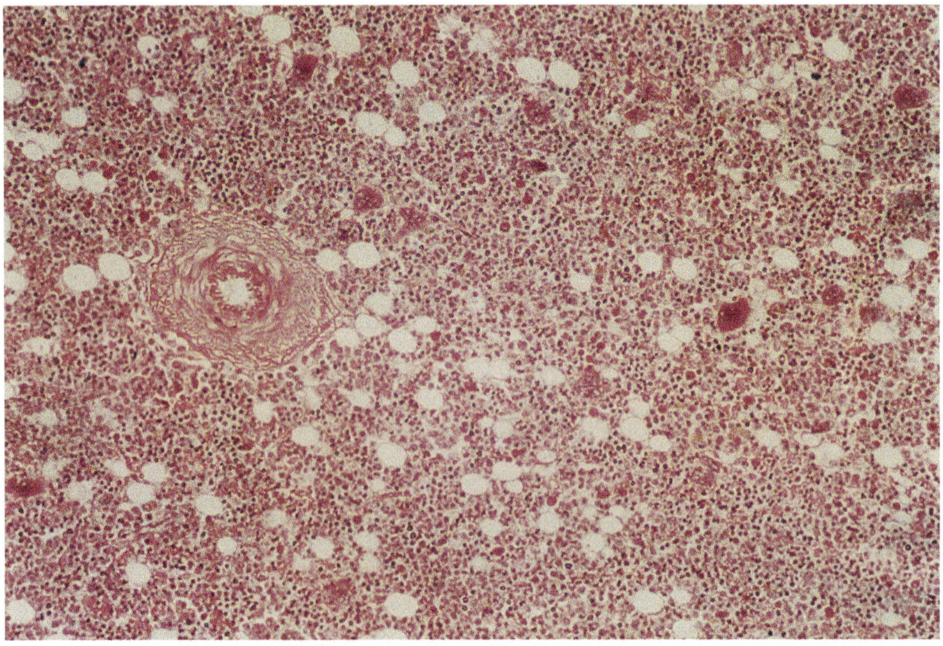

Bone marrow, shown here in a light micrograph, plays a fundamental role in immune response to infection by producing blood and immune cells. *© Astrid Kage/Science Source*

WORDS TO KNOW

ACQUIRED (ADAPTIVE) IMMUNITY The ability to resist infection that develops according to circumstances and is targeted to a specific pathogen. There are two types of acquired immunity, known as active and passive. Active immunity is either humoral, involving production of antibody molecules against a bacterium or virus, or cell-mediated, where T cells are mobilized against infected cells. Infection and immunization can both induce acquired immunity. Passive immunity is induced by injection of the serum of a person who is already immune to a particular infection.

ANTIBODIES Proteins found in the blood that help fight against foreign substances called antigens. Antigens, which are usually proteins or polysaccharides, stimulate the immune system to produce antibodies, or Y-shaped immunoglobulins. The antibodies inactivate the antigen and help remove it from the body. While antigens can be the source of infections from pathogenic bacteria and viruses, organic molecules detrimental to the body from internal or environmental sources also act as antigens. Genetic engineering and the use of various mutational mechanisms allow the construction of a vast array of antibodies (each with a unique genetic sequence).

ANTIGEN A substance, usually a protein or polysaccharide, that stimulates the immune system to produce antibodies, which inactivate the antigen and help remove it from the body. While antigens can be the source of infection by pathogenic bacteria and viruses, organic molecules detrimental to the body from internal or environmental sources also act as antigens.

CYTOKINE One of a family of small proteins that mediate an organism's response to injury or infection. Cytokines operate by transmitting signals between cells in an organism. Minute quantities of cytokines are secreted, each by a single cell type, to regulate functions in other cells by binding with specific receptors. Their interactions with the receptors produce secondary signals that inhibit or enhance the action of certain genes within the cell. Unlike endocrine hormones, which can act throughout the body, most cytokines act locally near the cells that produced them.

INNATE IMMUNITY Resistance against disease that an individual is born with, as distinct from acquired immunity, which develops with exposure to infectious agents.

LYMPHOCYTE A type of white blood cell, such as a B or T lymphocyte, that functions as part of the lymphatic and immune systems by stimulating antibody formation to attack specific invading substances.

MAJOR HISTOCOMPATIBILITY COMPLEX (MHC) The proteins that protrude from the surface of a cell that identify the cell as "self." In humans the proteins coded by the genes of the major histocompatibility complex (MHC) include human leukocyte antigens (HLAs), as well as other proteins. HLA proteins are present on the surface of most of the body's cells and are important in helping the immune system distinguish "self" from "nonself" molecules, cells, and other objects.

NEUTROPHIL A type of white blood cell that phagocytizes foreign microorganisms, releasing a bacteria-killing chemical known as lysozyme. Neutrophils are prominent in the inflammatory response.

PATHOGEN A disease-causing agent such as a bacterium, a virus, a fungus, or another microorganism.

nonself. The healthy immune system reacts to things identified as nonself and not to things identified as self.

Many organs in the body are regarded as part of the immune system because they produce, transport, coordinate, or help mature immune cells. The bone marrow is often considered first because it is the source of all blood and immune cells. The thymus is the developing ground for T cells, a type of lymphocyte, or white blood cell, that fights pathogens. In the thymus large numbers of unsuitable cells undergo apoptosis (programmed cell death) for each mature T cell that is produced.

One of the functions of the spleen is to store and release generalized immune cells to respond to infection. Other lymphoid organs, such as the tonsils, adenoids, and appendix, are placed strategically in the respiratory and digestive tracts to intercept infectious agents before they enter further into the body.

The lymphatic system is a complex network of vessels and nodes that transport lymph, a fluid similar to blood plasma. The lymph system connects the organs of the immune system with one another and with the rest of the body, carrying immune cells to their necessary locations. Lymph nodes are small compartments that provide space for immune cells to interact with antigens and begin their response. They also allow transfer of immune cells between the lymph system and the circulatory system. Unlike the

THE IMMUNE SYSTEM AND TATTOOS

In 2018 scientists discovered a potential new avenue for tattoo removal by studying the relationship between tattoos and the immune system. Tattoos are permanent because of how the tattoo needle and ink interact with the immune system. When the needle pierces the dermis (a deep layer of skin), the immune system sends macrophages to consume the foreign ink. Macrophages are a kind of white blood cell that the immune system uses to consume foreign bodies such as cancer cells.

Scientists have long thought that tattoos are permanent because the macrophages become full with ink and remain in the dermis. However, in an article published in 2018 in the *Journal of Experimental Medicine*, Anna Baranska and a team of researchers found evidence to the contrary. They used black mice to study the relationship between pigmentation and macrophages, finding that, whereas white mice contain cells that store pigments, in black mice these cells die off. Macrophages then consume the pigment particles, as they would any other foreign body. However, after the macrophages consume the pigment, they die and release it back into the system, contrary to previous scientific theories. The pigment is then consumed by new macrophages in a continuous cycle. This insight suggests a potential new way of removing tattoos by blocking the macrophages from responding to the pigment in tattoo ink.

blood, which is pumped around the body at high pressure by the heart, the lymph fluid is slow moving and at low pressure, lacking a central pump. The lymph fluid is extracted from the body's tissues by osmosis and then is transported around the body by the movement of muscles. Because of its slow-moving nature, lymph fluid can sometimes build up in the limbs, causing swelling and the possibility of infection. This is called lymphedema.

Anything that the immune system responds to, whether it is a microbe, protein, virus, or fragment of a pathogen, is called an antigen. The presence of antigens activates specific immune cells to destroy the pathogen and teach the immune system to recognize it in the future. There are two major kinds of immune cells: those that react generally to all pathogens and those that are keyed to a specific disease-causing agent. Generalized immune cells include neutrophils, which consume pathogens and kill them with powerful chemical granules and then send signals to other cells. Macrophages then arrive to consume the foreign bodies. Natural killer cells also use toxic granules to kill disease agents, responding to cells lacking the correct MHC proteins.

Lymphocytes, also known as white blood cells, are produced in the bone marrow and are present in the blood. From the bone marrow, certain lymphocytes known as T cells travel to an organ known as the thymus to mature. Lymphocytes are also carried around the body by the lymphatic system. Two major types of lymphocytes react to specific pathogens. B cells create antibodies, whereas T cells destroy invaders and coordinate the overall immune response. Antibodies are special markers that lock onto antigens and alert the T cells to destroy them. Cells use proteins called cytokines to communicate that they are injured and to organize immune cells.

After a pathogen has been detected and destroyed, a small number of antibodies and specialized T cells remain to guard against future attack. When that same pathogen is encountered again, the number of specialized cells multiplies to mount an immune response.

■ Impacts and Issues

The generalized immune system cells provide innate immunity, the ability to identify a foreign body and destroy it without having been exposed to it previously. Once the immune system has encountered a pathogen, activated its immune cells, and developed antibodies, the body is said to have developed acquired (or adaptive) immunity. Vaccines provide resistance from diseases that the body has not encountered by causing the production of antibodies. Thus, vaccines induce a kind of acquired immunity. Nursing infants also obtain antibodies and immune system proteins from their mothers when they breastfeed. This is widely recognized as one of the benefits of nursing because the immune system of infants is immature at birth.

One of the first bodily responses to infection or injury is inflammation, the familiar redness, swelling, heat, and pain associated with trauma. Inflammation is initiated locally by the blood vessels in the infected area. The activated vessels release fluids, which cause the swelling, as well as cytokines, which send signals to the immune system. This causes white blood cells of all types to rush to the area. The white blood cells begin acting on pathogens in their customary ways, identifying and consuming pathogens and creating antibodies. The cytotoxic (toxic to cells) chemicals present in neutrophils and other granulocytes are also responsible for reinforcing the inflammatory response. Inflammation can become harmful when it moves from a localized response to a systemic condition. Some heart problems, asthma, blood vessel disease, colitis (bowel disease), arthritis, fibromyalgia, septic shock, and nephritis (kidney disease) are all associated with excessive or inappropriate inflammation.

Disorders of the immune system can cause serious disease. Human immunodeficiency virus (HIV) is a well-known virus that attacks the helper T cells, which activate and manage immune response. Once levels of helper T cells fall to sufficiently low levels, the normal immune response breaks down, and the victim becomes more susceptible to opportunistic infections. Many types of autoimmune diseases are the result of the immune system attacking the body. Crohn's disease, type 1 diabetes, rheumatoid arthritis, multiple sclerosis, myasthenia gravis, celiac disease, and Addison's disease are among the serious conditions associated with misdirected immune response. It should be noted that some developmental processes and the destruction of cancer require the immune system to act on the self, so not all autoimmune responses are harmful.

Researchers have sought to harness the body's autoimmune responses to identify and attack tumors. For example, cancer researchers have developed a new form of immunotherapy known as chimeric antigen receptor (CAR) T cell therapy. In this increasingly common form of cancer treatment, medical professionals draw blood from a cancer patient, isolate T cells, and alter the T cells by adding CARs, which bind to cancer cell proteins. Once the CARs have been bound to the patient's T cells, technicians grow these altered cells in the laboratory. The CAR T cells are then infused in the patient. Once the cells are in the patient's bloodstream, the CARs allow the T cells to hunt down and destroy cancer cells.

The US Food and Drug Administration (FDA) approved CAR T cell therapy for two kinds of lymphoma, which are cancers of the blood, in 2017. While the newness of this revolutionary therapy makes it difficult for researchers to fully understand the drugs' effectiveness, these treatments have produced dramatic results in some patients who were otherwise deemed untreatable. As a result, medical professionals are hopeful that CAR T cell therapy might provide a breakthrough for a much broader range of cancer treatments using adoptive cell transfer (ACT), which involves altering a patient's immune cells to combat disease.

ACT may also have applications for treating diseases other than cancer, especially in patients who have weakened immune systems and need to fight off infections. As of 2018 researchers were actively investigating whether CAR T cells could be used to enhance the effectiveness of immune responses to other infectious pathogens. Evidence suggests, for example, that CAR T cells have the potential to kill HIV-1-infected cells that have evaded a person's endogenous immune response. Targeting the HIV viral envelope reduces the chances of unwanted side effects on healthy tissue. CAR T cells are not affected by HIV-1's activities to reduce the immune system's ability to recognize the pathogen as nonself. In their 2015 article in *Philosophical Transactions of the Royal Society B*, Carl H. June and Bruce L. Levine argued that research in ACT technology suggests "we are at the threshold of a golden era for adoptive T-cell therapy."

All organisms require defense from invasive pathogens. In humans and other vertebrates, the intricate and multilayered protection provided by the organs, cells, proteins, and chemicals of the immune system provide resistance to many kinds of attack. Even single-celled organisms use chemical substances to defend themselves. The proper function of the immune system is necessary for the health of the organism, avoiding both infection and autoimmune disease. Without the immune system, the body would be susceptible to endless attack, shortening the life span or even killing the individual.

See Also *Bacterial Disease; HIV; Vaccines and Vaccine Development; Viral Disease; Waterborne Disease*

BIBLIOGRAPHY

Books

Parham, Peter. *The Immune System.* 4th ed. New York: Garland Science, 2015.

Periodicals

Baranska, Anna, et al. "Unveiling Skin Macrophage Dynamics Explains Both Tattoo Persistence and Strenuous Removal." *Journal of Experimental Medicine* 215, no. 3 (2018): 1–19. This article can also be found online at http://jem.rupress.org/content/early/2018/03/05/jem.20171608 (accessed March 12, 2018).

Hale, Malika, et al. "Engineering HIV-Resistant, Anti-HIV Chimeric Antigen Receptor T Cells." *Molecular Therapy* 25, no. 3 (2017): 570–579. This article can also be found online at http://www.cell.com/molecular-therapy-family/molecular-therapy/fulltext/S1525-0016(17)30004-7 (accessed March 12, 2018).

June, Carl H., and Bruce L. Levine. "T Cell Engineering as Therapy for Cancer and HIV: Our Synthetic Future." *Philosophical Transactions of the Royal Society B* 370, no. 1680 (2015): 20140374. This article can also be found online at http://rstb.royalsocietypublishing.org/content/370/1680/20140374 (accessed March 12, 2018).

Websites

Bugl, Paul. "Immune System." University of Hartford, March 2001. http://uhaweb.hartford.edu/BUGL/immune.htm (accessed March 8, 2018).

"CAR T Cells: Engineering Patients' Immune Cells to Treat Their Cancers." National Cancer Institute. https://www.cancer.gov/about-cancer/treatment/research/car-t-cells (accessed March 8, 2018).

Corey, Lawrence. "Designing CAR T Cells for HIV: A Link between Cancer and Infectious Disease Therapy." International AIDS Society, 2017. http://www.iasociety.org/Web/WebContent/File/HIV_Cure_Forum_2017/Session%206_RT/2%20IS5-2_Corey.pdf (accessed March 8, 2018).

Kenneth T. LaPensee

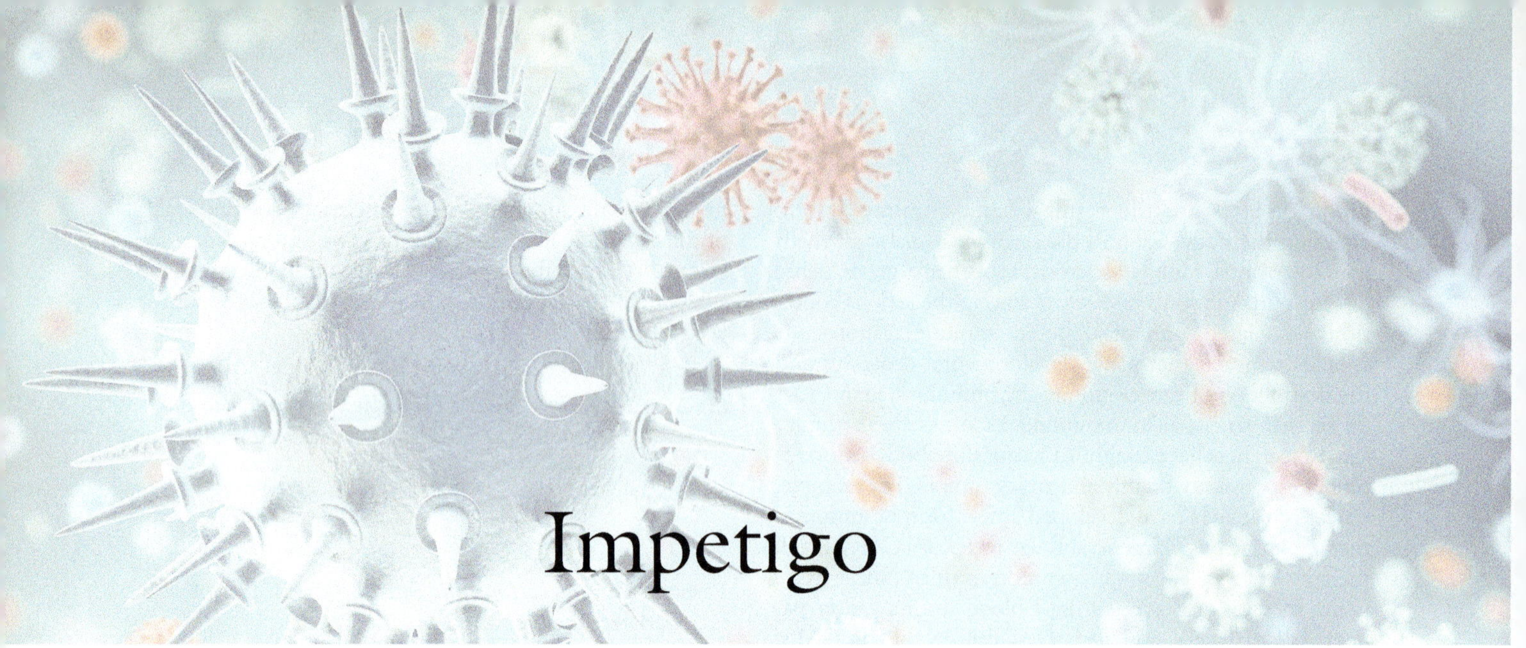

Impetigo

Introduction

Impetigo is a skin disorder characterized by crusting lesions that commonly occurs among young school-age children. Infection is due to either *Staphylococcus* or *Streptococcus* bacteria and occurs at sites of skin trauma such as bites, scratches, or cuts.

Symptoms present as tiny clusters of fluid-filled blisters that weep after bursting and form a crust. Fluids at these sites, as well as the nasal fluids of people who harbor the causative agent in their noses, carry infection and allow for easy transmission between people. Washing sores with antibacterial soap and covering them can prevent transmission of the bacteria.

Treatment with antibiotics is usually effective, and sores generally heal slowly without scarring. Prevention is achieved through good hygiene practices such as handwashing and treatment of other skin sores to prevent establishment of infection. Impetigo and its causative pathogens are found throughout the world.

WORDS TO KNOW

COLONIZATION The process of occupation and increase in number of microorganisms at a specific site.

FOMITE An object or a surface to which infectious microorganisms such as bacteria or viruses can adhere and be transmitted. Papers, clothing, dishes, and other objects can all act as fomites. Transmission is often by touch.

PATHOGEN A disease-causing agent, such as a bacterium, a virus, a fungus, or another microorganism.

Disease History, Characteristics, and Transmission

Impetigo is a skin disorder that results from bacterial infection, commonly by *Staphylococcus aureus* but also by *Streptococcus* bacteria. Infection usually occurs when the protective barrier of the skin is irritated or breached because of cuts, scratches, insect bites, or eczema.

The disease is one of the most common among children and is characterized by crusting skin lesions usually located around the nose, mouth, hands, and forearms. Symptoms begin as small pimple-like sores surrounded by reddened skin, which quickly develop into fluid-filled blisters. Once the blisters rupture, that patch of skin will continue to weep, and a yellowish crust will develop over four to six days. The lesions may vary slightly depending on the causative agent, but generally symptoms have the same presentation and will appear around two to three days after infection.

Impetigo is extremely contagious, and transmission occurs through contact with the infected site, nasal fluid, or fomites. Scratching may also spread the lesions.

Scope and Distribution

Those most commonly affected by impetigo are toddlers and schoolchildren between the ages of two and six, with peak incidence usually occurring in the hot and humid weather of the summer months. The disease tends to occur in small outbreaks. Epidemics are rare, although from September 1981 to February 1982, 20 infants became infected at a hospital nursery in Louisville, Kentucky. The nurse who was found to be the carrier of the infection was treated and removed from the nursery, and no further incidence of impetigo occurred there. All 20 of the infected infants recovered.

There is often no apparent source of infection for impetigo. This is largely because *S. aureus* is part of the human body's normal flora, which means that it is one of many bacteria that readily colonize areas of the human body without causing infection. *Staphylococcus* bacteria are commonly found on the skin's surface, nose, and mouth and cause infection when they enter open wounds at these sites.

Impetigo often follows a recent upper respiratory tract infection caused by *Streptococcus* bacteria, and people who suffer from cold sores may also have a higher chance of developing the disease.

Treatment and Prevention

The focus of treatment for impetigo is to cure the infection and to relieve symptoms. If the infection is limited to a small area, a topical antibiotic ointment will generally be sufficient. If this is not effective, oral antibiotics may be required. Healing will begin within a few days of treatment and sores generally clear within 10 days without severe scarring.

Prevention of impetigo may be achieved by maintaining good hygiene practices such as regular handwashing, bathing, and tending to skin injuries such as cuts, scrapes, bites, and rashes. To prevent spreading infection, infected sites should be covered and items such as linen and cutlery should not be shared.

EFFECTIVE RULES AND REGULATIONS

The Centers for Disease Control and Prevention (CDC), Coordinating Center for Infectious Diseases, Division of Bacterial and Mycotic Diseases, states that the spread of all types of GAS infection (group A streptococcal disease [strep throat, necrotizing fasciitis, impetigo]) can be reduced by good handwashing, especially after coughing and sneezing and before preparing foods or eating. People with sore throats should be seen by a doctor who can perform tests to find out whether the illness is strep throat. If the test result shows strep throat, the person should stay home from work, school, or day care until 24 hours after taking an antibiotic. All wounds should be kept clean and watched for possible signs of infection such as redness, swelling, drainage, and pain at the wound site. A person with signs of an infected wound, especially if fever occurs, should seek medical care. It is not necessary for all people exposed to someone with an invasive group A strep infection (e.g., necrotizing fasciitis or strep toxic shock syndrome) to receive antibiotic therapy to prevent infection. However, in certain circumstances antibiotic therapy may be appropriate. That decision should be made after consulting with your doctor.

Impacts and Issues

Although often widespread, impetigo generally poses little threat to communities, and treatment is readily available in developed countries. The ease of transmission between infected persons is heightened among

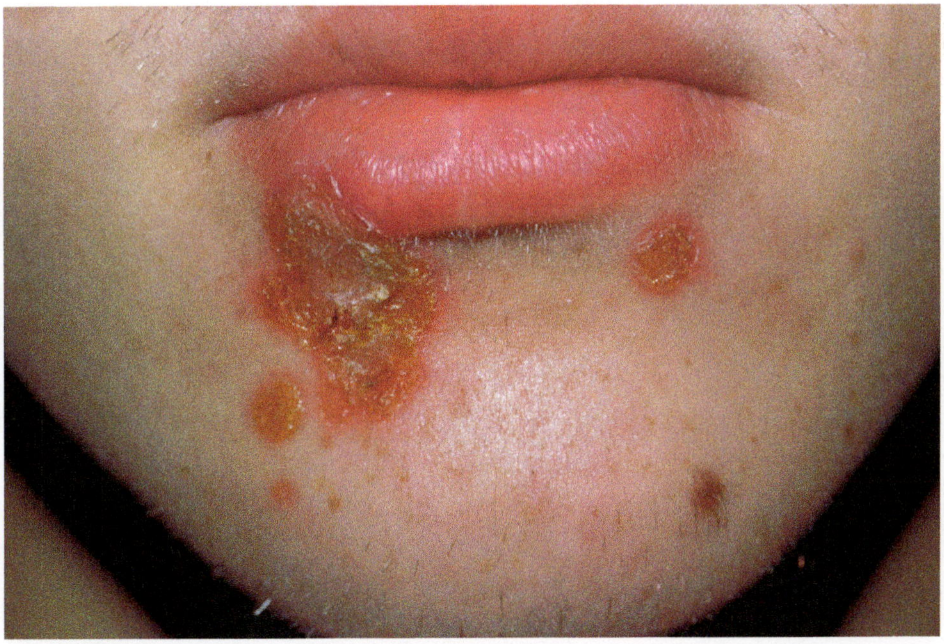

An impetigo lesion caused by the bacteria *Staphylococcus aureus* or *Streptococcus.* Impetigo is one of the most common diseases among children. © SCIENCE PHOTO LIBRARY/Getty Images

groups of young children where limiting contact can be difficult. In situations of outbreak among school groups, it is important that parents and teachers work together to ensure the infected children are appropriately and effectively treated while those not infected are successfully protected.

Evidence suggests that geography and climate will influence the primary infective organism causing impetigo. In developing nations and warmer climates, *Streptococcus* bacteria is the most common. In rare cases impetigo caused by *Streptococcus* bacteria can progress deeper than the skin. One such complication arising from infection by *Streptococcus* may lead to damage of the kidneys, heart, or other organs. This makes early detection and treatment important in these developing regions.

SEE ALSO *Bacterial Disease; Childhood Infectious Diseases, Immunization Impacts; Handwashing; Microorganisms;* Staphylococcus aureus *Infections; Strep Throat*

BIBLIOGRAPHY

Books

Bennett, John E., Raphael Dolin, and Martin J. Blaser. *Mandell, Douglas, and Bennett's Infectious Disease Essentials.* Philadelphia: Elsevier, 2016.

Bennett, John E., Raphael Dolin, and Martin J. Blaser. *Mandell, Douglas, and Bennett's Principles and Practice of Infectious Diseases.* 8th ed. Philadelphia: Elsevier, 2014.

Murray, Patrick R., Ken S. Rosenthal, and Michael A. Pfaller. *Medical Microbiology.* Philadelphia: Elsevier, 2015.

Wilson, Walter R., and Merle A. Sande. *Current Diagnosis & Treatment in Infectious Diseases.* New York: McGraw Hill, 2014.

Periodicals

Moore, S. Jason, et al. "Clinical Characteristics and Antibiotic Utilization in Pediatric Patients Hospitalized with Acute Bacterial Skin and Skin Structure Infection." *Pediatric Infectious Disease Journal* 33, no. 8 (2014): 825–828.

Nakashima, Allyn K., et al. "Epidemic Bullous Impetigo in a Nursery Due to a Nasal Carrier of *Staphylococcus aureus*: Role of Epidemiology and Control Measures." *Infection Control* 5, no. 7 (1984): 326–331.

Websites

Centers for Disease Control and Prevention (CDC), Coordinating Center for Infectious Diseases/Division of Bacterial and Mycotic Diseases. https://www.cdc.gov/ncezid/dfwed/mycotics/index.html (accessed March 8, 2018).

"Impetigo." Medline Plus, December 5, 2017. http://www.nlm.nih.gov/medlineplus/ency/article/000860.htm (accessed December 8, 2017).

"Impetigo: Guidance, Data and Analysis." Public Health England, July 1, 2014. https://www.gov.uk/government/collections/impetigo-guidance-data-and-analysis (accessed December 8, 2017).

Laura J. Cataldo

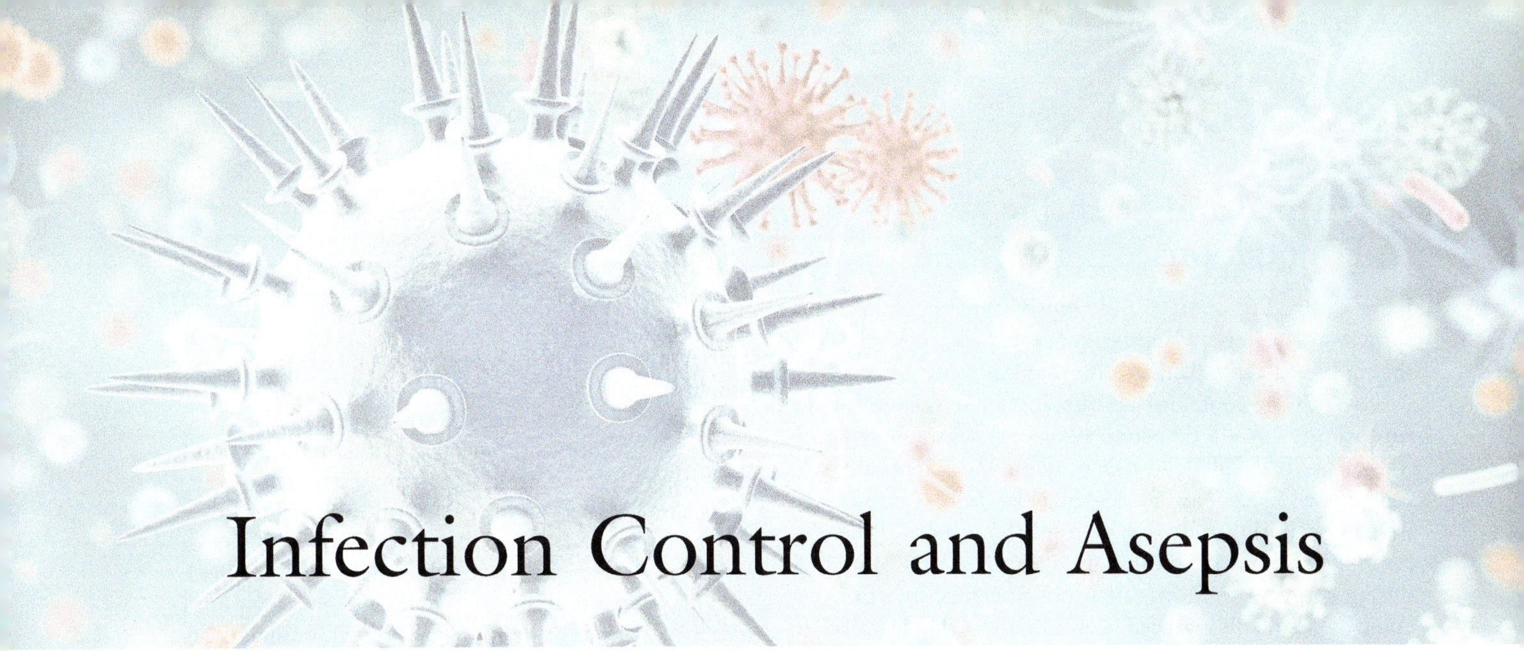

Infection Control and Asepsis

Introduction

Steps that are taken to reduce or prevent infection in health care settings are known as infection control. In 2014 more than 720,000 people in the United States acquired a nosocomial (hospital- or health care–related) infection, and 75,000 patients died, according to data from the US Centers for Disease Control and Prevention (CDC). Most hospitals have dedicated infection control practitioners whose job it is to oversee the infection control procedures as specified by the CDC and the Association for Professionals in Infection Control and Epidemiology (APIC). Infection control professionals (ICPs) are usually nurses, physicians, medical technologists, or epidemiologists. Their focus is on investigating and gathering data about existing infections to take the appropriate actions to contain infections and prevent future ones.

WORDS TO KNOW

ASEPSIS Without germs, more specifically microorganisms.

BIOFILM A population of microorganisms that forms following the adhesion of bacteria, algae, yeast, or fungi to a surface. These surface growths can be found in natural settings, such as on rocks in streams, and in infections, such as those that occur on catheters. Microorganisms can colonize living and inert natural and synthetic surfaces.

COHORTING The grouping of people with like infections or symptoms together to reduce the risk of transmission to others.

INFECTION CONTROL PROFESSIONAL (ICP) A nurse, doctor, laboratory worker, microbiologist, public health official, or other specialist in the prevention and control of infectious disease. ICPs develop methods to control infection and instruct others in their use. These methods include proper handwashing; correct wearing of protective masks, eye guards, gloves, and other specialized clothing; vaccination; monitoring for infection; and investigating ways to treat and prevent infection. Courses and certifications are available for those wishing to become ICPs.

ISOLATION Within the health community, precautions taken in the hospital to prevent the spread of an infectious agent from an infected or colonized patient to susceptible people. Isolation practices are designed to minimize the transmission of infection.

NOSOCOMIAL INFECTION An infection that is acquired in a hospital. More precisely, the US Centers for Disease Control and Prevention (CDC) in Atlanta, Georgia, defines a nosocomial infection as a localized infection or one that is widely spread throughout the body that results from an adverse reaction to an infectious microorganism or toxin that was not present at the time of admission to the hospital.

PATHOGENIC Causing or capable of causing disease.

STANDARD PRECAUTIONS The safety measures taken to prevent the transmission of disease-causing bacteria. These measures include proper handwashing; wearing gloves, goggles, and other protective clothing; proper handling of needles; and sterilization of equipment.

■ History and Scientific Foundations

Before infection control and asepsis were recognized, surgery was often a death sentence for patients. Until the mid-19th century, the death rate following surgeries was over 50 percent. Instead of being a life-saving measure, surgery was a desperate last resort when all other treatments had failed. British surgeon and scientist Joseph Lister (1827–1912) changed the role of surgery by demonstrating the value of infection control. When he applied a spray of disinfectant over a patient's wound during surgery, he showed that postoperative infections could be markedly reduced. Later this was shown to be due to the killing of bacteria present in the air of the operating room or on the clothing or gloves of health care providers. By killing the bacteria before or immediately after they contacted the wound, health care workers could minimize the infection. In the decades after Lister's method became popular, postoperative patient deaths dropped to less than 1 percent. This was the beginning of the modern concept of aseptic technique.

Asepsis is defined as the absence or removal of disease-causing (pathogenic) microorganisms. Compounds used to achieve asepsis are termed antiseptics. Asepsis is designed to leave a surface sterile, free from microorganisms, and is used in surgery and for procedures where surfaces of medical equipment such as instruments or wound dressings will come in contact with sterile areas of the body. Sanitization is sufficient for other surfaces in the health care setting, as well as at home and in the community, to prevent infections. Sanitization does not leave surfaces sterile but reduces the number of disease-causing microorganisms to an insignificant level.

The cornerstone of infection control involves breaking the cycle of infection and interrupting the transmission of disease-causing organisms. The concept of standard precautions is the infection control foundation for health care workers and is used universally in the developed world. Standard precautions assume that any patient's body fluid, tissue, or secretion could be potentially infectious until determined otherwise, and, along with handwashing, barrier protection such as latex (or a latex alternative) gloves, disposable gowns, and masks should be used as appropriate to avoid exposure to them. Likewise, barrier protections are used to prevent patients from being exposed to body fluids or surface disease-causing organisms that might be present on or in the health care worker.

Additional infection control measures are based on isolating or grouping together (cohorting) people with infectious diseases according to how the disease is spread. Isolation means setting apart a person with a known infection. Additional sets of precautions are used for people with documented infections and include airborne precautions, droplet precautions, and contact precautions. When airborne precautions are implemented, as with a person

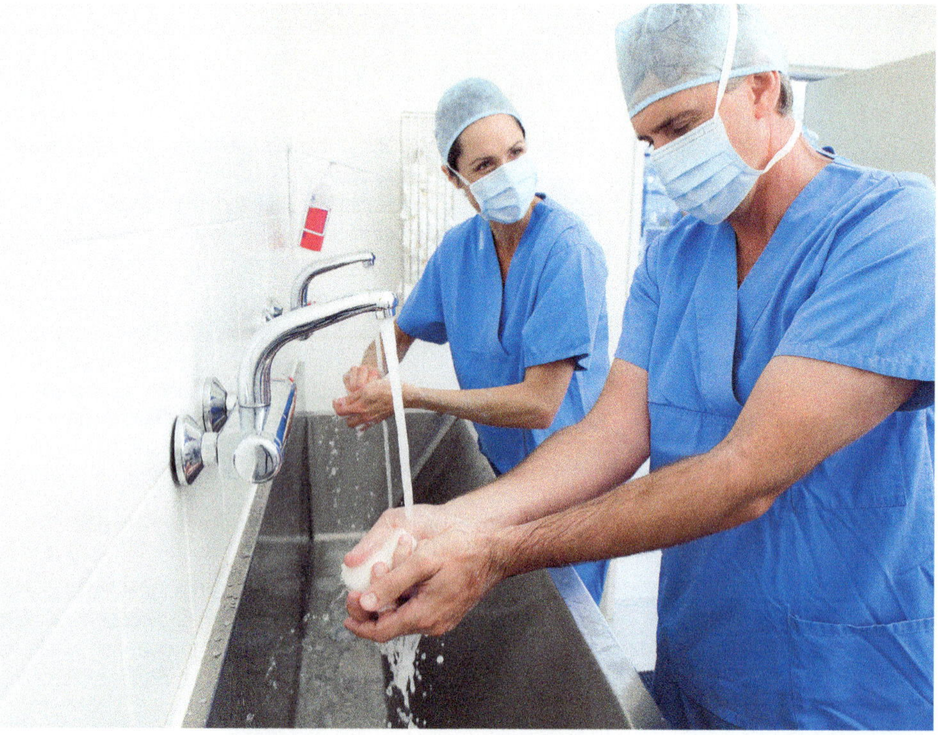

Infection control is an essential component of the practice of health care. Protective clothing and hand hygiene are two of the most common infection-control methods. *© Chris Ryan/Getty Images*

who has an active tuberculosis infection, negative-pressure airflow rooms ensure that the extremely small tuberculosis bacteria will not enter other patient rooms. Hospital staff and the patient also wear specialized masks to prevent the spread of tuberculosis. Droplet precautions are used for people with known or suspected diseases that can be spread through larger infectious particles released by coughing or sneezing, such as polio or measles. Gowns, masks, and gloves are usually worn by health care personnel and visitors when they are in the room of a patient with droplet precautions. Contact precautions are used with people who have infections that can be transmitted by direct or indirect skin-to-skin contact, such as wounds infected with resistant bacteria. Regardless of the type of specialized precautions implemented in people with infections, standard precautions are always additionally in effect.

Other key elements of infection control in the health care setting include disposing infectious waste, such as gloves and wound dressings, in separate containers that receive special handling and are labeled "biohazard"; disposing of needles, scalpels, and other sharp medical equipment in thick, labeled biohazard containers; limiting patient and visitor exposure; and using specialized housekeeping and laundry methods.

Asepsis has long been a valuable means of infection control. One of the first laboratory procedures a microbiology student learns is to wipe down the working surface with an alcohol solution before and after doing any work involving bacteria. This simple step kills most bacteria that are adhering to the work surface. This is because the alcohol dissolves the bacterial membrane. The membrane is composed mainly of phospholipids, or molecules that have water-loving (hydrophilic) ends and a central portion that lacks affinity for water (hydrophobic). This allows phospholipids to spontaneously associate with the hydrophilic portions oriented to the outside of the membrane and the hydrophobic regions buried inside. The result is a barrier that is vital for the structure and the survival of the bacteria. Alcohol, which is also hydrophobic, can induce hydrophobic portions of the phospholipids to associate with it instead of remaining an intact membrane. As a result, the bacterial membrane dissolves, killing the microbe. The simple act of wiping down a work surface prevents the spread of potentially harmful bacteria.

■ Applications and Research

Many infections are contagious and thus are capable of being spread from person to person or from another host to a person. People may even contaminate themselves and contract an infection. An example of the latter is the fecal-oral route, where hands soiled by feces during a bowel movement and that have not been properly cleaned come in contact with the mouth or other parts of the body. A common example is the infections that occur in day care facilities. Infants can handle their soiled diaper and subsequently put a hand in their mouth or another person's mouth. Another example is at the other end of the age spectrum. Elderly people who may be incontinent and whose attentiveness to their sanitary habits may have deteriorated can unknowingly transfer feces to the urinary tract through inadequate hygiene after a bowel movement. This route of transfer can also allow the fecal bacteria to enter the bloodstream. The subsequent blood infection (sepsis) can spread through the body quickly, lethally overwhelming the ability of the immune system to fight the infection.

A simple and time-tested way to minimize person-to-person transmission of microbes is handwashing. Proper handwashing is the most effective way to prevent the spread of infection. At home the use of household soap and vigorous scrubbing of the hands for 30 to 60 seconds has been shown to eliminate most microorganisms of concern from the hands. This is especially important for those who are involved in food preparation, as fecally acquired bacteria and viruses can contaminate food during handling. In a related step, the cleaning of cutting boards and utensils such as knives helps prevent transfer of microbes. For example, one of the main reasons for the millions of cases of food-borne contamination with the bacterium *Campylobacter jejuni* that occurs each year in the United States is not washing cutting boards used to process raw poultry before the board is used for another food. The bacteria sticking to the board are transferred to the other food that, if not cooked or undercooked, can cause illness when eaten.

In the hospital setting, handwashing is done according to CDC guidelines. These specify that health care providers wash their hands before and after seeing each patient and, if gloves have been worn, as the final step after the gloves have been removed and put in the proper disposal container. Many hospitals are equipped with an alcohol-based washstand at the foot of each patient bed or in the room. Handwashing using alcohol takes only seconds. The time savings can be important in a health care provider's busy schedule.

Various infection control procedures are in place in most hospitals to lessen the spread of infection. This is important for several reasons. First, bacteria that are resistant to most antibiotics are becoming more prevalent. An example is methicillin-resistant *Staphylococcus aureus* (MRSA). The prevalence of MRSA in hospitals increased from sporadic and rare in the early 1980s to over 90 percent of all clinical *S. aureus* isolates in hospitals in the United States and United Kingdom in 2006. Since then, with more stringent infection control measures, the number of MRSA infections has declined. In the United States the CDC reported a 54 percent decline in cases between 2005 and 2011, with nearly 31,000 fewer severe MRSA infections and 9,000 MRSA-related deaths. However, MRSA remains a problem, and infection control measures need to be maintained for a continued decline in cases. The fact that only a few antibiotics remain effective against MRSA makes control of the bacterium's presence and spread in a hospital critical for patient health and survival.

Clostridium difficile has also emerged as a concern in hospitals. The intestinal infections that cause a form of

STANDARD PRECAUTIONS

Standard precautions are an efficient way of minimizing the chance of transferring infectious microorganisms from patient to patient and from patients to health care providers. However, these precautions, such as handwashing, are effective only if they are used consistently. Even with widespread knowledge of the benefits of handwashing in reducing the spread of infection, it is still difficult to get people to regularly wash their hands. Studies continue to document a less than 50 percent rate of handwashing compliance among health care providers, particularly physicians, after finishing with one patient and before seeing another patient. The most common explanation is lack of time. Alcohol-based handwashing stations placed at patients' bedsides have helped raise awareness. Moreover, washing with an alcohol solution takes only a few seconds.

inflammation known as colitis, diarrhea, and abdominal cramps can be life-threatening for patients who are already ill, especially if their immune system is not working properly. In the Canadian province of Quebec, a series of outbreaks of *C. difficile* infection in hospitals killed almost 2,000 people between late 2006 and the beginning of 2016. The bacteria, which are excreted in feces, can end up on surfaces that someone subsequently touches, later passing the bacteria on to the patient. A 2015 investigative report by CBC News found that poor compliance with handwashing by hospital care staff was a factor in the spread of the infection.

A second reason for infection control is the emergence of new infectious viral and bacterial diseases that are easily spread from person to person. Examples include severe acute respiratory syndrome (SARS), avian influenza (bird flu), H1N1 influenza (swine flu), and Zika virus.

Infection control measures are also important because diseases that used to be rampant but have been under control for decades are reemerging as a significant health threat. One example is the form of tuberculosis caused by the bacterium *Mycobacterium tuberculosis.*

Research laboratories and hospitals often have a variety of infection control procedures in place. Depending on the organism being studied or encountered, most countries have a series of mandated safety controls, with more dangerous microbes requiring more stringent safety and infection control measures. One example is the use of filters in the ventilation system that trap bacteria and even particles as small as viruses. The filters prevent the movement of the microbes from the room to other parts of the building or outside.

Some work surfaces can be inside of an enclosed structure called a fume hood, which is separate from the rest of the lab. The fume hood can be open to the rest of the room. Even a semienclosed space cuts down on air movement. Fume hoods can also be completely enclosed in a glove box with attached plastic gloves into which the researcher slips his or her hands. Equipment and other items can be introduced into the chamber of the fume hood by a two-way door that does not allow air inside the fume hood to pass outside.

Even work surfaces may be designed for infection control. In the early 20th century, work surfaces in labs were made of wood. Cracks and crevasses in the surface of the wood were ideal breeding grounds for infectious bacteria. Modern lab surfaces are made of chemically resilient plastic that is smooth, watertight, and free of gaps. The same principle is used in operating theaters, where the floor is a single, crack-free unit made of material that can be easily cleaned.

Another infection control procedure in hospitals is the use of protective hand wear and clothing. This helps protect health care providers from contamination from patients. Discarding the protective gear when moving from patient to patient minimizes the chance that the health care provider will become a vehicle of transfer of an infection. The use of protective gear depends on the risk posed by a patient. For example, CDC guidelines indicate that if there is a reasonable chance that someone could be exposed to the splashing or spraying of blood (such as can occur in an Ebola infection, where copious bleeding can occur), a protective gown and perhaps a face mask should be worn. The gown may need to be made of a water-resistant material.

Highly infectious patients are often isolated from other patients in a hospital, and wards containing people who are particularly susceptible to infection (such as transplant recipients, whose immune system is usually deliberately suppressed to reduce the chance of rejection of the transplanted organ) may be in an area of the hospital that has less daily traffic. Contact precautions specify that such patients should be housed in a private room or with similarly affected people.

Infection control actions can also be taken in the community. An example is malaria. The disease is transmitted by mosquitoes, so steps to control mosquito populations, especially during the insect's breeding season, can help lessen the infection. Spraying prime breeding grounds with insecticide is a common strategy. In addition, more high-tech science approaches are being used. For example, in malaria-prone regions of Africa and in regions of North America that are susceptible to Zika virus, one program involves the release of sterile male mosquitoes. The males are unable to successfully mate with female mosquitoes, which reduce the numbers of the next generation. As malaria and other disease-causing viruses can be transmitted only by female mosquitoes, reduced numbers of new females mean less opportunity for the spread of malaria.

Another simple and effective infection control mechanism for insect-borne diseases is the use of mosquito netting over a bed during sleep. Organizations including WHO and World Vision conduct campaigns that solicit money for the purchase of mosquito netting and the delivery of the netting to rural villages in malaria-prone regions of Africa. This simple step saves many lives by preventing the mosquito-borne transmission of the infection.

The use of antimicrobial or antiviral agents can help overcome an infection and, in the case of vaccines, prevent someone from contracting an infection. An example of the power of a vaccine is polio. Prior to the 1950s, polio was a dreaded viral illness that paralyzed many children. After the introduction and refinement of two polio vaccines, polio has become a rare event. The Polio Eradication Initiative launched by the World Health Organization (WHO) in 1988 has been tremendously successful in reducing the global number of polio cases by over 99 percent. An ongoing program is on target to eliminate polio in a few remaining countries in Africa by 2018.

However, continued vigilance is necessary. During 2006 the interruption of the polio vaccination campaign in Nigeria due to a military conflict caused a renewed polio outbreak. The sporadic but troubling measles outbreaks in the United States in the 21st century also underscore the need for continued vigilance. Measles was viewed as a concern of the past because of the success of childhood vaccination. However, the resistance by some parents to vaccination has produced hot spots where the rate of non-vaccination is high enough that the whole population of the region is at risk. The consequence, according to CDC data, was 23 measles outbreaks in 2014 in areas such as California and Ohio. The latter was among Amish communities and involved 383 cases.

Even with vigilance, infection control can be difficult. An example is the use of antibiotics. From the 1940s to the 1960s, following the introduction of penicillin and the discovery or synthesis of new antibiotics, these agents were hugely successful at dealing with bacterial infections. But, as with the polio campaign, initial success does not guarantee long-term success. Bacteria have proven capable of adaptation to many of the antibiotics that have been introduced. This resistance can appear within only a few years and can spread. Strains of bacteria including enterococci and *Staphylococcus aureus* that are resistant to nearly all known antibiotics currently in use pose a challenge in patient care.

Antibiotic resistance can spread quickly through a bacterial population because the genetic information that specifies the protein involved in the resistance is often located on a piece of genetic material that is not part of the main chromosome but is more mobile. This means that the information is more capable of being transferred from one bacterium to another.

The hospital is a prime breeding ground for antibiotic resistance. The heavy use of antibiotics and disinfectants in hospitals imposes a selection pressure on bacteria. Those bacteria that can adapt to be resistant stand a better chance of surviving and thriving.

■ Impacts and Issues

Infection control and asepsis will always be fundamentally important measures in hospitals. One reason is evident from the prevalence of hospital-acquired (nosocomial) infections. According to the CDC, there are about 720,000 nosocomial infections in US hospitals every year, with about 75,000 proving to be fatal.

Infection control and asepsis are also becoming more important in the prevention of infections, as infectious diseases become more resistant and new diseases emerge. People are more at risk for infections, especially as the populations of many developed countries age. In general, the elderly are increasingly vulnerable to infections as their immune systems and overall resilience decline.

Traditionally, infection control strategies for bacterial disease have been geared toward the types of bacteria studied in the laboratory. Scientists now know, however, that bacteria that live and grow while floating in the lab growth medium are not at all like the populations found in the real world. Infections are often caused by bacteria that grow by adhering to surfaces. These so-called biofilms are more resistant to drugs that would easily kill their floating counterparts. This means that infection control strategies need to change to more realistically deal with the real world of biofilm-caused bacterial infections.

SEE ALSO *Airborne Precautions; Contact Precautions; Handwashing; Standard Precautions; Water-Borne Disease*

BIBLIOGRAPHY

Books

Amer, Fatma. *Hospital Infection Control, Part 1.* 3rd ed. Saarbrücken, Germany: Noor, 2017.

Buchanan, Charles M. *Antisepsis and Antiseptics.* 1895. London: Forgotten Books, 2017.

Websites

"*C. difficile* Control: Handwashing Practices Lax at Quebec Hospitals." CBC News, November 12, 2015. http://www.cbc.ca/news/canada/montreal/c-difficile-handwashing-quebec-hospitals-study-investigation-chart-1.3314788 (accessed December 6, 2017).

"*Clostridium difficile* Colitis—Overview." WebMD. https://www.webmd.com/digestive-disorders/tc/clostridium-difficile-colitis-overview#1 (accessed November 17, 2017).

"Healthcare-Associated Infections." Centers for Disease Control and Prevention, July 14, 2017. https://www.cdc.gov/hai/index.html (accessed November 17, 2017).

"Methicillin-Resistant *Staphylococcus aureus* (MRSA)." Centers for Disease Control and Prevention, July 6, 2017. https://www.cdc.gov/mrsa/tracking/index.html (accessed November 17, 2017).

Brian Hoyle

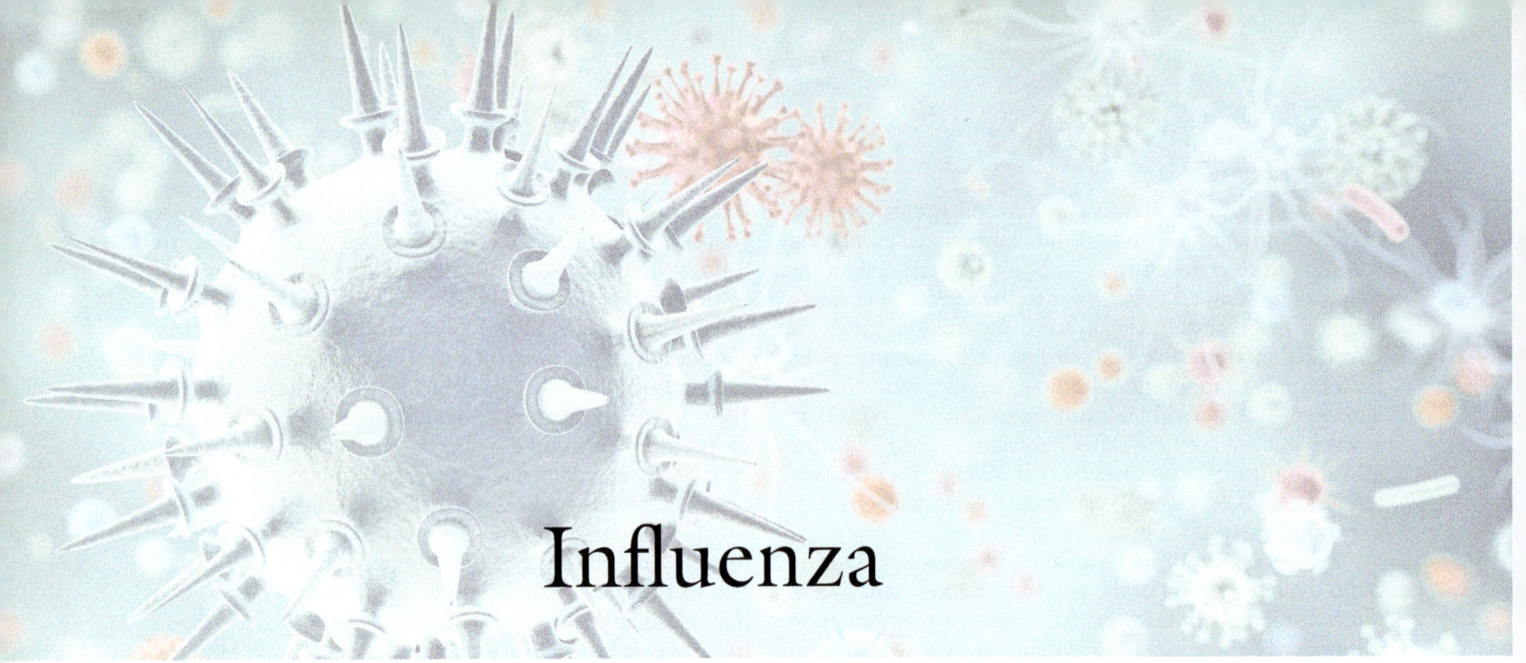

Influenza

Introduction

Influenza is a disease that has plagued humans for centuries. The medical writings of antiquity contain evidence that implicates influenza as the cause of a number of deadly epidemics. As early as 412 BCE, Greek physician Hippocrates (c. 460 BCE c.–375 BCE) wrote about the occurrence of epidemics that were likely caused by influenza. In addition, most medical historians agree that 12 influenza pandemics have occurred since the early 17th century.

A typical attack of influenza starts with high fever, chills, muscle aches, a dry cough, and a distinctly ill feeling. Soon a sore throat with nasal congestion and a runny nose develops, followed by a worsening cough. In healthy adults and children, a case of influenza lasts about a week. Many think the illness is nothing more than a particularly severe cold. However, influenza is caused by a different virus. A form of the influenza virus exists in nearly all animals, including domesticated birds and pigs, and these animal viruses bear a close genetic relationship to human influenza viruses. Influenza can be unpredictable and can kill healthy adults and children.

WORDS TO KNOW

ANTIGEN A substance, usually a protein or polysaccharide, that stimulates the immune system to produce antibodies. While antigens can be the source of infections from pathogenic bacteria and viruses, organic molecules detrimental to the body from internal or environmental sources also act as antigens.

ANTIGENIC SHIFT An abrupt and major genetic change (e .g., in genes coding for surface proteins of a virus).

DROPLET TRANSMISSION The spread of microorganisms from one space to another (including from person to person) via droplets that are larger than 5 microns in diameter. Droplets are typically expelled into the air by coughing and sneezing.

PANDEMIC An epidemic that occurs in more than one country or population simultaneously. *Pandemic* means "all the people."

STRAIN A subclass or a specific genetic variation of an organism.

Disease History, Characteristics, and Transmission

Most often influenza attacks the nose, throat, and lungs, but any part of the body can be infected. Sometimes influenza will cause abdominal pain, nausea, and diarrhea. Infants with influenza may develop a severe form of viral pneumonia. Influenza is unpredictable in how severe the disease may be in each individual.

Other diseases can take advantage of the weakened state of the body after a case of influenza and cause a secondary infection. Bacteria such as group A streptococcus, *Staph aureus*, and strep pneumonia are particularly efficient at causing a lethal pneumonia after influenza damages the lungs. About 10 percent of children will develop a secondary infection while recovering from influenza, and ear infections frequently afflict infants and young children just as they are trying to recover from the virus.

Influenza is highly contagious and primarily spreads person to person in virus-laden droplets produced by sneezing or coughing. Alternatively, the droplets land on a surface and contaminate the hands that, if not washed, carry the virus to the mouth or nose. School-age children are the main culprits in spreading influenza. Usually 10 to 40 percent of school-age children will get influenza in any one season. They swap the virus at school and bring it home to infect family members. Children are contagious before they even appear or feel ill, and the virus is present in nasal mucous and cough droplets for over a week after apparent recovery from influenza.

The microbiology of the influenza virus is quite complex. Influenza viruses consist of three different major types known as A, B, and C. Of the three types, only A and B cause significant disease in humans. Both A and B types cause the seasonal epidemics around the world, but at any one time there may be hundreds of different variations of each type circulating the globe. This multitude of subtly different varieties presents a challenge to the human immune system.

Both influenza A and B virus change their structure often enough such that the immune system can never develop long-lasting immunity. Influenza B virus changes much more slowly than influenza A and usually causes milder illness. However, influenza B can cause severe disease in young children, people over age 65, those with impaired immunity, or those with chronic lung or heart disease.

Influenza A generally causes more severe disease and is the most unpredictable. The yearly seasonal epidemics of the "flu" are primarily the result of influenza A. The virus has two specific proteins on its surface, which are important for infecting humans. These proteins, known as antigens, are called hemagglutinin (HA) and neuraminidase (NA). The HA and NA proteins vary in their chemical structure from year to year. This process, termed antigenic drift, results in virus particle proteins with subtle variations in structure. Eighteen different HA subtypes are known to exist, while there are 11 known NA subtypes. These slightly different proteins get different number designations, and the various influenza strains are named by the specific HA and NA proteins on the virus. The H3N1 virus contains HA protein 3 and NA protein 1.

Influenza vs. the Common Cold

Symptom	Influenza	Cold
Fever	Common (high)	Rare (low grade)
Chills	Common	Rare
Body aches	Severe	Slight or no
Headache	Common (severe)	Rare (mild)
Runny nose	Common	Common
Sneezing	Common	Common
Sore throat	Common	Common
Cough	Dry and hacking	Cough with mucus
Chest pain	Moderate to severe	Mild to moderate
Fatigue	Moderate to severe	Mild
Onset	Sudden	Slow

Influenza A employs an additional means of evading the immune system. When two different viral strains infect someone at the same time, the two viral variants will swap component genes and create yet another slightly different form of influenza. The new virus will contain some proteins of one variety of influenza A and some proteins of the other variety. This disordered way of making new virus particles extends to swapping genetic material with animal or bird influenza viruses. This process, termed antigenic shift, will sometimes create an influenza virus for which

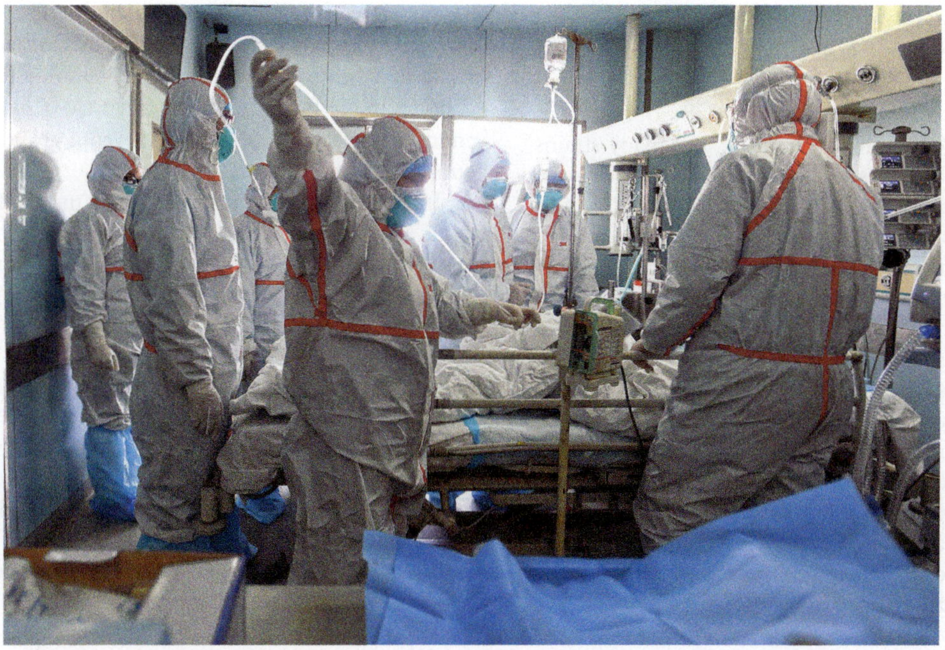

A patient is treated for H7N9 bird influenza in China in 2017. Bird influenza is one of many kinds of influenza virus, which exist in nearly all animals. *© STR/AFP/Getty Images*

humans have no immunity at all. A novel virus produced this way has the potential to spread worldwide, resulting in a pandemic.

Three influenza pandemics occurred in the 20th century. The influenza pandemic in 1918 killed at least 20 million people, and some experts think there were 50 million deaths within a period of 24 weeks. Nearly as many US soldiers died of influenza in 1918 as died in battle in all of World War I (1914–1918). In the United States, the 1957 pandemic resulted in 70,000 deaths, while in 1968 about 30,000 died. During influenza pandemics, a larger proportion of healthy adults die than during the yearly "flu season" outbreaks.

In the 21st century, a pandemic involving the H1N1 influenza virus killed as many as 575,400 people worldwide, including 12,469 in the United States, in the first year of circulation. The virus originated in pigs in Central Mexico in April 2009, leading to it becoming known as "swine flu." By June 2009 swine flu had spread to 74 countries and was declared a pandemic by the World Health Organization (WHO). Because H1N1 originated in animals and was a new genetic combination, humans had not developed an immunity to it. The pandemic caused an unusually high number of deaths among young adults, with approximately 80 percent of deaths occurring in people younger than 65. By the time the pandemic was declared over in August 2010, the virus had spread to over 200 countries, and more than 61 million people had been infected in the United States alone.

Treatment and Prevention

Drugs that have shown to be the most effective against influenza are adamantanes and neuraminidase inhibitors. The adamantanes, amantadine and rimantadine, treat only influenza A, while the neuraminidase inhibitors are used in treating both influenza A and B. Because the adamantanes have a limited spectrum, and many strains of influenza are now resistant to these drugs, they are no longer recommended for use in the United States. Both of these classes of medicines interfere with the ability of the influenza virus to make more virus particles. They either stop production of the viral genetic material or prevent the viral particles from escaping from infected cells to infect other cells. To help relieve symptoms or shorten the course of influenza, a person must take these drugs early in the course of influenza. Once the illness is established and new influenza virus particles have replicated, the medications are largely ineffective. Many of the symptoms of influenza are due to the damage the virus does to the body during the making of new virus particles, so stopping the virus early provides the greatest relief in symptoms.

Until effective medications became available to treat influenza, determining who had influenza rather than one of a similar multitude of viral respiratory illnesses was of little use. Treatment involved decreasing the fever, resting, and drinking plenty of fluids. This treatment is appropriate for most viral illnesses. However, because medications are now available, there is a difference whether the illness is a cold or the flu and why testing for influenza is often done.

Several rapid tests are available to detect the influenza virus. These tests use a sample of mucus taken from the nose or from the back of the throat. The tests are rapid, usually taking only five minutes, and will detect influenza virus accurately about 75 to 85 percent of the time if properly done.

Antibiotics are not effective treatment for influenza. Antibiotics are useful in the treatment of bacterial infections and have no benefit during viral illnesses. Antibiotics may be helpful if secondary bacterial infections develop during the course of influenza.

Drugs provide a treatment option unavailable in the past, but they do not provide the best option for control of influenza. As of 2018 the drugs approved for treatment of flu are oseltamivir (Tamiflu), zanamivir (Relenza), or peramivir (Rapivab). Oseltamivir is a neuraminidase inhibitor. It may be used to help prevent influenza in patients over one year of age or to treat influenza infections (A or B) in patients two weeks and older who have been symptomatic for no more than 48 hours. The drug is available only by prescription and comes as a capsule or an oral liquid. Although oseltamivir is generally safe, it may cause severe skin reactions or nervous system problems. Like oseltamivir, zanamivir is a neuraminidase inhibitor with similar uses and effects. Instead of being swallowed, it is given by oral inhalation. Permavir is also a neuraminidase inhibitor, but it is given by injection directly into the bloodstream as a single dose. Side effects are generally mild, but severe skin problems, delirium, and allergic reactions are possible. While these drugs are most effective if administered within 48 hours of the first symptoms, they may be useful in preventing complications of influenza even if given later in the course of the infection.

Influenza vaccination provides the most effective way to prevent the disease, but the influenza virus poses a challenge for vaccine development. Because the virus changes slightly each year and changes dramatically at unpredictable intervals, vaccines also need altering annually. Each year public health officials make an educated guess as to what will be the prevalent strains circulating in the next season, and vaccine preparation commences targeting those strains.

Influenza vaccines typically provide excellent protection when administered at least two weeks before exposure to the influenza virus, and vaccination is needed each year. The vaccine itself does not cause influenza, but depending on the exact form of vaccine administered, side effects may include soreness at the injection site, muscle aches, runny nose, or sore throat. Young children often need two doses of vaccine for full protection. In the United States the vaccine recommendations as of 2017 included people 65 years and older, those between six months and five years of age, and everyone with chronic health problems involving the lungs or heart.

In some cases, such as when the virus mutates after vaccines have been distributed, influenza vaccines can become less effective than normal. This occurred during the 2017–2018 flu season, leading to a particularly severe seasonal outbreak. The *Journal of Family Practice* alerted its readers to possible problems with influenza that season: "Good news and bad news on vaccine effectiveness. The good news: Circulating viruses were a close match to those contained in the vaccine. The bad news: Vaccine effectiveness at preventing illness was estimated to be just 34% against A (H3N2) and 56% against influenza B viruses. There has been no analysis of the relative effectiveness of different vaccines and vaccine types." Although the vaccine was less effective than might have been desired, it was still strongly recommended that everyone get the vaccine, as it gives some protection and will reduce the number of people who can spread the virus to others.

On January 12, 2018, Brenda Fitzgerald, director of the Centers for Disease Control and Prevention (CDC), cohosted a media briefing where she said that influenza was "widespread and intense" across the United States, but it was too soon to state the severity of this year's spread. On January 16 the *Los Angeles Times* reported that "California hospitals face a 'war zone' of flu patients—and are setting up tents to treat them."

■ Scope and Distribution

Every year about 35,000 deaths occur in the United States due to influenza. Most of these deaths occur among individuals older than 65, but more children die of influenza or its complications each year in the United States than all the deaths due to whooping cough and measles combined. In December 2017 the CDC raised its estimates of the number of global deaths attributable to influenza to between 291,000 and 646,000 each year, up from previous estimates of 250,000 to 500,000. For example, in 2002 an influenza outbreak started in Madagascar. Over a period of three months, 27,000 people developed influenza, and, despite rapid medical intervention, 800 deaths occurred.

■ Impacts and Issues

Unless a family member or close friend dies of influenza, many people do not really give much thought to the impact influenza has on their health and pocketbook. Influenza ranks far behind heart disease and cancer as a worldwide cause of death, yet its economic impact is considerable. Public health experts in 2017 estimated the total cost of influenza on the US economy to be $34.7 billion per year. These costs included direct medical expenses, lost wages, and lost productivity at work. For parents the cost often includes lost work while caring for the sick child and lost work if influenza is passed from child to parent.

A pandemic raises great concern for public health officials worldwide. Influenza pandemics generally occur several times a century but are unpredictable as to the exact timing. Each of the past four influenza pandemics (in 1918, 1957, 1968, and 2009) resulted from human influenza virus sharing genetic material with a bird or pig influenza virus. Human immune systems had never encountered the new virus, and everyone was susceptible to the new form of influenza. As a result, the new virus swept through countries throughout the globe.

The pandemic of 1918 deserves further explanation, as medical history warns that a similar event at some point in the future is highly likely. In the 1918 pandemic, about one-third of the world's population suffered a severe case of influenza, and nearly 3 percent of those infected with the virus died. An unusually high percentage of the young and healthy died during this pandemic. All current strains of influenza A virus are descended from the 1918 virus, but the current strains have weakened considerably. Now less than 0.1% of people die when infected by modern-day forms of influenza.

Given that the medical system has advanced since 1918, what would be the impact of a new, more lethal influenza virus? Public health experts predict an estimated 90,000 to 200,000 deaths, more than 700,000 hospital admissions, and about 40 million visits to doctors in the United States alone. The estimated economic impact exceeds $160 billion, not including the disruptions due to illness in the police, transportation workers, and health care workers themselves.

Since the late 1990s a particularly vicious strain of avian (bird) flu, known as H5N1 influenza, has caused many cases of disease and death in humans. Close contact with infected birds is required to catch this form of influenza. As of 2017 transmission of this virus from human to human did not readily occur. However, if this bird virus acquires the ability to infect humans from one person to another, a new pandemic could occur. Mild outbreaks of bird-to-human transmission continue, with the University of Minnesota's Center for Disease Research and Policy reporting new outbreaks of avian flu in the Netherlands and Italy in December 2017. The concern is that, as more strains of bird flu are reported, the risk that one of them will mutate to become dangerous to humans increases. The CDC and WHO recognize this possibility, and planning for the potential pandemic continues.

SEE ALSO *Droplet Precautions; H5N1 Virus; Influenza Pandemic of 1918; Influenza Pandemic of 1957; Influenza, Tracking Seasonal Influences and Virus Mutation; Pandemic Preparedness; Vaccines and Vaccine Development; Viral Disease*

BIBLIOGRAPHY

Books

Barry, John M. *The Great Influenza: The Story of the Deadliest Pandemic in History.* New York: Penguin, 2005.

Beers, Mark, ed. *The Merck Manual of Medical Information.* 2nd ed. London: Simon & Schuster, 2004.

Dehner, George. *Influenza: A Century of Science and Public Health Response.* Pittsburgh: University of Pittsburgh Press, 2012.

Scoones, Ian. *Avian Influenza: Science, Policy and Politics.* London: Earthscan, 2010.

Sipress, Alan. *The Fatal Strain: On the Trail of Avian Flu and the Coming Pandemic.* New York: Penguin, 2014.

Webster, Robert G., et al., eds. *Textbook of Influenza.* 2nd ed. Chichester, UK: Wiley-Blackwell, 2013.

Periodicals

Karlamangla, Soumya. "California Hospitals Face a 'War Zone' of Flu Patients—And Are Setting Up Tents to Treat Them." *Los Angeles Times* (January 16, 2018). This article can also be found online at http://www.latimes.com/local/lanow/la-me-ln-flu-demand-20180116-htmlstory.html (accessed January 17, 2018).

Rothman, Tiran. "The Cost of Influenza Disease Burden in U.S Population." *International Journal of Economics & Management Sciences* 6, no. 4 (2017). This article can also be found online at https://www.omicsonline.org/open-access/the-cost-of-influenza-disease-burden-in-us-population-2162–6359-1000443.pdf (accessed January 17, 2018).

Websites

"Influenza." World Health Organization. http://www.who.int/influenza/en/ (accessed January 17, 2018).

"Influenza (Flu)." Centers for Disease Control and Prevention, January 12, 2018. https://www.cdc.gov/flu/index.htm (accessed January 17, 2018).

"Seasonal Flu Death Estimate Increases Worldwide." Centers for Disease Control and Prevention, December 13, 2017. https://www.cdc.gov/media/releases/2017/p1213-flu-death-estimate.html (accessed January 17, 2018).

Lloyd Scott Clements
Sam Uretsky

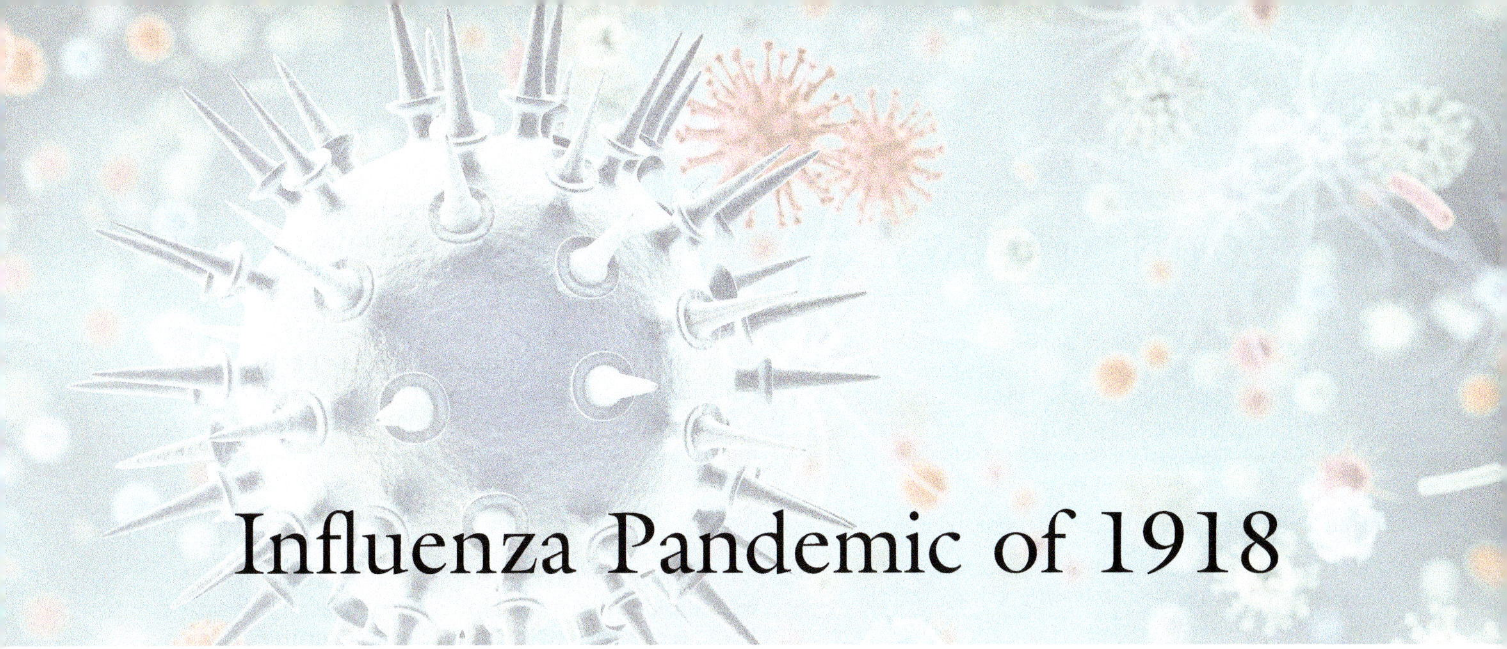

Influenza Pandemic of 1918

Introduction

Influenza ("flu" for short) is an infection of the lungs and bronchial tubes by an influenza virus. Common symptoms of flu include cough, muscle aches, vomiting, loss of appetite, and fever. Flu can also cause death, usually from respiratory failure and in people with weakened immune systems. The 1918 influenza pandemic, a global wave of flu infection that occurred from 1918 to 1919, was one of the deadliest infectious disease events in human history. A figure of 20 to 50 million deaths has traditionally been attributed to the pandemic, but in 2002 the *Bulletin of the History of Medicine* estimated that the toll was more likely between 50 and 100 million. The pandemic killed about 675,000 people in the United States, some 18 million in India (about 5 percent of the population at that time), and similar percentages elsewhere. The virus eventually evolved into less harmful forms.

The lethal 1918 influenza virus was re-created by US government scientists in 2005 for medical research purposes. There has been a number of flu outbreaks since 1918, but none have been anywhere near as deadly as that which occurred in 1918.

Disease History, Characteristics, and Transmission

Disease History

The exact origin of the virus strain that caused the 1918 flu pandemic is still a mystery. Although the flu was called the Spanish Flu at the time, it may have originated not in Spain but, like most new flu varieties, in Asia. Another hypothesis, based on epidemiological evidence, places the origin in the United States.

Normally, in the United States, about 5 to 20 percent of the population gets a symptomatic flu infection each year. One hundred thousand to 200,000 people are hospitalized with flu complications annually, and up to 36,000 people, mostly elderly, die. Similar figures apply to most countries of the world in proportion to population. In the 1918 pandemic, however, 25 to 40 percent of the world population contracted the flu and 2.5 to 5.0 percent of those people died. In the United States, about 2.5 percent died, resulting in about 675,000 deaths—about 10 times as many Americans as died in World War I (1914–1918). Two hundred thousand people died in the United States in October 1918 alone. Previous influenza outbreaks had death rates of about 0.1 percent in the United States, only 1/25th as high as the 2.5 percentage rate of 1918–1919.

The 1918 flu appeared 28 years after the pandemic of 1890, sweeping the world suddenly in September 1918. The flu was called Spanish Flu in the United States because it was especially deadly in Spain early in its history, killing as many as 8 million people. The 1918 flu was unique in that it was deadlier for young people than for the elderly: 99 percent of its victims were under age 65. Victims sometimes died within a few hours of infection. It should be noted that the great majority of those infected did not die. It struck rich, poor, and middle class alike, with similar death rates for all groups.

By late November 1918, the death rate from the flu was tapering off in the United States. By early 1919 the pandemic was over, both in the United States and most of the rest of the world.

Disease Characteristics

Influenza is an infection of the lungs and other parts of the respiratory tract (breathing organs) that is caused by a virus. Viruses are tiny clusters of molecules that are smaller than a cell. Each individual virus, called a virion or virus particle, consists of a sheath or covering called a capsid, which is made of proteins (a type of complex molecule basic to life). The capsid carries a core of ribonucleic acid (RNA) or, sometimes, deoxyribonucleic acid (DNA). A virus cannot live on its own but repro-

WORDS TO KNOW

ANTIGEN A substance, usually a protein or polysaccharide, that stimulates the immune system to produce antibodies. While antigens can be the source of infections from pathogenic bacteria and viruses, organic molecules detrimental to the body from internal or environmental sources also act as antigens.

CAPSID The protein shell surrounding a virus particle.

CREPITANT A crackling sound that accompanies breathing, a common symptom of pneumonia or other diseases of the lungs.

PANDEMIC An epidemic that occurs in more than one country or population simultaneously. *Pandemic* means "all the people."

RALES French term for a rattling sound in the throat or chest.

REASSORTMENT A condition resulting when two or more different types of viruses exchange genetic material to form a new, genetically different virus.

duces by attaching to a true cell such as a bacterium or human body cell and injecting its RNA or DNA into that cell. The cell is tricked into using the viral RNA or DNA to manufacture new virus particles, which can then infect other cells.

A global influenza pandemic occurs when a form of flu virus evolves that can be easily transmitted between human beings. There were three global flu pandemics in the 20th century (1918, 1957, and 1968) and another in 2009.

There are three basic types of flu virus, termed influenza A, B, and C. Influenza A viruses are the most common. They are also called avian viruses because the word *avian* means having to do with birds and these viruses are hosted by birds as well as by humans and some other mammals. The 1918 flu virus was an influenza A virus.

Each influenza A capsid consists of 11 different proteins. Two of these proteins tend to vary widely among flu strains. These are hemagglutinin (HA) and neuraminidase (NA). Strains of influenza A virus are named for which kinds of HA and NA protein they contain. For example, there are H1N1 flu viruses, H3N2 flu viruses, and dozens of others. The strain that caused the 1918 flu was an H1N1 virus. Not all H1N1 viruses are identical, as there are other proteins in the virus that can differ, and the H1 (HA number 1) protein itself can take on slightly different forms.

These differences are a matter of life and death. In the body the immune system fights viral infections by destroying virus particles and the cells that have been infected by them. It decides what cells or particles to destroy by detecting molecules that belong to the virus. These molecules are called antigens. The HA protein of an influenza A virus is an especially important antigen. When the body's immune system knows to attack a particular form of HA, it can effectively fight the virus bearing that form of HA. If a form of HA is unknown to the immune system, however, the virus is free to spread through the body while the immune system is learning how to identify it. If a person survives that variety of flu, they are permanently immune to it afterward because their immune system remembers it.

From about 1919 to 2005, the 1918 H1N1 flu strain was considered extinct. However, samples of the virus's RNA were recovered in the 1990s from an Inuit Eskimo woman who had died of the flu in 1918 in Alaska and whose body had been frozen in permafrost since that time, as well as from preserved laboratory samples of lung tissue of four US soldiers who died of flu in 1918. The full RNA sequence of the virus, which was reconstructed by scientists studying these samples and published in the journal *Science* in 2005, showed that the 1918 virus was probably transmitted directly from birds—which are a large natural reservoir of influenza A viruses—to human beings, unlike later pandemic influenzas, which are thought to have originated via reassortment. Reassortment can occur when two different (but related) viruses infect a single cell. Their RNA fragments, mixing inside the cell, can be reassembled into a new virus, a reassortant that contains RNA from both. The pandemic flu strains of 1957, 1968, and 2009 were probably reassortant viruses that mixed human flu viruses with avian flu viruses (and swine viruses in the case of the 2009 pandemic), but the 1918 flu was apparently a purely avian flu virus.

Re-creation of the 1918 flu virus has yielded some understanding of why this particular influenza A virus was so deadly. First, the virus replicates rapidly in the body's tissues. How it does so is not entirely understood, but research in the early 21st century revealed that the particular form of HA protein possessed by the 1918 virus was necessary to this rapid spreading. The HA protein is used by a flu virus to stick to host cells, and the form of HA protein possessed by the 1918 virus may be more efficient at doing this job. The 2009 pandemic, also caused by an H1N1 virus, contained an HA protein that was remarkably similar in structure to the 1918 virus, contributing to its rapid spread among those who had not been exposed to the 1918 virus. The 2009 virus had different genetic properties, however, resulting in much milder health effects.

The 1918 virus also spreads more widely in the body than most flu viruses. Most flu viruses use a molecule called trypsin to activate HA molecules and attach to cells. The trypsin must usually come from the cell being attacked. Lung cells are rich in trypsin, which is why flu viruses thrive in lung tissue. In contrast, the NA protein of the 1918 virus can activate the virus's own HA attachment molecule without help from cellular trypsin. The 1918 virus, therefore, was equipped to rapidly attack a wider variety of cells.

One popular theory for the deadliness of the 1918 virus is that it triggers an excessive immune response from the body. Excess amounts of the chemicals called interferons, cytokines, and chemokines are produced by the tissues attacked by the virus, and these substances themselves damage the tissues—an event called a "cytokine storm" by immunologists. Cells of the immune system also attack the tissues in response to these chemicals. In effect, the 1918 virus not only attacks the body but also tricks the body into attacking itself. This explains why the 1918 virus was most fatal to young adults—the population that has, on average, the strongest immune system.

In 2014, however, evolutionary biologist Michael Worobey and a team of researchers at the University of Arizona proposed an alternate theory for the high death toll associated with the 1918 flu. By looking at the genetic lineage of the virus, the scientists found that people born between 1880 and 1900—those aged 18 to 38 during the pandemic—had not been previously exposed to an H1 virus, while those born prior to 1880 or after 1900 had. Previous exposure to an H1 flu granted children and older adults partial immunity to the 1918 virus, while young adults had no protection against its worst health effects.

Disease Transmission

Flu virus is spread mostly through contact with droplets emitted during coughing and sneezing. It is also spread through direct skin contact. The contagious period, during which a person infected with the disease can spread virus particles to an uninfected person, is about one day before symptoms appear to five days after symptoms appear. Typically, about half of all flu infections are asymptomatic (the person does not feel sick). Whether this was true of the 1918 flu is not known because the viral nature of the disease was not understood until 1933, so asymptomatic cases could not be discovered.

The 1918 flu may have been more easily transmitted than later strains of flu because of the extreme number of virus particles probably produced in lung tissue of people who contracted it. Experiments in 2005 showed that 50 times more virus particles were released from human lung tissue growing in laboratory culture than were released when the tissue was infected by a modern H1N1 flu strain called the Texas virus. Mouse lungs infected with the 1918 virus contained 39,000 times more virus particles after four days than mouse lungs infected with the modern virus. However, a 2004 study published in *Nature* concluded from historical information that the transmissibility of the 1918 flu was "not large relative to many other infectious diseases."

Transportation systems such as ships and planes contribute to the global spread of viruses. The worldwide travel activity of troops during World War I probably helped the 1918 flu pandemic to occur by spreading the virus quickly between countries and continents. In the 21st century, commercial jet travel is the usual means of global flu transport.

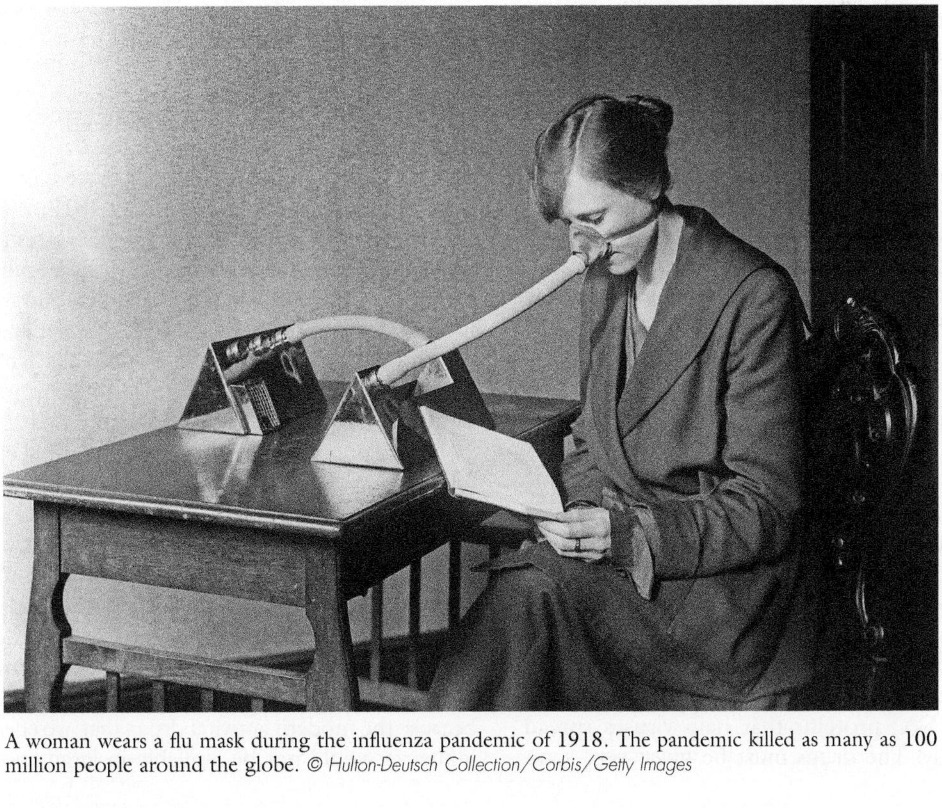

A woman wears a flu mask during the influenza pandemic of 1918. The pandemic killed as many as 100 million people around the globe. © *Hulton-Deutsch Collection/Corbis/Getty Images*

Scope and Distribution

H1N1 flu virus varieties are widespread in humans and pigs. However, a number of genetic differences distinguish the present-day strains of H1N1 from the deadly 1918 strain. As of 2018 the precise strain of H1N1 that caused the 1918 flu pandemic exists only in a few laboratories.

Treatment and Prevention

In 1918 the viral natural of influenza was not understood. No antiviral drugs had yet been discovered, and even antibiotics were not available. Antibiotics are drugs that kill bacteria; they are not useful directly against viral infections because they do not destroy virus particles, but they can help patients survive bacterial infections that may occur when the body is weakened by the primary, viral infection.

Influenza vaccines are now considered the best way to prevent flu. Each year a new dominant type of influenza reliably appears in Asia. Medical researchers identify the strain and produce a vaccine that is distributed in parts of the world that have not yet experienced the new virus strain. A vaccine is a preparation that contains antigens. After being trained on specific antigens by a vaccine, the body can attack a disease agent carrying those antigens as soon as it appears. In the case of a flu vaccine, the HA protein, which is harmless by itself, is often used as the antigen. Virus particles that have been damaged so that they cannot cause an infection are also used in vaccines.

International surveillance of new influenza viruses is coordinated by the World Health Organization's (WHO) Global Influenza Surveillance and Response System (GISRS), set up in 1952 as the Global Influenza Surveillance Network. Scores of medical institutions in 142 countries collect flu specimens and send them to six centers for analysis. WHO scientists study these samples each year to design vaccines for the northern and southern hemispheres, then send these vaccine designs to manufacturers for mass production. GISRS works well for the industrialized countries of the world, but, according to the US National Academy of Science, the network is not as effective in Africa and Asia. This leaves more people vulnerable to flu pandemic in those places.

In the early 21st century, vaccines are not the only tool for fighting a flu pandemic. Several antiviral drugs are available that would probably be effective against the 1918 virus or a similar virus. These drugs are designed to interfere with the functioning of one or more of the proteins a virus uses to reproduce. For instance, Relenza® and Tamiflu® are flu-specific drugs called neuraminidase inhibitors. They are designed to interfere with the action of the neuraminidase (NA) proteins that help viruses spread through the body. The drugs must be given very soon after infection to stop its spread; they do not kill the virus but slow its progress while the body's immune system actually kills the virus particles.

These drugs are relatively expensive to produce and not available as of 2018 in stockpiles large enough to treat the populations of whole countries. Therefore, despite the existence of effective antiviral drugs, WHO warns that a 1918-type flu pandemic could still be a global disaster.

Impacts and Issues

As described above, the 1918 flu virus is no longer extinct. In 2005 scientists at the US Centers for Disease Control and Prevention in Atlanta, Georgia, reconstructed live virus from RNA fragments recovered from tissue dating to the original pandemic. This caused some controversy. Most scientists agreed that prevention of a future flu pandemic could be aided by studying live 1918 virus. However, some also argued that resurrecting the 1918 virus itself created an unacceptable risk; if the virus were to escape from the laboratories that were using it to infect mice, monkeys, and tissue cultures, it could cause another global pandemic all by itself. Others argued that publishing the RNA information for the virus might enable sophisticated terrorists to re-create the virus as a weapon. An emergency meeting of the US National Science Advisory Board for Biosecurity was called before publication of the virus data in 2005, and the board decided that the benefits of the work outweighed the risks. While it may be unlikely that the 1918 flu will escape from captivity and cause a global pandemic, WHO and other expert groups warn that a new virus might evolve naturally with properties similar to those of the 1918 flu.

By 2018 an H5N1 virus causing a variety of avian flu had been circulating in Asia for several years and was a cause of international concern as it moved into Africa, Russia, and Europe. Between 2003 and 2017, WHO received reports of 860 confirmed cases of H5N1 resulting in 454 deaths. The present form of the virus, which was highly dangerous to humans, could only be contracted directly from birds or by intimate association of family members or health care providers with a person sick with avian flu. Only a few cases of limited human-to-human transmission by routine contact had been documented as of January 2018, making that form of H5N1 an unlikely candidate for a human pandemic. However, if the properties of this virus are modified by reassortment or mutation (always an ongoing process) so that it can spread quickly among humans, it is possible to cause a global pandemic with millions of casualties. In 2004 WHO estimated that such a pandemic would cause at least 2 to 7 million deaths worldwide and perhaps over 50 million—comparable to the 1918 pandemic. Such large numbers of deaths are possible because the modern antiviral drugs that are effective against influenza would not be available in large enough supply, and, although the US Food and Drug Administration approved an H5N1 vaccine for stockpiling in November 2013, it could not be manufactured in sufficient quantities to vaccinate enough of the population and prevent the pandemic.

PRIMARY SOURCE

Camp Devens Letter

SOURCE: *"Camp Devens Letter."* British Medical Journal *(December 22–29, 1979).*

INTRODUCTION: *The influenza pandemic of 1918 killed more people than any other epidemic in recorded history as of 2018, including the bubonic plague pandemic of the 14th century known as the Black Death. The flu moved too quickly for public health authorities to adequately respond. In both military and civilian life, hospital resources were strained by the sheer number of persons sick with influenza. Physicians and nurses were overwhelmed and in short supply. Quarantine measures were enacted but did little to stem the spread of the disease. Mortuaries were overcrowded. One US Army physician, known only as "Roy," documented his observations of the epidemic at the base hospital at Camp Devens, Massachusetts, in the letter below. The letter was found years later and resides in the archives at the University of Michigan.*

Camp Devens, Mass.
Surgical Ward No 16
29 September 1918
(Base Hospital)
My dear Burt,

It is more than likely that you would be interested in the news of this place, for there is a possibility that you will be assigned here for duty, so having a minute between rounds I will try to tell you a little about the situation here as I have seen it in the last week.

As you know I have not seen much Pneumonia in the last few years in Detroit, so when I came here I was somewhat behind in the niceties of the Army way of intricate diagnosis. Also to make it good, I have had for the last week an exacerbation of my old "ear rot" as Artie Ogle calls it, and could not use a Stethoscope at all, but had to get by on my ability to "spot" 'em thru my general knowledge of pneumonias. I did well enough, and finally found an old Phonendoscope that I pieced together, and from then on was all right. You know the Army regulations require very close locations etc.

Camp Devens is near Boston, and has about 50,000 men, or did have before this epidemic broke loose. It also has the Base Hospital for the Div. of the N. East. This epidemic started about four weeks ago, and has developed so rapidly that the camp is demoralized and all ordinary work is held up till it has passed. All assemblages of soldiers taboo.

These men start with what appears to be an ordinary attack of La Grippe or Influenza, and when brought to the Hosp. they very rapidly develop the most viscous type of Pneumonia that has ever been seen. Two hours after admission they have the mahogany spots over the cheek bones, and a few hours later you can begin to see the cyanosis extending from their ears and spreading all over the face, until it is hard to distinguish the coloured men from the white. It is only a matter of a few hours then until death comes, and it is simply a struggle for air until they suffocate. It is horrible. One can stand it to see one, two, or twenty men die, but to see these poor devils dropping like flies sort of gets on your nerves. We have been averaging about 100 deaths per day, and still keeping it up. There is no doubt in my mind that there is a new mixed infection here, but what I don't know.

My total time is taken up hunting rales, rales dry or moist, sibilant or crepitant or any other of the hundred things that one may find in the chest, they all mean but one thing here—Pneumonia—and that means in about all cases death.

The normal number of resident Drs. here is about 25 and that has been increased to over 250, all of whom (of course excepting me) have temporary orders—"Return to your proper Station on completion of work." Mine says "Permanent Duty," but I have been in the Army just long enough to learn that it doesn't always mean what it says. So I don't know what will happen to me at the end of this.

We have lost an outrageous number of nurses and Drs., and the little town of Ayer is a sight. It takes Special trains to carry away the dead. For several days there were no coffins and the bodies piled up something fierce, we used to go down to the morgue (which is just back of my ward) and look at the boys laid out in long rows. It beats any sight they ever had in France after a battle. An extra long barracks has been vacated for the use of the morgue, and it would make any man sit up and take notice to walk down the long lines of dead soldiers all dressed and laid out in double rows. We have no relief here, you get up in the morning at 5.30 and work steady till about 9.30 P.M., sleep, then go at it again. Some of the men of course have been here all the time, and they are TIRED.

If this letter seems somewhat disconnected, overlook it, for I have been called away from it a dozen times the last time just now by the Officer of the Day, who came in to tell me that they have not as yet found at any of the autopsies any case beyond the Red. Hepatitis stage. It kills them before they get that far.

I don't wish you any hard luck, Old Man, but I do wish you were here for a while at least. It's more comfortable when one has a friend about. The men here are all good fellows, but I get so damned sick of pneumonia that when I go to eat I want to find some fellow who will not "Talk Shop" but there ain't none nohow. We eat it, live it, sleep it, and dream it, to say nothing of breathing it 16 hours a day. I would be very grateful indeed if you would drop me a line or two once in a while, and I will promise you that if you ever get into a fix like this, I will do the same for you.

Each man here gets a ward with about 150 beds (mine has 168) and has an Asst. Chief to boss him, and you can imagine what the paper work alone is—fierce—and the Govt. demands all paper work be kept up in good shape. I have only four day nurses and five night nurses (female), a ward-master, and four orderlies. So you can see that we are busy. I write this in piecemeal fashion. It may be a long time before I can get another letter to you, but will try.

This letter will give you an idea of the monthly report which has to be in Monday. I have mine most ready now. My Boss was in just now and gave me a lot more work to do so I will have to close this.

Goodbye old Pal, "God be with you till we meet again"

Keep the Bouells open.
(Sgd) Roy.
Roy

SEE ALSO *Avian Influenza; H5N1 Virus; Influenza; Influenza Pandemic of 1957; Influenza, Tracking Seasonal Influences and Virus Mutation; Pandemic Preparedness; Viral Disease*

BIBLIOGRAPHY

Books

Corsby, Alfred W. *America's Forgotten Pandemic.* New York: Cambridge University Press, 2003.

Marrin, Albert. *Very, Very, Very Dreadful: The Influenza Pandemic of 1918.* New York: Knopf, 2018.

Opdycke, Sandra. *The Flu Epidemic of 1918: America's Experience in the Global Health Crisis.* New York, Routledge, 2014.

Pettit, Dorothy A., and Janice Bailie. *A Cruel Wind: Pandemic Flu in America, 1918–1920.* Murfreesboro, TN: Timberlane, 2008.

Spinney, Laura. *Pale Rider: The Spanish Flu of 1918 and How It Changed the World.* New York: Public Affairs, 2017.

Periodicals

Cohen, Jon. "Swine Flu Pandemic Reincarnates 1918 Virus." *Science* (March 24, 2010). This article is also available online at http://www.sciencemag.org/news/2010/03/swine-flu-pandemic-reincarnates-1918-virus (accessed January 16, 2018).

Johnson, Niall P. A. S., and Jeurgen Mueller. "Updating the Accounts: Global Mortality of the 1918–1920 'Spanish' Influenza Pandemic." *Bulletin of the History of Medicine* 76, no. 1 (2002): 105–115.

Koelle, Katia, et al. "Epochal Evolution Shapes the Phylodynamics of Interpandemic Influenza A (H3N2) in Humans." *Science* 314 (2006): 1898–1903.

Mills, Christina E., James M. Robins, and Marc Lipsitch. "Transmissibility of 1918 Pandemic Influenza." *Science* 432 (December 16, 2004): 904–906.

Taubenberger, Jeffery K., et al. "Reconstruction of the 1918 Influenza Virus: Unexpected Rewards from the Past" *mBio* 3, no. 5 (2012). This article can also be found online at http://mbio.asm.org/content/3/5/e00201-12.full (accessed January 16, 2018).

Tumpey, Terrence M., et al. "Characterization of the Reconstructed 1918 Spanish Influenza Pandemic Virus." *Science* 310 (October 7, 2005): 77–80.

Vergano, Dan. "Mystery of 1918 Flu That Killed 50 Million Solved?" *National Geographic* (April 29, 2014). This article can also be found online at https://news.nationalgeographic.com/news/2014/04/140428-1918-flu-avian-swine-science-health-science/ (accessed January 16, 2018).

Worobey, Michael, Andrew Rambaut, and Guan-Zhu Han. "Genesis and Pathogenesis of the 1918 Pandemic H1N1 Influenza A Virus." *Proceedings of the National Academy of Sciences of the United States of America* 111, no. 22 (June 2014): 8107–8112. This article can also be found online at http://www.pnas.org/content/111/22/8107.full (accessed January 16, 2018).

Websites

"Influenza." World Health Organization. http://www.who.int/influenza/en/ (accessed January 19, 2018).

"Influenza (Flu)." Centers for Disease Control and Prevention (January 19, 2018). https://www.cdc.gov/flu/ (accessed January 19, 2018).

"Pandemic Influenza Plan: 2017 Update." US Department of Health and Human Services. https://www.cdc.gov/flu/pandemic-resources/pdf/pan-flu-report-2017v2.pdf (accessed January 19, 2018).

Larry Gilman
Sam Uretsky

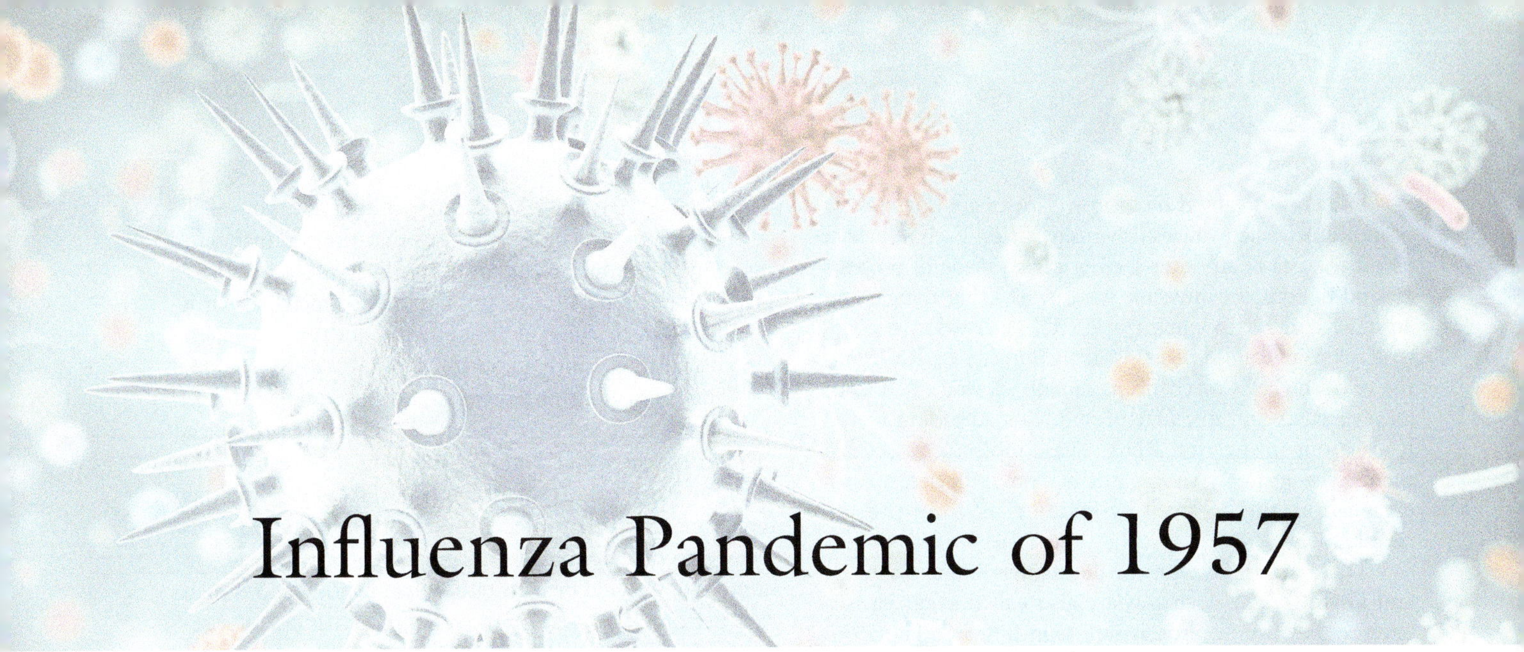

Influenza Pandemic of 1957

Introduction

Influenza ("flu" for short) is a viral infection of the respiratory system that is spread either by contact or by droplets of mucus or saliva ejected into the air by a cough or sneeze. Symptoms of flu include cough, muscle aches, vomiting, loss of appetite, fever, and, in extreme cases, death. Flu pandemics are defined as the emergence and worldwide spread of a new influenza virus to which most of the population has not developed an immunity. Three flu pandemics occurred in the 20th century—in 1918, 1957, and 1968—and another occurred in 2009. The 1957 influenza pandemic was the second-greatest influenza pandemic in the 20th century. It is estimated to have killed approximately 2 million people worldwide, including about 70,000 in the United States. A 2016 study in the *Journal of Infectious Diseases* placed the mortality rate from the 1957 pandemic at up to 1.5 million deaths above what would normally occur from the routine, seasonal rate of influenza.

Flu pandemics occur on average every 30 or 40 years, though research has cast doubt on the theory of a predictable pandemic cycle. The first influenza pandemic of the 20th century, in 1918, killed between 20 and 100 million people worldwide and about 675,000 in the United States. The third, in 1968, killed about 700,000 people worldwide and about 30,000 in the United States. The 2009 pandemic was much milder, resulting in an estimated 200,000 deaths worldwide and around 12,000 in the United States.

Disease History, Characteristics, and Transmission

The flu that caused the 1957 pandemic is called Asian flu because it was first detected in China in February 1957. US government experts could not decide at first whether a 1918-style disaster was in the making and did not want to alarm the public, so the US Surgeon General recommended that flu vaccinations be given only through ordinary doctor-patient channels. The pandemic did spread through the United States, however, starting in the late spring and peaking in October 1957. A second wave of infections, mostly affecting the elderly, occurred in January and February 1958. About 69,800 people died of the Asian flu in the United States. (A 2016 report from the Centers for Disease Control and Prevention noted that flu deaths in the United States ranged from 12,000 to 56,000 per year between 2010 and 2014. However, the US population was much smaller in 1957, so the death rate from the pandemic was relatively much higher than for a typical flu season.)

WORDS TO KNOW

CAPSID The protein shell surrounding a virus particle.

MUTATION A change in an organism's DNA that occurs over time and may render it less sensitive to drugs that are used against it.

PANDEMIC An epidemic that occurs in more than one country or population simultaneously. *Pandemic* means "all the people."

REASSORTMENT A condition resulting when two or more different types of viruses exchange genetic material to form a new, genetically different virus.

VIRION A mature virus particle consisting of a core of ribonucleic acid (RNA) or deoxyribonucleic acid (DNA) surrounded by a protein coat. This is the form in which a virus exists outside of its host cell.

Influenza is caused by a virus. Viruses are tiny clusters of molecules called virions or virus particles. Each influenza virion consists of an outer shell or capsid made of proteins (a kind of complex molecule used by all living things) and an inner core of ribonucleic acid (RNA). A virion attaches to a cell using capsid proteins. It then injects its RNA into the cell. The cell's mechanisms cannot tell viral RNA from its own RNA and manufacture proteins according to the instructions in the viral RNA. These molecules assemble themselves into new virus particles. New influenza viruses escape from the host cell by budding off from the cell membrane.

There are three types of flu, namely influenza A, B, and C. Influenza A viruses are also called avian viruses because they live in birds as well as in humans. The 1957 flu virus was an influenza A virus. Influenza A viruses are given code names to distinguish them. These names are based on 2 of the 11 proteins found in the capsid, hemagglutinin (HA) and neuraminidase (NA). HA and NA each occur in a variety of forms, which are given numbers by biologists. A virus having a type 2 HA protein and a type 2 NA protein is an H2N2 virus. The virus that caused the 1957 pandemic was an H2N2 virus.

Mutations occur in viral RNA, changing the capsid proteins in new viruses. When enough of these changes happen, the immune system's memory of its previous encounter with flu is no longer useful; the new, changed virus is not recognized as soon as it appears and so has a chance to cause an infection before the body destroys it. Viruses can also change by reassortment. Reassortment can happen when two different types of virus infect the same cell at the same time. The new viruses that the cell manufactures may contain RNA from both types. The 1957 H2N2 virus probably arose through reassortment of a virus originating in birds (an avian influenza) and a virus already easily transmitted among humans.

The flu is transmitted from person to person or, in some cases, from animal to person via microscopic droplets of fluid expelled by coughing, sneezing, or breathing. A 1957 World Health Organization (WHO) epidemiology report indicated that infectiousness of the influenza virus seemed to be determined primarily by contact with a large number of infected persons rather than considerations such as a person's age, sex, or race. A similar pattern was reported in 2017 in a Chinese report that found that the greatest risk of infection was related to contact with a high population of birds. The second greatest risk was associated with a dense population of humans.

A Canadian study of the mortality rates of the 1957 pandemic showed a unique trait in terms of mortality. While people who had a history of influenza exposure normally retained a limited resistance to influenza virus of the same type, people who survived one pandemic were more sensitive, and at greater risk, from another pandemic when the virus was of a different type. As a result, people who had been exposed to the influenza virus of 1918 had a higher than expected mortality rate when infected by the 1957 virus, even accounting for their greater age in 1957. The reason for this is not yet understood.

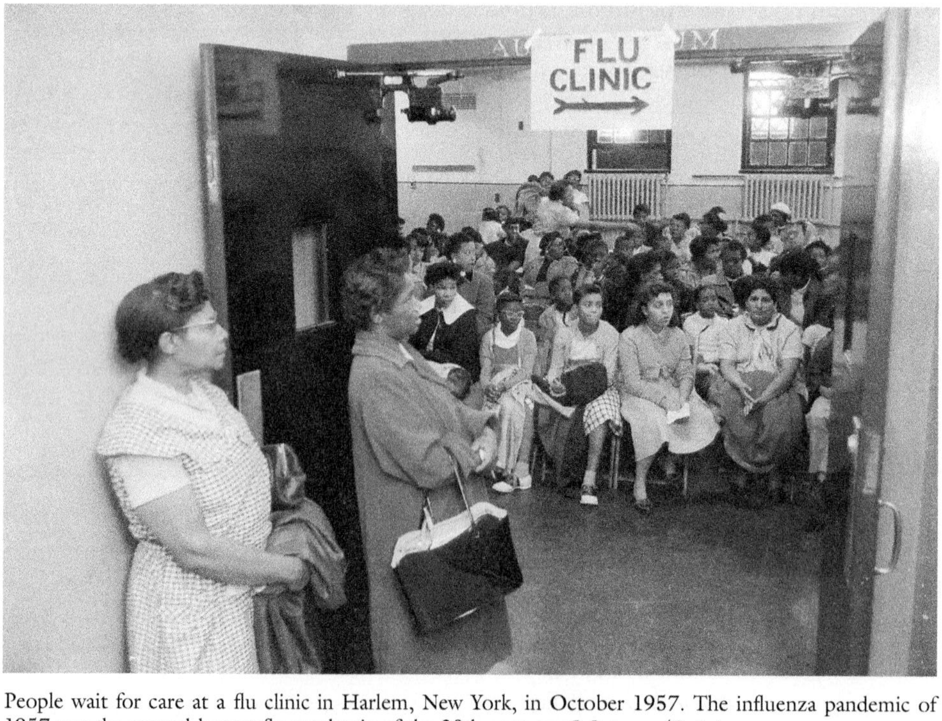

People wait for care at a flu clinic in Harlem, New York, in October 1957. The influenza pandemic of 1957 was the second-largest flu pandemic of the 20th century. *© Bettmann/Getty Images*

Scope and Distribution

As of 2018 the strain of H2N2 influenza A virus that caused the 1957 pandemic exists only in laboratory cultures. Other H2N2 viruses exist in the wild.

Treatment and Prevention

No antiviral drugs existed in 1957. A vaccine was created for this flu but was not available to most people. Treatment, as for the common cold, consisted mostly of rest, fluids, and staying warm. Antibiotics—drugs that kill only bacteria—were sometimes given to flu patients to fight secondary bacterial infections but could not treat the flu itself.

In the early 21st century, vaccination remains the first line of defense against any flu outbreak, but several antiviral drugs are available. Efforts are sometimes made to prevent the origin of 1957-type flu viruses by preventing people who have virus infections from working around or slaughtering birds while sick. The goal is to lessen the chances that reassortment will occur in cells infected by an avian virus from the birds and a virus already easily transmitted among humans.

Impacts and Issues

Unlike the flu pandemic of 1918, international strategies to report and respond to pandemic threats gave many nations advance warning of the new pandemic. Soon after the virus was identified in China, several nations were able to develop and produce vaccines to stem the spread of the illness. In addition to limited vaccination programs, many of the same quarantine techniques that were used to combat the 1918 pandemic were used again in 1957. Because children and families with young children were disproportionately affected, many schools and libraries closed temporarily to prevent the spread of the flu within local communities. Such measures helped limit the spread of the flu among children, but the disease reemerged in early 1958. Most of the victims of the "second wave" of the pandemic were elderly.

In 2005 it was found that quality-control kits containing live Asian flu virus had been sent to 6,000 labs in 19 countries. To prevent the reintroduction of the 1957 pandemic flu virus into the general population, efforts were overseen by WHO to track down and destroy all the virus samples. No outbreak occurred. In 2011 researchers from the National Institutes of Health warned that the H2N2 flu virus continued to circulate among birds and pigs and noted that most people under the age of 50 (most of whom were not alive during the 1957 pandemic) had little to no immunity against the subtype, leaving the world vulnerable to another deadly H2N2 pandemic similar to what occurred in 1957. The researchers urged public health officials to consider mass vaccinations against H2N2, but, as of early 2018, no such campaigns had been announced.

PRIMARY SOURCE

David Rex on the Influenza Pandemic of 1957

SOURCE: *Rex, David. "1957 Flu Pandemic." US Centers for Disease Control and Prevention. https://www.cdc.gov/publications/panflu/stories/1957_rex.html (accessed January 24, 2018).*

INTRODUCTION: *The Influenza Pandemic of 1957 affected millions of people around the world. Even those who did not become seriously ill were aware that they were living through an extraordinary time. In the following account, then college student David Rex describes what life was like on an Ohio college campus during the outbreak. Rex's account is part of a collection of oral stories collected by the US Centers for Disease Control and Prevention.*

In the fall of 1957, I was a freshman at the College of Wooster in Wooster Ohio. For some reason, I took the flu shot for the first time. It may be that I was encouraged to do so by the school doctor. However, I was one of the few who did.

Later that fall I was in class and began to have flu-like symptoms that were fairly mild; aches, temperature, and other symptoms. I returned to my dorm room and fell asleep without dinner. I slept until late morning, missing class and breakfast. I still had some mild symptoms, but the aches and elevated temperature were gone. I felt well enough to go to lunch and then on to my afternoon classes. I noticed that the dining room was not as full as usual. Later, in class, I also noticed a lot of students missing.

By the next day, I had no symptoms at all. However, there were even fewer students in the dining room and classrooms, and several professors were also missing. My girlfriend was quite sick and through her I learned that her roommates and a large number of dorm mates were in bed very ill, too. Eventually over 80% of the student body was "hospitalized" in the dorms. The few like me, who were not ill, began delivering meals, checking for students with serious symptoms, and making reports to the health center. The center staff made visits to the dorms on a regular basis, but depended on us "well ones" to point out those sick students who needed the most assistance.

Throughout the state of Ohio (and I believe most of the nation) schools, churches, public meetings were all cancelled. However, the closing of our college and another Presbyterian college required a meeting of the Synod of

Ohio, and since such meetings were all cancelled, "officially" we remained open.

Fortunately, despite the high morbidity rate, I don't believe we had any deaths.

SEE ALSO *Avian Influenza; H5N1; Influenza; Influenza Epidemic of 1918; Influenza, Tracking Seasonal Influences and Virus Mutation; Viral Disease*

BIBLIOGRAPHY

Books

Dehner, George. *Influenza: A Century of Science and Public Health Response.* Pittsburgh: University of Pittsburgh Press, 2012.

Goldsmith, Connie. *Influenza: The Next Pandemic?* Minneapolis: Twenty-First Century Books, 2007.

Periodicals

Check, Erika. "Heightened Security after Flu Scare Sparks Biosafety Debate." *Nature* 432 (2005): 943.

Gagnon, Alain, et al. "Pandemic Paradox: Early Life H2N2 Pandemic Influenza Infection Enhanced Susceptibility to Death during the 2009 H1N1 Pandemic." *MBio* 9, no. 1 (January 16, 2018): 1–15. This article can also be found online at http://mbio.asm.org/content/9/1/e02091-17.full.pdf (accessed January 22, 2018).

Lu, Lu, Andrew J. Leigh Brown, and Samantha J. Lycett. "Quantifying Predictors for the Spatial Diffusion of Avian Influenza Virus in China." *BMC Evolutionary Biology* 17 (January 13, 2017): 1–14. This article can also be found online at https://bmcevolbiol.biomedcentral.com/articles/10.1186/s12862-016-0845-3 (accessed January 22, 2018).

McNeil, Donald G., Jr. "The Next Flu Pandemic Will Appear When You Least Expect It." *New York Times* (December 8, 2017). This article can also be found online at https://www.nytimes.com/2017/12/08/health/next-flu-pandemic.html (accessed January 22, 2018).

Viboud, Cécile, et al. "Global Mortality Impact of the 1957–1959 Influenza Pandemic." *Journal of Infectious Diseases* 213, no. 5 (March 1, 2016): 738–745. This article can also be found online at https://academic.oup.com/jid/article/213/5/738/2459470 (accessed January 22, 2018).

Websites

"Epidemiological Notes: Influenza." World Health Organization, 1957. http://www.who.int/iris/handle/10665/211117 (accessed January 20, 2018).

"Estimating Seasonal Influenza-Associated Deaths in the United States." Centers for Disease Control and Prevention, December 9, 2016. https://www.cdc.gov/flu/about/disease/us_flu-related_deaths.htm (accessed January 22, 2018).

"National Strategy for Pandemic Flu." US Department of Homeland Security, July 6, 2009. https://www.dhs.gov/national-strategy-pandemic-flu (accessed January 22, 2007).

"Pandemic Influenza." Centers for Disease Control and Prevention, January 2, 2018. https://www.cdc.gov/flu/pandemic-resources/index.htm (accessed January 22, 2018).

"Pandemic Influenza." US Department of Health and Human Services. https://www.hhs.gov/about/agencies/oga/global-health-security/pandemic-influenza/index.html (accessed January 22, 2018).

Larry Gilman
Sam Uretsky

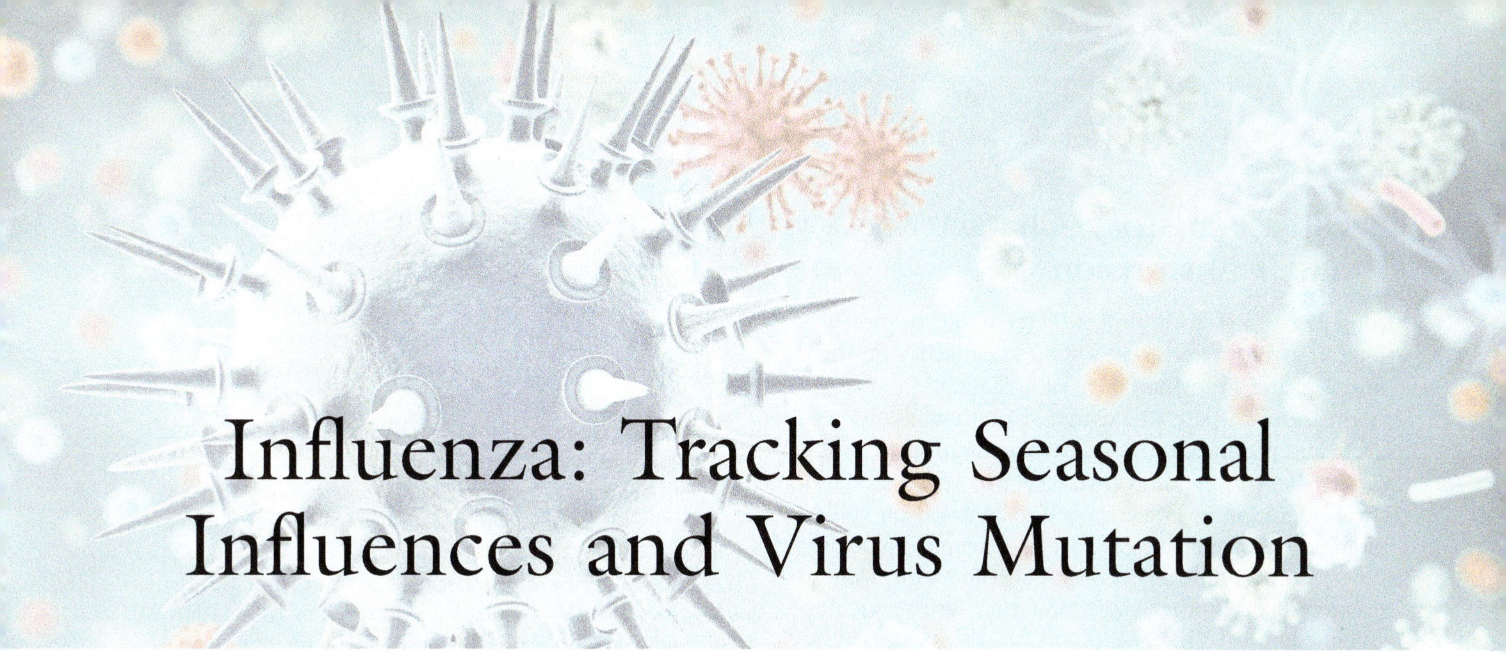

Influenza: Tracking Seasonal Influences and Virus Mutation

Introduction

Due to influenza's contagious nature, potential for serious complications, and high mortality rates, public health agencies around the world have developed systems for tracking influenza epidemics. These systems have allowed agencies to mount defensive measures such as immunization and educational programs to help prevent influenza infections and slow the virus's spread. By tracking seasonal influences and viral mutations, the World Health Organization (WHO) and national public health agencies aim to prevent major influenza epidemics, during which severe illness and death occur, mainly among the elderly and people with compromised immune systems.

An important element of influenza tracking is monitoring the viral strains that are being transmitted. There are two main types of influenza virus, A and B. These strains are undergoing constant genetic change, either as a result of antigenic drift or antigenic shift. Antigenic drift occurs as people develop antibodies that protect against the virus, and the virus makes corresponding changes to resist these antibodies. Antigenic shift occurs only in influenza A when a major change in the virus suddenly occurs, often as a result of the virus being transferred from an animal population to a human population. By tracking changes in the virus, public health officials better anticipate which strains to guard against, including when trying to anticipate which strain is mostl likely to be most prevalent during the next flu season and should be vaccinated against.

Since 1997 WHO has operated FluNet, an online system that tracks data supplied by the world's various National Influenza Centres (NICs), which belong to the Global Influenza Surveillance and Response System (GISRS). FluNet provides information about influenza infections by country and region, with detailed information about which strains of influenza are infecting how many people in which parts of the world. In the United States, the Centers for Disease Control and Prevention (CDC) conducts surveillance of influenza incidence and mortality.

WORDS TO KNOW

ANTIGENIC DRIFT The gradual accumulation of mutations in genes, such as in gene coding for surface proteins, over a given period.

ANTIGENIC SHIFT An abrupt and major genetic change, such as in gene coding for surface proteins of a virus.

COHORTING The practice of grouping people with similar infections or symptoms together to reduce transmission to others.

EPIDEMIC From the Greek *epidemic*, meaning "prevalent among the people," it is most commonly used to describe an outbreak of an illness or a disease in which the number of individual cases significantly exceeds the usual or expected number of cases in any given population.

REASSORTMENT A condition resulting when two or more different types of viruses exchange genetic material to form a new, genetically different virus.

PANDEMIC An epidemic that occurs in more than one country or population simultaneously. *Pandemic* means "all the people."

PROSTRATION A condition marked by nausea, disorientation, dizziness, and weakness caused by dehydration and prolonged exposure to high temperatures; also called heat exhaustion or hyperthermia.

Disease History, Characteristics, and Transmission

Influenza is an acute viral disease of the respiratory tract. It is characterized by fever, headache, myalgia (muscle aches), prostration, nasal inflammation and discharge, sore throat, and cough. Cough can often be severe and protracted, but other manifestations are usually self-limiting, with recovery in two to seven days. The recognition of influenza is usually based on epidemiological characteristics as part of a general epidemic. Otherwise it is difficult to distinguish influenza from a severe cold or another viral respiratory disease such as viral pneumonia. Viral pneumonia can also be caused by influenza virus, although gastrointestinal tract symptoms (nausea, vomiting, diarrhea) have been reported in about 25 percent of children in school outbreaks.

The spread of influenza virus is predominantly airborne among crowded populations in confined spaces, especially school buses and barracks. Transmission may also occur by indirect contact, as the influenza virus may persist for hours, particularly in cold and dry weather. The viral incubation period is short, usually one to three days. Influenza is communicable for about three to five days after onset in adults and up to a week in young children.

There are three types of influenza virus currently recognized: types A, B, and C. Type A includes three subtypes (H1N1, H2N2, and H3N2), which have been associated with widespread epidemics and pandemics. Type B has been associated with regional or widespread epidemics. Type C is typically associated with sporadic cases and minor localized outbreaks. The viral type is determined by the antigenic properties of two relatively stable structural proteins, the nucleoprotein and the matrix protein.

The emergence of a completely new subtype, the process known as antigenic shift, occurs at unpredictable intervals and only with type A viruses. Viruses characterized by antigenic shift are responsible for the pandemics that result from the unpredictable recombination (new combinations of genetic material) of human and swine or avian (usually duck) antigens. Relatively minor antigenic changes (known as "drift") of type A and type B viruses occur constantly, necessitating periodic (almost annual) reformulation of influenza vaccine. Pandemics have occurred in 1889, 1918, 1957, and 1968, all caused by influenza A strain antigenic shifts. A more recent pandemic occurred in 2009 and 2010 as a result of a unique combination of genetic changes in the virus. An estimated 203,000 people died as a result, though the virus killed fewer people than in earlier outbreaks, such as the pandemic of 1918, which killed some 50 million people.

Scope and Distribution

Once an epidemic is underway, case attack rates range from 10 to 20 percent in the general population and can range up to 50 percent in confined populations such as boarding schools, military bases, and nursing homes. Influenza epidemics caused by type A viruses, type B viruses, or both occur in the United States al-

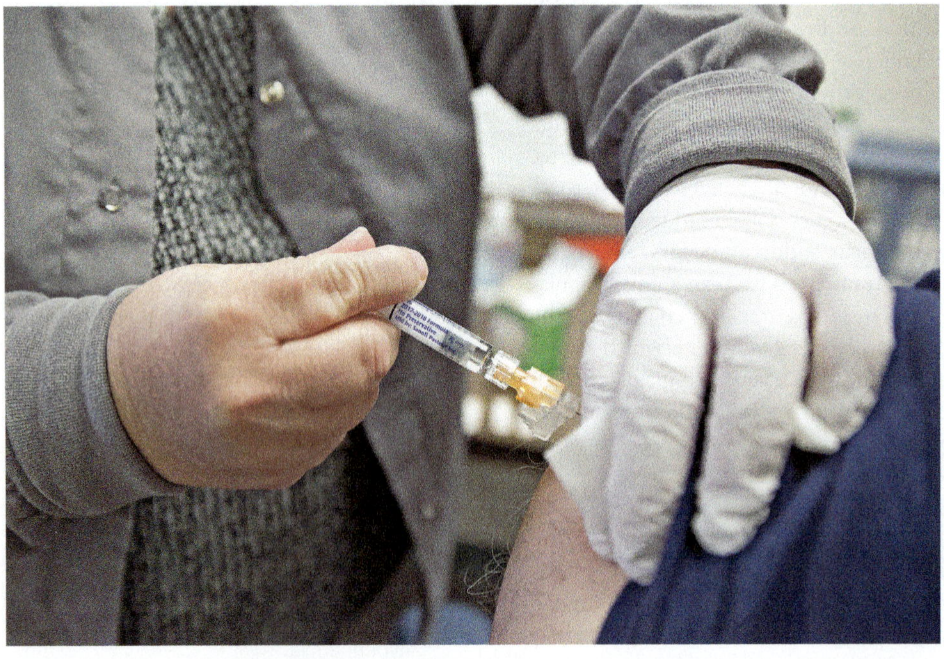

Flu shots deliver an influenza vaccination. While vaccination is the most effective means of preventing influenza, the virus changes often, meaning vaccines need to be altered each year. © *Daniel Acker/ Bloomberg/Getty Images*

most every year. In temperate zones epidemics usually occur in winter. In the tropics they often occur during the rainy season, but outbreaks or sporadic cases may occur in any month. Influenza also occurs naturally in swine, horses, mink, and seals and in many domestic and wild bird species all over the world. Transmission between species and reassortment (exchanging genetic material inside a host) of influenza A viruses have been reported to occur between swine, humans, ducks, and turkeys. The human influenza viruses responsible for the 1957 and 1968 pandemics contained gene segments closely related to those of avian influenza viruses.

Humans are the primary reservoir for human infections, though mammalian reservoirs such as swine and avian reservoirs such as ducks are likely sources of new human subtypes thought to emerge through genetic reassortment. New virulent subtypes cause pandemic influenza by spreading through a population that has little or no immunity because of lack of exposure to the new viral surface antigens.

When a new viral subtype appears, all children and adults are equally susceptible except for individuals who have lived through earlier epidemics of the same subtype. Infection produces immunity to the specific infecting virus, but the duration of immunity depends on the degree of antigenic drift and the number of previous infections. Flu vaccines produce responses that are specific for the included viruses and also boost responses to related strains to which the individual has been previously exposed. Attack rates tend to be age specific. People who have lived long enough to experience earlier epidemics of the same subtype usually have at least partial immunity years later, and this partial immunity protects them from closely related subtypes.

■ Treatment and Prevention

Treatment

Because any outbreak of influenza has important and sometimes catastrophic implications, all cases must be reported to local health authorities to assist disease surveillance. The identity of the disease agent by viral subtype as determined by laboratory testing should be provided, if possible. Although annual vaccination is the primary strategy for preventing complications of influenza virus infections, the CDC notes that antiviral medications with activity against influenza viruses can be effective for the chemoprophylaxis and treatment of influenza.

Five licensed influenza antiviral agents are available in the United States: Tamiflu® (oseltamivir), Relenza® (zanamivir), Rapivab® (Peramivir), amantadine, and rimantadine. However, the flu viruses that make humans sick are highly resistant to amantadine and rimantadine, so these two medications are not recommended to prevent or treat influenza. These treatments should be started within 48 hours of the onset of symptoms. Influenza A virus resistance to amantadine and rimantadine can emerge rapidly during treatment. On the basis of antiviral testing conducted at the CDC and in Canada that indicated high levels of resistance, the CDC recommends that neither amantadine or rimantadine be used for the treatment or chemoprophylaxis of influenza A in the United States until susceptibility to these antiviral medications has been reestablished among circulating influenza A viruses. Oseltamivir may cause delirium in some pediatric patients.

Because influenza is usually self-limiting in healthy adults under age 65, the CDC generally advises against personal stockpiling of the drugs. Federal and state health authorities and health care institutions are creating stockpiles of antiviral influenza medications for people at greatest risk for complications from influenza. A potential consequence of personal stockpiling is depletion of existing supplies of antivirals so that they will not be available to those people who most need them. In addition, widespread personal stockpiling and inappropriate use of antivirals (for example, as a daily regimen regardless of the degree of influenza risk) might compound the risk for influenza by creating conditions for the emergence of resistant strains of influenza. Widespread resistance to oseltamivir could be catastrophic in the event of an avian flu pandemic on the scale of the 1918 pandemic.

Prevention

Influenza vaccination remains the cornerstone for the control and treatment of influenza, and antiviral influenza medications should serve as an adjunct to vaccine. In addition, public and health care personnel need to be trained to avoid unprotected coughs and sneezes and to use proper handwashing techniques. Patient isolation is impractical in most cases because of the viral incubation period during which victims are infectious without symptoms. However, during an epidemic it would be desirable to isolate patients, especially infants and children, by putting them in the same room (known as cohorting) during the first five to seven days of illness.

Immunization may provide 70 to 80 percent protection against infection in healthy young adults when the vaccine antigen closely matches circulating viruses. Vaccine programs have been less successful in preventing disease but have reduced the hospitalization of people over age 65 for complications such as pneumococcal pneumonia by 30 to 50 percent. The CDC recommends that influenza vaccination for the elderly be supplemented with immunization against pneumococcal pneumonia. Immunization can benefit any individual, but it should especially be considered for emergency responders, people performing essential services, and military personnel.

Influenza vaccine should be provided each year before influenza is expected in the community (November through March in the United States). Travelers should be immunized according to the seasonal patterns of influenza

SMART THERMOMETERS

In 2014 the US Food and Drug Administration (FDA) approved a new tool for tracking influenza called a smart thermometer. The digital thermometer immediately uploads data about a person's body temperature to the internet, allowing public health officials to track spikes in fever that are likely associated with cases of the flu. By 2018 some half a million of these web-connected thermometers were in use in the United States, according to Kinsa, the manufacturer of the devices. With an estimated 25,000 daily readings from the thermometers, Kinsa claims it can more accurately track influenza epidemics than traditional mechanisms for doing so, such as the reporting that the US Centers for Disease Control and Prevention (CDC) relies on.

According to a 2018 *New York Times* article on the new influenza-tracking technology, Kinsa's analysis of the 2017–2018 flu season differed from the CDC's. Data from the smart thermometers indicated that Missouri and Iowa were the hardest-hit states, whereas the Southeast, New England, and New York were largely spared. The CDC, by contrast, considered the flu to be widespread throughout the United States, with no specific states or regions identified as hot spots. While smart thermometers demonstrate how technology can help improve influenza tracking, Kinsa's product had not been analyzed for accuracy as of early 2018.

in various parts of the world. The single dose suffices for people with prior exposure to influenza A and B. Two doses of vaccine one month apart are required for younger people with no previous immunization history. Routine immunization programs should be directed primarily at those with the greatest risk of serious complications or death and those who might spread infection to them, such as health care personnel and household contacts of high-risk people.

Tracking

Influenza is a disease that is under surveillance by WHO, which recommends the following procedures:

1. Report any influenza epidemics, including the viral subtype, to WHO.
2. Submit prototype strains to one of the WHO Collaborating Centres for Reference and Research on Influenza. Throat secretion specimens, aspirates, and paired blood samples may also be sent to any WHO-recognized national influenza center.
3. Conduct epidemiological studies and promptly identify viruses at the national health agencies.
4. Ensure sufficient commercial or governmental facilities for the production of adequate quantities of vaccine and programs for vaccine administration to high-risk people and essential personnel. In view of the seriousness of the threat of an avian flu pandemic, some nations add the stockpiling of adequate supplies of antiviral medications to this list of national health agency responsibilities.

As of 2018 WHO recognized five Collaborating Centres for Reference and Research on Influenza: the CDC; the UK National Institute for Medical Research in London; the Victorian Infectious Diseases Reference Laboratory in Melbourne, Australia; the National Institute for Infectious Diseases in Tokyo, Japan; and the National Institute for Viral Disease Control and Prevention in Beijing, China. These centers collect information from nearly 150 influenza-tracking institutions located in more than 110 countries. The network monitors which influenza strains are most prevalent, where they are infecting people, how they are being transmitted, and whether they are susceptible to vaccines.

■ Impacts and Issues

The tracking and prevention of influenza are closely related. Once data have been collected, they are analyzed by public health officials to understand which strains are most prevalent, where they are most prevalent, how they are spreading, and which are the most severe. Officials use the data and analysis to determine which strains of the influenza virus should be used to create that year's flu vaccine. In September of each year, officials decide the composition of a vaccine for the northern hemisphere, and in February they decide the southern hemisphere's vaccine. The timing of these decisions ensures that the vaccines are available in time for each hemisphere's annual flu season. However, much about the flu vaccine is uncertain, as expert predictions about which strains to inoculate against are sometimes wrong due to unforeseeable factors.

Publicity regarding the possibility of another avian flu epidemic on the scale of the 1918 pandemic stimulated many members of the public to purchase, privately stockpile, and consume pharmaceutical products, especially oseltamivir, as a way to ward off a supposed imminent outbreak of H5N1 influenza in the first decade of the 21st century. This consumption amounted to a waste of valuable antiviral supplies and has increased the probability of the emergence of resistant viral strains.

During treatment drug-resistant viruses may emerge late in the course of therapy and be transmitted to others. Therefore, the cohorting of people on antiviral therapy should be considered, especially in closed populations with many high-risk individuals. Antibiotics should be administered only if patients develop bacterial complications. However, if government agencies are to ask individuals to forgo private stockpiles of antivirals, governments must ensure adequate supplies of antivirals for the public in case of a severe outbreak of type A influenza. In the case of a severe outbreak, aggregations of people in emergency shelters should be avoided, as this will favor outbreaks of the disease if the virus is introduced.

According to CDC analysis of the 31 flu seasons previous to 2007, the deaths attributed to influenza averaged 23,607 per year. However, the average per year for 1997–2007 was higher (32,743). The 2017–2018 flu season, described as severe by the US Public Health Service, has been dominated by the H3N2 influenza strain, which is linked to more severe illnesses, especially among adults over the age of 65 and children younger than 5.

SEE ALSO *H5N1; Influenza; Pandemic Preparedness; Public Health and Infectious Disease*

BIBLIOGRAPHY

Books

Heymann, David L. *Control of Communicable Diseases Manual.* 20th ed. Washington, DC: American Public Health Association, 2014.

Periodicals

"Estimates of Deaths Associated with Seasonal Influenza—United States, 1976–2007." *Morbidity and Mortality Weekly Report* 59, no. 33 (August 27, 2010): 1057–1062.

McNeil, Donald G., Jr. "'Smart Thermometers' Track Flu Season in Real Time." *New York Times* (January 16, 2018). This article can also be found online at https://www.nytimes.com/2018/01/16/health/smart-thermometers-flu.html (accessed March 13, 2018).

Websites

"Antiviral Drugs." Centers for Disease Control and Prevention, January 24, 2018. http://www.cdc.gov/flu/professionals/treatment (accessed March 11, 2018).

"Increased Antiviral Medication Sales before the 2005–06 Influenza Season—New York City." Centers for Disease Control and Prevention, March 16, 2006. http://www.cdc.gov/mmwr/preview/mmwrhtml/mm5510a3.htm (accessed March 11, 2018).

"Influenza Pandemics." The History of Vaccines, 2018. https://www.historyofvaccines.org/content/articles/influenza-pandemics (accessed March 11, 2018).

"Influenza Surveillance and Monitoring." World Health Organization. http://www.who.int/influenza/surveillance_monitoring/en/ (accessed March 11, 2018).

Kenneth T. LaPensee

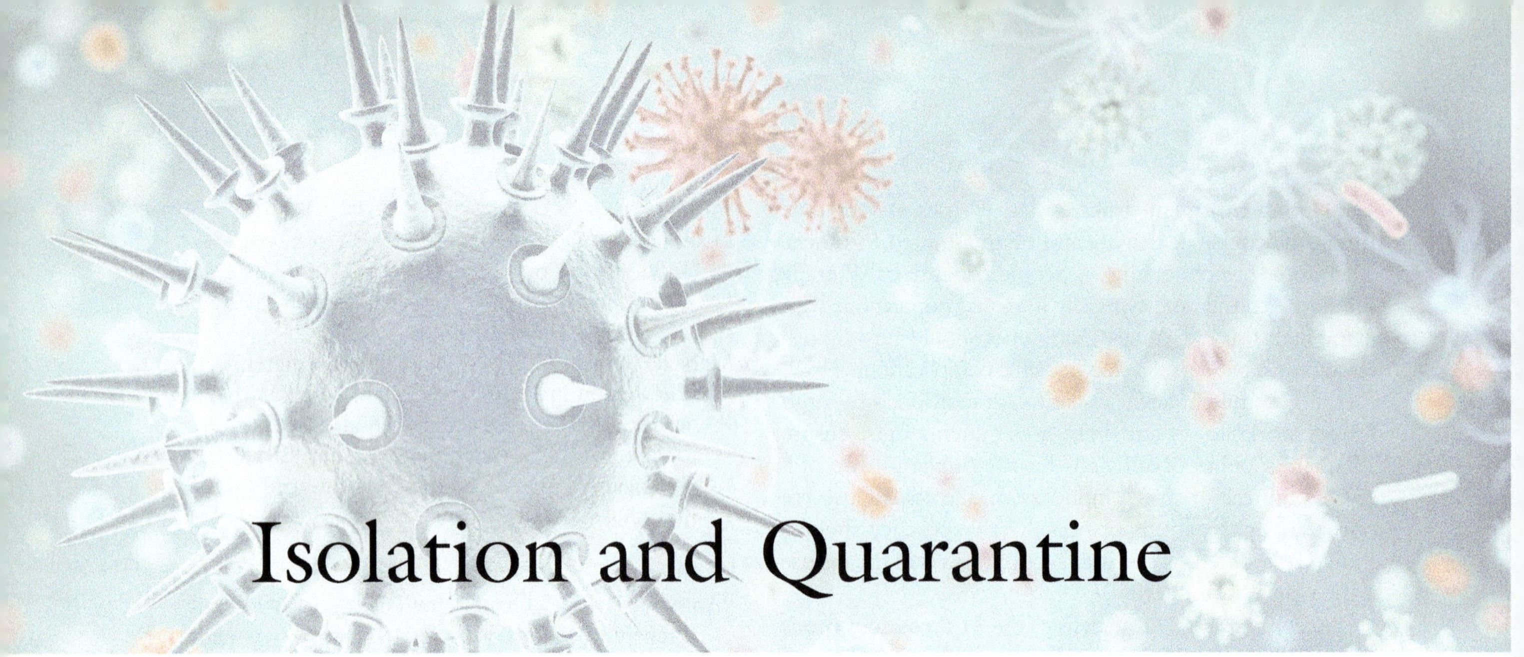

Isolation and Quarantine

■ Introduction

Isolation and quarantine are two strategies that can be used to control the spread of a disease that is contagious. Both approaches minimize the exposure of other people to infected persons.

Isolation and quarantine are not the same. Isolation is more common than quarantine and is used for someone who is known to have a disease. Quarantine is used for someone who has been exposed to a disease or disease-causing agent but who is not currently displaying symptoms and who may not necessarily become ill.

Isolation and quarantine may be voluntary. During a voluntary quarantine, people may elect to remain at home, forgo public gatherings, and curtail travel on airplanes, buses, trains, and other forms of public transit. However, if an outbreak involves a disease that is judged by public health authorities to be a severe contagious threat, isolation or quarantine may be imposed by law. In the United States only disease threats that are listed in an executive order by the president qualify for government-imposed quarantine.

WORDS TO KNOW

CONTAGIOUS A disease that is easily spread among a population, usually by casual person-to-person contact.

EXECUTIVE ORDER Presidential orders that implement or interpret a federal statute, administrative policy, or treaty.

NONGOVERNMENTAL ORGANIZATION (NGO) A voluntary organization that is not part of any government; often organized to address a specific issue or perform a humanitarian function.

■ History and Scientific Foundations

The concept of quarantine dates back to the 14th century, when ships arriving in Venice, Italy, from regions where plague was occurring were required to anchor in the harbor for 40 days before the crew was permitted to go ashore. The word *quarantine* is derived from the Italian *quaranta giorni*, meaning 40 days.

In the United States federal legislation governing the imposition of quarantine was first enacted in 1878 in response to outbreaks of yellow fever. Then the quarantine powers of the federal government were minimal and did not override state and local government public health practices. The federal government assumed more responsibility for quarantine in 1892 in response to cholera outbreaks.

While states continue to have powers to issue quarantines for illnesses within their borders, the federal government has been responsible for quarantine on a national scale since the implementation of the 1944 Public Health Service Act. In 1967 federal responsibility for the imposition and enforcement of quarantine was transferred to the US Centers for Disease Control and Prevention (CDC), where it has remained. The Division of Global Migration and Quarantine (DSMQ) is responsible for the nationwide system of quarantine stations. As of 2017 there were 20 stations located at various ports of entry to the United States.

Both quarantine and isolation are designed to protect the larger community from people known to be infected with a contagious disease deemed to be a public health threat (isolation) or people who have had contact with someone who has become ill with the disease and so who may themselves be infected while not yet displaying symptoms (quarantine). Those in isolation can be treated while at the same time minimizing the chance that the disease will spread. People under quarantine can be monitored for symptoms of the diseases. If symptoms do not appear within a certain time (10 days is typical, as voluntary compliance with a quarantine becomes difficult after that), then the quarantine can be lifted.

■ Applications and Research

Isolation and quarantine are public health responses to an illness outbreak. Isolation is more common and is practiced daily in most hospitals, particularly since the appearance and increasing prevalence of tuberculosis and disease-causing bacteria that are resistant to multiple antibiotics. Examples include methicillin-resistant *Staphylococcus aureus* (MRSA), vancomycin-resistant enterococci (VRE), and carbapenem-resistant *Enterobacteriaceae* (CRE). Many hospitals post warnings restricting visitation to a ward room housing a patient with a contagious infection.

■ Impacts and Issues

Quarantine can affect civil liberties. Imposed quarantines may restrict freedoms of movement and assembly. Schools, restaurants, businesses, means of transit, and public spaces may be closed. The degree to which civil liberties are curtailed in response to an epidemic may be controversial, and, whenever possible, quarantine is a voluntary measure. In the event of an imposed quarantine, government entities, law enforcement, media, and public health organizations should provide as much information as possible to those affected by a quarantine.

Isolation and quarantine can also affect an individual's privacy, because out of necessity the community will need to know who is being contained. This lack of privacy can even include revealing a person's medical history. Thus, isolation and quarantine are considered carefully and not undertaken without a demonstrated and immediate need to do so.

In the United States an executive order of the president identifies quarantinable diseases and authorizes government action to implement quarantines, restrict travel, and detain persons to stop the spread of certain infectious diseases. Executive Order 13295 lists cholera, diphtheria, infectious tuberculosis, plague, smallpox, yellow fever, and viral hemorrhagic fevers (such as Ebola, Marburg, and others) as quarantinable. In 2003, following an outbreak in Asia, severe acute respiratory syndrome (SARS) was added to the list. The growing threat of H5N1 virus and possible pandemic influenza prompted the Department of Health and Human Services (HHS) to request its addition to the list. On July 31, 2014, US President Barack Obama amended Executive Order 13295, identifying severe acute respiratory syndromes as quarantinable in the United States.

Increased movement of peoples worldwide through migration, travel, or war has prompted the need for better international protocols for preventing the spread of infectious diseases. Quarantine across national borders is problematic, sometimes complicated by war, political tensions, different languages, differences in the delivery of health care or in managing outbreaks, and legal systems. In the late 20th and early 21st centuries, national governments

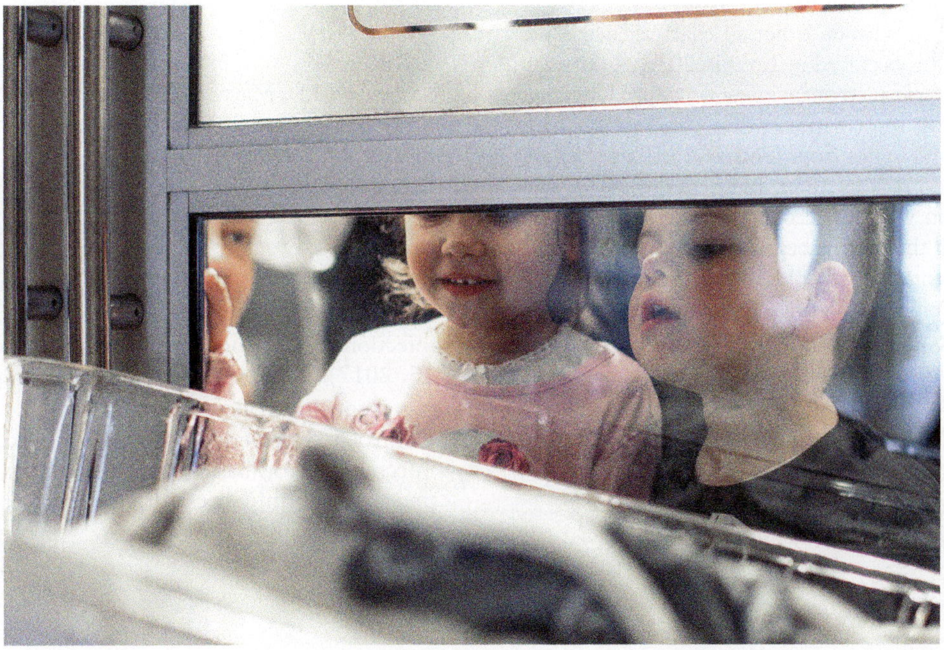

Newborn babies are sometimes held in quarantine for the first hours after their birth. This practice allows health care professionals to monitor their health and ensure that they have not been exposed to any infectious diseases. *© Petri Oeschger/Getty Images*

EFFECTIVE RULES AND REGULATIONS

In the United States [42 U.S.C. 247d] Sec. 319(a) of the Public Health Service Act allows the Health and Human Services (HHS) Secretary to declare a public health emergency and "take such action as may be appropriate to respond," including quarantine, prevention of disease, treatment recommendations, and research, if "the Secretary determines, after consultation with such public health officials as may be necessary, that (1) a disease or disorder presents a public health emergency; or (2) a public health emergency, including significant outbreaks of infectious diseases or bioterrorist attacks, otherwise exists, the Secretary may take such action as may be appropriate to respond to the public health emergency, including making grants, providing awards for expenses, and entering into contracts and conducting and supporting investigations into the cause, treatment, or prevention of a disease or disorder as described. Any such determination of a public health emergency terminates upon the Secretary declaring that the emergency no longer exists, or upon the expiration of the 90-day period beginning on the date on which the determination is made by the Secretary, whichever occurs first. Determinations that terminate under the preceding sentence may be renewed by the Secretary (on the basis of the same or additional facts), and the preceding sentence applies to each such renewal. Not later than 48 hours after making a determination under this subsection of a public health emergency (including a renewal), the Secretary shall submit to the Congress written notification of the determination."

and international agencies have worked to develop a global network of disease reporting. Increased communication about outbreaks of infectious diseases help nations prepare for disease threats and enact preventive measures within their own borders. The World Health Organization (WHO) and other nongovernmental organizations (NGOs), such as Doctors Without Borders, also report and respond to infectious disease outbreaks. International agencies and NGOs typically work with national and local governments to implement disease treatment and prevention strategies, including recommendations of isolation or voluntary or imposed quarantine.

Isolation and quarantine is not an exact science. The latest example of this occurred in Texas in 2016. A nurse in a Texas hospital contracted an infection caused by the Ebola virus during the treatment of a patient who had come to the United States from Liberia—then a site of an ongoing Ebola outbreak in Africa. In a series of errors, the patient's condition was not recognized. Even after Ebola was identified and the patient began receiving treatment, a breach in the hospital's protocol for the handling of infectious diseases deemed especially dangerous exposed the nurse to the infection. The patient ultimately died. The nurse recovered and successfully sued the hospital, arguing that the hospital's policy did not adequately protect her. As of 2017 the hospital denied the claim of negligence.

SEE ALSO *Contact Precautions; Influenza Pandemic of 1918; Personal Protective Equipment; Standard Precautions*

BIBLIOGRAPHY

Books

Delort, Anne-Marie, and Pierre Amato. *Microbiology of Aerosols.* New York: Wiley-Blackwell, 2017.

Flynn, Laura. *All about Infection Control.* Guelph, ON: Mediscript Communications, 2017.

Kumar, Sandeep, and Jane C. Benjamin. *Pathogenic Bacteria in Bioaerosol of Hospitals: Importance of Airborne Pathogen in Hospital.* New York: Lambert Academic, 2013.

Periodicals

Fast, Shannon M., Marta C. González, and Natasha Markuzon. "Cost-Effective Control of Infectious Disease Outbreaks Accounting for Societal Reaction." *PLOS One* 8 (2015): 211–223.

Websites

"Infection Control." Centers for Disease Control and Prevention. https://www.cdc.gov/infectioncontrol/index.html (accessed November 15, 2017).

"Transmission-Based Precautions." Centers for Disease Control and Prevention. https://www.cdc.gov/infectioncontrol/basics/transmission-based-precautions.html (accessed November 15, 2017).

Brian Hoyle

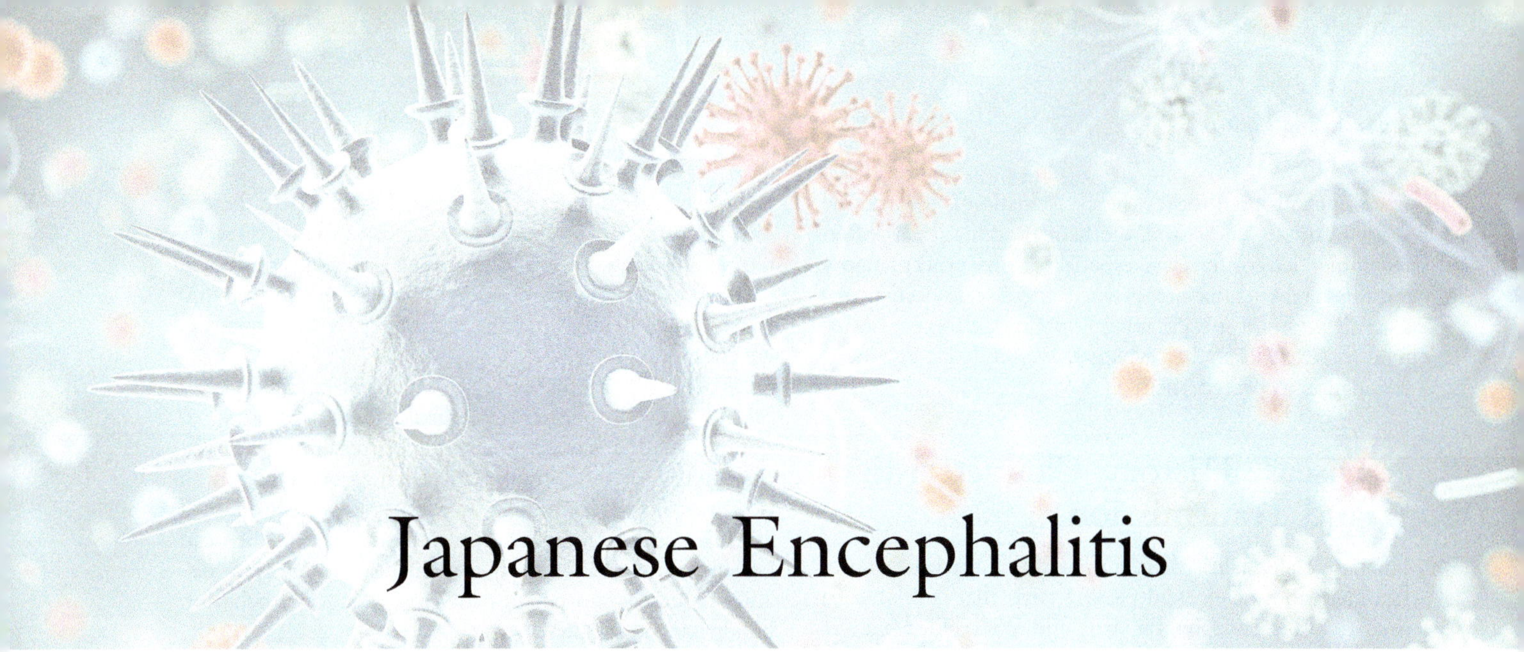

Japanese Encephalitis

Introduction

Encephalitis is an inflammation of the brain that is most often caused by a virus. Japanese encephalitis (JE) is a type of encephalitis caused by the Japanese encephalitis virus (JEV). It is the leading cause of viral encephalitis in many countries of Southeast Asia and the Western Pacific islands, but the infection is relatively rare in the Western Hemisphere. About 30,000 to 60,000 cases are reported annually, with roughly 20 to 30 percent of those cases resulting in death.

The infection is brought on by mosquitoes within the genus *Culex*, and the JEV is a flavivirus, a genus of viruses in the family *Flaviviridae* that also includes the dengue virus, West Nile virus, yellow fever virus, and Zika virus. Although only a minority of JE cases include symptoms—which include headache, seizures, and paralysis—the disease is potentially fatal, and there can be long-lasting disability among survivors.

There is no cure for Japanese encephalitis, but there are vaccines available. Countries that vaccinate their populations against JEV, such as Japan, tend to have fewer cases

WORDS TO KNOW

ACUTE INFECTION An infection of rapid onset and of short duration that either resolves or becomes chronic.

ANTIBODIES Proteins found in the blood that help fight against foreign substances called antigens. Antigens, which are usually proteins or polysaccharides, stimulate the immune system to produce antibodies, or Y-shaped immunoglobulins. The antibodies inactivate the antigen and help remove it from the body. While antigens can be the source of infections from pathogenic bacteria and viruses, organic molecules detrimental to the body from internal or environmental sources also act as antigens. Genetic engineering and the use of various mutational mechanisms allow the construction of a vast array of antibodies (each with a unique genetic sequence).

ARTHROPOD-BORNE DISEASE A disease caused by one of a phylum of organisms characterized by exoskeletons and segmented bodies.

ENCEPHALITIS A type of acute brain inflammation, most often due to infection by a virus.

ENDEMIC Present in a particular area or among a particular group of people.

INCUBATION PERIOD The time between exposure to a disease-causing virus or bacterium and the appearance of symptoms of the infection. Depending on the microorganism, the incubation time can range from a few hours, such as with food poisoning due to *Salmonella*, to a decade or more, such as with acquired immunodeficiency syndrome (AIDS).

MORBIDITY From the Latin *morbus*, "sick," it refers to both the state of being ill and the severity of the illness. A serious disease is said to have high morbidity.

RESERVOIR The animal or organism in which a virus or parasite normally resides.

of encephalitis than those where vaccination is less routine—for example, India and Vietnam. Vaccination is often recommended for travelers, especially if they expect lengthy stays in rural endemic areas (where the disease occurs consistently within a specific region/locality). People who intend to reside in an area where JEV is endemic also need vaccination to protect themselves.

Disease History, Characteristics, and Transmission

Japanese encephalitis virus is a flavivirus, a type of single-stranded ribonucleic acid (RNA) virus that is related to the St. Louis encephalitis virus and West Nile virus. It was first medically documented in Japan in 1871. The incubation period of JEV is 5 to 15 days, and people with symptoms will usually have a history of exposure to mosquitoes in an endemic area in Asia. Most JEV infections are subclinical—that is, the infected person has no symptoms or only mild symptoms, such as headache, fever, and chills.

One person in 250 will develop acute symptoms of JEV, including headache, neck stiffness, muscle pain and spasm, stupor, disorientation and confusion, vomiting, tremor, seizures (especially in children), difficulty moving (often leading to paralysis), swelling around the brain, and even coma and death. Japanese encephalitis can be difficult to distinguish from the other types of viral encephalitis; tests of blood or cerebrospinal fluid can give a definitive diagnosis. The mortality rate among the symptomatic cases is between 10 and 30 percent and is higher where there is limited access to intensive care facilities, which may be required if paralysis leads to breathing or feeding problems. The World Health Organization (WHO) states that 10,000 to 15,000 deaths occur each year from Japanese encephalitis.

WHO reports that at least 30 percent of clinical cases of JEV result in permanent neurologic or psychiatric sequelae, where a sequela is a condition resulting from disease, injury, or other trauma in which an acute condition becomes more complicated, eventually resulting in a chronic condition. Survivors of Japanese encephalitis can be left with a variety of sequelae, including long-term disabilities such as movement problems, changes in behavior, blindness, and seizures.

Because intensive care is often needed in Japanese encephalitis to help the patient feed and breathe, there may also be various complications arising from the bacterial infections, such as pneumonia and urinary tract infection, that are common to any patient requiring incubation for breathing, elimination, or nutrition.

Japanese encephalitis is an arthropod-borne virus and is transmitted through the bite of the mosquito genus *Culex*, which breeds within grasses, fallow rice fields, ponds, and ditches, primarily by the species *Culex tritaeniorynchus.* The disease tends to occur mainly in rural areas but is also in urban areas with suitable conditions. Mosquitoes become infected with JEV through feeding on natural animal reservoirs of JEV, which are wild birds and domestic pigs. Once JEV has been transmitted to a human host through a mosquito bite, it may spread through the body and reach

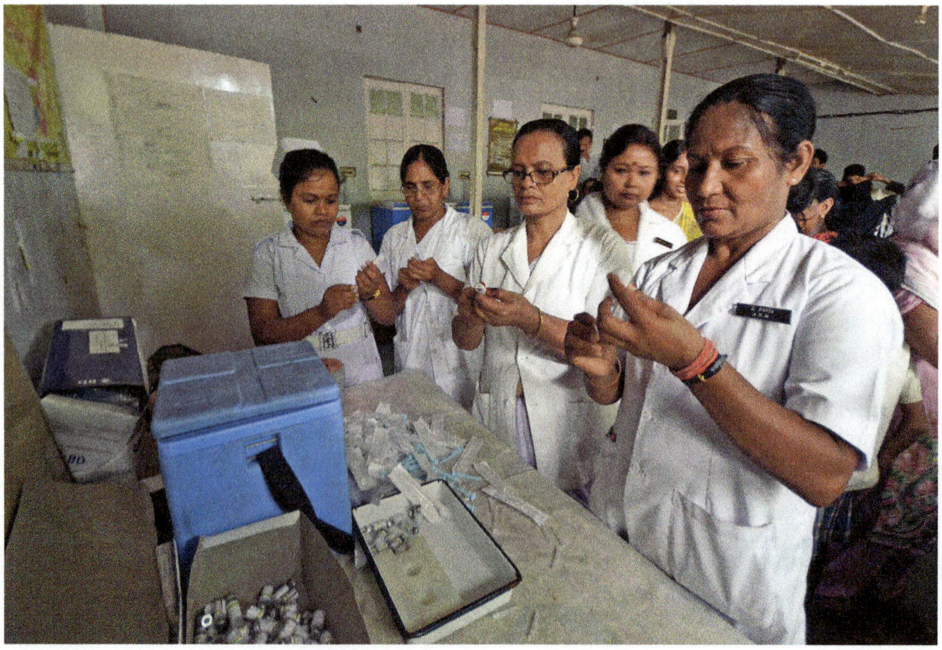

Health care workers in India prepare to give vaccinations against Japanese encephalitis. Transmitted by mosquitoes, the Japanese encephalitis virus is common in Asia and the western Pacific. *© Pacific Press/LightRocket/Getty Images*

the brain. The transmitting mosquitoes prefer to bite humans outdoors and are at their most active during dusk and the early morning hours (but are also active mid-afternoon and at night). JEV cannot be transmitted via direct person-to-person contact.

Scope and Distribution

Children and the elderly are the most likely to develop the symptomatic form of Japanese encephalitis. The disease is endemic in the countries of the Indian subcontinent, Southeast Asia, and northeastern Asia, including Japan. It is transmitted by *Culex* mosquitoes living in rural rice-growing and pig-farming regions or breeding in flooded rice fields, marshes, and standing water around rice fields. Research has shown that most people in endemic areas have been exposed to JEV, even though they may not have had any symptoms of encephalitis. The rate of symptomatic disease in an endemic area is estimated at about 1 per 150,000 people.

Japanese encephalitis is seasonal, as might be expected from a disease transmitted by mosquitoes whose activity depends on temperature. In temperate regions it occurs from June to September; in the subtropics the season is extended from April to October; and in tropical regions Japanese encephalitis occurs all year.

In the United States, just 12 cases were recorded between 1978 and 1993, and these were among expatriates, travelers, or military personnel returning from parts of the world where Japanese encephalitis is endemic. As of 2018 the rate of infection among US citizens remained at less than one case per year. In endemic areas those living in rural areas continue to be most at risk; the disease tends to occur less frequently in towns and cities. In general, the risk of travelers contracting JEV infection is low, but much depends on where they are residing and the length of potential exposure.

The diagnosis for JEV is difficult at times because its symptoms are not specific to only this malady. A person with symptoms of encephalitis (fever, lowered level of consciousness, neurological problems, and seizures) should be tested for JEV, especially if he or she is traveling in or has recently traveled to areas known to contain the disease. Diagnosis is usually confirmed with a sample of cerebrospinal fluid (in which specific antibodies are present), a lumbar puncture (also called a spinal tap), or a blood sample.

Treatment and Prevention

As of early 2018 there were no specific antiviral drugs effective against JEV. Treatment of Japanese encephalitis involves supportive treatment dealing with the symptoms of the disease. For instance, anticonvulsant drugs can be used to treat seizures. If neurological problems such as paralysis set in, intensive care is often needed to provide feeding and airway support.

DISEASE IN DEVELOPING NATIONS

In 2005, after an unusually heavy monsoon season, an epidemic of Japanese encephalitis occurred in India's most populous state, Uttar Pradesh. The outbreak soon spread into the neighboring state of Bihar and eventually crossed the border into Nepal. Officials in overcrowded hospitals filled every available space with Japanese encephalitis patients. Some families with children suffering from the disease even camped outside hospitals, hoping to gain access to treatment. After running out of oxygen masks, one Indian hospital fashioned makeshift oxygen masks out of cardboard rolled into cones. The outbreak resulted in more than 5,000 Japanese encephalitis cases and approximately 1,300 deaths, mostly among children.

There are a number of vaccines against JEV, some of which are only available in Asia. As of early 2018, there were four primary types of vaccines in use. These four vaccines are inactivated mouse brain–based vaccines, inactivated cell-based vaccines, live attenuated vaccines, and live chimeric vaccines. Vaccines are relatively expensive, primarily due to the necessity of providing three doses.

If a traveler is sleeping in a rural area where JEV is endemic, avoiding mosquito exposure is crucial. Bed nets treated with the proven mosquito repellent and insecticide DEET (N,N-diethyl-meta-toluamide) are recommended. It is best to avoid the outdoors during the evenings and at night and to stay in well-screened rooms. However, only certain *Culex* species transmit JEV, and only a small number of these mosquitoes are infected. Among those travelers who are infected with a JEV-bearing mosquito bite, only 1 in 50 to 1 in 1,000 will become ill with JEV.

Impacts and Issues

Although travelers are still considered at low risk of contracting Japanese encephalitis, Western interest in vacations to Asia has been on the increase in recent years. Therefore, there are potentially more people at risk of exposure. Advice on precautions and prevention changes frequently, so those traveling to countries such as Vietnam, Japan, India, or almost anywhere in Asia are recommended to seek travel health advice from their physician prior to departure. Vaccination may or may not be recommended, depending on the traveler's specific plans, but advice on reducing exposure to mosquitoes should always be heeded. WHO generally recommends immunization for JEV for any region of Asia where the disease is recognized as a public health problem.

There is a clear need for improved and cheaper vaccines against JEV, which could enable whole at-risk populations to be protected. Areas where vaccination is routine, such as China, Korea, and Japan, have tended not to have the epidemics that still occur in India, Nepal, and Myanmar, where vaccination is not yet the norm. In May 2006 WHO adopted a 10-year strategy to increase immunization coverage worldwide for several preventable diseases, including Japanese encephalitis. WHO is building on this effective strategy as the organization moves into 2018 and beyond.

As of 2018 vaccines using inactivated adjuvants (ingredients that create a stronger than normal immune response in the body), various types of viral strains, and genetically engineered substances are being considered. Advanced clinical trials of potential new preventions are being held based on these vaccines. In the meantime, it appears that the range of JEV may be extending and may continue to do so with global warming and increased frequency of international travel.

There have been two outbreaks of Japanese encephalitis in Australia: one in 1995 on islands in the Torres Strait and another in 1998 on the Cape York Peninsula. In 2004 JEV was found in mosquitoes on the Cape York Peninsula, indicating an ongoing risk from Japanese encephalitis. As of 2016 many outbreaks of JEV have occurred in the northern region of the Chiang Mai Valley in Thailand. Sporadic outbreaks have been found in and around the cities of Bangkok and Phitsanulok, in the central region of the country, and scattered about in its southern section.

See Also *African Sleeping Sickness (Trypanosomiasis); Arthropod-Borne Disease; Climate Change and Infectious Disease; Mosquito-Borne Diseases; St. Louis Encephalitis; West Nile*

BIBLIOGRAPHY

Books

Berger, Stephen. *Japanese Encephalitis: Global Status.* Los Angeles: GIDEON Informatics, 2015.

Prüss-Üstün, Annette, et al. *Preventing Disease through Healthy Environments: Towards an Estimate of the Environmental Burden of Disease.* Geneva: World Health Organization, 2016.

Tan, Tina Q., John P. Flaherty, and Melvin V. Gerbie. *The Vaccine Handbook: A Practitioner's Guide to Maximizing Use and Efficacy Across the Lifespan.* New York: Oxford University Press, 2018.

Turtle, Lance, et al. "Japanese Encephalitis Virus Infection." In *Viral Infections of the Human Nervous System*, edited by Alan C. Jackson, 271–293. Basel, Switzerland: Springer, 2013.

Periodicals

Connor, Bradley, and William B. Bunn. "The Changing Epidemiology of Japanese Encephalitis and New Data: The Implications for New Recommendations for Japanese Encephalitis Vaccine." *Tropical Disease, Travel Medicine and Vaccines* 3, no. 14 (August 1, 2017). This article can also be found online at https://tdtmvjournal.biomedcentral.com/articles/10.1186/s40794-017-0057-x (accessed February 15, 2018).

Websites

Ellerington, Alina. "Japanese Encephalitis." Encephalitis Society, December 2017. https://www.encephalitis.info/japaneseencephalitis?gclid=Cj0KCQiA_JTUBRD4ARIsAL7_VeU9jpuLE074M7r78ZxAUvongEtvtrzzHLkH19KNR9SHV-6MDT2Ps5IaAqaDEALw_wcB (accessed February 15, 2018).

"Japanese Encephalitis." World Health Organization. http://www.who.int/immunization/research/development/japanese_encephalitis/en/ (accessed February 15, 2018).

"Selective Vaccinations: Japanese Encephalitis." International Association for Medical Assistance to Travelers, September 20, 2016. https://www.iamat.org/country/thailand/risk/japanese-encephalitis (accessed February 15, 2018).

"Travelers' Health: Japanese Encephalitis." Centers for Disease Control and Prevention, November 24, 2015. https://wwwnc.cdc.gov/travel/diseases/japanese-encephalitis (accessed February 15, 2018).

Susan Aldridge
William Arthur Atkins

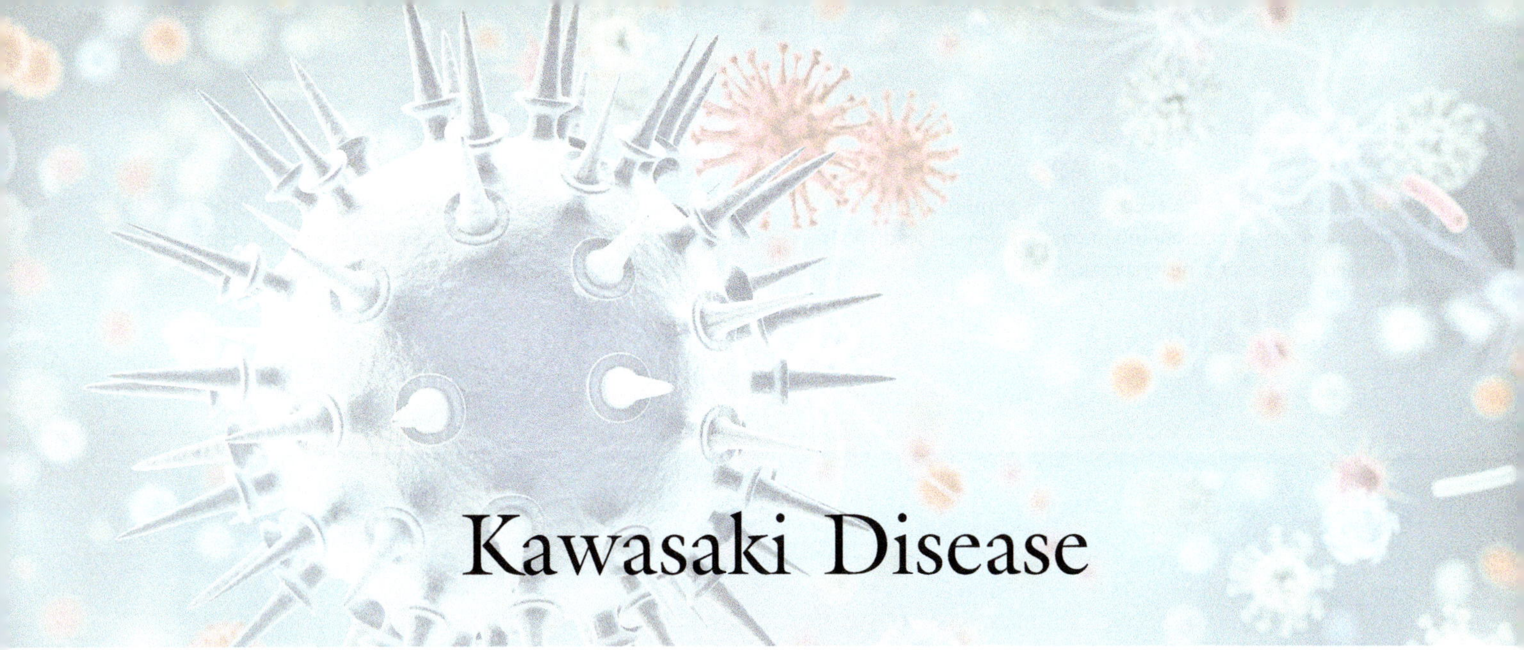

Kawasaki Disease

Introduction

Kawasaki disease, also referred to as Kawasaki syndrome, is a disease of unknown cause that can affect children of any age but tends to be most prevalent in children younger than five. It is a form of vasculitis (an inflammation of the arteries). The disease causes acute symptoms including fever, rash, swelling, irritations in the eyes and around the mouth, and red or peeling hands and feet.

In more serious cases, Kawasaki disease can lead to heart complications such as congestive heart failure, along with coronary artery dilation and aneurysms (thinned, weakened areas of arteries), both of which increase the risk of heart attacks. Kawasaki is a leading cause of acquired heart disease in children, with around 25 percent of children with untreated Kawasaki disease developing aneurysms.

Kawasaki disease occurs worldwide, with a higher occurrence in East Asia than in other parts of the world. It is treatable using an administration of aspirin and gamma globulin (a group of proteins in blood plasma that contains many antibodies). Because the risk of heart complications is enhanced when treatment is delayed or not given, treatment is vital to prevent complications. Because its causes are unknown, there is no known way to prevent contracting Kawasaki disease.

Disease History, Characteristics, and Transmission

Kawasaki disease was first described by Tomisaku Kawasaki (1925–) in Japan in 1967. The disease mostly affects children and has become the most common cause of heart disease in children from developed countries. The cause of this disease is unknown. The incidence of Kawasaki disease is also higher in Japan, South Korea, and Taiwan and greatest in individuals of East Asian and Pacific Island descent. This suggests that there may be a genetic component that predisposes individuals to the disease.

After acquiring Kawasaki disease, patients develop acute (rapid-onset) symptoms. These include inflammation of arteries, organs, and tissues; fever; rash; swelling of the hands and feet; swollen lymph nodes; irritation and inflammation of the mouth, lips (often cracked), and tongue (called strawberry tongue); red eyes; and red palms of the

WORDS TO KNOW

ANTIBODIES Proteins found in the blood that help fight against foreign substances called antigens. Antigens, which are usually proteins or polysaccharides, stimulate the immune system to produce antibodies, or Y-shaped immunoglobulins. The antibodies inactivate the antigen and help remove it from the body. While antigens can be the source of infections from pathogenic bacteria and viruses, organic molecules detrimental to the body from internal or environmental sources also act as antigens. Genetic engineering and the use of various mutational mechanisms allow the construction of a vast array of antibodies (each with a unique genetic sequence).

GAMMA GLOBULIN A group of soluble proteins in the blood, most of which are antibodies that can mount a direct attack on pathogens and can be used to treat various infections.

PREVALENCE The actual number of cases of disease (or injury) that exist in a population.

hands and soles of the feet. Chronic symptoms include coronary artery dilatation and aneurysms, which lead to an increased chance of a heart attack.

Because the cause of the disease is unknown, little is known about the transmission of Kawasaki disease. However, it is known that the disease is not contagious.

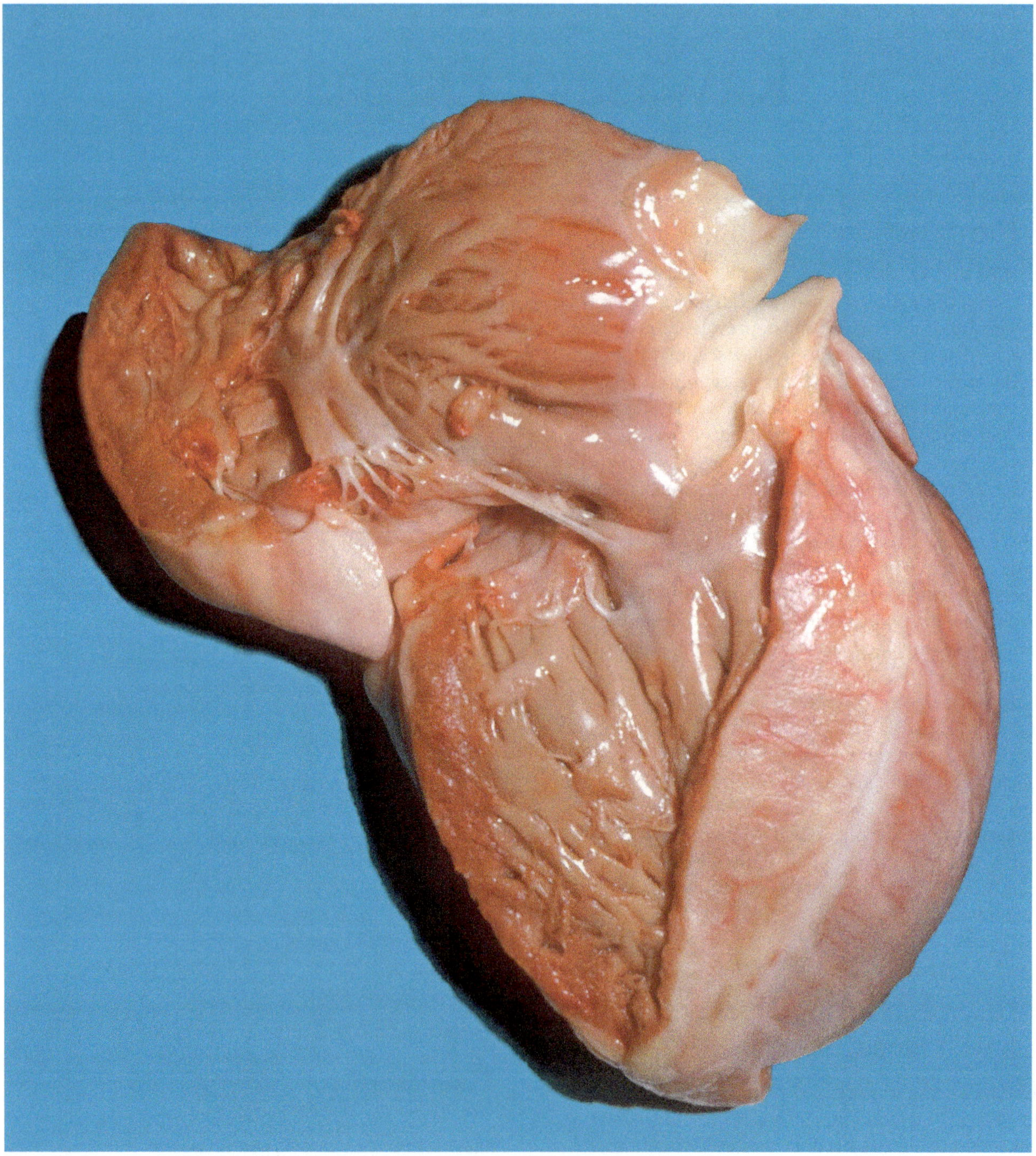

Kawasaki syndrome can affect children of any age but tends to be most prevalent in children younger than five. The disease causes acute symptoms, including fever, rash, swelling, and, in more serious cases, heart complications. © *Biophoto Associates/Science Source*

Scope and Distribution

Kawasaki disease was first diagnosed in Japan, and the highest incidence of this disease remains in East Asia. However, Kawasaki disease occurs worldwide. In the United States, around 9 to 19 people out of 100,000 develop the disease.

Children under age five are at greatest risk of developing Kawasaki disease. In 2000 (the last year data was available) 77 percent of all children in the United States being treated for Kawasaki disease were under age five. However, older children, including teenagers, also develop the disease. Worldwide, cases of Kawasaki disease are uncommon before six months. This is perhaps related to the protective action of maternal antibodies.

Incidence of Kawasaki disease also appears to be influenced by sex and race. Males tend to be more prone to developing the disease, as are children of East Asian or Pacific Island descent, especially people of Japanese descent.

Most incidences of Kawasaki disease occur during winter or early spring.

Treatment and Prevention

In 2017 the American Heart Association (AHA) published updated treatment guidelines for Kawasaki disease. The AHA stated that the goal of treatment was to prevent or reduce damage to the arteries. Treatment should begin as soon as possible after diagnosis, ideally no longer than 10 days after onset of the illness.

People who are in the acute phase of Kawasaki disease require hospitalization, during which time they are treated with aspirin and a high dose of intravenous gamma globulin (IVIG). IVIG treatment contains antibodies and comes from donor plasma. This treatment is given for 10 to 12 hours and acts primarily to lower the risk of heart complications. Aspirin is also administered every six hours for both its anti-inflammatory action and to lower fever. Depending on the outcome of treatment, aspirin may be prescribed for six to eight weeks after the acute phase of the disease or indefinitely.

After treatment, patients should be monitored. The severity of the disease will indicate how long the patient needs to be monitored. Someone with no heart complications may only need a year of monitoring, while someone with severe heart complications may need to be monitored indefinitely. Monitoring includes assessing heart health and checking to see if the patient has inducible myocardial ischemia (blocking of the coronary arteries). People who have had Kawasaki disease should stay physically active to keep their heart healthy.

Women who have had moderate to severe heart complications from the disease should avoid certain oral contraceptives (birth control pills) and should work with a team of physicians, including a cardiologist, throughout any subsequent pregnancy and delivery. Successful pregnancies in women who have had giant aneurysms from Kawasaki disease have been reported, as well as many successful pregnancies in women who had less severe heart complications.

In the majority of cases where treatment is given within 10 days after disease onset, recovery from acute symptoms is complete and heart problems are unlikely. However, the risk of developing heart problems increases the longer the patient goes without treatment, and some patients do not respond well to treatment.

Although recovery from the acute symptoms of Kawasaki disease is possible without treatment, the risk of heart problems is significant. Untreated Kawasaki disease increases the likelihood of heart problems and other complications such as arthritis, meningitis, and death. Because the cause of this disease is unknown, there is no definitively known way to prevent contracting it.

Symptoms of Kawasaki Disease

Phase 1

A fever of 102.2°F (39.0°C) or higher that lasts for more than three days
Red eyes with no discharge
Rash on the genitals and trunk of the body
Red, swollen tongue and red, swollen, and cracked lips
Red, swollen skin on soles of feet and palms of hands
Swollen lymph nodes (especially in the neck)
Irritability

Phase 2

Peeling skin on hands and feet
Diarrhea
Vomiting
Abdominal pain
Joint pain

Phase 3

Diminishing symptoms, unless complications develop

SOURCE: Mayo Clinic

Impacts and Issues

Kawasaki disease is the leading cause of acquired heart problems in children less than five years of age who live in developed countries. It achieved this distinction after the incidence of scarlet fever (along with the rheumatic heart disease that often accompanied it) dropped dramatically as a result of the introduction of antibiotics in the 1940s.

Because there is no current prevention against contracting Kawasaki disease, it is important that patients be identified and treated as soon as possible. The risk of heart disease and other medical complications increases when treatment is not administered or when treatment is delayed.

This is another reason why rapid administration of treatment is necessary. Determining the cause of the disease would increase the likelihood of being able to control and prevent Kawasaki disease. Research has been conducted since the disease was first diagnosed in 1967. However, the specific cause for the disease remains unknown. In addition, it remains unknown whether the disease is caused by reaction to a chemical or toxin or is a classic infectious disease of bacterial or viral origin. Current research points to an infectious trigger for the disease, but many scientists believe that certain genes play a role.

SEE ALSO *Childhood-Associated Infectious Diseases, Immunization Impacts; Demographics and Infectious Disease; Immune Response to Infection*

BIBLIOGRAPHY

Books

Saji, Ben Tsutomu, et al., eds. *Kawasaki Disease: Current Understanding of the Mechanism and Evidence-Based Treatment.* Tokyo: Springer, 2017.

Periodicals

McCrindle, Brian W., et al. "Diagnosis, Treatment, and Long-Term Management of Kawasaki Disease: A Scientific Statement for Health Professionals from the American Heart Association." *Circulation* 135, no. 17 (2017): e927–e999. This article can also be found online at http://circ.ahajournals.org/content/135/17/e927.short (accessed February 5, 2018).

Pinches, Helene, et al. "Asymptomatic Kawasaki Disease in a 3-Month Old Infant." *Pediatrics* 138, no. 2 (2016): e1–4. This article can also be found online at http://pediatrics.aappublications.org/content/pediatrics/138/2/e20153936.full.pdf (accessed February 5, 2018).

Principi, Nicola, Donato Rigante, and Susanna Esposito. "The Role of Infection in Kawasaki Syndrome." *Journal of Infection* 67, no. 1 (July 2013): 1–10. This article can also be found online at http://www.journalofinfection.com/article/S0163-4453(13)00077-7/abstract (accessed February 5, 2018).

Saguil, Aaron, and Matthew Fargo. "Diagnosis and Management of Kawasaki Disease." *American Family Physician* 91, no. 6 (March 15, 2015): 365–371. This article can also be found online at https://www.aafp.org/afp/2015/0315/p365.html (accessed February 5, 2018).

Uehara, Ritei, and Ermias D. Belay. "Epidemiology of Kawasaki Disease in Asia, Europe, and the United States." *Journal of Epidemiology* 22, no. 2 (2012): 79–85. This article can also be found online at https://www.jstage.jst.go.jp/article/jea/22/2/22_JE20110131/_article/-char/ja/ (accessed February 5, 2018).

Websites

"Kawasaki Disease." US National Library of Medicine—Genetics Home Reference, January 30, 2018. https://ghr.nlm.nih.gov/condition/kawasaki-disease#statistics (accessed February 5, 2018).

"Kawasaki Syndrome." Centers for Disease Control and Prevention, December 13, 2013. https://www.cdc.gov/kawasaki/ (accessed February 5, 2008).

"Kawasaki Syndrome." US Department of Health & Human Services—National Heart, Lung, and Blood Institute. https://www.nhlbi.nih.gov/health-topics/kawasaki-disease (accessed February 5, 2018).

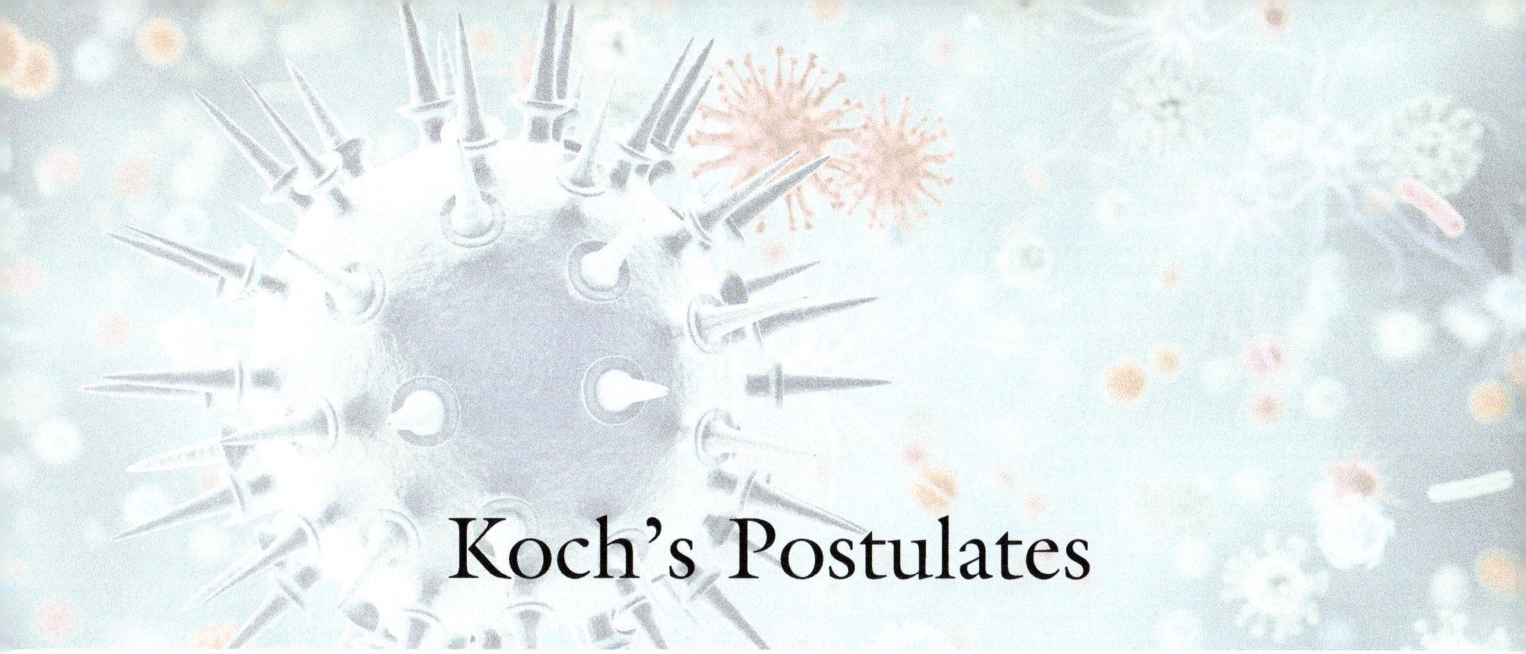

Koch's Postulates

Introduction

Koch's postulates are a set of principles that guide scientific efforts to establish the cause of an infectious disease. Koch's postulates are named after the German physician Robert Koch (1843–1910), who was the first scientist to identify several important pathogens (disease-causing agents). The postulates propose that a series of observational and experimental conditions must be satisfied before it is concluded that a particular microorganism causes a certain disease.

Because of advances in microbiology during the 20th and 21st centuries, Koch's postulates have been revised, but they remain relevant to modern research. For example, they have been extended to include nonliving molecular causes of disease such as prions (proteins that are infectious).

History and Scientific Foundations

Robert Koch was a German medical researcher. He is famous not only for formulating Koch's postulates but also for using them to identify the pathogens that cause some of the deadliest diseases afflicting humankind, including anthrax, cholera, and tuberculosis. Along with French physician Louis Pasteur (1822–1895), Koch is considered one of the pioneers of bacteriology (the study of bacteria). Working at home in an improvised laboratory, without assistance from any university, rich patron, or government agency, Koch proved that anthrax is caused by a bacterium. This was the first time that a disease was shown to be caused by a specific microorganism. Koch received a Nobel Prize in Medicine in 1905.

Koch's postulates are four rules for deciding whether the scientific evidence warrants concluding that a certain microorganism is the cause of a disease. They are as follows:

1. The organism must be found in all animals that have the disease, not present in healthy animals.

WORDS TO KNOW

CULTURE A single species of microorganism that is isolated and grown under controlled conditions. German bacteriologist Robert Koch first developed culturing techniques in the late 1870s. Following Koch's initial discovery, medical scientists quickly sought to identify other pathogens. In the 21st century bacteria cultures are used as basic tools in microbiology and medicine.

ETIOLOGY The study of the cause or origin of a disease or disorder.

PATHOGEN A disease-causing agent, such as a bacterium, a virus, a fungus, or another microorganism.

PRIONS Proteins that are infectious. Indeed, the name *prion* is derived from "proteinaceous infectious particles." The discovery of prions and confirmation of their infectious nature overturned a central dogma that infections were caused only by intact organisms, particularly microorganisms such as bacteria, fungi, parasites, or viruses. Because prions lack genetic material, the prevailing attitude was that a protein could not cause disease.

ULCER An open sore on the inside or outside of the body that is accompanied by disintegration or necrosis of the surrounding tissue.

CHALLENGES TO KOCH'S POSTULATES

In the years since the proposal and general acceptance of Koch's postulates, they have proven to have a number of limitations. For example, infectious organisms such as the bacterium *Mycobacterium leprae*, some viruses, and prions cannot be grown in artificial laboratory media. Additionally, the postulates are fulfilled for a human disease–causing microorganism by using test animals. Although a microorganism can be isolated from a human, the subsequent use of the organism to infect a healthy person is unethical. Fulfillment of Koch's postulates requires the use of an animal that mimics the human infection as closely as possible.

Another limitation of Koch's postulates concerns instances where a microorganism that is typically part of the normal flora of a host becomes capable of causing disease when introduced into a different environment in the host (e.g., *Staphylococcus aureus*) or when the host's immune system is malfunctioning (e.g., *Serratia marcescens*).

Despite these limitations, Koch's postulates remain useful in clarifying the relationship between microorganisms and disease.

2. It must be possible to isolate the organism from a diseased animal and grow it in pure culture (a nonliving nutritional medium in a container).
3. It must then be possible to infect a healthy animal with the organisms grown in culture.
4 The organism must then be isolated again from the experimentally infected animal.

In the late 19th century Koch's students used the principles that were later named in his honor to quickly identify the bacteria that cause bubonic plague, diphtheria, gonorrhea, leprosy, syphilis, tetanus, typhoid, and several other diseases.

Scientists have noted that the power of Koch's postulates as an aid to science comes not from their rigid application but from their encouragement of a spirit of scientific rigor. They serve as guidelines rather than as absolute rules for collecting the scientific evidence that will prove the cause of a given disease. Exceptions to Koch's postulates are numerous; for example, many pathogens, including those that cause giardiasis, polio, and acquired immunodeficiency syndrome (AIDS), can be carried asymptomatically, which violates the first postulate. That is, these pathogens can sometimes live and reproduce in an individual without making that individual sick. Koch's original first postulate has, therefore, been clarified in practice to: "The organism must be found in all animals that have the disease." Also, not all pathogens can grow in pure culture, as the second postulate requires; viruses and prions, for example, can only reproduce with the help of living cells.

Impacts and Issues

One modern example of fulfilling Koch's postulates involves Australian physician Barry Marshall (1951–) and his work with the bacterium *Helicobacter pylori.* Marshall, a gastroenterologist, studied the bacteria in the 1980s, after a colleague noticed that *H. pylori* was present in the stomachs of patients with gastrointestinal ulcers but not in patients without ulcers. Marshall set out to determine if *H. pylori* caused stomach ulcers, and he eventually succeeding in growing it in the laboratory. Lacking human test subjects, Marshall first determined that his stomach was without disease, then infected himself by drinking a mixture containing *H. pylori.* After about a week, Marshall began vomiting, and an endoscopy (examination with a thin, flexible, camera-mounted cable) proved he had developed severe inflammation in the lining of his stomach, from which *H. pylori* was recovered. By satisfying Koch's postulates, Marshall had proven that *H. pylori* could cause disease in humans. This revolutionized the treatment of stom-

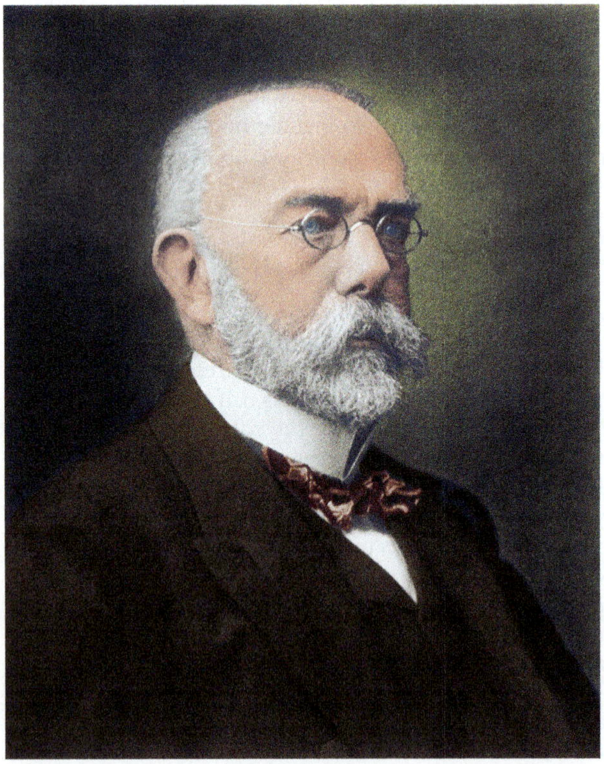

Robert Koch was a German scientist who won the 1905 Nobel Prize and helped establish the science of bacteriology. With Friedrich Loeffler, he formulated Koch's postulates, four criteria for determining a causative relationship between a microbe and a disease. *© Science Source*

ach ulcers, which had previously been attributed to stress and excess stomach acid. By the mid-1990s scientists recognized that stomach ulcers were caused by an infectious agent and could successfully be treated with antibiotics. In 2005 Marshall was awarded the Nobel Prize for his discovery.

Koch's postulates were also cited in the 1980s in a long and acrimonious debate in which American virologist Peter Duesberg (1936–) and a few others disagreed with a majority of other scientists over whether AIDS is in fact caused by the human immunodeficiency virus (HIV). Duesberg had long maintained that HIV does not cause AIDS (he believed AIDS was caused by recreational and other drugs). For some years he argued that HIV had not been shown to be the cause of AIDS according to the standards of Koch's postulates. In the mid-1990s, however, many researchers indicated that all of Koch's postulates had finally been fulfilled and that HIV had indeed been proved to be the cause of AIDS.

New infectious diseases are emerging at the rate of about one per year, but it is often difficult to discover the cause of a particular infectious disease. Koch's postulates, therefore, remain relevant in the 21st century. For example, the authors of a 2016 article in the *New England Journal of Medicine* used Koch's postulates, along with other criteria, to argue that the Zika virus, a new virus that emerged in early 2015, can cause birth defects in the children of infected mothers.

SEE ALSO *Bacterial Disease; Culture and Sensitivity;* Helicobacter pylori

BIBLIOGRAPHY

Books

Nester, Eugene W. *Microbiology: A Human Perspective.* 8th ed. New York: McGraw-Hill, 2016.

Periodicals

Byrd, Allyson L., and Julia A. Segre. "Adapting Koch's Postulates." *Science* 351, no. 6270 (January 15, 2016): 224–226. This article can also be found online at http://science.sciencemag.org/content/351/6270/224 (accessed January 16, 2018).

Nelson, Andrew, et al. "Polymicrobial Challenges to Koch's Postulates: Ecological Lessons from the Bacterial Vaginosis and Cystic Fibrosis Microbiomes." *Innate Immunity* 18, no. 5 (2012): 774–783. This article can also be found online at http://journals.sagepub.com/doi/pdf/10.1177/1753425912439910 (accessed January 16, 2018).

Rasmussen, Sonja A., et al. "Zika Virus and Birth Defects—Reviewing the Evidence for Causality." *New England Journal of Medicine* 374, no. 20 (May 19, 2016): 1981–1987. This article can also be found online at http://www.nejm.org/doi/full/10.1056/NEJMsr1604338#t=article (accessed January 16, 2018).

Tabrah, Frank L. "Koch's Postulates, Carnivorous Cows, and Tuberculosis Today." *Hawaii Medical Journal* 70, no. 7 (2011): 144–148. This article can also be found online at https://www.ncbi.nlm.nih.gov/pmc/articles/PMC3158372/ (accessed January 16, 2018).

Websites

Markel, Howard. "The Day We Discovered the Cause of the 'White Death.'" PBS NewsHour, March 24, 2015. https://www.pbs.org/newshour/health/march-24-1882-robert-koch-announces-his-discovery-of-the-cause-of-tuberculosis (accessed January 16, 2018).

Larry Gilman
Claire Skinner

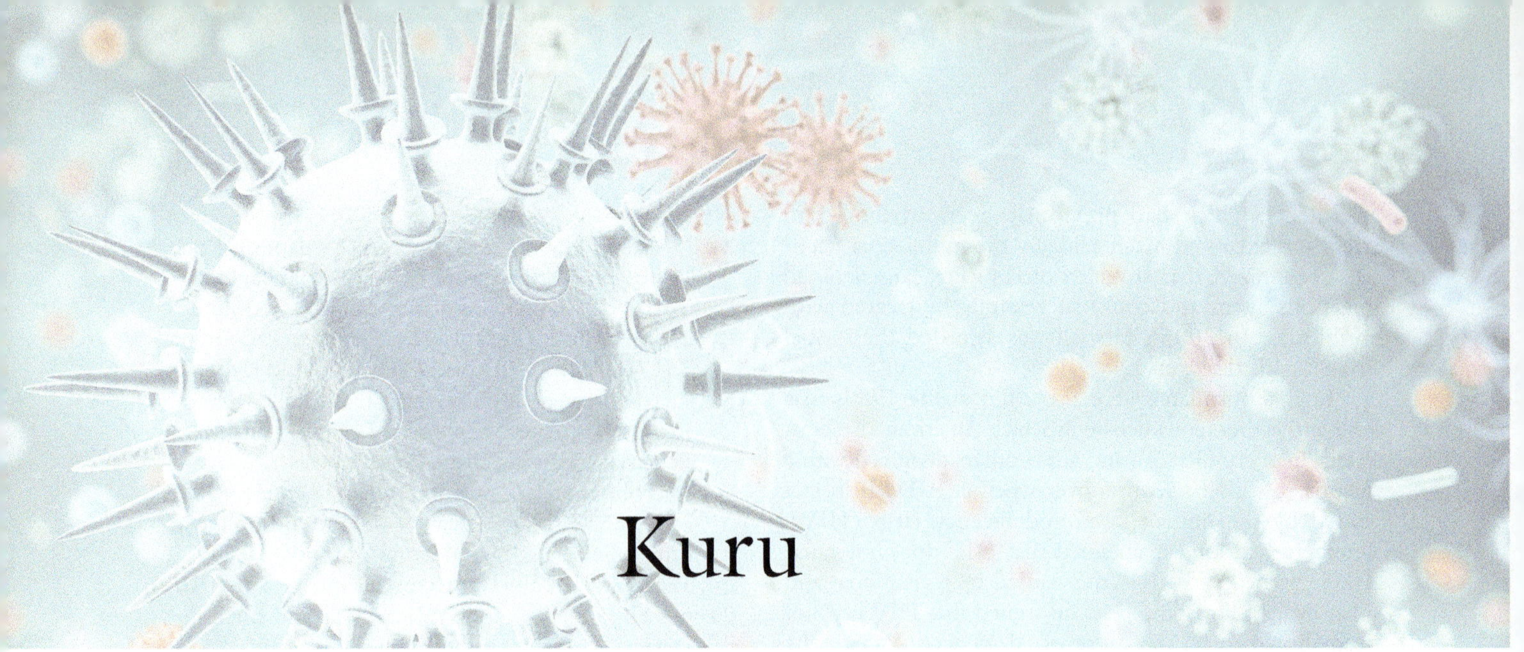

Kuru

Introduction

Kuru is a progressive, fatal brain disease that was discovered in the 1950s by American physician Carleton Gajdusek (1923–2008) among the Fore people of the eastern highlands of New Guinea. The name *kuru*, which means "trembling with fear" in the Fore dialect, refers to the tremor that is characteristic of the disease.

WORDS TO KNOW

EMERGING DISEASE A new infectious disease such as severe acute respiratory syndrome (SARS) or West Nile virus, as well as a previously known disease such as malaria, tuberculosis, or bacterial pneumonia that is appearing in a new form that is resistant to drug treatments.

ENCEPHALOPATHY Any abnormality in the structure or function of the brain.

INCUBATION PERIOD The time between exposure to a disease-causing virus or bacterium and the appearance of symptoms of the infection. Depending on the microorganism, the incubation time can range from a few hours, such as with food poisoning due to *Salmonella*, to a decade or more, such as with acquired immunodeficiency syndrome (AIDS).

PRIONS Proteins that are infectious. Indeed, the name *prion* is derived from "proteinaceous infectious particles." The discovery of prions and confirmation of their infectious nature overturned a central dogma that infections were caused only by intact organisms, particularly microorganisms such as bacteria, fungi, parasites, or viruses. Because prions lack genetic material, the prevailing attitude was that a protein could not cause disease.

Gajdusek won the Nobel Prize in medicine in 1976 for his research, which suggested that the disease was linked to the ritualistic handling or consumption of human brain tissue during funeral ceremonies. Kuru is one of a group of rare brain diseases called the transmissible spongiform encephalopathies (TSEs), which include Creutzfeldt-Jakob disease (CJD). Postmortem studies show that TSEs lead to the development of tiny holes in brain tissue, giving it a spongy appearance. After the Fore stopped the funeral practices that led to the spread of kuru, the disease disappeared.

Disease History, Characteristics, and Transmission

Kuru affected the cerebellum, which is the area at the base of the brain that controls coordinated movement. Accordingly, the symptoms of kuru included ataxia, or unsteadiness, tremor, stiffness, rigidity, and slurred speech. People with kuru did not usually suffer from memory loss or dementia until a later stage of the disease, or at all, although mood changes were common. Eventually, victims of kuru would become unable to stand or eat and would slip into a comatose state. Death from starvation or pneumonia would usually occur between three and nine months after the onset of symptoms.

Transmission of kuru occurred by exposure to infected brain tissue. The Fore custom was to remove the brains of the deceased during a funeral, possibly for ritualistic cooking and eating. The task of handling the brain fell to female relatives who were probably infected through cuts or sores on their skin or by consuming tissue. The women could also transmit the infection to their children through unwashed hands over the next several weeks. Once the disease entered the Fore food chain, it reached epidemic proportions.

TSEs such as kuru and CJD are unusual because the infective agent is a kind of infectious protein called a prion

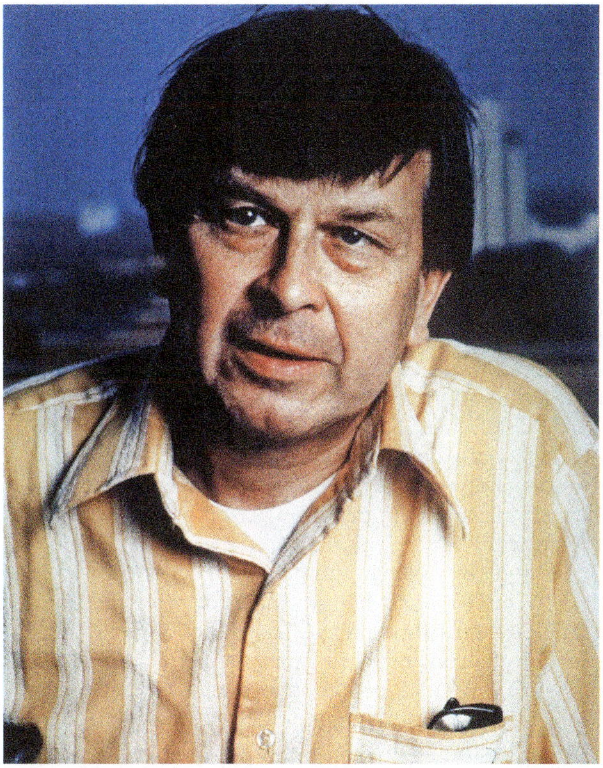

American physician Carleton Gajdusek discovered kuru—a progressive, fatal brain disease—among the Fore people of New Guinea. Gajdusek won the Nobel Prize for his research, which suggested that the disease was linked to the ritualistic handling or consumption of human brain tissue during funeral ceremonies. © *NLM/Science Source*

rather than a bacterium or virus. The long incubation time of kuru, which can be up to 40 years, meant that new cases continued to appear even as the funerary practices were abolished and the disease was no longer spread.

Scope and Distribution

Kuru was confined to the Fore people who lived in the eastern highlands of New Guinea. They were isolated from Western civilization and from other natives by mountainous terrain, and the disease has never been found elsewhere. Women and children of either sex seemed to be most at risk in the early years. Later, when adults who were exposed as children began to develop the disease, it affected men and women equally. During the 1950s and 1960s, it reached epidemic proportions and wiped out the population of many Fore villages.

Treatment and Prevention

There is no treatment for Fore or any TSE. Prevention of kuru required cessation of the funerary practices that allowed exposure to the infective prion. After the Fore ceased these practices in 1959, occasional cases still arose because of the long incubation time of the disease. The disease was first described in 1957, and the Fore people said that it had appeared only a few years before this. No one knows how kuru first arose. It is possible that a TSE crossed the species barrier from an animal with a similar disease and was spread by the consumption of the infected tissue.

Impacts and Issues

Kuru has both cultural and scientific significance. Decimated Fore populations in the 20th century endured upheaval to their communities and customs. Because more women than men died from the disease, Fore men were sometimes executed by village rulers to even out the population. Scientists initially assumed the disease was triggered by a genetic susceptibility, prompting the Australian government to restrict the movements of the Fore in an attempt to prevent intermarriage with islanders considered not susceptible. After Gajdusek discovered that kuru was caused by an infectious agent, the custom of honoring the dead by cannibalizing their tissue and brains ceased out of necessity.

Kuru might have remained as no more than a medical curiosity had it not turned out to be a TSE. The infective agent in all TSEs, including CJD, is neither a bacterium or a virus but an entity known as a prion, which is best described as an infectious protein. A prion is an abnormally shaped version of a protein that occurs naturally in the brain. When a normal prion protein comes into contact with the abnormal version, it is converted into the abnormal version and can go on to corrupt other normal prion protein molecules. This cascade of damage then spreads throughout the brain.

Interest in kuru was heightened with the emergence of variant CJD in the United Kingdom in the mid-1990s. The clinical course of kuru resembles that of variant CJD rather than classical CJD. Both are spread through consumption of exposure to infected tissue, and both may have arisen in the population in a similar way. Kuru could have started from a TSE from an unknown animal host. Variant CJD is the human form of bovine spongiform encephalopathy, a TSE of cattle thought to have started when scrapie, a sheep TSE, entered cattle feed. Therefore, although TSEs are rare, it is worthwhile to study their pathology, as circumstances could conspire to allow the emergence of a new type of this fatal brain disease.

PRIMARY SOURCE

How a History of Eating Human Brains Protected This Tribe from Brain Disease

SOURCE: *Kaplan, Sarah. "How a History of Eating Human Brains Protected This Tribe from Brain*

Disease." Washington Post *(June 11, 2015). This article can also be found online at https://www.washingtonpost.com/news/morning-mix/wp/2015/06/11/how-a-history-of-eating-human-brains-protected-this-tribe-from-brain-disease/?utm_term=.b0e8ce36e2f4 (accessed January 9, 2017).*

INTRODUCTION: *This article from the* Washington Post *examines how a genetic mutation present in the Fore people of Papua New Guinea may offer new insights into prion diseases.*

The sickness spread at funerals.

The Fore people, a once-isolated tribe in eastern Papua New Guinea, had a long-standing tradition of mortuary feasts—eating the dead from their own community at funerals. Men consumed the flesh of their deceased relatives, while women and children ate the brain. It was an expression of respect for the lost loved ones, but the practice wreaked havoc on the communities they left behind. That's because a deadly molecule that lives in brains was spreading to the women who ate them, causing a horrible degenerative illness called "kuru" that at one point killed 2 percent of the population each year.

The practice was outlawed in the 1950s, and the kuru epidemic began to recede. But in its wake it left a curious and irreversible mark on the Fore, one that has implications far beyond Papua New Guinea: After years of eating brains, some Fore have developed a genetic resistance to the molecule that causes several fatal brain diseases, including kuru, mad cow disease and some cases of dementia.

The single, protective gene is identified in a study published Wednesday in the journal *Nature*. Researchers say the finding is a huge step toward understanding these diseases and other degenerative brain problems, including Alzheimer's and Parkinson's.

The gene works by protecting people against prions, a strange and sometimes deadly kind of protein. Though prions are naturally manufactured in all mammals, they can be deformed in a way that makes them turn on the body that made them, acting like a virus and attacking tissue. The deformed prion is even capable of infecting the prions that surround it, reshaping them to mimic its structure and its malicious ways.

The prions' impact on their hosts is devastating and invariably fatal. Among the Fore, the prions riddled their victims' brains with microscopic holes, giving the organ an odd, spongy texture. In cattle, prions cause mad cow disease—they are responsible for the epidemic in Britain of the late '80s and '90s that required hundreds of thousands of cattle to be destroyed. They have been linked to a bizarre form of fatal insomnia that kills people by depriving them of sleep. And they're the source of the degenerative neurological disorder Creutzfeldt-Jakob disease (CJD), characterized by rapid dementia, personality changes, muscle problems, memory loss and eventually an inability to move or speak.

The vast majority of prion-diseases are "sporadic," seemingly appearing without cause. But a lead author of the *Nature* study, John Collinge, said in an interview with *Nature* that a portion of cases are inherited from one's parents, and an even smaller percentage are acquired from consuming infected tissue. Variant CJD, often called the "human mad cow disease," is caused by eating beef from infected cows.

Prions are especially insidious because there's no way of stopping them, science writer D.T. Max, author of a book on prions and fatal familial insomnia, told NPR in 2006. In the hierarchy of pathogens, they're even more elusive and difficult to quash than a virus. They can't be treated with antibiotics or radiation. Formalin, usually a powerful disinfectant, only makes them more virulent. The only way to clean a prion-contaminated object is with massive amounts of extremely harsh bleach, he said. But that technique isn't helpful in treating a person who has already been infected.

The study by Collinge and his colleagues offers a critical insight into ways that humans might be protected from the still-little-understood prions. They found it by examining the genetic code of those families at the center of the Fore's kuru epidemic, people who they knew had been exposed to the disease at multiple feasts, who seemed to have escaped unscathed.

When the researchers looked at the part of the genome that encodes prion-manufacturing proteins, they found something completely unprecedented. Where humans and every other vertebrate animal in the world have an amino acid called glycine, the resistant Fore had a different amino acid, valine.

"Several individuals right at the epicenter of the epidemic, they have this difference that we have not seen anywhere else in the world," Collinge told *Nature*.

That minute alteration in their genome prevented the prion-producing proteins from manufacturing the disease-causing form of the molecule, protecting those individuals from kuru. To test whether it might protect them from other kinds of prion disease, Collinge—the director of a prion research unit at University College London—and his team engineered the genes of several mice to mimic that variation.

When the scientists re-created the genetic types observed in humans—giving the mice both the normal protein and the variant in roughly equal amounts—the mice were completely resistant to kuru and to CJD. But when they looked at a second group of mice that had been genetically modified to produce only the variant protein, giving them even stronger protection, the mice were resistant to every prion strain they tested—18 in all.

"This is a striking example of Darwinian evolution in humans, the epidemic of prion disease selecting a single genetic change that provided complete protection against an invariably fatal dementia," Collinge told Reuters.

The Fore aren't the only people to demonstrate prion resistance. More than a decade ago, Michael Alpers — a specialist on kuru who has studied the Fore since the 1960s and was a co-author of the *Nature* study—conducted similar research on prion protein genes in humans worldwide. In a study published in *Science*, he found that people as far-flung as Europe and Japan exhibited the genetic protection, indicating that cannibalism was once widespread and that prehistoric humans probably dealt with waves of kuru-like epidemics during our evolution.

But the gene found in the Fore is special because it seems to render mutant prion-producing proteins (the kind that would be passed down from one's parents, causing inherited prion diseases) incapable of producing any kind of prion whatsoever. It also stops the wild-type protein —the phenotype that most people have—from making malformed prions.

Scientists say that the benefits of this discovery don't stop at prion diseases, which are relatively rare—only about 300 cases are reported each year in the United States. According to Collinge, the process involved in prion diseases —prions changing the shape of the molecules around them and linking together to form long chains called "polymers" that damage the brain—is probably responsible for the deadly effects of all kinds of degenerative brain illnesses: Alzheimer's, Parkinson's and dementia chief among them.

According to the World Health Organization, there are 47.5 million people worldwide living with dementia. An additional 7.7 million are diagnosed each year.

If Collinge and his colleagues can understand the molecular mechanisms by which prions do their work—and how the prion-resistant gene stops them—they might better understand the misshapen proteins that are afflicting millions with those other degenerative brain illnesses.

Eric Minikel, a prion researcher at the Broad Institute in Cambridge, Mass., who was not involved in the study, was impressed by the finding.

SEE ALSO *Bovine Spongiform Encephalopathy (Mad Cow Disease); Creutzfeldt-Jakob Disease; Prion Disease*

BIBLIOGRAPHY

Books

Gajdusek, D. Carleton. *Journal of Further Explorations in the Kuru Region and in the Kukukuku Country, Eastern Highlands of Eastern New Guinea and of a Return to West New Guinea: December 25, 1963 to May 4, 1964.* Victoria, Australia: Leopold Classic Library, 2016.

Liberski, Pawel P., ed. *Prion Diseases.* New York: Springer, 2017.

Wilson, Walter R., and Merle A. Sande. *Current Diagnosis & Treatment in Infectious Diseases.* Vol. 2. New York: McGraw Hill, 2014.

Periodicals

Radford, Anthony, and Roy Scragg. "Discovery of Kuru Revisited: How Anthropology Hindered Then Enhanced Kuru Research." *Health and History* 15, no. 2 (2013): 29–52.

Websites

Khan, Zartash Zafar. "Kuru." Medscape, February 17, 2016. http://www.emedicine.com/med/topic1248.htm (accessed December 8, 2017).

"Kuru Information Page." National Institute of Neurological Disorders and Stroke, February 14, 2007. https://www.ninds.nih.gov/Disorders/All-Disorders/Kuru-Information-Page (accessed December 8, 2017).

Laura J. Cataldo

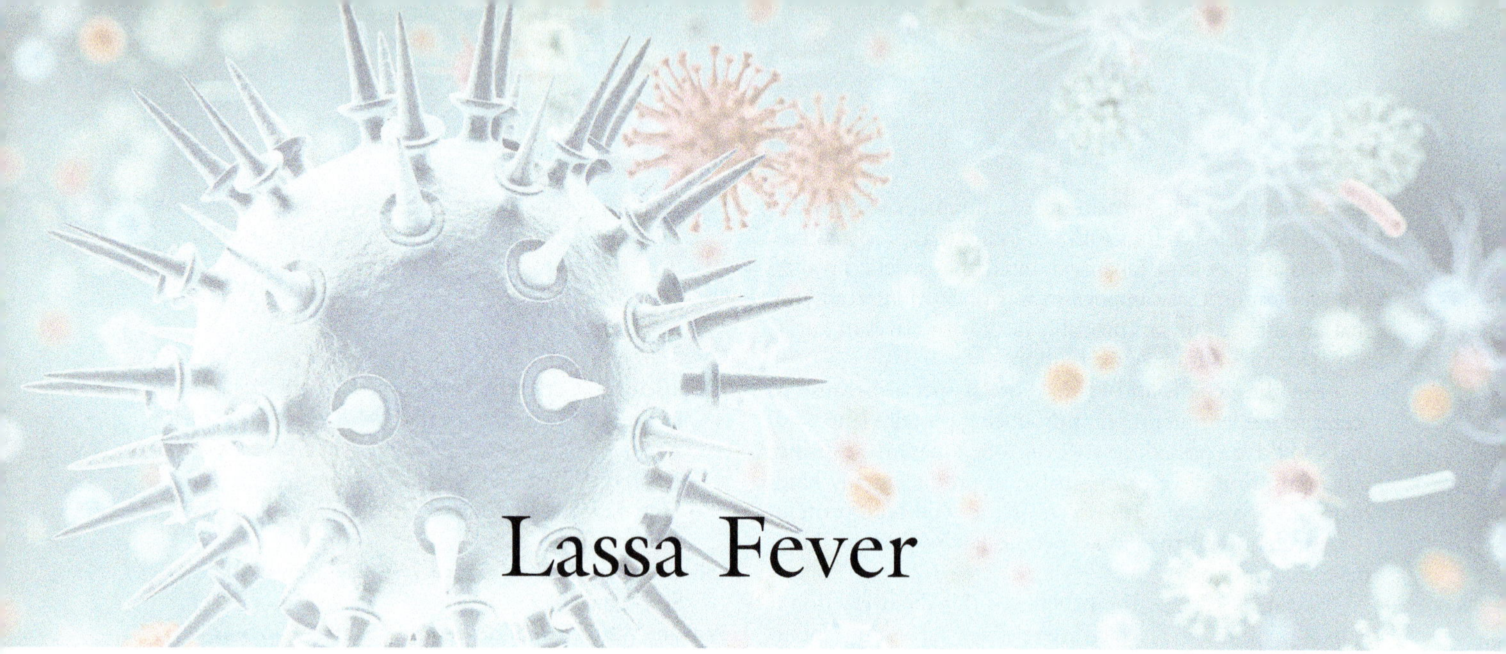

Lassa Fever

Introduction

Lassa fever is an animal-borne (zoonotic) virus that is transmitted via contact with contaminated urine or feces of the Natal multimammate rat (*Mastomys natalensis*). Rural regions of the West African countries Nigeria, Sierra Leone, Guinea, and Liberia, known as the "Lassa belt," experience intermittent outbreaks of Lassa fever.

According to the World Health Organization (WHO), following infection with Lassa virus, 80 percent of people remain symptom free or develop mild symptoms, while the remaining 20 percent develop a more severe illness. Symptoms increase in severity as infection progresses, with neurological problems and sometimes death occurring in the later stages. Lassa fever is treated via antiviral drugs in addition to symptom management. As no vaccine is available, prevention methods focus on avoiding contaminated food and other materials, avoiding rats, and taking precautions while in close contact with infected people.

Progress has been made in the treatment and prevention of Lassa fever. Work is also underway to improve diagnostic testing for the disease, as well as to create a human vaccine for the virus.

WORDS TO KNOW

ENDEMIC Present in a particular area or among a particular group of people.

RESERVOIR The animal or organism in which the virus or parasite normally resides.

SPECIAL PATHOGENS BRANCH A group within the US Centers for Disease Control and Prevention whose goal is to study highly infectious viruses that produce diseases within humans.

ZOONOSES Diseases of microbiological origin that can be transmitted from animals to people. The causes of the diseases can be bacteria, viruses, parasites, or fungi.

Disease History, Characteristics, and Transmission

Lassa fever was first described in the 1950s, although the virus responsible for the infection was not identified until 1969, when missionary nurses in Nigeria died from an infection caused by a virus identified as the Lassa virus. Lassa virus is a member of the Arenaviridae family and is transmitted to humans via contact with infected urine or droppings of certain species of rats.

Rats from the genus *Mastomys* are the reservoirs of Lassa virus. They are efficient hosts due to their high frequency of breeding and large number of offspring. Furthermore, they tend to colonize human habitats, increasing the chances of human exposure. *Mastomys* rats become infected with Lassa virus but do not become ill from it. Humans become infected following exposure to infected rat excreta, either directly or indirectly.

The virus is primarily transmitted when humans touch objects or eat food that is contaminated with rat excreta or when excreta comes in contact with cuts and sores. In addition, inhaling small particles of excreta in the air transmits the virus, as does consuming infected rats as food. According to Giovanni Lo Iacono and his coauthors of a 2014 study published in *PLOS Neglected Tropical Diseases*, about 20 percent of the time, Lassa fever is also transmitted between humans. This occurs following contact with infected body fluids such as blood, excretions, secretions, and tissues from infected humans.

Lassa fever is asymptomatic or mild in 80 percent of infected people. However, the remaining 20 percent experience severe disease in which many organs within the body are affected. Symptoms include fever, aches, vomiting, diarrhea, conjunctivitis (inflammation and redness of the conjunctiva of the eye), facial swelling, protein in the urine, and mucosal (mucous membranes such as in the nose and mouth) bleeding. Symptoms increase in severity as the isease progresses, leading to neurological problems such as hearing loss, tremors, and coma in the later stages. Symptoms usually take one to three weeks to appear and generally last for one to four weeks. According to the US Centers for Disease Control and Prevention (CDC), mortality rates have been estimated to be 1 percent in total and between 15 and 20 percent in hospitalized patients. In fatal cases death usually occurs within two weeks following the arise of symptoms. The disease is especially fatal in pregnant women in the last trimester.

Scope and Distribution

Lassa fever occurs predominantly in West Africa during the dry season (November to April). While it is endemic in certain countries, namely Guinea, Liberia, Sierra Leone, and Nigeria, the disease may exist in adjoining countries due to the wide distribution of the host rodent species. Between 1969 and 2017, there were seven imported cases from West Africa reported in the United States.

The CDC reports an annual infection rate of between 100,000 and 300,000 in West Africa and an annual death rate of about 5,000. As disease surveillance for Lassa fever is not uniformly undertaken, these estimates are rudimentary and subject to error. Lassa fever tends to be restricted to the rural regions of West Africa, particularly in areas where humans live in close proximity to the rats that are the main reservoir of the virus. Infections have also occurred as a consequence of laboratory exposure elsewhere in the world.

PREVENTION PROGRAMS

Control of Lassa fever has been set back by civil unrest within endemic countries such as Guinea, Liberia, and Sierra Leone. However, peace initiatives have led to steps being taken by these three countries to develop prevention and coping strategies for Lassa virus. These developments have been led by the Mano River Union Lassa Fever Network, which works to enhance diagnostic testing, improve clinical management, and perform environmental control. The Mano River Union Lassa Fever Network is supported by the health ministries of Guinea, Liberia, and Sierra Leone; the World Health Organization; and other government entities and groups.

The people who tend to be most at risk of infection with Lassa virus are those who reside in areas with high densities of *Mastomys* rats or those who come in contact with infected humans. Therefore, populations living in rural areas where rat populations are high, as well as hospital staff in these areas, are at the greatest risk. However, hospital staff greatly reduce their risk by taking preventive measures including standard and isolation precautions to avoid contact with the virus.

In addition, according to Iacono and colleagues, "infants, children, young adults, and pregnant women are disproportionately impacted by LF [Lassa fever]."

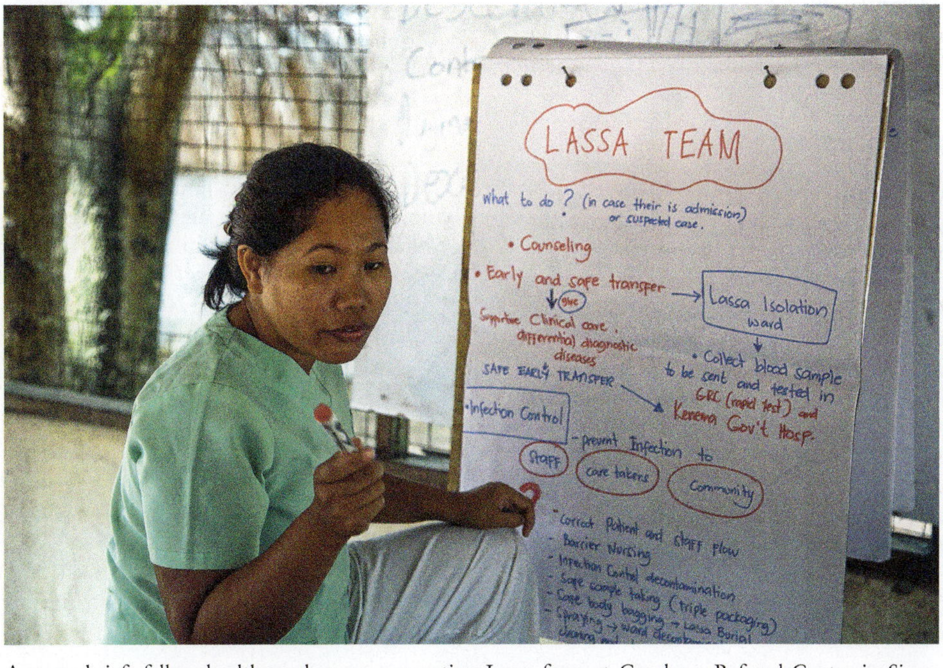

A nurse briefs fellow health workers on preventing Lassa fever at Gondama Referral Centre in Sierra Leone in 2014. Lassa fever is an animal-borne virus that is transmitted via contact with contaminated rat urine or feces. © *Lam Yik Fei/Getty Images*

Treatment and Prevention

Lassa fever is treated using the antiviral drug ribavirin. This drug has been shown to be effective against early stages of Lassa fever but does not appear to be as effective if given during the later stages of the illness. In addition to drug treatment, patients should receive supportive care. This includes caring for fever symptoms and maintaining fluid and electrolyte balance, along with blood pressure and oxygenation levels.

There is no vaccine for Lassa fever, but there is ongoing work to create one. A 2017 study published in *Human Vaccines and Immunotherapies* showed that a vaccine has been developed that fully protects nonhuman primates called cynomolgus macaques from Lassa fever. The authors wrote that the success of the vaccine in primates may indicate that a similar vaccine could work for humans.

Until the vaccine is tested and approved for human usage, prevention consists mainly of avoiding contact with potentially contaminated materials. Contamination from rat excreta can be avoided by discouraging rats from human living quarters through removing garbage from the home, keeping cats, and maintaining clean living quarters. Furthermore, keeping food stored in rodent-proof containers prevents food from becoming contaminated with infected rat excreta. Those in close contact with infected people, such as family members and health care workers, should wear gloves, gowns, face shields, and masks to prevent exchange of blood and body fluids.

Complete eradication of *Mastomys* is unlikely to occur due to their high prevalence in endemic areas. Therefore, avoidance rather than eradication appears to be the most effective way of preventing infection via rat excreta. To achieve avoidance, good hygiene practices, including storing food in rat-safe containers, are being promoted within infected communities.

Impacts and Issues

The symptoms of Lassa fever are common to a variety of viral fevers, and thus diagnosis is difficult and often requires diagnostic testing that can be both expensive and time consuming. Therefore, improved testing procedures would lead to increased accuracy of diagnosis and a more accurate idea of infection prevalence.

A poorly managed Lassa fever outbreak in January 2018 in Nigeria inspired members of the editorial board of the Nigerian paper the *National* to call out the government in an editorial. The editorial board argued that the government needed to better supply health care workers with hand sanitizer and protective clothing and equipment and hospitals with reliable running water and electricity. Lack of medical supplies, coupled with unreliable water and electric sources, in Lassa fever–affected communities contributes to the spread of the disease.

Exportation of Lassa fever, as well as diseases such as malaria and typhoid, occurs when travelers pass through endemic areas and become infected. This creates the threat that these diseases will become introduced to areas previously unaffected.

The Lassa virus is also considered a potential candidate for use as an agent of bioterrorism.

See Also *Airborne Precautions; Animal Importation; Antiviral Drugs; Malaria; Rapid Diagnostic Tests for Infectious Diseases; Travel and Infectious Disease; Typhoid Fever; Vaccines and Vaccine Development; War and Infectious Disease*

BIBLIOGRAPHY

Books

Singh, Sunit K., and Daniel Ruzek, eds. *Viral Hemorrhagic Fevers.* Boca Raton, FL: CRC, 2016.

Periodicals

"Another Lassa Fever Outbreak." *National* (January 23, 2018). http://thenationonlineng.net/another-lassa-fever-outbreak/ (accessed January 24, 2018).

Cashman, Kathleen A., et al. "A DNA Vaccine Delivered by Dermal Electroporation Fully Protects Cynomolgus Macaques against Lassa Fever." *Human Vaccines and Immunotherapies* 13, no. 12 (2017): 2902–2911. This article can also be found online at http://www.tandfonline.com/doi/full/10.1080/21645515.2017.1356500?scroll=top&needAccess=true (accessed January 24, 2018).

Iacono, Giovanni Lo, et al. "Using Modelling to Disentangle the Relative Contributions of Zoonotic and Anthroponotic Transmission: The Case of Lassa Fever." *PLOS Neglected Tropical Diseases* (January 8, 2015). This article can also be found online at http://journals.plos.org/plosntds/article?id=10.1371/journal.pntd.0003398 (accessed January 24, 2018).

Mylne, Adrian Q. N., et al. "Mapping the Zoonotic Niche of Lassa Fever in Africa." *Transactions of the Royal Society of Tropical Medicine and Hygiene* 109, no. 8 (August 1, 2015): 483–492. This article can also be found online at https://academic.oup.com/trstmh/article/109/8/483/1910156 (accessed January 24, 2018).

Websites

"Lassa Fever." Centers for Disease Control and Prevention (CDC), June 2, 2015. https://www.cdc.gov/vhf/lassa/ (accessed January 24, 2018).

"Lassa Fever." World Health Organization (WHO), July 2017. http://www.who.int/mediacentre/factsheets/fs179/en/ (accessed January 24, 2018).

Legionnaires' Disease (Legionellosis)

■ Introduction

Legionellosis refers to a disease caused by the bacteria *Legionella*. Most commonly the responsible organism is *Legionella pneumophila*.

The bacteria usually reside in freshwater creeks, ponds, and lakes. They can also be present in the water supply inside buildings, where they have entered the air via tiny water droplets from ventilation or water ducts.

There are two forms of legionellosis. The first is a more severe pneumonia that is known as Legionnaires' disease. The second includes a milder type of pneumonia and is called Pontiac fever.

■ Disease History, Characteristics, and Transmission

Legionellosis was first apparent in July 1976. At that time an outbreak of pneumonia occurred during an American Legion convention being held at the Bellevue-Stratford Hotel in Philadelphia, Pennsylvania. During the outbreak 221 veterans were sickened. Thirty-four of these people eventually died of the infection, which was later dubbed Legionnaires' disease.

The disease outbreak caused national alarm. It was feared to be the start of an epidemic of swine flu, which at

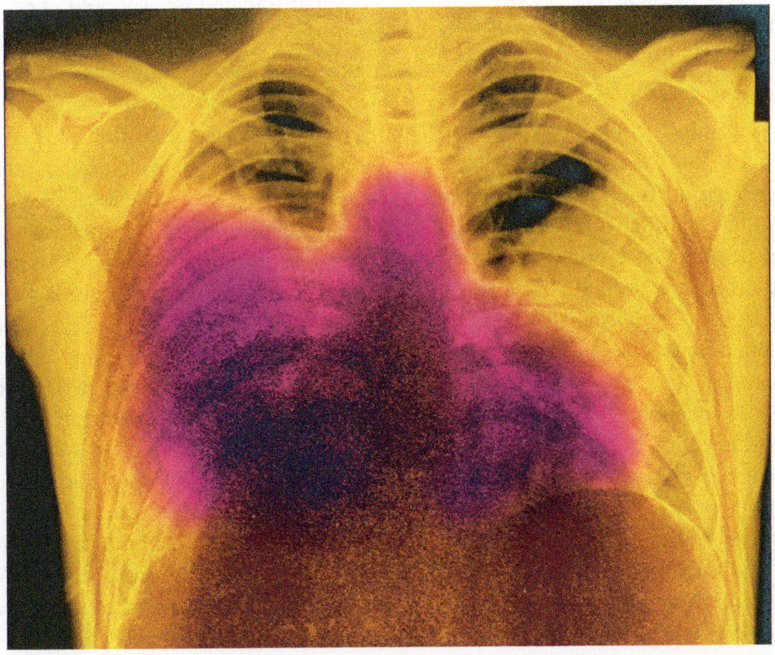

Lung inflammation caused by the bacterium *Legionella*. Commonly found in freshwater environments, the bacterium can sometimes be found in showerheads, hot tubs, and plumbing systems. © BSIP/UIG/Getty Images

WORDS TO KNOW

BIOFILM A population of microorganisms that forms following the adhesion of bacteria, algae, yeast, or fungi to a surface. These surface growths can be found in natural settings, such as on rocks in streams, and in infections, such as those that occur on catheters. Microorganisms can colonize living and inert natural and synthetic surfaces.

OPPORTUNISTIC INFECTION An infection that occurs in people whose immune systems are diminished or are not functioning normally. Such infections are opportunistic insofar as the infectious agents take advantage of their hosts' compromised immune systems and invade to cause disease.

the time was affecting Asia. However, an investigation conducted by the US Centers for Disease Control and Prevention (CDC) determined that the Philadelphia outbreak was due to a newly discovered bacterium, eventually named *L. pneumophila*.

The outbreak was traced to bacteria growing in the hotel's cooling tower. Later investigators showed that the bacterium is capable of growth as a surface-adherent structure called a biofilm. It is likely that bits of the biofilm broke off and were sucked into the hotel's ventilation system and that the bacteria were inhaled. Other outbreaks have been traced to biofilms growing on showerheads and in contaminated drinking water.

Legionellosis is an example of an opportunistic infection, or an infection caused in some people by a bacterium that normally is not harmful. For example, studies have determined that 5 to 10 percent of Americans carry *Legionella* antibodies even though they have not developed legionellosis. However, in people whose immune systems are less capable of fighting off an infection, the bacteria can cause disease. Pneumonia due to *Legionella* is responsible for 2 to 15 percent of all pneumonia cases in US hospitals, according to the CDC.

Most cases of legionellosis (over 90 percent) are caused by *L. pneumophila*. *L. micdadei* and *L. dumoffi* can also cause legionellosis, especially in people who are immunocompromised. Other organs that can be infected include the lymph nodes, the brain, the kidney, the liver, the spleen, bone marrow, and the lining around the heart.

The equipment most often involved in outbreaks of legionellosis are cooling towers, humidifiers, respiratory therapy equipment, whirlpool spas, showers, and faucets.

Some people who are infected contract Pontiac fever, an illness that appears suddenly but does not persist long.

Approximately 6,000 Americans acquire Legionnaires' disease every year. The death rate is about 10 percent. The people who are the most likely to become ill are over age 50. The risk is greater for those with diminished immune system function due to illness, diabetes, cigarette smoking, or immunosuppressing drugs. Legionnaires' disease can occur in children but is not normally considered a childhood disease. Children who are at risk are those who are on a respirator to assist with breathing and those whose immune systems are impaired due to recent surgery or drug treatment. Curiously, those infected with the human immunodeficiency virus (HIV) or who have developed acquired immunodeficiency syndrome (AIDS) do not appear to be at higher risk than others. However, when people with HIV/AIDS contract the disease, their symptoms are often more severe.

Legionnaires' disease is caused by inhaling *Legionella* suspended in minute water droplets or by aspirating *Legionella* bacteria, which occurs when particles bearing the bacteria escape the gag reflex and fall directly into the respiratory tract. The bacteria can be naturally found in bodies of freshwater and whirlpool spas (the source of the first outbreak of Pontiac fever), where they can be dispersed into the air by the action of wind and waves. In addition, the bacteria growing within biofilms in stagnant water at the intake of air-conditioning cooling towers, humidifiers, faucets, showerheads, and even the water misters in supermarket produce departments can slough off and be carried on water droplets. Person-to-person transmission has not been demonstrated.

When inhaled or aspirated, *Legionella* bacteria enter the lungs. Normally, as bacteria enter the lungs, they are engulfed and dissolved by cells called alveolar macrophages. However, *Legionella* are able to grow and divide inside the macrophages. Eventually the infected macrophages burst, releasing the bacteria, which infect other macrophages and continue the cycle of infection.

The symptoms of legionellosis develop 2 to 10 days after inhalation of the bacteria. At first the symptoms include a feeling of tiredness, headache, fever, chills, muscle aches, and loss of appetite. A fever of up to 104°F (40°C) can develop. A dry and hacking cough also develops and can change to a cough that involves the release of bloody mucus. Pneumonia affects breathing in about 50 percent of people and can cause chest pain in about 30 percent of those who get the infection. Some people develop a decreased heart rate, which can be dangerous when combined with the decreased breathing capability of the lungs.

In addition, legionellosis can involve other areas of the body. Less common complications include diarrhea, nausea with vomiting, abdominal pain, kidney failure, impaired urine production (which allows the buildup of toxic byproducts of body processes), and diminished mental capacity.

Pontiac fever is a milder form of legionellosis that does not involve the lower respiratory tract. The symptoms, which are flu-like and which typically appear within two days of exposure to the bacteria, include fever, headache, muscle aches, and fatigue. The infection passes within a few days. Often, infected persons do not seek medical treatment.

■ Scope and Distribution

Legionellosis can occur almost anywhere in the world. An outbreak occurred between August and October 2017 in Anaheim, California. Most of the illnesses were linked to the Disneyland amusement park. Bacteria from a contaminated cooling system in the park sickened 15 people and killed 2.

■ Treatment and Prevention

Cases of legionellosis that occur as part of an outbreak are usually diagnosed more quickly than isolated cases. Diagnosis is complicated by the fact that the early symptoms and appearance of the chest in an X-ray are similar to other types of bacterial or viral pneumonia. Prompt diagnosis and treatment results in a better prognosis for people with legionellosis. Death occurs about 5 percent of the time for previously healthy individuals and almost 25 percent of the time for people who were already ill or whose immune system was impaired when they contracted the disease. In severe cases that require mechanical assistance for breathing and kidney function, the death rate can be over 65 percent.

Legionellosis can be diagnosed by detecting antibodies to *L. pneumophila* produced by the immune system. A number of tests use the antibodies to detect the bacteria. For example, the antibodies can be linked to a fluorescent probe, and when samples are treated with the fluorescent antibody, *L. pneumophila* will appear as bright objects upon microscopic examination. Other tests can detect the presence of protein components of the bacteria in the urine or the presence of the bacterial genetic material in urine and other body fluid.

Because legionellosis is caused by bacteria, it is treated with antibiotics. As the bacteria reproduce inside host cells, the antibiotics must be capable of penetrating into the host cells. Typically, levofloxacin or azithromycin are used. Prompt antibiotic therapy leads to a complete recovery in most cases.

Legionellosis is prevented by keeping ductwork, pipes, cooling towers, showerheads, and other potential breeding spots clean and free of stagnant water. In reality, this sort of vigilance can be difficult to maintain unless a mandated and inspection schedule is imposed and documentation required.

REAL-WORLD RISKS

The US Centers for Disease Control and Prevention stated:

- About 6,000 cases of Legionnaires' disease were reported in the United States in 2015. However, because Legionnaires' disease is likely underdiagnosed, this number may underestimate the true incidence.
- About one out of every 10 people who get sick from Legionnaires' disease will die.
- People can get Legionnaires' disease or Pontiac fever when they breathe in small droplets of water in the air that contain Legionella.
- In general, people do not spread Legionnaires' disease to other people. However, this may be possible in rare cases.
- Legionella is found naturally in freshwater environments such as lakes and streams. It can become a health concern when it grows and spreads in human-made water systems.
- Keeping *Legionella* out of water systems in buildings is key to preventing infection.

As of 2017 there was no vaccine for legionellosis.

■ Impacts and Issues

In the aftermath of the Philadelphia outbreak, regulations governing the cleaning and monitoring of air-conditioning systems in public places were changed to minimize the development of *L. pneumophila*.

Legionellosis has the most impact in places where people gather and which are ventilated or have shower facilities. Examples include indoor recreation centers, pools, spas, hotels, and hospitals. The latter is especially important because ill people are even more susceptible to the infection. Construction workers can also be at increased risk because the bacteria may be dispersed into the air during excavation of a site.

In contrast to diseases such as bacterial meningitis and AIDS, there is no indication that poorer regions of the world are any more at risk than the wealthier developed world. Indeed, the association of legionellosis with facilities such as hospitals and hotels has made the disease more of a problem in developed countries.

See Also *Opportunistic Infection; Water-Borne Disease*

BIBLIOGRAPHY

Books

Delort, Anne-Marie, and Pierre Amato, eds. *Microbiology of Aerosols.* Hoboken, NJ: Wiley, 2017.

Kumar, Sandeep, Jane C. Benjamin, and Shubhra Shukla. *Pathogenic Bacteria in Bioaerosol of Hospitals: Important of Airborne Pathogen in Hospital.* New York: Lap Lambert Academic, 2013.

Periodicals

Fast, Shannon M., Marta C. González, and Natasha Markuzon. "Cost-Effective Control of Infectious Disease Outbreaks Accounting for Societal Reaction." *PLOS One* 8 (2015): 211–223.

Websites

"Infection Control." Centers for Disease Control and Prevention, January 7, 2016. https://www.cdc.gov/infectioncontrol/index.html (accessed November 15, 2017).

"Legionella (Legionnaires' Disease and Pontiac Fever)." Centers for Disease Control and Prevention, June 1, 2017. https://www.cdc.gov/legionella/fastfacts.html (accessed November 15, 2017).

Legionella.org. http://www.legionella.org/ (accessed December 7, 2017).

Brian Hoyle

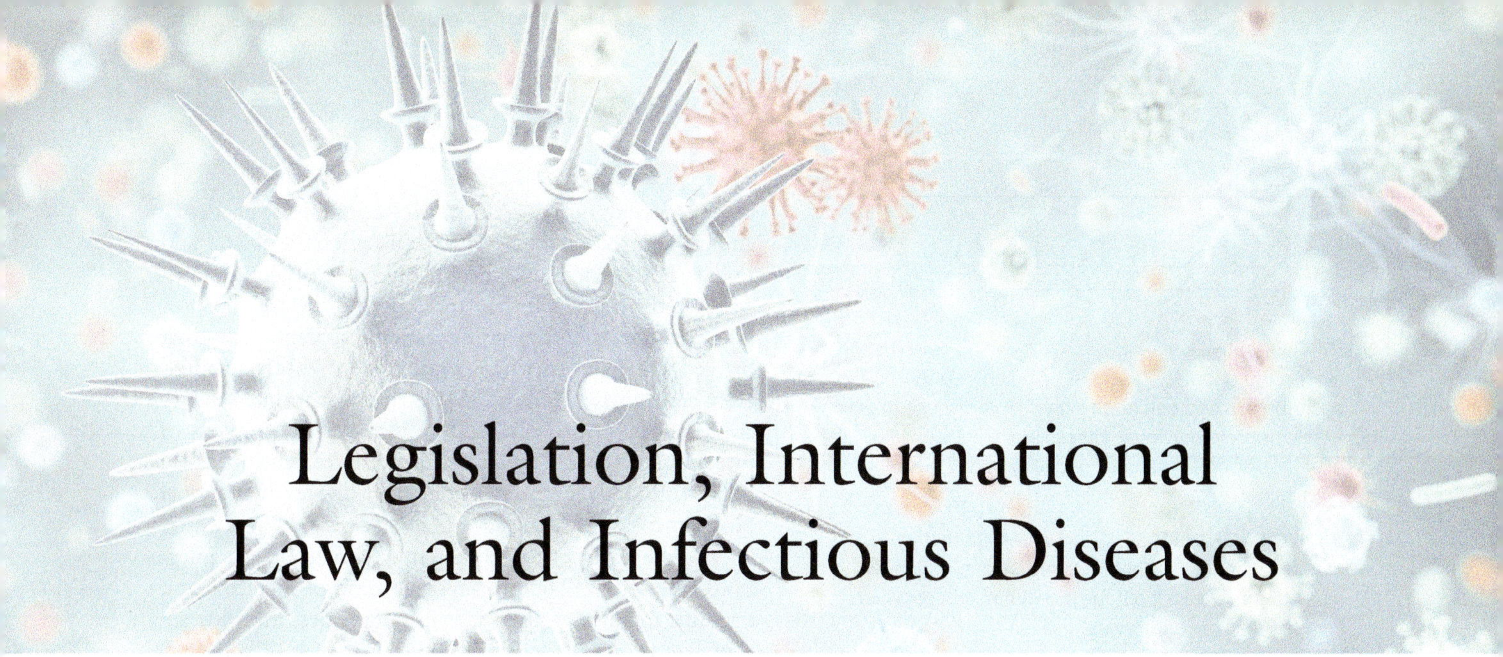

Legislation, International Law, and Infectious Diseases

■ Introduction

While national infectious disease laws and legislation are essential, globalization demands increasingly international solutions because epidemic diseases do not respect national boundaries. International cooperation among national governments and between governments and international nongovernmental agencies (NGOs) is facilitated by a basic set of international public health and infectious disease laws.

The body of international infectious disease law is composed of different types of agreements among nations, including treaties, accords, conventions, and agreements. In addition, nations may contribute to international infectious disease law by participating in international organizations such as the United Nations (UN), World Trade Organization (WTO), and World Bank. Furthermore, several nations may sponsor or aid the missions of various NGOs, agreeing to let their members assess and respond to infectious disease outbreaks within their national borders.

■ History and Policy Response

The earliest attempts at systematized government responses to epidemic disease arose out of the persistent threat of plague in Europe. Quarantine, or the confinement of people who have been exposed to a disease but do not show symptoms of the disease, was widely used to control epidemic plague. From the time of the Black Death, during which one-third of Europe's population perished from the plague, those who could afford to leave densely plague-infested cities often retreated to residences in the countryside. This exodus from the cities may have saved some from being exposed but also helped spread the disease. After the Black Death, many small municipalities forbade entry to those fleeing the cities. In rural Italy a Catholic priest wrote the Vatican asking for a decree permitting monasteries to close their doors on plague victims and refugees. Instead, the church viewed plague as punishment for people's sins and instructed non-cloistered orders of lower-level clergy across Europe to minister and aid the sick.

When epidemic plague struck England in 1665, the royal government left the city. The mayor and alderman were left in charge of governing the city through the epidemic. Isolation and quarantine were again employed. Businesses, public spaces, restaurants, and inns were closed. Churches, however, remained open, undermining the efficacy of the health laws. The city government hired physicians and regulated burial practices, criminalizing the dumping of bodies into the River Thames. Some plague-infested inns and public houses were ordered burned. When the plague escaped the confines of London to the village of Eyam, the villagers isolated the sick and quarantined the village. Nearly 75 percent of its inhabitants died, but surrounding villages were largely spared from the epidemic.

The often-conflicting laws, which were the result of a lack of understanding about disease transmission, proved limitedly effective against plague. While it was never epidemic in London after the Great Fire of 1666, plague continued to arise periodically in European cities until the late 18th century. The disappearance of epidemic plague was less a victory for infectious disease law and more likely the result of diminishing numbers of its vector, black rats and their plague-carrying fleas. When epidemic cholera hit Europe in the 1830s, officials looked to the historical example of public health measures and laws enacted to combat plague as a foundation.

The genesis of modern infectious disease law is often traced to the cholera pandemic in Europe from 1829 to 1851. From 1816 to 1826, a cholera pandemic spread through India, Southeast Asia, and China. Three years after the pandemic subsided in China, it reached parts of Europe. In 1831 and 1832, cholera was epidemic in several of Europe's major cities. In 1849 cholera again spread through several European, and then US, cities. Many historians note that the period was one of rapidly increasing immigration and trade, a dangerous situation for infectious

WORDS TO KNOW

EPIDEMIC From the Greek *epidemic*, meaning "prevalent among the people," it is most commonly used to describe an outbreak of an illness or a disease in which the number of individual cases significantly exceeds the usual or expected number of cases in any given population.

GERM THEORY OF DISEASE A fundamental tenet of medicine that states that microorganisms, which are too small to be seen without the aid of a microscope, can invade the body and cause disease.

ISOLATION Within the health community, the precautions taken in the hospital to prevent the spread of an infectious agent from an infected or colonized patient to susceptible people. Isolation practices are designed to minimize the transmission of infection.

LATENT INFECTION An infection already established in the body but not yet causing symptoms or having ceased to cause symptoms after an active period.

PANDEMIC An epidemic that occurs in more than one country or population simultaneously. *Pandemic* means "all the people."

QUARANTINE The practice of separating from the general population people who have been exposed to an infectious agent but have not yet developed symptoms. In the United States, this can be done voluntarily or involuntarily by the authority of states and the federal Centers for Disease Control and Prevention.

VECTOR Any agent that carries and transmits parasites and diseases. Also, an organism or a chemical used to transport a gene into a new host cell.

disease. Medicine and modern scientific research were newly emerging, but scientific knowledge of disease had limitedly progressed in the preceding century. The cholera epidemics prompted substantial change in medicine, public health, and infectious disease law.

In 1854 John Snow (1813–1854) identified polluted public water supplies as the source of cholera. Snow advocated radical changes in sanitation and water safety, persuading the London city government to approve construction of new water systems and enact laws protecting the water supply. Sanitation and hygiene laws, championed by the growing sanitation and public health movement, helped reduce incidence of cholera and other waterborne diseases.

In 1851 the First International Sanitary Conference convened in Paris, France. Cholera identification and prevention was a primary concern of the attendees. Pandemic cholera spurred diplomacy between nations. England and France both sent public health officials to medical academies and hospitals abroad to study the disease and possible treatments. Infectious disease and sanitation laws that proved effective in one location were often adopted elsewhere. From 1851 to 1900, 10 international sanitary conferences met to discuss the international impacts of infectious disease. Eight international conventions were drafted, though few were adopted into force by national governments.

By the dawn of the 20th century, science drove infectious disease law. The professionalization of medicine and scientific training of physicians in universities, the wide acceptance of germ theory, and the discovery of antisepsis revolutionized public health. Infectious disease laws became more effective as researchers were better able to identify the sources of disease and understand how diseases spread. By the outbreak of World War I (1914–1918), international agencies already operated to assess sanitation conditions and identify and treat disease outbreaks across national borders. The Red Cross and Pan American Sanitary Bureau helped draft international conventions on infectious disease prevention. International treaties and agreements outlined infectious disease controls associated with trade and immigration. National governments had passed laws outlining effective isolation and quarantine measures, adopted food safety regulations, instituted comprehensive health screening for arriving immigrants and restricted entry to healthy individuals, and established national public health agencies.

After World War II (1939–1941), the availability of antibiotics and the rapid development of modern vaccines again changed the ways in which health officials were able to respond to diseases. International agreements provided for the sharing and distribution of vaccines and antibiotics. The founding of the UN created a global organizational structure for international public health programs and laws. WHO was created on July 22, 1946, to promulgate international public health regulations and promote public health laws worldwide.

Since the 1960s economic and trade organizations have played an increasing role in international infectious disease laws. Free trade agreements often carry requirements that exports will meet quality and safety standards or that nations can decline imports if they pose a general health threat. Trade agreements on agricultural, animal, and food products typically stipulate regulations for disease testing, hygienic packaging, safe handling, and inspection. Sometimes trade agreements contain public health provisions, such as aid for combating endemic parasites or infectious diseases.

Even with the rise of trade organizations and the formation of the UN and WHO, public health laws remain uneven throughout the world. Most international public health laws are nonbinding or difficult to enforce without total cooperation by participating nations. UN and trade organization member nations have full national sovereignty, meaning they reserve the power to adopt and enforce laws within their national borders. Adding to the inequalities in national health care systems, sanitation systems, and resources for combating diseases, some nations do not recognize international infectious disease conventions or do not participate in WHO-led anti-disease programs. International infectious disease conventions sometimes fail completely in conflict-torn nations, often areas where infectious disease monitoring, prevention, and response are needed most. NGOs, such as the International Red Cross and Médecins Sans Frontières (Doctors Without Borders), are often effective at responding to epidemic disease in these regions.

■ Impacts and Issues

In the 21st century, laws that govern response to infectious diseases are increasingly international. Increased migration and trade have expanded the reach of once-localized diseases. While globalization has aided in the spread of some diseases, it has also opened new channels for combating infectious disease. Once the exclusive domain of local and national governments, laws governing reporting and responding to infectious diseases are increasingly international.

Infectious Disease Response, Civil Liberties, and Medical Privacy in the United States

The expansion of scientific research capabilities and computerized information systems has aided the global fight against infectious disease. Researchers and public health officials are better able to identify, study, respond to, and communicate about disease outbreaks. However, disease prevention and containment measures can impede personal civil liberties or affect personal privacy.

US Executive Order 13295 provides for government authority to detain, seize, apprehend, quarantine, or isolate people potentially sickened by or exposed to cholera, diphtheria, emerging pandemic influenza, infectious tuberculosis, plague, severe acute respiratory syndrome (SARS), smallpox, yellow fever, and viral hemorrhagic fevers. States have passed varying forms of the Model State Emergency Health Powers Act (MSEHPA), outlining state and local

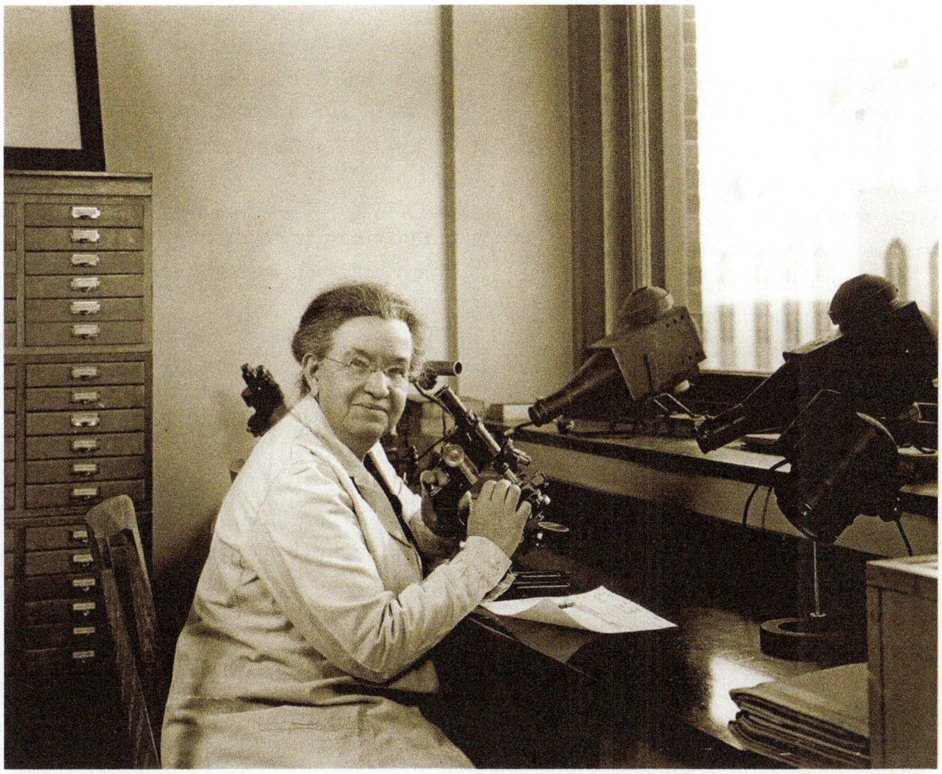

Florence Rena Sabin was an American medical scientist whose work led to the passage of the Sabin health laws. The law signaled a critical change in public health policy by mandating stringent regulations regarding infectious disease, milk pasteurization, and sewage disposal. © *National Library of Medicine/Science Source*

SABIN HEALTH LAWS

Florence Sabin (1871–1953) was the first woman to graduate from the Johns Hopkins Medical School. She then became the first woman appointed to a full professorship at Johns Hopkins and was elected the first woman president of the American Association of Anatomists. After becoming the first lifetime woman member of the National Academy of Sciences, Sabin ultimately expanded her work to include research on understanding the pathology and immunology of tuberculosis.

Sabin's methods of blood analysis became important indicators of various disease states, and her work was important in attempts to combat tuberculosis. Near the end of World War II (1939–1945), Sabin was called on to chair a study on public health practices in her home state of Colorado. As part of her work, she studied the effects of water pollution and the prevention of brucellosis in cattle, At the time brucellosis, especially in infants, often resulted from exposure to contaminated and unpasteurized milk from diseased cows.

The result of Sabin's work was the passage of the Sabin health laws, which signaled a critical change in public health policy. The Sabin health bills mandated stringent regulations regarding infectious disease, milk pasteurization, and sewage disposal.

epidemic disease response plans and powers. Some critics assert that governments can too greatly encroach on freedoms of travel and association when responding to epidemic disease by instituting quarantines or isolation orders.

Several nations have responded to concerns about personal privacy by passing laws safeguarding patients' personal information. In the United States, concerns of medical privacy were addressed through the passage of the Health Insurance Portability and Accountability Act (HIPAA) in 1996. The primary aim of the legislation was to protect access to private health insurance for workers who lose or change their employment. However, the legislation also contains several provisions on privacy and security. Under HIPAA, a patient's health status, medical history, payment history for medical services, and private identifying information must be protected. While insurers still have access to some of this information to facilitate payment of patient claims, patients have greater control over how much information insurers may obtain and doctors may release. Patients must be notified of any use of their personal health information or sign a waiver.

While patient privacy advocates applaud the legislation, several researchers have asserted that HIPAA hampers the ability to conduct needed avenues of research, especially those that formerly involved studying past patient medical charts. Furthermore, some researchers have noticed a drop in follow-up survey responses, complicating research on recovery and relapse.

HIPAA does not affect the reporting of notifiable diseases to federal and state health officials. The US Centers for Disease Control and Prevention (CDC) National Electronic Disease Surveillance System (NEDSS) is also unaffected as individually identifiable health information is available for public health research use without consent but cannot include personal identifiers such as name or address.

Fighting Epidemic Disease across National Borders

There is no universally accepted international body of law. Thus, international anti-infectious disease regulation is typically the result of participation in UN initiatives by member nations or through voluntary cooperative efforts governed by treaty. Not all nations participate in or acknowledge the authority of various international laws governing infectious diseases. Other nations participate in some programs and treaties while opting out of others.

Problems may also arise when national legal systems are in conflict with international law mandates. For example, many international laws are based on the assumption that national governments have broad power over local police, health officials, and health care facilities. The United States often adapts international regulations to fit within its system of federalism, which delegates significant powers to state and local governments. While laws governing patient privacy or federal quarantine orders apply to the whole nation, states may enact supplemental public health laws. In contrast, many other nations have centralized public health and health care systems that are only governed at the national level.

As infectious disease threats, treatment options, and prevention mechanisms change, so too must international law governing disease response. On July 25, 1951, WHO member states adopted the International Sanitary Regulations, later renamed the International Health Regulations (IHR), to "ensure the maximum protection against the international spread of disease with minimum interference with world traffic." IHR guidelines require that nations notify other countries about disease outbreaks within their borders, maintain accurate records about such outbreaks, establish public health protocols at national points of entry and exit (such as border crossings or airports), and base substantial restrictions on trade for disease prevention on scientific evidence of a public health concern. Nations may require vaccine certificates or health screenings of travelers and immigrants and may adopt hygiene, disinfection, isolation, or quarantine protocols at points of entry as needed. Diseases that the IHR guidelines currently address include cholera, yellow fever, plague, smallpox, polio, SARS, and new strains of human influenza.

Many aspects of the IHR remain difficult to enforce. Member nations have adopted several provisions of the IHR while abandoning others. National laws governing reporting of diseases are sometimes not as stringent, or nations have failed to report epidemics. The annual World Health Assembly approved revised IHR in May 2005, addressing these issues and updating the list of targeted diseases to include new threats such as SARS and pandemic influenza. The revised regulations, which were accepted by the United States in December 2006, took effect in June 2007.

See Also *CDC (Centers for Disease Control and Prevention); Economic Development and Disease; Isolation and Quarantine; World Health Organization (WHO)*

BIBLIOGRAPHY

Books

Amer, Fatma. *Hospital Infection Control.* Part 1. 3rd ed. Saarbrücken, Germany: Noor, 2017.

Fidler, David P. *International Law and Infectious Diseases.* Oxford, UK: Clarendon, 1999.

Websites

"International Health Regulations (IHR)." World Health Organization. http://www.who.int/topics/international_health_regulations/en/ (accessed December 11, 2017).

Adrienne Wilmoth Lerner
Brian Hoyle

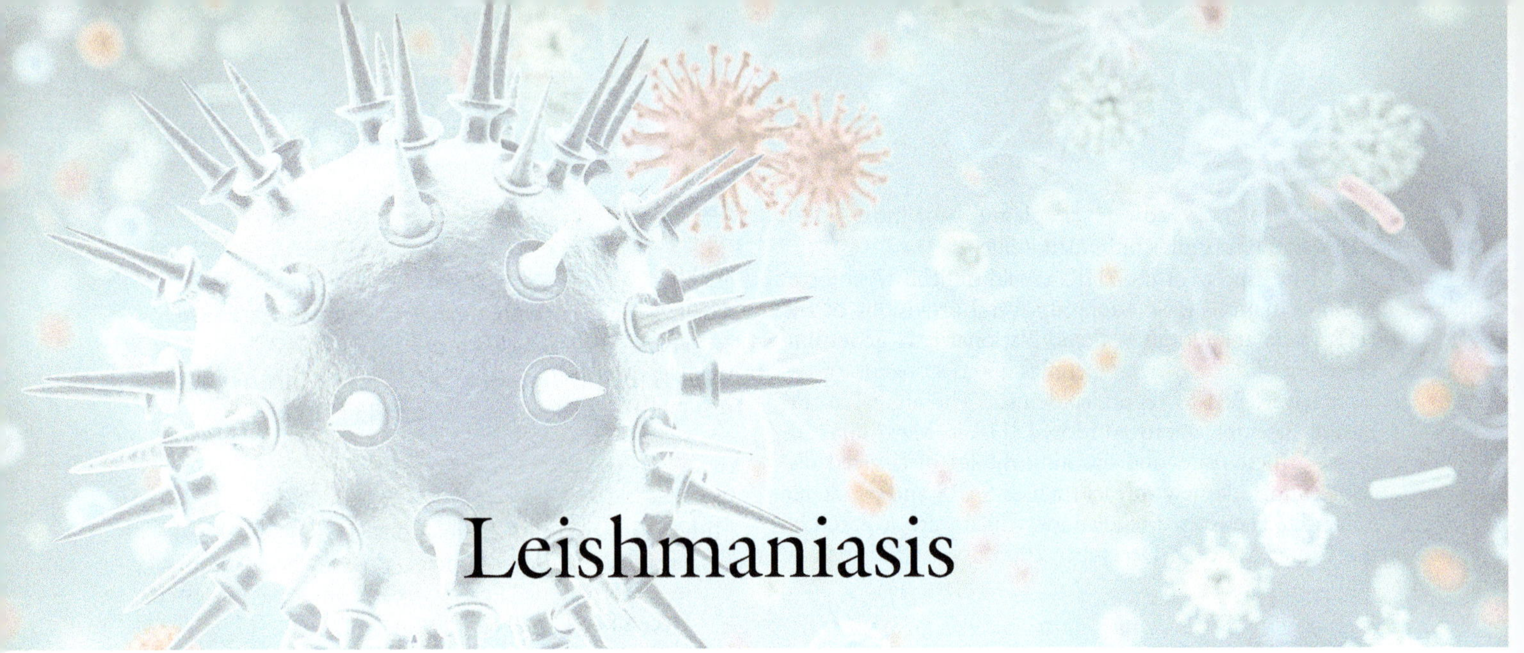

Leishmaniasis

Introduction

Leishmaniasis (LEASH-ma-NIGH-a-sis) is a parasitic disease caused by a protozoan of the genus *Leishmania* and spread by the bite of a female phlebotomine sand fly. According to the World Health Organization (WHO), the disease is endemic in 97 countries worldwide, and about 1 million cases occur each year, causing as many as 30,000 deaths.

Leishmaniasis usually affects impoverished people living in tropical and subtropical regions frequently exposed to the sand fly. Signs and symptoms vary depending on the form of infection, but mild cases present with skin sores on the face, arms, and legs that eventually heal with treatment. The more severe cases of visceral leishmaniasis affect organs such as the spleen and liver and are almost always fatal within two years if left untreated.

Treatment with drugs is usually quite effective if administered prior to significant immune damage, but, in the majority of cases, severe scarring is often unavoidable. There is no vaccine or drug available for the prevention of leishmaniasis, however, minimizing contact with the sand fly vector significantly reduces the risk of infection.

WORDS TO KNOW

CUTANEOUS Pertaining to the skin.

PROTOZOA Single-celled, animal-like microscopic organisms that live by taking in food rather than making it by photosynthesis and must live in the presence of water. (Singular: protozoan.) Protozoa are a diverse group of single-celled organisms, with more than 50,000 different types represented. The vast majority are microscopic, many measuring less than 5 one-thousandth of an inch (0.005 millimeters), but some, such as the freshwater Spirostomun, may reach 0.17 inches (3 millimeters) in length, large enough to enable it to be seen with the naked eye.

VECTOR Any agent that carries and transmits parasites and diseases. Also, an organism or a chemical used to transport a gene into a new host cell.

VISCERAL Pertaining to the viscera. The viscera are the large organs contained in the main cavities of the body, especially the thorax and abdomen; for example, the lungs, stomach, intestines, kidneys, or liver.

Disease History, Characteristics, and Transmission

One of the first clinical descriptions of leishmaniasis appeared in 1756, although the disease has been referenced as far back as the 7th century BCE. The name *leishmaniasis* was given to the disease in 1901 when a Scottish doctor identified the causative organism as being the protozoa *Leishmania*.

Leishmaniasis has several forms, each with varying symptomatic presentation and clinical severity. Cutaneous leishmaniasis (CL) is the most common form. It is characterized by skin sores over the face, arms, and body, which may be painful or painless. Glands near the sores may be swollen. The sores usually develop within a few weeks of infection and may leave severe scarring.

Visceral leishmaniasis (VL), commonly known as kala-azar, is the most serious form of the disease. It affects organs, such as the liver and spleen, and presents symptoms such as persistent chronic fever, fatigue, scaly/gray skin, weight loss, anemia, and enlarged spleen or liver. In developing countries this form of leishmaniasis may have a 100 percent fatality rate within two years if untreated. A related condition, post-kala-azar dermal leishmaniasis (PKDL), occurs in as many as half of all successfully treated VL patients and produces large, swollen lesions on the face and body. PKDL is rarely fatal but may appear as late as 10 years after VL treatment and can last for several months. It is also thought to serve as a reservoir for VL, allowing the disease to survive and reemerge even after extensive eradication campaigns.

Mucocutaneous leishmaniasis (ML) often occurs if the cutaneous (skin) form is untreated. In this form of the disease, the skin sores spread and may cause partial or total destruction of mucous membranes found in the nose, mouth, and throat. These mucosal sores often leave patients with severe facial deformities.

Leishmaniasis is transmitted by the bite of about 30 species of the phlebotomine sand fly, which are most active between dusk and dawn. Only female sand flies are capable of spreading the disease after infecting themselves by ingesting host blood containing the protozoa. Hosts of the parasite include dogs, foxes, jackals, and rodents. After 4 to 25 days within the sand fly, the protozoan transforms and completes its life cycle after being reinjected into a new host. Transmission is possible between humans through blood transfusions or the use of contaminated needles.

■ Scope and Distribution

The WHO estimates that there are at least 12 million cases of leishmaniasis globally. It is found in 97 countries around the world and is most common in tropical and subtropical regions of Africa, South America, and Asia. Each year there are between 600,000 and 1 million new cases of cutaneous leishmaniasis and between 200,000 and 400,000 cases of visceral leishmaniasis, according to WHO.

The geographic distribution of the disease is limited by the suitability of habitat for sand flies, their ability to remove blood from the host and transfer it to another, and the role the flies play in completing the life cycle of the infecting protozoa. WHO reports that over 90 percent of new cases of leishmaniasis (both CL and VL) occur in just 13 countries: Afghanistan, Algeria, Bangladesh, Bolivia, Brazil, Columbia, Ethiopia, India, Iran, Peru, South Sudan, Sudan, and Syria. Also according to WHO, as of 2015, of all new cases of VL, approximately 90 percent occur in just seven countries: Brazil, Ethiopia, India, Kenya, Somalia, South Sudan, and Sudan. These regions offer tropical and subtropical climates and provide the perfect conditions for phlebotomine sand flies to live, breed, and successfully transmit the disease.

People at greatest risk of contracting leishmaniasis are those living, working, or visiting those areas where sand flies are found. There is a notably higher incidence of infection in rural areas than in urban areas, though the number of urban infections has steadily increased in the early 21st century. Poverty and a lack of sufficient shelter or sanitary facilities are among the most significant risk factors for high rates of leishmaniasis infection. Transmission between pregnant women and unborn children is possible but rare, and contaminated blood or needles can also spread the disease.

Leishmaniasis rarely occurs in the United States, but some cases of skin sores arising from cutaneous leishmania-

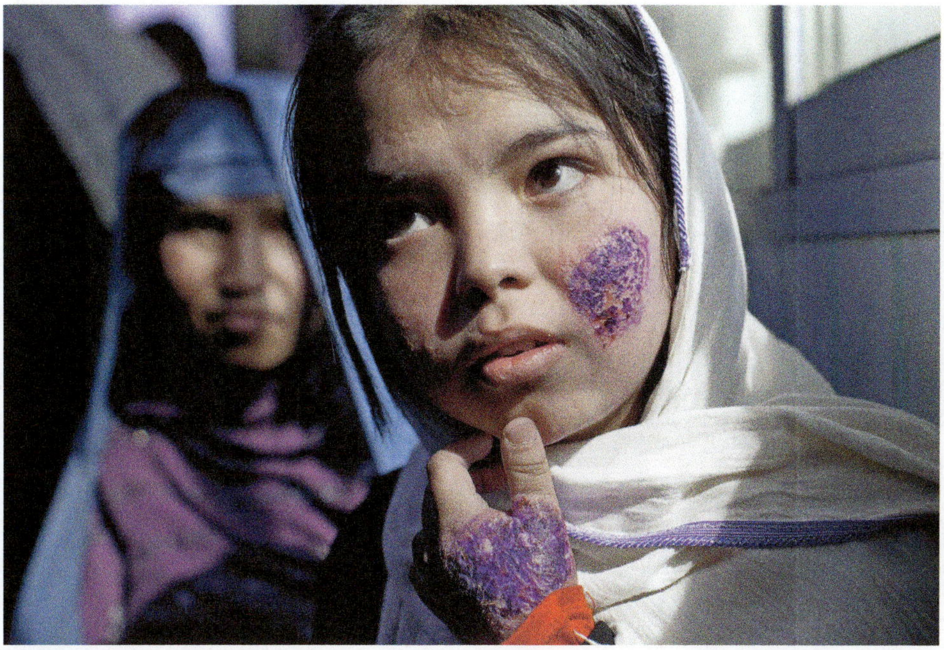

A girl waits to be treated at a specialized clinic for leishmaniasis in Kabul, Afghanistan. Transmitted by sand flies, leishmaniasis can cause severe scarring, often on the face. *© Paula Bronstein/Getty Images*

sis have been reported in rural areas of Texas and Oklahoma. Scientists have become increasingly concerned about the growing prevalence of the disease in North America, particularly among soldiers and travelers who have visited endemic countries. As of 2018 no cases of visceral leishmaniasis have been reported in humans the in United States, but the parasite has been discovered in a number of North American canine populations.

■ Treatment and Prevention

Leishmaniasis is caused by parasitic infection, and treatment with drugs is usually effective if applied prior to immune system damage. Traditionally, leishmaniasis was treated with a class of antiparasitic drugs known as pentavalent antimonials. However, by the 1980s reports began to surface out of India that some strains of the parasite had developed a resistance to antimonials, and the drugs were causing severe side effects, including cardiac toxicity and pancreatitis. As a result, treatments began to shift toward other options. Since the 1990s the most common treatments have been miltefosine (an oral medication originally developed as a cancer treatment), liposomal amphotericin B (an intravenous medication), or a combination of the two. In August 1997 liposomal amphotericin B was the first drug approved for the treatment of visceral leishmaniasis by the US Food and Drug Administration, and miltefosine was licensed for use in 2014.

The sores caused by cutaneous leishmaniasis may lead to unsightly scarring if not treated, and severe cases of mucocutaneous leishmaniasis may require reconstructive surgery to repair damage to facial tissues. In some cases of drug-resistant visceral leishmaniasis, it may be necessary to remove the patient's spleen. Because the disease is parasitic, there may be reactivation of infection after the initial signs and symptoms disappear. Previous infection does not provide any form of immunity against future infection.

Although several vaccines are in clinical trials as of 2018, there is no vaccine or drug available to prevent leishmaniasis. Transmission may be avoided by limiting exposure to the sand fly vector that carries the disease. Sand flies are most active from dusk to dawn, and it is best to limit outdoor activities during these times in areas where the disease occurs. Protective clothing, such as long-sleeved shirts and long pants, can reduce the amount of exposed skin and prevent fly bites. If the sleeping area is not well screened or air-conditioned, a bed net that has been soaked in or sprayed with insecticide should be used. Dogs and rodents should be kept away from sleeping areas. When exposure to sand flies is unavoidable, it is beneficial to use a strong insect repellent and spray sleeping areas with insecticides, if possible.

In addition to undertaking individual prevention, governments may implement public health measures. In 2005 the governments of Bangladesh, India, and Nepal launched a campaign to eliminate (reduce incidence below 1 case per 10,000 population) visceral leishmaniasis by 2015. In 2014 the deadline was extended to 2017, and two new countries, Bhutan and Thailand, joined the campaign. Efforts included expansive training of health care professionals in the recognition of VL symptoms, implementation of rapid-

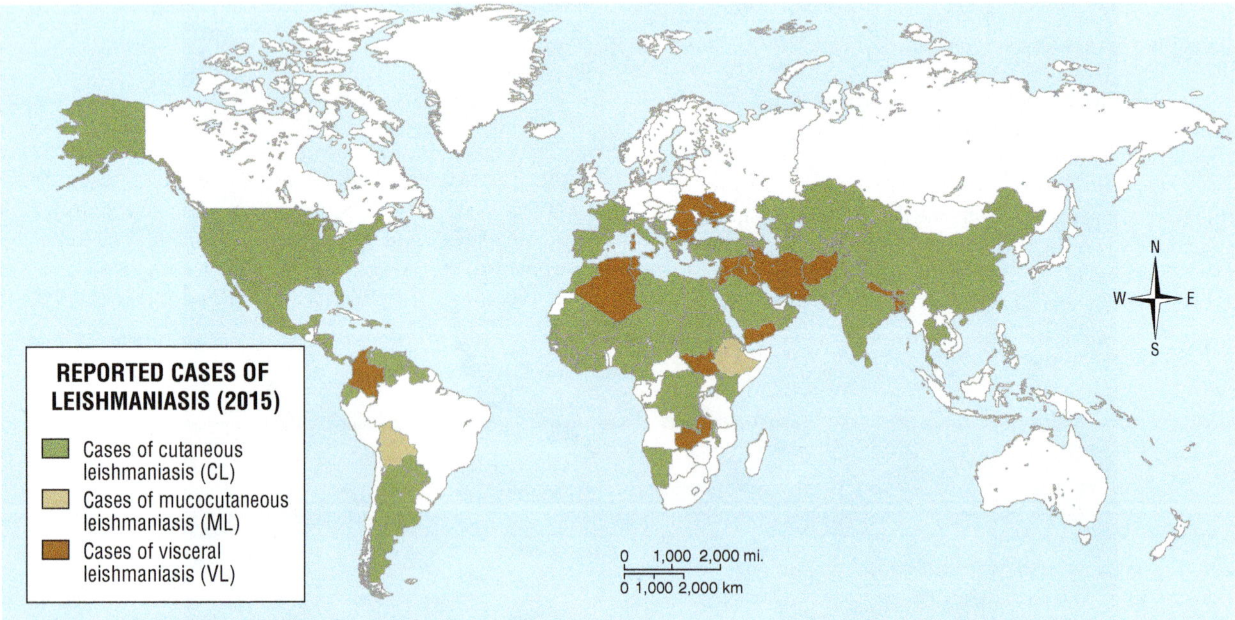

SOURCE: Adapted from "Unveiling: The Neglect of Leishmaniasis." World Health Organization. 2015. Available from: http://www.who.int/leishmaniasis/Unveiling_the_neglect_of_leishmaniasis_infographic.pdf?ua=1

response testing, and vector control through the use of bed nets and insecticides. As of December 2017, Bangladesh in particular had shown significant progress in combatting the disease, reducing the number of annual VL cases from 9,300 in 2006 to 159 in 2016, according to WHO.

A related international effort at eliminating VL around the globe by 2020, led by WHO, was launched in 2012. In 2014 WHO announced a partnership with Gilead, a US producer of liposomal amphotericin B, to provide 445,000 vials of the drug to areas most affected by VL. In 2016 the two groups signed another agreement to provide an additional 380,400 vials to health care providers throughout Southeast Asia and East Africa. Increased use of the treatment was credited with helping to substantially reduce the spread of the disease in countries such as India, Bangladesh, and Nepal, which reported decreases in new cases in 2016 of 61 percent, 67 percent, and 46 percent, respectively, from 2005 levels.

While avoidance of the vector is helpful in preventing individual cases, a reduction in animals harboring infection will have a greater impact on preventing the spread of disease. Public awareness is important to ensure that communities are working toward the same goal and following similar guidelines to reduce sand fly populations and animal reservoirs.

■ Impacts and Issues

The impacts of a widespread condition such as leishmaniasis are evident at the community level and also across countries and continents. One of the significant physical effects of leishmaniasis infection is the severe scarring caused by the sores that develop on the face, legs, and arms. In some communities affected by the disease, social prejudices exist toward people with these unattractive scars, and in some situations people with disabling disfigurations become social outcasts. This may cause division within communities and may eventually lead to social breakdown.

On a larger scale, human-caused environmental changes are having an impact on natural habitats and, as a result, are increasing the risk of human exposure to the sand fly vector. Activities, such as dam building, mining, deforestation, irrigation, and conversion of land to cultivation, permanently alter the conditions under which the vectors exist naturally and create new opportunities for vector contact. Although the disease was previously limited to poverty-stricken rural areas, leishmaniasis has also successfully adapted to the urban environment. The movement of large groups from rural to urban areas, in addition to worldwide urbanization, is also adding to this effect.

When war breaks out in areas where leishmaniasis is endemic, the disease can have an international impact. Massive movements of refugees from war-torn areas to crowded, often unsanitary camps in neighboring countries can help spread the disease to populations and areas that were not previously at risk of an outbreak. During the Syrian Civil War beginning in 2013, for example, the number of cutaneous leishmaniasis cases in Syria nearly doubled, from around 23,000 cases per year to over 40,0000 as widespread environmental degradation and the breakdown of public health services and prevention efforts led to a proliferation of sand flies. As more than 4 million Syrian refugees fled across the country's borders, receiving countries began to report an increase in leishmaniasis infections. In Lebanon, which had just six cases of CL between 2000 and 2012, there were 1,033 cases of CL in 2013 alone. Several hundred cases of CL were also reported in Turkey and Jordan.

The deployment of foreign troops to endemic countries also places those soldiers at increased risk of contracting the disease, despite extensive measures taken to prevent sand fly contact. The deployment of US troops to Iraq and Afghanistan in the early 21st century resulted in 2,040 reported cases of leishmaniasis and an unknown number of unreported, asymptomatic, or misdiagnosed cases between 2001 and 2016, according to the US Department of Defense. Soldiers fighting in the region dubbed the disease "Baghdad Boil." When these foreign soldiers return to their home countries, they potentially create a portal of entry for the parasite to move into previously unaffected zones, thus aiding the worldwide spread of leishmaniasis. While these countries generally are able to implement stringent preventative measures among their troops to protect them from infection, there remains a potential risk of spreading the disease to new areas.

Coinfection of human immunodeficiency virus (HIV) and leishmaniasis is another concern. HIV infection increases the risk of leishmaniasis infection, while leishmaniasis causes an increase in the progression of HIV to acquired immunodeficiency syndrome (AIDS). Patients with HIV also respond poorly to traditional treatments for leishmaniasis, resulting in much higher rates of disease relapse or death. In Europe the primary way in which leishmaniasis is transmitted is thought to be through sharing of intravenous needles, which also significantly raises the risk of contracting HIV. WHO considers coinfection of HIV and leishmaniasis to be a significant concern because it could lead to spread of the disease into previously nonendemic areas. In 1998 WHO and UNAIDS implemented the Programme for the Surveillance and Control of Leishmaniasis to monitor leishmaniasis/HIV coinfection, improve response capability, and ensure that epidemics are detected and contained.

See Also *AIDS (Acquired Immunodeficiency Syndrome); Blood Supply and Infectious Disease; Emerging Infectious Diseases; HIV; Host and Vector; Parasitic Diseases; War and Infectious Disease; World Health Organization (WHO)*

BIBLIOGRAPHY

Books

Kumar, Awanish. *Leishmania and Leishmaniasis.* New York: Springer, 2013.

Satoskar, Abhay R., and Ravi Durvasula, eds. *Pathogenesis of Leishmaniasis: New Developments in Research.* New York: Springer, 2014.

Periodicals

Du, Rebecca, et al. "Old World Cutaneous Leishmaniasis and Refugee Crises in the Middle East and North Africa." *PLOS Neglected Tropical Diseases* 10, no. 5 (May 26, 2016). This article can also be found online at http://journals.plos.org/plosntds/article?id=10.1371/journal.pntd.0004545 (accessed February 3, 2018).

Gillespie, Portia M., et al. "Status of Vaccine Research and Development of Vaccines for Leishmaniasis." *Vaccine* 34, no. 26 (June 2016): 2992–2995. This article can also be found online at https://www.sciencedirect.com/science/article/pii/S0264410X16002899 (accessed February 3, 2018).

Lindoso, José Angelo Lauletta, et al. "Leishmaniasis–HIV Coinfection: Current Challenges." *HIV/AIDS* 8 (2016): 147–156. This article can also be found online at https://www.ncbi.nlm.nih.gov/pmc/articles/PMC5063600/ (accessed February 3, 2018).

Stahlman, Shauna. "Incident Diagnoses of Leishmaniasis, Active and Reserve Components, U.S. Armed Forces, 2001–2016." *Medical Surveillance Monthly Report* 24, no. 2 (February 2017): 2–7. This article can also be found online at https://health.mil/MSMRArchives (accessed February 3, 2018).

Steverding, Dietmar. "The History of Leishmaniasis." *Parasites & Vectors* 10, no. 82 (2017). This article can also be found online at https://parasitesandvectors.biomedcentral.com/articles/10.1186/s13071-017-2028-5 (accessed February 2, 2018).

Websites

"Leishmaniasis." Centers for Disease Control and Prevention. https://www.cdc.gov/parasites/leishmaniasis/index.html (accessed February 3, 2018).

"Leishmaniasis." European Centre for Disease Prevention and Control. https://ecdc.europa.eu/en/leishmaniasis (accessed February 3, 2018).

"Leishmaniasis." World Health Organization. http://www.who.int/leishmaniasis/en/// (accessed February 2, 2018).

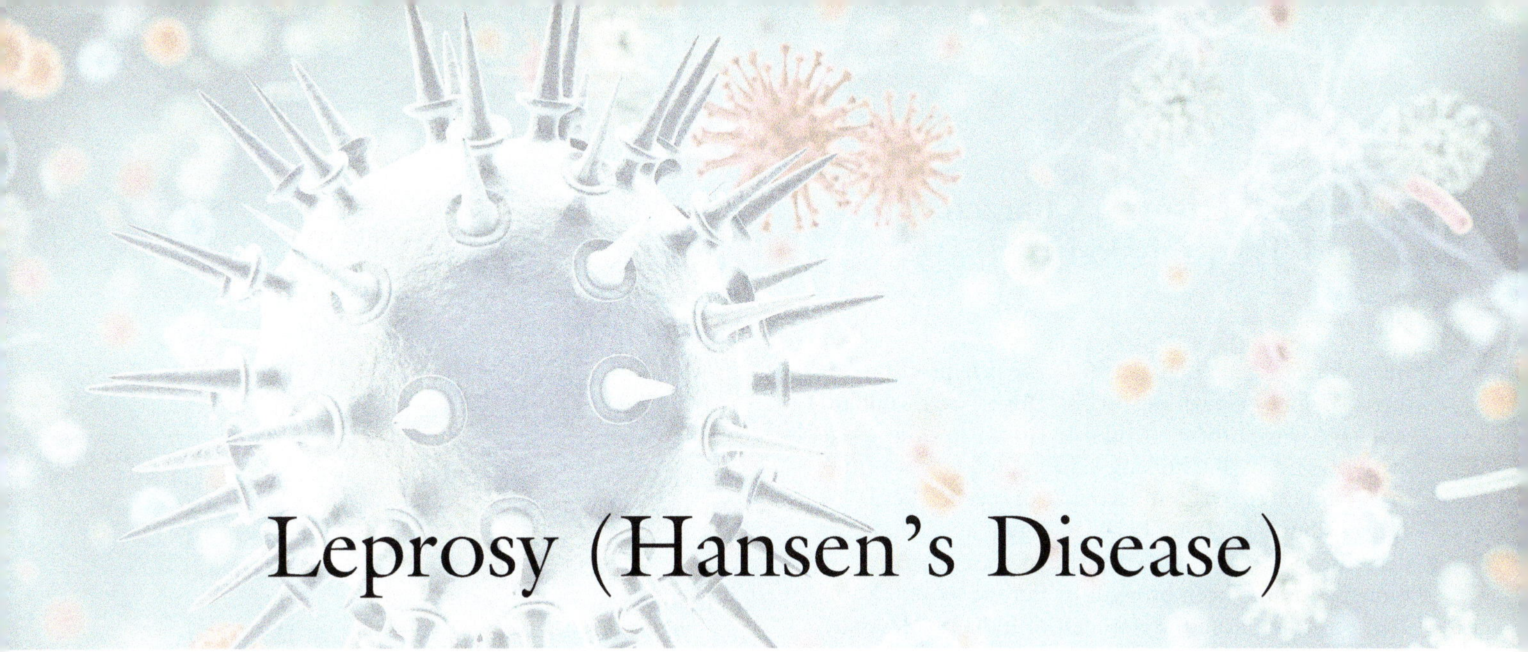

Leprosy (Hansen's Disease)

Introduction

Leprosy, also known as Hansen's disease, is a chronic disease caused by infection with the bacillus *Mycobacterium leprae* or the closely associated *Mycobacterium lepromatosis*. The disease was greatly feared for many centuries because of the extreme disfigurement it can cause. It is widely known in the 21st century from references to *tzaraath* in the Hebrew Bible, translated as "leprosy," though it probably included a wide range of skin diseases. When diagnosed soon after infection, leprosy is treatable by combination drug therapy. Eradication campaigns successfully eliminated leprosy as a public health problem in 2000, according to the World Health Organization (WHO), but cases continue to occur. In 2016 WHO launched a new campaign against leprosy that focused on preventing disabilities caused by the disease.

Leprosy does not, as is commonly assumed, cause fingers, toes, and noses to drop off. This is a side effect of the disease's attack on the peripheral nerves. Loss of sensation makes patients unable to respond to minor injuries and infections in their fingers, toes, and elsewhere, and it is these secondary causes that lead to the characteristic loss of body parts. Leprosy more commonly causes puffy, deforming lesions on the face and elsewhere, skin discoloration, ulcers, and swelling, among other symptoms.

WORDS TO KNOW

ALLELE Any of two or more alternative forms of a gene that occupy the same location on a chromosome.

CULTURE A single species of microorganism that is isolated and grown under controlled conditions. German bacteriologist Robert Koch first developed culturing techniques in the late 1870s. Following Koch's initial discovery, medical scientists quickly sought to identify other pathogens. In the 21st century bacteria cultures are used as basic tools in microbiology and medicine.

DROPLET TRANSMISSION The spread of microorganisms from one space to another (including from person to person) via droplets that are larger than 5 microns in diameter. Droplets are typically expelled into the air by coughing and sneezing.

ENDEMIC Present in a particular area or among a particular group of people.

ERADICATION The process of destroying or eliminating a microorganism or disease.

LATENT A condition that is potential or dormant, not yet manifest or active.

MULTIDRUG THERAPY The use of a combination of drugs against infection, each of which attacks the infective agent in a different way. This strategy can help overcome resistance to anti-infective drugs.

RESISTANCE Immunity to an antibiotic or another drug, developed within a species, especially bacteria, via evolution. For example, in bacteria, resistance involves the acquisition of genetic mutations that render the bacteria invulnerable to the action of antibiotics.

■ Disease History, Characteristics, and Transmission

History

According to genetic data, *M. leprae* first probably infected human populations in East Africa over 100,000 years ago. From there the disease spread to other parts of the world by hitchhiking on repeated waves of human migration. Written accounts of leprosy began to appear about 1550 BCE, when Egyptian documents describe what seems to be the disease. Leprosy is thought to have been brought to Europe by Greek soldiers returning from the conquest of India by Alexander the Great (356 BCE–323 BCE). It is first mentioned explicitly in Roman records dating to 62 BCE, coinciding with the return of troops from western Asia.

Particularly in the Middle Ages, when Arab invasions and the Crusades brought renewed rates of leprosy to Europe from Africa and the Middle East, the disease was intensely feared throughout Europe. People afflicted by leprosy were called *lepers*, a term now disfavored as it implies social stigma. By the 1100s approximately 19,000 asylums or leper houses had been established by monks and nuns to isolate and care for the victims of the disease. People with leprosy not confined to the leper houses were required to give warning of their approach by sounding a wooden clapper. They were also forbidden to enter churches, inns, mills, or bakeries; to touch or dine with people without leprosy; or to walk on narrow pathways where people coming the other way might have to touch them. Thanks to these stringent isolation measures, or possibly because of reduced frequency of the genes causing vulnerability to leprosy, the disease slowly decreased in Europe and had become rare there by the 1600s.

Leprosy was probably spread to West Africa by European traders or colonialists, as the variety found there closely resembles that found in Europe. From West Africa it was brought to the Caribbean and South America by the slave trade in the 18th century. The European variety is the one found in North America and was introduced by colonialism and emigration. In the 1700s and 1800s, for example, immigrants from Scandinavia, where a leprosy epidemic was occurring at the time, brought the disease with them to the midwestern United States.

In 1873 Norwegian physician Gerhard Henrik Armauer Hansen (1841–1912) showed that leprosy is caused by a bacillus, later named *M. leprae.* Although Hansen did not identify the objects he saw in his microscope as bacteria, he noted that he found the same objects in the tissues of all people suffering from the disease. Initially, his discovery was given little attention. In 1879 he shared tissue samples with German physician Albert Neisser (1855–1916), who identified the bacteria and attempted to claim credit for their discovery.

Despite the identification of *M. leprae* as the cause of leprosy, progress on creating a treatment for the disease was slow. Until about 1940 treatment was by injection of oil derived from the chaulmoogra nut, a traditional remedy. Numerous injections forced the oil under the skin, a painful procedure, though modern-day physicians do not assume that this treatment resulted in significant, permanent benefit. In 1921 the US Public Health Service built a re-

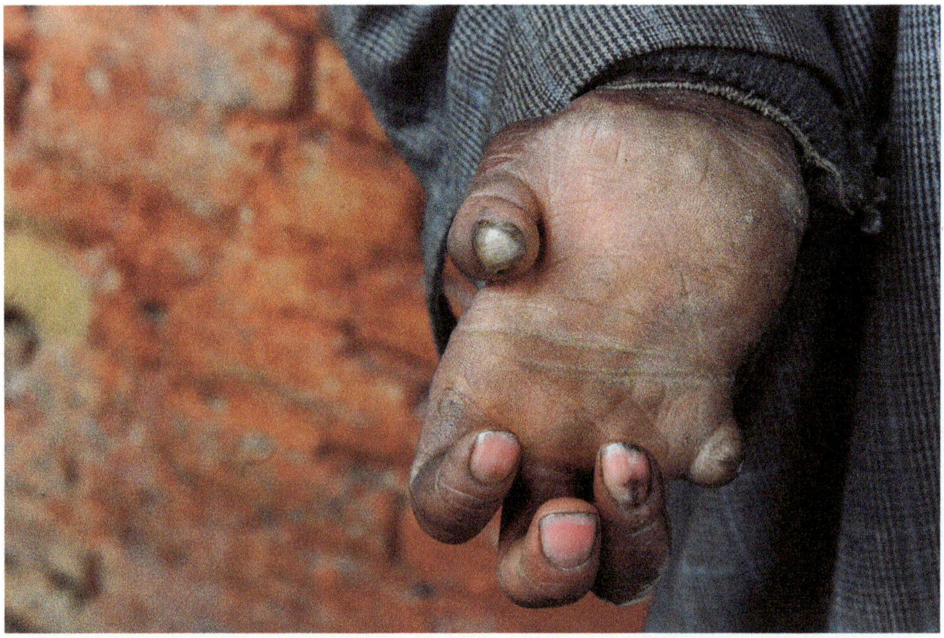

A patient with leprosy holds out his hand at a leprosy hospital in Srinagar, India. Leprosy, which is also known as Hansen's disease, can cause extreme disfigurement. © TAUSEEF MUSTAFA/AFP/Getty Images search and live-in treatment center for leprosy in Carville, Louisiana. Carville researchers announced the discovery of an effective anti-leprosy drug, Promin, in 1941. However, Promin, a sulfone drug, still required numerous painful injections.

In the 1950s another drug, dapsone, became available in pill form. Dapsone was highly effective, but *M. leprae* began to evolve resistance to the drug over the next decade. Given alone, it would not have remained effective for more than a few decades. In the 1970s the first multidrug therapy (MDT) for leprosy was developed, blending dapsone with other drugs to prevent the development of resistance. In 1981 WHO endorsed an MDT regimen consisting of dapsone, rifampicin (also known as rifampin), and clofazimine. This mixture continues to be used in the 21st century. Like the drug cocktails used to fight human immunodeficiency virus (HIV), MDT for leprosy exploits the fact that it is more difficult for a microorganism to evolve resistance to several agents at once than to evolve resistance to each agent separately or in series.

For years an obstacle to a fuller scientific understanding of *M. leprae* was the idea that it was impossible to grow the bacillus in pure culture (a prepared medium) in the laboratory. Also, its population-doubling time in tissue is the longest of any known bacterium, from 13 to 20 days (compared to about 20 minutes for *Escherichia coli*, the dominant bacterium in the human digestive tract). Until the early 1970s, *M. leprae* was not known to thrive in any laboratory animal. It grew only in humans and, in relatively small numbers, in the foot pads of mice. In 1971, however, researchers discovered that the nine-banded armadillo, a mammal native to South America and found across the southern United States, can be infected with *M. leprae.* Having acquired the disease from human sources, many armadillos in the wild have leprosy. As of 2017 about 5 percent of armadillos showed symptoms of the disease, but just over 20 percent were likely infected with *M. leprae.*

In 2008 scientists working to sequence the *M. leprae* genome discovered a second bacterium that causes leprosy in humans, *M. lepromatosis.* According to David M. Scollard in a 2016 article in the *American Journal of Tropical Medicine and Hygiene*, "microbiologically, *M. lepromatosis* is very similar to *M. leprae*: both are acid-fast, noncultivable, and have the ability to infect peripheral nerves." The genetic difference between the two species is 9 percent. While initial research indicated *M. lepromatosis* might cause a more severe form of leprosy, further study has not borne this out. In fact, there is no known practical difference between the two strains in terms of how they are diagnosed, how they are treated, their symptoms, or their mortality rates.

Characteristics

M. leprae and *M. lepromatosis* are rod-shaped bacteria about 1 to 8 micrometers long and 0.2 to 0.5 micrometers wide. Bacteria of the genus Mycobacterium are characterized by an unusually thick, multilayered cell wall, which helps make them resistant to antibiotics. Both the bacterium that causes tuberculosis (*Mycobacterium tuberculosis*) and those that cause leprosy are in this genus.

M. leprae and *M. lepromatosis* infect the mucus membranes, nerves, and skin. They tend not to invade deeper tissues because they thrive at temperatures slightly lower than that of the body core. The armadillo's low body temperature is thought to be one reason *M. leprae* can infect that species as well as humans. *M. leprae* and *M. lepromatosis* have an affinity for nerve cells, which is why loss of feeling can be a symptom of leprosy.

According to analysis published in *Nature Communications* in 2018, strains of *M. leprae* show evidence of hypermutation that "could be detrimental and ultimately lethal," as well as a growing drug resistance to antibiotics commonly used to treat leprosy. According to Andrej Benjak and his colleagues, "Drug resistance is alarming for leprosy control." While the link between hypermutation has not been definitively established, the authors urged "further experimentation in order to establish their [the mutations'] true role and contribution to antimicrobial resistance."

Leprosy causes a spectrum of disease, from mild to severe. Progression of the disease is slow, with incubation times of a few years to 30 years. About 90 percent of people with leprosy experience loss of temperature sensation of some part of the body, such as the fingers, as their first symptom. In other words, the patient cannot sense hot and cold with parts of his or her body. This often happens before any lesions or spots appear. Next, the ability to sense pain is lost and then the ability to sense deep pressure. The inability to sense pain allows otherwise trivial injuries or irritations to go unchecked, often leading to infections, injuries, and loss of tissue. The progress of leprosy is divided into four stages:

1. Intermediate leprosy. In this early, mildest form, some spots (lesions) may appear on the skin. Patients with low susceptibility may defeat the infection without assistance at this stage.
2. Tuberculoid leprosy. Large, pale spots called macules may appear on the skin. These lesions lack sensation. Nerves are infected and may thicken and cease to function.
3. Borderline leprosy. In this stage, skin lesions are present and numerous. They may now take the form of protruding nodules or sunken lesions that are sometimes described as appearing punched out.
4. Lepromatous leprosy. This is the most developed and severe form of the disease. Lesions are numerous and more severe (that is, more protruding or deeper set) than in the earlier stages. The eyes may become involved, leading to pain, light sensitivity, glaucoma, and blindness. The testicles may atrophy. Deepening nerve damage may lead to

SCIENTIFIC, POLITICAL, AND ETHICAL ISSUES

The stubbornness of the leprosy stigma was underlined in Japan in 2001, when a court ruled that the Japanese government owed millions of dollars in compensation to leprosy patients who had been confined and abused in leper colonies since the 1950s. The colonies, or centers, were established under the 1953 Leprosy Prevention Law (repealed in 1996), which forced all people with leprosy, including children, to move to those locations. According to a Japanese government commission that studied the leper colonies, patients were sterilized (surgically rendered unable to have children), forced to have abortions, and treated as research subjects. Infanticide was also practiced. All this continued for decades after outpatient treatment with anti-leprosy drugs became available in 1960. "For 60 years, I was not treated as a human," one former patient, Mamoru Kunimoto, said. The fact that the government apologized rather than disputing the court's ruling, he said, "has given me back my humanity."

partial paralysis. Any of the three earlier stages of leprosy may regress to less severe stages, but not this stage.

For purposes of treatment, leprosy is separated into two types, paucibacillary and multibacillary. In paucibacillary leprosy there are no more than five skin lesions on the patient, and the number of *M. leprae* or *M. lepromatosis* bacteria in the body is small, approximately less than 1 million. No *M. leprae* appear in a skin smear, which involves making a small cut in the most prominent lesion, scraping tissue from it, placing the sample on a microscope slide stained with a substance that highlights the presence of *M. leprae* or *M. lepromatosis*, and examining the sample to see if any of the bacteria are present. Most leprosy infections are of this type. In multibacillary leprosy a skin smear is positive, and there are more than five lesions. All more severe and advanced cases of leprosy are in the multibacillary category.

Transmission

The mode of transmission of leprosy remains uncertain. Most experts state that the disease is probably transmitted by mucus and saliva droplets produced by sneezing and coughing. People who have close contact with people with active, untreated infection are at risk for contracting the disease and so, more generally, is anyone living in a country where the disease is endemic. Experts speculate that insect bites, some animals, and bacilli in soil may also spread the disease, but none of these routes has been proved.

Only about 10 percent of the human population is vulnerable to infection by *M. leprae* and *M. lepromatosis.* Of those people, only about half will develop detectable disease. Susceptibility to infection by *M. leprae* and *M. lepromatosis* has been shown to be associated with a person's genetic makeup, namely the possession of certain alleles (alternative forms of a gene) for a specific area of human deoxyribonucleic acid (DNA) also shared by the Parkinson's disease gene PARK2 and its coregulated gene PACRG. The mechanism by which these alleles make people more susceptible to leprosy is not yet known.

■ Scope and Distribution

In many countries leprosy has been virtually eliminated, with 30 countries reporting no new cases in 2015. However, infections continue to occur in over 100 countries. As of 2015 the countries with the highest rates of new cases were India, which reported approximately 60 percent of the world's new cases; Brazil, which reported 13 percent of new cases globally; and Indonesia, which accounted for 8 percent of new cases. Other countries with high rates of infection included Sri Lanka, the Philippines, Nepal, Myanmar, Bangladesh, Tanzania, Nigeria, Mozambique, Madagascar, Ethiopia, and the Democratic Republic of the Congo. Brazil had the world's highest per capita leprosy rate. As many as 2 million people worldwide were disabled by leprosy as of 2017, according to the US Centers for Disease Control and Prevention (CDC).

■ Treatment and Prevention

Prevention of leprosy was traditionally through isolation of victims from the uninfected. Conventional antibiotics such as penicillin have never been effective against *M. leprae* and *M. lepromatosis.* In the 1940s the drug dapsone was shown to be effective in treating leprosy. While this represented a breakthrough in combatting leprosy, dapsone started to become less effective in the 1960s, as *M. leprae* and *M. lepromatosis* demonstrated increasing resistance to the drug. In response, researchers developed an MDT that combined the use of dapsone with rifampicin and clofazimine, which proved highly effective. Dapsone, the primary drug in this combination, inhibits bacterial growth by preventing the formation of folic acid. Rifampicin acts by inhibiting the bacterial enzyme ribonucleic acid (RNA) polymerase, which is needed for cell functioning. It is always used in combination with another drug. The third drug, clofazimine, inhibits bacterial growth by binding to DNA and thus interfering with transcription and replication.

For paucibacillary leprosy, a two-drug MDT consisting of dapsone and rifampicin is given for six months. For multibacillary leprosy, the full three-drug MDT is given for two years. MDT is given out in calendar-marked blister packs to patients, who must take the pills at home on a regular schedule.

Impacts and Issues

International efforts to eliminate leprosy have been under way since 1991, when the 49th World Health Assembly, the body that governs WHO, resolved to eliminate leprosy as a public health problem by 2000. This initiative defined elimination of the disease as reducing the worldwide prevalence rate to less than 1 in 10,000 people. In 1999 WHO formed the Global Alliance for the Elimination of Leprosy, based in India, with a strategy of early detection, MDT treatment, and eliminating the stigma attached to people with leprosy. The global elimination goal was met in 2000, but rates remained significantly higher in several countries.

Novartis, the US-based company that makes the three anti-leprosy drugs, entered into a partnership with the Global Alliance for the Elimination of Leprosy in 2000, supplying the MDT drugs at no cost and agreeing to do so until 2020. In 2016 WHO sought to reenergize global anti-leprosy efforts through the launch of its Global Leprosy Strategy 2016–2020, the goal of which "is to further reduce the global and local leprosy burden, thereby aiming for zero children with leprosy-affected disabilities, a reduction of new patients diagnosed with leprosy-related deformities to less than one per million population, and a repeal of all laws that allow discrimination of leprosy patients."

The impact of leprosy on the infected symptomatic individual has historically been severe. Furthermore, isolation and shunning of people with Hansen's disease (a name intended to reduce social stigma associated with the term *leprosy*, although both terms are correct) did not end with the Middle Ages. Loss of one's job, social standing, family position, and the like continue to be common consequences in many societies for persons with leprosy.

In 2006 researchers discovered that the drugs being given for the acquired immunodeficiency syndrome (AIDS) virus, which had infected about 38 million people in the undeveloped world, could make silent, or asymptomatic, leprosy become symptomatic. Patients on AIDS drugs reported ulcers or loss of sensation in the toes and fingers as their latent (dormant) leprosy became active. This was something of a medical paradox, as AIDS, which weakens the immune system, does not cause latent leprosy to become active, though the treatment for AIDS can.

Finally, as with all drug treatments for infectious disease, the evolution of drug resistance by *M. leprae* is a concern. Resistance to all major anti-leprosy drugs has been reported worldwide, particularly for dapsone. However, reports of relapse after MDT have been rare, and resistance to leprosy drugs is not yet considered a major problem.

SEE ALSO *Bacterial Disease; Contact Precautions*

BIBLIOGRAPHY

Books

Demaitre, Luke. *Leprosy in Premodern Medicine: A Malady of the Whole Body.* Baltimore, MD: Johns Hopkins University Press, 2009.

Gould, Tony. *A Disease Apart: Leprosy in the Modern World.* New York: St. Martin's, 2005.

Periodicals

Benjak, Andrej, et al. "Phylogenomics and Antimicrobial Resistance of the Leprosy Bacillus *Mycobacterium leprae.*" *Nature Communications* 9 (2018): 352. This article can also be found online at https://www.nature.com/articles/s41467–017-02576-z (accessed February 16, 2018).

Cole, S. T., et al. "Massive Gene Decay in the Leprosy Bacillus." *Nature* 409 (February 22, 2001): 1007–1011. This article can also be found online at https://www.nature.com/articles/35059006 (accessed February 9, 2018).

McNeil, Donald G., Jr. "Worrisome New Link: AIDS Drugs and Leprosy." *New York Times* (October 24, 2006). This article can also be found online at http://www.nytimes.com/2006/10/24/health/24lepr.html (accessed February 9, 2018).

Mira, Marcelo T., et al. "Susceptibility to Leprosy is Associated with PARK2 and PACRG." *Nature* 427 (2004): 636–640.

Monot, Marc, et al. "On the Origin of Leprosy." *Science* 308 (June 2005): 1040–1042.

Scollard, David M. "Infection with *Mycobacterium lepromatosis.*" *American Journal of Tropical Medicine and Hygiene* 95, no. 3 (September 2016): 500–501. This article can also be found online at https://www.ncbi.nlm.nih.gov/pmc/articles/PMC5014247/ (accessed February 12, 2018).

Wong, Alia. "When the Last Patient Dies." *Atlantic* (May 27, 2015). This article can also be found online at https://www.theatlantic.com/health/archive/2015/05/when-the-last-patient-dies/394163/ (accessed February 9, 2018).

Websites

"Hansen's Disease (Leprosy)." Centers for Disease Control and Prevention, February 10, 2017. https://www.cdc.gov/leprosy/ (accessed February 9, 2018).

"Leprosy." World Health Organization, January 2018. http://www.who.int/mediacentre/factsheets/fs101/en/ (accessed February 9, 2018).

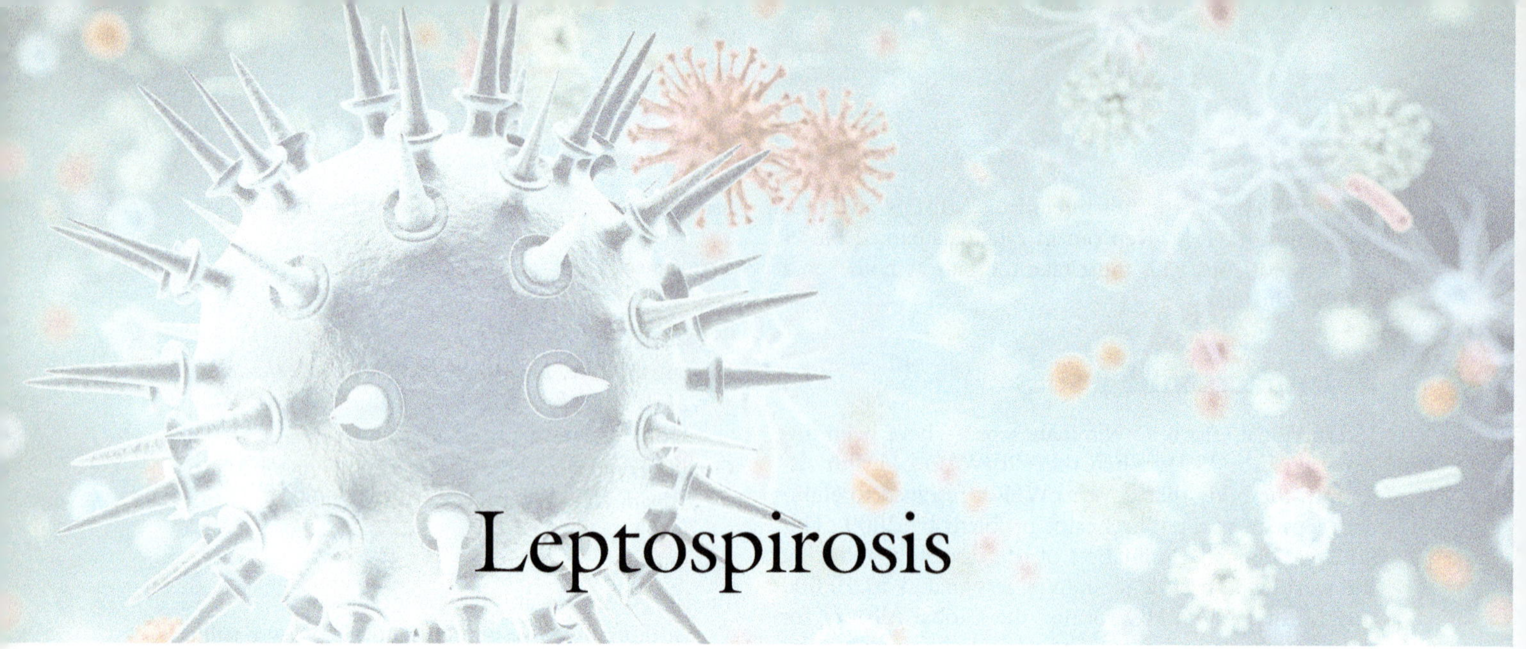

Leptospirosis

Introduction

Leptospirosis is a disease that is caused by bacteria from the genus *Leptospira*. It is considered an emerging disease and is found worldwide. Leptospirosis often goes undiagnosed because its symptoms are similar to those of a number of other diseases, including influenza. For this reason, the prevalence of the disease is unknown. In the 2010s the World Health Organization (WHO) called for more research into the disease and its burden on communities.

Infection occurs when humans come in contact with freshwater, soil, or vegetation that is contaminated with the urine of an infected animal. The bacteria pass from the urine into the human body via mucosal linings, such as the linings of the eyes, nose, or mouth; through broken skin; or orally, when food or water is ingested. Illness typically develops within 10 days and is characterized by fever, aches, vomiting, diarrhea, and jaundice. Treatment with antibiotics leads to successful recovery, although in some cases a second phase can occur with more severe symptoms. During this second phase, known as Weil's disease, patients suffer more severe symptoms that may include kidney failure, liver failure, or meningitis. Weil's disease occurs in around 5 to 10 percent of cases. People who die from leptospirosis usually have developed Weil's disease.

Leptospirosis occurs mainly in the tropics, although it is a worldwide disease found both in rural and urban regions of developed and developing countries. According to WHO, there are vaccines for this disease, but none are commercially available. Prevention efforts focus on avoiding contact with anything that may have been contaminated with the bacteria. Risk is highest for people who work or spend time outdoors, in fresh water, or with animals.

WORDS TO KNOW

JAUNDICE A condition in which a person's skin and the whites of the eyes are discolored a shade of yellow due to an increased level of bile pigments in the blood as a result of liver disease. Jaundice is sometimes called icterus, from a Greek word for the condition.

LEPTOSPIRE Also called a leptospira, any bacterial species of the genus *Leptospira*. Infection with leptospires causes leptospirosis.

WEIL'S DISEASE Named after German doctor Adolf Weil (1848–1916), a severe form of leptospirosis or seven-day fever, which is a disease caused by infection with the corkscrew-shaped bacillus *Leptospira interrogans*.

Disease History, Characteristics, and Transmission

Leptospirosis was first recognized in 1886 by German scientist Adolf Weil (1848–1916). The cause of the disease was not identified until about the 1920s, when both Japanese and German scientists discovered that bacteria were responsible. Leptospirosis is caused by leptospires, which are disease-causing bacteria in the genus *Leptospira*. The primary agent causing leptospirosis is *Leptospira interrogans*.

Scope and Distribution

Leptospirosis most commonly occurs in the tropics, although it is present in temperate regions as well. It thrives in warm temperatures and moist conditions and is transmitted by wild and domestic animals, including rodents, dogs, cattle, horses, and pigs. Therefore, people who spend a great deal of time outdoors, or with animals, are more likely to contract leptospirosis.

At-risk populations include subsistence farmers, pastoralists (people who care for livestock), and people who live in poor, urban environments. Sewer workers, military personnel, and veterinarians are also at risk, as are people taking part in outdoor recreational activities, such as camping or water sports, because they are more likely to come in contact with urine-contaminated water.

Leptospirosis occurs worldwide but tends to be underreported in most countries because it is often overlooked during diagnosis. This is due to the similarities between symptoms of leptospirosis and those of other tropical diseases. As a result, the global prevalence of this disease is unknown. In a 2015 article for *PLOS Neglected Tropical Diseases*, Mathieu Picardeau wrote that "the limitations of surveillance systems in low-income tropical countries likely contribute to an underestimation of [leptospirosis's] burden. This is the case for numerous countries in Africa, for example, where there is increasing evidence that leptospirosis accounts for a significant proportion of nonmalarial fever cases."

■ Treatment and Prevention

Patients with leptospirosis can recover without treatment, although recovery may take several months, and lack of treatment can lead to complications. Treatment is usually administered as soon as possible and involves a course of antibiotics. A range of antibiotics can be used for mild leptospirosis, including doxycycline, ampicillin, and amoxicillin. In severe cases intravenous penicillin G is the drug of choice. Recovery can take from three days to several weeks. In most cases recovery is complete. More severe complications arise when the patient does not receive antibiotics or if the patient develops the second phase of the illness.

PREVENTIVE MEASURES TO TAKE AGAINST DISEASE

A fact sheet published by the World Health Organization (WHO) outlined numerous ways to prevent leptospirosis, stating, "Risk of infection is minimized by avoiding contact with animal urine, infected animals or a contaminated environment. Measures to prevent transmission of leptospirosis include the following:

- Wearing protective clothing (boots, gloves, spectacles, aprons, masks).
- Covering skin lesions with waterproof dressings.
- Preventing access to, or giving adequate warning about, water bodies known or suspected to be contaminated (pools, ponds, rivers). Try to avoid wading or swimming in potentially contaminated water.
- Washing or showering after exposure to urine splashes or contaminated soil or water.
- Washing and cleaning wounds.
- Avoiding or preventing urine splashes and aerosols, avoiding touching ill or dead animals, or assisting animals in giving birth.
- Strictly maintaining hygienic measures during care or handling of all animals.
- Where feasible, disinfecting contaminated areas (scrubbing floors in stables, butcheries, abattoirs, etc.).
- Consuming clean drinking-water.

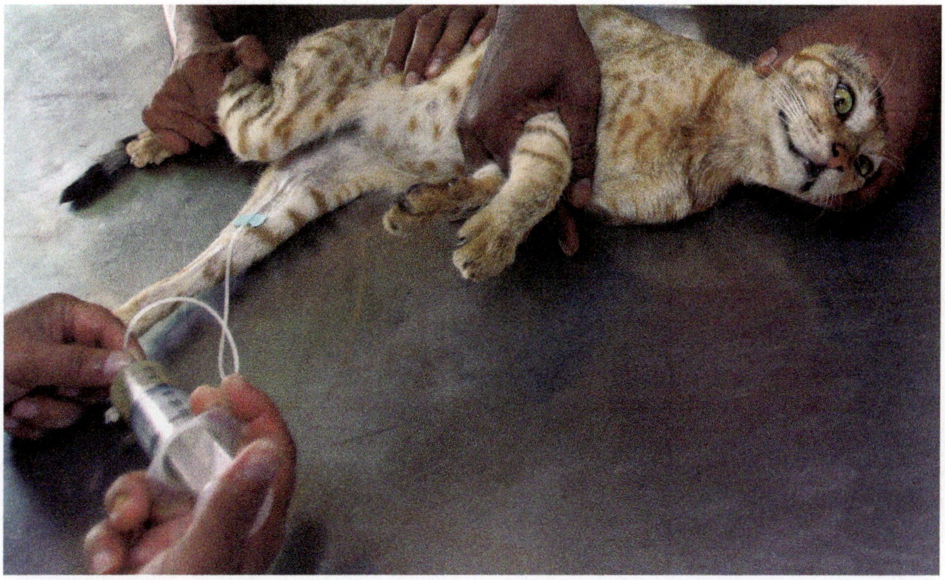

Cats, such as the one being treated here at a hospital in Mumbai, India, are among the various wild and domestic animals infected with leptospirosis. © *Kunal Patil/Hindustan Times/Getty Images*

Prevention is best achieved by avoiding contaminated water, soil, or vegetation, particularly in areas with infected or potentially infected animals. Clothing such as boots or waders can provide protection during recreational activities, and gloves can provide protection when handling animals. Taking antibiotics while traveling through infected areas may also help prevent severe infections from developing if people become contaminated.

■ Impacts and Issues

Leptospirosis is becoming more common. Because this disease occurs in both developed and developing countries and in both urban and rural areas, it has become globally important.

Despite the high likelihood of recovery following treatment, there is still a significant mortality rate for leptospirosis. This is largely because the disease is hard to recognize, which delays diagnosis. In addition, due to the lack of a commercially available vaccine, avoidance of the bacteria remains the best prevention method. However, avoidance depends on the maintenance of rigorous sanitation methods, which is not always possible in developing countries or in countries experiencing war or other social upheavals. Therefore, contamination still occurs frequently.

The chance of exposure to contaminated sources is exacerbated during floods, outdoor activity, or in animal-populated regions. In 1995 widespread flooding in Nicaragua spread the bacteria, and more than 2,000 people contracted leptospirosis. At least 13 of those with the disease died. Two years later nine Americans became infected while white-water rafting in Costa Rica. In addition, growing rat populations, especially in urban areas, increase public exposure to leptospirosis when water systems and sewers become contaminated. This may explain the higher levels of leptospirosis seen in Germany between 1962 and 2003. Experts are concerned that leptospirosis rates may continue to increase due to extreme weather events caused by climate change and the development of wilderness areas home to wildlife with the disease.

According to a 2015 study led by Federico Costa and published in *PLOS Neglected Tropical Diseases,* an estimated 1,030,000 people contract leptospirosis each year, with approximately 58,900 dying of the disease. Men in their 20s had the highest morbidity rate. Costa and his coauthors stated that the "majority of leptospirosis cases and deaths occur in tropical regions; 73% of the world's leptospirosis cases and deaths occur in countries situated between the Tropics of Cancer and Capricorn." In addition, a 2015 study led by Paul R. Torgerson and published in *PLOS Neglected Tropical Diseases* noted that, "because most cases [of leptospirosis] are reported in young adult males, it can have a substantial economic impact in low and middle income countries."

SEE ALSO *Bacterial Disease; Emerging Infectious Diseases; Meningitis, Bacterial; Personal Protective Equipment; Travel and Infectious Disease; War and Infectious Disease; Water-borne Disease*

BIBLIOGRAPHY

Books

Adler, Ben, ed. *Leptospira and Leptospirosis.* Berlin: Springer-Verlag, 2016.

Bennett, John E., Raphael Dolin, and Martin J. Blaser. *Mandell, Douglas, and Bennett's Principles and Practice of Infectious Diseases.* 8th ed. Philadelphia: Elsevier/Saunders, 2015.

Guerrant, Richard L., David H. Walker, and Peter F. Weller. *Tropical Infectious Diseases: Principles, Pathogens and Practice.* 3rd ed. Philadelphia: Elsevier/Saunders, 2011.

Periodicals

Chiu, C. H. et al. "Leptospirosis and Depression: A Nationwide Cohort Analysis." *Journal of Clinical Psychiatry* 78, no. 4 (April 2017): e398–e403. This article can also be found online at https://www.ncbi.nlm.nih.gov/pubmed/28297597 (accessed January 19, 2018).

Costa, Federico, et al. "Global Morbidity and Mortality of Leptospirosis: A Systematic Review." *PLOS Neglected Tropical Diseases* (September 17, 2015). This article can also be found online at http://journals.plos.org/plosntds/article?id=10.1371/journal.pntd.0003898 (accessed January 19, 2018).

Guerra, Marta A. "Leptospirosis: Public Health Perspectives." *Biologicals* 41, no. 5 (September 2013): 295–297. This article can also be found online at http://www.sciencedirect.com/science/article/pii/S1045105613000687 (accessed January 19, 2018).

Picardeau, Mathieu. "Leptospirosis: Updating the Global Picture of an Emerging Neglected Disease." *PLOS Neglected Tropical Diseases* (September 24, 2015). This article can also be found online at http://journals.plos.org/plosntds/article?id=10.1371/journal.pntd.0004039 (accessed January 19, 2018).

Torgerson, Paul R., et al. "Global Burden of Leptospirosis: Estimated in Terms of Disability Adjusted Life Years." *PLOS Neglected Tropical Diseases* (October 2, 2015). This article can also be found online at http://journals.plos.org/plosntds/article?id=10.1371/journal.pntd.0004122 (accessed January 19, 2018).

Turkan, Togal, et al. "Intensive Care of a Weil's Disease with Multiorgan Failure." *Journal of Clinical Medicine Research* 2, no. 3 (June 2010): 145–149. This article can also be found online at https://www.ncbi.nlm.nih.gov/pmc/articles/PMC3104646/ (accessed January 19, 2018).

Websites

"Leptospirosis." Centers for Disease Control and Prevention, October 13, 2017. https://www.cdc.gov/leptospirosis/index.html (accessed January 19, 2018).

"Leptospirosis." World Health Organization, August 13, 2012. http://www.wpro.who.int/mediacentre/factsheets/fs_13082012_leptospirosis/en/ (accessed January 19, 2018).

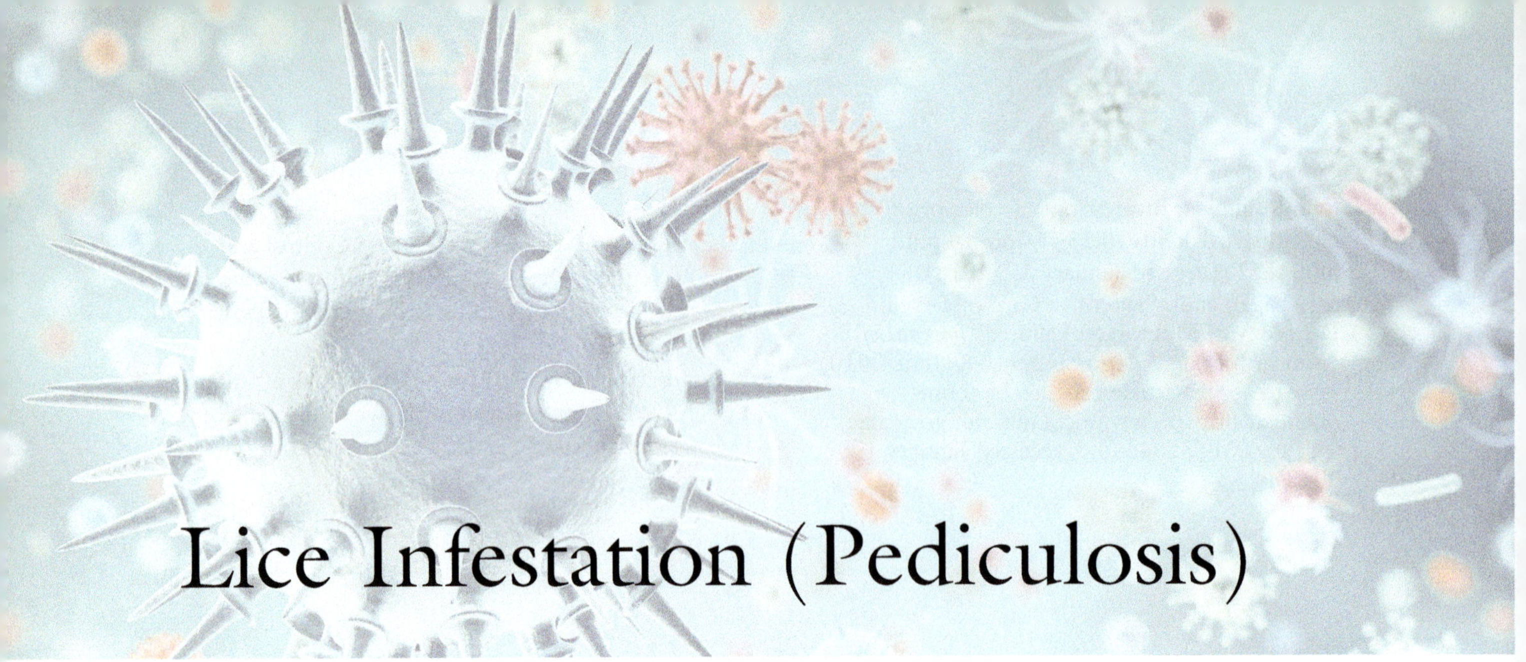

Lice Infestation (Pediculosis)

Introduction

Of the many parasites that can infest humans, one of the most common is the louse, a wingless insect. There are several types of lice that infect humans, usually classified as one of three species. These are the head louse (*Pediculus humanus capitis*), which infests only the head; the body louse (*Pediculus humanus corporis*), which lives in clothing near the skin; and the crab louse or pubic louse (*Phthirus pubis*), which mostly infests the groin. Infestation with lice is called pediculosis (ped-ih-q-LO-sis). Some biologists have argued that the head louse and body louse may be different varieties of a single species. Head and body lice can interbreed in captivity but do not do so on the human body.

WORDS TO KNOW

PARASITE An organism that lives in or on a host organism and that gets its nourishment from that host. The parasite usually gains all the benefits of this relationship, while the host may suffer from various diseases and discomforts or show no signs of the infection. The life cycle of a typical parasite usually includes several developmental stages and morphological changes as the parasite lives and moves through the environment and one or more hosts. Parasites that remain on a host's body surface to feed are called ectoparasites, while those that live inside a host's body are called endoparasites. Parasitism is a highly successful biological adaptation. There are more known parasitic species than nonparasitic ones, and parasites affect just about every form of life, including most all animals, plants, and even bacteria.

Disease History, Characteristics, and Transmission

Human lice can exist only on human beings; they die in about 24 hours if they are removed from the body. Lice also infest humans' nearest evolutionary cousins, chimpanzees and gorillas, but these lice belong to a different species than those that infest humans. As apes and humans continued to evolve over the last few million years, lice evolved along with them.

The female head or body louse lays several eggs a day. Lice eggs are called nits (the source of the word *nitpick*) and are cemented to the hair or, in the case of body lice, to clothing fibers. The eggs take 7 to 10 days to hatch. A female louse can start laying eggs 7 to 10 days after hatching. A louse bites through the skin to suck blood from its host about five times a day.

On a healthy host, lice can cause itching, rash, fever, headaches, and fatigue but are rarely life-threatening. However, body lice can act as carriers of more serious diseases. Three types of disease can be transmitted by body lice to the humans they bite, namely relapsing fever (caused by the bacterium *Borrelia recurrentis*), trench fever (caused by the bacillus *Bartonella quintana*), and—most seriously—typhus (caused by *Rickettsia prowazekii*).

Lice spread by crawling from one host to another or through the transfer of eggs. The majority of head lice are spread by head-to-head contact or, more rarely, by coming into contact with objects that have picked up eggs from the hair, such as combs, pillows, hats, hair ties, and the like. Body lice are spread through body contact or shared clothing and bedding. Pubic lice are spread primarily through sexual contact or other body contact.

Scope and Distribution

Lice infestation has been common in most populations throughout history. Dead lice and eggs have been found on Egyptian mummies and Roman bodies buried under volcanic ash at Pompeii. About 6 to 12 million people acquire head lice in the United States each year; smaller numbers acquire body or pubic lice.

The head louse is still found worldwide at all levels of society. Head lice are extremely common in developing countries. In Western industrialized countries, outbreaks are often associated with schoolchildren. The CDC estimated in 2015 that 6 to 12 million head lice infestations occur in children ages 3 to 11 each year.

With the Industrial Revolution and the spread of bathing technology through much of the modern world—including indoor plumbing, soap, shampoo, laundry machines, and detergent—the body louse has become less common. In the 21st century human body lice are found mostly in situations where poor hygiene, overcrowding, and wearing the same clothing for extended periods are more common.

Treatment and Prevention

Lice infestation is diagnosed through the identification of live louse nymphs or adults on a person's scalp or hair. The two methods of treating lice infestation are pesticides (chemicals that kill insects or other pests) and physical removal of the lice via lice combs. The pesticides most often used are permethrin and pyrethrins, which are available over the counter. Prescription treatments include malathion, ivermectin lotion, or spinosad topical suspension. In cases where these remedies have failed, lindane shampoo may be prescribed. Lindane shampoo must be used with care, however, because it is highly toxic if swallowed and can cause damage to the nervous system, including the brain. However, as is common with pesticides, heavily exposed populations of lice have evolved resistance to these chemicals. The National Pediculosis Association (NPA) advises against the use of pesticides on any person with preexisting illnesses such as severe asthma, epilepsy, cancer, or acquired immunodeficiency syndrome (AIDS). Fine-toothed steel combs can also be used to remove head lice and nits from hair.

In addition to treating the heads of those affected, it is important to treat the living environment to prevent reinfestation. Combs and brushes should be soaked in water of at least 130°F (54°C) for a minimum of 5 to 10 minutes. Clothes and bedding of those affected by lice infestation should be dry-cleaned or washed in hot water and dried using high heat. Carpets and rugs should be vacuumed thoroughly.

To prevent head lice infestation, it is important to avoid head-to-head contact. Although it is not the most common method of transmittal, lice can be spread by sharing clothing, hair accessories, and bedding. School-age children should be taught to avoid these practices. To prevent body lice infestation, it is important to bathe and change into clean clothes at least once a week and to avoid sharing clothing or linens with anyone who may be suffering from lice infestation.

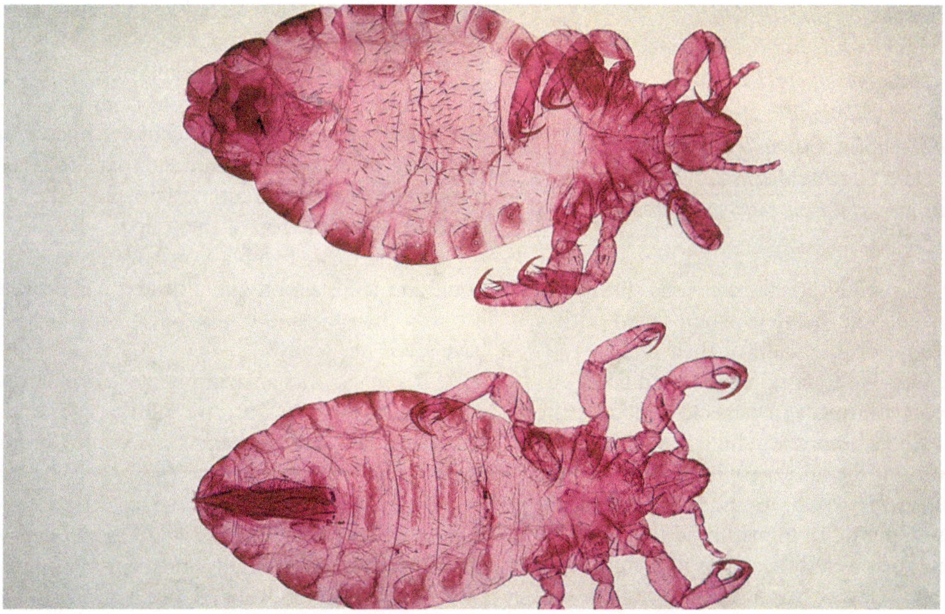

Close-up of a human body louse. Other varieties of lice include head lice and pubic lice. © *AFIP/Science Source*

Impacts and Issues

As of 2017 lice and louse-borne disease remained a problem for homeless and poor inner-city populations in industrialized countries such as the United States, France, Holland, and Russia.

Wars and social breakdown can lead to large outbreaks of lice, as can any condition where people exist in crowded areas without access to sanitation and clean clothing. A large outbreak of typhus occurred in several refugee camps in Burundi in 1997 where most of the inhabitants were louse-infested. In 2015 several cases of louse-borne relapsing fever, a bacterial disease transmitted by lice, were confirmed in Europe among refugees from northeastern Africa, who were believed to have contracted body lice during their journey to Europe. The diagnosis of cases in Italy, the Netherlands, and Switzerland led to calls for awareness of the condition and its symptoms and greater attention to the living conditions of at-risk populations.

The safety of the pesticides used in standard anti-lice products is questioned by the NPA, which has campaigned for the use of fine-toothed combs as the treatment of choice in removing lice. Some individuals can have allergic reactions to the pesticides used to treat pediculosis.

PRIMARY SOURCE

An Expert Approach

SOURCE: *Henn, Steve. "The Key to Keeping Lice at Bay? A Lot of Hot Air."* All Things Considered. *National Public Radio, April 9, 2012. https://www.npr.org/2012/04/09/150299564/the-key-to-keeping-lice-at-bay-a-lot-of-hot-air (accessed November 14, 2017).*

INTRODUCTION: *In the following transcript from National Public Radio, entomologist and parasitologist Dale Clayton discusses what happened when his own children contracted head lice.*

Even researchers who study lice for a living—Ph.D.s in entomology—can become helpless when faced with a live, fertile louse loose on the scalp of their child.

"My wife and I couldn't get rid of the head lice," says Dale Clayton, a co-evolution and parasite expert at the University of Utah who's been researching lice for decades. "Here I am supposed to be an expert on lice—and there are not many of us in the world, by the way—completely clueless about how to get rid of human head lice."

When Clayton's kids were little, they—like millions of others—got lice, and Clayton spent weeks combing and picking and shampooing to get them out.

"Even then it was already pretty well known that lice were evolving resistance to many of the shampoos that are available in drugstores and grocery stores and so on," says Clayton, so he made it his mission to build a better louse trap.

"The first attempt was to take pigeon lice—and I am not making this up—and put them in my hair and then put on my mother's bonnet hair dryer and see if it had any effect on them—if it killed them," he says.

It didn't. But one thing you should know about Clayton is that he's not crazy—he just knows a lot about lice. For example, he knew that pigeon lice could never survive and breed on a human head.

Airing Them Out

So when Clayton moved his lab from Oxford, England, to Utah and his lice started dying off, that got him thinking.

"It's quite arid here," he says. "We couldn't keep lice alive on our birds, and we couldn't figure out why for a few months."

Then it came to him: Sudden changes in climate can kill lice, and lice get most of their moisture from the air. If you suck all the moisture out of a louse, you can dry it out, desiccate it, kill it.

A bunch of dead lice may have been bad for Clayton's research, but as a parent who was sick of nit-picking, he saw an opportunity: He imagined building a machine that could kill these annoying little bugs by the thousands.

"We tried a bunch of different approaches to drying out lice," he says. He tried hair dryers, bonnets from beauty parlors and handhelds; he tried those wall-mounted hand blowers you see in bathrooms; he even tried a leaf blower.

"At one point, we infested my kids with head lice—male lice only so they couldn't breed—and treated them in the lab," Clayton says. "They're in college now, but they like to tell that story to shock their friends."

Eventually, he and a team of engineers built the LouseBuster. It looks like an old canister vacuum cleaner, but instead of sucking air in, it blows hot air out. On the end of it there's an attachment that looks a bit like an overgrown plastic porcupine with 28 little nozzles that direct air along the top of the scalp.

Getting treated with a LouseBuster takes about half an hour, and it feels a bit like a heated head massage. It kills lice *and* their eggs, the nits. Sheri Nacht says it also may have saved her sanity.

"It's magic. It's amazing because nothing else kills the eggs," she says. "If you can't kill the eggs and you don't find every last one of them, then you're starting all over again."

Today, Clayton's company sells the LouseBuster to nurses, schools and hospitals, and it leases it to salons with names like Nitless Noggins and Hair Whisperers. Clayton doubts his invention will ever make him rich, but he says it has at least allowed him to scratch his entrepreneurial itch.

SEE ALSO *Parasitic Diseases; Typhoid Fever; Typhus*

BIBLIOGRAPHY

Books

Gratz, Norman. *Vector- and Rodent-Borne Diseases in Europe and North America: Distribution, Public Health Burden, and Control.* Cambridge, UK: Cambridge University Press, 2006.

Periodicals

Brody, Jane E. "That Dreaded Nemesis, Head Lice." *New York Times* (June 2, 2015): D5. This article can also be found online at https://well.blogs.nytimes.com/2015/06/01/new-tactics-for-battling-head-lice/ (accessed November 14, 2017).

Elston, Dirk M. "Drugs Used in the Treatment of Pediculosis." *Journal of Drugs in Dermatology* 4, no. 2 (March–April 2005): 207–211.

Land, Stephanie. "Kids Shouldn't Be Sent Home for Lice, but Schools Can't Ignore the Issue Either." *Washington Post* (October 24, 2017). This article can also be found online at https://www.washingtonpost.com/news/parenting/wp/2017/10/24/easing-up-on-the-no-nit-policy-at-schools-hurts-low-income-families/?utm_term=.8e360f99b675 (accessed November 14, 2017).

Websites

"Parasites—Lice—Body Lice." Centers for Disease Control and Prevention. https://www.cdc.gov/parasites/lice/body/index.html (accessed November 14, 2017).

"Welcome to Headlice.org." National Pediculosis Association. 2007. http://www.headlice.org/ (accessed November 14, 2017).

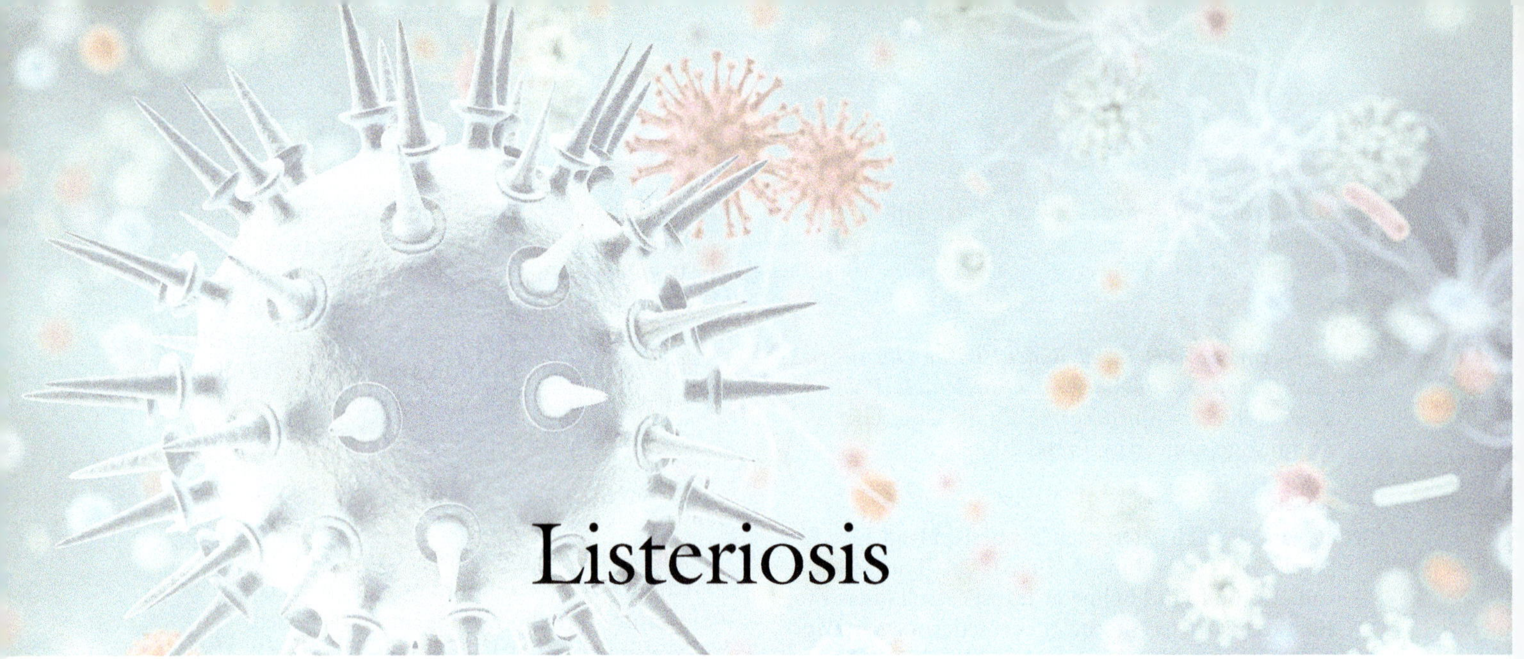

Listeriosis

Introduction

Listeriosis is an infection that is caused by eating food that is contaminated by the bacterium *Listeria monocytogenes.* The infection, which can be serious, primarily affects pregnant women, infants, and immunocompromised people.

Disease History, Characteristics, and Transmission

The bacterium *L. monocytogenes* is a normal inhabitant of soil and water. Vegetables can become contaminated with the bacterium if soil or manure clings to them. Humans can then become infected if the contaminated vegetables are not properly washed before eating.

Foods other than vegetables also can become contaminated because animals such as cattle can harbor the bacterium without any ill effects. Meat and dairy products may become contaminated unknowingly. Infection can result if the meat is eaten raw or cooked improperly or if unpasteurized milk is consumed. Other foods that can be contaminated by *L. monocytogenes* include cheeses (particularly those made with unpasteurized milk) and processed meats that remain unrefrigerated long enough (within a day) for contaminating bacteria to multiply. In contrast to some bacterial infections, where a large number of living bacteria need to be consumed to cause illness, relatively few *L. monocytogenes* need to be eaten to cause listeriosis.

Symptoms of listeriosis include flu-like fever, nausea, and vomiting, as well as abdominal cramping, diarrhea, and headache. The symptoms may appear within a few days after eating contaminated foods but also can appear two to three months later. In people whose immune systems are compromised, the infection can progress to a lethal blood infection (sepsis) or brain infection. Infections during pregnancy can lead to infection of the newborn, as well as to miscarriage, stillbirth, or premature birth.

WORDS TO KNOW

IMMUNOCOMPROMISED Having an immune system with reduced ability to recognize and respond to the presence of foreign material.

PASTEURIZATION A process in which fluids such as wine and milk are heated for a predetermined time at a temperature below the boiling point of the liquid. The treatment kills any microorganisms that are in the fluid but does not alter the taste, appearance, or nutritive value of the fluid.

SEPSIS A bacterial infection in the bloodstream or body tissues. This is a very broad term covering the presence of many types of microscopic disease-causing organisms. Sepsis is also called *bacteremia.* Closely related terms include *septicemia* and *septic syndrome.*

Scope and Distribution

Listeriosis has become a significant health threat. In the United States the Centers for Disease Control and Prevention (CDC) estimated in 2017 that 1,600 people are sickened with listeriosis each year. Of these, about 260 die, representing a mortality (death) rate of about 16 percent.

Pregnant women and people over 65 years old are more likely to acquire listeriosis than are other adults. Immunocompromised individuals, who cannot as easily fight off infections, are also susceptible to listeriosis. Proper functioning of the immune system may be impaired by certain diseases, including diabetes, cancer, kidney disease, and acquired immunodeficiency syndrome (AIDS), as well as by advanced age and certain drugs, such as those taken by transplant patients to reduce the likelihood of transplant rejection. Listeriosis also can occur in individuals whose immune systems are functioning normally, but the infection is usually not nearly as serious.

Treatment and Prevention

L. monocytogenes is easily killed by pasteurization, a process during which a product is held at a certain temperature for a certain length of time to kill most bacteria without altering the chemistry or taste of the product. However, some foods can become contaminated after they have been processed but before they are packaged for sale. Delicatessen-style meat and hot dogs are two common examples. The bacteria can remain alive and capable of causing infection during transport, sale, and consumption.

Many common-sense precautions can prevent listeriosis. Thoroughly cooking beef, pork, and poultry is sufficient to kill any *L. monocytogenes* that may contaminate the product. Washing vegetables removes bacteria. When storing food, uncooked meat should not be allowed to come into contact with vegetables, food that is already cooked, or prepared foods. All items used in the preparation of uncooked foods should be thoroughly washed before reuse to avoid transferring *L. monocytogenes* to other foodstuffs. While cheeses made from unpasteurized milk (such as Brie, Camembert, and feta) are preferred by some people, and the consumption of unpasteurized milk is sometimes advocated as a healthy alternative, there is a risk to these practices, as they increase the likelihood of exposure to the bacteria. Finally, prepared foods should be eaten promptly because *L. monocytogenes*, in contrast to most other disease-causing bacteria, can slowly grow at temperatures above 39°F (4°C). A malfunctioning refrigerator can also create conditions in which the bacteria can grow.

Government agencies such as the US Food and Drug Administration (FDA) and the US Department of Agriculture (USDA) monitor food regularly to reduce contamination of food by the *Listeria* bacterium and other infectious agents. Food monitoring and plant inspection are key assessment and prevention tools. Recalls can also be issued for contaminated or suspect food.

Impacts and Issues

Listeriosis can be a serious infection, and, in the case of pregnant women, it can lead to miscarriage, stillbirth, premature delivery, or infection in the newborn. Although pregnant women in the United States are not routinely tested for infection with the bacteria that causes listeriosis, many health care providers recommend that pregnant women avoid consuming unpasteurized milk products and ready-to-eat deli-type meat products unless they are reheated until steaming hot.

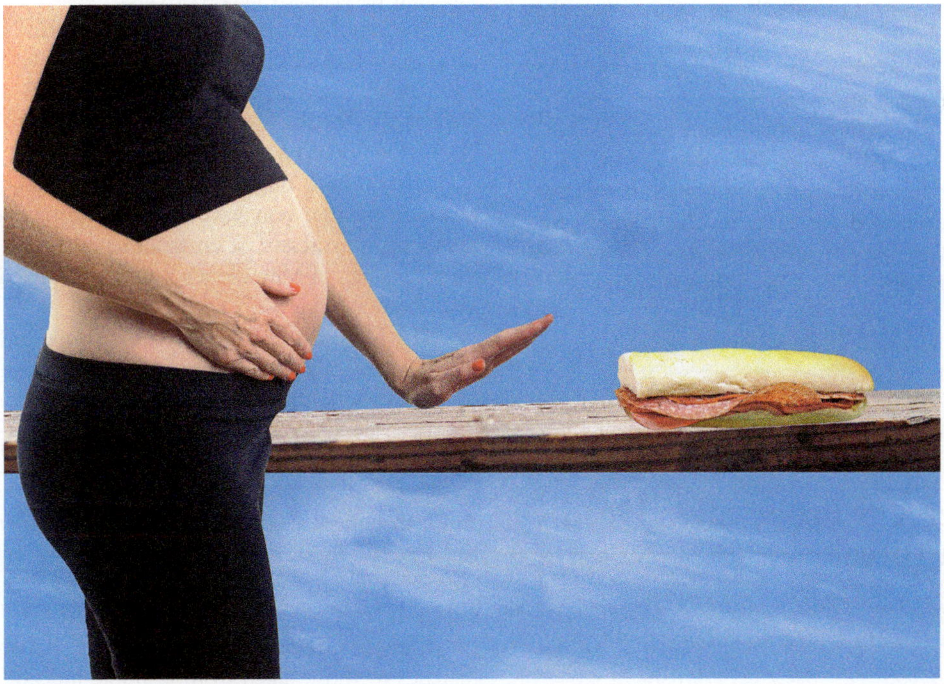

Listeriosis, a type of food poisoning often spread by processed foods such as cold cuts, is particularly dangerous for pregnant women. Dangers of listeriosis in pregnant women include miscarriage and stillbirth. *© FtLaudGirl/Getty Images*

From 1996 to 2002 the rate of listeriosis cases in the United States fell by 35 percent. This decrease was attributed to aggressive sampling and testing programs by government meat inspectors and education designed to raise awareness about the dangers of *L. monocytogenes*, especially among at-risk groups such as pregnant women. In the years since, the lowered rate has been maintained. In 2017 the CDC estimated 1,600 cases of listeriosis, with 260 deaths attributed to the infection. The US Food Safety and Inspection Service (FSIS) established regulations in 2003 for plants that make or process ready-to-eat meat and poultry products. The regulations have been updated frequently, such as in 2015, when guidelines for delicatessens selling meat or poultry products or salads susceptible to contamination by *Listeria* were released. The updates reflect scientific developments, as well as developments in food processing technology. The rule also encourages plants to install new technologies to eliminate or reduce the growth of *L. monocytogenes.*

The latter is important, as the machinery used in the processing of some foods can be difficult to clean. Without regular and dedicated cleaning, *L. monocytogenes* can become established in the machinery and contaminate food. In 2016 a food processing facility in Pasco, Washington, was identified as the source of a listeriosis outbreak linked to contaminated frozen foods. Conditions at the plant had deteriorated to the point where regular cleaning of the machinery could not eliminate the bacterial growth. The plant was closed for over six months for cleaning.

In January to March 2016, an outbreak caused by contaminated bagged salad sold by Dole resulted in a nationwide recall and a four-month closure of the plant that was involved.

Researchers are working on "smart packaging" that may help reduce the sale and consumption of contaminated foods. One type of packaging incorporates molecules that recognize surface components of *L. monocytogenes.* These molecules are combined with other molecules that change color in the presence of the bacterium. This color change can alert consumers that the product is contaminated. As of 2017 the technology was still in the research and development stage.

PRIMARY SOURCE

Dole under US Probe after Deadly Listeria Outbreak

SOURCE: *Baertlein, Lisa. "Dole under U.S. Probe after Deadly Listeria Outbreak." Reuters, April 29, 2016. https://www.reuters.com/article/us-dole-food-listeria/dole-under-u-s-probe-after-deadly-listeria-outbreak-idUSKCN0XQ2N2 (accessed November 20, 2017).*

INTRODUCTION: *LOS ANGELES (Reuters)—Dole Food Co Inc [DFCI.UL] said on Friday the US Department of Justice was investigating a deadly Listeria monocytogenes outbreak linked to packaged salad products from its processing plant in Springfield, Ohio.*

Dole, the world's largest fruit and vegetable producer, said in a statement the agency recently contacted the company and "we will be ... cooperating with the DOJ to answer questions and address any concerns."

Listeria, a common bacterium that can be either harmless or pathogenic, can enter a processing facility via raw produce or other materials, and form colonies. Thirty-three people in the United States and Canada fell ill in the outbreak from May 2015 to February 2016. All were hospitalized and four died.

Dole said on Jan. 22 it had temporarily suspended operations at the Springfield plant. It also issued recalls on all salad products packaged at the facility.

The plant reopened on April 21.

Plant officials found evidence of Listeria contamination there as early as July 2014, Food Safety News (FSN) reported on Friday.

A Food and Drug Administration (FDA) inspection report obtained by FSN and reviewed by Reuters on Friday showed that Dole's tests of surfaces at the plant came back positive for Listeria on nine separate occasions in 2014 and 2015.

Dole said in its statement that the report dealt with issues that had already been corrected.

The report, dated Feb. 5, said the plant's third-party laboratory had notified Dole about positive Listeria test results from internal samples taken on Jan. 5 and 7. But it did not say whether testing was done to determine whether the bacteria posed a threat.

"If you have ongoing, persistent contamination, that can indicate that you have a sanitation problem," Craig Hedberg, a professor of environmental health sciences at the University of Minnesota's School of Public Health, said in a phone interview on Friday.

The FDA inspected the plant five times in January and February 2016. Product samples collected at various stages of salad processing on Jan. 16 tested positive for Listeria monocytogenes, a strain that can cause severe illness, the report said.

On Jan. 26, Dole told inspectors the company was aware that the Canadian Food Inspection Agency (CFIA) had found Listeria monocytogenes in four salad product samples collected by the agency earlier that month, according to the report.

The samples found by FDA and CFIA were genetic matches to those taken from multiple individuals who fell ill during the outbreak.

See Also *Bacterial Disease; Food-Borne Disease and Food Safety*

BIBLIOGRAPHY

Books

Cramer, Michael M. *Food Plant Sanitation: Design, Maintenance, and Good Manufacturing Practices.* 2nd ed. Boca Raton, FL: CRC, 2016.

Kazemi, Samaneth. *Stress Response in Listeria Monocytogenes.* London: Lambert Academic, 2017.

Ryser, Elliot T., and Elmer H. Marth. *Listeria, Listeriosis, and Food Safety.* 3rd ed. Boca Raton, FL: CRC, 2007.

Periodicals

Addady, Michal. "FDA Says Processing Plant Linked to Massive Listeria Outbreak Is Impossible to Clean." *Fortune* (May 15, 2016). This article can also be found online at http://fortune.com/2016/05/15/frozen-food-listeria/ (accessed November 20, 2017).

Biji, K. B., et al. "Smart Packaging Systems for Food Applications: A Review." *Journal of Food Science Technology* 52 (October 2015): 6125–6135.

Charlier, Caroline, et al. "MONOLISA: A Grim Picture of Listeriosis." *Lancet Infectious Diseases* 17 (May 2017): 464–466.

Websites

"Listeria (Listeriosis)." Centers for Disease Control and Prevention. https://www.cdc.gov/listeria/index.html (accessed November 20, 2017).

"Listeria Monocytogenes: Policy, Procedures, Guidance." United States Department of Agriculture, June 11, 2015. https://www.fsis.usda.gov/wps/portal/fsis/topics/regulatory-compliance/listeria (accessed November 20, 2017).

Brian Hoyle

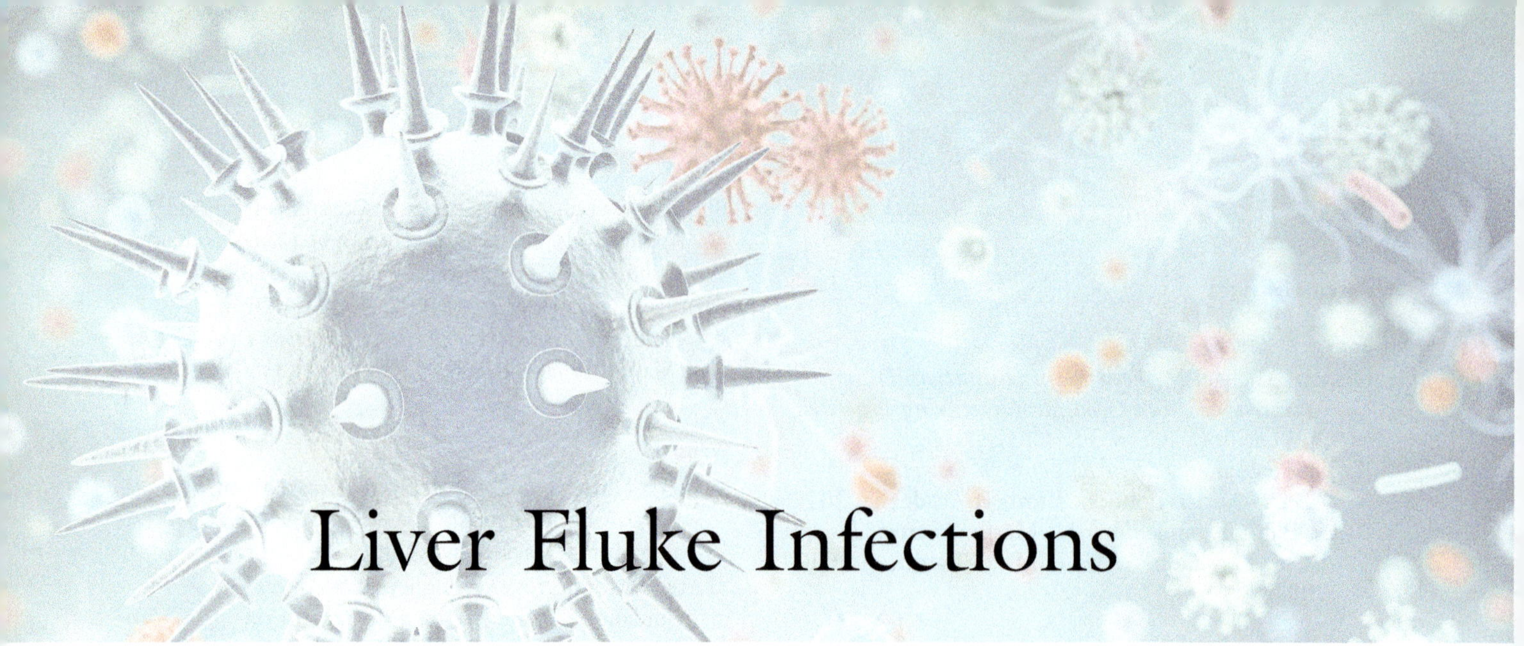

Liver Fluke Infections

■ Introduction

Liver fluke infections are the result of infestation by liver flukes, a type of flat parasitic worm known as a helminth. Liver fluke infections are zoonotic, meaning they originate in domestic and wild animals before being transmitted to humans. There are various types of liver fluke infections caused by different kinds of liver flukes. Among the most widely reported liver fluke infections are clonorchiasis, which is caused by infection with *Clonorchis sinensis*; opisthorchiasis, which results from infection with *Opisthorchis viverrini* or *O. felineus;* and fascioliasis, which is caused by *Fasciola hepatica*.

Although each infection is caused by different species of flukes, they share similarities in characteristics and transmission. Humans become infected after drinking contaminated water or eating raw or undercooked food with cysts containing parasitic forms of the flukes. These cysts open in the digestive system and release the parasites.

Most liver fluke infections are asymptomatic, but in more severe cases patients experience acute or chronic symptoms. Mild cases result in tiredness, fever, aches, swollen liver, abdominal pain, and rash. Symptoms of chronic forms include exacerbated versions of the acute symptoms with possible diarrhea, nausea, swelling of the face, block-

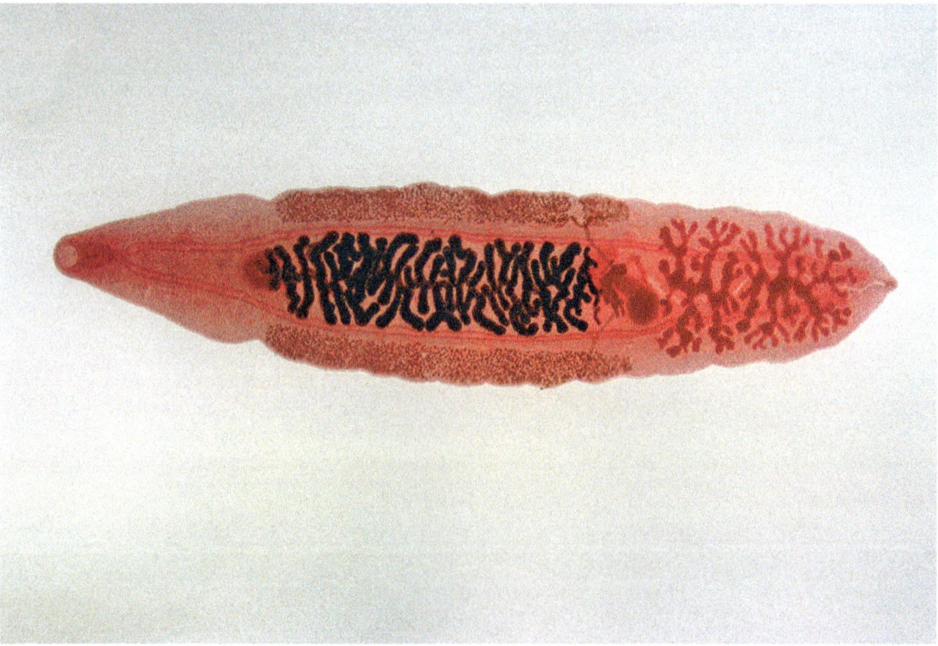

Liver fluke infections are the result of infestation by parasitic worms known as liver flukes. People become infected when they ingest the cysts containing parasitic forms of the flukes, often by drinking contaminated water or eating undercooked food that contains the cysts. *© Eric V. Grave/Science Source*

age of the bile ducts, and sometimes complications such as migration of flukes to other regions in the body. Certain forms of chronic liver fluke infection, including clonorchiasis, are associated with cancer. Administration of any anthelmintic drug is usually effective, with recovery likely to occur.

Liver fluke infections occur worldwide but are concentrated primarily in Eastern Europe and Asia, including Russia and other former Soviet states. Prevalence is highest in China, Thailand, and South Korea. Some 35 million people are believed to be infected with liver flukes worldwide, about 15 million of them Chinese.

Disease History, Characteristics, and Transmission

Liver flukes belong to a specific group of parasitic worms known as flukes or trematodes. There are various kinds of trematodes that cause the different kinds of liver fluke infections. While the infections produce similar symptoms, the trematodes differ in terms of their structure, geographic distribution, and means of transmission.

Fascioliasis is caused by one species of fluke from the genus *Fasciola*, known as *F. hepatica*, or the sheep liver fluke. The life cycle of this fluke begins as the eggs are released from the animal host's feces into water. Larvae from the eggs infect snails, and the snails release larvae onto vegetation. The larvae form cysts containing infective parasites, and humans ingest the cysts while eating the vegetation, such as watercress. Once ingested, the cysts break open in the human digestive tract, and the flukes enter the liver and destroy tissue.

Opisthorchiasis is caused by several species of fluke from the genus *Opisthorchis*. These include *C. sinensis*, *O. viverrini*, and *O. felineus*. These flukes have a life cycle similar to that of the sheep liver fluke, but rather than being encysted on plants, they are encysted inside fish. Humans then consume the fish and become infected. Transmission of clonorchiasis occurs similarly by consuming raw, salted, pickled, smoked, marinated, dried, partially cooked, or otherwise incompletely cooked fish tainted with *C. sinensis* larvae.

WORDS TO KNOW

ANTHELMINTIC DRUGS Medicines that rid the body of parasitic worms.

ASYMPTOMATIC A state in which an individual does not exhibit or experience symptoms of a disease.

CYST A closed cavity or sac or the dormant stage of life of some parasites when they live inside an enclosed area, covered by a tough outer shell.

HELMINTH A representative of various phyla of wormlike animals.

LARVAE Immature forms (wormlike in insects; fishlike in amphibians) of an organism capable of surviving on its own. Larvae do not resemble the parent and must go through metamorphosis, or change, to reach the adult stage.

PARASITE An organism that lives in or on a host organism and gets its nourishment from that host. The parasite usually gains all the benefits of this relationship, whereas the host may suffer from various diseases and discomforts or show no signs of the infection. The life cycle of a typical parasite usually includes several developmental stages and morphological changes as the parasite lives and moves through the environment and one or more hosts. Parasites that remain on a host's body surface to feed are called ectoparasites, whereas those that live inside a host's body are called endoparasites. Parasitism is a highly successful biological adaptation. There are more known parasitic species than nonparasitic ones, and parasites affect just about every form of life, including most all animals, plants, and even bacteria.

TREMATODES Also called flukes, a type of parasitic flatworm. In humans flukes can infest the liver, lung, and other tissues.

ZOONOTIC A disease that can be transmitted between animals and humans. Examples of zoonotic diseases are anthrax, plague, and Q fever.

Scope and Distribution

Liver fluke infections occur worldwide, though the distribution of fascioliasis and opisthorchiasis differs. Fascioliasis is global in distribution, occurring in both temperate and tropical regions. *F. hepatica* infections have been reported in Europe, the Middle East, and Asia. *F. gigantica* infections have been reported in Asia, Africa, and Hawaii. In general, fascioliasis is closely connected to regions where sheep and cattle are raised. Sheep and cattle are natural hosts for liver flukes and thus are likely to transmit the parasite to humans in close contact with the animals or their water supply.

Opisthorchiasis occurs in areas of Asia and Europe. In particular, *O. viverrini* infections have been reported from northeastern Thailand, Laos, and Kampuchea. *O. felineus* infections have been reported mostly in Europe and Asia. *O. sinensis* infections are present throughout most of China.

Clonorchiasis is most common in humans and dogs in Asia, most frequently in China, Korea, and Vietnam.

In China health officials reported a 75 percent increase in the number of cases of liver fluke from 2001 to 2004. Since then liver fluke has remained prevalent and is a constant presence. The cause of the increase was attributed to an increased desire to consume raw or undercooked seafood and meat, both of which are a source of liver flukes. Because of this increase in infections, there has also been an increase in the number of cases in which a liver disorder has developed due to the flukes.

Treatment and Prevention

Treatment for liver fluke infections is achieved through administration of medications. There are several effective drugs, including triclabendazole, praziquantel, bithionol, albendazole, and mebendazole. Treatment of infection caused by *F. hepatica* usually involves triclabendazole or bithionol. Use of praziquantel has been ineffective in some cases and is thus not recommended by the US Centers for Disease Control and Prevention (CDC) for treating *F. hepatica* fluke infections.

Opisthorchiasis and clonorchiasis fluke infections can be effectively treated using praziquantel, which is the preferred treatment as suggested by the CDC. These medications act to eradicate the parasite. Praziquantel works by paralyzing the flukes' attachment apparatus, which disables them from remaining attached to the host's blood vessels. This leads to the death of the parasites, and eventually the infection dissipates.

On occasion treatment using the previously mentioned drugs may cause side effects such as diarrhea, dizziness, or headache. However, full recovery is likely to occur following treatment. In some cases liver damage resulting from the attachment of flukes to tissue may make patients vulnerable to other infections. Treatment may be required for several days or weeks depending on the type of fluke causing the infection.

As of 2018 there was no vaccine against liver fluke, although a vaccine for livestock was advocated as a means of reducing transmission. A vaccine candidate has been tested on rodents, with encouraging evidence of protection from infection. Other animal models have been explored, but avoidance of these parasites remains the best method of prevention. Avoidance can be achieved by boiling or purifying drinking water, ensuring freshwater fish and vegetation are cooked thoroughly prior to consumption, and eradicating or controlling snails, as they are an intermediate host for flukes.

Impacts and Issues

Liver flukes are transmitted to humans via consumption of raw meat, fish, and vegetation. Therefore, the food habits of humans have strong implications for the prevalence of liver fluke infections.

F. hepatica often infects livestock such as sheep, cattle, and pigs. This creates issues for the beef, lamb, and pork industries, as the flukes can do extensive damage to the animals and act as a source of infection for human populations. Prevention of liver fluke infection in livestock requires routine worming of animals, as well as the implementation of snail control methods such as exclusion of animals from snail-infested regions and drainage of water bodies containing snails. The disease is likely to occur in wet areas where snails are present. The flukes cannot be present if snails are absent.

Incidence of liver flukes is greatest in areas that lack adequate sanitation and water purification resources. Increased sanitation practices, including proper disposal and treatment of human and livestock wastes, prevention of water source contamination by fecal matter, and safer food storage and preparation practices, could dramatically reduce the occurrence of disease caused by all helminths. However, the World Health Organization (WHO) notes that more than 1 billion people worldwide do not have access to clean water. Coupled with a diet rich in the foods that most often carry liver flukes, unsanitary conditions make liver flukes difficult to prevent in underdeveloped regions.

According to WHO, modernization, urbanization, and changes in eating habits have helped reduce incidence of liver fluke infections in many parts of the world. However, infections persist in less developed areas, especially in Asia. In response, WHO launched the Collaborating Centre for Research and Control of Opisthorchiasis in Thailand in 2008. Rather than focusing only on treatment, as previous efforts had largely relied on, this initiative sought to produce "a multi-sectoral, multi-disciplinary, community-based control model, with a focus on school children and education for awareness." In the village of Lawa, where the initiative was focused, liver fluke inflections declined precipitously, from 67 percent of the local population to 16 percent over a three-year period. The project was subsequently expanded nationwide and even to Thailand's neighbors.

In 2016 the government of Thailand began another campaign that focused on ensuring the cooking of fish at community meals and dissuading people from defecating near water sources. As of mid-2017 the campaign had produced positive results in terms of reduced numbers of cases of infection, with infections in some regions dropping from 70 percent of people to less than 1 percent.

PRIMARY SOURCE

Thailand Uses Integrated Ecosystems Health Approach to Beat Cancer-Causing Disease

SOURCE: *"Thailand Uses Integrated Ecosystems Health Approach to Beat Cancer-Causing*

Disease." World Health Organization, December 15, 2017. http://www.who.int/neglected_diseases/news/fbti_thailand_uses_integrated_ecosystems_health_approach/en/ (accessed January 5, 2018).

INTRODUCTION: *The following report describes a successful campaign operated by the World Health Organization (WHO) and the Thai government to test new methods for combatting opisthorchiasis in a rural area of Thailand. The project's success has led WHO to consider launching similarly integrated approaches to combat infectious diseases.*

15 December 2017 | Geneva—The pain grew from worse to intense. At one point it became so bad that Surawat, a fisherman and head of a family of four, could hardly lift a straw broom. After protracted episodes of acute abdominal pain, Surawat's wife decided to take him to the nearest health clinic of the village in Chonnabot District (Khon Kaen Province) – although distance always deterred Surawat.

On examination, the doctor ordered stool tests and imaging of the abdomen. The diagnosis was clear: Surawat was suffering from a foodborne infection caused by the parasite *Opisthorchiasis viverrini* (opisthorchiasis)—adult flukes that live in the bile ducts. The infection, if left untreated, can cause cancer of the liver.

Surawat was lucky. His condition was treatable. He was prescribed 25 milligram-praziquantel tablets and had to take them three times a day for three consecutive days. The doctor explained to Surawat and his wife that eating traditional raw fish (koi pla) could be one of the major reasons for his infection.

Opisthorchiasis in Thailand was widespread about 60 years ago. With the implementation of a national programme and along with rapid industrialization and urbanization, including changes in life-style and food habits, the prevalence of *O. viverrini* infection decreased considerably.

But the scenario remains different in rural northeastern Thailand, where many people still live off traditional agriculture and fisheries and where opisthorchiasis remains an important public health problem. For the government, it was clear that previous control strategies had sustainably decreased the level of infection in this part of the country.

Ecosystems approach

In 2008 the WHO Collaborating Centre for Research and Control of Opisthorchiasis (Southeast Asian liver fluke disease) at Khon Kaen University in discussion with Thai authorities introduced the EcoHealth/One Health approach—known as the Lawa Lake Project—an integrated eco-systems approach involving a multisectoral, multi-disciplinary, community-based control model, with a focus on school children and education for awareness. Among other materials, local health officials have also introduced a school curriculum of colourful cartoons that aim to teach children about the risks of consuming raw foods.

The approach has contrasted with past conventional "top-down" medical and public health interventions programmes which Thailand carried in the past, focusing on treatment alone.

There have been a number of different initiatives over the years that focused on health promotion, awareness campaigns, and education campaigns on "safe cooking", among others, with support from different organizations besides the Ministry of Health: the United States Agency for International Development (USAID), the German Society for International Cooperation (GTZ) and Mahidol University of Thailand.

Results

The results of the Lawa Lake project have been outstanding: the prevalence of liver fluke infection in Lawa village declined from 67% to 16% over three years with minimal re-infection (Sripa et al., 2015).

The success was a result of not only access to medicines, treatments and ecosystem monitoring but most importantly of innovative education methods and tools to generate awareness about transmission of liver fluke and on sustainable and eco-friendly tools to prevent infection in the communities.

The strength of the Lawa Project, which makes this initiative worth implementing in other areas and countries, is its multiple components to control foodborne diseases:

- **Manual of liver fluke control strategies**: Development of a manual on liver fluke control, to guide the community-based activities and school initiatives, as well as the hospital awareness campaigns.
- **Technical training for liver fluke control**: Development of specific training on liver fluke for hospital staff and volunteers. These trainings prepare them to monitor and report cases and prepare health recommendations accordingly to the communities.
- **Community-based treatment and intensive education**: Special treatment programmes with intensive education, targeting different age groups including not only children but also adults, and utilizing media and technological tools to get better reach and engage communities.
- **School-based information, education and communication and science curriculum**: Liver fluke disease was incorporated in the science curriculum at local schools to expand the impact of the awareness campaigns through children.
- **Disease surveillance and environmental monitoring**: Programmes that strengthen

surveillance and monitoring are crucial to measure and help estimate the prevalence and burden of liver fluke disease, as well as contributing to research in which environmental conditions favour the infection or presence of the trematode.

Success and hope

The success of the project has gone beyond the initially selected villages and has now expanded to the whole country with a focus on rural and high prevalence areas, and internationally to neighbouring countries.

The Lawa Project has also become a model of how to address foodborne disease control activities and programmes. It harmonizes efforts of different stakeholders to avoid duplication and provides a bottom-up approach with a focus on disease awareness and education. Part of the education campaign focuses on getting people to use proper toilets, and avoid defecating in the lake, which reduces the number of fluke eggs.

The burden of opisthorchiasis has decreased in the past few years in Thailand as a result of the collective efforts of the Lawa Project, public initiatives and other activities, but significant efforts are still required.

SEE ALSO *Food-Borne Disease and Food Safety; Helminth Disease; Lung Fluke (Paragonimus) Infection; Opportunistic Infection; Parasitic Diseases*

BIBLIOGRAPHY

Books

Sripa, Banchob, and Paul J. Brindley. *Asiatic River Fluke: From Basic Science to Public Health.* New York: Elsevier, 2018.

Periodicals

Lim, Jae Hoo. "Liver Flukes: The Malady Neglected." *Korean Journal of Radiology* 12, no. 3 (May–June 2011): 269–279. This article can also be found online at https://www.ncbi.nlm.nih.gov/pmc/articles/PMC3088844/ (accessed January 4, 2018).

Samiphak, Sara, and S. Leonard Syme. "The Battle of Worldviews: A Case Study of Liver Fluke Infection in Khon Kaen, Thailand." *Journal of Evidence-Based Integrative Medicine* 22, no. 4 (2017): 902–908. This article can also be found online at http://journals.sagepub.com/doi/full/10.1177/2156587217723497 (accessed January 4, 2018).

Websites

"Clonorchiasis." World Health Organization. http://www.who.int/foodborne_trematode_infections/clonorchiasis/en/> (accessed January 5, 2018).

"Fascioliasis (Fasciola Infection)." Centers for Disease Control and Prevention, January 10, 2013. https://www.cdc.gov/parasites/fasciola/index.html (accessed January 5, 2018).

"Opisthorchiasis." Centers for Disease Control and Prevention, December 14, 2017 https://www.cdc.gov/dpdx/opisthorchiasis/index.html (accessed January 5, 2018).

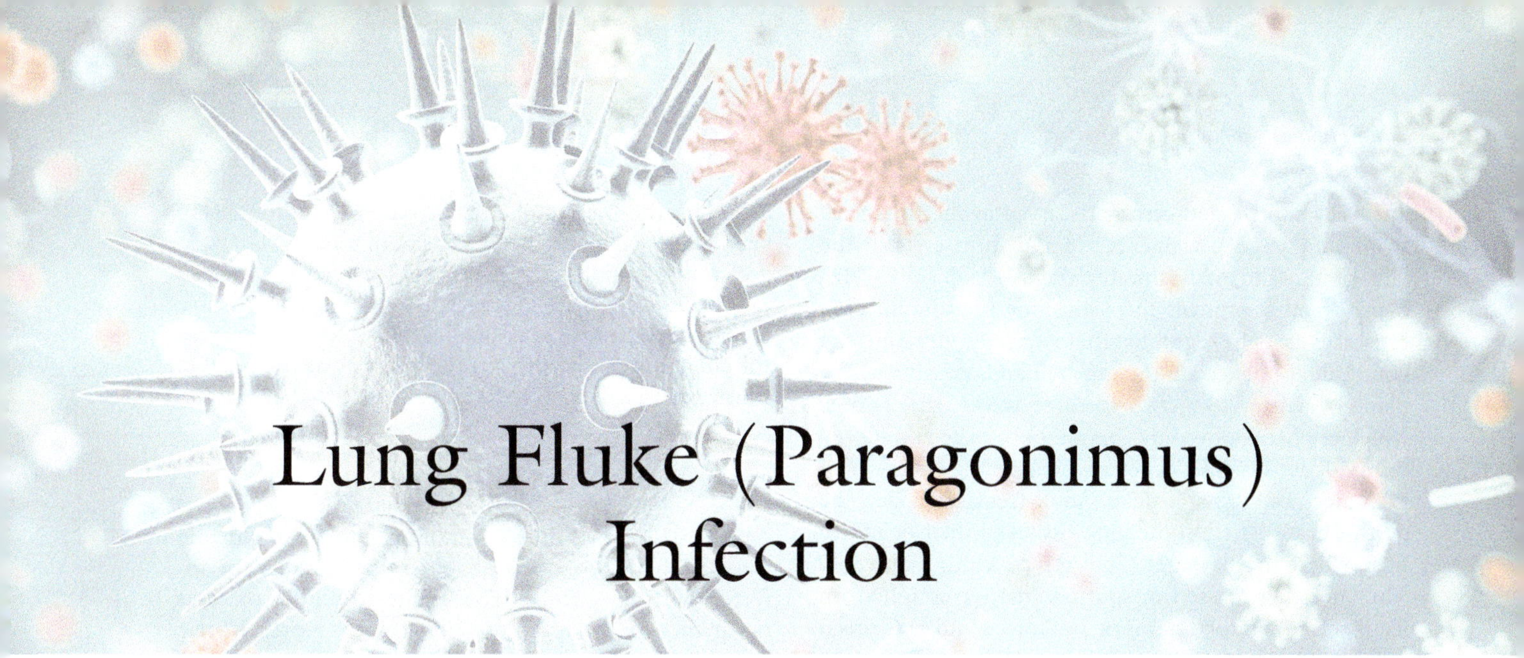

Lung Fluke (Paragonimus) Infection

Introduction

Lung fluke infection, or paragonimiasis, is a potentially serious illness that is caused by over 30 species of trematodes (parasitic flatworms) of the genus *Paragonimus.* Among the more than 10 species reported to infect humans, the most common is *P. westermani*, found in tropical and subtropical regions of Asia.

Lung flukes are not transmitted from person to person. Humans contract paragonimiasis when they eat inadequately cooked or pickled flesh that is infected. Most reported cases result from consuming raw freshwater crabs or crayfish. However, some species of lung fluke occur only in domestic or wild animals. Humans can contract the illness from consuming the raw flesh of these creatures. *Paragonimus* infect wild boars, wild and domestic canids, wild and domestic felids, raccoons, mongooses, rats, and weasels.

Disease History, Characteristics, and Transmission

The first human paragonimiasis case was observed in an autopsy in Taiwan in 1879. Until the last quarter of the 20th century, however, the public health importance of lung fluke infections was underestimated. Both snails and crustaceans serve as intermediate hosts of the parasitic flatworms that cause paragonimiasis. Lung fluke eggs hatch in freshwater into miracidia (early-stage larvae), which penetrate the snails. The miracidia develop

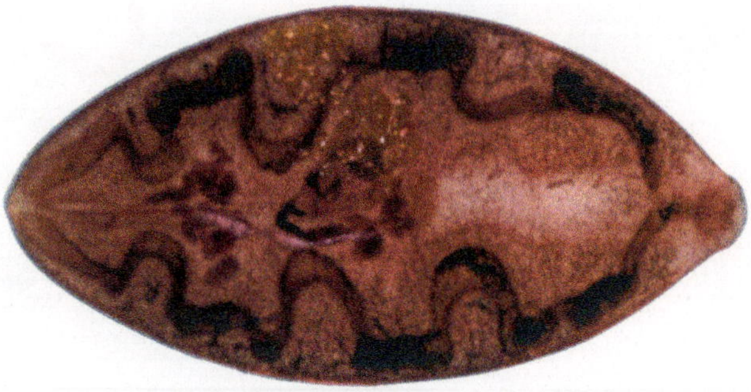

Lung flukes belong to the genus *Paragonimus.* If left untreated, symptoms of lung fluke infection can last for years or even decades. © *Visuals Unlimited, Inc./Dr. Robert Calentine/Getty Images*

into very short-tailed cercariae (larvae in the final free-swimming stage) that penetrate and form cysts in the gills or muscles of freshwater crayfish and crabs. Humans or other animals then consume the raw infected crustaceans. The eggs hatch in the duodenum; the young flukes penetrate the gut wall and, eventually, the pleural cavity. Within two to three weeks, the worms, which are hermaphroditic (having both male and female reproductive organs), penetrate beneath the lungs where they meet and cross-fertilize. Adult trematodes become partly encapsulated in the lung tissues of their definitive host, where they lay eggs. The eggs pass into the alveoli. They are then passed in sputum (matter coughed up from the respiratory tract) or swallowed and are passed later in feces. Eggs that reach water hatch and begin the cycle again. The time from infection to oviposition is 65 to 90 days.

Lung fluke infections can be serious illnesses. Onset of symptoms generally occurs between 6 and 10 weeks after infection. A classic symptom is bloody sputum, in which eggs can be found. Other symptoms include cough, difficulty breathing, diarrhea, abdominal pain, fever, and hives. The infection is often mistaken for pulmonary tuberculosis. The parasite can migrate from the lungs to other organs, including the brain and striated muscles. Although the brain is affected in less than 1 percent of patients with paragonimiasis, lung flukes that become localized in the brain can create major neurological symptoms, including double vision and seizures that resemble those seen in epilepsy. Infections can persist for years, with some cases reported in which people suffered for 20 to 40 years.

Scope and Distribution

As of 2017 more than 22 million people worldwide were estimated by tropical disease specialists to be infected with lung fluke. The greatest number of cases occur in China, Japan, the Philippines, North Korea, Taiwan, Laos, Thailand, and Vietnam. The majority of cases in this region are caused by *Paragonimus westermani*, also known as Asian lung fluke. In some parts of China, as much as 30 percent of the population has antibodies associated with *Paragonimus westermani* infection. Human infections with *P. heterotremus* are well known in Thailand and with *P. pulmonalis* in the Far East. *P. africanus* and *P. uterobilateralis* are distributed among humans in West Africa. *P. mexicanus* affects people in parts of Central and South America.

Lung Fluke Life Cycle

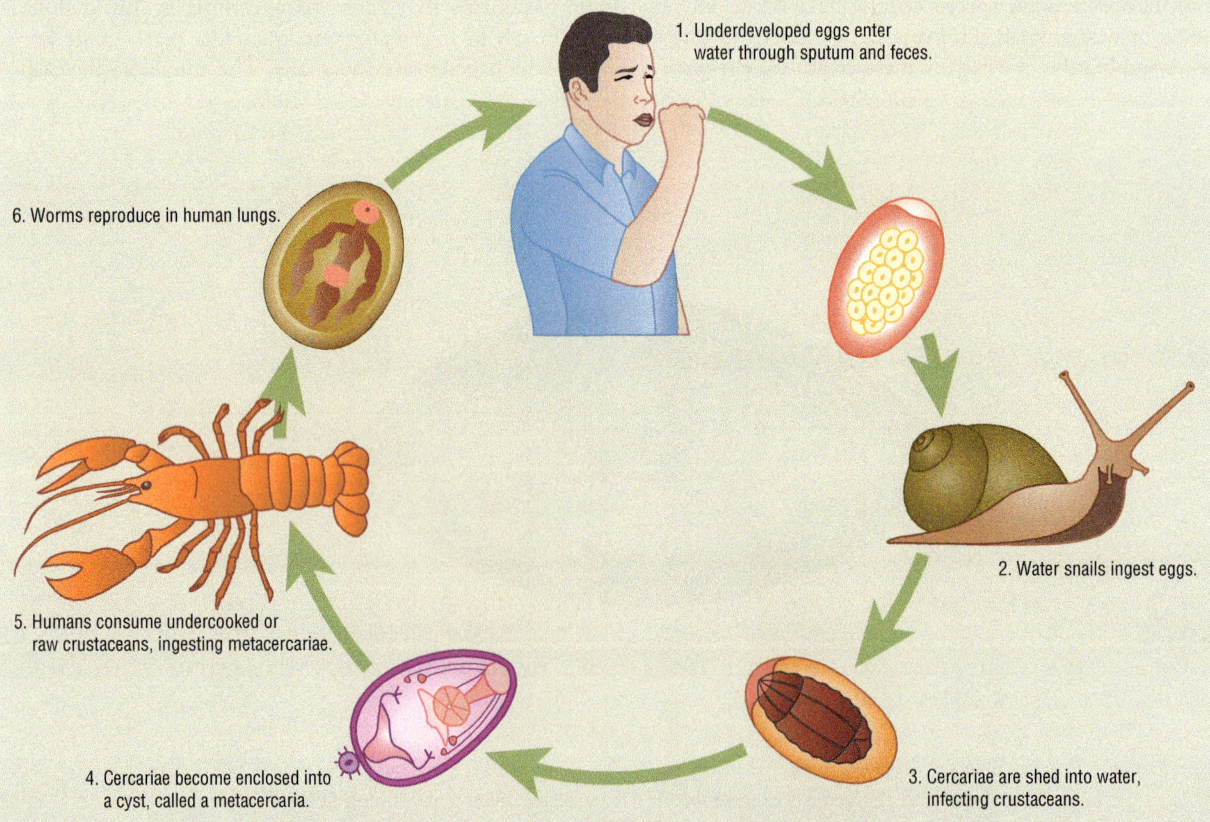
1. Underdeveloped eggs enter water through sputum and feces.
2. Water snails ingest eggs.
3. Cercariae are shed into water, infecting crustaceans.
4. Cercariae become enclosed into a cyst, called a metacercaria.
5. Humans consume undercooked or raw crustaceans, ingesting metacercariae.
6. Worms reproduce in human lungs.

One lung fluke, *Paragonimus kellicotti*, is native to the United States and is found in rivers that are part of the Mississippi River drainage basin. Between 1984 and 2010, 16 cases of paragonimiasis caused by *Paragonimus kellicotti* were reported. Ten of these cases were in Missouri. The consumption of undercooked crayfish, the primary crustacean host for *Paragonimus kellicotti*, is the primary cause of cases of paragonimiasis in the United States. *Paragonimus kellicotti* is also prevalent in the freshwater snail *Pomatiopsis lapidaria*. Mammalian hosts for *Paragonimus kellicotti* include cats, dogs, coyotes, sheep, skunks, and raccoons.

WORDS TO KNOW

ALVEOLI An alveolus (alveoli is plural) is a tiny air sac located within the lungs. The exchange of oxygen and carbon dioxide takes place within these sacs.

ANTIBODIES Proteins found in the blood that help fight against foreign substances called antigens. Antigens, which are usually proteins or polysaccharides, stimulate the immune system to produce antibodies, or Y-shaped immunoglobulins. The antibodies inactivate the antigen and help remove it from the body. While antigens can be the source of infections from pathogenic bacteria and viruses, organic molecules detrimental to the body from internal or environmental sources also act as antigens. Genetic engineering and the use of various mutational mechanisms allow the construction of a vast array of antibodies (each with a unique genetic sequence).

DEFINITIVE HOST The organism in which a parasite reaches reproductive maturity.

INTERMEDIATE HOST An organism infected by a parasite while the parasite is in a developmental, not sexually mature form.

OVIPOSITION Ovum is Latin for "egg." To oviposition is to position or lay eggs, especially when done by an insect.

PLEURAL CAVITY The lungs are surrounded by two membranous coverings, the pleura. One of the pleura is attached to the lung, the other to the ribcage. The space between the two pleura, the pleural cavity, is normally filled with a clear lubricating fluid called pleural fluid.

TREMATODES Also called flukes, a type of parasitic flatworm. In humans flukes can infest the liver, lung, and other tissues.

Treatment and Prevention

Paragonimiasis is usually diagnosed based on the identification of eggs from the parasites in the sputum of the affected person. It is less frequently diagnosed based on the identification of eggs in the patient's stool. These tests, however, require that the infection is far enough along for eggs to be present, which can take as long as three months following initial infection with the parasite. A blood test can also identify antibodies that are produced in the body following infection by *Paragonimus*. Increased counts of white blood cells called *eosinophils* can also be suggestive of a parasitic infection. Other diagnostic technology, such as X-rays or computerized tomography (CT) scans, may also be used to evaluate damage to organs.

Once diagnosed paragonimiasis is treated with antiparasite medications. The preferred treatment is praziquantel tablets, which are taken three times a day for two days. Praziquantel stops worms from developing or multiplying in the body. Triclabendazole tablets are an alternative drug. In cases where the brain is affected, corticosteroids to reduce swelling or medications to control seizures may be required. Surgery may also be needed to reduce swelling in the brain.

The best method of avoiding paragonimiasis infection is to only consume properly cooked food. Cooking crustaceans at 131°F (55°C) for five minutes will kill the parasites.

Impacts and Issues

Paragonimiasis once tended to be limited to regions where the appropriate crustaceans formed part of the human diet in one culinary delicacy or another. However, the rise of global cuisine has contributed to the spread of lung flukes. In 2006 two people who consumed live, imported, freshwater crabs in an Orange County, California, restaurant contracted paragonimiasis. In 2011 a case was confirmed in a US resident and traced to imported live crabs that he had consumed at a sushi restaurant in California two years earlier. In the 2010s the trend of consuming live crabs in martinis raised new paragonimiasis concerns.

The invasion of non-native species into American and Canadian waters poses a further threat to human health. The mitten crab, *Eriocheir sinensis*, was first spotted in fisheries on the West Coast in 1992 and on the East Coast in 2005. As of 2017 the crabs were also common in the Great Lakes and the Chesapeake Bay. This Yellow Sea native is a Chinese delicacy, and crabs were imported live to markets in Los Angeles and San Francisco before California outlawed their possession. A female can carry from

250,000 to 1 million eggs. The crabs, adept on land, climb easily over levees as they migrate upstream. Mitten crabs can carry lung fluke, though no infected crabs have been detected in North American waters.

Proposals to eradicate paragonimiasis on a larger scale have faced many challenges. One proposal involves using chemical agents to control snail populations in water sources where lung flukes are common. However, these chemicals have been found to harm other organisms, and researchers fear they could have long-ranging detrimental effects on ecosystems. Moreover, snail populations have proven resilient to many chemicals, with those that survive quickly repopulating affected areas. Another proposed solution, the introduction of other species to control snail populations, faces scrutiny over fears that the introduction of new species, particularly non-native species, could quickly disrupt ecosystems.

SEE ALSO *Helminth Disease; Parasitic Diseases*

BIBLIOGRAPHY

Books

Peters, Wallace, and Geoffrey Pasvol. *Atlas of Tropical Medicine and Parasitology.* 6th ed. London: Elsevier Mosby, 2007.

Periodicals

Boland, Jennifer M., et al. "Pleuropulmonary Infection by *Paragonimus westermani* in the United States: A Rare Cause of Eosinophilic Pneumonia after Ingestion of Live Crabs." *American Journal of Surgical Pathology* 35, no. 5 (May 2011): 707–713.

Diaz, James H. "Paragonimiasis Acquired in the United States: Native and Nonnative Species." *Clinical Microbiology Reviews* 26, no. 3 (July 2013): 493–504.

Websites

"Paragonimiasis." World Health Organization. http://www.who.int/foodborne_trematode_infections/paragonimiasis/en/ (accessed November 14, 2017).

"Paragonimus Westermani–Lung Fluke." Parasites in Humans. http://www.parasitesinhumans.org/paragonimus-westermani-lung-fluke.html (accessed November 14, 2017).

"Parasites–Paragonimiasis (also known as Paragonimus Infection)." Centers for Disease Control and Prevention. https://www.cdc.gov/parasites/paragonimus/index.html (accessed November 14, 2017).

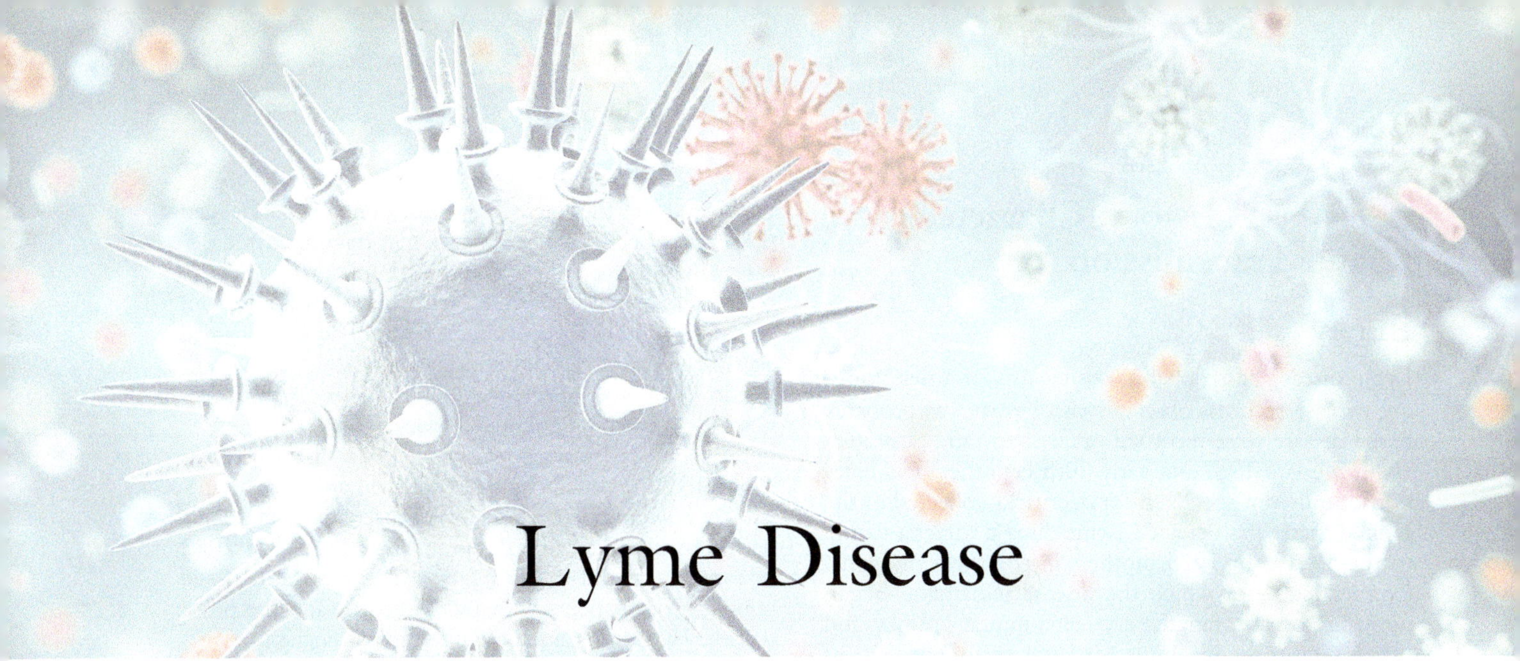

Lyme Disease

Introduction

Lyme disease is a bacterial infection caused by the spirochete (corkscrew-shaped bacterium) *Borrelia burgdorferi*. It is transmitted to humans through the bites of several kinds of ticks, including blacklegged ticks (*Ixodes scapularis*) and the western blacklegged tick, also known as the "deer tick" (*Ixodes pacificus* in the United States and *Ixodes ricinus* in Europe).

Initial Lyme disease syndromes may include a localized infection that can produce the distinctive skin rash erythema migrans, along with fever, headache, aches, tiredness, and swollen lymph nodes. Left untreated, the disease may cause arthritis, facial palsy, and heart problems, including palpitations and an irregular heartbeat, as well as continued rashes, pain and swelling in the joints and tendons, and neck pain, among other symptoms.

The disease is treated using antibiotics. Most people respond well to treatment, but some do not. Some patients report lingering symptoms and may be diagnosed with post-treatment Lyme disease syndrome (PTLDS).

WORDS TO KNOW

BABESIOSIS An infection of the red blood cells caused by *Babesia microti*, a form of parasite (parasitic sporozoan).

ENDEMIC Present in a particular area or among a particular group of people.

GRANULOCYTE Any cell containing granules (small, grain-like objects). The term is often used to refer to a type of white blood cell (leukocyte).

HOST An organism that serves as the habitat for a parasite or possibly for a symbiont. A host may provide nutrition to the parasite or symbiont, or it may simply provide a place in which to live.

NYMPH In aquatic insects, the larval stage.

SPIROCHETE A bacterium shaped like a spiral. These spiral-shaped bacteria live in contaminated water, sewage, soil, and decaying organic matter, as well as inside humans and animals.

SPOROZOAN The fifth phylum of the kingdom Protista, known as Apicomplexa, comprises several species of obligate intracellular protozoan parasites classified as sporozoa or sporozoans because they form reproductive cells known as spores. Many sporozoans are parasitic and pathogenic species, such as *Plasmodium falciparum, Plasmodium malariae, Plasmodium vivax, Toxoplasma gondii, Pneumocystis carinii, Cryptosporidium parvum,* and *Cryptosporidium muris.* The sporozoa reproduction cycle has both asexual and sexual phases. The asexual phase is schizogony (from the Greek, meaning "generation through division"), in which merozoites (daughter cells) are produced through multiple nuclear fissions. The sexual phase is sporogony (i.e., generation of spores) and is followed by gametogony, or the production of sexually reproductive cells termed *gamonts.*

VECTOR Any agent that carries and transmits parasites and diseases. Also, an organism or a chemical used to transport a gene into a new host cell.

■ Disease History, Characteristics, and Transmission

History

Lyme disease has probably existed for centuries. Judging by case records, observations of what was probably Lyme disease were recorded in Germany and Scandinavia in the late 19th and early 20th centuries. Examination of museum specimens of deer ticks collected in the United States has detected Lyme disease bacteria dating to the 1940s. In 1975 mothers in the town of Lyme, Connecticut—for which the disease is named—began noticing arthritis, fatigue, erythema migrans rashes, and other symptoms in about 50 local children. Two of these women, Judith Mensch and Polly Murray, began tracking the cases by recording dates and locations. Several of the children recalled being bitten by a tick just before becoming ill. Murray called rheumatologist Allan C. Steere, who, along with fellow rheumatologist Stephen E. Malawista, investigated the cases. They concluded that a tick-borne pathogen was to blame for the disease.

Thus, by 1976 the existence of Lyme disease was recognized, and its transmission by ticks was known. However, the specific pathogen causing the disease was still unknown. In 1981 Willy Burgdorfer, working at the US National Institute of Allergy and Infectious Diseases (NIAID) of the US National Institutes of Health (NIH), was studying the transmission of Rocky Mountain spotted fever (RMSF) by ticks. Studying the microorganisms found in blacklegged ticks (one of two US tick varieties that transmit Lyme disease), Burgdorfer noticed a hitherto unknown variety of corkscrew-shaped bacterium (spirochetes) in fluids from two ticks. Within a year this bacterium had been named *Borrelia burgdorferi* in Burgdorfer's honor.

In 1982 other researchers found *B. burgdorferi* in deer ticks. By combining cultured *B. burgdorferi* bacteria with blood samples from people with Lyme disease, it was shown that the patients' blood contained an antibody specific to *B. burgdorferi.* This showed that the blood donors had been infected with *B. burgdorferi.* Finally, in 1983 researchers found *B. burgdorferi* in blood and tissue samples from patients with Lyme disease, and the proof that the bacterium caused the disease was clinched.

Characteristics and Transmission

Lyme disease is caused by the spirochete *B. burgdorferi*, a member of the phylum Spirochaetes. Spirochetes are corkscrew- or helix-shaped bacteria. *B. burgdorferi* are about 0.2 to 0.5 μm wide, are 3 to 18 μm long, and are built with a double-layered structure like a long, blunt-ended corkscrew nested within a slightly larger corkscrew of the same shape. In the space between the two layers are flagella (long, hairlike filaments attached to a rotating base embedded in the outer cell wall). Many types of bacteria have flagella, but normally the flagella protrude into the bacterium's environment and are used for propulsion like tiny outboard propellers. A spirochete uses a different strategy: its internal flagella

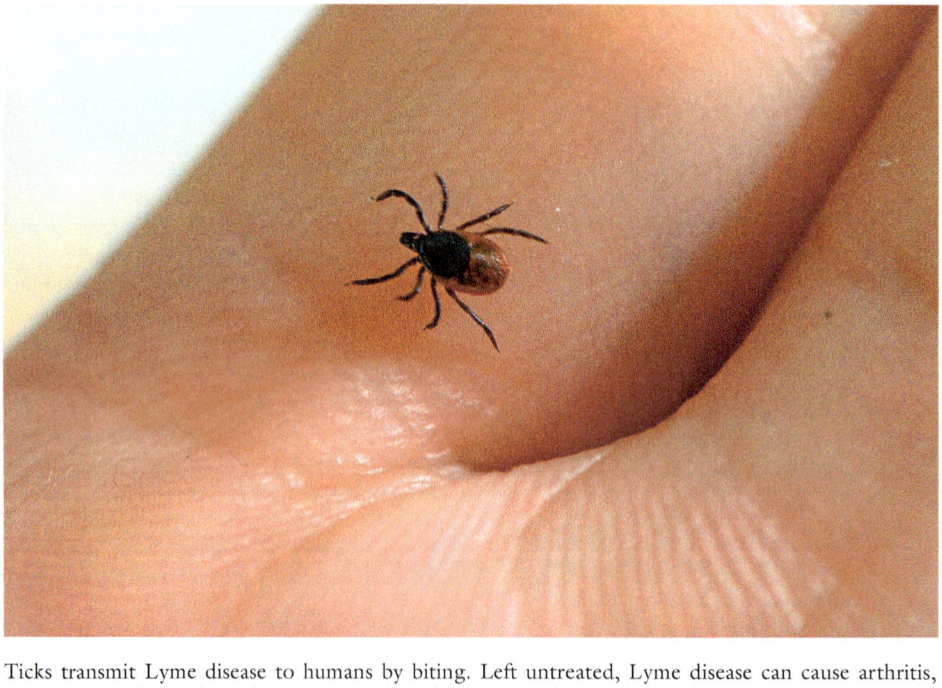

Ticks transmit Lyme disease to humans by biting. Left untreated, Lyme disease can cause arthritis, meningitis, and neurological symptoms such as depression and Bell's facial palsy. *© BERTRAND GUAY/AFP/Getty Images*

wrap lengthwise around the inner layer of the bacterium, forcing it into its characteristic corkscrew shape. As the flagella rotate, they cause the whole shape of the bacterium to change as if it were rotating on its axis. Just as an actual corkscrew is driven into a cork by rotating, a spirochete progresses through the medium in which it is embedded. Its corkscrewing mode of locomotion gives it a mobility advantage over other bacteria in more viscous (thicker, stickier) media.

Both syphilis (a chronic, contagious disease that is usually venereal and often congenital) and Lyme disease are caused by spirochetes. There are three common species of *B. burgdorferi*: *Borrelia garinii*, *Borrelia afzelli*, and *Borrelia burgdorferi* sensu stricto (meaning "in the strict sense"). Together these three are known as *Borrelia burgdorferi* sensu lato ("in the wide sense") or simply as *Borrelia burgdorferi*. *B. burgdorferi* sensu stricto is the only Lyme strain found in the United States as of early 2018. Three other, less common species of *Borrelia burgdorferi* sensu lato ("in the broad sense") have been discovered to cause Lyme disease in Africa, Asia, and Europe.

Lyme disease is a vector-borne disease, meaning it is transmitted to human beings by an intermediate host (in this case, a tick), not directly from other human beings. Although far from the most common infectious disease in the United States, it is the most common vector-borne disease, accounting for over 95 percent of reported vector-borne illness cases. The vector for Lyme disease is the deer tick, and the transmission of Lyme disease to humans is intimately involved with the life cycle of both the *B. burgdorferi* spirochete and the tick.

In the spring tick eggs lying on the ground hatch, producing tick larvae. Each larva attaches to a small mammal, usually a mouse. Ticks attach firmly to the skin and feed on their host by sucking blood. The larval tick ingests *B. burgdorferi* from its mouse host and becomes infected; this infection does not sicken the tick. In the fall and winter, the larva drops off the mouse and becomes dormant, attaching itself to vegetation. The next spring it molts and becomes a nymph-stage tick. The nymph attaches to a deer, mouse, or human host (its preferred host is the deer) and bites the host, transmitting Lyme disease. The tick develops to an adult form throughout the summer, living on the host. In this stage it mates. In the fall it drops off its host and lays eggs in leaf litter on the ground (about 3,000 eggs per laying female), beginning a new two-year cycle. This is the basic ecology of Lyme disease in the northeastern and north-central United States.

Scope and Distribution

Ticks that carry Lyme disease can be found in the United States, as well as some parts of Europe and Asia.

Lyme disease is a larger problem in the United States than elsewhere in the world, with about 300,000 likely diagnosed and treated new cases reported each year. However, most experts agree that the disease is greatly underreported and that the true number of new cases is probably closer to 300,000 per year. From 2008 to 2015, there were 275,589 cases of Lyme disease reported to the US Centers for Disease Control and Prevention (CDC).

According to the CDC, as of 2015 there were 14 US states in which Lyme disease was most commonly found: Connecticut, Delaware, Maine, Maryland, Massachusetts, Minnesota, New Hampshire, New Jersey, New York, Pennsylvania, Rhode Island, Vermont, Virginia, and Wisconsin. The disease was present in other states (especially ones bordering the 14 states listed above) but was less common.

The CDC reports that on average the rates of Lyme disease are increasing in the United States (for example, there were approximately 15,000 cases in 1995 and approximately 35,000 in 2015) and the geographic range of the tick that carries the disease is expanding as well. The latter is likely in response to global climate change.

Treatment and Prevention

To diagnose Lyme disease, physicians take into account the patient's symptoms and assess whether the patient has been in a location where he or she could have come into contact with Lyme-disease-carrying ticks. Blood tests may also be taken to assess if the patient has Lyme disease; the presence of Lyme disease antibodies in the blood may indicate that the patient has Lyme disease.

Symptoms of early untreated Lyme disease include the classic "bull's-eye" rash, headaches, fatigue, fever, and achy joints. Symptoms of late untreated Lyme disease include a continuation of early Lyme disease symptoms or an escalation in their severity. Other symptoms include arthritis and heart complications, or Lyme carditis.

One reason why Lyme disease may produce such varied symptoms is that the ticks that transmit it are also host to numerous other pathogens and can serve as vectors for such disorders as babesiosis (infection of the red blood cells caused by the parasitic sporozoan *Babesia microti*) and human granulocytic ehrlichiosis (an infection of white blood cells caused by a species of bacteria in the *Ehrlichia* genus). When more than one pathogen infects a person at a time, the result is called coinfection.

Lyme disease is treated primarily with antibiotics. If Lyme disease is diagnosed early—such as when a physician notes that a patient reporting a tick bite has the characteristic rash and/or flu-like symptoms—treatment is a course of oral antibiotics, most often doxycycline (for 10 to 21 days), cefuroxime axetil (14 to 21 days), or amoxicillai (14 to 21 days). Most people respond well to treatment and recover fully. New evidence suggests that just 10 days of doxycycline may be just as effective in treating Lyme disease as a longer course of the drug.

Continuing antibiotic treatment is not recommended for people who suffer from post-treatment Lyme disease syndrome (PTLDS). Symptoms of PTLDS include fatigue, headaches, and aches after a course of antibiotic treatment. Previously, some physicians treated people with PTLDS with antibiotics for long periods of time. However, this is not recommended. According to the CDC, "Studies funded by the NIH have not shown that people who received prolonged courses of antibiotics do better in the long run than people treated with placebo. Furthermore, long-term antibiotic or alternative treatments for Lyme disease have been associated with serious complications," including inflammation of the gallbladder, bacterial infections such as bacterial infection of the blood, and death. Researchers are working to develop an appropriate treatment for people with PTDLS, who report a low quality of life.

Lyme disease is prevented by avoiding infected ticks. From April through September, caution should be taken when in outdoor areas where Lyme-disease-infected ticks are endemic. The CDC states that it is best to "avoid wooded and brushy areas with high grass and leaf litter" and to "walk in the center of the trail." Light-colored clothing makes it easier to spot ticks and remove them before they bite. Wearing long-sleeved shirts, tucking pants into socks, and applying insect repellents containing DEET (N,N,diethyl-meta-toluamide) or clothes treated with permethrin can decrease the chances of a tick bite. Taking a shower and checking your body for ticks two hours or less after spending time outside in an area where Lyme disease is endemic is recommended. Check clothes, pets, and outdoor accessories (such as picnic blankets, hiking boots, and backpacks) for ticks. Place clothes in the dryer on high heat for at least 10 minutes to kill ticks. If clothes need to be laundered, wash them in hot water to kill ticks.

Promptly removing a tick that has attached to the body is important because *B. burgdorferi* usually does not infect the host until 36 to 48 hours after tick attachment. Ticks should be removed by gripping them right next to the skin with tweezers and pulling. The body of the tick should never be squeezed or irritated by heat or chemicals while the tick is attached, as this will drive its stomach contents into the skin and increase the chances of infection.

Many of the ticks acquired by people engaged in outdoor activity in the northeastern United States are dog ticks (*Dermacentor variabilis*), which cannot transmit Lyme disease. The Lyme-transmitting deer tick *Ixodes scapularis* is notably smaller than a dog tick. Even if one is bitten by a tick, it is not necessary to seek treatment for Lyme disease unless flu-like symptoms or the characteristic erythema migrans rash appear.

As of early 2018, no vaccine for Lyme disease was available.

■ Impacts and Issues

Lyme disease has become the most common vector-borne inflammatory disease in the United States thanks to changing human activities. In the 19th century, the central and northeastern United States were largely deforested, and deer populations were eliminated or greatly reduced by hunting and habitat loss over large areas. After food production shifted elsewhere, these regions have largely reforested, and deer populations, along with the ticks that infest them, have rebounded. At the same time, greater numbers of human beings have been brought into contact with ticks by living in suburban developments and enjoying outdoor recreations such as hiking.

LYMErix, a vaccine for Lyme disease that is 79 percent effective, was placed on the market in 1999. It was withdrawn in 2002, however, because of low sales. Low demand was caused by a combination of the vaccine's high cost ($50 per inoculation), its inconvenience (three shots were needed over a year), and fears that the vaccine might trigger permanent arthritis or neurological problems. The effectiveness of the vaccine diminishes over time; therefore, people who received the vaccine before 2002 were no longer immune to the disease in 2017. That year efforts to create a safe and effective Lyme disease vaccine were underway.

Lyme disease is a notoriously contentious subject, dividing patient advocacy groups from many physicians. This is partially because Lyme disease has no definitive, predictable course. Some infected people show no symptoms; others show symptoms, are debilitated for a time, and are successfully treated; and still others are left with permanent disabilities from the disease. Disagreements, often angry, persist on whether long-term Lyme infection exists, what its symptoms and proper treatment are (if any), and whether Lyme disease is diagnosed too much or too little.

PRIMARY SOURCE

Dangerous Unproven Treatments for 'Chronic Lyme Disease' Are On the Rise

SOURCE: *Sun, Lena H. "Dangerous Unproven Treatments for 'Chronic Lyme Disease' Are on the Rise."* Washington Post *(June 15, 2017). This article can also be found online at https://www.washingtonpost.com/news/to-your-health/wp/2017/06/15/dangerous-unproven-treatments-for-chronic-lyme-disease-cause-are-on-the-rise/?utm_term=.c43eaa9624a2 (accessed February 6, 2018).*

INTRODUCTION: *In the following article, the author summarizes reports that show that administering antibiotics to people suffering from post-treatment Lyme disease syndrome (PTLDS) for months or years does not eliminate PTLDS*

> *symptoms. Such treatment can also be dangerous to patients. PTLDS is sometimes referred to as "chronic Lyme disease," although the latter term is not recommended by the Centers for Disease Control and Prevention.*

An increasing number of Americans with medically ambiguous symptoms are being misdiagnosed with "chronic Lyme disease" and prescribed dangerous and often expensive treatments that do not work, according to a new report.

In some instances, patients have died after receiving intensive, long-term and inappropriate courses of intravenous antibiotics that led to septic shock. In other cases, misdiagnosis caused dangerous delays in treatment of a patient's actual underlying condition.

These incorrect diagnoses have existed for years. But public health officials and clinicians say they are alarmed because of the increasing severity and scope of some treatments in recent years, said Christina Nelson, a medical epidemiologist and author of a report released Thursday by the Centers for Disease Control and Prevention.

Many of the various treatments, including courses of intravenous antibiotics lasting months and years, have no evidence of effectiveness. Studies have shown that prolonged courses of intravenous antibiotics can often result in serious harm, including death.

Unorthodox alternative therapies include intravenous infusions of hydrogen peroxide, electromagnetic frequency treatments, garlic supplements, even stem cell transplants.

Chronic Lyme disease is a diagnosis that some health-care providers use to describe patients with a variety of symptoms such as fatigue, generalized pain, and neurological symptoms.

It's a confusing term because it's been used to mean many different things. Some practitioners have used the diagnosis to describe lingering symptoms after infection with the bacteria *Borrelia burgdorferi* that causes Lyme disease. Others use the catchall term to describe patients with subjective symptoms but no evidence of ever having been infected with the tick-borne illness.

Many of these patients have experienced significant debilitation from their symptoms and failed to find relief after seeing conventional medical practitioners. As a result, some turn to alternative medicine clinics or practitioners who sometimes identify themselves as Lyme disease specialists, or "Lyme literate" doctors, who may subject patients to a host of unproven treatments, the report said.

Typical symptoms of true Lyme disease include fever, headache, fatigue and a skin rash that may have a characteristic bull's eye shape. If left untreated, infection can spread to joints, the heart and nervous system. The recommended treatment is generally a two-to-four-week course of antibiotics. The CDC estimates about 300,000 people are diagnosed with Lyme each year, and the numbers have been on the rise.

Federal health officials don't know the number of people who undergo treatments for chronic Lyme disease or the complications that result from such treatments. But based on information received in the past three years from state and local health departments, and from clinicians who have treated patients who have become very sick as a result of these treatments, "we really have a sense that both the treatment and scope are broadening," Nelson said.

"Health-care providers are seeing the fallout," she said. "These treatments are really dangerous. This is just the tip of a very large iceberg that no one is talking about."

One woman in her 50s with progressive weakness, swelling and tingling in her extremities was eventually diagnosed with amyotrophic lateral sclerosis, or ALS. She sought a second evaluation and was told she had chronic Lyme disease. She received seven months of intensive antimicrobial treatment—including drugs that were antifungal agents not recommended for treating Lyme disease—but her weakness worsened. She developed an intractable *C. difficile* infection, with severe abdominal cramps and diarrhea that persisted for more than two years.

The woman eventually died from complications related to ALS, said Nelson, who had spoken with the patient.

"She ended up spending a lot of money on these treatments, as well as time and effort, and that took away from her other life experiences," Nelson said.

The CDC is trying to raise awareness about the dangers of misdiagnosis and unproven treatments. The report focuses on the serious bacterial infections associated with prolonged antibiotic treatment. While antibiotics are effective for many conditions, unnecessary antibiotics provide no benefit and actually put patients at risk for serious harm, especially if used for extended periods. The drugs kill beneficial bacteria and allow drug-resistant ones to dominate, and intravenous treatments can introduce new infections.

Neither the CDC nor the National Institutes of Health recommends using the diagnosis "chronic Lyme disease," for several reasons, Nelson said. The diagnosis is often based on clinical judgment, with no objective evidence of Lyme disease, such as standard laboratory testing for Lyme bacteria or even a history of possible tick exposure in an area with endemic Lyme disease.

Clinicians who call themselves "Lyme literate" are often self-anointed; there is no special training program and no requirement to be board certified in infectious disease, Nelson said.

In addition to the woman with ALS, the CDC report describes four other cases that highlight the severity and scope of the harm caused by unproven treatments for chronic Lyme disease. All five patients developed serious complications; two patients died.

- A woman in her late 30s with fatigue and joint pain was prescribed multiple courses of oral antibiotics. Despite that treatment, her symptoms worsened, and she was put on three months of intravenous antibiotics. She got sicker, developed fever and rash and was hospitalized in intensive care. As her condition worsened, she received more powerful intravenous antibiotics and was put on a ventilator. She died of septic shock related to a bloodstream infection.

- An adolescent girl who had years of muscle and joint pain, backaches, headaches and lethargy, received a diagnosis of chronic fatigue syndrome. She sought a second opinion from an alternative medicine clinic and was given a diagnosis of chronic Lyme disease. After eight months of oral and intravenous antibiotics, she had no improvement. One week after antibiotics were stopped, the alternative clinic recommended she receive a dose of a different antibiotic intravenously. That same day, she was rushed to a hospital emergency department with a high fever and signs of septic shock. She was hospitalized in intensive care and later found to have a catheter-associated bacterial infection. She received broad-spectrum antibiotics to treat the infection and was discharged after several weeks.
- A woman in her late 40s received multiple insect bites and developed a flulike illness with pain in her arms, legs and back. One year after her symptoms began, she received a diagnosis of Lyme disease based on the standard laboratory test. She was treated with two four-week courses of oral doxycycline, which is recommended for patients with arthritis associated with untreated Lyme infection. She later developed fatigue and cognitive difficulties. Two years after her initial diagnosis, she was told she had chronic Lyme disease based on results of unvalidated tests. She received multiple courses of oral and intravenous antibiotics for more than a year. She developed back pain and shortness of breath, and was hospitalized twice after a catheter-related infection spread to her back and spine. After treatment for that infection, her back pain eventually improved.
- A woman in her 60s with a low white blood cell count and degenerative arthritis received intravenous immunoglobulin, or antibodies, every three weeks for more than 10 years. She developed an antibiotic-resistant staph infection in her back that turned into an abscess next to her spine that required surgery to drain.

SEE ALSO *Arthropod-Borne Disease; Climate Change and Infectious Disease; Emerging Infectious Diseases; Mosquito-Borne Disease; Rocky Mountain Spotted Fever; Vector-Borne Disease; Zoonoses*

BIBLIOGRAPHY

Books

Barbour, Alan G. *Lyme Disease: Why It's Spreading, How It Makes You Sick, and What to Do about It.* 2nd ed. Baltimore: Johns Hopkins University Press, 2015.

Fallon, Brian A., and Jennifer Sotsky. *Conquering Lyme Disease: Science Bridges the Great Divide.* New York: Columbia University Press, 2017.

Periodicals

Berende, Anneleen, et al. "Randomized Trial of Longer-Term Therapy for Symptoms Attributed to Lyme Disease." *New England Journal of Medicine* 374 (2016): 1209–1220. This article can also be found online at http://www.nejm.org/doi/full/10.1056/NEJMoa1505425 (accessed February 6, 2018).

Marzec, Natalie S., et al. "Serious Bacterial Infections Acquired during Treatment of Patients Given a Diagnosis of Chronic Lyme Disease—United States." *Morbidity and Mortality Weekly Report* 66, no. 23 (June 16, 2017): 607–609. This article can also be found online at https://www.cdc.gov/mmwr/volumes/66/wr/mm6623a3.htm (accessed February 6, 2018).

Nelson, Christina A., et al. "Incidence of Clinician-Diagnosed Lyme Disease, United States, 2005–2010." *Emerging Infectious Diseases* 21, no. 9 (September 2015): 1625–1631. This article can also be found online at https://www.ncbi.nlm.nih.gov/pmc/articles/PMC4550147/ (accessed February 6, 2018).

Rebman, Alison W., et al. "The Clinical, Symptom, and Quality-of-Life Characterization of a Well-Defined Group of Patients with Posttreatment Lyme Disease Syndrome." *Frontiers in Medicine* 4 (December 14, 2017). This article can also be found online at https://www.frontiersin.org/articles/10.3389/fmed.2017.00224/full?&u (accessed February 6, 2018).

Websites

"Lyme Borreliosis (Lyme Disease)." World Health Organization. http://www.who.int/ith/diseases/lyme/en/ (accessed February 6, 2018).

"Lyme Disease." Centers for Disease Control and Convention, January 19, 2018. https://www.cdc.gov/lyme/index.html (accessed February 6, 2018).

"Lyme Disease." National Institute of Allergy and Infectious Diseases, April 6, 2016. https://www.niaid.nih.gov/diseases-conditions/lyme-disease (accessed February 6, 2018).